ENDOCRINOLOGY OF PREGNANCY

CONTEMPORARY ENDOCRINOLOGY

P. Michael Conn, SERIES EDITOR

9. ***Endocrinology of Pregnancy*** edited by *FULLER W. BAZER,* 1998
8. ***Clinical Management of Diabetic Neuropathy,*** edited by *ARISTIDIS VEVES,* 1998
7. ***Gastrointestinal Endocrinology,*** edited by *GEORGE H. GREELEY, JR.,* 1998
6. ***G Proteins, Receptors, and Disease,*** edited by *ALLEN M. SPIEGEL,* 1998
5. ***Natriuretic Peptides in Health and Disease,*** edited by *WILLIS K. SAMSON AND ELLIS R. LEVIN,* 1997
4. ***Endocrinology of Critical Diseases,*** edited by *K. PATRICK OBER,* 1997
3. ***Diseases of the Pituitary:*** *Diagnosis and Treatment,* edited by *MARGARET E. WIERMAN*, 1997
2. ***Diseases of the Thyroid,*** edited by *LEWIS E. BRAVERMAN,* 1997
1. ***Endocrinology of the Vasculature,*** edited by *JAMES R. SOWERS,* 1996

Endocrinology of Pregnancy

Edited by

Fuller W. Bazer, PhD

Department of Animal Science and Institute of Biosciences and Technology, Texas A&M University,
College Station, TX

Springer Science+Business Media, LLC

For additional copies, pricing for bulk purchases, and/or information about other Humana titles, contact Humana at the above address or at any of the following numbers: Tel: 973-256-1699; Fax: 973-256-8341; E-mail: humana@humanapr.com or visit our website at http://humanapress.com

This publication is printed on acid-free paper. ∞
ANSI Z39.48-1984 (American National Standards Institute)
Permanence of Paper for Printed Library Materials.

Cover design by Patricia F. Cleary.

10 9 8 7 6 5 4 3 2 1

Endocrinology of pregnancy/edited by Fuller W. Bazer
p. cm.—(Contemporary endocrinology; 9)
Includes index.
ISBN 978-1-4612-7291-5 ISBN 978-1-4612-1804-3 (eBook)
DOI 10.1007/978-1-4612-1804-3
1. Obstetrical endocrinology. I. Bazer, Fuller Warren, 1938–
II. Series: Contemporary endocrinology (Totowa, NJ) ; 9.
[DNLM: 1. Pregnancy—physiology. 2. Hormones—physiology. WQ 205 E566 1998]
RG558.5.E532 1998
573.6' 719—dc21
DNLM/DLC
for Library of Congress

98-3059
CIP

PREFACE

Endocrinology of Pregnancy is appropriate and timely for the Contemporary Endocrinology series. Over the past two decades, significant advances in our understanding of signals from the conceptus (embryo and its associated extra-embryonic membranes) responsible for the establishment and maintenance of pregnancy have been realized. Attention has turned from interactions between the immune and reproductive systems that would "destroy" the conceptus to the theory of immunotropism whereby immune cells produce growth factors that enhance fetal–placental growth. In fact, we now recognize that cytokines and lymphokines, once thought to be unique to immune cells, are expressed by cells of the uterus and/or fetal–placental tissues, and thus have been added to the list of growth factors that contribute to the successful outcome of a pregnancy. Each of these growth factors complement the effects of steroid hormones and must act through a receptor that is appropriately expressed within the pregnant uterus or maternal system.

There is considerable "crosstalk" between the maternal and fetal–placental systems that influence behavior, physiology, and endocrinology of organ systems and development of the mammary glands to ensure continued nutrition to the offspring during postnatal development. Another set of key signals are those that lead to parturition, final maturation of the fetus/neonate, and bonding between offspring and mother.

This volume provides the reader with a comprehensive treatise on the "Endocrinology of Pregnancy" in both primate and subprimate mammals. The aim was to address key mechanisms associated with the establishment, maintenance, and termination of a successful pregnancy and, in so doing, to provide a solid base of information for use by both research scientists and clinicians with interests in factors that affect pregnancy. Each of the contributors has based the information in their respective chapters on research from their laboratories and from the laboratories of their colleagues.

Fuller W. Bazer, PhD

CONTENTS

CONTRIBUTORS

EUGENE D. ALBRECHT, PHD, *Bressler Research Laboratories, Department of Obstetrics, Gynecology and Reproductive Sciences, University of Maryland, Baltimore, MD*

RUSSELL V. ANTHONY, PHD, *Animal Reproduction and Biotechnology Lab, Department of Physiology, Colorado State University, Fort Collins, CO*

FULLER W. BAZER, PHD, *Department of Animal Sciences and Institute of Biosciences and Technology, Texas A&M University, College Station, TX*

JEFFERY A. BOWEN, PHD, *Department of Veterinary Anatomy and Public Health, Texas A&M University, College Station, TX*

DAVID L. BUCHANAN, MS, *Department of Veterinary Biosciences, University of Illinois, Urbana, IL*

ROBERT C. BURGHARDT, PHD, *Department of Veterinary Anatomy and Public Health, Texas A&M University, College Station, TX*

BEVERLY S. CHILTON, PHD, *Department of Cell Biology and Biochemistry, Texas Tech University, Health Sciences Center, Lubbock, TX*

KRISTOF CHWALISZ, MD, PHD, *Fertility Control and Hormone Therapy Research, Research Laboratories of Schering Aktiengesellschaft, Schering AG, Berlin, Germany*

CHRISTOPHER B. COHICK, PHD, *Department of Physiology, University of Kansas Medical Center, Kansas City, KS*

ALAN J. CONLEY, PHD, *Department of Population Health and Reproduction, School of Veterinary Medicine, University of California, Davis, CA*

PAUL S. COOKE, PHD, *Department of Veterinary Biosciences, University of Illinois, Urbana, IL*

B. ANNE CROY, DVM, PHD, *Department of Biomedical Sciences, University of Guelph, Ontario Veterinary College, Guelph, Ontario, Canada*

GERALD R. CUNHA, PHD, *Department of Anatomy, University of California, San Francisco, CA*

GUOLI DAI, DVM, PHD, *Department of Physiology, University of Kansas Medical Center, Kansas City, KS*

HEIDI E. ENGELHARDT, PHD, *Department of Animal and Poultry Sciences, University of Guelph, Ontario, Canada*

MICHAEL D. FANNING, PHD, *Animal Reproduction and Biotechnology Lab, Department of Physiology, Colorado State University, Fort Collins, CO*

ROBERT E. GARFIELD, PHD, *Department of Obstetrics and Gynecology, University of Texas Medical Branch, Galveston, TX*

RODNEY D. GEISERT, PHD, *Department of Animal Science, Oklahoma State University, Animal Science Building, Stillwater, OK*

JOHN P. HEARNE, PHD, *Wisconsin Regional Primate Research Center, University of Wisconsin, Madison, WI*

SHERI A. HILD-PETITO, PHD, *BioQual, Inc., Rockville, MD*

STUART HOOPER, PHD, *Department of Physiology, Monash University, Clayton, Victoria, Australia*

Takeshi Kurita, PhD, *Department of Anatomy, University of California, San Francisco, CA*
Rongti Liang, PhD, *Reproduction and Biotechnology Lab, Department of Physiology, Colorado State University, Animal Fort Collins, CO*
Sean W. Limesand, MS, *Reproduction and Biotechnology Lab, Department of Physiology, Colorado State University, Animal Fort Collins, CO*
Dennis B. Lubahn, PhD, *Departments of Biochemistry and Child Health, University of Missouri, Columbia, MO*
Ronald R. Magness, PhD, *Department of Obstetrics and Gynecology, Meriter Hospital/Park, Madison, WI*
Heiner Müller, PhD, *Department of Physiology, University of Kansas Medical Center, Kansas City, KS*
William C. Okulicz, PhD, *Department of Obstetrics and Gynecology, University of Massachusetts, Worcester, MA*
Kyle E. Orwig, PhD, *Department of Physiology, University of Kansas Medical Center, Kansas City, KS*
Kevin G. Osteen, PhD, *Department of Obstetrics and Gynecology, Vanderbilt University, Nashville, TN*
Troy L. Ott, PhD, *Center for Animal Biotechnology, Texas A&M University, College Station, TX*
Gerald J. Pepe, PhD, *Department of Physiology, Eastern Virginia Medical School, Norfolk, VA*
Marta Piva, PhD, *Division of Molecular Biology and Biochemistry, University of Missouri, Kansas City, MO*
Jeffrey W. Pollard, PhD, *Albert Einstein College of Medicine, Bronx, New York*
Tom E. Porter, PhD, *Department of Animal Sciences, University of Maryland, College Park, MD*
Ch. V. Rao, PhD, *Department of OB/GYN, University of Louisville, Health Sciences Center, Louisville, KY*
Virginia C. Rider, PhD, *Division of Molecular Biology and Biochemistry, University Missouri, Kansas City, MO*
George Saade, PhD, *Department of Obstetrics and Gynecology, University of Texas Medical Branch, Galveston, TX*
David O. Sherwood, PhD, *Department of Molecular & Integrated Physiology, University of Illinois, Urbana, IL*
Michael J. Soares, PhD, *Department of Physiology, University of Kansas Medical Center, Kansas City, KS*
Thomas E. Spencer, PhD, *Center for Animal Biotechnology, Texas A&M University, College Station, TX*
Richard L. Stouffer, PhD, *Oregon Regional Primate Research Center, Beaverton, OR*
Philippa F. Whitelaw, PhD, *Department of Biomedical Sciences, University of Guelph, Ontario, Canada*
Gary L. Williams, PhD, *Animal Reproduction Laboratory, Agricultural Research Station, Texas A&M University, Beeville, TX*
I. R. Young, PhD, *Department of Physiology, Monash University, Wellington Road, Clayton, Victoria, Australia*

1 Endocrinology of the Transition from Recurring Estrous Cycles to Establishment of Pregnancy in Subprimate Mammals

Fuller W. Bazer, PHD, *Troy L. Ott*, PHD
and Thomas E. Spencer, PHD

CONTENTS

INTRODUCTION

Pregnancy is established and maintained in subprimate mammals in response to a series of interactions among the conceptus (embryo and associated membranes), uterus, and/or ovarian corpus luteum (CL). These interactions prevent functional and structural regression of the CL, or luteolysis. This chapter describes aspects of the endocrinology of recurring estrous cycles in ruminants, swine, horses, cats, dogs, and rodents, but the primary focus is on signaling for maternal recognition of pregnancy. During the peri-implantation period, pregnancy recognition signals from the conceptus to the maternal system are antiluteolytic and/or luteotrophic. The functional life-span of the CL is controlled by release of prostaglandin $F_{2\alpha}$ (PGF) from the uterus and/or ovaries, whereas pregnancy recognition signals from the trophoblast may act in a paracrine or endocrine manner to interrupt endometrial or intraovarian production of luteolytic PGF (antiluteolytic) or the effect may be directly on the CL (luteotropic). The primary focus of this chapter is pregnancy recognition signals in subprimate mammals, which prevent luteolysis and ensure maintenance of an intrauterine environment that supports events associated with establishment and maintenance of pregnancy.

THE ESTROUS CYCLE AND LUTEOLYSIS

Ruminants

ESTROUS CYCLE. Ruminants are spontaneously ovulating, polyestrous mammals. Cattle, sheep, and goats exhibit recurring estrous cycles with average lengths of 21, 17, and 20 d, respectively *(see 1–3* for reviews). Although cattle are not seasonal breeders, the breeding seasons for both sheep (*Ovis aries*) and goats (*Capra hircus*) are affected by season (photoperiod). In general, sheep and goats are short-day breeders with regular estrous cycles occurring from late summer through midwinter. Sheep have been extensively used as a model to study regulation of the estrous cycle and pregnancy recognition in ruminants.

Estrus, the period of sexual receptivity, marks the beginning of each estrous cycle and lasts about 30 h in sheep. Ewes ovulate spontaneously 24–27 h after the onset of estrus in response to an estrogen-induced discharge of luteinizing hormone (LH) and follicle-stimulating hormone (FSH) from the anterior pituitary. Following ovulation and during metestrus, d 1–4 after onset of estrus, theca and granulosa cells of the follicle differentiate into luteal cells under the influence of LH, a process termed luteinization, and give rise to the CL. The CL begins to secrete progesterone on about d 4, marking the beginning of diestrus, and reaches its maximum size and functional activity between d 7 and 14 *(3)*.

Progesterone from the CL suppresses gonadotropin-releasing hormone (GnRH) pulse frequency, behavioral estrus and circulating levels of LH and FSH. Therefore, Graafian follicles, which form during diestrus, do not ovulate. Primary functions of progesterone are to maintain the myometrium in a quiescent state and provide an endometrial environment conducive to conceptus growth and development. Ovarian follicles grow and regress during the estrous cycle, a phenomenon termed "follicular waves," but progesterone from the CL suppresses ovulation until after luteolysis has occurred during proestrus. Increases in estradiol-17β in ovarian venous blood on d 3, 9, and 14 correspond to successive nonovulatory and ovulatory follicular waves *(4)*. In pregnant ewes, these nonovulatory waves of follicular growth and atresia continue until about d 60. Changes in circulating estrogens associated with nonovulatory follicular waves may affect endometrial function, but such effects have not been characterized.

LUTEOLYSIS. The estrous cycle of ruminants is dependent on the uterus because the endometrium produces the luteolysin, PGF. Progesterone exposure during the early to midluteal phase of the estrous cycle is essential for initiation of endometrial PGF production and luteolysis. Progesterone increases phospholipid stores *(5)* and prostaglandin synthase activity necessary for the conversion of arachidonic acid to PGF *(6)*. Administion of exogenous progesterone to cyclic ewes during metestrus, prior to the endogenous rise in progesterone production, decreases interestrous intervals, whereas administration of the progesterone receptor antagonist mifepristone (RU38486) during the early luteal phase delays onset of endometrial PGF production and luteolysis *(7)*. Therefore, exposure of the endometrium to progesterone for 10–12 d, as occurs during diestrus, not only prepares the uterus for establishment of pregnancy, but also activates mechanisms for endometrial production of luteolytic PGF in the event that pregnancy is not established.

In ewes, the CL regress between d 15 and 16 postestrus in response to pulsatile release of PGF by the uterus. If ewes are hysterectomized during the active life of the CL, luteolysis does not occur, and CL life-span is prolonged to about 5 mo, the duration of normal pregnancy *(8,9)*. In ruminants, an intimate anatomical relationship between the uterine branch of the ovarian vein and the ovarian artery is required for countercurrent exchange of luteolytic PGF from the uterine venous drainage to the ovarian artery. This anatomical arrangement allows delivery of high concentrations of PGF directly from the uterus to the CL during luteolysis. If the PGF enters the peripheral circulation, >80% is metabolized, and thus inactivated in one pass through the lungs. McCracken et al. *(10)* demonstrated that [^{3}H]PGF is transferred from the utero-ovarian vein to the ovarian artery and, therefore, to the CL by a local route. Uterine PGF is also transported from the lymphatic drainage to the ovarian artery *(11,12)*. Injection of ewes with exogenous PGF causes premature luteolysis *(13)*, and immunization of ewes against PGF blocks luteolysis *(14,15)*. Uterine-derived PGF binds to receptors on luteal cells and initiates intracellular events, which terminate production of progesterone and initiate cell death. Luteolytic effects of PGF have been attributed to:

1. Decrease in luteal blood flow;
2. Reduction in LH receptors;
3. Uncoupling of LH receptor from adenyl cyclase;
4. Activation of protein kinase C (PKC);
5. Influx of high levels of calcium; and/or
6. Activation of a cytotoxic cascade *(see 16)*.

Concentrations of PGF in the uterine vein increase during luteolysis concomitant with pulsatile secretion of PGF by the endometrium. Luteolysis in ewes does not require a decrease in LH receptors or withdrawal of basal LH support. The CL must be exposed to approximately five pulses of PGF over a 25-h period to undergo complete luteolysis. Preluteolytic pulses of PGF are released into the utero-ovarian vein on d 13 and 14 in both cyclic and pregnant ewes; however, luteolytic pulses of PGF on d 15 and 16 occur only in cyclic ewes preceded by a rise in circulating levels of estradiol *(13)*. In pregnant ewes, the antiluteolytic signal from the conceptus abrogates pulsatile release of PGF *(17)*.

Pulsatile release of PGF by the ruminant uterus occurs in response to oxytocin (OT) binding to its receptors on uterine endometrial cells and activating the phosphatidyl inositol-diacylglycerol-PKC second messenger system *(18)*). OT is synthesized and secreted by large luteal cells *(19)*, and also released from the posterior pituitary *(20)*. In large luteal cells, the OT gene is transcribed on d 0–4 postestrus *(21)*, OT mRNA is translated to OT peptide to about d 7, and stores of OT and its neurophysin in luteal cells are highest on d 10–12 *(22)*. Thus, CL contains finite stores of OT that are not replenished later in the estrous cycle or during pregnancy. Secretion of luteal OT can be stimulated by a PGF agonist *(22)*. During the peri-luteolytic period, >95% of PGF pulses coincide with pulses of OT *(20)*. Low-amplitude pulses of PGF from the uterus stimulate large luteal cells to release OT from secretory granules, which induces pulsatile release of PGF *(22)*. Major pulses of PGF occur at 4–5 h intervals on d 14–16, and uterine release of about 5 pulses of PGF/25 h results in complete luteolysis *(13)*. The mechanism resulting in synchronous pulsatile release of OT from CL on each ovary and from the posterior pituitary in ewes is unknown *(20)*. Control of OT release by hormones other than PGF or prostaglandin E_2 (PGE) is possible, but such a factor has not been defined.

Immunization of ewes against OT extends CL life-span and interestrous interval *(22,23))*, as does the administration of an oxytocin receptor (OTR) antagonist to ewes and goats *(24)*. Likewise, chronic systemic infusion of OT prevents OTR formation in the endometrium during late diestrus and blocks luteal regression in cyclic ewes *(22)*. During the luteolytic period, most PGF pulses are coincident with pulses of OT. However, only one-half of the OT pulses result in a pulse of PGF, suggesting that OT is responsible for coordinating luteolytic events. The PGF pulse frequency may be less than that for OT because of the time required for replenishment of pools of phospholipids from which arachidonic acid can be mobilized for either the time required for OTR recycling or the synthesis of PGF. Luteal OT is released before development of endometrial responsiveness to OT, and temporal release of OT from CL and posterior pituitary is not different between cyclic and pregnant ewes *(25)*. Pulsatile release of OT and PGF between d 15 and 17 continues until the CL is depleted of its finite stores of OT. Therefore, OT-induced release of luteolytic pulses of PGF from the uterus is dependent on the presence of endometrial OTR.

Expression of OTR mRNA increases between d 13 and 14 in the endometrial epithelium, and OTR protein, which is low or undetectable between d 4 and 13, increases rapidly between d 14 and estrus *(26)*. The OTR is initially expressed on lumenal (LE) and superficial glandular epithelia (GE) on d 14, but expression extends to caruncular stroma and deep GE by d 16, and is abundant in all endometrial cell types during estrus. During the estrous cycle, expression of OTR on the LE and superficial GE appears to be responsible for pulsatile release of PGF and luteolysis. Regulation of OTR gene expression occurs at the level of transcription, and is primarily influenced by the ovarian hormones, estrogen, and progesterone *(23,27,28)*.

Uterine secretion of luteolytic pulses of PGF in sheep is dependent on effects of progesterone, estrogen, and OT on the uterine LE *(see 23)*. In sheep, expression of estrogen receptor (ER) and OTR represents the default state, since endometrium of long-term ovariectomized and anestrus ewes expresses these receptors. The effects of progesterone on uterine expression of ER and OTR in long-term ovariectomized ewes are complex. Progesterone acts on the LE to increase phospholipid stores (arachidonic acid source) and cyclooxygenase enzyme activity necessary for conversion of arachidonic acid to PGF. Therefore, without progesterone stimulation, uteri expressing ER and OTR are unable to produce PGF in response to OT. When long-term ovariectomized ewes are treated with progesterone, endometrial expression of ER and OTR is suppressed. However, progesterone eventually downregulates PR to allow upregulation of ER and OTR, and OT-induced pulsatile release of PGF *(27)*. Thus, progesterone is critical for luteolysis as well as pregnancy by ensuring the potential for uterine release of luteolytic PGF in the absence of a viable conceptus and, at the same time, maintaining a uterine environment that will support growth and differentiation of the conceptus in the absence of luteolysis.

McCracken et al. *(13)* proposed that the ovarian steroid hormones, estrogen and progesterone, regulate OTR gene expression in the endometrial epithelium. Progesterone inhibits endometrial OTR synthesis for 10–12 d; a phenomenon termed the "progesterone block" to endometrial OTR formation. However, continuous exposure of the endometrium to progesterone downregulates expression of progesterone receptor (PR), particularly in the endometrial LE. In the absence of sufficient PR, the endometrial epithelium expresses ER, responds to estrogen, and upregulates expression of OTR *(28)*. The initial increases in OTR occur in cyclic ewes when ER increases and PR decreases in the endometrial epithelium. The rapid increases in OTR occur when circulating progesterone decreases to basal levels and follicular estrogens increase during late diestrus, proestrus, and estrus *(13,28,29)*.

Progesterone prevents increases in ER and OTR during the early to midluteal phase of the ovine estrous cycle, but the precise molecular mechanism remains unknown. Progesterone most likely suppresses ER gene expression to prevent estrogen induction of OTR gene expression. When ovariectomized ewes are treated with progesterone for 10–12 d, ER and OTR gene expression increases and oxytocin-induced PGF release occurs *(28,30,31)*. Loss of the "progesterone block" to ER and OTR formation following chronic exposure of the endometrial epithelium to progesterone in cyclic ewes may result from progesterone-induced negative autoregulation of endometrial PR gene expression. This would permit estrogen to increase OTR expression *(28)*. Alternatively, increases in OTR expression may occur with loss of PR expression and be independent of the effects of estrogen.

Estrogen upregulates OTR gene expression, whereas OT, acting through OTR, induces pulsatile release of PGF. Estrogen also enhances postreceptor events mediated by OT to ensure a PGF pulse frequency necessary for luteolysis. Destruction of developing follicles and immunization of ewes against estrogen delay luteolysis *(32)*. In the absence of estrogen, OT cannot adequately stimulate uterine PGF release to induce luteolysis in ewes *(33)*. Similarly, administration of a GnRH agonist every 3 d to prevent development of steroidogenically competent ovarian follicles in cows prevents luteolysis for at least 45 d *(34)*. Moreover, endometrial expression of OTR increases when progesterone is low relative to estrogen in ovariectomized ewes *(30,35)*. Administration of estradiol-17β benzoate on either d 11 or 12 of the estrous cycle causes premature luteolysis in sheep and cattle *(28,36)*. The effects of estrogen are to induce endometrial ER and OTR expression *(28,36,37)*. Administration of a pharmacological dose of estradiol benzoate (750 μg, im) to cyclic ewes on d 9 or 10 of the estrous cycle sequentially upregulates ER mRNA, ER protein, and then OTR protein in the endometrial LE *(28,36)*.

Results from in vivo studies clearly indicate that progesterone progressively suppresses expression of PR in the endometrial LE and, therefore, loses its ability to suppress endometrial expression of ER and OTR during mid- to late diestrus. Moreover, a preponderance of evidence suggests that estrogen induces expression of OTR in the LE and superficial GE, which are responsible for production and release of luteolytic PGF. Recent reports on the tissue- and cell-type-specific expression of ER, PR, and OTR in ovine endometrium support the model of McCracken et al. *(13)* for regulation of OTR gene expression during the estrous cycle by progesterone and estrogen *(24,25,28,29)*. In cyclic ewes, endometrial ER expression is maximal during estrus and metestrus (d 0–5) owing to high levels of estrogen secreted by ovarian follicles and very low levels of circulating progesterone. In the absence of occupied PR, interactions between estrogen and ER induces OTR expression in all cell types of the endometrium. Although OTR expression is high, circulating OT is low or absent, and pulsatile secretion of PGF by the endometrium is absent during early to middiestrus (d 6–12), because the "progesterone block" prevents expression of endometrial ER and OTR. However, when chronic progesterone exposure downregulates expression of PR in the LE and superficial GE by d 13, increases in ER and then OTR gene expression result in activation of the luteolytic mechanism. During luteolysis (d 14–17), estrogen from maturing ovarian follicles further stimulates endometrial ER and OTR expression to ensure that OT from the CL and posterior pituitary stimulates pulsatile release of luteolytic PGF to terminate CL function. This is followed by estrus, mating, and another opportunity for establishment of pregnancy.

Rodents

Estrous Cycle. Laboratory rodents are nonseasonal, spontaneously ovulating, polyestrous mammals. The estrous cycle lasts 4–5 d. Moreover, the timing and completion of physiological events during the estrous cycle are under photoperiodic control. The lengths of the various phases of the estrous cycle are defined on the basis of the cytology of vaginal smears *(38)*. Proestrus lasts for 12–14 h, estrus 25–to 27 h, metestrus 6–8 h, and diestrus 55–57 h. In these species (rats, mice, and hamsters), the CL secretes progesterone for approx 2 d, but does not become fully functional. The estrous cycle of rodents is atypical, lacking a true luteal phase and consists of recurrent estrous cycles of short duration, which ensure numerous opportunities for mating and establishment of pregnancy.

During the estrous cycle of the rat, three or more generations of CL may be present on the ovary *(39)*. During diestrus, newly formed CL attains maximal size, which is maintained through metestrus of the following cycle. These CL regress abruptly during diestrus of the second cycle, which is accompanied by apoptosis, degeneration of the blood supply, leukocytic infiltration, and increased activity of 20α-hydroxy steroid dehydrogenase (20α-HSD) *(38)*. Although PGF is luteolytic in rodents, the underlying mechanisms of luteolysis in rodents is not well-understood *(16)*. The CL of unmated rodents is considered nonfunctional, since they do not secrete sufficient quantities of progesterone to permit a uterine decidual reaction. Progesterone is metabolized by 20α-HSD in the CL to 20α-hydroxy progesterone (20α-OHP), which is an inactive metabolite *(40)* that will not support pregnancy or a uterine decidual reaction. As secretion of luteal 20α-OHP declines during diestrus, a new ovulation ensues.

Swine

Estrous Cycle. The pig is a spontaneously ovulating, polyestrous, litter-bearing species. Gilts (nonparous females) reach puberty between 4 and 9 mo of age, depending on breed, nutrition, and housing conditions (*see 41,42* for reviews). The estrous cycle averages 21 d (range 18–24 d). Length of gestation for commercial breeds is 114 d. Just prior to estrus, the vulva often swells and develops a reddened appearance (this is especially apparent in gilts), and the gilt exhibits restlessness and increased attempts to mount other females. Estrus females will often seek out the male (boar), and will allow mounting by boars and by other females. Estrus females exhibit a characteristic posture on mounting with ears laid back on the neck and legs locked (lordosis response). Presence of the boar facilitates estrus detection in females owing to pheremones produced by the boar. However, estrus detection can be accomplished by moving through the pen and applying firm pressure with both hands on the female's back just over the pelvis, inciting the lordosis response. Estrus typically lasts for 40–60 h with gilts exhibiting shorter and sows longer periods of estrus.

Estrus is a behavioral response to the physiological actions of estrogen secreted from developing follicles. Estrogen from developing follicles increases just prior to behavioral estrus, which stimulates the ovulatory surge of LH. The number of ova ovulated ranges from 8–10 for the first postpubertal estrus to 15–20 for mature sows (parous females). Progesterone begins to increase in the peripheral circulation starting at about d 3 postovulation, reaching maximum levels (20–40 ng/mL) between d 6 and 14 postestrus. Progesterone then rapidly declines between d 15 and 18, coincident with increasing estrogen, as the next wave of follicles is recruited to mature. Estrogen concentrations peak approx 2 d prior to the next estrus period. Prolactin concentrations are greatest during periods of maximal estrogen production and remain elevated during estrus. Levels of relaxin remain low during the estrous cycle.

Luteolysis. Endocrine requirements for luteolysis in pigs have not been clearly delineated (*see 43,44* for reviews). However, luteolysis occurs during late diestrus following stimulation of the uterine endometrium by progesterone for 10–12 d. The uterine luteolysin in pigs is PGF. Hysterectomy extends the estrous cycle and CL function by removing the source of PGF *(44)*. The CL of pigs is refractory to luteolytic effects of PGF until about d 12 of the estrous cycle because of low numbers of luteal receptors for PGF *(45)*. Luteolysis occurs when pulsatile release of PGF into the uterine venous drainage begins on about d 15 or 16 of the estrous cycle *(46)*.

In ruminants, OT from the CL binds uterine OTR to elicit pulses of PGF, but the mechanism is not well-defined for pigs. The CL of pigs contains only low levels of OT and vasopressin *(47,48)* and undetectable levels of OT mRNA *(49)*, and the role of these neuropeptides of ovarian and/or posterior pituitary origin in luteolysis has not been established. Recent results indicate that the endometrium is a source of OT that may be involved in luteolysis *(50)*, but the role of endometrial OT remains to be defined. Exogenous OT decreases interestrous interval when administered to cyclic gilts between d 10 and 16 postestrus, but not when administered to ovarian-intact hysterectomized gilts, suggesting that the effect of OT is uterine-dependent *(44)*. The endometrium of pigs contains receptors for OT and lysine vasopressin *(51)*, but only responds to OT with increased secretion of PGF *(52,53)*, whereas both peptides stimulate IP turnover *(54)*.

In pigs, like ruminants, OT is thought to act through the G-protein-coupled OTR to stimulate phospholipase C activity and phosphatidylinositol hydrolysis, resulting in elevation of intracellular calcium and diacylglycerol concentrations, thereby activating PKC. This in turn results in activation of phospholipase A_2 and release of arachidonic acid, which then serves as a substrate for prostaglandin biosynthesis *(see 44)*. Concentrations of OT increase in the peripheral circulation during luteolysis *(see 53)*. In addition, OT-induced increases in circulating concentrations of $PGF_{2\alpha}$ metabolite (PGFM) are reduced in pregnant gilts compared to cyclic gilts *(44,53)* or in gilts made pseudopregnant by injection of exogenous estrogen from d 11–15 postestrus *(53)*. Prostaglandins, however, are thought to be critical for establishment of pregnancy in the pig, because inhibition of prostaglandin synthesis results in pregnancy failure *(43)* and basal peripheral concentrations of PGFM are elevated in pregnant gilts on d 12 *(44,53)*.

Horses

Estrous Cycle. Mares exhibit considerable variability with respect to their reproductive cycle (*see 55–57* for reviews). Mares are seasonally polyestrous, with onset of cyclicity occurring in the late winter months in the Northern Hemisphere. In general, ovarian activity is inhibited by decreasing day lengths (photoperiod), although the response is not as acute as for other seasonal breeders, often lagging several months after the solstice. Another complicating factor is that behavioral estrus is often not accompanied by ovulation nor is ovulation accompanied by behavioral estrus. The effects of photoperiod are thought to be regulated by melatonin from the pineal gland. The mare typically exhibits a 21–22 d estrous cycle, although variability in length of estrus and diestrus is common. Prolonged estrus, short estrus, and variability in the length of diestrus occur most frequently around the transition into and out of the breeding season with May to July being the most fertile period in the Northern Hemisphere. Since considerable pressure is placed on mares to foal near January 1 (the arbitrary birth date for all foals born in a given year), artificial lengthening of the photoperiod, specifically delaying sunset, is often used to hasten the onset of cyclicity in this species.

Estrus in the mare can last from 3–7 d, and is accompanied by swelling and reddening of the vulva resulting from high levels of follicular estrogen. During estrus, the vulva becomes covered with a thin layer of mucus, and the cervix dilates several centimeters. The mare will frequently assume a posture associated with urination, i.e., the tail head is raised and deviated, and the clitoris repeatedly exposed by rhythmic contractions of the vulva (termed "winking").

Ovulation takes place after the oocyte undergoes the first meiotic division, typically 24–48 h before the end of behavioral estrus. Ovulation is preceded by a protracted increase and then decrease in serum LH concentrations, over a period of up to 10 d. This is in contrast to the short-lived ovulatory surge of LH, which precedes ovulation in many mammalian species. Multiple ovulations are somewhat common, but secondary ovulations typically occur within 48 h of the initial ovulation. Additional ovulations during the luteal phase have been described for the mare, but the physiology of these late ovulations has not been defined. Secretion of FSH parallels that of LH with an initial increase during late estrus/early diestrus and the second increaseoccurring during mid-diestrus.

Progesterone production begins about 24 h after ovulation, with maximal secretion occurring between d 6 and 18–20 postestrus. Progesterone concentrations during this period range from 4–8 ng/mL, but decline rapidly at the end of diestrus when there is an increase in uterine release of PGF.

Luteolysis. The uterine endometrium of mares releases PGF, which results in luteolysis, but neither the pattern of release of PGF required for luteolysis nor endocrine regulation of uterine production of luteolytic PGF is established. It is known that cervical stimulation of OT release via the Ferguson reflex stimulates uterine secretion of PGF *(58)* and that administration of exogenous OT stimulates uterine release of PGF in mares *(59)*. The CL of mares, however, is responsive to luteolytic effects of PGF after about d 5 postovulation.

Rabbits

Estrous Cycle. The rabbit doe is polyestrous from puberty at 3–5 mo of age for 1–3 yr of her reproductive life *(see 60,61)*. Photoperiod, temperature, and nutrition can influence cyclicity in wild species. However, in modern production systems, rabbits will reproduce year round, especially if exposed to long day lengths (> 12 h light/d) *(see 60,61)*. At puberty (typically when the doe reaches 70–80% of her mature body weight), the ovaries commence production of waves of follicular growth. Mature follicles persist on the ovary for 7–10 d before they undergo atresia and are replaced by another wave of follicles, which secrete high levels of both estrogen and inhibin. Estrogen stimulates sexual receptivity, and inhibin suppresses additional follicular growth by blocking FSH secretion. During this period of growth and atresia of follicles, the doe remains receptive to the buck and will exhibit lordosis when mounted by other does or bucks. Does, ovulating in response to mating with sterile bucks, undergo a 16–18 d pseudopregnancy that is analogous to diestrus in animals that spontaneously ovulate. Receptive does are identified by examining the vulva, which will be red and swollen and by the presence of "chinning" behavior *(see 60,61)*.

The rabbit is an induced ovulator that ovulates in response to mating or mechanical stimulation of the perineal or vaginal area *(see 61)*. Mating stimulates broad-based neural input into the hypothalamus, which results in a large episode of GnRH secretion, a subsequent ovulatory surge of LH, and ovulation 9–12 h postcoitum (pc). The ovulatory LH surge increases cholesterol mobilization in the ovary, resulting in increased production of 20α-OHP by the ovarian interstitial cells. The 20α-OHP is the principal mating-induced progestin, and levels of 20α-OHP increase within 10–60 min pc, peak at 4–6 h (200–300 ng/mL), and return to below basal levels by 9–12 h pc. Concentrations of LH peak at 1–2 h, and FSH at 2–3 h pc, and both return to premating levels within 6–12 h pc. Levels of LH are low throughout pregnancy, whereas a second peak of FSH occurs at 1–2 d of pregnancy (probably related to development of the next wave of follicles). This second surge of FSH may result from the decrease in inhibin concentrations following ovulation. After this second surge, FSH remains low throughout the remainder of pregnancy *(see 61)*. Testosterone in ovarian plasma and estradiol output increase about threefold by 90–120 min pc and return to below basal levels by 12 h pc. At mating, plasma prolactin levels decrease and return to normal in about 30 min, suggesting that mating blocks prolactin release from the pituitary. Plasma prolactin levels increase again 3–4 d pc and remain elevated during the first one-half to two-thirds of gestation *(see 60)*. In addition to its role in lactation, prolactin appears to be important in steroidogenesis and functioning of the rabbit ovary *(see 61)*.

OT levels increase in response to mating, parturition, and lactation. A second release of OT occurs about 5 h pc, and may be involved in uterine and oviductal contractions responsible for transport of the second wave of spermatozoa that enter the oviduct.

Luteolysis. In the rabbit, which lacks a luteal phase of the estrous cycle, CL regression occurs at the end of pregnancy or pseudopregnancy. Prostaglandins are produced by the ovary, blastocysts, and endometrium, and administration of exogenous PGF can induce luteolysis *(see 60,62,63)*. The uterus synthesizes prostaglandins, and hysterectomy delays, but does not block, luteolysis in pseudopregnant does *(see 62)*. The CL can synthesize PGF, PGE, and 6-keto-prostaglandin $F_{2\alpha}$, suggesting that intraovarian mechanisms for luteolysis may be similar to those for humans and rodents. Concentrations of PGF are elevated in uterine venous plasma and in ovarian tissue during luteolysis. However, it is not certain that these increases initiate luteal regression, because progesterone production declines prior to detectable increases in PGF. Purified PGE reductase from CL of pseudopregnant rabbits possess both PGE-9-keto-reductase and 20α-HSD activity, suggesting that both progesterone and PGE are substrates *(64)*. This suggests that prostaglandin and steroid metabolism are tightly linked, and that PGE reductase may be a key enzyme in the luteolytic cascade in rabbits *(64)*.

The CL from pseudopregnant does become responsive to exogenous PGF around d 12. However, CL from pregnant does are responsive as early as d 7, but become unresponsive by d 15. These results suggest that the conceptus affects the CL prior to maternal recognition of pregnancy on d 12, and that the effect renders the CL initially more sensitive and later more resistant to PGF *(62)*. Whether this dual effect results from altered sensitivity of the CL to PGF or altered metabolism of PGF remains to be determined.

Immune cells participate in luteolysis in several species. Interestingly, in contrast to sham-operated control rabbits, splenectomy on d 7 of pseudopregnancy extends luteal life-span, suggesting a role for immune cells in luteolysis *(65)*. Treatment of rabbits with the immunosuppressant methylprednisolone drastically reduced macrophage (70%) and T-lymphocyte (>90%) numbers and luteal cell class II antigen expression, but did not increase the duration of pseudopregnancy *(66)*. Therefore, a role for the immune system in initiating luteolysis in rabbits remains to be demonstrated.

Cats

Estrous Cycle. The cat is a seasonally polyestrous, induced ovulator with onset of cyclicity occurring as early as 4 mo and as late as 21 mo of age depending on breed, photoperiod, and level of nutrition *(see 67,68)*. Cats are long-day breeders with litters being born in the spring and summer months. In the Northern Hemisphere, cats exhibit seasonal anestrus from about October to January, whereas in the tropics cats exhibit sexual activity year round. In the absence of mating, estrus can last for 2–10 d or more (average 7 d). During this period, females vocalize and exhibit characteristic "treading" with hind legs, rub against objects, and accept mounting by males. Interestrous periods, lasting for 3–14 d (average 10 d), separate periods of estrus, and are characterized by low estrogen levels and nonreceptivity to mating.

Rapid growth of ovarian follicles and increased secretion of estradiol occur over a 2–3 d period prior to estrus. At the onset of estrus, circulating levels of estradiol-17β increase from proestrus levels of 5–20 to 40–100 pg/mL *(67)*. At estrus, the ovaries contain an average of five preovulatory follicles and an average of 4.3 ova are ovulated *(see 67)*. The queen ovulates in response to mating-induced activation of a neuroendocrine reflex, which releases a pulse of GnRH from the hypothalamus. This surge of GnRH results in a pulse of LH as early as 5 min pc, peaks at 20 min, and returns to basal levels by 1 h *(68)*. However, it is important to point out that onset of estrus and the capacity to release an LH surge in response to copulation do not necessarily coincide *(69,70)*. In addition, cats may ovulate in the absence of cervical stimulation. Lawler et al. *(71)* diagnosed noncoital ovulation in cats housed in the same room, but restricted from physical contact, and found that 7 of 20 queens had elevated progesterone, indicative of ovulation, one to six times during a 9-mo sampling period.

The LH surge following mating varies in amplitude (10 to >100 ng/mL) and duration (1–24 h), and increases with number of copulations *(70)*. With self-paced matings during a 2-h period, estradiol-treated ovariectomized cats exhibited peak LH values of 600–2000 ng/mL, which remained above basal levels for 2–4 h *(60)*. Multiple matings on successive days of estrus ensure ovulation in all females, but $<150\%$ of estrus queens ovulate after a single copulation *(68,72)*.

Luteolysis. Feline CL is resistant to exogenous PGF even late in gestation *(see 68)*. However, production of PGF by the fetal-placental unit and endometrium increases during the last half of pregnancy and reaches a plateau around d 45. There is a sharp increase in PGF secretion just before parturition, which decreases rapidly thereafter *(68)*. Administration of high levels of PGF after d 40 will induce abortion, but the mechanism is not known *(67,68)*.

Dog

Estrous Cycle. The dog is monestrous and ovulates once or twice per year, starting at 7–12 mo of age *(67,72)*. Follicles grow and begin to secrete estradiol and inhibin at the end of anestrus. This period is associated with a transient increase in LH and a slight reduction in FSH just prior to proestrus. Ovarian inhibin suppresses FSH levels during proestrus as estrogen increases to 50–100 pg/mL. Proestrus typically lasts 7 d, but can range from 3 d to 3 wk. A bloody discharge from the vagina is common during proestrus, and the vaginal and perineal areas increase in size and turgidity. An LH surge (5–20 ng/mL) around the onset of estrus is accompanied by decreasing concentrations of estrogen, increasing concentrations of progesterone, and an increase in sexual receptivity toward the male for mating. The role of GnRH in regulating LH and FSH secretion in the bitch has not been studied in detail. The LH surge lasts 2–3 d and is associated with increased concentrations of FSH, which peak shortly after the LH surge and return to basal levels in 1–2 d. Ovulation typically occurs 48 h after the LH surge; however, its relation to the onset of estrus is variable *(67)*. During anestrus, LH concentrations are low, but remain pulsatile *(73)*, and FSH levels are 5 to 10 times higher than during proestrus *(73)*. Oocytes undergo ovulation at the germinal vesicle stage and achieve metaphase II in the isthmus of the oviduct. Mature oocytes remain fertilizable for 2–3 d and spermatozoa remain viable in the female reproductive tract for 6–7 d. Fertilization takes place approx 4 d after the LH surge. Morulae/blastocysts enter the uterus around d 9 and 10 and implantation occurs around d 16–18 post-LH surge.

The length of the luteal phase in nonpregnant and pregnant bitches is similar. The luteal phase is marked by a lack of sexual receptivity and increasing concentrations of progesterone to peak values of 15–90 ng/mL between d 10 and 40 post-LH surge, which then gradually decline to term *(see 67,73)*. The interval from the LH surge to parturition is typically 64–66 d. Estrogen levels gradually increase during the latter half of gestation and are thought to be critical for development of the mammary glands. Prolactin concentrations gradually increase from d 30–40 of gestation and peak 1–2 d prior to parturition (50–60 ng/mL). Prolactin is luteotropic during pregnancy, and suppression of prolactin with a dopamine agonist can suppress progesterone production early in pregnancy and cause luteolysis late (> d 30) in pregnancy. Prolactin may regulate the length of anestrus by affecting gonadotropin secretion or ovarian responsiveness to gonadotrophins *(73,74)*. Relaxin, which may be the only pregnancy-specific hormone in dogs, peaks during the latter third of gestation and remains detectable for 1–2 mo after parturition *(75)*. Relaxin is produced by both the ovary and the pregnant uterus *(75)*.

Luteolysis. In the nonpregnant bitch, luteolysis is protracted, progesterone concentrations gradually decrease at the end of the luteal phase to below 1 ng/mL, and remain at low levels for weeks to months before the next ovarian follicular phase is initiated *(73)*. At the end of pregnancy, there is rapid luteolysis, which is thought to result from inadequate gonadotrophin support *(76)*. Frequent administration of PGF over several days is luteolytic in the bitch. However, hysterectomy does not prolong the life-span of the CL *(see 77)*, which suggests that luteolysis in the bitch is uterine-independent.

PREGNANCY RECOGNITION SIGNALS

Ruminants

Introduction. An ovulatory surge of LH coincident with onset of estrus (d 0) initiates events that culminate in ovulation about 30 h later. With maturation of the CL, concentrations of progesterone in peripheral blood are maximum in mid-diestrus (d 12–14), and in cyclic females, luteolysis is induced by pulsatile release of PGF from endometrial epithelium during late diestrus (d 15 and 16). The antiluteolytic signal for pregnancy recognition in ruminants is interferon tau (IFNτ) produced by mononuclear cells of the embryonic trophectoderm *(see 17)*. The IFNτ exerts a paracrine, antiluteolytic effect on the endometrium to inhibit endometrial production of luteolytic pulses of PGF. Other conceptus and/or uterine products secreted during early pregnancy, e.g., PGE and platelet-activating factor (PAF), may exert secondary luteal protective effects *(see 17)*. Results from studies of sheep will be used to describe mechanisms affecting endometrial responsiveness to progesterone, estrogen, and OT in ruminants, since the mechanism for pregnancy recognition is similar, if not identical, for sheep, cattle, and goats.

Structure of IFNτ Genes. τ Interferons are a subclass of the 172 amino acid ω interferons. Ovine IFNτ (OIFNτ) was initially termed Trophoblastin or Protein X and then Ovine Trophoblast Protein-1 (oTP-1 and bTP-1), because it was the first major protein secreted by trophectoderm of the peri-implantation ruminant conceptus *(see 17)*. Following cDNA cloning and amino acid sequencing, these proteins were identified as Type I interferons and later given the Greek letter designation tau (τ) by the International Interferon Society *(78)*. The IFNτ were confirmed as functional interferons based on their potent antiviral *(79)*, antiproliferative *(80)*, and immunomodulatory *(see 81,82)* activities.

Support for IFNτ as a distinct IFN gene subtype came from the high amino acid sequence homology of IFNτ across ruminant species and apparent unique role in the establishment of pregnancy *(see 17,78)*. The IFNτ of cattle and sheep is generated from multiple mRNAs approx 1 kb in length, which probably arose from multiple genes. The functional significance of multiple IFNτ isoforms is equivocal, since individual oIFNτ isoforms, produced using recombinant DNA technology, are sufficient to extend CL function when injected into the uterine lumen of cyclic ewes, cows, and goats *(see 17)*.

Southern blotting of ovine and bovine genomic DNA detects 4–5 IFNτ genes, using probes designed to distinguish between IFNω and IFNτ *(see 78)*. The IFNτ genes were also identified in related ruminants, including musk ox, gazelle, and giraffe. Using those same probes, Leaman and Roberts *(83)* did not detect IFNτ genes in the horse, pig, llama, dolphin, mouse, rabbit, or human, and they suggested that IFNτ genes diverged from IFNω genes 40–80 million years ago. The oIFNτ and bovine IFNτ (bIFNτ) cDNAs share a greater degree of homology than bIFNτ does with bIFNω. This cross-species homology and presence within a limited subset of mammals (Artiodactyla) strongly implicate evolutionary divergence of IFNτ from IFNω. This is manifest as a unique mechanism for maternal recognition of pregnancy that relies on massive production of IFNτ during a defined period of early pregnancy.

Like other Type I interferon genes, IFNτ genes are intronless. A 585-bp open reading frame codes for a 195 amino acid preprotein containing a 23 amino acid signal sequence, which is cleaved to yield a mature protein of 172 amino acids. Secreted forms of ovine IFNτ are not glycosylated, although one of the sequenced genes contains a potential *N*-glycosylation site (AsnThrThr) *(83,84)*. Bovine IFNτ transcripts contain a potential site for *N*-glycosylation at Asn78, and multiple glycosylation variants are present in the secreted proteins *(83)*. Peri-implantation goat conceptuses also express multiple isoforms of a caprine IFNτ that crossreact with antisera to oIFNτ and bIFNτ *(see 17)*. Both *N*-glycosylated and nonglycosylated forms of caprine IFNτ are secreted by goat conceptuses. Genes for cIFNτ and oIFNτ share >95% identity *(83)*. Within the coding region, oIFNτ and bIFNτ transcripts exhibit approx 90% identity, and their inferred amino acid sequences share ~80% identity *(78)*. The predicted amino acid sequence identity between bIFNτ and bIFNαI and IFNω is ~50 and 72%, respectively *(78,83)*.

The IFNτ composite surface profile and predicted relative hydrophilicity profile both support a conserved three-dimensional structure for α and τ interferons *(85,86)*. Pontzer et al. *(87)* demonstrated that a synthetic peptide corresponding to the carboxyl-terminus (aa 139–172) of oIFNτ blocked the antiviral activity of oIFNτ, recombinant bIFNα, and recombinant hIFNα, but did not block the activity of recombinant bIFNγ. A synthetic peptide corresponding to the amino-terminus (aa 1–37) of oIFNτ only blocked antiviral activity of oIFNτ without affecting antiviral activity of the IFNα. These results suggest that the C-terminus may contain a receptor binding epitope common to Type I IFNs, whereas the amino-terminus may mediate the unique and characteristic biologic activities of IFNτ. This is supported by the observation that human IFNα displaces oIFNτ from ovine endometrial receptors *(see 17)*. Interestingly, the amino-terminus peptide of oIFNτ has been reported to have antiluteolytic agonist activity *(88)*.

The IFNτ are only ~30% identical to IFNβ; however, IFNα, β, and τ are all believed to act through the Type I interferon receptor. Competition for the same receptor dictates that portions of the epitope involved in receptor binding of IFNτ are shared by IFNα, β, and ω *(85)*. If the locations of hydrophobic residues between IFNτ and IFNβ are compared, they are 75% identical, and it is the hydrophobic residues that appears to influence protein folding critically *(85)*.

Molecular modeling based on the crystal structure of murine IFNβ suggests that five regions of helical structure (designated A–E) are connected by loop regions in an antiparallel arrangement thought to provide IFNτ with a three-dimensional structure remarkably similar to that for IFNβ, IL-1, IL-4, growth hormone, and granulocyte-macrophage colony-stimulating factor (GM-CSF) *(85,86)*. Although the precise packing of the helical regions is not known, they are thought to form a four-helical bundle motif, which mediates receptor binding. This model is especially appealing because it brings previously identified functional domains of oIFNτ into close proximity.

The 5′ (about 93% to −400; *83*) and 3′ (about 92%) noncoding regions of the ovine and bovine IFNτ genes share a high degree of cross-species conservation. Within the 100 bases upstream of the transcription start site, the degree of conservation is >90% among bovine, ovine, caprine, and musk ox. The apparent divergence from related IFNαI and IFNω genes supports the unique quantitative and qualitative pattern of IFNτ gene expression. Structures of the IFNτ gene promoters have been reviewed extensively *(see 78)*. The IFNτ genes share considerable within- and cross-species homology up to position −400. A consensus IFNτ promoter contains interferon-stimulated response elements (ISREs) and putative interferon regulatory factor 1 (IRF-1) binding hexamers, although the arrangements of these motifs differ from the viral response elements present in other Type I IFNs. The functional consequence of these motifs is poor virus inducibility of the IFNτ genes *(see 78)*.

Perhaps most interesting is the cross-species sequence identity of IFNτ promoters to approx −400 bases upstream of the transcription start site, since promoters of other Type I IFNs typically diverge beyond −150 bp *(83)*. Because IFNτ promoter constructs are expressed in uninduced cells of trophoblast origin (JAR and BeWo), but not in nontrophoblast cells, it is postulated that trophoblast cell-specific factors activate transcription of the IFNτ genes via distal enhancer elements *(78,83)*. Nephew et al. *(84)* provided evidence for such an element in a report that presented sequence data for four additional oIFNτ genes. Only one of those genes (clone 010) was expressed during the period of maternal recognition of pregnancy at levels comparable to those for oIFNτ. The promoter region of this gene (to −175) is >95% identical to the oTP-p7 gene. Clone 010 had an AP-1-like regulatory element starting at −929, suggesting that factors (i.e., cytokines) that affect AP-1 enhancer activity, such as GM-CSF, may regulate oIFNτ gene expression *(89)*. There is evidence that GM-CSF is expressed by the ovine endometrium during early pregnancy, and that addition of GM-CSF to culture medium containing ovine conceptuses results in an approximate doubling of antiviral activity secreted into the culture medium (indicator of oIFNτ production; *89*). These results support the idea that the growing family of cytokines resident in the uterus during early pregnancy may influence maternal recognition of pregnancy signaling and subsequent fetal/placental development.

The structural relatedness of the IFNτ of domestic ruminants is supported by their cross-species functional relatedness. Early experiments demonstrated that trophoblastic vesicles from sheep could extend the interestrous interval when placed into the uterine lumen of cattle *(90)*. Purified recombinant oIFNτ (roIFNτ) suppressed OT-induced uterine PGF production, and extended the interestrous interval in cattle as well *(91)*. In goats, twice-daily intrauterine injections of 100 μg roIFNτ from d 14–18 postestrus extended CL function by approx 8 d *(92)*.

Type I IFN Receptors. Ovine IFNτ binds to a receptor with an apparent mol wt of 100 kDa in ovine endometrial membrane preparations, and can be competitively displaced by recombinant bovine and human α_i IFNs *(see 93)*. The human Type I IFN receptor, present on essentially all human cell types, is a 95–100 kDa transmembrane glycoprotein generated from a 2.7-kb mRNA encoding a 65-kDa protein with 15 potential asparagine-linked glycosylation sites *(see 78)*. Binding of IFNτ to ovine endometrium does not stimulate increases in cAMP, cGMP, or IP turnover *(see 17)*. However, IFNτ is assumed to activate a signal transduction system similar, if not identical to that of IFNα and other Type I IFNs.

IFNτ Suppresses Transcription of the Ovine ER Gene. Molecular mechanisms whereby IFNτ suppresses ER gene transcription have not been defined, but they likely involve the Type I IFN receptor signal transduction system and several members of the Type I IFN-induced transcription factor family. The Type I IFN transcription factor family includes interferon-stimulated gene factor-3 (ISGF3), IRF-1, IRF-2, interferon consensus sequence binding protein (ICBSP), and lymphoid-specific IRF (LSIRF) *(94,95)*. The ICBSP and LSIRF are unique to cells of lymphoid lineage. In contrast, ISGF3, IRF-1, and IRF-2 represent a transcription factor network that regulates expression of IFN-inducible genes in several cell types *(see 94)*. The ISGF3 transcription factor complex is composed of four proteins that are dissociated and normally located in the cytoplasm. Binding of a Type I IFN to its receptor immediately activates latent tyrosine kinases, JAK1 and tyk2, which phosphorylate tyrosine residues of STAT1 (p84), STAT1a (p91), and STAT2 (p113) *(94)*. These three phosphoproteins then bind a fourth DNA binding protein, p48, and the multimeric protein complex is transported to the nucleus. This ISGF3 transcription factor complex binds to an ISRE present in the promoter/enhancer region of IFN-responsive genes and increases rates of gene transcription. The IRF-1 gene contains an ISRE and is upregulated by Type I IFNs. IRF-1 is a positive-acting transcription factor that binds to an interferon regulatory factor element (IRF-E) and increases gene transcription. The IRF-E is often contained within the larger ISRE. Although the IRF-1 protein can bind to an ISRE containing an IRF-E and activate transcription, the ISGF3 transcription factor complex can only bind to an ISRE. Transcription of the IRF-2 gene is increased by IRF-1, and then IRF-2 then acts as a negative regulator of transcription factor that binds to IRF-E to silence gene transcription. The IRF-2 can displace IRF-1 binding, from IRF-E and silence activities of other transcription factors, such as Sp1 *(94)*. This yin-yang interaction between IRF-1 and IRF-2 regulates induction and repression of Type I IFN-responsive gene expression.

IFNτ and Expression of Receptors for Sex Steroids. PR and ER are among the proteins for which transcription is affected by Type I interferons. In endometrial adenocarcinoma cells, levels of ER and PR protein are increased by IFNα_{2b}, whereas IFNα enhances levels of PR, but not ER in AE-7 endometrial cancer cells *(see 96,97)*. In human breast cancer tissue and human and rabbit endometrium, IFNα increases ER expression. The amounts of mRNA for both PR and ER were not measured in the above studies, but effects of IFNα were probably owing to increased transcription of the PR and/or ER genes. Organization of the rabbit PR and human PR and ER genes has been described, but functional ISREs have not been characterized in the 5′-flanking regions of these genes. Computer-assisted analyses of these regions for homology to the consensus ISRE sequence indicated putative ISREs in rabbit PR (-2976 and -2605), human PR (-1324), and human ER (-1838) genes with the transcription initiation site as (+1). Furthermore, it was demonstrated that intrauterine injections of oIFNτ in ovariectomized ewes prevents development of endometrial sensitivity to OT only when progesterone replacement therapy is provided, which strongly suggests that antiluteolytic effects of oIFNτ are dependent on the presence of progesterone and endometrial PR *(see 96,97)*.

High-affinity, low-capacity oIFNτ binding sites (presumably Type I IFN receptors) are present in endometrial membranes, and human IFNα will displace oIFNτ from those receptors *(see 93)*. Unoccupied Type I receptor numbers are similar for cyclic and pregnant ewes on d 8 and 12, but decrease thereafter *(see 93)*. Recombinant oIFNτ and recombinant bovine IFNα_1I (rbIFN$_\alpha$) may interact differently with Type I IFN receptors, since antiluteolytic activity of roIFNτ is at least sevenfold greater than that of rbIFNα_1I *(see 93)*.

Antiluteolytic Activity of IFNτ. The unique biological effect of IFNτ is its antiluteolytic activity. Ovine IFNτ is secreted between d 10 and 21 of pregnancy, the period of maternal recognition of pregnancy, by mononuclear trophoblast cells. Secretion of oIFNτ appears to be developmentally regulated, because it begins on about d 10 and increases as conceptuses change morphologically from spherical (312 ng/mL uterine flush), to tubular (1380 ng), and then to filamentous (4455 ng) forms on d 12–13. Successful transfer of embryos to cyclic ewes can occur as late as d 12, i.e., 48–72 h prior to the luteolytic period *(8)*. Thus, secretion of oIFNτ begins prior to the luteolytic period to prevent the pulsatile release of PGF. Intrauterine infusions of either highly purified oIFNτ or roIFNτ from d 12–14 of the cycle extend the interestrous interval and life-span of the CL. Therefore, IFNτ alone is assumed to be the antiluteolytic pregnancy recognition factor produced by ruminant conceptuses. IFNτ is not detectable in the uterine venous drainage or uterine lymphatic drainage *(see 97)*, and because of this, its antiluteolytic effects are assumed to be local on the endometrial epithelium. Intrauterine injections of roIFNτ into cyclic sheep, cattle, and goats abrogate development of the luteolytic mechanism *(see 34,97)*.

During the luteolytic period, expression of OTR increases in endometrial epithelium of cyclic ewes. Using endometrium from d 15 of the estrous cycle when OTR is present, Vallet et al. *(98)* demonstrated that oIFNτ does not compete with OTR for its receptor, inhibit OT stimulation of endometrial inositol phosphate metabolism, or inhibit OT stimulation of endometrial PGF secretion. Rather, the endometrium of cyclic ewes must be exposed to IFNτ from d 11 or 12 to d 14, (i.e., 2–3 d before OTR increase in endometrial LE of cyclic ewes), to block expression of OTR and OT induction of inositol phospholipid metabolism and luteolytic pulses of PGF *(see 32,94)*. During early pregnancy, endometrial OTR is very low and OT cannot elicit pulsatile release of PGF by the uterus. However, basal secretion of PGF is actually higher during early pregnancy than during the cycle in ewes *(see 97)*.

Estrogen and progesterone are the regulators of OTR gene expression in the endometrium *(23)*. During pregnancy recognition, secretion of these hormones by the ovary is the same for both cyclic and pregnant ewes. Therefore, IFNτ could regulate expression of ER and/or PR gene expression to suppress OTR formation *(see 97)*. If IFNτ stabilized or upregulated PR gene expression in the endometrial epithelium, progesterone could continue to suppress ER and OTR formation. Alternatively, IFNτ could block the increase in ER gene expression, which is a prerequisite for OTR formation and luteolysis in cyclic ewes. Recent evidence strongly supports the hypothesis that IFNτ blocks transcription of the ER and OTR genes *(99)*.

Endometrial ER and PR gene expression is regulated in a tissue- and cell-type-specific manner, which differs during the estrous cycle and early pregnancy *(see 31)*. Endometrial ER mRNA is lower in pregnant ewes than cyclic ewes between d 13 and 16 of the estrous cycle *(96,100)*. Moreover, ER mRNA and protein are low or undetectable in LE and shallow GE in the endometrium of ewes during early pregnancy. Doses of either exogenous OT or estrogen, which initiate luteolysis in cyclic ewes and cows, fail to induce luteolysis in pregnant ewes or in ewes receiving intrauterine injections of oIFNτ, because ER and OTR are absent or very low in the endometrium of pregnant ewes *(see 28,32)*.

In both cyclic and pregnant ewes, progesterone negatively autoregulates expression of its own receptor in the endometrial epithelium, and PR is not detectable in the endometrial LE after d 6–8 *(28)*. Thus, pregnancy does not stabilize or upregulate PR gene expression in the endometrium. Moreover, intrauterine injections of roIFNτ did not prevent PR downregulation in response to continuous exposure of the endometrium to progesterone for 12 d. However, roIFNτ did block increases in endometrial ER mRNA and protein and OTR density *(28)*. Therefore, the major antiluteolytic effects of oIFNτ are to prevent increases in ER and OTR gene expression in the endometrial LE during maternal recognition of pregnancy.

Transcription rates of the ER and OTR genes are twofold lower in the endometrium of pregnant ewes compared to cyclic ewes as well as cyclic ewes receiving intrauterine injections of roIFNτ between d 11 and 14 compared to ewes receiving control proteins *(99)*. Given that ER, OTR, mRNA, and protein are absent in pregnant ewes and cyclic ewes receiving intrauterine injections of roIFNτ, IFNτ most likely suppresses transcription of the ER gene in the endometrial epithelium, which prevents increases in OTR gene expression *(31,99)*. Molecular mechanisms whereby IFNτ suppresses ER gene transcription have not been defined, but likely involve the Type I IFN receptor signal transduction system and several members of the Type I IFN-induced transcription factor family *(see 96)*.

IFNτ is assumed to activate the Type I IFN signal transduction system in the ovine endometrium. Since production of oIFNτ is developmentally regulated and produced in massive quantities for an extended period, i.e., much longer than the period of IFNα induced by a viral infection, one may hypothesize that IFNτ activates expression of large amounts of IRF-2. If the ovine ER gene contains a functional IRF-E, IRF-2 could silence transcription of the ER gene, which would be expected as long as a high IRF-2:IRF-1 ratio was maintained. Silencing ER gene transcription in lumenal and superficial glandular epithelium of the ovine endometrium may block ER and OTR gene transcription and abrogate the luteolytic mechanism. Progesterone from the CL could continue to act on PR-positive stroma and deep glandular epithelium to suppress ER and OTR expression in those cells to complete induction of the antiluteolytic mechanism.

The hypothesis that IRF-2 negatively regulates ER and OTR gene transcription is supported by the fact that the trophectoderm must produce IFNτ prior to development of the endometrial luteolytic mechanism. That is, IFNτ would first activate transcription of IRF-1 and then IRF-2. This would require sequential IRF-1 gene activation and translation, followed by another round of transcriptional and translational activity to produce IRF-2, a process requiring 24–48 h. Recent results (Spencer and Bazer, unpublished data) are consistent with the hypothesis that endometrium exposed to serum proteins (control) expressed low levels of IRF-1 in compact stroma and midglandular epithelium and IRF-2 in midglandular epithelium, but not in the lumenal or superficial glandular epithelium at 1, 3, 6, 12, 24, 48, 72, 96, or 120 h posttreatment on d 11. However, endometrium exposed to roIFNτ expressed abundant IRF-1 in lumenal and superficial glandular epithelium at 12 and 24 h postinjection, and abundant IRF-2 in those same cells between 24 and 120 h. Collectively, these results indicate that roIFNτ induces transient expression of IRF-1, which induces expression of IRF-2. Furthermore, IRF-2 may then suppress expression of IRF-1, as well as ER and OTR. The length of time required for induction of expression of IRF-1 and then IRF-2 is consistent with results from early embryo transfer experiments, which demonstrated that the conceptus must be present in the uterus 48–72 h prior to development of the luteolytic mechanism in order to block expression of ER and OTR by lumenal and superficial glandular epithelium.

CATTLE. bIFNτ exhibits immunological identity with oIFNτ, has high amino acid sequence identity with oIFNτ, and possesses potent antiviral activity *(see 78)*. Secretion of bIFNτ is maximal between d 16 and 19 of pregnancy, but can be detected from d 12 until at least d 38 of pregnancy *(see 34,96)*. During maternal recognition of pregnancy, ovarian follicular development is suppressed on the ovary bearing the CL, but not the contralateral ovary *(see 33)*. This effect may support the antiluteolytic mechanism by suppressing follicular development and reducing secretion of estradiol that could enhance uterine secretion of luteolytic PGF. Endometrial OTR are low in pregnant compared to cyclic cows during the luteolytic period (563 ± 117 vs 18 ± 5 fmol/mg protein) *(see 34)*. bIFNτ likely inhibits synthesis of endometrial ER and OTR to abrogate uterine production of luteolytic pulses of PGF.

Intrauterine infusion of bCSP in cyclic cows between d 15 and 21 increased the interestrous interval from 23–24 d to 30–39 d and inhibited uterine production of PGF in response to exogenous estradiol *(see 34)*. Bovine endometrium contains an inhibitor of prostaglandin biosynthesis, recently identified as linoleic acid, that is active during the estrous cycle and pregnancy *(see 34)*. However, the inhibitory activity was greatest between d 16 and 31 of pregnancy. It was shown that bovine conceptus secretory proteins (bCSP) stimulated endometrial production of linoleic acid. As suggested for the ewe, PGE produced by the bovine conceptus may play a luteal protective role, but this has not been established. Bovine conceptuses also produce limited quantities of progesterone, androstenedione, and estradiol as well as 5β-reduced androgens and progestins, but their role(s) in the establishment and maintenance of pregnancy is not known *(see 96)*.

GOAT. Pregnancy recognition in goats occurs around d 17, and goat conceptuses secrete cIFNτ between d 16 and 21. Caprine IFNτ can be immunoprecipitated with antiserum to oIFNτ and is assumed to be the antiluteolytic protein in goats *(see 96)*. Pulsatile release of OT and PGF is suppressed in pregnant goats between d 10–12 and estrus or d 20 of pregnancy, suggesting that antiluteolytic mechanisms in goats are similar to those for ewes and cows *(see 96)*. Intrauterine injection of roIFNτ in goats extended the interestrous interval by >8 d *(92)*.

MODEL OF IFNτ ACTION ON BOVINE ENDOMETRIAL EPITHELIAL CELLS. The IFNτs are assumed to induce the same receptor-mediated transduction signals as other Type I IFNs. Antiluteolytic mechanisms induced by IFNτ suppress transcription of ER and OTR genes, as well as regulate lipid metabolism within the bovine endometrium to increase linoleic acid release and inhibit synthesis of PGF *(see 34)*. Treatment of mouse Balb/c (clone A31) cells with inhibitors of fatty acid cyclooxygenase or lipoxygenase enzymes results in amplification of ISGF-3α. Arachidonic acid metabolism may be redirected from cyclooxygenase- and lipoxygenase-catalyzed transformations to an alternative pathway, such as epoxygenase for catabolism of arachidonic acid. An epoxygenase derivative may affect activation or formation of the ISGF-3α transcription factor complex by IFNs to enhance IFN-induced gene expression. Reduced utilization of arachidonic acid for prostaglandin synthesis may increase its availability for alternative pathways and enhance IFNτ-induced gene expression. Consistent with this idea is the increase in free linoleic acid in endometrial microsomes during early bovine pregnancy, which competitively inhibits cyclooxygenase enzyme activity *(34)*. Linoleic acid is also a precursor for arachidonic acid. Thus, lipid metabolism in early pregnancy is an important area for investigation since essential fatty acids (e.g., linoleic and arachidonic acids) can amplify receptor signal transduction pathways to affect gene expression *(see 34)*.

Induced Endometrial Proteins. During the peri-implantation period, the ruminant conceptus is bathed in endometrial secretions (histotroph), which nourish and sustain it. Histotroph contains a complex mixture of proteins, carbohydrates, sugars, lipids, and ions *(see 46)*. Changes in the quantitative and qualitative pattern of endometrial protein production in cyclic and pregnant ruminants have provided clues to the identity and function of the protein components of histotroph and their roles in establishment of pregnancy. IFN-induced proteins are well characterized in immune responses *(see 101)*; however, IFN-induced proteins in the uterus are less well defined. The receptor for IFNτ in the uterus has not been cloned, but is thought to be the Type I IFN receptor that mediates effects of IFNα, β, and ω *(see 93)*. Likewise, the second messenger system activated by IFNτ binding to its receptor has not been characterized, but it is assumed to be similar to the JAK/STAT pathway activated by IFNα *(see 94)*.

Effects of oIFNτ on *de novo* synthesis and secretion of proteins by endometrium in vitro were to increase secretion of 11 proteins and decrease secretion of six proteins *(102)* in response to treatment with oIFNτ (5 μg/mL). Only two of these secretory proteins, β_2-microglobulin in sheep *(103)* and ubiquitin crossreactive protein in cattle *(104)* have been identified, but their functions remain to be determined. Another secreted protein, identified by its size (~70 kDa) and acidic pI (~4.0), has been used as a marker for IFN action on the endometrium, although the identity and function of the 70-kDa protein are unknown *(102)*. The most recently reported pregnancy-associated protein is granulocyte chemokine produced by bovine endometrium *(105)*. In addition, IFNs affect expression of numerous intracellular proteins, but only a few of these have been examined in the pregnant ruminant uterus.

Endometrial 2′,5′-oligoadenylate synthetase enzyme (2′,5′-A) activity increased in response to pregnancy or IFNτ in ruminants *(106)*. In the IFN-induced antiviral state, this enzyme catalyzes the production of oligomers of adenine, which activate a latent endoribonuclease to degrade invading viral as well as cellular RNA. The role of the 2′,5′-A enzyme in pregnancy remains undetermined. Another IFN-induced protein expressed in the pregnant ruminant uterus is the Mx protein *(107,108)*. The Mx proteins are monomeric GTPases that possess antiviral activity *(see 96)*. Charleston and Stewart *(107)* recently cloned a cDNA for ovine Mx that shared 80 and 73% amino acid sequence identity with human MxA and mouse Mx1, respectively. The Mx mRNA abundance was greater in the pregnant uterine horn of unilaterally pregnant ewes on d 13 (mating = d 0) compared to the nonpregnant uterine horn, suggesting a local effect of the conceptus on Mx expression. Intrauterine injection of either human IFNα or oIFNτ also increased endometrial oMx mRNA abundance in cyclic ewes *(107,108)*.

Interestingly, cyclic ewes express substantial amounts of Mx mRNA, particularly in the endometrial LE and shallow GE (*108;* Ott and Bazer, unpublished observations). In cyclic ewes, steady-state levels of endometrial Mx mRNA were greatest when both endometrial progesterone receptors and circulating progesterone concentrations were maximal. Immunohistochemical analysis of cyclic and pregnant ovine and bovine uteri using an antibody against human MxA indicated the presence of immunoreactive Mx *(108)*. The Mx levels were greatest during the period of maximal IFNτ production in sheep (d 12–17) and cattle (d 15–21). Pregnancy resulted in a marked increase in steady-state levels of Mx expression in ewes. This increase was first evident at d 13 of pregnancy. By d 17 of pregnancy, Mx expression in the LE was greater than for any day of the estrous cycle. Expression was also strong in the shallow GE, deep GE, and throughout the stroma and myometrium. Stromal and myometrial expression of Mx, however, was not detected in uterine tissues from cyclic ewes. Interestingly, Mx expression continued to be strong at d 25 of pregnancy in sheep, well beyond the period of maximal production of oIFNτ (d 15–17). Ott et al. *(109)* detected low levels of immunoreactive IFN during this period; however, this IFN has not been characterized. In addition, the half-life of Mx protein is long, being detectable for 2 wk following a single exposure to IFN in humans. At d 25 of pregnancy, Mx expression was confined primarily to the LE and shallow GE with minimal expression in the stroma and myometrium (Ott and Bazer, unpublished results).

Intrauterine injections of roIFNτ from d 11–15 resulted in strong induction of Mx expression throughout the endometrium and myometrium, whereas ewes receiving ovine serum proteins had only a weak hybridization signal in the LE *(108)*. Taken together, these results indicate that Mx induction is a major response to pregnancy in the cow and ewe, and that Mx expression may be regulated by progesterone during the cycle. The role of Mx in establishment and maintenance of pregnancy remains to be determined, but it may serve a role in the uterus as an antiviral protein, a steroid-and/or IFNτ-dependent regulator of secretion, and/or a component of the antiluteolytic pathway.

In cattle, pregnancy results in increased levels of an endometrial prostaglandin synthesis inhibitor (EPSI) recently identified as linoleic acid *(see 34)*. Linoleic acid acts as a competitive inhibitor of arachidonic acid for the enzyme cyclooxygenase to reduce endometrial prostaglandin production. The mechanism whereby bIFNτ increases endometrial production of linoleic acid has not been determined. A similar EPSI has not been identified in ovine endometrium, and this is supported by the fact that basal PGF levels are actually higher in pregnant than cyclic ewes. In addition, enhanced phospholipase A_2 (PLA) inhibitory activity in early pregnancy, as well as increased expression of lipocortin and/or annexin families of proteins in response to oIFNτ, warrants investigation *(see 32)*. The inhibitors of PLA may suppress PGF secretion by binding Ca, and preventing phospholipid-PLA binding, or inhibiting PLA activity directly. In general, it is becoming increasingly clear that IFNτ mediates maternal recognition of pregnancy in ruminants by altering protein and lipid metabolism in the endometrium using many of the same pathways IFN uses to affect the immune system. Endometrial proteins induced by IFNτ in sheep (β_2-microglobulin *[103]*) and cattle (12- and 28-kDa ubiquitin-like proteins *[see 102]*) may be important markers of gene expression in response to early activated transcription factors that bind to ISREs in target genes. Detailed studies of genes induced by IFNτ (12-and 28-kDa proteins, and 2′,5′-oligoadenylate synthetase *[106]*, Mx protein *[106,107]*, and IRF-1/IRF-2) (Spencer and Bazer, unpublished results), or inhibited by IFNτ (estradiol and OT receptors) are necessary to elucidate intracellular mechanisms responsible for decreased endometrial secretion of PGF.

Experimental results from studies of IFNτ and IFNα suggest that local intracellular responses to IFNτ account for its antiluteolytic effects. In cattle, cyclooxygenase is inhibited owing to IFNτ-induced mobilization of free linoleic acid as a consequence of increased phospholipase or lipase activities associated with the IFNτ receptor signal transduction pathway. Regulation of phospholipases (e.g., PLC and PLA_2) is an integral part of hormonal signal transduction systems (e.g., OT). The increase in free linoleic acid may redirect arachidonic acid metabolism from prostaglandins and leukotrienes to epoxygenase derivatives. This proposed alteration in arachidonic acid metabolism could result from competitive inhibition of the cyclooxygenase enzyme by linoleic acid. Epoxygenase derivatives and linoleic acid have synergistic effects on IFN-stimulated gene expression through activation of transcription factors by tyrosine kinase. Alterations in IFNτ-regulated gene expression change secretion of prostaglandins by increasing annexins and lipases or inhibiting expression of ER and OTR. The combined effects would be coordinated attenuation of secretion of luteolytic PGF.

Rodents

Maternal Recognition of Pregnancy in Rodents. Gestation in rodents last 20–22 d, and functional CL must be maintained until d 17 *(110)*. The transition in rodents (i.e., rats, mice, and hamsters) from recurrent estrous cycles to pregnancy is dependent on maintenance of progesterone production by the CL, the main source of progesterone throughout pregnancy. Replacement therapy with progesterone alone is sufficient to maintain pregnancy in ovariectomized rats *(110,111)*. In addition to lacking a true luteal phase during the estrous cycle, rodents do not exhibit a change in source of progesterone from the CL to the placenta. Thus, maternal recognition of pregnancy in rodents involves activation of nonfunctional CL of the cycle into functional CL of pregnancy.

Sterile mating or cervical stimulation of rodents during estrus results in pseudopregnancy, and the activated CL secretes progesterone for 12–14 d. Function of the CL past 12 d is dependent on the presence of viable conceptuses within the uterus. A successful pregnancy in rats requires active progesterone secretion from the CL until at least d 17–18. Therefore, establishment and maintenance of pregnancy in rodents requires two separate endocrine events *(see 16)*. The first endocrine event is a surge of prolactin from the pituitary that is produced via activation of a neural reflex arc in response to either mating or cervical manipulation *(see 112)*. In rats, artificial stimulation of the cervix or mating result in both diurnal and nocturnal surges of prolactin that last throughout pregnancy or pseudopregnancy *(see 112)* in rats. The increase in prolactin is necessary for maintenance of active CL and progesterone secretion. Injections of prolactin will maintain the CL in cycling rats, injection of an inhibitor of prolactin (PRL) secretion, e.g., ergocornine, terminates pseudopregnancy *(see 16)*. Therefore, the luteotrophic effects of PRL during early pregnancy are required to convert the nonfunctional CL of the estrous cycle into functional CL of pregnancy or pseudopregnancy.

The luteotrophic actions of PRL on the CL during early pregnancy are complex. Enhanced secretion of PRL increases the number of LH receptors to enhance steroidogenesis *(113)*. Recently, PRL was demonstrated to suppress 20α-HSD activity in the CL to reduce conversion of progesterone to 20α-OHP. A reciprocal relationship exists between plasma levels of progesterone and 20α-OHP during pregnancy *(114)*. The activity of 20α-HSD in rat CL is suppressed by PRL during the luteal phase, but 20α-HSD activity increases at the end of pseudopregnancy *(115)*. Moreover, the diurnal surges of PRL in response to mating also cease between d 12 and 14 postmating in both pregnant and pseudopregnant rodents. Serum concentrations of progesterone during early pregnancy are similar to those of pseudopregnant rodents. However, serum concentrations of progesterone decline around d 11 of pseudopregnancy, but increase to about twice the values for pseudopregnancy and are maintained at those levels until the end of gestation on d 20 *(116)*.

The second endocrine event required for the maintenance of pregnancy in rodents is dependent on implantation and development of normal conceptuses. In pregnant rodents, the placenta and decidua produce PRL-like hormones, which sustain the luteotrophic actions of PRL on the CL to ensure production of progesterone during the middle and late stages of pregnancy *(117)*.

Rodent Decidual PRL-Like Proteins. Implantation in rodents involves the transformation of stromal cells into decidual cells, a process termed decidualization. The presence of decidual cells affects the production of progesterone by the CL *(see 118)*. Thus, a complex relationship exists between decidual and ovarian signals. Progesterone from CL is essential for decidualization, which is responsible for continued production of progesterone by CL during pregnancy. In the mouse and rat, decidualization produces two uniquely different cell populations depending on the relative position of the cells to the implantation site. The initial site of decidualization in the antimesometrial endometrium forms the antimesometrial decidua, or decidua capsularis. Subsequently, decidualization of the mesometrial stromal cells forms the mesometrial decidua or decidua basalis, which is characterized by small, loosely packed fibroblast-like and binucleated cells. These decidual cells have apparent endocrine functions, and secrete α_2-macroglobulin and numerous growth factors *(119)*. In contrast, the antimesometrial decidua is formed by giant polyploid cells, which are closely packed and secrete numerous hormones, including follistatin, activin, transforming growth factors-β (TGF-β), PRL-like protein B (PLP-B), and decidual PRL-like protein (dPRP) *(119,120)*.

Hormones produced by the antimesometrial decidua sustain luteal production of progesterone and reduce the ability of follicles to aromatize androgens and estradiol *(118)*. The main luteotropic hormone of the decidua is a PRL-like protein. Although decidual tissue also expresses PLP-B, it is produced in very low amounts compared to dPRP mRNA *(see 121)*. Cloning of the dPRP cDNA confirmed that it is a member of the PRL family *(see 122)*. The dPRP gene is located on rat chromosome 17 along with other members of the rat PRL gene family. This PRL-like protein is approx 28 kDa and serves as an excellent marker for induction of decidualization as well as antimesometrial decidual cell formation. Decidual PRP binds to PRL receptors on luteal cell membranes and suppresses 20α-HSD, which stimulates secretion of progesterone. Moreover, dPRP binds receptors in the mesometrial decidua and upregulates expression of α_2-macroglobulin. Thus, dPRP acts on both the ovary and the decidua.

Rodent Placental PRL-Like Molecules or Placental Lactogens. Placental lactogens (PLs) are found in a variety of subprimate mammals, including rodents. However, the only clear physiological roles for these PLs have been established in rodents. In the rat, seven members of the PRL gene family are expressed by trophoblast cells of the placenta: placental lactogen-I (PL-I), PL-I variant (PL-Iv), PL-I mosaic (PL-Im), PL-II, PRL-like protein A (PLP-A), PLP-B, and PLP-C *(see 40,123)*. The initial members of this family (PL-I and PL-II) were identified by their biological activities, which are similar to those of pituitary PRL, including maintenance of CL functions and stimulation of mammary gland growth *(124)*. The remaining members of the placental PRL-like family of PL were identified by copurification with known members or during the course of cloning their cDNAs *(125)*. As mentioned previously, two members of the PRL gene family are expressed in the uterus, dPRP and PLP-B. Although dPRP is expressed exclusively by antimesometrial decidual cells, PLP-B appears to be expressed both in the placenta and decidua *(126)*.

Placental Lactogens. All seven members of the rodent PRL-like hormone family have been characterized, and their cDNAs cloned. In both rats and mice, the PL genes are clustered with PRL and dPRP on either chromosome 17 or 13. As reviewed by Shiota et al. *(40)*, these results support the concept that placental and decidual members of the PRL family arose from PRL gene duplication.

The PL-I, PL-Iv, and PLP-A display molecular heterogeneity owing to differences in glycosylation. Mouse PL-I is comprised of five different glycoproteins (36.5–42 kDa) with a common 29-kDa core protein *(127)*. The PL-Iv is secreted predominantly as a 33-kDa species, whereas PLP-A is a glycoprotein synthesized as two distinct species (29 and 33 kDa). The PLP-B is a glycoprotein with mol wt of 24–30 kDa. The PLP-C is secreted as a 25-kDa nonglycosylated form and a 29-kDa glycosylated form. The cDNA of PL-Im has an open reading frame of 687 bp encoding 229 amino acids with two putative *N*-glycosylation sites. The PL-Im is highly homologous to the other six members of the rat PL family, and is over 90% homologous with PL-I and PL-Iv. Detailed comparisons of PL nucleotide sequences suggest that PL-Im is a mosaic structure of PL-I and PL-Iv. The predicted structure of PL-Im protein contains the 20 conserved amino acids with that of the other six family members. Shiota et al. *(40)* constructed an evolutionary dendrogram based on the nucleotide sequence homologies of PL family members. The midpregnancy-specific PLs (PL-I and PL-Im) appear to be derived from the late-pregnancy-specific PL-II, with PL-Im being placed between PL-Iv and PL-I. The unique structure of the PL-Im cDNA suggests that it may be a principal factor in the molecular evolution of PLs. The PL-II is not a glycoprotein, suggesting that the evolution of PL genes was accompanied by a process that produced molecular diversity with respect to glycoresidues *(40)*.

Expression of the PL Family During Trophoblast Cell Morphogenesis. The most striking feature of the PL family is that its members are expressed in cell-, positional-, and temporal-specific patterns, which provide excellent markers of trophoblast cell differentiation *(see 126)*. The PL family can be divided into two categories based on their expression during gestation: midpregnancy (PL-I) and late-pregnancy (PL-Iv, PL-Im, PL-II, PLP-A, PLP-B, PLP-C). The PL-I is expressed by mural trophoblast giant cells of the implanting blastocyst, and later extends to specific compartments of the choriovitelline and chorioallantoic placenta. The initial pattern of PL-I expression appears to be developmentally regulated by implantation and formation of trophoblast giant cells between d 4 and 5, whereas termination of PL-I expression is coordinated with loss of the choriovitelline placenta. Between d 10 and 12 of gestation in the rat, PL-II expression is initiated and PL-I expression is terminated. During this period, both PL-I and PL-II are expressed by trophoblast giant cells, but cellular and molecular mechanisms governing expression of these genes are not known. During midgestation, the primary source of PL-I and PL-II is trophoblast giant cells of the choriovitelline placenta. During d 13 and 14 of gestation, the choriovitelline placenta degenerates, PL-I expression ends, and PL-II expression by trophoblast giant cells of the chorioallantoic placenta begins. The PL-II is expressed initially in trophoblast giant cells of the junctional zone and then trophoblast giant cells of the labyrinth zone during late gestation.

Expression of PLP-A, PLP-C, and PL-Iv increases in cells of the chorioallantoic placental junctional zone just after midgestation. During mid- to late gestation, expression of these three genes increases, but remains confined to spongiotrophoblast cells and some trophoblast giant cells of the junctional zone. Although PLP-B expression is restricted to spongiotrophoblast cells, its temporal expression is similar to that for PLP-A, PLP-C, and PL-Iv. Collectively, knowledge of expression of these members of the placental PRL family provides cell-specific and temporal-specific landmarks of trophoblast cell differentiation *(see 126)*. It is clear that the other two cell types of the rodent placenta, glycogen cells and syncytial cells, do not express members of the placental PRL family.

Factors Regulating Production of PLs by Trophoblast Cells. Factors regulating production of PLs by trophoblast cells are not well known. The ontogeny of PL-I expression appears to be a developmentally programmed event linked to trophoblast cell differentiation during the peri-implantation period *(see 126)*. In the mouse, PL-I gene expression appears to be regulated by the number of conceptuses and by the pituitary gland *(see 125)*. Similarly, factors affecting PL-II gene expression include the number of conceptuses, genotype of the conceptuses, pituitary via growth hormone (GH), ovarian steroids, and the nutritional status of the mother. However, the molecular mechanisms regulating the shift from mid- to late-pregnancy-specific PLs is not known. The shift from PL-I to PL-II expression is temporally associated with degeneration of the choriovitelline placenta between d 13 and 14 of gestation. Therefore, mechanisms regulating trophoblast and placental cell differentiation most likely affect expression of PLs. Estrogen and progesterone are factors involved in the cytodifferentiation of placental tissues. Moreover, the decidua and placenta produce a variety of growth factors and cytokines, which may act as either autocrine or paracrine regulators of trophoblast cell differentiation and, thus, PL gene expression. Epidermal growth factor (EGF), insulin-like growth factor, and insulin have been reported to stimulate PL release in vitro by rat placental cells. Other growth factors, including TGF-β, IL-1, colony-stimulating factor-one (CSF-1), and tumor necrosis factor-α (TNF-α), also function as regulators of trophoblast cell growth, differentiation, and degeneration. Therefore, the cytokine milieu provided by placental and maternal sources may directly affect PL gene expression in trophoblast cells, or indirectly affect programmed PL expression by altering growth, differentiation, and degeneration of placental cells *(40)*. Shiota and coworkers *(40)* suggest that both intraplacental changes and the maternal endocrinological milieu are involved in the shift of midpregnancy-specific PLs to PL-II.

Physiological Function of Placental Lactogens. Since members of the rat placental PRL-like family display structural and functional similarity to PRL and diurnal surges of PRL cease when secretion of PLs starts, the proposed function of PLs is to replace pituitary PRL. In support of this contention, PL-I, PL-Iv, PL-Im, and PL-II bind PRL receptors and activate the JAK-STAT signal transduction pathway similar to other members of the cytokine superfamily *(128)*. In contrast, PLP-A, PLP-B, and PLP-C do not bind to PRL receptors, and their activities are largely unknown. In rodents, proposed physiological roles of PL are:

1. Maintenance of progesterone secretion by CL during pregnancy;
2. Development of the mammary gland during pregnancy; and
3. Control of maternal metabolic functions *(see 40)*.

In rats, PRL secretion is essential for maintenance of progesterone secretion by CL throughout pseudopregnancy. However, in the pregnant rat, removal of the anterior pituitary after midgestation does not affect luteal function, and pregnancy is maintained *(110)*. Thus, pituitary PRL is not necessary after d 6 of gestation in rodents. Given their

PRL-like activity and their ontogeny during pregnancy, PLs are likely placental luteotrophic factors during mid- to late pregnancy in rodents. Galosy and Talamantes *(129)* recently offered direct evidence for the luteotropic actions of mouse PL-I and PL-II during midpregnancy. Moreover, factors from both pituitary and placental sources appear to regulate the ontogeny and production of PLs by trophoblast cells.

The number of PRL receptors increase in the liver during pregnancy *(130)*. Moreover, ovine PL stimulates glycogen synthesis in fetal rat hepatocytes *(131)*, and PRL affects the growth and proliferation of neonatal and adult rat islet β-cells *(132)*. Collectively, these results indicate a role for PRL and members of the placental PRL-like family in maternal metabolic function. As reviewed by Thodarson and Talamantes *(124)*, PLs play a role in mammary gland development and function during pregnancy in a variety of subprimate mammals. In addition, PRL has also been implicated in the control of maternal behavior and direct actions on the central nervous system.

Swine

Estrogens. Uterine PGF is luteolytic, and estrogens produced by conceptuses between d 11 and 12 of gestation provide the initial signal for maternal recognition of pregnancy in swine (*see 43* for review). A second period of estrogen production occurs between d 15 and 30 of pregnancy *(see 133)*. Injection of exogenous estrogen (estradiol valerate, 5 mg/d) on d 11–15 of the estrous cycle will result in CL maintenance for a period equivalent to or slightly longer than pregnancy. This condition is referred to as pseudopregnancy *(see 133)*.

Whereas a single injection of estradiol on either d 9.5, 11, 12.5, 14, 15.5, or 14–16 resulted in interestrous intervals of about 30 d *(see 43)*. Estradiol must be administered to gilts on d 11 and d 14-16 or daily from d 11–15 to obtain interestrous intervals of >60 d. This suggests that two phases of estradiol, similar to that produced by conceptuses on d 11–13 and d 15–30, are necessary for prolonged secretion of PGF into the uterine lumen. Estradiol may induce receptors for maternal hormones, e.g., prolactin, or conceptus secretory proteins, which influence exocrine (into the uterine lumen) secretion of PGF. The first estrogen signal may induce those receptors, and the second estrogen signal may be required to replenish those receptors. Administration of estradiol on d 9 advances the uterine secretory response in pregnant gilts, which leads to conceptus death by d 16. An explanation for this "induced" conceptus death is not available, but it may result from ansynchrony between development of the conceptus and uterine environment *(see 133)*.

Estradiol may affect maintenance of CL by acting directly on luteal cells to increase receptors for LH and/or prolactin; however, this has not been clearly established *(see 43,133)*. Maintenance of CL occurs in hysterectomized pigs, because the source of PGF is removed and basal LH support is available. A luteotrophic hormone, produced by the conceptus, should have a systemic effect, but the pig requires the presence of at least two conceptuses in each uterine horn to establish pregnancy. Maternal recognition of pregnancy in pigs probably results from local antiluteolytic effects of estradiol of conceptus origin on the endometrium to allow PGF to be sequestered in the uterine lumen.

Prolactin. Estrogen induces endometrial receptors for prolactin in pigs, and prolactin acts on the endometrium to induce calcium cycling across the epithelium *(see 43,133)*. Endometrial concentrations of progesterone (estimate of progesterone receptor numbers) decreases between d 14 (20 pmol/mg DNA) and d 20 (2 pmol/mg DNA) of the estrous cycle. Similarly, concentrations of endometrial ER decrease from d 12 (1.5 pmol/mg DNA) to d 20 (< 0.5 pmol/mg DNA) *(see 133)*. However, endometrial concentrations of progesterone remain stable (10–15 pmol/mg DNA) between d 14 and 20 of pregnancy, whereas concentrations of estradiol decrease to < 0.25 pmol/mg DNA during the same period. Changes in PR, PR mRNA, or ER mRNA in cyclic and pregnant pigs have not been reported; therefore, one can only speculate that changes in endometrial concentrations of progesterone are related to endometrial PR. Estrogen and prolactin can interact to increase PR and endometrial secretion of progesterone-induced proteins *(see 17)*. It is possible that combined effects of prolactin and estrogen, which stabilize endometrial PR and initiate downregulation of the ER, may be influenced by γ and/or α IFNs secreted by porcine trophoblast *(134)*.

Endocrine–Exocrine Theory of Pregnancy Recognition in Pigs. The theory of maternal recognition of pregnancy in pigs has been reviewed extensively *(see 133)*. The major assumptions are that the uterine endometrium secretes PGF and that the conceptuses secrete estrogens, which are antiluteolytic. The present theory is that in cyclic gilts, PGF is secreted in an endocrine direction, toward the uterine vasculature, and transported to the CL to exert its luteolytic effect. However, in pregnant pigs, the direction of secretion of PGF is exocrine, into the uterine lumen, where it is sequestered to exert its biological effects *in utero* and/or be metabolized to prevent luteolysis. Mean concentrations, peak frequency, and peak amplitude of PGF in utero-ovarian vein plasma are lower in pregnant and estrogen-induced pseudopregnant gilts than in cyclic gilts. On the other hand, uterine flushings from pseudopregnant and pregnant gilts have significantly higher amounts of PGF than those from cyclic gilts. These results indicate that PGF is released primarily into the uterine venous drainage (endocrine) in cyclic gilts, but into the uterine lumen (exocrine) in pregnant and pseudopregnant pigs, and that secretion of PGF is not inhibited during either pregnancy or pseudopregnancy.

A perfusion device that allows one to discriminate between release of PGF from the luminal and myometrial sides of the endometrium was used to demonstrate that endometrium from cyclic pigs secretes PGF primarily from the myometrial side (endocrine) and that pregnant gilts secrete PGF primarily from the luminal side (exocrine) *(see 133)*. The transition from endocrine to exocrine secretion occurs between d 10 and 12 of pregnancy, which is temporally associated with initiation of estrogen secretion by elongating pig conceptuses. Estrogens, either secreted by the conceptus or injected, induce a transient release of calcium into the uterine lumen within 12 h. Reuptake of that calcium by endometrial and/or conceptus tissues occurs about 12 h after concentrations of calcium in uterine secretions reach maximum values. The switch in direction of endometrial secretion of PGF from an endocrine to an exocrine orientation is closely associated with this period of release and reuptake of calcium by the endometrium in pregnant and pseudopregnant gilts. When endometrium from d 14 cyclic gilts was treated with the calcium ionophore A23187 (induces calcium flux across epithelial membranes), secretion of PGF changed from an endocrine toward an exocrine direction. These results suggest that induction of calcium cycling across endometrial epithelium is associated with redirection of secretion of PGF *(see 43,133)*.

Trophoblast IFNs. Pig conceptus secretory proteins (pCSP) recovered from culture medium of d 15 conceptuses have antiviral activity owing to secretion of both α (25%) and γ (75%) IFNs *(see 134)*. Intrauterine infusion of pCSP on d 12–15 of the estrous cycle had no effect on interestrous interval or temporal changes in concentrations of progesterone in plasma *(see 133)*. The pCSP do stimulate endometrial production of PGE, which may influence the establishment and maintenance of pregnancy *(see 133)*. Inhibition of secretion of prostaglandins between d 12 and 20 after mating results in pregnancy failure in pigs *(see 43,133)*. Available results indicate that estrogens of blastocyst origin are essential for maternal recognition of pregnancy in pigs, and that pCSP, including IFNs, play other roles during early pregnancy in pigs.

Horses

Pregnancy Recognition in Mares. The uterine luteolytic substance in mares is PGF and the conceptus appears to inhibit production of PGF by the uterine endometrium *(see 133,135)*. In cycling mares, PGF concentrations in uterine venous plasma and uterine flushings increase between d 14 and 16 when luteolysis occurs and plasma progesterone levels decline. The amount of PGF bound by luteal receptors is maximal on d 14 of the estrous cycle and d 18 of pregnancy. Since CL of mares can respond to circulating PGF during pregnancy, the conceptus must evoke an antiluteolytic mechanism. Pregnant mares have little PGF in uterine fluids, PGF in uterine venous plasma is reduced, and PGFM in peripheral plasma has no episodic pattern of release *(see 133,135)*. In the presence of the conceptus, endometrial production of PGF in response to cervical stimulation and exogenous oxytocin is markedly reduced, indicating the absence/reduction of endometrial receptors for OT in mares during early pregnancy *(see 133,135)*.

Estrogens. The equine conceptus migrates between uterine horns 12–14 times/d on d 12–18 of pregnancy *(see 135)* to inhibit endometrial PGF production and protect the CL. Thus, the equine conceptus does suppress PGF production by the endometrium, but the agent has not been identified. The equine conceptus also produces increasing amounts of estradiol between d 8 and 20 of gestation. A similar trend, but of greater magnitude, was found for estrone. Attempts to prolong CL life-span in mares by injection of estrogens have been inconsistent *(see 135)*.

Conceptus Proteins. Horse conceptuses secrete three major proteins between d 12 and 14 of pregnancy with mol wt of >400,000, 50,000, and 65,000. However, the role(s) of these proteins is not known *(see 135)*. Estrogens and/or conceptus secretory proteins may provide the maternal recognition of pregnancy signal in the mare by directly or indirectly inhibiting endometrial production of luteolytic pulses of PGF.

Rabbits

Pregnancy Recognition. The rabbit has a duplex uterus with two cervices, and the male deposits semen into the anterior vagina. Multiple ova are ovulated from each ovary approx 10 h pc, and the eggs remain fertilizable for about 6 h. Fertilization occurs in the ampullary oviduct near the isthmus with the first sperm apparent in the oviduct within 30 min of mating. Fertilization usually occurs 1–2 h postovulation in the distal ampulla near the isthmus of the oviduct. The fertilized ova arrive in the uterus 3 d postovulation, and implantation occurs on d 7 postfertilization during the blastocyst stage of conceptus development. Distribution of the blastocysts is approximately equal in the two uterine horns; however, blastocysts cannot migrate between the two uterine horns. Embryonic mortality is high in the rabbit, ranging between 60 and 70%, with the majority of losses occurring before d 15 of gestation.

The rabbit has a hemochorial placenta with discoid villous distribution. The rabbit placenta is not, however, a significant source of progesterone, and the CL is required for pregnancy to go to term. Following sterile mating, CL forms and persists for 14–16 d without support from conceptus products *(see 136)*. For both pseudopregnant and pregnant does, progesterone begins to increase 2 d after mating to maximal levels of 12–20 ng/mL between d 6 and 8 pc. Between d 8 and 10 pc, progesterone profiles of pregnant and pseudopregnant does begin to diverge with levels declining rapidly after d 12 to basal levels between d 16 and 18 of pseudopregnancy. Pregnant does exhibit elevated progesterone levels, which begin to decline 3–4 d prior to parturition (kindling).

In the rabbit, maternal recognition of pregnancy occurs after implantation between d 10 and 12 of gestation *(see 137)*. Estrogen and a placental luteotropin interact to maintain progesterone production until term (28–35 d). Estrogen from developing follicles is required for luteal progesterone production for the first 10–12 d of pregnancy, but not to term. Rabbit luteal cells contain LH receptors; however, LH does not appear to be the stimulus for progesterone production in vivo *(138)*. Rather, estrogen exerts a luteotrophic effect, which results from uncoupling progesterone production from cyclic AMP (cAMP) allowing progesterone production to proceed autonomously *(139)*. In estradiol-withdrawn does, however, human chorionic gonadotropin (hCG)-stimulated luteal cAMP accumulation, and both hCG and cAMP stimulated progesterone production. Estrogen's effect does not result from progesterone production being maximal and thus unable to respond further to hCG and cAMP, but results from a specific uncoupling of cAMP from progesterone production *(139)*.

Production of a placental luteotrophin is necessary for luteal progesterone production to term, and exogenous estrogen will not support progesterone production in does hysterectomized during late pregnancy. The luteotrophic effect of the placenta is apparently not a result of increased concentrations or affinity of luteal estrogen receptors. Rabbit placentae secrete immunoreactive GnRH-like activity; however, this activity is not present in the uterine vein at concentrations greater that those of estrus rabbits, suggesting a local site of action for this placental product *(140)*. Therefore, there does not appear to be a direct effect of a placental GnRH-like factor on luteal progesterone production in the rabbit.

A putative placental luteotrophic factor was characterized with a mol wt >6–8 kDa *(see 136)*. Addition of this factor to luteal cell cultures enhanced progesterone production approximately threefold, and cotreatment with estrogen resulted in a sixfold stimulation of progesterone production. Marcinkiewicz and Bahr *(141)* also reported a rabbit placental luteotrophin that is acidic, trypsin- and heat-sensitive, and > 12–14 kDa. This factor stimulated production of progesterone 1.5-fold by luteal explants in the presence of estrogen. Although this effect appeared to be specific, since muscle cell extract had no effect, the amount of placental extract (200 μg/mL incubation medium) necessary to achieve this modest increase was large. Overall, these two groups appear to have identified a similar, if not the same factor, with the only difference being the apparent sensitivity to heat, which could be explained by differences in experimental techniques. The identity of this luteotropic activity remains to be determined. More recently, rabbit placental giant cells were shown to contain immunoreactive chorionic gonadotropin, and cytotrophoblast cells were demonstrated to contain immunoreactive PL/PRL. However, the identity, regulation, and function of these proteins have not been determined *(142,143)*.

Cat

Pregnancy Recognition. The cat has a bipartite uterus, and the male deposits semen in the anterior vagina at ejaculation. Ovulation takes place 25–50 h pc (about 24–36 h after the LH peak) with frequent matings reducing the time to ovulation. Fertilization takes place in the oviduct, up to 48 h after ovulation. The embryo enters the uterus at the blastocyst stage, 4–6 d postovulation, hatches on d 11, and begins implanting by d 12 and 13. The cat has an endotheliochorial-type placenta with zonary villous distribution. Following mating, plasma progesterone concentrations increase from about d 3 to maximal levels (15–90 ng/mL) between d 10 and 40 of pregnancy, or d 13 and 30 of pseudopregnancy. Pseudopregnancy typically lasts 40 d and gestation ranges between 56 and 71 d, averaging 63–65 d. By d 30, circulating levels of progesterone are significantly higher in pregnant than in pseudopregnant queens. Level of physical activity, litter size, and nutritional status can all affect duration of gestation.

The placenta does not appear to be a significant source of progesterone during gestation in cats. Ovariectomy on d 45 results in a rapid decline of progesterone concentrations and abortion 6–9 d postsurgery *(144)*. Prolactin levels increase during the latter third of gestation, peak just prior to parturition (5–10 ng/mL), and are elevated during lactation, especially in response to suckling. Prolactin is thought to be an important luteotrophin in late gestation *(145)*. Relaxin is produced by the fetal-placental unit and increases to peak levels of 5–10 ng/mL during the latter half of gestation *(146)*. Relaxin is thought to work in concert with progesterone to keep the uterus quiescent and to facilitate parturition by softening the connective tissues of the pelvis. Following parturition, queens experience a period of lactational anestrus and resume cycling 2–3 wk after weaning kittens.

Dog

Pregnancy Recognition. Fertilization takes place 2–5 d after ovulation in the bitch, and embryos enter the uterus at the blastocyst stage around d 10 *(146)*. Embryos remain free-floating in the uterus until hatching and implantation around d 16. The dog has endotheliochorial placentation with zonary villous distribution. The ovary is the primary source of progesterone, and ovariectomy or hypophysectomy at any stage of pregnancy results in abortion. Since CLs of pregnancy and pseudopregnancy have similar life-spans, there is no known requirement for signaling between the conceptus and maternal system for CL maintenance or pregnancy recognition.

SUMMARY AND CONCLUSIONS

The transition from recurring estrous cycles to pregnancy requires highly orchestrated interactions among the conceptus, uterus, and ovaries. Although this chapter has highlighted some of the species differences in the mechanisms of pregnancy recognition, many commonalities exist. All mammalian pregnancies require the continued actions of progesterone on maternal physiology (whether from the CL or placenta). Strategies to accomplish this range from direct conceptus support of luteal function (luteotropic) as occurs in primates and rodents, to conceptus-mediated signals, which abrogate the uterine luteolytic mechanism (antiluteolytic) as occurs in domestic ruminants, horses, and pigs, to tailoring the length of diestrus to the length of pregnancy as occurs in cats and dogs. Ensuring the continued production of progesterone is only half of the picture, however. The ability of progesterone to downregulate its receptor ensures cyclicity in many species and necessitates that the conceptus alter uterine gene expression to maintain a progestational uterus. In ruminants, the conceptus accomplishes this by blocking the cyclic upregulation of estrogen and OT receptors. The effects of the conceptus on uterine gene expression are only beginning to be unraveled in other species. This area of research should prove to be quite exciting as technical advances provide us with a clearer picture of biochemical communications between the peri-implantation conceptus and the uterus.

REFERENCES

1. Jainudeen MR, Hafez ESE (1993) Cattle and buffalo, In: Reproduction in Farm Animals, 6th ed. (Hafez ESE, ed.), Lea & Febiger, Philadelphia, pp. 315–329.
2. Jainudeen MR, Hafez ESE (1993) Sheep and goats, In: Reproduction in Farm Animals, 6th ed. (Hafez ESE, ed.), Lea & Febiger, Philadelphia, pp. 330–342.
3. Hansel W, Convey EM (1983) Physiology of the estrous cycle. J Anim Sci 57 (suppl):404–424.
4. Baird DT, Land RB, Scaramuzzi RJ, Wheeler AG (1976) Endocrine changes associated with luteal regression in the ewe; The secretion of ovarian oestradiol, progesterone, and androstenedione and uterine prostaglandin $F_{2\alpha}$ throughout the estrous cycle. J Endocrinol 69:275–286.
5. Boshier DP, Fairclough RJ, Holloway H (1987) Assessment of sheep blastocyst effects on neutral lipids in the uterine caruncular epithelium. J Reprod Fertil 79:569–573.
6. Eggleston DL, Wilken C, Van Kirk EA, Slaughter RG, Ji TH, Murdoch WJ (1990) Progesterone induces expression of endometrial messenger RNA encoding for cyclooxygenase (sheep). Prostaglandins 39:675–683.
7. Morgan GL, Geisert RD, McCann JP, Bazer FW, Ott TL, Mirando MA, Stewart M (1993) Failure of luteolysis and extension of the interoestrus interval in sheep treated with the progesterone antagonist mifepristone (RU 486). J Reprod Fertil 98:451–457.
8. Moor RM, Rowson LEA (1964) Influence of the embryo and uterus on luteal function in the sheep. Nature 201:522–523.
9. Wiltbank JN, Casida LE (1956) Alteration of ovarian activity by hysterectomy. J Anim Sci 15: 134–140.
10. McCracken JA, Carlson JC, Glew ME, Goding JR, Baird DT, Green K, Samuelson B (1972) Prostaglandin F-2 alpha identified as a luteolytic hormone in sheep. Nature 238:129–134.
11. Staples LD, Whylie PA (1984) Contribution of the utero-ovarian lymphatic network to the control of corpus luteum function in the ewe, In: Reproduction in Sheep (DR Lindsay, DT Pearce, eds.), University Press, England, pp. 122–124.
12. Heap RB, Fleet IR, Hamon M (1985) Prostaglandin F-2 alpha is transferred from the uterus to the ovary in sheep by lymphatic and blood vascular pathways. J Reprod Fertil 74:645–656.
13. McCracken JA, Schramm W, Okulicz WC (1984) Hormone receptor control of pulsatile secretion of $PGF_{2\alpha}$ from the ovine uterus during luteolysis and its abrogation in early pregnancy. Anim Reprod Sci 7:31–55.
14. Scaramuzzi RJ, Baird DT (1976) The oestrus cycle after active immunization against prostaglandin F-2 alpha. J Reprod Fertil 46:39–47.
15. Fairclough RJ, Smith JF, McGowan LT (1981) Prolongation of the oestrus cycle in cows and ewes after passive immunization with PGF antibodies. J Reprod Fertil 62:213–219.
16. Niswender GD, Nett TM (1994) Corpus luteum and its control in infraprimate species, In: The Physiology of Reproduction (E Knobil, JD Neill, eds.), Raven, New York, pp. 781–816.
17. Bazer FW, Spencer TE, Ott TL, Johnson HM Cyt (1995) Cytokines and pregnancy recognition, In: Immunobiology of Reproduction (JS Hunt, ed.), Springer-Verlag, New York, pp. 37–56.
18. Silvia WJ, Raw RE (1993) Regulation of pulsatile secretion of prostaglandin F2 alpha from the ovine uterus by ovarian steroids. J Reprod Fertil 98:341–347.
19. Wathes DC, Denning Kendall PA (1992) Control of the synthesis and secretion of ovarian oxytocin in ruminants. J Reprod Fertil 45 (Suppl):39–52.
20. Hooper SB, Watkins WB, Thorburn GD (1986) Oxytocin, oxytocin associated neurophysin, and prostaglandin $F_{2\alpha}$ concentrations in the utero-ovarian vein of pregnant and nonpregnant sheep. Endocrinology 119:2590–2597.
21. Jones DSC, Flint APF (1986) Oxytocin-neurophysin mRNA in the corpus luteum of the sheep during the oestrus cycle and in pregnancy. J Endocrinol 111 (Suppl 1):140.
22. Silvia WJ, Lewis GS, McCracken JS, Thatcher WW, Wilson L Jr (1991) Hormonal regulation of uterine secretion of prostaglandin $F_{2\alpha}$ in ruminants. Biol Reprod 45:655–663.
23. Wathes DC, Lamming GE (1995) The oxytocin receptor, luteolysis and the maintenance of pregnancy. J Reprod Fertil 49 (Suppl):53–67.
24. Jenkin G (1992) The interaction between oxytocin and prostaglandin $F2\alpha$ during luteal regression and early pregnancy in sheep. Reprod Fertil Dev 4:321–328.
25. Rhodes L, Nathanielsz PW (1990) Myometrial activity and plasma progesterone and oxytocin concentrations in cycling and early pregnant ewes. Biol Reprod 42:834–841.

26. Stevenson KR, Riley PR, Stewart HJ, Flint APF, Wathes DC (1994) Localization of oxytocin receptor mRNA in the ovine uterus during the oestrus cycle and early pregnancy. J Mol Endocrinol 12:93–105.
27. Vallet JL, Lamming GE, Batten M (1990) Control of endometrial oxytocin receptor and uterine response to oxytocin by progesterone and oestradiol in the ewe. J Reprod Fertil 90:625–634.
28. Spencer TE, Ing NH, Ott TL, Mayes JS, Becker WC, Watson GH, Mirando MA, Bazer FW (1995) Intrauterine injection of ovine interferon-τ alters oestrogen receptor and oxytocin receptor expression in the endometrium of cyclic ewes. J Mol Endocrinol 15:203–220.
29. Wathes DC, Hamon M (1993) Localization of oestradiol, progesterone and oxytocin receptors in the uterus during the oestrus cycle and early pregnancy of the ewe. J Endocrinol 138:479–491.
30. Beard AP, Lamming GE (1994) Oestradiol concentration and the development of the uterine oxytocin receptor and oxytocin-induced $PGF_{2\alpha}$ release in ewes. J Reprod Fertil 100:469–475.
31. Spencer TE, Mirando MA, Mayes JS, Watson GH, Ott TL, Bazer FW (1996) Effects of interferon-tau and progesterone on oestrogen stimulated expression of receptors for oestrogen, progesterone and oxytocin in the endometrium of ovariectomized ewes. Reprod Fertil Dev 8:843–853.
32. Flint APF, Sheldrick EL (1986) Ovarian oxytocin and maternal recognition of pregnancy. J Reprod Fertil 76:831–839.
33. Zhang J, Weston PG, Hixon JE (1991) Influence of estradiol on the secretion of oxytocin and prostaglandin $F_{2\alpha}$ during luteolysis in the ewe. Biol Reprod 45:395–403.
34. Thatcher WW, Meyer MD, Danet-Desnoyers G (1995) Maternal recognition of pregnancy. J Reprod Fertil (Suppl. 49):15–28.
35. Beard AP, Hunter MG, Lamming GE (1994) Quantitative control of oxytocin-induced $PGF_{2\alpha}$ release by progesterone and oestradiol in ewes. J Reprod Fertil 100:143–150.
36. Hixon JE, Flint APF (1987) Effects of luteolytic dose of oestradiol benzoate on uterine oxytocin receptor concentrations, phosphoinositide turnover and prostaglandin F-2α secretion in sheep. J Reprod Fertil 78:457–467.
37. Ing NH, Fleming JGW, Newton GR, Bazer FW (1996) Estrogen up-regulates expression of its receptor gene in sheep endometrium. Biol Reprod 50 (Suppl 1):118.
38. Freeman ME, Smith MS, Nazian SJ, Neill JD (1994) Ovarian and hypothalamic control of the daily surges of prolactin secretion during pseudopregnancy. Endocrinology 94:875–882.
39. Long JA, Evans HM (1922) The estrous cycle of the rat and its associated phenomena. Mem Univ Calif 6:1–148.
40. Shiota K, Hirosawa M, Hattori N, Itonori S, Miura R, Noda K, Takahashi M, Ogawa T (1994) Structural and functional aspects of placental lactogens (Pls) and ovarian 20α-hydroxysteroid dehydrogenase (20α-HSD) in the rat. Endocrine 41 (Suppl):S43–S56.
41. Dziuk PJ (1977) Reproduction in pigs, In: Reproduction in Farm Animals, 3rd ed. (Cole HH, Cupps PT, eds.), Academic, New York, pp. 456–473.
42. Anderson LL (1993) Pigs, In: Reproduction in Farm Animals, 6th ed. (Hafez ESE, ed.), Lea & Febiger, Philadelphia, pp. 343–360.
43. Geistert RD, Zavy MT, Moffatt RJ, Blair RM, Yellin T (1990) Embryonic steroids and the establishment of pregnancy in pigs. J Reprod Fertil 40 (Suppl):293–305.
44. Mirando MA, Prince BC, Tysseling KA, Carnahan KG, Ludwig TE, Hoagland TA, Crain RC (1995) A proposed role for oxytocin in regulation of endometrial prostaglandin $F_{2\alpha}$ secretion during luteolysis in swine. Adv Exp Med Biol 395:421–433.
45. Gadsby JE, Balapure AK, Britt JH, Fitz FA (1990) Prostaglandin F2α receptors on enzyme-dissociated pig luteal cells throughout the estrous cycle. Endocrinology 126:787–795.
46. Bazer FW (1989) Establishment of pregnancy in sheep and pigs. Reprod Fertil Dev 1:237–242.
47. Pitzel L, Welp K, Holtz W, Konig A (1994) The content of oxytocin and vasopressin in the corpus luteum of the pig. Acta Endocrinol 105 (Suppl 264):140,141.
48. Einspanier R, Pitzel L, Wuttke W, Hagendorff G, Preuβ WD, Kardanlinou E, Scheit KH (1986) Demonstration of mRNAs for oxytocin and prolactin in porcine granulosa and luteal cells. FEBS Lett 204:37–40.
49. Choy VJ, Watkins WB (1988) Arginine vasopressin and oxytocin in the porcine corpus luteum. Neuropeptides 11:119–123.
50. Trout WE, Smith GW, Gentry PC, Galvin JM, Keisler DH (1995) Oxytocin secretion by the endometrium of the pig during maternal recognition of pregnancy. Biol Reprod 52 (Suppl 1):189.
51. Soloff MS, Swartz TL (1974) Characterization of a proposed oxytocin receptor in the uterus of the rat and sow. J Biol Chem 249:1376–1381.

52. Gross TS, Lacroix MC, Bazer FW, Thatcher WW, Harney JP (1988) Prostaglandin secretion by perifused porcine endometrium: further evidence for an endocrine versus exocrine secretion of prostaglandins. Prostaglandins 35:327–341.
53. Edgerton LA, Kaminski MA, Silvia WJ (1996) Changes in uterine secretion of prostaglandin $F_{2\alpha}$ in response to oxytocin during the estrous cycle, early pregnancy, and estrogen-induced pseudopregnancy in swine. Biol Reprod 55:657–662.
54. Mirando MA, Leen MPJM, Beers S, Harney JP, Bazer FW (1990) Endometrial inositol phosphate turnover in pigs is reduced during pregnancy and estradiol-induced pseudopregnancy. J Anim Sci 68:4285–4291.
55. Stabenfeldt GH, Hughes JP (1977) Reproduction in horses, In: Reproduction in Domestic Animals, 3rd ed. (Cole HH, Cupps PT, eds.), Academic, New York, pp. 401–427.
56. Hafez ESE (1993) Horses, In: Reproduction in Farm Animals, 6th ed. (Hafez ESE, ed.), Lea & Febiger, Philadelphia, pp. 361–384.
57. Irvine CHG (1995) The nonpregnant mare: A review of some current research and of the last 25 years of endocrinology, In: Equine Reproduction IV, Biol Reprod Monograph Series (Bazer FW, Sharp DC, eds.), 1:343–360.
58. Zavy MT, Vernon MW, Sharp DC, Bazer FW (1984) Endocrine aspects of early pregnancy in pony mares: a comparison of uterine luminal and peripheral plasma levels of steroids during the estrous cycle and early pregnancy. Endocrinology 115(1):214–219.
59. Goff AK, Pontbriand D, Sirois J (1987) Oxytocin stimulation of plasma 15 keto-13,14-dihydroprostaglandin F2α during the oestrous cycle and early pregnancy in the mare. J Reprod Fertil (Suppl) 35:253–260.
60. Rowlands IW, Weir BJ (1984) Mammals: Non-primate eutherians, In: Marshall's Physiology of Reproduction, Vol. 1 (Lamming GE, ed.), Churchill Livingston, New York, pp. 455–658.
61. Ramirez VD, Beyer C (1994) The neuroendocrine control of the rabbit ovarian cycle, In: The Physiology of Reproduction, Vol. 2 (Knobil E, Neill JD, eds.), Raven, New York, pp. 585–612.
62. Marcinkiewiz JL, Moy ES, Bahr JM (1992) Change in responsiveness of rabbit corpus luteum to prostaglandin F-2α during pregnancy and pseudopregnancy. J Reprod Fertil 94:305–310.
63. Miller JB, Pawlak CM (1994) Characterization and physiological variation in prostaglandin, prostacyclin, and thromboxane synthesis by corpora lutea, non-luteal and uterine tissues during pseudopregnancy in the rabbit. Life Sci 54(5):341–353.
64. Wintergalen N, Thole HH, Galla HJ, Schlegel W (1995) Prostaglandin-E2 9-reductase from corpus luteum of pseudopregnant rabbit is a member of the aldo-keto reductase superfamily featuring 20 alpha-hydroxysteroid dehydrogenase activity. Eur J Biochem 234(1):264–270.
65. Nariai K, Kanayama K, Endo T, Tsukise A (1995) Effects of splenectomy on luteolysis in pseudopregnant rabbits. J Vet Med Sci 57(3):503–505.
66. Seiner SJ, Schramm W, Keyes PL (1992) Effect of treatment with methylprednisolone on duration of pseudopregnancy and on macrophages and T lymphocytes in rabbit corpora lutea. J Reprod Fertil 96(1):347–33.46.
67. Chaffaux ST (1993) Reproduction of the cat and dog. In: Reproduction in Mammals and Man (Thibault C, Levasseur M-C, Hunter RHF, eds.), Ellipses, Paris, pp. 695–713.
68. Tsutsui T, Stabenfeldt G (1993) Biology of ovarian cycles, pregnancy and pseudopregnancy in the domestic cat. J Reprod Fertil 47 (Suppl):29–35.
69. Johnson LM, Gay VL (1981) Luteinizing hormone in the cat II Mating-induced secretion. Endocrinology 109(1): 247–252.
70. Banks DH, Stabenfeldt G (1982) Luteinizing hormone release in the cat in response to coitus on consecutive days of estrus. Biol Reprod 26:603–611.
71. Lawler DF, Johnston SD, Hegstad RL, Keltner DG, Owens SF (1993) Ovulation without cervical stimulation in domestic cats. J Reprod Fertil 47 (Suppl):57–61.
72. Wildt DE, Chan SYW, Seager SWJ, Chakraborty PK (1981) Ovarian activity, circulating hormones, and sexual behavior in the cat. I. Relationships during the coitus-induced luteal phase and the estrous period without mating. Biol Reprod 25:15–28.
73. Concannon PW (1993) Biology of gonadotrophin secretion in adult and prepubertal female dogs. J Reprod Fertil 47 (Suppl):3–27.
74. Jeffcoate IA (1993) Endocrinology of anoestrous bitches. J Reprod Fertil 47 (Suppl):69–76.
75. Steinetz BG, Goldsmith LT, Hasan SH, Lust G (1990) Diurnal variation of serum progesterone, but not relaxin, prolactin, or estradiol-17 beta in the pregnant bitch. Endocrinology 127(3): 1057–1063.

76. Hoffmann B, Schneider S (1993) Secretion and release of luteinizing hormone during the luteal phase of the oestrous cycle in the dog. J Reprod Fertil 47 (Suppl):85–91.
77. Concannon PW, McCann JP, Temple M (1989) Biology and endocrinology of ovulation, pregnancy and parturition in the dog. J Reprod Fertil 39 (Suppl):3–25.
78. Roberts RM, Cross JC, Leaman DW (1992) Interferons as hormones of pregnancy. Endocr Rev 13:432–452.
79. Pontzer CH, Torres BA, Vallet JL, Bazer FW, Johnson JM (1988) Antiviral activity of the pregnancy recognition hormone ovine trophoblast protein-one. Biochem Biophys Res Commun 152:801.
80. Pontzer CH, Bazer FW, Johnson HM (1991) Antiproliferative activity of a pregnancy recognition hormone, ovine trophoblast protein-1. Cancer Res 51:5304–5309.
81. Skopets B, Li J, Thatcher WW, Roberts RM, Hansen PJ (1992) Inhibition of lymphocyte proliferation by bovine trophoblast protein-1 (type I trophoblast interferon) and bovine interferon-α1. Vet Immunol Immunopathol 12:201–205.
82. Tuo WT, Ott TL, Bazer FW (1993) Natural killer cell activity of lymphocytes exposed to ovine, type I, trophoblast interferon. Am J Reprod Immunol 29:26–34.
83. Leaman DW, Roberts RM (1992) Genes for the trophoblast intererons in sheep, goat, and musk ox and distribution of related genes among mammals. J Interferon Res 12:1–11.
84. Nephew KP, Whaley AE, Christenson RK, Imakawa K (1993) Differential expression of distinct mRNAs for ovine trophoblast protein-1 and related sheep type I interferons. Biol Reprod 48: 768–778.
85. Jarpe MA, Johnson HM, Bazer FW, Ott TL, Curto EV, Krishna NR, Pontzer CH (1991) Predicted structural motif of IFN tau. Protein Engineering 7:863–867.
86. Senda T, Saitoh S, Mitsui Y, Li J, Roberts RM (1995) A three-dimensional model of interferon-τ. J Interferon Cyto Res 15:1053–1060.
87. Pontzer CH, Ott TL, Bazer FW, Johnson HM (1990) Localization of an antiviral site on the pregnancy recognition hormone, ovine trophoblast protein 1. Proc Natl Acad Sci USA 87(15): 5945–5949.
88. Schalue TK (1992) Effects of intrauterine infusion of synthetic peptide fragments corresponding to ovine trophoblast interferon (oTIFN) on oxytocin-induced endometrial inositol phosphate turnover in ewes. Biol Reprod 46 (Suppl. 1):70.
89. Imakawa K, Helmer SD, Nephew KP, Meka CSR, Christenson RK (1993) A novel role for GM-CSF: enhancement of pregnancy specific interferon production, ovine trophoblast protein-1. Endocrinology 132:1869–1871.
90. Heyman Y, Camous S, Fevre J, Meziou W, Martal J (1984) Maintenance of the corpus luteum after uterine transfer of trophoblastic vesicles to cyclic cows and ewes. J Reprod Fertil 70:533–540.
91. Meyer MD, Hansen PJ, Thatcher WW, Drost M, Badinga L, Roberts RM, Li J, Ott TL, Bazer FW (1995) Extension of corpus luteum lifespan and reduction of uterine secretion of prostaglandin F2 of cows in response to recombinant interferon-tau. J Dairy Sci 78:1921–1931.
92. Newton GR, Ott TL, Woldesenbet S, Shelton AH, Bazer FW (1996) Biochemical and immunological properties of related small ruminant trophoblast interferons. Theriogenology 46:703–716.
93. Li J, Roberts RM (1994) Interferon-τ and interferon-α interact with the same receptors in bovine endometrium. J Biol Chem 269:13,544–13,550.
94. Darnell JE Jr, Kerr IM, Stark GW (1994) Jak-STAT pathways and transcriptional activation in response to IFNs and other extracellular signaling proteins. Science 264:1415–1421.
95. Matsuyama T, Grossman A, Mittrucker H-W, Siderovski DP, Kiefer F, Kawakami T, Richardson CD, Taniguchi T, Yoshinaga SK, Mak TW (1995) Molecular cloning of LSIRF, a lymphoid-specific member of the interferon regulatory factor family that binds the interferon-stimulated response element (ISRE). Nucleic Acids Res 23:2127–2136.
96. Spencer TE, Ott TL, Bazer FW (1996) Interferon tau: Pregnancy recognition signal in ruminants. Proc Exp Biol Med 213:215–229.
97. Bazer FW, Spencer RE, Ott TL (1996) Placental interferons. Am J Reprod Immunol 35:297–308.
98. Vallet JL, Gross TS, Fliss MFV, Bazer FW (1989) Effects of pregnancy, oxytocin, ovine trophoblast protein-1 and their interactions on endometrial production of prostaglandin $F_{2\alpha}$ in vitro in perifusion chambers. Prostaglandins 38:113–124.
99. Spencer TS, Bazer FW (1996) Ovine interferon tau suppresses transcription of the estrogen receptor and oxytocin receptor genes in the ovine endometrium. Endocrinology 137:1144–1147.

100. Ott TL, Zhou Y, Mirando MA, Stevens C, Harney JP, Ogle TF, Bazer FW (1993) Changes in progesterone and oestrogen receptor mRNA and protein during maternal recognition of pregnancy and luteolysis in ewes. J Mol Endocrinol 10:171–183.
101. Pestka AJ, Langer JA (1987) Interferons and their actions. Ann Rev Biochem 56:727–777.
102. Vallet JL, Bazer FW, Roberts RM (1987) The effect of ovine trophoblast protein-one on endometrial protein secretion and cyclic nucleotides. Biol Reprod 37:1307–1316.
103. Vallet JL, Barker PJ, Lamming GE, Skinner N, Huskisson NS (1991) A low molecular weight endometrial secretory protein which is increased by ovine trophoblast protein-1 is a β2-microglobulin-like protein. J Endocrinol 130:R1–R4.
104. Austin KJ, Ward SK, Teixeira MG, Dean VC, Moore DW, Hansen TR (1996) Ubiquitin cross-reactive protein is released by the bovine uterus in response to interferon during early pregnancy. Biol Reprod 54:600–606.
105. Teixieira MG, Austin KJ, Perry DJ, Dooley VD, Johnson GA, Hansen TR (1996) Granulocyte chemotactic protein-2 is a pregnancy-associated uterine chemokine. Biol Reprod 54 (Suppl 1):104.
106. Short EC, Geisert RD, Helmer SD, Zavy MT, Fulton RW (1991) Expression of antiviral activity and induction of 2′,5′-oligoadenylate synthetase by conceptus secretory proteins enriched in bovine trophoblast protein-1. Biol Reprod 44:261–268.
107. Charleston B, Stewart HJ (1993) An interferon-induced Mx protein: cDNA sequence and high-level expression in the endometrium of pregnant sheep. Gene 137:327–331.
108. Ott TL, Wiley AA, Spencer TE, Bartol FF, Bazer FW (1995) Uterine expression of interferon-induced Mx in cyclic and pregnant ewes. Biol Reprod 52 (Suppl. 1):143.
109. Ott TL, Mirando MA, Davis MA, Fliss MFV, Bazer FW (1989) Characterization of a second period of immunoreactive ovine trophoblast protein-one secretion in sheep. J Anim Sci 67 (Suppl. 1):370.
110. Heap RB, Perry JS, Challis JRG (1973) Hormonal maintenance of pregnancy, In: Handbook of Physiology, section 7: Endocrinology, vol. 1, part 2 (Greep RO, Astwood EB, Geiger SR, eds.), Williams and Wilkins Co., Baltimore, pp. 217–260.
111. Csapo AI, Wiest WG (1969) An examination of the quantitative relationship between progesterone and the maintenance of pregnancy. Endocrinology 85:735–746.
112. Freeman ME (1994) The neuroendocrine control of the ovarian cycle of the rat, In: The Physiology of Reproduction, 2nd ed. (Knobil E, Neill JD, eds.), Raven, New York, pp. 613–658.
113. Richards JS, Williams JL (1976) Luteal cell receptor content for prolactin (PRL) and luteinizing hormone (LH). Regulation by LH and PRL. Endocrinology 99:1571–1581.
114. Hashimoto I, Henricks DM, Anderson LL, Melampy RM (1968) Progesterone and pregn-4-en-20α-ol-3-one in ovarian venous blood during various reproductive states in the rat. Endocrinology 82:333–341.
115. Matsuda J, Noda K, Shiota K, Takahashi M (1990) Participation of ovarian 20α-hydroxysteriod dehydrogenase in luteotrophic and luteolytic processes during rat pseudopregnancy. J Reprod Fertil 1990; 88:467–478.
116. Pepe GJ, Rothchild I (1974) A comparative study of serum progesterone levels in pregnancy and in various types of pseudopregnancy in the rat. Endocrinology 95:275–279.
117. Soares MJ, Julian JA, Glasser SR (1985) Trophoblast giant cell release of placental lactogens: temporal and regional characteristics. Dev Biol 107:520–526.
118. Gibori G (1994) The decidual hormones and their role in pregnancy recognition, In: Endocrinology of Embryo-Endometrium Interactions (Glasser SR, Mulholland J, Psychoyos A, et al., eds.), Plenum, New York, pp. 217–222.
119. Gu Y, Gibori G (1995) Isolation, culture and characterization of the two cell subpopulations forming the rat decidua: differential gene expression for activin, follistatin, and decidual prolactin-related protein. Endocrinology 136:2451–2458.
120. Gu Y, Srivastava RK, Ou J, Krett NL, Mayo KE, Gibori G (1995) Cell-specific expression of activin and its two binding proteins in the rat decidua: role of α_2-macroglobulin and follistatin. Endocrinology 1995; 136:3815–3822.
121. Gu Y, Soares MJ, Srivastava, Gibori G (1994) Expression of decidual prolactin-related protein in the rat decidua. Endocrinology 1994; 135:1422–1427.
122. Roby KF, Deb S, Gibori G, Szpirer C, Levan G, Kwok SCM, Soares MJ (1993) Decidual prolactin-related protein identification, molecular cloning, and characterization. J Biol Chem 268:3136–3142.
123. Ogren L, Talamantes F (1994) The placenta as an endocrine organ: polypeptides, In: The Physiology of Reproduction, 2nd ed. (Knobil E, Neill JD, eds.), Raven, New York, pp. 875–945.

124. Thodarson G, Talamantes F (1987) Role of the placenta in mammary gland development and function, In: The Mammary Gland (Neville C, Daniel CW, eds.), Plenum, New York, pp. 459–498.
125. Soares MJ, Faria TN, Roby KF, Deb S (1991) Pregnancy and the prolactin family of hormones: coordination of anterior pituitary, uterine and placental expression. Endo Rev 12:402–423.
126. Soares MJ, Faria TN, Hamlin GP, Lu X-J, Deb S (1993) Trophoblast cell differentiation: expression of the placental prolactin family, In: Trophoblast Cells: Pathways for Maternal-Embryonic Communication (Soares MJ, Handwerger S, Talamantes FJ, eds.), Springer-Verlag, New York, pp. 45–67.
127. Talamantes FJ, Masaaki Y, Thordarson G, Southard J, Ogren L (1993) Mouse placental lactogens: characterization and regulation of expression in trophoblast cells, In: Trophoblast Cells: Pathways for Maternal-Embryonic Communication (Soares MJ, Handwerger S, Talamantes FJ, eds.), Springer-Verlag, New York, pp. 163–168.
128. Cohick CB, Dai G, Xu L, Deb S, Kamei T, Levan G, Szpirer C, Szpirer J, Kwok SCM, Soares MJ (1996) Placental lactogen-I variant utilizes the prolactin receptor signal transduction pathway. Mol Cell Endocrinol 116:49–58.
129. Galosy SS, Talamantes F (1995) Luteotropic actions of placental lactogens at midpregnancy in the mouse. Endocrinology 136:3993–4003.
130. Kelly PA, Djane J, P-Vinay MC, Edery M (1991) The prolactin/growth hormone receptor family. Endocr Rev 12:235–251.
131. Freemark M, Handwerger S (1984) Ovine placental lactogen stimulates glycogen synthesis in fetal rat hepatocytes. Am J Physiol 246:E21–24.
132. Brelje TC, Sorenson RL (1991) Role of prolactin versus growth hormone on islet B-cell proliferation in vitro: implication for pregnancy. Endocrinology 128:45–57.
133. Bazer FW (1992) Mediators of maternal recognition of pregnancy in mammals. Proc Soc Exp Biol Med 199:373–384.
134. La Bonnardiere C, Martinat-Botte F, Terqui M, Lefevre F, Zouari K, Martal J, Bazer FW (1991) Production of two species of interferon by Large White and Meishan pig conceptuses during the peri-attachment period. J Reprod Fertil 91(2):496–478.
135. Sharp DC, McDowell KJ, Weithenauer J, Thatcher WW (1989) The continuum of events leading to maternal recognition of pregnancy in mares. J Reprod Fertil (Suppl) 37:101–107.
136. Gadsby JE (1989) Control of corpus luteum function in the pregnant rabbit. J Reprod Fertil 37 (Suppl):45–54.
137. Nowak RA, Bahr JM (1983) Maternal recognition of pregnancy in the rabbit. J Reprod Fertil 69: 623–627.
138. Keyes PL, Kostyo JL, Towns R (1994) The autonomy of the rabbit corpus luteum. J Endocrinol 143(3):423–431.
139. Townson DH, Keyes PL, Kostyo JL (1995) Estrogen uncouples steriodogenesis from 3′,5′-cyclic adenosine monophosphate regulation in the rabbit corpus luteum. Biol Reprod 53(3):718–723.
140. Nowak RA, Bahr JM (1987) Secretion of a gonadotrophin-releasing hormone-(GnRH)like factor by the rabbit fetal placenta in vitro. Placenta 8:299–304.
141. Marcinkiewicz JL, Bahr JM (1993) Identification and preliminary characterization of luteotropic activity in the rabbit placenta. Biol Reprod 48:403–408.
142. Grunder C, Hrabe de Angelis M, Kirchner C (1993) Placental lactogen-like proteins in the rabbit placenta. Anat Embryol 188(4):395–399.
143. Grunder C, Hrabe de Angelis M, Kirchner C (1994) Chorionic gonadotropin-like proteins in the obplacental giant cells of the rabbit. Cell Tissue Res 278(3):573–578.
144. Verstegen JP, Onclin K, Silva LDM, Wouters-Ballman P, Delahaut P, Ectors F (1993) Regulation of progesterone during pregnancy in the cat: studies on the roles of corpora lutea, placenata and prolactin secretion. J Reprod Fertil 47 (Suppl):165–173.
145. Tsutsui T, Stabenfeldt GH (1993) Biology of ovarian cycles, pregnancy and pseudopregnancy in the domestic cat. J Reprod Fertil (Suppl) 47:29–35.
146. Concannon PW, McCann JP (1989) Biology and endocrinology of ovulation, pregnancy and parturition in the dog. J Reprod Fertil (Suppl) 39:3–25.

2 Endocrinology of the Transition from Menstrual Cyclicity to Establishment of Pregnancy in Primates

Richard L. Stouffer, PHD *and John P. Hearn,* PHD

CONTENTS

INTRODUCTION

An important feature of ovarian function in mammalian species is the development of the corpus luteum from the ovulatory follicle and its subsequent role in producing hormonal factors, notably progesterone, that are essential to the initiation and maintenance of intrauterine pregnancy. In some species, including primates, the functional life-span of the corpus luteum during the ovarian cycle is sufficient to permit timely movement of the early embryo through the oviduct, preparation of the uterus for implantation, and actual embryo invasion of the endometrium. However, the regression of the corpus luteum near the end of the menstrual cycle (~2 wk postovulation) typically occurs before the developing placenta can initiate local mechanisms (e.g., progesterone production) to keep the uterus in a continued quiescent, supportive state throughout gestation. Thus, a critical interval in early pregnancy occurs when the early conceptus signals the mother (i.e., maternal recognition of pregnancy) that intrauterine pregnancy is eminent or occurring, and that extended luteal function is necessary. Luteal function may be extended throughout pregnancy or, in primate species, until the time when the essential activities are replaced by placental functions (i.e., the luteal–placental shift).

Considering the importance of these processes, it is unfortunate that our understanding of the early events in maternal recognition of pregnancy in primates is so limited. A major factor is the apparent differences between primate and nonprimate (e.g., ruminants *[1]*) species that have ovarian cycles characterized by long luteal phases in: (1) the mechanisms controlling the regression of the corpus luteum at the end of a nonfertile cycle, and (2) the processes whereby the conceptus signals the mother that a fertile cycle has occurred and extended luteal function is required. In many nonprimate species, the regression of the corpus luteum is controlled by prostaglandin $F_{2\alpha}$ ($PGF_{2\alpha}$) secreted by the uterus toward the end of the ovarian cycle *(2,3)*; this luteolytic signal is either prevented or neutralized when an early embryo is present in the uterus. The mechanism of luteolysis is not known in primates, but it is clear that the demise of the corpus luteum is not the result of a luteolytic signal from the uterus, since hysterectomy does not alter cyclic ovarian function in women or monkeys (for review *see 4*).

Investigators proposed "self-destruct" mechanisms *(5)*, whereby substances synthesized within the primate ovary or corpus luteum initiate luteolysis near the end of the menstrual cycle. Research on this problem has focused on two types of substances, estrogen and $PGF_{2\alpha}$, but a physiologic role for either local factor in regression of the primate corpus luteum remains unsubstantiated *(4)*. Reports of direct effects of estrogens on primate luteal cells are countered by evidence that exogenous estrogen is luteolytic only when treatment suppresses pituitary luteotropic support (i.e., circulating luteinizing hormone (LH) levels). Whether the primate corpus luteum contains estrogen receptor-mediated pathways typical of other estrogen target tissues, such as the uterus, is also unclear *(6)*. Likewise, antigonadotropic effects of $PGF_{2\alpha}$ on primate luteal cells in vitro support a direct action on the corpus luteum, but protocols administering PG synthesis inhibitors either systemically or locally did not extend the life-span of the corpus luteum *(see 4)*. Nevertheless, intraluteal infusion of $PGF_{2\alpha}$, but not other PGs, will cause premature luteolysis in monkeys. Although $PGF_{2\alpha}$ remains the leading candidate as a local luteolysin, any number of peptide/protein factors recently localized to primate luteal tissue could interact with various cell types in the corpus luteum to cause luteal regression *(4,7)*.

Although the processes limiting the functional life-span of the primate corpus luteum in the nonconceptive cycle are unclear, it is well established that the "rescue" *(5)* of the corpus luteum from its impending demise in the fertile cycle is owing to an additional luteotropic signal, chorionic gonadotropin (CG), derived from the peri-implantation embryo *(8)*. In this chapter, we consider the embryo-maternal interactions during implantation and early pregnancy, using a New World (marmoset) and an Old World (rhesus) monkey for comparisons with the human. These three species conform to a basic primate pattern, but there are variations (e.g., in the timing of the first release of CG, the onset of the luteal-placental shift, and the duration of CG production during pregnancy) that may provide insight into the evolution of mechanisms of maternal recognition in primates. This chapter summarizes the recent advances in the field, building on the framework of earlier reviews on the corpus luteum and pregnancy initiation in women and nonhuman primates *(4,9,10)*, while hopefully stimulating the reader to new avenues of investigation.

THE DEVELOPMENT OF EMBRYONIC SIGNALS: CG

The primate embryo enters the uterus by late d 3 to early d 4 postovulation, having reached the morula stage of development. Allowing some variation, it is generally believed that embryo attachment occurs on d 7–9 postovulation in macaques and humans, but somewhat later on d 11–12 in marmosets *(9)*. In all cases, implantation occurs after expansion of the blastocyst and "hatching" from the surrounding zona pellucida. There is evidence the early preimplantation embryo produces potential signals, e.g., early pregnancy factor *(11)*, platelet-activating factor *(12)*, Schwangershafts protein *(13)*, and histamine-releasing factor *(14)* that maternal tissues may recognize. However, there is a lack of evidence to date that these signals exist in primates and/or are essential for pregnancy to proceed. Therefore, we will concentrate on the regulation, secretion, and biological actions of the one embryonic factor, CG, recognized as essential for early pregnancy in primate species.

Chorionic Gonadotropin (CG)

CG is structurally related to the gonadotropins, follicle-stimulating hormone (FSH) and LH, that are secreted by the anterior pituitary and regulate gonadal structure–function *(15,16)*. They are glycoprotein hormones consisting of two subunits, α and β, that associate noncovalently to form a heterodimer. Within a species (i.e., the human), the α-subunits are virtually identical, whereas the β-subunits differ for each hormone. Nevertheless, the β-subunits contain varying degrees of homology; human LHβ and CGβ demonstrate remarkable similarity (85% homology) in the first 114 amino acids, but CGβ is unique from the other β-subunits owing to the presence of a 24–31 amino acid extension at the C-terminus. The hormones are all glycosylated with N-linked complex carbohydrates, which confer heterogeneity to each hormone. CG is also the most heavily glycosylated with four O-linked carbohydrates on the serine-rich C-terminus extension of the β-subunit. The structures of the oligosaccharides on these hormones differ depending on the tissue of origin; LHα and β-subunits bear sulfated *N*-acetyl-glucosamine and galactosamine resides on nonreduced termini of oligosaccharide chains, whereas hCGα- and β-oligosaccharides contain terminal sialic acid residues and no sulfate. Thus, some steps in the synthesis and sulfation of oligosaccharides for gonadotropic hormones appear tissue-specific. This is important, since the number and structure of oligosaccharides influences markedly the hormone's circulating half-life and, hence, bioactivity.

Following the detection and isolation of highly purified preparations of gonadotropins, particularly hCG from pregnancy urine *(17)*, numerous immunologic and chemical approaches were employed to characterize the structure–function relationships that reflect receptor binding and biologic activity *(18–20)*. More recently, Lapthorn and associates *(21)* reported the three-dimensional structure of hCG, showing that each of its two subunits has a similar topology. The heterodimer is stabilized by a segment of the β-subunit, which wraps around the α-subunit and is covalently linked like a seatbelt by the disulfide bond Cys26-Cys110. This remarkable feature appears essential for receptor binding as well as subunit association. The elucidation of disulfide bridges and the tertiary folding of hCG revealed, surprisingly, that the glycoprotein hormones are members of a superfamily of endocrine/paracrine factors, including nerve growth factor (NGF), transforming growth factor- (TGF) β and platelet-derived growth factor (PDGF), that contain a cysteine knot. The striking structural similarity between PDGF and hCG "β-core" molecule (a polypeptide consisting of β6–40 and 55–92 amino acids) suggests that this circulating molecule, viewed previously as a degradation product of hCG, could have a biologic function.

Because of the relative abundance of mRNAs for CGα and β in the placenta, the complementary DNAs for the α- and β-subunits of hCG were among the first hormone sequences to be cloned *(16,22)*. The CGα- and CGβ-genes were identified soon thereafter. Because of the similarity in amino acid composition between α-subunits, it is not surprising that only one single-copy gene was detected and localized to chromosome 6q 21.1–23. The α gene has a classical structure of four exons with its most distinguishing feature, compared to other glycoprotein hormone genes, a large 6.4-kb first intron separating the promoter and first exon. In contrast, the organization of the human LHβ- and CGβ-genes is very complex. Investigators *(23)* reported multiple copies of structurally related β-genes arranged in a cluster on chromosome 19q 13.3. Recent analyses indicate that the gene on the far right of the cluster encodes LHβ, whereas the six remaining genes encode CGβ-like proteins. It remains unclear which CGβ-genes are functional, or if their activities or regulation vary during pregnancy. Unlike in vitro studies on CG-producing cell lines, Bo and Boime *(24)* observed that every gene was actively transcribing in vivo, but with different levels of expression: GGβ5 > 3 = 8 > 7 > 1 or 2. The LHβ-gene in the cluster was not active in the placenta. Characterization of these genes facilitated efforts to identify the factors controlling transcription and CG production, as well as molecular approaches to produce recombinant gonadotropins *(25)* or hybrids *(26,27)* for research and clinical applications. Similar efforts for nonhuman primate CGs have been very slow despite their obvious importance. However, recombinant macaque FSH and LH (but not CG) are now available (National Hormone and Pituitary Program, NIDDK, NIH, Rockville, MD), and the cDNA sequences for baboon and marmoset α and β CGs were recently reported *(28)*. Vervet monkey and baboon CG have been partially purified and characterized *(29)*. It is currently believed that the primate CGβ-gene evolved from an ancestral LHβ-like gene, through a single base pair (bp) deletion in exon III and a 2-bp insertion that extended the translated region through the C-terminal region *(16)*. Since the mature peptide of marmoset CGβ possesses the extended C-terminus *(28)*, the CGβ-gene must have evolved prior to the divergence of Old World and New World monkeys (~40 million yr ago).

CG Secretion

Although CG secretion appears to be a characteristic of pregnancy in all primates, the patterns and peak levels vary among apes, and Old World and New World monkeys. Peak CG concentrations are highest in women, about 10 times lower in apes (e.g., chimpanzees), and 100- to 1000-fold less in baboons, macaques, and marmosets (Fig. 1 *[10]*). Likewise, three different patterns of CG are typically observed during gestation. Although CG is first detected around the time of implantation in all primates, among humans and apes, CG levels peak in the first trimester, then decline, but remain at substantial levels throughout gestation. However, in baboons and macaques, CG levels decline to near or below the limits of detection by midpregnancy. In New World monkeys, CG levels do not peak until midpregnancy and decline just before parturition.

The exact time when CG is first produced by the conceptus remains unresolved. CG is first detected in the peripheral blood of primates around the time of implantation, but rigorous review of the data suggests that CG is not definitively measurable until 2–3 d after embryo attachment in vivo (Table 1 *[30]*). Studies in rhesus monkeys suggest that "rescue" of the corpus luteum, as judged by a rise in serum progesterone levels, occurs on d 9 postovulation when CG is detectable in the utero-ovarian vein, but not in the peripheral circulation *(31)*. These data led to the hypothesis that CG could pass directly by a uterine-ovarian portal system to the ovary, where it stimulates luteal function before becoming detectable in peripheral blood. An anatomical basis for a local veno-arterial pathway was demonstrated in the rhesus monkey *(32)*, but its physiologic significance, particularly for countercurrent exchange of CG, has not been demonstrated.

With the advent of assisted reproductive technologies, a few investigators have examined directly CG expression by primate embryos during in vitro culture. There is one report that mRNA for β-hCG was detectable by *in situ* hybridization in three of seven eight-cell human embryos *(33)*. These were triploid embryos, the normality of which may be questioned (as may be that of many "spare" human embryos available for experimentation). The suggestion that transcription and possibly expression of CG, or at least the β-subunit,

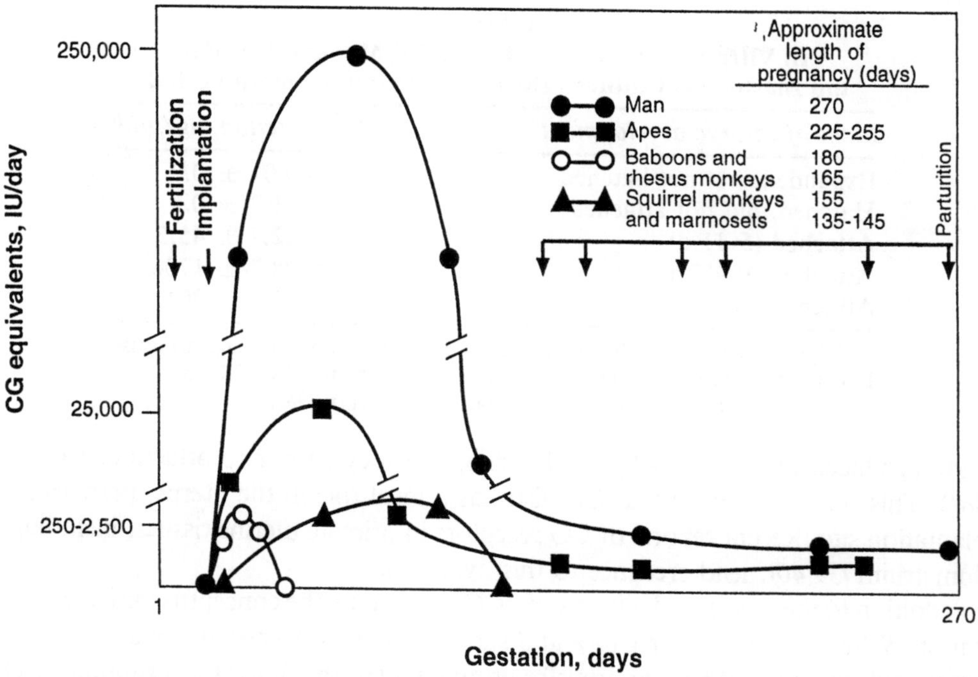

Fig. 1. The patterns and quantities of chorionic gonadotropin excreted during gestation by a variety of primate species. The time scale in the upper right corner denotes the approximate duration of pregnancy and parturition (arrows) for these species. Adapted from the review by Hodgen and Itskovitz *(10)*.

Table 1
Estimated Day, Before or After Embryo Attachment, of the First Detection of CG In Vivo (in Peripheral Blood) and In Vitro (in Culture Media) in Various Primate Species[a]

	Days before (−) and after (+) embryo attachment when CG was first measurable	
Species	*In Vivo*	*In Vitro*
Human	+2 to 5	−2 onwards
Chimpanzee	+3 to 4	Unknown
Baboon	+3 to 4	0 onwards
Rhesus monkey	+3 to 4	−2 onwards
Marmoset	+3 to 6	−1 onwards

[a] Adapted from the review by Seshagiri et al. *(30)*; the reader is encouraged to review this paper for further information and pertinent references.

is attained at this early stage even before any clear specialization of cell lineage requires further investigation. When marmoset embryos recovered by surgical flushing of the uterus *(34)* or human embryos produced by in vitro fertilization *(35–37)* are grown in culture, there is little or no evidence for detectable CG, as measured by bioassay or immunoassay, respectively, in the incubation medium until the time of attachment. Thereafter, an exponential rise in levels occurs for several days; thus, substantial CG expression is characteristic of embryo attachment and/or postattachment development. Such expression can occur independent of the normal uterine epithelium, indeed, on plastic or fibroblastic monolayers. Data from the rhesus monkey suggest that in some primate species, CG is

Table 2
In Vitro Secretion of CG by Rhesus Monkey Morulae and Blastocysts Cultured During the Periattachment Period[a]

Stage of embryo development	*CG secretion, ng/mL[b]*
Expanded, but not hatched	≤0.01 ± 0.0
Hatched, but not attached	1.7 ± 0.5
Attached (5–11 d)	122.7 ± 45.5
Attached (10–17 d)	5108.7 ± 1706
Attached (16–40 d)	317.0 ± 201

[a]Spent media from different timepoints were analyzed using a mouse Leydig cell bioassay; values expressed as equivalent to hCG CR125.
[b]Adapted from the article by Seshagiri and Hearn *(38)*.

already produced in low levels by the hatching blastocyst prior to attachment (Table 2 *[9,38]*). This finding suggests that CG also has a local role in the uterus, perhaps at the implantation site. Recent reports of CG receptors in primate uterine tissues, including the endometrium *(39,40)*, lend credence to this hypothesis.

In addition to the amount, the forms of hCG secreted by the conceptus may vary during gestation. When hCG and its free α- and β-subunits were measured in women undergoing in vitro fertilization (IVF) embryo transfer protocols *(41)*, the free β-hCG subunit was first detected approx 6.5 d after oocyte retrieval. However, dimer hCG was not detectable until 8 d after egg collection. After d 9, the rise in total β-hCG (dimer and β-subunit) was owing primarily to dimer hCG; by d 22, β-subunit comprised only 5% of total β-hCG. This phenomenon may be related to the differentiation of the trophoblast. It is hypothesized that the immature trophoblast produces β-subunit in excess of the α-subunit; only as the cytotrophoblast starts to differentiate is α-subunit produced in sufficient quantities to match β-subunit production. By the later stages of the first trimester and again at term pregnancy when CG levels are declining, there is a relative excess of α-subunit. Thus, there is evidence for independent regulation of subunit production, but its physiologic relevance remains to be determined. The comparison of hCG and subunit levels may have clinical relevance to monitoring for complications in early pregnancy. It is reported that in some patients who lost their pregnancy, a transient increase in CG levels was owing predominantly to free β-hCG *(10)*.

Regulation of CG Secretion

The complexity and dynamics of the placenta, as well as the difficulty in obtaining normal tissues particularly in early pregnancy, have hindered efforts to establish the mechanisms controlling CG synthesis and secretion. Recent studies on human placenta from the first, second, and third trimesters, and particularly on several CG-producing cell lines, have aided in identifying (1) potential endocrine or local factors that regulate CG production and (2) intracellular transcription factors or regulatory DNA elements that control the CGα- and β-genes *(22)*. A more difficult issue is clearly establishing which factors play a physiologic role and their interaction in controlling the dynamics of CG production throughout pregnancy.

Some of the proposed modulators of CG production by human placental cells are categorized in Table 3 *(22)*. An intriguing scenario arises from evidence that hormones originally observed in the hypothalamus (i.e., GnRH) and ovary (inhibin, activin, progesterone) and considered regulators of pituitary gonadotropin secretion also are potential

Table 3
Hormonal and Local Factors that Modulate CG Synthesis and Secretion

Modulator	*Effect*[a]
GnRH, gonadotropin-releasing hormone	+
EGF, epidermal growth factor	+
Activin	+
IL-6, interleukin-6	+
IL-1, interleukin-1	+
MCSF, macrophage colony-stimulating factor	+
GABA, γ-aminobututyric acid	+
Retinoic acid	+
Glucocorticoids	+
DHEA, dehydroepiandrosterone	+
TGF-β, transforming growth factor-β	−
Dopamine	−
Inhibin	−
Progesterone	−
IGF-1, insulin-like growth factor 1	±
Testosterone	±
Estrogens	±

[a] Stimulates (+), inhibits (−), or has little effect (±) on CG production in a variety of experimental models. Adapted from the review by Jameson and Hollenberg *(22)*; the reader is encouraged to review this paper for further information and references.

modulators of placental CG production. There is evidence that GnRH (or a similar factor) is produced by *(42)* and putative GnRH receptors are detectable in *(43)* placental tissue. However, placental GnRH mRNA levels do not vary significantly during pregnancy *(42)*, suggesting that other factors are involved in the decline in CG production after the first trimester. The placenta also contains mRNA for the α- and β-subunits of inhibin/activin, and inhibin production has been demonstrated *(44)*. In agreement with their antagonistic actions in many systems, (1) exogenous activin potentiates GnRH-stimulated release from placental cultures, whereas (2) inhibin decreases basal CG release and blocks activin's stimulation of GnRH-mediated CG release *(45)*. Thus, inhibin-related proteins and GnRH may interact to regulate CG production by the placenta. However, steroids (particularly progesterone) may also play an important role in regulating CG production. It is noteworthy that CG production in many primates declines in conjunction with the luteal–placental shift when placental concentrations of progesterone approach maximal levels. However, these findings await interpretation in the context of placental expression of receptors for inhibin-related peptides and steroids, an area that has yet to receive much attention. Nevertheless, the evidence suggests that the placenta contains all the factors or similar analogs to those produced by the hypothalamic–pituitary–gonadal axis, which regulate LH/FSH secretion. These factors may act in a paracrine or autocrine manner, with additional input from other hormones (e.g., glucocorticoids) or local growth factors/cytokines (e.g., epidermal growth factor [EGF]) to regulate placental CG production. However, the majority of studies supporting this concept were performed with term placental cultures, so the effects of these factors on CG production in early pregnancy remain unclear.

Using morula and blastocyst-stage embryos recovered by uterine flushing, Hearn and colleagues *(9,46)* now have evidence that a GnRH-responsive system of CG secretion is potentially operational around the time of implantation in marmosets and rhesus monkeys. GnRH was localized by immunocytochemistry to the preimplantation embryo, and there were measurable quantities of GnRH in media samples from cultured macaque embryos around the time of hatching (32–52 pg/mL), which increased with time post-attachment (62–130 pg/mL). Incubation of blastocyst-stage embryos with a GnRH agonist ($DTrp^6$, Pro^9-NHET-GnRH) enhanced CG secretion, whereas an antagonist (Nal-Glu GnRH) diminished CG secretion. Interestingly, incubation with either the GnRH agonist or antagonist reduced embryo attachment, perhaps by disruption of early embryo differentiation. These results suggest that there is a relationship, either direct or indirect, between GnRH and CG production in primate peri-implantation blastocysts. Moreover, disruption of this relationship may prevent timely embryonic development and embryo attachment. Unconfirmed reports that preattachment primate embryos also produce inhibin *(47)* and steroids *(48,49)* suggest that all factors involved in hypothalamo–pituitary–gonadal control of gonadotropin secretion are present at the time of initial CG secretion around implantation. Further studies on early embryos, particularly as available from nonhuman primates for in vivo and in vitro manipulation, are critical to understand better embryonic differentiation and to elucidate the intraembryonic signals important for successful maternal recognition of pregnancy. Indeed, such embryonic signals could be exploited for control of fertility (e.g., blockade of implantation) or clinical treatment of early pregnancy dysfunction.

MATERNAL RESPONSE TO CG: CORPUS LUTEUM RESCUE

It is widely accepted that CG secreted by the implanting embryo is responsible for "rescue" of the corpus luteum from its impending demise and extended luteal function in early pregnancy. In the 1970s, investigators reported that (1) passive immunization of monkeys with anti-LH/CG antiserum prior to the luteal–placental shift caused a rapid decline in serum progesterone levels and pregnancy termination in monkeys *(50)*, and (2) active immunization with modified forms of CG or its β-subunit produced infertility in baboons *(51)* and women *(52)*, despite normal ovulatory cycles. In an elegant study, Thau and Sundaram *(53)* showed that the antifertility effect of CG antibodies in macaques was owing to prevention of extended luteal function in early pregnancy, which could be overcome by administration of a progestin until placental progesterone production began as expected. Moreover, there are numerous reports that exogenous CG acutely increases progesterone production and extends the life-span of the corpus luteum of the menstrual cycle in women *(54)*, and Old World *(55)* and New World *(56)* monkeys. After development of specific immunoassays for CG, investigators employed longer treatment regimens of urinary *(57)* or, more recently, recombinant *(58)* hCG to mimic the patterns and levels of endogenous CG in early pregnancy. When such an hCG treatment regimen was initiated in rhesus monkeys at the expected time of implantation (d 8–10 post-LH surge) in the luteal phase (Fig. 2 *[57]*), the changes elicited were characteristic of early pregnancy:

1. The temporal response, levels, and patterns of progesterone secretion were remarkably similar,
2. The life-span of the corpus luteum was extended (e.g., timely menses did not occur); and
3. Nonsteroidogenic activities, such as relaxin production (discussed later), were enhanced.

Thus, CG in the absence of other embryonic factors is capable of rescuing the corpus luteum of early pregnancy. Treatment of nonhuman primates with hCG offers a valuable

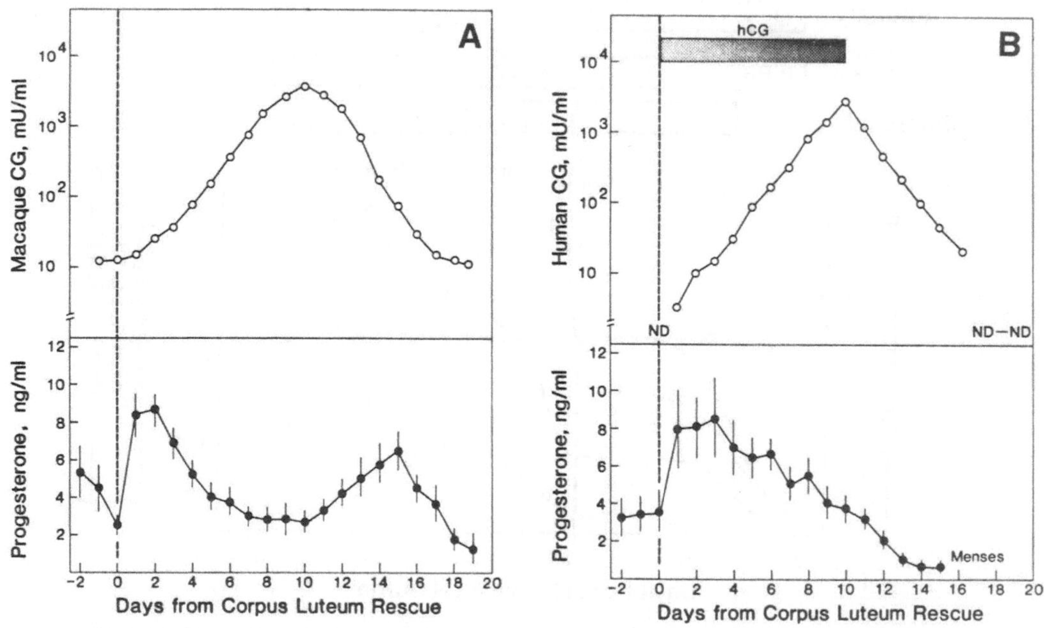

Fig. 2. Composite of progesterone and CG levels circulating in rhesus monkeys during actual early pregnancy (**A**) or during administration of increasing doses of urinary hCG for 10 d (**B**) to simulate the pattern of CG in macaques during normal pregnancy. Data (mean ± SEM) are normalized to the day of rescue of the corpus luteum (d 0). Note the temporal relationship between progesterone and CG patterns. The second peak in circulating progesterone on d 16 of normal pregnancy is of placental origin. Reproduced with permission *(57)*.

model for studying the responses of the primate corpus luteum to CG, as well as the mechanisms in CG action in early pregnancy.

Changes in Maternal Hormones in Response to CG

Although the promotion of luteal progesterone production is a salient feature of maternal recognition of pregnancy, the patterns and duration of progesterone secretion by the corpus luteum in early pregnancy vary between primate species. In women, serum progesterone levels increase above midluteal phase concentrations in parallel with rising hCG levels for several days and remain elevated for 2–3 wk; the luteal-placental shift does not occur until approximately the sixth wk of pregnancy. In the rhesus monkey, CG exposure leads to an initial rise in progesterone concentrations, but after a short interval of 2–4 d, levels decline despite a continued increase in circulating CG (Fig. 3). The luteal-placental shift occurs by the end of the third wk of gestation in macaques. In contrast, circulating progesterone levels in marmosets at pregnancy initiation are simply maintained at concentrations similar to those at midluteal phase of the cycle; the time of the luteal-placental shift during gestation in this species of New World monkeys has not been experimentally defined.

More recently, investigators determined that the primate corpus luteum produces at least three other potential hormones, and that their patterns of secretion in response to CG (either endogenous CG in early gestation or exogenous CG in simulated early pregnancy) are not necessarily comparable to that for luteal progesterone production. First, the corpus luteum of women and Old World monkeys produces significant amounts of another

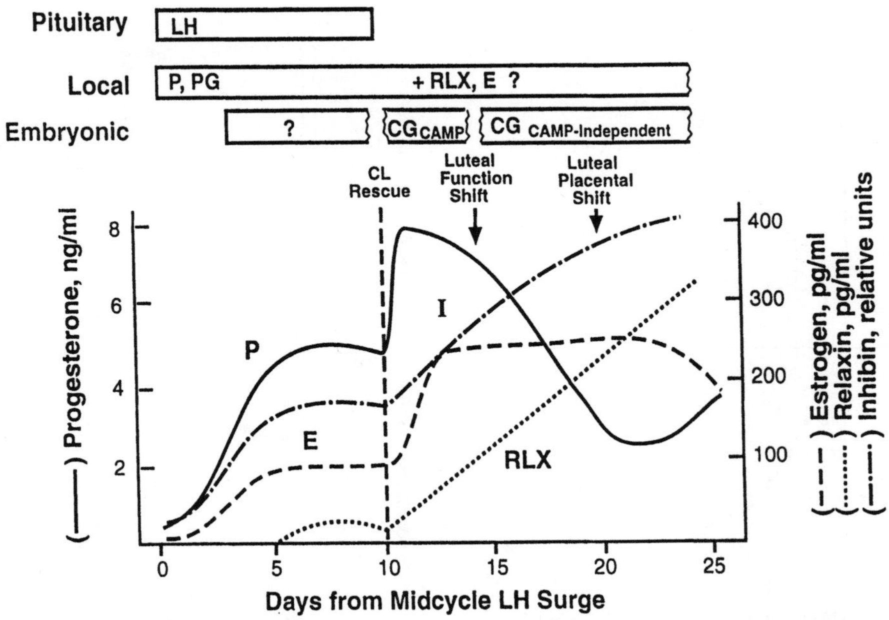

Fig. 3. Schematic of the changes in circulating levels of progesterone (P), estrogen (E), relaxin (RLX), and inhibin (I) during the luteal phase of the fertile menstrual cycle in rhesus monkeys. The recognized or proposed (?) roles of pituitary hormones (LH), embryonic hormones (CG), and local ovarian factors (P, E, RLX, I, prostaglandins [PGs]) in controlling luteal function are summarized. Adapted from the review by Stouffer et al. *(113)*.

class of steroids, the estrogens *(59)*. CG exposure increases circulating estradiol and estrone levels, and concentrations remain elevated in macaques even when progesterone levels begin to decline (Fig. 3). Second, the primate corpus luteum of the menstrual cycle produces very little if any of the peptide hormone relaxin, except for small amounts late in the luteal phase *(60–62)*; however, CG exposure in actual *(60,62)* or simulated *(54,63)* pregnancy markedly increases circulating relaxin levels, which continue to rise even after progesterone concentrations decline (Fig. 3). Third, the corpus luteum of women and nonhuman primates is apparently unique, compared to nonprimate species, in its ability to produce significant amounts of inhibin *(64–66)*. Inhibin is a 32-kDa dimeric protein composed of an α-subunit and one of two related β-subunits (βA and βB) *(67)*. With the development of specific immunoassays, evidence from women suggests that inhibin B (α-βB) —presumably arising from the developing follicle(s)—circulates in the follicular phase, whereas inhibin A (α-βA) circulates in a pattern similar to that for progesterone in the luteal phase *(68)*. Exogenous CG causes a significant increase in inhibin A, not inhibin B, levels *(69)*, and secretion of inhibin A paralleled that of hCG in women *(70,71)*. That the corpus luteum is the primary source of inhibin in early pregnancy is confirmed by evidence from women lacking endogenous luteal function where circulating inhibin levels failed to rise through 4–6 wk of pregnancy (maintained by steroid replacement), compared to normal women. By 8 wk, i.e., after the luteal–placental shift, inhibin levels were identical in both groups *(66)*.

Thus, CG not only "rescues" the corpus luteum near the end of the fertile cycle and extends its progestational function, but it also promotes (e.g., inhibin) or begins (e.g., relaxin) new luteal activities even when progesterone secretion may be declining. One can consider early pregnancy the final interval of luteal differentiation in primates—a process that starts with the LH surge at ovulation and ends with CG secretion postimplantation. Although it is generally believed that progesterone of luteal origin is the indispensable factor for pregnancy initiation in women and macaques *(72,73)*, definitive studies are needed to evaluate the possible roles of other luteal products, including estrogen, relaxin, and inhibin, in facilitating early gestation in primate species.

Mechanism of CG Action

In every primate species studied, research supports the concept that pituitary LH and placental CG share a common receptor that regulates luteal cells at least in part via a cyclic AMP- (cAMP) mediated pathway. The macaque corpus luteum contains a single population of receptors that bind hLH (but not nonprimate LH preparations *[74]*) and hCG with equally high affinity ($K_d \approx 10^{-10}$ *M*) throughout the luteal phase of the menstrual cycle and during CG exposure simulating early pregnancy *(75–77)*. Moreover, both hLH and hCG stimulate adenylate cyclase and cAMP production by macaque luteal membranes *(78)* and enhance progesterone secretion by dispersed luteal cells during short-term incubations in vitro *(79)*. Similar results were obtained with preparations of human luteal tissue *(80,81)*. Since the effects of administered hCG closely resemble those of pituitary LH, hCG is used routinely in place of hLH in clinical and research situations to promote a number of ovarian events, including meiotic maturation of oocytes, ovulation, and the development and function of the corpus luteum *(82,83)*. The widespread use of hCG is predicated on its relative abundance from pregnancy urine. With the generation of recombinant gonadotropins, LH preparations may be the choice in some situations *(84)*, particularly because of its shorter half-life compared to CG. Owing to limited quantities, studies have never determined whether exogenous LH is capable of mimicking CG's action in early pregnancy. Again, with increased availability of recombinant LH preparations, this issue could be resolved.

In view of their common mechanisms, it remains unclear why or how the production of another LH-like hormone, i.e., CG, rescues the primate corpus luteum in early pregnancy. In both women and monkeys, LH is secreted by the pituitary in an episodic manner and the frequency of LH pulses slows during the mid- to late-luteal phase of the menstrual cycle (*see* ref *4*). However, studies indicate that varying the LH pulse frequency within the range observed over the duration of the menstrual cycle (1 pulse every 60–90 min to 1 pulse/8 h) does not alter the functional life-span of the corpus luteum. In particular, maintenance of high-frequency endogenous LH pulses (via GnRH treatment) or regular exogenous LH treatment (3–4 injections/d) does not prevent timely luteal regression in monkeys *(85,86)* or women *(87)*. These observations suggest that a decrease in pituitary LH support is not the primary cause for the demise of the corpus luteum at the end of the menstrual cycle.

It is unknown whether CG prevents some luteolytic signal from occurring in the fertile cycle or provides a quantum increase in luteotropic support that prevents the luteolytic process. Because of differences in secretion patterns and circulating half-life of LH and CG, there are qualitative then quantitative differences in the gonadotropin milieu in early pregnancy. The intermittent pulses of LH translate into intervals of gonadotropin support and withdrawal during the mid- to late-luteal phase, which correlate positively with luteal steroidogenic activity (Fig. 4, *[57]*). Since CG has a much longer half-life than LH in the bloodstream and is produced in exponentially increasing amounts by the developing trophoblast, CG circulates continuously and in rising levels until obscuring any remaining vestige of LH pulses *(88)*. Thus, the conceptus offers uninterrupted (as opposed to episodic) and increasing levels of luteotropic support for the corpus luteum. Whether such

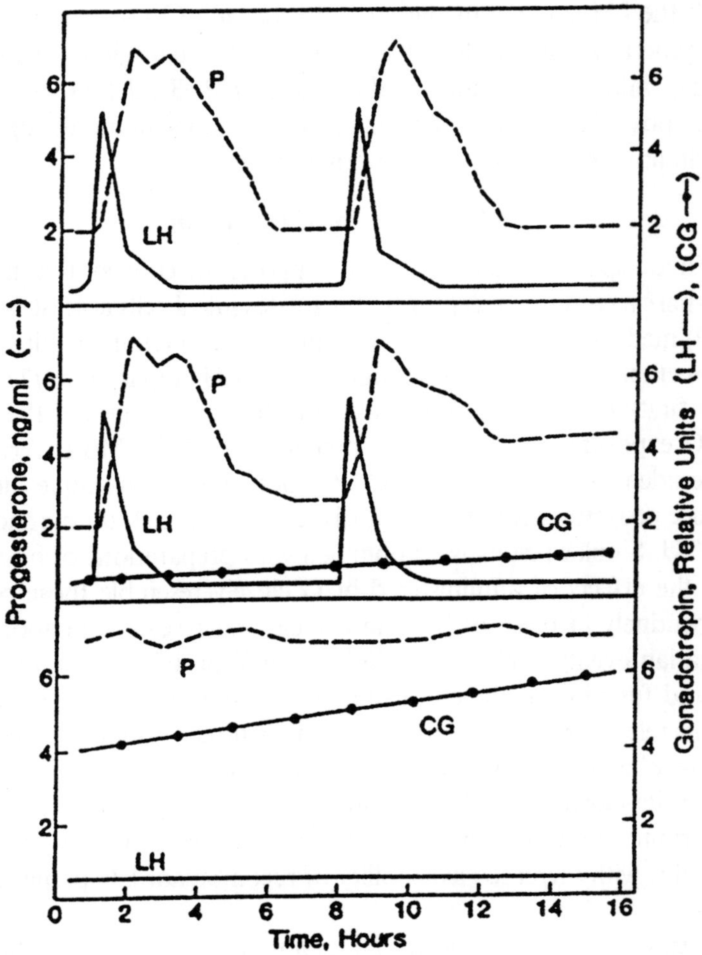

Fig. 4. Schematic representation of progesterone (P) and gonadotropin (LH and CG) levels circulating in rhesus monkeys during the mid- to-late-luteal phase of the menstrual cycle **(A)** and as postulated following initial (d 1) and 3 d of CG exposure during rescue of the corpus luteum in the fertile cycle **(B,C)**. Whereas LH is secreted in intermittent pulses, the implanting conceptus secretes increasing amounts of CG, which circulate for long intervals owing to its protracted half-life. Whether qualitative and/or quantitative differences in the pattern of gonadotropin secretion are sufficient to explain the rescue of the corpus luteum by an LH-like hormone is unknown. Adapted from the review by Stouffer et al. *(57)*.

qualitative and quantitative differences in circulating gonadotropins are primary factors in the rescue of the corpus luteum in early pregnancy awaits investigation. Alternatively, there may be critical differences in the cellular actions of CG vs LH that facilitate luteal function and differentiation. Although LH and CG are believed to share the same receptor sites, there is evidence that the duration of CG action is longer than that of LH, in terms of enhanced steroidogenesis, which correlates with differences in the rate of receptor movement or turnover in cell membranes following binding of CG vs LH (Fig. 5). However, these studies were performed on luteal cells/membranes from nonprimate species *(see 89)*. A recent study analogous to that demonstrating differences in the steroidogenic response of nonprimate cells to ovine LH and CG failed to extend the concept of disparate actions of gonadotropins to the monkey in which both LH and CG are endogenous

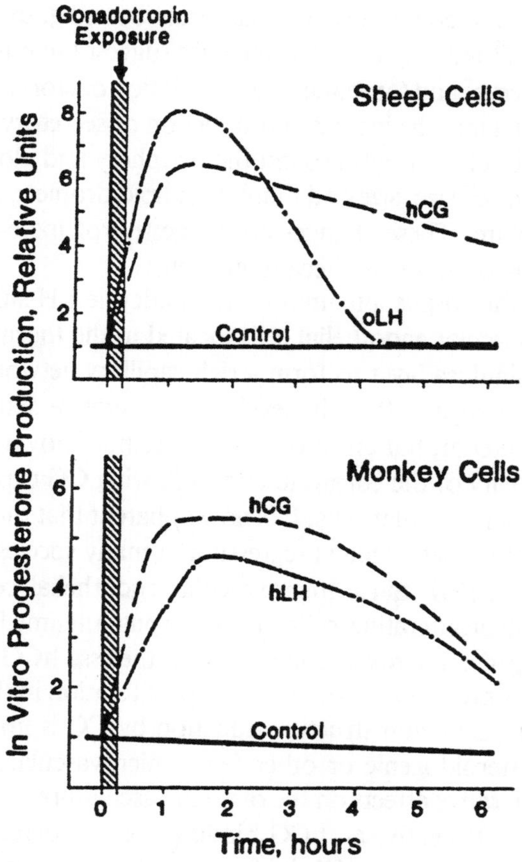

Fig. 5. The patterns of progesterone produced by luteinized cells from sheep (top panel) or monkeys (bottom panel) following a 15-min exposure to LH or hCG. Whereas experiments suggest qualitative differences between the dynamics of LH and hCG in nonprimates *(89)*, analogous experiments have yet to demonstrate differences in primate species where both gonadotropins are endogenous hormones *(90)*. Reproduced with permission *(115)*.

hormones (Fig. 5 *[90]*). These experiments emphasize the need to use primate systems since: (1) primate gonadotropins differ from those of nonprimates (e.g., oLH vs hLH) in glycosylation and sulfation, which may influence receptor binding characteristics, and (2) LH/CG receptors in monkeys and women are unique in their relative specificity for primate gonadotropins *(74)*. Further studies are needed on human and nonhuman primate tissue to determine whether the actions of LH and CG differ and contribute to the rescue of the corpus luteum in early pregnancy.

To date, most studies on CG action have focused on acute responses; little is known about subsequent effects on cellular parameters, including luteal structure or differentiation and hormone production. Such studies are hindered by difficulties in procuring tissues from early pregnancy either from women for ethical reasons or from nonhuman primates because of logistical problems in confirming pregnancy onset. Again, models simulating early pregnancy via exogenous CG treatment have provided novel opportunities. Morphologic and fine structural studies, particularly in the rhesus monkey *(91)*, identified rapid and remarkable changes in luteal tissue during implantation. Structural changes in the granulosa lutein cells comprising the bulk of the endocrine tissue included: increased granular endoplasmic reticulum, reduced number and size of lipid droplets, increased size of the Golgi complex, increased numbers of membrane-bound granules, and development of microvillus-lined intracellular spaces. The changes suggest the rapid utilization of existing steroid precursor reserves and/or reduced accumulation or storage of steroid precursors for progesterone synthesis and the increased production of secretory proteins. In contrast, structural changes in theca lutein cells around the periphery and along the vascular channels included increases in cell size, size and number of lipid droplets, and amount of agranular endoplasmic reticulum. These changes are suggestive of increased steroid precursor accumulation and steroidogenesis by theca lutein cells.

The development of the corpus luteum after the midcycle LH surge includes an angiogenic process as microvascular endothelial cells located in the thecal layer proliferate and invade the avascular granulosa layer to form a rich capillary network among the luteinizing endocrine cells. Data suggest that the level of proliferative activity varies during the life-span of the corpus luteum, but until recently, it was not known whether the increased mass and endocrine activity of the corpus luteum following CG exposure involved hyperplasia of endocrine or microvascular cells. It is now apparent that there is a marked decline in cell proliferation at the onset of luteal regression in many species, including the rhesus monkey *(92)* and human *(93)*. Since microvascular endothelial cells comprise the vast majority (≥ 85-95%) of proliferating cells in the corpus luteum, luteolysis may involve early events influencing the microvasculature. Nevertheless, hCG treatment simulating early pregnancy does not prevent the decline in cell proliferation in the corpus luteum *(92)*. Thus, the rescue of corpus luteum structure–function by CG is not likely attributable to proliferation of either steroidogenic or other (e.g., microvascular) cell types. However, CG may have nonproliferative effects on the ovarian vasculature to increase blood flow or endothelial cell function. Recently, an hCG binding site was detected on gonadal endothelial cells *(94)*; whether this "receptor" site functions to transport CG from the blood to the interstitial space where it can interact with receptors on luteal cells or to transduce CG action directly in endothelial cells remains to be determined. In the absence of extended or enhanced hyperplasia, it is likely that CG exposure promotes the differentiation of luteal cells to produce and secrete steroids and peptides more efficiently.

Limited evidence suggests that CG exposure results in divergent changes in the expression of the mRNAs and proteins involved in steroid and peptide hormone production by the primate corpus luteum. Benyo et al *(95)* reported that 7 d of hCG treatment simulating early pregnancy markedly stimulated mRNA levels for low-density lipoprotein (LDL) receptor in the macaque corpus luteum, whereas mRNA for P450 side-chain cleavage ($P450_{scc}$) was only minimally stimulated and that for 3β-hydroxysteroid dehydrogenase (3β-HSD) was not different from that of control corpora lutea (d 16 of the cycle). These data suggest that hCG transiently stimulates progesterone production in the monkey corpus luteum by enhancing uptake and availability of cholesterol sources (i.e., LDL) for existing steroidogenic systems, not by stimulating key enzymatic (e.g., $P450_{scc}$ and 3β-HSD) steps. However, earlier time-points need to be evaluated, since recent immunocytochemical studies observed increased staining for $P450_{scc}$ and 3β-HSD in macaque luteal tissue after 1–3 d of CG exposure *(96)*. By day 6 of exposure, enzyme expression may be declining in monkeys following the transient rise in circulating progesterone in response to CG in these species (Fig. 2). Whether a more robust, prolonged expression of components in the steroidogenic system occurs in apes or women, where CG levels are much higher and where luteal progesterone production occurs for a longer interval, is unknown.

Despite modest effects of CG on mRNAs for $P450_{scc}$ and 3β-HSD, 7 d of treatment markedly increased that encoding P450 aromatase ($P450_{arom}$) in the macaque corpus

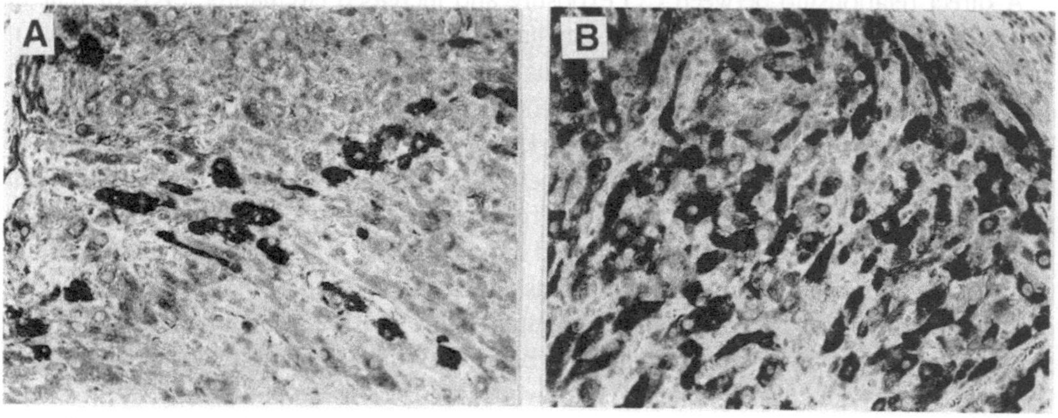

Fig. 6. Immunohistochemical localization of cytochrome P450 17α hydroxylase/17,20 lyase ($P450_{C17}$, **[A]**) and P450 aromatase ($P450_{arom}$, **[B]**) in the macaque corpus luteum. Specific $P450_{C17}$ staining was evident in luteal cells around the periphery of the corpus luteum and along the vascular tracts penetrating the tissue. In contrast, $P450_{arom}$-stained luteal cells were scattered throughout the luteal parenchyma, but not along the vascular tracts. A heterogeneous staining pattern was apparent with some cells staining intensely for $P450_{arom}$ and others intermediately or lightly stained. The data are consistent with a two-cell model for estrogen production by the primate corpus luteum, whereby putative theca luteal cells along the periphery produce androgen that is aromatized to estrogens by centrally located granulosa luteal cells *(96)*.

luteum *(95)*. However, it is unlikely that increased aromatase expression is the only reason for enhanced estrogen synthetic capacity, since Ellinwood et al. *(59)* noted that total estrogen (estradiol plus estrone) synthesized from radiolabeled androgens did not differ between macaque luteal tissue from midluteal phase of the cycle and d 23–27 of pregnancy. Since tissue levels of androgen (androstenedione, not testosterone) were markedly elevated, they concluded that increased estrogen production resulted primarily from increased luteal androgen production. The divergence in progesterone vs estrogen production by the corpus luteum of early pregnancy reflects the changing circulating patterns of these steroids, since elevated estrogen levels continue, whereas progesterone levels fall after their transient rise (Fig. 3). Immunocytochemical studies on both the human *(97,98)* and monkey *(96)* corpus luteum localized aromatase and 3β-HSD to the same cell type, the granulosa luteal cells, within the tissue. Therefore, one cannot attribute the divergence in estrogen vs progesterone synthesis to different responses of two cell types to CG. Nevertheless, heterogeneity in function and hormone responsiveness likely exists within the granulosa luteal cell population *(99)*. Likewise, it appears that cell–cell interaction analogous to the two-cell model in the follicle is operating for estrogen production by the human *(97)* and macaque *(96)* corpus luteum. Immunocytochemical localization (Fig. 6) suggests that presumptive theca luteal cells around the periphery and vascular infoldings are the primary site of P450 17α-hydroxylase/lyase for androgen production, whereas the granulosa luteal cells in the central parenchyma contain the $P450_{arom}$ catalyzing the conversion of androgen to estrogen. Since CG exposure produces morphologic changes suggestive of increased steroid precursor accumulation and steroidogenesis by theca luteal cells, it seems likely that enhanced androgen synthesis *(59)* provides additional substrate for estrogen production by luteal tissue in early pregnancy. To date, there have been very few studies on different luteal cell populations within the primate corpus luteum (for review, *see 7*), especially during CG exposure in actual or simulated early pregnancy.

A direct relationship between CG exposure and increased circulating levels of relaxin during actual or simulated early pregnancy has been recognized for several years (Fig. 3), but the cellular and molecular mechanisms whereby CG stimulates luteal cell relaxin expression remain obscure *(100)*. The recent identification and sequencing of the two human relaxin genes *(101,102)* producing H1 and H2 relaxin, and the availability of recombinant peptides and antibodies have permitted considerable progress. In nonhuman primates *(103)*, the great apes also have two relaxin genes, whereas the baboon and rhesus monkey have only one relaxin gene as found in nonprimates. Both relaxin genes are functional in the human and chimpanzee, whereas only the equivalent of the H2 human relaxin gene is functional in the gorilla and orangutan. Only the H2 gene, unlike that for H1 relaxin, was shown by Northern analysis to be expressed by the human corpus luteum of the menstrual cycle and pregnancy *(104)*. Two transcripts were identified, both prevalent in the late-luteal phase of the cycle and the smaller one dominant in pregnancy. Thus, transcriptional or posttranscriptional control of relaxin expression appears to occur in the corpus luteum, but whether CG directly regulates these processes is unknown.

Earlier studies on women *(54)* and monkeys *(57)* given exogenous CG to simulate pregnancy initiation suggested there was a delay of several days before relaxin secretion increased. However, when recently developed homologous RIAs and ELISAs were employed, this delay was markedly reduced *(63,105)*, suggesting the reported phenomenon was primarily an artifact related to assay sensitivity. Nevertheless, there are no reports of acute stimulation of relaxin mRNA or protein production by CG using primate luteal tissue/cells in vitro. Exposure of macaque luteal cells to hCG or cAMP had no effect on cell content or media levels of relaxin during 8 h of incubation *(106)*. In cultures of human luteinized granulosa cells, hCG exposure immediately stimulated progesterone production, but relaxin secretion increased only after 10–24 d in the presence of hCG *(107)*. Thus, granulosa/luteal cells may need to undergo further differentiation before relaxin secretion can be detected. There is little doubt that CG is the critical factor in a sequence of events leading to increased luteal relaxin production in early pregnancy, but further studies are needed to elucidate the mechanisms involved in this process.

The corpus luteum of women and macaques *(6)* contains progesterone receptors, and it was suggested that progesterone is a local factor critical for subsequent luteal production of relaxin *(100)*. However, recent studies in rhesus monkeys, using a 3β-HSD inhibitor to reduce circulating progesterone levels to a minimum (<0.1 ng/mL, with premature onset of menses), indicate that acute (3-d) deprivation at midluteal phase of the cycle and chronic (9-d) deprivation throughout hCG treatment did not alter the patterns or levels of relaxin circulating during simulated early pregnancy *(58,63)*. Moreover, Schmidt et al. *(108)* reported that a woman with homozygous familial hypobeta-lipoproteinemia had appreciably lower progesterone levels, but normal relaxin levels during gestation. These studies suggest that progesterone is not a major regulator of relaxin production by the primate corpus luteum. However, intraluteal progesterone levels were not measured, so one cannot rule out that sufficient progesterone remained to act locally to regulate relaxin expression. Nevertheless, other paracrine or autocrine factors, such as prostaglandins *(109)*, warrant investigation.

Any evaluation of CG action in early pregnancy must consider the dynamics of LH/CG receptor-effector systems in primate luteal cells during chronic CG exposure. Researchers have reported the loss or "downregulation" of gonadotropin receptors and diminished or "desensitized" gonadotropin-stimulated adenylate cyclase activity in luteal tissue from nonprimate species following in vivo administration of a large bolus of LH or CG *(57)*. However, the scenario in primate luteal tissue during exposure to rising CG levels appears somewhat different, at least in a macaque model simulating early pregnancy. First, CG exposure did **not** result in downregulation or loss of LH/CG receptors *per se*. Rather, there was remarkable constancy of the **total** receptor population, with the numbers of unoccupied receptors declining and of CG-occupied receptors increasing with the duration and level of CG exposure *(110)*. Nevertheless, the functional capacity of these receptors after 3–6 d of CG exposure is questionable, since their affinity for gonadotropin decreased fivefold. Second, by 3 d of CG exposure, the ability of luteal membranes to produce cAMP in response to gonadotropins was severely impaired, and by d 6, gonadotropin stimulation was lost *(111)*. However, nonhormonal activators, such as forskolin, and paracrine factors, such as prostaglandin (PG) E_2 and I_2, continued to stimulate cAMP production throughout CG exposure. Thus, the various membrane components of the adenylate cyclase system were functional and capable of transducing signals from PG receptors, but **not** from gonadotropin receptors, after the initial stages of CG exposure.

These data, and more limited data obtained from corpora lutea of women *(112)* and rhesus monkeys *(113)* during actual early pregnancy, suggest that homologous desensitization of the adenylate cyclase system occurs in the primate corpus luteum during CG exposure. The functional, if not physical, uncoupling of gonadotropin receptors from cAMP production could be an important step in the transient progestational response of the corpus luteum to CG in early pregnancy (Fig. 3). However, the molecular events leading to desensitization, their relevance to the dynamics of luteal function in early pregnancy, and the possible involvement of cAMP-independent effector systems (e.g., the phosphoinositol-protein kinase C pathway *[114]*) in CG action in luteal tissue are unknown. Likewise, the involvement of the latter or gonadotropin-independent (e.g., PG-stimulated) cAMP-mediated events in luteal activities that persist in early pregnancy, such as relaxin secretion, awaits investigation.

SUMMARY

The establishment of early pregnancy in primates is distinctly different from that in nonprimate species. It depends on different mechanisms, particularly the synthesis and secretion of CG by the peri-implantation embryo and the recognition of this hormone by the corpus luteum (Fig. 7), which promotes continued luteal progesterone production until the time of the luteal–placental shift. The past decade has witnessed a marked increase in our knowledge of the structure–function of CG, and the cellular composition and activities of the corpus luteum. However, little is known about the processes regulating CG expression in the implanting embryo, the mechanisms whereby CG prevents the usual regression of the corpus luteum at the end of the ovarian cycle and promotes further luteal differentiation in early pregnancy, or the importance, if any, of luteal relaxin, inhibin-related peptides, and estrogens (or androgens) in facilitating gestation. Further investigations, using molecular, cellular, and whole-animal approaches, are required to elucidate the embryo–maternal interactions that are critical for successful pregnancy initiation in primates. Manipulation of these interactions should have relevance to future modalities for controlling fertility and for alleviating specific types of infertility, such as recurrent miscarriage and early pregnancy wastage.

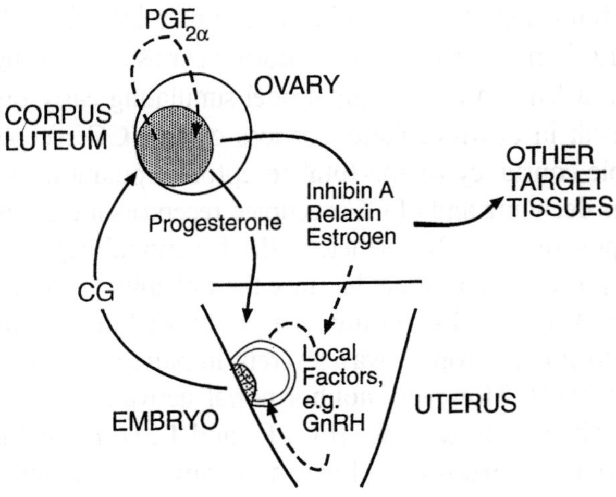

Fig. 7. Current perspective on the endocrine and local mechanisms activated during rescue of the corpus luteum at the start of pregnancy in primate species. Solid lines indicate established, whereas dotted lines indicated proposed, pathways. Embryo-derived CG, perhaps regulated by locally produced GnRH or other factors, prevents the typical regression of the corpus luteum at the end of the nonfertile ovarian cycle. CG may prevent the action of the putative local luteolysin PGF_{2a}, at least in some species. Therefore, the corpus luteum continues to produce progesterone, which sustains intrauterine pregnancy until the luteal–placental shift. CG also promotes the production of other steroid (e.g., estrogen) and protein (e.g., relaxin, inhibin A) hormones whose actions in the uterus may facilitate gestation. Adapted from review by Webley and Hearn *(9)*.

ACKNOWLEDGMENTS

The authors acknowledge the important contributions of many collaborators in spects of research performed in their laboratories. Program support for R. L. S. was provided by NIH RR00163 and HD18185, and for J. P. H. by NIHRR-00167. Research support for R. L. S. (NIH RO1 HD20869 and 22408) and to J. P. H. (NIH Women's Health Initiative Supplement) is also acknowledged. The generous donation of urinary and recombinant hCG for R. L. S.' studies by Ares Advanced Technology, Inc. is appreciated.

REFERENCES

1. Roberts RM, Xie S, Mathialagan N (1996) Maternal recognition of pregnancy. Biol Reprod 54: 294–302.
2. Niswender GD, Juengel JL, McGuire WJ, Belfiore CJ, Wiltbank MC (1994) Luteal function: The estrous cycle and early pregnancy. Biol Reprod 50:239–247.
3. Michael AE, Abayasekara DRE, Webley GE (1994) Cellular mechanisms of luteolysis. Mol Cell Endocrinol 99:R1–R9.
4. Stouffer RL (1988) Perspectives on the corpus luteum of the menstrual cycle and early pregnancy. Semin Reprod Endocrinol 6:103–113.
5. Knobil E (1973) On the regulation of the primate corpus luteum. Biol Reprod 8:246–258.
6. Stouffer RL, Duffy DM (1995) Receptors for sex steroids in the primate corpus luteum. New insight into gonadotropin and steroid action. Trends Endocrinol Metab 6:83–89.
7. Stouffer RL, Brannian JD (1993) The function and regulation of cell populations composing the corpus luteum of the ovarian cycle, In: The Ovary (Adashi EY, Leung PCK, eds.), Raven, New York, pp. 245–259.

8. Tullner WW (1974) Comparative aspects of primate chorionic gonadotropins, In: Contributions to Primatology (Kuhn H, Luckett WP, Noback CK, Schultz AH, Starck D, Szalay FS, eds.), Karger, Basel, pp. 235–257.
9. Webley GE, Hearn JP (1994) Embryo-maternal interactions during the establishment of pregnancy in primates, In: Oxford Reviews of Reproduction Biology (Charlton HM, eds.), Oxford-University Press, Oxford, UK, pp. 1–32.
10. Hodgen GD, Itskovitz J (1988) Recognition and maintenance of pregnancy, In: The Physiology of Reproduction (Knobil E, Neill J, eds.), New York, Raven, pp. 1995–2021.
11. Morton H, Rolfe B, Clunie GJA, Anderson MJ, Morrisson J (1977) An early pregnancy factor detected in human serum by the rosette inhibition test. Lancet i:394–397.
12. O'Neill C (1985) Examination of causes of early pregnancy associated thrombocytopenia in mice. J Reprod Fertil 73:567–577.
13. Sinosich MJ, Ferrier A, Saunders DM (1985) Monitoring of postimplantation embryo viability following successful in vitro fertilization and embryo transfer by measurements of placental proteins. Fertil Steril 44:70–74.
14. Cocchiara R, Di Trapani G, Azzolina A, Albeggiani G, Ciriminna R, Cefalu E (1987) Isolation of a histamine releasing factor from human embryo culture medium after in vitro fertilization. Hum Reprod 2:341–344.
15. Stockell Hartree A, Renwick AGC (1992) Molecular structures of glycoprotein hormones and functions of their carbohydrate components. Biochem J 287:665–679.
16. Layman LC (1991) The genetics of gonadotropin genes and the GnRH/GAP gene. Semin Reprod Endocrinol 9:22–33.
17. Pierce JG, Parsons TF (1981) Glycoprotein hormones: structure and function. Ann Rev Biochem 50:465–495.
18. Lustbader JW, Yarmush DL, Birken S, Puett D, Canfield RE (1993) The application of chemical studies of human chorionic gonadotropin to visualize its three-dimensional structure. Endocr Rev 14:291–311.
19. Ryan RJ, Charlesworth MC, McCormick DJ, Milius RP, Keutmann HT (1988) The glycoprotein hormones: recent studies of structure-function relationships. FASEB J 2:2661–2669.
20. Combarnous Y (1992) Molecular basis of the specificity of binding of glycoprotein hormones to their receptors. Endocr Rev 13:670–691.
21. Lapthorn AJ, Harris DC, Littlejohn A, Lustbader JW, Canfield RE, Machin KJ, Morgan FJ, Isaacs NW (1994) Crystal structure of human chorionic gonadotropin. Nature 369:455–461.
22. Jameson JL, Hollenberg AN (1993) Regulation of chorionic gonadotropin gene expression. Endocr Rev 14:203–220.
23. Boorstein WR, Vamvakopoulos NC, Fiddes JC (1982) Human chorionic gonadotropin β-subunit is encoded by at least eight genes arranged in tandem and inverted pairs. Nature 300:419–422.
24. Bo M, Boime I (1992) Identification of the transcriptionally active genes of the chorionic gonadotropin beta gene cluster in vivo. J Biol Chem 267:3179–3184.
25. Shoham Z, Insler V (1996) Recombinant technique and gonadotropins production: new era in reproductive medicine. Fertil Steril 66:187–201.
26. Campbell RK, Dean-Emig DM, Moyle WR (1991) Conversion of human choriogonadotropin into a follitropin by protein engineering. Proc Natl Acad Sci USA 88:760–764.
27. Fares FA, Suganuma N, Nishimori K, LaPolt PS, Hsueh AJW, Boime I (1992) Design of a long-acting follitropin agonist by fusing the C-terminal sequence of the chorionic gonadotropin β subunit to the follitropin β subunit. Proc Natl Acad Sci USA 89:4304–4308.
28. Simula AP, Amato F, Faast R, Lopata A, Berka J, Norman RJ (1995) Luteinizing hormone/chorionic gonadotropin bioactivity in the common marmoset (*Callithrix jacchus*) is due to a chorionic gonadotropin molecule with a structure intermediate between human chorionic gonadotropin and human luteinizing hormone. Biol Reprod 53:380–389.
29. Mwenda JM, Bambra CS, Tarara RP (1990) Studies with human, baboon, and vervet monkey chorionic gonadotrophins. J Med Primatol 19:715–724.
30. Seshagiri PB, Terasawa EI, Hearn JP (1996) Secretion of chorionic gonadotrophin by the peri-implantation embryo of rhesus and marmoset monkeys, with its possible relationship to embryo-derived GnRH, In: Current Concepts in Fertility Regulation and Reproduction (Puri, CP, Van Look PFA, eds.), Wiley Eastern, New Delhi, pp. 395–410.
31. Meyer RK (1972) Chorionic gonadotropin, corpus luteum function and embryo implantation in the rhesus monkey. Acta Endocrinol (Suppl) 166:214–217.

32. Ginther OJ, Dierschke DJ, Walsh SW, Del Campo CH (1974) Anatomy of arteries and veins of uterus and ovaries in rhesus monkeys. Biol Reprod 11:205–219.
33. Bonduelle ML, Dodd R, Liebaers I, Steirteghem AV, Williamson R, Akhurst R (1988) Chorionic gonadotrophin-β mRNA, a trophoblast marker, is expressed in human 8-cell embryos derived from tripronucleate zygotes. Hum Reprod 3:909–914.
34. Hearn JP, Hodges JK, Gems S (1988) Early secretion of chorionic gonadotrophin by marmoset embryos in vitro and in vivo. J Endocrinol 119:249–255.
35. Dokras A, Sargent IL, Ross C, Gardner RL, Barlow DH (1991) The human blastocyst: morphology and human chorionic gonadotrophin secretion in vitro. Hum Reprod 6:1143–1151.
36. Hay DL, Lopata A (1988) Chorionic gonadotrophin secretion by human embryos in vitro. J Clin Endocrinol Metab 67:1322–1324.
37. Hay DL, Lopata A (1990) Factors modifying early hCG production of the human blastocyst in vitro. Assisted Reprod Technol Androl 1:9–23.
38. Seshagiri PB, Hearn JP (1993) In-vitro development of in-vivo produced rhesus monkey morulae and blastocysts to hatched, attached, and post-attached blastocyst stages: morphology and early secretion of chorionic gonadotropin. Hum Reprod 8:279–287.
39. Reshef E, Lei ZM, Rao C, Pridham DD, Chegini N, Luborsky JL (1990) The presence of gonadotropin receptors in nonpregnant human uterus, human placenta, fetal membranes, and decidua. J Clin Endocrinol Metab 70:421–430.
40. Toth P, Li X, Rao CV, Lincoln SR, Sanfilippo SJ, Spinnato JA, Yussman MA (1994) Expression of functional human chorionic gonadotropin/human luteinizing hormone receptor gene in human uterine arteries. J Clin Endocrinol Metab 79:307–315.
41. Hay DL (1985) Discordant and variable production of human chorionic gonadotropin and its free α- and β-subunits in early pregnancy. J Clin Endocrinol Metab 61:1195–1200.
42. Kelly AC, Rodgers A, Dong K, Barrezueta NX, Blum M, Roberts JL (1991) Gonadotropin-releasing hormone, chorionic gonadotropin gene expression in human placental development. DNA Cell Biol 10:411–422.
43. Iwashita M, Evans MI, Catt KJ (1986) Characterization of a gonadotropin-releasing hormone receptor site in term placenta, chorionic villi. J Clin Endocrinol Metab 62:127–133.
44. Petraglia F, Sawchenko P, Lim AT, Rivier J, Vale W (1987) Localization, secretion, action of inhibin in human placenta. Science 237:187–189.
45. Petraglia F, Vaughan J, Vale W (1989) Inhibin, activin modulate the release of gonadotropin-releasing hormone, human chorionic gonadotropin, progesterone from cultured human placental cells. Proc Natl Acad Sci USA 86:5114–5117.
46. Hearn JP, Terasawa E, Becker RA (1996) Endocrine regulation of embryo implantation in primates: the relationship between gonadotropin releasor hormone and chorionic gonadotropin. XVIth Congress of the International Primatological Society and XIXth Conference of the American Society of Primatologists (Madison, WI, Aug 11–16) Abstract #230.
47. Phocas I, Sarandakou A, Rizos D, Dimitriadou F, Mantzavinos T, Zourlas PA (1992) Secretion of α-immunoreactive inhibin by human pre-embryos cultured in vitro. Hum Reprod 7:545–549.
48. Edgar DH, James GB, Mills JA (1993) Steroid secretion by human early embryos in culture. Hum Reprod 8:277,278.
49. Sengupta J, Talwar D, Paria BC, Ghosh D (1989) Is there any delta^5-3β hydroxysteroid dehydrogenase activity in preimplantation embryo of rhesus monkey? Indian J Exp Biol 27:417–420.
50. Prahalada S, Venkatramaiah M, Rao AJ, Moudgal NR (1975) Termination of pregnancy in macaques (Macaca radiata) using monkey antiserum to ovine LH. Contraception 12:137–147.
51. Stevens VC (1973) Immunization of female baboons with hapten-coupled gonadotropins. J Obstet Gynecol 42:496–506.
52. Talwar GP, Sharma NC, Dubey SK (1976) Isoimmunization against hCG with conjugates of processed β-subunit of the hormone and tetanus toxoid. Proc Natl Acad Sci USA 73:218–222.
53. Thau RB, Sundaram K (1980) The mechanisms of action of an antifertility vaccine in the rhesus monkey: reversal of the effects of antisera to β-oLH by medroxyprogesterone acetate. Fertil Steril 33:317–320.
54. Quagliarello J, Goldsmith L, Steinetz B, Lustig DS, Weiss G (1980) Induction of relaxin secretion in nonpregnant women by human chorionic gonadotropin. J Clin Endocrinol Metab 51:74–77.
55. Surve AH, Harrington FE, Elton RL (1973) Effect of chorionic gonadotropin on corpus luteum of the monkey. Proc Soc Exp Biol Med 144:963–968.

56. Hearn JP, Webley GE (1987) Regulation of the corpus luteum of early pregnancy in the marmoset monkey: local interactions of luteotrophic and luteolytic hormones in vivo and their effects on the secretion of progesterone. J Endocrinol 114:231–239.
57. Stouffer RL, Ottobre JS, VandeVoort CA (1987) Regulation of the primate corpus luteum during early pregnancy, In: The Primate Ovary (Stouffer RL, eds.), Plenum New York, pp. 207–220.
58. Duffy DM, Hutchison JS, Stewart DR, Stouffer RL (1996) Stimulation of primate luteal function by recombinant hCG and modulation of steroid, but not relaxin, production by an inhibitor of 3β-hydroxysteroid dehydrogenase during simulated early pregnancy. J Clin Endocrinol Metab 81: 2307–2313.
59. Ellinwood WE, Stanczyk FZ, Lazur JJ, Novy MJ (1989) Dynamics of steroid biosynthesis during the luteal-placental shift in rhesus monkeys. J Clin Endocrinol Metab 69:348–355.
60. Stewart DR, Celniker AC, Taylor CA, Jr., Cragun JR, Overstreet JW, Lasley BL (1990) Relaxin in the peri-implantation period. J Clin Endocrinol Metab 70:1771–1773.
61. Steinetz BG, Randolph C, Mahoney CJ (1992) Serum concentrations of relaxin, chorionic gonadotropin, estradiol-17β, and progesterone during the reproductive cycle of the chimpanzee (*Pan troglodytes*). Endocrinology 130:3601–3607.
62. Stewart DR, Stouffer R, Overstreet JW, Hendrickx A, Lasley BL (1993) Measurement of peri-implantational relaxin concentrations in the macaque using a homologous assay. Endocrinology 132:6–12.
63. Duffy DM, Stouffer RL, Stewart DR (1995) Dissociation of relaxin and progesterone secretion from the primate corpus luteum by acute administration of a 3β-hydroxysteroid dehydrogenase inhibitor during the menstrual cycle. Biol Reprod 53:447–453.
64. Smith KB, Lunn SF, Fraser HM (1990) Inhibin secretion during the ovulatory cycle and pregnancy in the common marmoset monkey. J Endocrinol 126:489–495.
65. Nozaki M, Watanabe G, Taya K, Katakai Y, Wada I, Sasamoto S, Oshima K (1990) Changes in circulating inhibin levels during pregnancy and early lactation in the Japanese monkey. Biol Reprod 43:444–449.
66. Santoro N, Schneyer AL, Ibrahim J, Schmidt CL (1992) Gonadotropin and inhibin concentrations in early pregnancy in women with and without corpora lutea. Obstet Gynecol 79: 579–585.
67. Mather JP, Woodruff TK, Krummen LA (1992) Paracrine regulation of reproductive function by inhibin and activin. Proc Soc Exp Biol Med 201:1–15.
68. Groome NP, Illingworth PJ, O'Brien M, Pai R, Rodger FE, Mather JP, McNeilly AS (1996) Measurement of dimeric inhibin B throughout the human menstrual cycle. J Clin Endocrinol Metab 81:1401–1405.
69. Illingworth PJ, Reddi K, Smith K, Baird DT (1990) Pharmacological "rescue" of the corpus luteum results in increased inhibin production. Clin Endocrinol 33:323–332.
70. Illingworth PJ, Groome NP, Duncan WC, Grant V, Tovanabutra S, Baird DT, McNeilly AS (1996) Measurement of circulating inhibin forms during the establishment of pregnancy. J Clin Endocrinol Metab 81:1471–1475.
71. Rombauts L, Verhoeven G, Meuleman C, Koninckx PR, Poncelet E, Franchimont P (1996) Dimeric inhibin A and α-subunit immunoreactive material in maternal serum during spontaneous and in vitro fertilization pregnancies. J Clin Endocrinol Metab 81:985–989.
72. Trounson A (1992) Development of the technique of oocyte donation and hormonal replacement therapy: is oestrogen really necessary for the establishment and maintenance of pregnancy. Reprod Fertil Dev 4:671–679.
73. Ghosh D, De P, Sengupta J (1994) Luteal phase ovarian oestrogen is not essential for implantation and maintenance of pregnancy from surrogate embryo transfer in the rhesus monkey. Hum Reprod 9:629–637.
74. Cameron JL, Stouffer RL (1981) Comparisons of the species specificity of gonadotropin binding to primate and nonprimate corpora lutea. Biol Reprod 25:568–572.
75. Cameron JL, Stouffer RL (1982) Gonadotropin receptors of the primate corpus luteum. I. Characterization of ^{125}I-labeled human luteinizing hormone and human chorionic gonadotropin binding to luteal membranes from the rhesus monkey. Endocrinology 110:2059–2067.
76. Cameron JL, Stouffer RL (1982) Gonadotropin receptors of the primate corpus luteum: II. Changes in available LH and CG binding sites in macaque luteal membranes during the nonfertile menstrual cycle. Endocrinology 110:2068–2073.

77. Ottobre JS, Ottobre AC, Stouffer RL (1984) Changes in available gonadotropin receptors in the corpus luteum of the rhesus monkey during simulated early pregnancy. Endocrinology 115: 198–204.
78. Eyster KM, Stouffer RL (1985) Characterization of the adenylate cyclase system in the nonhuman primate (*Macaca mulatta*) corpus luteum. II. Sensitivity to gonadotropins, other hormones and nonhormonal activators. Endocrinology 116:1552–1558.
79. Stouffer RL, Nixon WE, Gulyas BJ, Hodgen GD (1977) Gonadotropin-sensitive progesterone production by rhesus monkey luteal cells in vitro: A function of age of the corpus luteum during the menstrual cycle. Endocrinology 100:506–512.
80. Rao CV, Griffin LP, Carman FR, Jr. (1976) Gonadotropin receptors in human corpora lutea of the menstrual cycle and pregnancy. Am J Obstet Gynecol 128:146–153.
81. Marsh JM, LeMaire WJ (1974) Cyclic AMP accumulation and steroidogenesis in the human corpus luteum: effect of gonadotropins and prostaglandins. J Clin Endocrinol Metab 38:99–106.
82. Dukelow WR (1979) Human chorionic gonadotropin: induction of ovulation in the squirrel monkey. Science 206:234,235.
83. Thornton SJ, Pantos C, Speirs A, Johnston I (1990) Human chorionic gonadotropin to oocyte retrieval interval in in vitro fertilization—how critical is it. Fertil Steril 53:177–179.
84. Aladin Chandrasekher Y, Hutchison JS, Zelinski-Wooten MB, Hess DL, Wolf DP, Stouffer RL (1994) Initiation of periovulatory events in primate follicles using recombinant and native human luteinizing hormone to mimic the midcycle gonadotropin surge. J Clin Endocrinol Metab 79: 298–306.
85. Hutchinson JS, Zeleznik AJ (1985) The corpus luteum of the primate menstrual cycle is capable of recovering from a transient withdrawal of pituitary gonadotropin support. Endocrinology 117: 1043–1049.
86. Zelinski-Wooten MB, Hutchison JS, Aladin Chandrasekher Y, Wolf DP, Stouffer RL (1992) Administration of human luteinizing hormone (hLH) to macaques after follicular development: Further titration of LH surge requirements for ovulatory changes in primate follicles. J Clin Endocrinol Metab 75:502–507.
87. Soules MR, Steiner RA, Clifton DK, Bremner WJ (1986) The effects of inducing a follicular phase gonadotropin secretory pattern in normal women during the luteal phase. Fertil Steril 47:45–53.
88. Monfort SL, Hess DL, Hendrickx AG, Lasley BL (1989) Absence of regular pulsatile gonadotropin secretion during implantation in the rhesus macaque. Endocrinology 125:1766–1773.
89. Niswender GD, Schwall RH, Fitz TA, Farin CE, Sawyer HR (1985) Regulation of luteal function in domestic ruminants: New concepts. Rec Prog Horm Res 41:101–151.
90. Molskness TA, Zelinski-Wooten MB, Hild-Petito SA, Stouffer RL (1991) Comparison of the steroidogenic response of luteinized granulosa cells from rhesus monkeys to luteinizing hormone and chorionic gonadotropin. Biol Reprod 45:273–281.
91. Booher C, Enders AC, Hendrickx AG, Hess DL (1981) Structural characteristics of the corpus luteum during implantation in the rhesus monkey (*Macaca mulatta*). Am J Anat 160:17–36.
92. Christenson LK, Stouffer RL (1996) Proliferation of microvascular endothelial cells in the primate corpus luteum during the menstrual cycle and simulated early pregnancy. Endocrinology 137:367–374.
93. McClure N, Macpherson AM, Healy DL, Wreford N, Rogers PAW (1994) An immunohistochemical study of the vascularization of the human Graafian follicle. Hum Reprod 9:1401–1405.
94. Ghinea N, Hai MTV, Groyer-Picard M, Milgrom E (1994) How protein hormones reach their target cells. Receptor-mediated transcytosis of hCG through endothelial cells. J Cell Biol 125: 87–97.
95. Benyo DF, Little-Ihrig L, Zeleznik AJ (1993) Noncoordinated expression of luteal cell messenger ribonucleic acids during human chorionic gonadotropin stimulation of the primate corpus luteum. Endocrinology 133:699–704.
96. Sanders SL, Stouffer RL (1995) Localization of steroidogenic enzymes in macaque luteal tissue during the menstrual cycle and simulated early pregnancy: Immunohistochemical evidence supporting the two-cell model for estrogen production in the primate corpus luteum. Biol Reprod 56: 1077–1087.
97. Sasano H, Okamoto M, Mason JI, Simpson ER, Mendelson CR, Sasano N, Silverberg SG (1989) Immunolocalization of aromatase, 17α-hydroxylase and side-chain-cleavage cytochromes P450 in the human ovary. J Reprod Fertil 85:163–165.
98. Sasano H, Mori T, Sasano N, Nagura H, Mason JI (1990) Immunolocalization of 3β-hydroxysteroid dehydrogenase in human ovary. J Reprod Fertil 89:743–751.

99. Brannian JD, Shiigi SM, Stouffer RL (1991) Differential uptake of fluorescent-tagged low density lipoprotein by cells from the primate corpus luteum: Isolation and characterization of subtypes of small and large luteal cells. Endocrinology 129:3247–3253.
100. Bryant-Greenwood GD, Schwabe C (1994) Human relaxins: chemistry and biology. Endocr Rev 15:5–26.
101. Hudson P, Haley J, John M, Cronk M, Crawford R, Haralambidis J, Tregear G, Shine J, Niall H (1983) Structure of a genomic clone encoding biologically active human relaxin. Nature 301: 628–631.
102. Hudson P, John M, Crawford R, Haralambidis J, Scanlon D, Gorman J, Tregear G, Shine J, Niall H (1984) Relaxin gene-expression in human ovaries and the predicted structure of a human preprorelaxin by analysis of cDNA clones. EMBO J 3:2333–2339.
103. Evans BA, Fu P, Tregear GW (1994) Characterization of primate relaxin genes. Endocr J 2:81–86.
104. Ivell R, Hunt N, Khan-Dawood F, Dawood MY (1989) Expression of the human relaxin gene in the corpus luteum of the menstrual cycle and in the prostate. Mol Cell Endocrinol 66:251–255.
105. Stewart DR, Overstreet JW, Celniker AC, Hess DL, Cragun JR, Boyers SP, Lasley BL (1993) The relationship between hCG and relaxin secretion in normal pregnancies vs peri-implantation spontaneous abortions. Clin Endocrinol 38:379–385.
106. Ottobre AC, Ramsey KR, Ottobre JS (1991) Acute versus chronic effects of human chorionic gonadotrophin on relaxin secretion in rhesus monkeys. J Reprod Fertil 91:313–320.
107. Gagliardi CL, Goldsmith LT, Saketos M, Weiss G, Schmidt CL (1992) Human chorionic gonadotropin stimulation of relaxin secretion by luteinized human granulosa cells. Fertil Steril 58: 314–320.
108. Schmidt CL, Goldsmith LT, Carr BR, Weiss G, Parker CR, Jr., Illingworth DR (1988) Peripheral relaxin levels during pregnancy in a woman with homozygous familial hypobetalipoproteinemia. Fertil Steril 50:815–817.
109. Seki K, Uesato T, Kato K (1987) Serum relaxin concentrations in women following the administration of 16,16-dimethyltransdelta^2-PGE$_1$ methyl ester during early pregnancy. Prostaglandins 33: 739–742.
110. Ottobre JS, Stouffer RL (1986) Receptors for chorionic gonadotropin in the corpus luteum of the rhesus monkey during simulated early pregnancy: Lack of down-regulation. Endocrinology 119: 1594–1602.
111. VandeVoort CA, Molskness TA, Stouffer RL (1988) Adenylate cyclase in the primate corpus luteum during chorionic gonadotropin treatment simulating early pregnancy: Homologous versus heterologous desensitization. Endocrinology 122:734–740.
112. Hagstrom H, Hahlin M, Bennegard-Eden B, Bourne T, Hamberger L (1996) Regulation of corpus luteum function in early human pregnancy. Fertil Steril 65:81–86.
113. Stouffer RL, Ottobre JS, Molskness TA, Zelinski-Wooten MB (1989) The function and regulation of the primate corpus luteum during the fertile menstrual cycle, In: Development of Preimplantation Embryos and Their Environment (Yoshinaga K, Mori T, eds.), Alan R. Liss, New York, pp. 129–142.
114. Houmard BS, Guan Z, Stokes BT, Ottobre JS (1994) The effects of gonadotropin on the phosphatidylinositol pathway in the primate corpus luteum. Mol Cell Endocrinol 104:113–120.
115. Stouffer RL (1990) Corpus luteum function and dysfunction. Clin Obstet Gynecol 33:668–689.

3 Role of Cytokines in the Pregnant Uterus of Interstitial Implanting Species

Jeffrey W. Pollard, PHD

CONTENTS

INTRODUCTION

The uterus undergoes profound, reversible remodeling coupled with differentiation of resident cell types and invasion by hematopoietic cells during pregnancy. It is the only adult tissue to exhibit such plasticity, making it a uniquely approachable system to study events controlling differentiation and development. These include the preparation of the uterus to receive the implanting blastocyst, the decidualization of the uterine stroma in response to this implanting blastocyst, the coordinated development of the maternal aspect of the placenta with fetal development, the expulsion of the conceptus at parturition, and the remodeling of the uterus in preparation for the next pregnancy. The overall regulators of all these events are the ovarian sex steroid hormones, estrogen and progesterone (P_4), in whose absence pregnancy cannot proceed. Each of these steroid hormones acts through a nuclear transcription factor receptor. Induced null mutations in the genes for the estrogen (ERKO) and progesterone receptor (PRKO) in mice, support the view that both estradiol-17β (E_2) and P_4 act directly in the uterus. In both null mutants, a uterus develops; however, it is estrogen-insensitive and hypoplastic in the ERKO mouse *(1)* and progesterone-insensitive and hyperplastic in the PRKO mouse *(2)*. Despite these direct effects of the ovarian steroid hormone/receptor complexes on gene transcription and given the complexity of the physiological responses to sex steroid hormones, many of these responses are thought to be mediated through the secondary actions of growth factors/cytokines whose local synthesis is directly or indirectly regulated by the steroid hormones *(3)*. It is the action of these factors in the uterus that is the subject of this chapter, with a particular emphasis on their function in the interstitial implanting species, mouse and human. The literature in this field is now immense, and since there are many recent reviews *(4–11)*, the author does not intend to provide lists of cytokines nor their sites of synthesis and action. Furthermore, because cytokines, especially leukemia inhibitory factor (LIF), colony stimulating factor-1 (CSF-1), and interleukin-6 (IL-6), are released by many cells (including those of the reproductive tract) in response to cell culture and the consequent removal from the constraints imposed from the surrounding extracellular matrix, interpretation of cell-culture experiments is extremely problematic. Thus, this chapter will focus on in vivo experiments in mice aimed at determining the actions of these cytokines in the pregnant uterus. In humans, where in vivo manipulations are impossible, parallels from the animal studies will be drawn when relevant. This chapter will also concentrate on the roles of hematopoietic or immune class cytokines synthesized in the uterus. For the action of more classical growth factors and the older literature on hematopoietic cytokines, the reader is referred to Chapter 4 of this vol. and the previous reviews by this author *(3,4,7,12)*.

UTERINE PREPARATION FOR IMPLANTATION

Progesterone synthesized as a consequence of copulation in Murids, or during the menstrual cycle in humans, causes the epithelial cells that had been previously stimulated to proliferate by E_2, to exit the cell cycle and differentiate in preparation for blastocyst attachment *(13,14)*. In the mouse, P_4 slightly stimulates stromal cell proliferation and primes the uterine stromal cells to respond to E_2 with a wave of cell division *(13)*. The beginning of P_4 synthesis coincides in the mouse with morula entering the uterus and their differentiation into blastocysts *(15,16)*. A further 1.5 d elapse before the blastocyst hatches from its zona pellucida and the uterine epithelial cells become receptive to its attachment. In Murids, and it is presumed in humans, a low concentration of E_2 is required for the final preparation of the epithelium for blastocyst attachment *(17,18)*. If this E_2 is not forthcoming, for example as a result of ovariectomy, the blastocyst enters a state of delay, which can be broken by treatment of the animal with a nidatory dose of E_2 *(19)*. Following attachment of the blastocyst to the apical surface of antimesometrial luminal epithelium in rat and mouse, a signal is transduced that causes the underlying stroma to begin the process of decidual transformation, which propagates both outward and mesometrially to surround completely the invading blastocyst, which by this time has progressed to the egg cylinder stage. Once such a state is achieved, implantation can be considered complete.

In preparation for implantation, there has been considerable debate over whether the sex steroid hormone-regulated mitogenic events are direct actions of these hormones or are mediated by cytokines and growth factors (reviewed in *20*). Cytokines can transactivate steroid hormone receptors to become transcriptionally active in the absence of hormone *(21,22)*. Similarly, E_2 and P_4 acting alone or synergistically can induce the expression of many growth factors *(4,6,9)*. For example, epidermal growth factor (EGF) expression and that of its receptor (EGFR), is regulated by E_2 *(23–26)*. In the absence of E_2, EGF can stimulate uterine epithelial cell proliferation in vivo *(27)* and transcriptionally transactivate the estrogen receptor (ER) in vitro *(22)*, probably by altering its state of phosphorylation *(28)*. Recent studies with ERKO mice showed that this EGF action on uterine epithelial cell proliferation is absolutely dependent on a functional ER *(29)*, suggesting that EGF acts in vivo via the transactivation of the ER. However, there is debate over the cellular site of action of EGF, since there have been conflicting reports over whether the EGFR is expressed in the uterine epithelium or only in the underlying stroma *(23,30)*. Furthermore,

Table 1
The Mouse Uterine Epithelium: a Cytokine Factory

Cytokine	*Hormonal regulation*	*Phenotype of null mutation in ligand or receptor gene*	*Reference*
CSF-1	E_2P_4	Macrophage deficiency Increased embryonic loss Mammary gland deficiency (ligand only)	*(52,61)*
GM-CSF	E_2	NRP[a] (ligand and receptor)	*(54,144)*
IL-1	E_2P_4	NRP (receptor only)	*(82,217)*
IL-6	E_2	NRP (ligand only)	*(161,217,218)*
LIF	E_2	Implantation failure Placental deficiency (ligand and receptor)	*(83,84)*
TGF-β1	E_2P_4	Embryonic lethal (ligand only)	*(35,105)*
TNF-α	E_2P_4	NRP (ligand and receptor)	*(67,69,191)*

[a]NRP: no phenotype reported.

although EGF can mimic E_2 action, it is not certain that it is the physiological mediator of E_2 in the uterus. Nevertheless, these studies on EGFR interactions, together with those demonstrating activation of the ER by the protein kinases C and A and the MAP kinase pathway *(21,31,32)*, together with the modification of ER activity by phosphorylation *(28)*, indicate that cytokines and hormone receptors can undergo a process of crosstalk that influences physiological response to hormone in target tissue.

Little is known of the action of P_4 in inhibiting the proliferation of the uterine epithelium, stimulating proliferation in the stroma, and in preparing the uterus for implantation. Several cytokines are synthesized in the uterus, particularly the uterine epithelium, under the influence of P_4 (Table 1). These include transforming growth factor-β1 (TGF-β1) and tumor necrosis factor-α (TNF-α) *(33–35)*, whose action in certain contexts can inhibit cell proliferation, but there is no direct evidence that this is the case in the uterus. In fact, TNF-α has been proposed to mediate uterine cell death at menstruation after P_4 concentrations have dropped *(9)*, and TNF-α instilled into the uterine lumen of mice induces endothelal cell death *(36)*. Recent evidence has shown that fibroblast growth factor (FGF) can synergize with P_4 to stimulate cell proliferation in cultured stromal cells from rats *(37)*, and this is consistent with FGF and FGF receptor (FGFR) expression in the uterine stromal cells *(37,38)*. This is reviewed in greater detail in Chapter 4 of this vol. Nevertheless, there is little physiological evidence that any of these growth factors play an essential role in the P_4 regulation of uterine cell proliferation.

The uterine epithelium is a major site of cytokine synthesis (Table 1 *[4]*). Several of these cytokines influence the development of the preimplantation mouse or rat embryo in culture *(see 39)*. Furthermore, coculture of preimplantation embryos with uterine epithelial cells enhances their in vitro growth, suggesting the effects of paracrine factors. Both EGF and TGF-α stimulate the rate of blastocoele formation in cultured embryos *(40)*, and antisense EGFR oligonucleotides inhibit the rate of their development *(41,42)*. EGFRs are expressed in preimplantation embryos from the four-cell *(43)* until the blastocyst stage, at which stage their expression appears to be regulated by the maternal steroid hormonal environment. EGFR expression is decreased in delayed blastocysts and increased on release of delay by E_2 treatment of the mother *(44)*. An important role for EGFR in embryonic development at the implantation stage was shown by targeted disruption of the EGFR gene in mice. In certain genetic strains, this results in peri-implantation failures owing to degeneration of the inner cell mass *(45)*. Interestingly, despite the cell-culture experiments described above, preimplantation embryos lacking EGFR develop normally, and lethality is only observed after implantation is initiated *(45)*.

Several EGFR ligands are synthesized in the uterus, including EGF, TGF-α, amphiregulin, and hepain-binding (HB)-EGF *(46–49)*. TGF-α is expressed in the preimplantation embryo *(41)*; however, targeted disruption of the TGF-α gene does not compromise fertility of homozygous mutants, indicating that this ligand does not play an essential autocrine or paracrine role in implantation *(50)*. Other candidate EGFR ligands include amphiregulin, EGF, and HB-EGF. EGF is expressed in the uterine epithelium at d 1 of pregnancy, followed by a decline with re-expression at the time of implantation *(26)*. HB-EGF is expressed in the uterine epithelium under the influence of E_2 *(47–49)*, and later in the uterine stroma under the influence of P_4 and E_2 *(47–49)*. Amphiregulin on the other hand is regulated solely by P_4 and is expressed in the uterine epithelium at the time of implantation and, after blastocyst attachment, in the luminal epithelium specifically at the site of attachment *(51)*. Amphiregulin, therefore, is a prime candidate as a ligand for the EGFR expressed in the blastocyst, and if it is, it emphasizes the close maternal–fetal interaction occurring at implantation.

Several other cytokines synthesized by the uterine epithelium also effect preimplantation embryonic development in culture *(15,39)*. Interestingly, many of these were originally characterized as hematopoietic cytokines. They include granulocyte-macrophage colony-stimulating factor (GM-CSF), CSF-1, LIF, IL-1, and TNF-α, all of whose synthesis is regulated by ovarian sex steroid hormones in the uterus *(6,52–57)*. However, many of the experiments of the effects of cytokines on embryonic development in vitro were performed in nonoptimized media *(39)*. Using an optimized medium that allows a high rate of development of zygotes into blastocysts, Bhatnagar et al. *(58)* showed that CSF-1 at physiologic concentrations promotes the rate of differentiation and the rate of trophectodermal cell proliferation. This is consistent with, in both mouse and humans, the maternal expression of CSF-1 and the expression of CSF-1 receptor (CSF-1R) transcripts in the preimplantation embryo *(59,60)*. However, detailed studies with a CSF-1 null mutant mouse, osteopetrotic (*csfm^{op}*), indicates that the absence of CSF-1 in vivo has only a minimal effect on implantation rates *(61,62)*. This, however, can be reconciled with the culture data, because CSF-1-treated embryos had similar rates of implantation to those untreated control embryos when transferred to pseudopregnant females, despite their enhanced growth and differentiation rate *(58)*.

The impact of cytokines on embryonic development need not necessarily be positive. TNF-α, for example, reduces the rate of inner cell mass (ICM) proliferation in cultured preimplantation embryos *(63)*, an effect that could be reversed by treatment with antisense oligonucleotides directed against the TNF-α p60 receptor that is expressed in the embryo *(64,65)*. This may have physiological consequences, because in diabetic rats, the uterine concentration of TNF-α is significantly elevated *(66)*, and this elevation may negatively influence embryonic development and explain the embryopathologies associated with diabetes. Ovarian steroid hormone regulated expression of TNF-α in uterine epithelium is found in normal pregnancies in both human and mouse *(34,67–69)*, suggesting that a fine regulation over uterine TNF-α concentration is required for pregnancy to proceed normally.

Blastocysts capable of implanting and developing to term can be obtained at high frequency after culture in chemically defined, cytokine-free media *(70)*. This suggests that if cytokines play an important role in this phase of development, most of them are embryonically synthesized *(41)*. However, the rate of embryonic development is slower and the number of cell divisions reduced in culture *(70)*. Thus, it is possible that maternally synthesized cytokines, in both the oviduct and uterus, play a role in maternal to embryo communication, perhaps helping to synchronize the rate of embryonic development with the maternal preparation for implantation *(39)*. Therefore, perturbation of these cytokine balances in pathological conditions might result in embryopathy and/or failure of implantation. This contention is supported because addition of cytokines, such as CSF-1, to the mouse at inappropriate times during the preimplantation period can result in disruption of normal pregnancy *(71)*, or conversely, treatment of mice during the preimplantation period with GM-CSF or TNF-α can promote pregnancy in abortion-prone mice *(72)*.

Cytokines have also been implicated in the process of implantation itself *(4,11,20,73)*. As discussed above, the evidence for the involvement of the EGF family of growth factors in embryonic growth coincidental with implantation is compelling. Simón et al. using an IL-1R antagonists showed inhibition of blastocysts attachment to the uterine epithelium and a disruption of implantation *(74)*. IL-1 stimulates prostaglandin E_2 (PGE_2) production by cultured uterine stromal cells through the activation of cyclooxygenase *(75,76)*. Since prostaglandins are thought to be involved in regulating the decidual response *(77)*, this may be the mechanism of IL-1 action during implantation. However, although IL-1, probably largely synthesized by macrophages, but also by the uterine epithelium, is detected in the mouse and human uterus, there are disputes regarding whether it is expressed during the implantation period *(53,78–81)*. Furthermore, mice homozygous for a null mutation in the IL-1R type 1 (the IL-1 signaling) receptor gene had normal implantation rates and pregnancies *(82)*. This shows that pregnancy can proceed in the absence of IL-1 signaling and suggests the data from Simón et al. *(74)* are either owing to differences in response because of mouse strain, or more likely, that the IL-1R antagonists used had some unknown side effect that inhibited implantation. These experiments on the IL-1R type 1 null mutant mice call into question the importance of IL-1 in pregnancy in both mice and humans.

A complete inhibition of implantation was observed in mice lacking LIF caused by an induced null mutation *(83)*. In mice, LIF is synthesized under the influence of E_2 at estrus and in a discrete burst by the glandular epithelium at the time of implantation *(84)*. Recent studies in humans show an elevation of LIF expression in the uterine epithelium during the secretory phase *(85–89)*, whereas LIF receptor (LIFR) and its coreceptor protein gp130 are expressed in luminal, but not glandular epithelium during the secretory phase *(85)*. Similar patterns of LIFR expression have been found in the mouse uterus (Stewart, personal communication). This suggests a model whereby nidatory E_2 stimulates the P_4-primed uterine epithelium (glandular in mouse, and luminal and glandular in human) to synthesize LIF, which then activates the LIF receptor in luminal epithelial cells causing these cells to become receptive to the implanting blastocyst and competent to transmit the signal to the underlying stroma to induce decidualization (Fig. 1). LIF, therefore, is an essential intrauterine mediator of E_2 action during pregnancy.

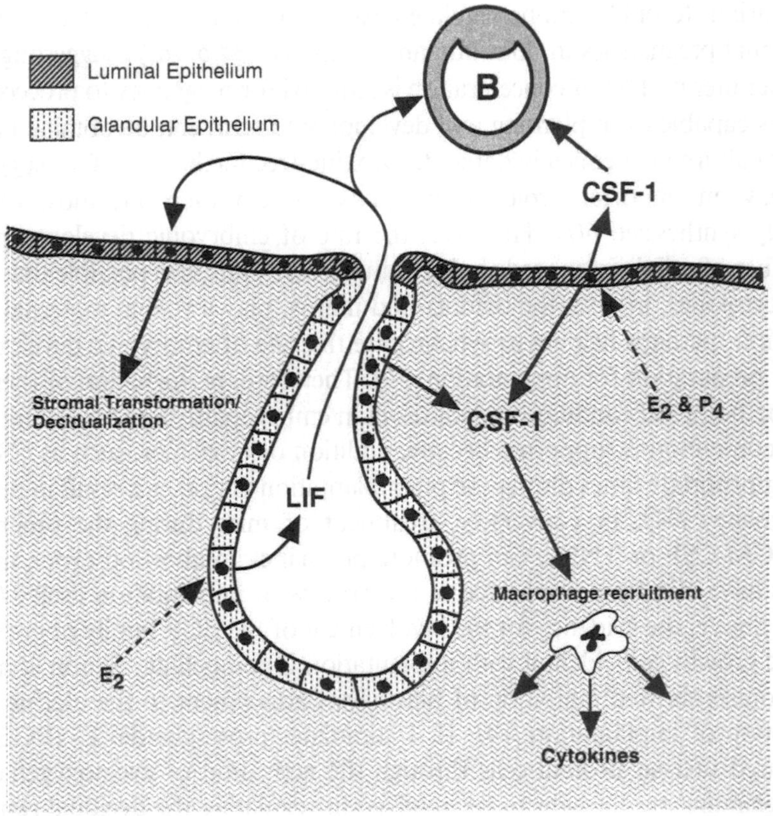

Fig. 1. Cytokine synthesis by the uterine epithelium. LIF is synthesized by the glandular epithelium in response to E_2. Receptor-bearing cells are found in the blastocyst (B) and on the luminal epithelium. A null mutation in the LIF gene results in failure of the uterus to decidualize and of the epithelium to allow blastocyst attachment. Implantation, therefore, is disrupted. The synthesis of CSF-1 by both the luminal and glandular epithelium is regulated by the synergistic actions of E_2 and P_4. Receptors are located in the blastocyst and in stromal macrophages. A null mutation in the CSF-1 gene results in a diminished number of recruitment of macrophages to the uterus. Although both LIF and CSF-1 affect preimplantation embryonic development in culture, the development of embryos in vivo is only marginally affected in the respective null mutant.

DECIDUALIZATION

In mice and rats, attachment of the blastocyst to the uterine epithelium triggers the underlying stroma to decidualize. This process spreads out and around the invading embryo, eventually surrounding it entirely. The decidua differentiates into a primary and secondary zone, and into mesometrial and antimesometrial areas, as the former becomes progressively more vascularized. The decidua capsularis eventually regresses by apoptosis, whereas the mesometrial decidua basalis contributes the maternal component to the placenta. During these processes, the rates of cell division are extremely high *(90)* equaling those documented anywhere else in the organism. In humans, a rather similar process occurs, except that during the menstrual cycle, cells begin to decidualize even in the absence of any embryo and there is no obvious orientation to implantation *(11)*.

Many growth factors have been shown to be synthesized in decidual cells of both Murids and humans *(3)*. They include members of the TGF-β gene superfamily. For example, activin β_A is expressed from d 5–7 and more mesometrially from d 6–9½ of pregnancy in mice *(91)*. TGF-β1 is expressed preferentially in the secondary decidua *(35,91,92)*, β2 in the mesometrial decidua, and by d 8.5 of pregnancy, principally in the uterine epithelium *(91–94)*, whereas TGF-β3 is localized in the myometrium *(94)*. TGF-βs are known to be involved in extracellular matrix formation, and in the regulation of cell proliferation and death. Experimentally, TGF-β2 has been shown to induce apoptosis in uterine stromal cells in culture *(95)*, and in vivo, this molecule may regulate decidual regression either as part of the ongoing developmental program, in the decidual regression during menstruation, or as a result of a failed implantation. Based on suppression of cytotoxic T-lymphocyte assays, Clark and coworkers have also suggested that decidual TGF-β2 (or β2-like molecule) could play a role in inhibiting the rejection of the allogeneic fetus during the early period of implantation before the formation of the placenta *(96–98)*. However, there appear to be few T-cells in the mouse decidua *(99)*.

Many growth factor receptors are expressed on decidual cells, including those for EGF, CSF-1, and c-kit *(23,59,100,101)*. Ligands for these receptors are synthesized either in the adjacent epithelium or by the decidual cells themselves. Thus, TGF-α *(46,102,103)* and HB-EGF *(48)* are expressed in the decidua, while CSF-1 is synthesized in the uterine epithelia *(52)*. However, mice nullizygous for the genes SF/c-kit, CSF-1, and TGF-α do not have apparent defects in the decidua *(50,61,104)*, whereas TGF-β1 nullizygous mice only reach adulthood if on a strict immunosuppressed background, and to date, the effects on decidualization have not been reported *(105)*. Consequently, the only information available about function of these growth factors is through expression studies or cell-culture experiments. For example, Casey et al. showed that TGF-β stimulated parathyroid hormone synthesis by human endometrial cells *(106)*. The physiological role for such responses, however, is unknown.

PLACENTATION

Placentation in interstitial implanting species is characterized by trophoblastic invasion establishing a direct contact between fetal cells and the maternal circulation. Diploid trophoblast also differentiates into endocrine cells, either syncytiotrophoblast cells in humans or giant cells in Murids, that interface directly with the maternal circulation and/or tissue. In addition, there are also several other forms of phenotypically distinguishable trophoblast cells in humans. These include trophoblast of the villous column (intermediate trophoblast), the extravillous trophoblast, and the intra-arterial trophoblast *(11)*. Many growth factors have been documented to be synthesized by these cells, and their expression of growth factor receptors has also been well described *(3,7,11)*. For example, the rapid proliferation of cytotrophoblast in vivo is accompanied by the autocrine actions of insulin-like growth factor II (IGF-II) and platelet-derived growth factor (PDGF) *(107–109)*. PDGF-α and β receptors have been detected in cytotrophoblast *(109,110)* and PDGF in human *(111,112)* placenta. However, others have failed to confirm these expression patterns for PDGF in humans *(11)*. In contrast, expression of IGF-II, its receptor, and IGF binding proteins in the human *(107,108,113,114)* and mouse *(115)* placenta have been well documented. Furthermore, IGF-II has 5′-splice variants unique to the human placenta, suggesting placental specific promoter usage *(116)*. Genetic studies in mice strongly support roles for IGF-II in placental growth, since IGF-II nullizygous mice have small placentae *(117)*, and mice nullizygous for IGF-II type II receptor (cation-independent mannose-6-phosphate receptor), the nonsignaling receptor that is thought to be involved in regulating the IGF-II concentration by sequestering it, have larger placentae because growth continues throughout pregnancy *(118)*. However, in in vitro cultures of trophoblast derived from the ectoplacental cone of mice, IGF-I stimulates DNA synthesis, but IGF-II promotes transformation into giant cells *(115)*.

Genetic studies in mice have also shown an essential role in placentation for hepatocyte growth factor/scatter factor (HGF), since the labyrinthine layer of the placenta has a reduced number of trophoblast cells and a disorganized structure in mice nullizygous for the HGF receptor, c-met *(119)*. These data are consistent with the HGF stimulation of trophoblastic cell proliferation *(120)*. Interestingly, mice nullizygous for *c-met* also display incomplete muscle development, but this effect could be dissociated from the placental defect by targeted mutation of a single tyrosine in the cytoplasmic tyrosine kinase domain of the c-met receptor, indicating that the downstream signaling molecules are different in trophoblast and myoblast *(121)*. HGF, however, does not appear to be derived from the uterus, but from the placenta and allantois at midpregnancy *(119,120)*.

Several CSFs and their receptors have been documented to be expressed in human and mouse placenta, including CSF-1R, granulocyte-macrophage colony stimulating factor receptor (GM-CSFR), and granulocyte colony stimulating factor receptor (G-CSFR) *(7,11, 100)*. In mice, high levels of expression of CSF-1R are seen in giant trophoblastic cells with lower levels in spongiotrophoblast and little to no expression in labyrinthine trophoblast *(83,100,122,123)*. High-affinity CSF-1 binding to isolated mouse trophoblast has been demonstrated *(124)*. In humans, immunohistochemical studies show that CSF-1R is expressed in both syncytiotrophoblast and cytotrophoblasts with particularly high expression in trophoblast of the villous column *(125)*, and these data have been confirmed by Western blotting *(126)*. The results of Joki et al. *(127)*, however, differ in some aspects from these observations, because although in confirmation of these reports *(126)*, they detected strong immunostaining for CSF-1R of cytotrophoblast of the villous columns, they also found expression only in late first trimester syncytiotrophoblast with no expression in term syncytiotrophoblast or in villous cytotrophoblast. It is not clear why there are differences in these results, but it may relate to the antibody used. Using an entirely different set of anti-CSF-1R antibodies, Shorter confirmed our original observations (personal communication), and this is consistent with the expression of CSF-1R mRNA in second and third trimester placenta *(128)* and high affinity binding of radioiodinated CSF-1 to term trophoblast *(129)*. Expression, however, of CSF-1R mRNA is lower in third trimester than first trimester *(125)*. In humans, this placental CSF-1R mRNA is initiated from a trophoblast-specific promoter *(130,131)*.

In humans, CSF-1 expression persists throughout pregnancy in the uterine epithelium, and is also detected in first trimester villous column trophoblast and cytotrophoblast *(132)*. Expression in trophoblast is lost by the second trimester *(132)* consistent with a peak of CSF-1 protein being detected in the endometrium and placenta during first trimester. CSF-1 expression is detected in the villous core in second and third trimester trophoblast possibly in Hofbauer and endothelial cells *(132,133)*. This might be the source of the high circulating concentrations of CSF-1 in fetal serum at birth *(134)*. Purified first trimester extravillous trophoblast also expresses CSF-1 and CSF-1R and secretes CSF-1 into the media (Pollard and Fisher, unpublished observations). In mice, CSF-1 is not expressed in the placenta, but only in the uterine epithelium, and CSF-1 concentrations increase logarithmically through pregnancy *(52,135)*.

Expression of GM-CSF and G-CSF and their receptors have been relatively well documented in the cyto- and syncytiotrophoblast of human placentae *(11,136–140)*. GM-CSF is expressed in the endometrial uterine lumenal epithelium and lymphoid cells *(141)*, while G-CSF is detected in macrophages *(139)*.

CSF-1 and GM-CSF have been reported to stimulate the incorporation of ^{3}H-thymidine into isolated mouse trophoblast *(129,142)*. This measure of cell proliferation, however, is flawed in cytokine-stimulated cells because of changing specific activities of thymidine pools. Drake and Head *(143)* have shown that this increased incorporation is not associated with cytokinesis in mice. Furthermore, even small amounts of contamination of these trophoblast cultures with macrophages, which respond to these cytokines by proliferation, can confound the interpretation of results. GM-CSF appears to promote syncytialization in isolated human trophoblast *(124)*. Thus, an interpretation of these data is that GM-CSF promotes differentiation of trophoblast leading either to endo-reduplication of DNA in mice or conversion of trophoblast to syncytia in human. However, mice nullizygous for the entire GM-CSF/IL-5/IL-3 signaling pathway appear to be fully fertile *(144)*. Similarly, mice nullizygous for CSF-1 display only a small amount of embryonic wastage *(61)*.

Very high levels of expression of *c-kit*, a member of the class III transmembrane tyrosine kinase receptor, has been detected in spongiotrophoblast of the mouse, with the ligand, Steel factor, expressed in the adjacent labyrinthine layer and in the uterus *(59, 60,145–147)*. In contrast, no *c-kit* expression was detected in any human trophoblast populations, although it was detected in some hematopoietic cells, including, uniquely, macrophages *(11)*. Steel factor is expressed in cytotrophoblast, syncytiotrophoblast, and extravillous trophoblast *(148)*. In mice there is a long allelic series of mutants in both the *W* (*c-kit*) and *SL* (*Steel*) genes. Although null mutants in both ligand and receptor genes are embryonic lethals, this is usually regarded as the consequence of fetal anemia and no placental defects have yet been reported in these mutants *(104,149)*.

LIF not only seems to have a role in implantation, but also in placental development. Targeted disruption of the LIFR gene in mice results in placentae where there is a lack of the characteristic demarcation of trophoblastic zones and presence of intraplacental fluid-filled spaces. Despite these gross abnormalities, some embryos could be carried to term *(150)*. In humans, LIFR mRNA is abundant in first trimester trophoblast *(151)*, while in both humans and mice, LIF appears to be expressed in the uterine epithelium, and in humans, it is present in some unidentified decidual cells *(84,85)*. Thus, uterine LIF appears to act in a paracrine fashion affecting placental development.

The placenta, in addition to providing nutrients to the embryo, is also an endocrine organ synthesizing both steroid and polypeptide hormones. Several in vitro experiments suggest that cytokines regulate syntheses of these peptide hormones. For example, in cultured trophoblast, EGF, FGF, LIF, IL-6 and CSF-1 all stimulate human chorionic gonadotropin (hCG) production *(124,152–155)*; IGF-1, EGF, IL-6, and GM-CSF stimulate placental lactogen production *(124,153,154,156)*, whereas IL-1 stimulates aromatase activity *(157)*. In contrast, TGF-β1 inhibits trophoblast differentiation and expression of hCG and human placental lactogen (hPL) *(158)*, although Graham et al., have reported that TGF-β1 stimulates trophoblast differentiation *(159)*.

The amplitude of the stimulatory effects of these cytokines are modest, and caution needs to be exercised in interpreting the data. Cytokines can alter global rates of protein synthesis, increase the viability of cells and cause a greater percentage of cells to differentiate. For example, the action of CSF-1 on hCG production is associated with conversion of the cells to form syncytia *(160)*, suggesting that the increased hormone production is indirectly related to the action of CSF-1 on trophoblastic differentiation. In contrast, in the study of Stephanou and Handwerger *(153)*, IL-6 increased hPL expression in trophoblast, and the hPL promoter was shown to contain NF1-IL-6 DNA binding sites, which in BeWo choriocarcinoma cells mediated transcriptional activation by IL-6, as determined by a CAT reporter assay. The results of these assays suggest a direct effect of IL-6 on hPL transcription, which may have biological relevance. IL-6 nullizygous mice, however, appear to be completely fertile *(161)*.

During pregnancy in mice lacking CSF-1, the mammary glands display a relative failure to grow out into the fat pad, compared to wild-type mice, and the result is a failure to lactate *(162)*. The placenta synthesizes several lactogenic factors, and the growth of the mammary gland is proportional to the number of placentae. Thus, we proposed that CSF-1 may regulate the placenta to synthesize a lactogenic factor that enhances mammary gland outgrowth during pregnancy *(162,163)*. The identity of this putative factor(s) remains to be determined. Nevertheless, this hypothesis does emphasize the interrelationship between the mother and fetus, and suggests that in cases where a null mutation in a cytokine or its receptor gene does not result in obvious histological malformations, there may be a failure in function that could be reflected in either a maternal or a fetal phenotype. Caution, therefore, needs to be exercised in overinterpreting the lack of an overt phenotype as a lack of a role for a cytokine in placental function. In fact, in cases where there is strong uterine and/or placental expression of a cytokine and/or receptor and gene ablation is associated with embryonic lethality, experiments should be conducted exploiting the tetraploid aggregation technique of Nagy and colleagues *(164)* to determine whether the requirement for the cytokine is embryonic or placental. This was recently performed to demonstrate that the placental defects in a *mash*2 nullizygous mouse was owing to a lack of expression in trophoblast *(165)*.

Trophoblast can also be highly invasive, a property that is essential for successful pregnancy. These events are precisely controlled, since aberrations in these processes can lead to pathologies, such as pre-eclampsia, which is associated with a shallow invasion *(11)*. This invasion is characterized by specific expression of metalloproteinases as well as adhesion molecules involved in both cell-to-cell and cell-to-substratum interactions *(166,167)*. These processes have been studied extensively in human trophoblast because of the ability to obtain pure populations for analysis in vitro *(11)*. Both IL-1 and EGF stimulated trophoblast invasion *(168,169)* in a matrigel invasion assay. Cytotrophoblast expresses IL-1 type 1 receptors, and IL-1 is synthesized by trophoblast and the uterus. In cultured trophoblast, IL-1 induced the 92-kDa type IV collagenase that is implicated in trophoblast invasion *(168,170)*. EGFRs are also expressed on cytotrophoblast, but in contrast to IL-1, EGF appears to be largely, if not entirely, maternally derived *(169,171)*. CSF-1 induces expression of $\alpha 5$ integrin and fibronectin in cytotrophoblast; molecules that are characteristic of invading trophoblast (Coutifaris, personal communication). CSF-1 and CSF-1R are coexpressed in these cells during the first trimester *(125,132)*. From these results, it seems likely that maternal- and fetal-derived cytokines influence trophoblast invasion, perhaps providing localized regulation of the extent of invasion. In this regard, it is interesting to note that TGF-β1, synthesized in the uterus, inhibits trophoblast invasion as assessed by matrigel invasion assay *(172)*.

HEMATOPOIETIC CELLS

During pregnancy, there is a fluctuating population of hematopoietic cells in the uterus. These include eosinophils, mast cells, macrophages, lymphocytes, and uterine natural killer (NK) (u-NK) cells. Considerable differences exist between Murids and humans in these populations. For example, in the human stroma, there are lymphoid aggregates associated with the glands that are absent in Murids. Human decidua is rich in macrophages *(173)*, whereas these are almost entirely excluded from the decidua in rats and mice *(174)*. The uterine hematopoietic cells undoubtedly have classical immune functions preventing infection following mating *(99)*. However, these immunological events in the uterus have to be counterbalanced against the generation of a host-vs-graft reaction to the allogenic fetus. The regulation of humoral immune responses by cytokines makes it certain that such molecules will be involved in regulating the action of immune cells at the maternal–fetal interface *(175)*. Wegmann et al. have also suggested that pregnant females are biased toward humoral rather than cell-mediated immunity, and have postulated that the utero–placental unit preferentially synthesizes Th2 cytokines, such as IL-10 and IL-4, that are responsible for this tilting toward the humoral immune response *(176,177)*. IL-10 has been shown to be synthesized both by mouse and human trophoblast *(177,178)*. In addition to immune functions, it has been suggested that uterine hematopoietic cells, particularly macrophages, have trophic roles in embryonic development through their synthesis of cytokines *(179)*.

Among the best studied of the uterine hematopoietic cells are macrophages *(174,180)*. The exact function(s) of these cells is unknown. However, they are likely to have immunological functions, both acting as accessory cells for immune responses and phagocytozing invading organisms. They also synthesize many cytokines, including IL-1, TGF-β, and TNF-α, that may influence embryonic development and/or resident uterine cells *(181)*. In turn, the uterine epithelium in response to sex steroid hormones synthesizes GM-CSF and CSF-1, the two cytokines that have been documented to regulate proliferation and differentiation of cells of the mononuclear phagocytic lineage *(52,54)*. GM-CSF is synthesized on the first day of pregnancy, but only if the female has mated with intact males *(182)*. The factor in semen that induces uterine GM-CSF synthesis appears to be TGF-β1, which, in turn, is synthesized in the seminal vesicles *(182)*. CSF-1 mRNA is induced by E_2, and to a greater extent by P_4 and E_2 once pregnancy has been initiated *(52)*. At implantation, uterine CSF-1 concentrations are elevated about fivefold, but thereafter increase through pregnancy to reach about 1000 times the concentration detected in nonpregnant uterus by term *(135)*. Studies of mice with null mutations in the GM-CSF and CSF-1 genes indicate that CSF-1 is the major regulator of the mononuclear phagocytic lineage in most tissues of the body *(144,183,184)*. Consistent with this is a significant depletion of macrophages in the uterus of CSF-1 null mutant mice during the estrus cycle and during pregnancy *(61)*. However, CSF-1 cannot be the only cytokine that regulates macrophage recruitment, since in CSF-1 nullizygous mice, there are always some macrophages present in the uterus, and in estrus, these approach 35% of the normal density (Zhu and Pollard, unpublished observations). Furthermore, during early pregnancy in the CSF-1 null mutant mice, macrophages are recruited into the metrial gland, where they reside until they disappear as pregnancy progresses, indicating that although CSF-1 is required for their viability, another factor recruits them into the uterus at this stage *(61)*. Chemotactic chemokines, such as RANTES, macrophage inflammatory protein (MIP1α), and β, have been detected in the uterus, and these, together with cytokines, such as TNF-α, interferon γ (IFNγ), and TGF-β1, may have important roles in these macrophage population dynamics *(181)*.

Interestingly, cultured macrophages are both chemokinetic and chemotactic to CSF-1, but the chemotaxis is ablated by TNF-α without affecting chemokinesis *(185)*. Thus, uterine CSF-1 may recruit macrophages into the tissue because of its high local concentration, causing a gradient along which macrophages are chemoattracted. Once in the appropriate place, TNF-α, also synthesized by the uterine epithelium *(186)*, may serve to stop the chemotaxis, but without inhibiting macrophage mobility. Consistent with this role for CSF-1, instillation of this growth factor into the uterine lumen resulted in recruitment of macrophages *(180)*. However, concern has to be expressed about this experiment, since effects were obtained with concentrations of CSF-1 below the physiologically relevant range. GM-CSF instilled into the uterus also results in macrophage recruitment *(87)*. Thus, in the mouse, it seems likely that GM-CSF, CSF-1, as well as other cytokines and chemokines recruit macrophages at estrus and, as soon as P_4 predominates, GM-CSF expression is inhibited and CSF-1 expression is stimulated, which further recruits and maintains the viability of uterine macrophages. Similar patterns of expression of CSF-1 and population dynamics of macrophages *(173)* in the human uterus suggest that this growth factor plays such a role in this species *(132)*.

There is considerable interaction between cytokines in regulating the function of macrophages. GM-CSF and CSF-1 appear to have opposing effects on cultured bone marrow macrophages. GM-CSF upregulates MHC class II expression, whereas CSF-1 inhibits the basal level of MHC class II expression in untreated macrophages, as well as suppresses the elevation of MHC class II expression induced by GM-CSF and IFNγ *(188)*. Similarly, the ratio of GM-CSF to CSF-1 dictates the immunostimulatory or immunosuppressive actions of lung macrophages *(189)*. Macrophages isolated from pregnant mouse uteri are immunosuppressive *(190,191)*, and placental macrophages, developing in high concentrations of CSF-1, have a relative inability to present antigens compared to other systemic macrophages *(192)*. Thus, the very high uterine concentrations of CSF-1 may tip the balance from immunologically active macrophages to those that play trophic and/or scavenging functions in the developing placenta. These interactions among GM-CSF, CSF-1, IFNγ, and TNF-α in regulating macrophage behavior might, in part, explain their effects on the alteration of rates of abortion in certain mouse strains when high concentrations of these cytokines are administered systemically *(98,193,194)*. These effects are discussed in detail in Chapter 12 of this vol. Despite the dramatic effects on macrophage phenotypes by GM-CSF and CSF-1, mice nullizygous for either gene loci undergo normal embryo implantation, and pregnancy does not appear to be dramatically affected by the absence of these cytokines *(62,144)*. However, no experiments have yet been performed that examine the ability of these mice to constrain infections of the utero-placental unit.

In uterine tissue, mast cells are increased in number at implantation *(195)* probably as a consequence of locally synthesized steel factor (c-kit ligand) *(60)*, the major lineage regulator of these cells. However, in an elegant experiment using *W/W*^{V} mice, Wordinger et al. showed that implantation, decidualization, and pregnancy progressed normally in the absence of mast cells *(104)*.

In mice, there is a population of u-NK cells in the metrial gland *(196)*, which in culture, at least, express several cytokines, including CSF-1, IL-6, GM-CSF, and IL-1 *(196)*. Similar cells are found through the decidua in humans *(197)*. In mice in which the population of u-NK cells has been depleted, the metrial glands are absent, there are malformations of maternal vessels, and the placentae are small and exhibit various pathologies, including aberrant trophoblast proliferation *(198)*. These data strongly suggest that u-NK cells produce trophic cytokines that are especially involved in the establishment of the placental vasculature.

Another potent group of immune activators are the IFNs, especially IFNγ, usually synthesized by T-cells and acting on macrophages. Apart from antiviral functions, these molecules can also exert strong inhibitory actions on cell proliferation. A special class of

IFN, τ, has been documented in ruminant pregnancies *(199)*. IFNτ, secreted at extremely high concentrations by trophoblast, is involved in the maternal recognition of pregnancy, and its biology is discussed extensively in other chapters of this volume. An IFNτ-like molecule has recently been reported for the human placenta, but is detected only at low concentration and this report has not been confirmed *(200)*. IFNγ, however, appears to be synthesized in first trimester human placenta, mostly by the syncytiotrophoblast *(201,202)* and by unidentified cells in the mouse *(203)* with high concentrations detected immediately postimplantation *(177)*. IFNγ receptor, in addition to being localized on macrophages, is detected in the villous and extravillous cytotrophoblast *(11,204)* and, in one unconfirmed report *(11)*, in syncytiotrophoblast *(202)*. In mouse, this receptor is expressed in the spongiotrophoblastic and labyrinthine trophoblastic regions *(205)*. Garcia-Lloret et al. have reported that TNF-α and IFNγ can induce apoptotic cell death of human cytotrophoblast and that this effect can be ameliorated by EGF *(206)*. IFNγ upregulates MHC class I expression in placenta *(207)* and in cultured trophoblast *(208,209)*, where it effected partial protection from lysis by NK cells, suggesting a possible immuno-protective role for the fetus of this cytokine *(11)*. IFNγ therefore exerts powerful immunological and antiviral effects, and its presence in the utero–placental unit probably protects against viral infection during the course of pregnancy and may serve to regulate trophoblast cell proliferation.

In the cycling and early pregnant human uterus, IFNγ is synthesized by T-cells associated with lymphocytic aggregates at the base of the glands in the basalis region *(210)*. This IFNγ is postulated to inhibit glandular epithelial proliferation and has been shown to upregulate uterine epithelial expression of HLA-DR *(8,9,212,213)*. The presence of IFNγ will also determine the activation state of macrophages, and Chen et al. *(205)* have shown that uterine macrophage IFNγR mRNA expression is upregulated at the onset of pregnancy and remains high until term. IFNγ also induces a downregulation of the CSF-1R, altering macrophage responsiveness to CSF-1 *(211)*. IFNγ activation may, therefore, enhance the phagocytic activity of these cells during the remodeling of the pregnant uterus *(181)*.

IFNα has been detected in human placenta *(214)*. Cultured human trophoblast synthesize biologically active IFNα and IFNβ in response to GM-CSF, PDGF, and to a much greater extent to viral infection, with invasive trophoblast having the most pronounced response *(126)*. Interestingly, trophoblast expression of both CSF-1R and EGF-R is downregulated by IFNα/β *(126)*.

Pregnancy is beset by a number of immunological problems; sperm and bacteria need to be removed postmating, viral and bacterial infections need to be limited (for example, cytomegalovirus and *Listeria monocytogenes* infections are common complications of human pregnancy), whereas the allogenic fetus needs to be protected. Elaborate mechanisms are in place to achieve these ends. Cytokine synthesis both by resident uterine cells together with the varying populations of hematopoietic cells in the uterus and the placenta undoubtedly play a role in these mechanisms. Thus, the utero–placental unit may be tilted toward synthesizing Th2 cytokines to limit cell-mediated immunity *(176)*, and perturbations in the balance of these cytokines may have important ramifications for the success of pregnancy. Several mouse model systems have been employed that show both the beneficial and harmful effects of systemic applications of cytokines *(71,98,194,215,216)*. Such models are described in other chapters of this vol. To date, however, dissection of the immunological roles of uterine cytokines in controlling infections during pregnancy using mice mutants in various aspect of their immune response have not been performed. Such experiments are likely to reveal unusual aspects of the immunology of the utero–placental interface.

SUMMARY

Many ovarian steroid hormone actions are mediated by locally synthesized cytokines/growth factors. These factors influence all stages of pregnancy, and some have critical, nonredundant roles, such that their absence results in termination of pregnancy. The uterine luminal and glandular epithelium is a major source of these hormonally regulated cytokines, and therefore, the epithelium plays a pivotal role during pregnancy in the translation of steroid hormone signals. An immediate experimental challenge is to define the molecular mechanisms of this steroid hormonal regulation. Such knowledge will allow us to modify the local uterine expression of the cytokine using transgenic mouse technology so that a definitive role(s) *in utero* can be ascribed to particular cytokines. Mouse genetics has already provided significant information about the causal role of some cytokines during pregnancy. Spatial and temporal targeted mutagenesis and expression of genes in the mouse reproductive system will begin to unravel the roles of cytokines and their intracellular effectors.

Remarkably, many of the uterine cytokines were originally identified because of their activities on the lymphoid and myeloid blood cell compartments, even though within the utero–placental unit their targets are not necessarily hematopoietic cells. Their synthesis in the uterus and placenta suggests that, in addition to other roles, they regulate uterine hematopoietic cells to resist infection without rejecting the allogenic fetus.

In the final analysis, mouse experimentation needs to be translated to the human. Significant advances have been made in culturing defined, pure trophoblast populations and in obtaining decidualization in culture. In these respects, experimentation in humans is in advance of that with the mouse. Despite their pitfalls, these culture systems will allow molecular analysis of the action of the cytokines. These findings, with those derived from genetic studies, should profoundly increase our understanding of the local regulation of pregnancy, and enhance our ability to provide therapeutics to enhance fertility, limit premature abortion, and restrict the pathogenicity of organisms, such as HIV, *Listeria,* and cytomegalovirus.

ACKNOWLEDGMENTS

This work was supported by NIH grants HD/AI 30280 and the Albert Einstein Core ancer Grant P30-CA13330. The author is a Monique Weill-Caulier Scholar. The author wishes to thank P. Cohen and R. Lee for helpful comments on this manuscript.

REFERENCES

1. Couse JF, Curtis SW, Washburn TF, Eddy EM, Schomberg DW, Korach KS (1995) Disruption of the mouse oestrogen receptor gene: resulting phenotypes and experimental findings, In: Nuclear receptors in cell growth, death and inflammation (Chapman KE, Green S, eds.), Roche, Manchester, pp. 929–935.
2. Lydon JP, DeMayo FJ, Funk CR, Mani SK, Hughes AR, Montgomery CA, Shyamala G, Conneely OM, O'Malley BW (1995) Mice lacking progesterone receptor exhibit pleiotropic reproductive abnormalities. Genes Dev 9:2266–2278.
3. Cohen PE, Pollard JW (1996) Cytokines and growth factors in reproduction, In: Reproductive Immunology (Bronson RA, Alexander NJ, Anderson D, Branch DW, Kutteh WH, eds.), Blackwell, pp. 52–102.
4. Pollard JW (1990) Regulation of polypeptide growth factor synthesis and growth factor-related gene expression in the rat and mouse uterus before and after implantation. J Reprod Fertil 88: 721–731.

5. Simmen FA, Simmen RCM (1991) Peptide growth factors and proto-oncogenes in mammalian conceptus development. Biol of Reprod 44:1–5.
6. Brigstock DR (1991) Growth factors in the uterus: steroidal regulation and biological actions, In: Bailliere's Clinical Endocrinology and Metabolism. Bailliere, Tindall, pp. 791–808.
7. Pollard JW, Pampfer S, Daiter E, Arceci RJ (1991) Cytokines at the maternal fetal interface: Colony stimulating factor-1 as a paradigm for the maternal regulation of pregnancy, In: Uterine and Embryonic Factors in Early Pregnancy (Strauss JF, Lyttle CR, eds.), Plenum, New York, pp. 107–118.
8. Tabibzadeh S (1994) Role of cytokines in endometrium and at the fetomaternal interface. Reprod Med Rev 3:11–28.
9. Tabibzadeh S (1994) Cytokines and the hypothalamic-pituitary-ovarian-endometrial axis. Hum Reprod Update 9:947–967.
10. Giudice LC (1994) Growth factors and growth modulators in human uterine endometrium: their potential relevance to reproductive medicine. Fertil Steril 61:1–17.
11. Loke YW, King A (1995) Human Implantation. Cambridge University Press, Cambridge, UK.
12. Pollard JW (1991) Lymphohematopoietic cytokines in the female reproductive tract. Curr Opinion Immunol 3:772–777.
13. Martin L, Finn CA, Trinder G (1973) DNA synthesis in the endometrium of progesterone-treated mice. J Endocrinol 56:303–307.
14. Martin L, Das RM, Finn CA (1973) The inhibition by progesterone of uterine epithelial proliferation in the mouse. J Endocrinol 57:549–554.
15. Kidder GM. The genetic program for preimplantation development. Dev Genetics 13:319–325.
16. McCormack JT, Greenwald GS (1974) Progesterone and oestradiol-17β concentrations in the peripheral plasma during pregnancy in the mouse. J Endocrinol 62:101–107.
17. Finn CA (1965) Oestrogen and the decidual cell reaction of implantation in mice. J Endocrinol 62:223–229.
18. Finn CA, Martin L (1972) Endocrine control of the timing of endometrial sensitivity to a decidual stimulus. Biol Reprod 7:82–86.
19. Paria BC, Huet-Hudson YM, Dey SK (1993) Blastocyst's state of activity determines the "window" of implantation in the receptive mouse uterus. Proc Natl Acad Sci USA 90:10,159–10,162.
20. Cullingford TE, Pollard JW (1994) Growth factors as mediators of sex-steroid hormone action in the uterus during the pre-implatation period, In: Protooncogenes and Growth Factors in Steroid Hormone-Induced Growth Differentiation (Kohn SA, Stancel GM, eds.), CRC, New York, pp. 13–30.
21. Kato S, Endoh H, Masuhiro Y, Kitamoto T, Uchiyama S, Sasaki H, Masushige S, Gotoh Y, Nishida E, Kawashima H, Metzger D, Chambon P (1995) Activation of the estrogen receptor through phosphorylation by mitogen-activated protein kinase. Science 270:1491–1494.
22. Ignar-Trowbridge DM, Nelson KG, Bidwell MC, Curtis SW, Washburn TF, McLachlan JA, Korach KS (1992) Coupling of dual signaling pathways: Epidermal growth factor action involves the estrogen receptor. Proc Natl Acad Sci USA 89:4658–4662.
23. Das SK, Tsukamura H, Paria BC, Andrews GK, Dey SK (1994) Differential expression of epidermal growth factor receptor (EGF-R) gene and regulation of EGF-R bioactivity by progesterone and estrogen in the adult mouse uterus. Endocrinology 134:971–981.
24. Gardner RM, Verner G, Kirkland JL, Stancel GM (1989) Regulation of uterine epidermal growth factor (EGF) receptors by estrogen in the mature rat and mouse during estrous cycle. J Steroid Biochem 32:339–343.
25. Mukku VR, Stancel GM. Regulation of epidermal growth factor receptor by estrogen. J Biol Chem 260:9820–9824.
26. Huet-Hudson YM, Chakraborty C, De SK, Suzuki Y, Andrews GK, Dey SK (1990) Estrogen regulates the synthesis of epidermal growth factor in mouse uterine epithelial cells. Mol Endocrinol 4:510–523.
27. Nelson KG, Takahashi T, Bossert NL, Walmer DK, McLachlan JA (1991) Epidermal growth factor replaces estrogen in the stimulation of female genital-tract growth and differentiation. Proc Natl Acad Sci USA 88:21–25.
28. LeGoff P, Montano MM, Schodin DJ, Katzenellenbogen BS (1994) Phosphorylation of the human estrogen receptor. J Biol Chem 269:4458–4466.
29. Curtis SW, Washburn T, Sewall JC, DiAugustine R, Lindzey J, Couse JF, Korach KS (1996) Physiological coupling of growth factor and steroid receptor signaling pathways: estrogen recep-

tor knockout mice lack estrogen-like response to epidermal growth factor. Proc Natl Acad Sci USA 93:12,626–12,630.
30. Bossert NL, Nelson KG, Ross KA, Takahashi T, McLachlan JA (1990) Epidermal growth factor binding and receptor distribution in the mouse reproductive tract during development. Dev Biol 142:75–85.
31. Cho H, Katzenellenbogen BS (1993) Synergistic activation of estrogen receptor-mediated transcription by estradiol and protein kinase activators. Mol Endocrinol 7:441–452.
32. Ince BA, Montano MM, Katzenellenbogen BS (1994) Activation of transcriptionally inactive human estrogen receptors by cyclic adenosine 3′,5′-monophosphate and ligands including antiestrogens. Mol Endocrinol 8:1397–1406.
33. Hunt JS. Endocrine regulation of tumor necrosis factor-α. Reprod Fertil Dev 5:141–153.
34. Terranova PF, Hunter V, Roby KF, Hunt JS (1995) Tumor necrosis factor-α in the female reproductive tract. PSEMB 209:325–342.
35. Tamada H, McMaster MT, Flanders KC, Andrews GK, Dey SK (1990) Cell type-specific expression of transforming growth factor-β1 in the mouse uterus during the peri-implantation period. Mol Endocrinol 4:965–972.
36. Shalaby MR, Laegried WW, Ammann AJ, Liggitt HD (1989) Tumor necrosis factor-α associated uterine endothelial injury in vivo. Lab Invest 61:564–570.
37. Piva M, Flieger O, Rider V (1996) Growth factor control of cultured rat uterine stromal cell proliferation is progesterone dependent. Biol of Reprod 55:1333–1342.
38. Wordinger RJ, Moss AE, Lockard T, Gray D, Chang I-FC, Jackson TL (1992) Immunohistochemical localization of basic fibroblast growth factor within the mouse uterus. J Reprod Fertil 96:141–152.
39. Pampfer S, Arceci RJ, Pollard JW (1991) Role of colony stimulating factor-1 (CSF-1) and other lympho-hematopoietic growth factors in mouse preimplantation development. BioEssays 13: 535–540.
40. Dardik A, Schultz RM (1991) Blastocoel expansion in the preimplantation mouse embryo: stimulatory effect of TGF-α and EGF. Development 113:919–930.
41. Adamson ED (1993) Activities of growth factors in preimplantation embryos. J Cell Biochem 53: 280–287.
42. Brice EC, Wu J-X, Muraro R, Adamson ED, Wiley LM (1993) Modulation of mouse preimplantation development by epidermal growth factor receptor antibodies, antisense RNA, and deoxyoligonucleotides. Dev Genetics 14:174–184.
43. Wiley LM, Wu J-X, Harari I, Adamson ED (1992) Epidermal growth factor receptor mRNA and protein increase after the four-cell preimplantation stage in murine development. Dev Biol 149: 247–360.
44. Paria BC, Das SK, Andrews GK, Dey SK (1993) Expression of the epidermal growth factor receptor gene is regulated in mouse blastocysts during delayed implantation. Proc Natl Acad Sci USA 90:55–59.
45. Threadgill DW, Dlugosz AA, Hansen LA, Tennenbaum T, Lichti U, Yee D, LaMantia C, Mourton JA, Yuspa SH, Coffey RJ, Magnuson T (1995) Targeted disruption of mouse EGF receptor: effect of genetic background on mutant phenotype. Science 269:230–234.
46. Tamada H, Das SK, Andrews GK, Dey SK (1991) Cell-type-specific expression of transforming growth factor-α in the mouse uterus during the peri-implantation period. Biol Reprod 45:365–372.
47. Zhang Z, Funk C, Roy D, Glasser S, Mulholland J (1994) Heparin-binding epidermal growth factor-like growth factor is differentially regulated by progesterone and estradiol in rat uterine epithelial and stromal cells. Endocrinology 134:1089–1094.
48. Zhang Z, Funk C, Glasser SR, Mulholland J (1994) Progesterone regulation of heparin-binding epidermal growth factor-like growth factor gene expression during sensitization and decidualization in the rat uterus: effects of the antiprogestin, ZK 98.299. Endocrinology 135:1256–1263.
49. Wang X-N, Das SK, Damm D, Klagsbrun M, Abraham JA, Dey SK (1994) Differential regulation of heparin-binding epidermal growth factor-like growth factor in the adult ovariectomized mouse uterus by progesterone and estrogen. Endocrinology 135:1264–1271.
50. Luetteke NC, Qiu TH, Peiffer RL, Oliver P, Smithies O, Lee DC (1993) TGFα deficiency results in hair follicle and eye abnormalities in targeted and waved-1 mice. Cell 73:263–278.
51. Das SK, Chakraborty I, Paria BC, Wang X-N, Plowman G, Dey SK (1994) Amphiregulin is an implantation specific and progesterone-regulated gene in the mouse uterus. Mol Endocrinol 9:691–705.

52. Pollard JW, Bartocci A, Arceci RJ, Orlofsky A, Ladner MB, Stanley ER (1987) Apparent role of the macrophage growth factor, CSF-1, in placental development. Nature 330:484–486.
53. De M, Sanford TR, Wood GW (1992) Interleukin-1, interleukin-6, and tumor factor α are produced in the mouse uterus during the estrous cycle and are induced by estrogen and progesterone. Dev Biol 151:297–305.
54. Robertson SA, Mayrhofer G, Seamark RF (1992) Uterine epithelial cells synthesize granulocyte-macrophage colony-stimulating factor and interleukin-6 in pregnant and nonpregnant mice. Biol Reprod 46:1069–1079.
55. Tabibzadeh S (1991) Ubiquitous expression of TNF-α/cachectin immunoreactivity in human endometrium. Am J Reprod Immunol 26:1–4.
56. Chen H-L, Yang Y, Hu X-L, Yelavarthi KK, Fishback JL, Hunt JS (1991) Tumor necrosis factor-alpha mRNA and protein are present in human placental and uterine cells at early and late stages of gestation. Am J Pathol 139:327–335.
57. Yelavarthi KK, Chen H-L, Yang Y, Cowley Jr. BD, Fishback JL, Hunt JS. (1991) Tumor necrosis factor-α mRNA and protein in rat uterine and placental cells. J Immunol 146:3840–3848.
58. Bhatnagar P, Papaioannou VE, Biggers JD (1995) CSF-1 and mouse preimplantation development in vitro. Development 121:1333–1339.
59. Arceci RJ, Pampfer S, Pollard JW (1992) Role and expression of colony-stimulating factor-1 and steel factor receptors and their ligands during pregnancy in the mouse. Reprod Fertil Dev 4:619–632.
60. Arceci RJ, Pampfer S, Pollard JW (1992) Expression of CSF-1/c-*fms* and SF/c-*kit* mRNA during preimplantation mouse development. Dev Biol 151:1–8.
61. Pollard JW, Hunt JW, Wiktor-Jedrzejczak W, Stanley ER (1991) A pregnancy defect in the osteopetrotic (*op/op*) mouse demonstrates the requirement for CSF-1 in female fertility. Dev Biol 148:273–283.
62. Cohen PE, Zhu L, Pollard JW (1997) The absence of CSF-1 in osteopetrotic ($csfm^{op}/csfm^{op}$) mice disrupts estrous cycles and ovulation. Biol Reprod 56:110–118.
63. Pampfer S, Moulaert B, Vanderheyden I, Wuu Y-D, De Hertogh R (1994) Effect of tumour necrosis factor α on rat blastocyst growth and glucose metabolism. J Reprod Fertil 101:199–206.
64. Pampfer S, Vanderheyden I, Vesela J, De Hertogh R (1995) Neutralization of tumor necrosis factor α (TNFα) action on cell proliferation in rat blastocysts by antisense oligodeoxyribonucleotides directed against TNFα p60 receptor. Biol Reprod 52:1316–1326.
65. Pampfer S, Wuu Y-D, Vanderheyden I, De Hertogh R (1994) Expression of tumor necrosis factor-α (TNFα) receptors and selective effect of TNFα on the inner cell mass in mouse blastocysts. Endocrinology 134:206–212.
66. Pampfer S, Vanderheyden I, Wuu Y-D, Baufays L, Maillet O, De Hertogh R (1995) Possible role for TNF-α in early embryopathy associated with maternal diabetes in the rat. Diabetes 44:531–536.
67. Roby KF, Hunt JS (1994) Mouse endometrial tumor necrosis factor-α messenger ribonucleic acid and protein: localization and regulation by estradiol and progesterone. Endocrinology 135: 2780–2789.
68. Tabibzadeh S, Zupi E, Babaknia A, Liu R, Marconi D, Romanini C (1995) Site and menstrual cycle-dependent expression of proteins of the tumour necrosis factor (TNF) receptor family, and BCL-2 oncoprotein and phase-specific production of TNFα in human endometrium. Hum Reprod 10:277–286.
69. Hunt JS (1993) Expression and regulation of the tumour necrosis factor-α in the female reproductive tract. Reprod Fertil Dev 5:141–153.
70. Erbach GT, Lawitts JA, Papaioannou VE, Biggers JD (1994) Differential growth of the mouse preimplantation embryo in chemically defined media. Biol Reprod 50:1027–1033.
71. Tartakovsky B, Goldstein O, Brosh N (1991) Colony-stimulating factor-1 blocks early pregnancy in mice. Biol Reprod 44:906–912.
72. Tartakovsky B, Ben-Yair E (1991) Cytokines modulate preimplantation development and pregnancy. Dev Biol 146:345–352.
73. Hunt JS, Roby KF (1994) Implantation factors. Clin Obstet Gynecol 37:635–645.
74. Simón C, Frances A, Piquette GN, El Danasouri I, Zurawski G, Dang W, Polan ML (1994) Embryonic implantation in mice is blocked by interleukin-1 receptor antagonist. Endocrinology 134:521–528.
75. Bany BM, Kennedy TG (1995) Interleukin-1α regulates prostaglandin production and cyclooxygenase activity in sensitized rat endometrial stromal cells in vitro. Biol Reprod 53:126–132.

76. Frank GR, Brar AK, Jikihara H, Cedars MI, Handwerger S (1995) Interleukin-1β and endometrium: an inhibitor of stromal cell differentiation and possible autoregulator of decidualization in humans. Biol Reprod 52:184–191.
77. Yee GM, Squires PM, Cejic SS, Kennedy TG (1993) Lipid mediators of implantation and decidualization. J Lipid Mediators 6:525–534.
78. Simón C, Piquette GN, Frances A, Polan ML (1994) Localization of interleukin-1 type receptor and interleukin-1β in human endometrium throughout the menstrual cycle. J Clin Endocrinol Metab 77:549–555.
79. Simón C, Piquette GN, Frances A, Westphal LM, Heinrichs WL, Polan ML (1993) Interleukin-1 type I receptor messenger ribonucleic acid expression in human endometrium throughout the menstrual cycle. Fertil Steril 59:791–796.
80. Simón C, Frances A, Piquette G, Hendrickson M, Milki A, Polan ML (1994) Interleukin-1 system in the materno-trophoblast unit in human implantation: Immunohistochemical evidence for autocrine/paracrine function. J Clin Endocrinol Metab 78:847–854.
81. McMaster MT, Newton RC, Dey SK, Andrews GK (1992) Activation and distribution of inflammatory cells in the mouse uterus during the preimplantation period. J Immunol 148:1699–1705.
82. Abbondanzo SJ, Cullinan EB, McIntryre K, Labow MA, Stewart CL (1996) Reproduction in mice lacking a functional type 1 IL-1 receptor. Endocrinology 137:3598–3601.
83. Stewart CL, Kaspar P, Brunet LJ, Bhatt H, Gadi I, Köntgen F, Abbondanzo SJ (1992) Blastocyst implantation depends on maternal expression of leukaemia inhibitory factor. Nature 359:76–79.
84. Bhatt H, Brunet LJ, Stewart CL (1991) Uterine expression of leukemia inhibitory factor coincides with the onset of blastocyst implantation. Proc Natl Acad Sci USA 88:11,408–11,412.
85. Cullinan EB, Abbondanzo SJ, Anderson PS, Pollard JW, Lessey BA, Stewart CL (1996) Leukemia inhibitory factor (LIF) and LIF receptor expression in human endometrium suggests a potential autocrine/paracrine function in regulating embryo implantation. Proc Natl Acad Sci USA 93: 3115–3120.
86. Arici A, Engin O, Attar E, Olive DL (1995) Modulation of leukemia inhibitory factor gene expression and protein biosynthesis in human endometrium. J Clin Endocrinol Metab 80:1908–1915.
87. Vogiagis D, Marsh MM, Fry RC, Salamonsen LA (1996) Leukaemia inhibitory factor in human endometrium throughout the menstrual cycle. J Endocrinol 148:95–102.
88. Charnock-Jones DS, Sharkey AM, Fenwick P, Smith SK (1994) Leukaemia inhibitory factor mRNA concentration peaks in human endometrium at the time of implantation and the blastocyst contains mRNA for the receptor at this time. J Reprod Fertil 101:421–426.
89. Kojima K, Kanzaki H, Iwai M, Hatayama H, Fujimoto M, Inou T, Horie K, Nakayama H, Fujita J, Mori T (1994) Expression of leukemia inhibitory factor in human endometrium and placenta. Biol Reprod 50:882–887.
90. Das RM, Martin L (1978) Uterine DNA synthesis and cell proliferation during early decidualization induced by oil in mice. J Reprod Fertil 53:125–128.
91. Manova K, Paynton BV, Bachvarova RF (1992) Expression of activins and TGFβ1 and β2 RNAs in early postimplantation mouse embryos and uterine decidua. Mech Dev 36:141–152.
92. Lea RG, Flanders KC, Harley CB, Manuel J, Banwatt D, Clark DA (1992) Release of transforming growth factor (TGF)-beta 2-related suppressor factor from postimplantation murine decidual tissue can be correlated with the detection of a subpopulation of cells containing RNA for TBF-beta 2. J Immunol 148:778–787.
93. Cheng H-L, Schneider SL, Kane CM, Gollnick SO, Grande C, Thompson D, Pietrzak E, Tomasi TB (1993) TGF-β2 gene and protein expression in maternal and fetal tissues at various stages of murine development. J Reprod Immunol 25:133–148.
94. Das SK, Flanders KC, Andrews GK, Dey SK (1992) Expression of transforming growth factor-β isoforms (β2 and β3) in the mouse uterus: Analysis of the periimplantation period and effects of ovarian steroids. Endocrinology 130:3459–3466.
95. Moulton BC (1994) Transforming growth factor-β stimulates endometrial stromal apoptosis *in vitro*. Endocrinology 134:1055–1060.
96. Lea RG, Clark DA (1993) Effects of decidual cell supernatants and lymphokines on murine trophoblast growth in vitro. Biol Reprod 48:930–935.
97. Clark DA, Flanders KC, Hirte H, Dasch JR, Coker R, McAnulty RJ, Laurent GJ (1997) Characterization of murine pregnancy decidua transforming growth factor beta. I. Transforming growth factor beta 2-like molecules of unusual molecular size released in bioactive form. Biol Reprod 52:1380–1388.

98. Clark DA (1992) Cytokines, decidua and early pregnancy. ORRB 16:83–111.
99. Parr, MB, Parr EL (1996) Immunoglobulins in the female genital tract, In: Reproductive Immunology (Bronson RA, Alexander NJ, Anderson D, Branch DW, Kutteh WH, eds.), Blackwell Science, Cambridge, pp. 275–308.
100. Regenstreif LJ, Rossant J (1989) Expression of the c-*fms* proto-oncogene and of the cytokine, CSF-1, during mouse embryogenesis. Dev Biol 133:284–294.
101. Brown MJ, Zogg JL, Schultz GS, Hilton FK (1989) Increased binding of epidermal growth factor at preimplantation sites in mouse uteri. Endocrinology 124:2882–2888.
102. Bonvissuto AC, LaLa PK, Kennedy TG, Nygard K, Lee DC, Han VKM (1992) Induction of transforming growth factor-α gene expression in rat decidua is independent of the conceptus. Biol Reprod 46:607–616.
103. Han VKM, Hunter ESIII, Pratt RM, Zendegul JB, Lee DC (1987) Expression of rat transforming growth factor alpha mRNA during development occurs predominately in the maternal decidua. Mol Cell Biol 7:2335–2343.
104. Wordinger RJ, Jackson FL, Morril A (1986) Implantation, deciduoma formation and live births in mast cell-deficient mice (W/W^v). J Reprod Fertil 77:471–476.
105. Shull MM, Doetschman T (1994) Transforming growth factor-beta 1 in reproduction and development. Mol Reprod Dev 39:239–246.
106. Casey ML, Mibe M, Erk A, MacDonald PC (1992) Transforming growth factor-β_1 stimulation of parathyroid hormone-related protein expression in human uterine cells in culture: mRNA levels and protein secretion. J Clin Endocrinol Metab 74:950–952.
107. Ohlsson R, Holmgren L, Glaser A, Szpecht A, Pfeifer-Ohlsson S (1989) Insulin-like growth factor 2 and short-range stimulatory loops in control of human placental growth. EMBO J 8:1993–1999.
108. Fant M, Munro H, Moses AC (1986) An autocrine/paracrine role for insulin-like growth factors in the regulation of human placental growth. J Clin Endocrinol Metab 63:499–505.
109. Holmgren L, Claesson-Welsh L, Heldin CH, Ohlsson R (1992) The expression of PDGF α- and β-receptors in subpopulations of PDGF-producing cells implicates autocrine stimulatory loops in the control of proliferation in cytotrophoblasts that have invaded the maternal endometrium. Growth Factors 6:219–231.
110. Holmgren L, Glaser A, Pfeifer-Ohlsson S, Ohlsson R (1991) Angiogenesis during human extraembryonic development involves the spatiotemporal control of PDGF ligand and receptor gene expression. Development 113:749–754.
111. Orr-Urtreger A, Lonai P (1992) Platelet-derived growth factor-A and its receptor are expressed in separate, but adjacent cell layers of the mouse embryo. Development 115:1045–1058.
112. Goustin AS, Betsholtz C, Pfeifer-Ohlsson S, Persson H, Rydnert J, Bywater M, Holmgren G, Heldin C-H, Westermark B, Ohlsson R (1985) Coexpression of the sis and myc proto-oncogenes in developing human placenta suggests autocrine control of trophoblast growth. Cell 41:301–312.
113. Ohlsson R, Larsson E, Nilsson O, Wahlstrom T, Sundstrom P (1989) Blastocyst implantation precedes induction of insulin-like growth factor II gene expression in human trophoblasts. Development 106:555–559.
114. Zhou J, Bondy C (1992) Insulin-like growth factor-II and its binding proteins in placental development. Endocrinology 131:1230–1240.
115. Kanai-Azuma M, Kanai Y, Kurohmaru M, Sakai S, Hayashi Y (1993) Insulin-like growth factor (IGF)-I stimulates proliferation and migration of mouse ectoplacental cone cells, while IGF-II transforms them into trophoblastic giant cells *in vitro*. Biol Reprod 48:252–261.
116. Shen S-J, Daimon M, Wang C-Y, Jansen M, Ilan J (1988) Isolation of an insulin-like growth factor II cDNA with a unique 5′ untranslated region from human placenta. Proc Natl Acad Sci USA 85:1947–1951.
117. Dechiara TM, Robertson EJ, Efstratiadis A (1997) Parental imprinting of the mouse insulin-like growth factor II gene. Cell 64:849–859.
118. Lau MM, Stewart CE, Liu Z, Bhatt H, Rotwein P, Stewart CL (1994) Loss of the imprinted IGF2/ cation-independent mannose 6-phosphate receptor results in fetal overgrowth and perinatal lethality. Genes Dev 8:2953–2963.
119. Schmidt C, Bladt F, Goedecke S, Brinkmann V, Zschiesche W, Sharpe M, Gherardi E, Birchmeier C (1995) Scatter factor/hepatocyte growth factor is essential for liver development. Nature 373: 699–702.
120. Uehara Y, Kitamura N (1996) Hepatocyte growth factor/scatter factor and the placenta. Placenta 17:97–101.

121. Maina F, Casagranda F, Audero E, Simeone A, Comoglio PM, Klein R, Ponzetto C (1996) Uncoupling of Grb2 from the met receptor in vivo reveals complex roles in muscle development. Cell 87:531–542.
122. Arceci RJ, Shanahan F, Stanley ER, Pollard JW (1989) Temporal expression and location of colony-stimulating factor 1 (CSF-1) and its receptor in the female reproductive tract are consistent with CSF-1-regulated placental development. Proc Natl Acad Sci USA 86:8818–8822.
123. Hume DA, Monkley SJ, Wainwright BJ (1995) Detection of c-fms protooncogene in early mouse embryos by whole mount *in situ* hybridization indicates roles for macrophages in tissue remodelling. Br J Haematol 90:939–942.
124. Garcia-Lloret MI, Morrish DW, Wegmann TG, Honore L, Turner AR, Guilbert LJ (1994) Demonstration of functional cytokine-placental interactions: CSF-1 and GM-CSF stimulate human cytotrophoblast differentiation and peptide hormone secretion. Exp Cell Res 214:46–54.
125. Pampfer S, Daiter E, Barad D, Pollard JW (1992) Expression of the colony-stimulating factor-1 receptor (c-*fms* proto-oncogene product) in the human uterus and placenta. Biol Reprod 46:48–57.
126. Aboagye-Mathiesen G, Toth FD, Zdravkovic M, Ebbesen P (1996) Functional characteristics of human trophoblast interferons. Am J Reprod Immunol 35:309–317.
127. Jokhi PP, Chumbly G, King A, Gardner L, Loke YW (1993) Expression of the colony stimulating factor-1 receptor (c-fms product) by cells at the human uteroplacental interface. Lab Invest 68: 308–320.
128. Hoshina M, Nishio A, Bo M, Biome I, Mochizuki M (1985) The expression of oncogene fms in human chorionic tissue. Acta Obstet Gynaecol Jpn 37:2791–2798.
129. Athanassakis-Vassiliadis I, Papamatheakis J, Vassiliadis S (1993) Specific CSF-1 binding on murine placental trophoblasts and macrophages serves as a link to placental growth. J Receptor Res 13: 739–751.
130. Visvader J, Verma IM (1989) Differential transcription of exon 1 of the human c-*fms* gene in placental trophoblasts and monocytes. Mol Cell Biol 9:1336–1341.
131. Roberts WM, Shapiro LH, Ashmun RA, Look AT (1992) Transcription of the human colony-stimulating factor-1 receptor gene is regulated by separate tissue-specific promoters. Blood 79:586–593.
132. Daiter E, Pampfer S, Yeung YG, Barad D, Stanley ER, Pollard JW (1992) Expression of colony stimulating factor-1 in the human uterus and placenta. J Clin Endocrinol Metab 74:850–858.
133. Kanzaki H, Yui J, Iwai M, Imai K, Kariya M, Hatayama H, Mori T, Guilbert LJ, Wegmann TG (1992) The expression and localization of mRNA for colony-stimulating factor (CSF)-1 in human term placenta. Hum Reprod 7:563–567.
134. Roth P (1991) Colony-stimulating factor 1 levels in the human newborn infant. J Pediatr 119: 113–116.
135. Bartocci A, Pollard JW, Stanley ER (1986) Colony stimulating factor-1 specifically accumulates in the uterus during pregnancy. J Exp Med 164:956–961.
136. Loke YW, King A, Gardner L, Carter NP (1992) Evidence for the expression of granulocyte-macrophage colony-stimulating factor receptors by human first trimester extravillous trophoblast and its response to this cytokine. J Reprod Immunol 22:33–45.
137. Saito S, Fukunaga R, Ichijo M, Nagata S (1994) Expression of granulocyte colony-stimulating factor and its receptor at the fetomaternal interface in murine and human pregnancy. Growth Factors 10:135–143.
138. Uzumake H, Okabe T, Sasaki N, Hagiwara K, Takaku F, Tobita M, Yasukawa K, Ito S, Umezawa Y (1989) Identification and characterization of receptors for granulocyte colony-stimulating factor on human placenta and trophoblastic cells. Proc Natl Acad Sci USA 86:9323–9326.
139. Shorter SC, Vince GS, Starkey PM (1992) Production of granulocyte colony-stimulating factor at the materno-foetal interface in human pregnancy. Immunology 75:468–474.
140. Scheffler JE, Fleissner LC, Seelig GF, Nagabhushan TL, Trotta PP (1990) Characterization of the human granulocyte-macrophage colony-stimulating factor receptor from placenta, In: Hematopoiesis (Clark SC, Golde DW, ed.), Alan R. Liss, New York, pp. 107–115.
141. Kanzaki H, Crainie M, Lin H, Yui J, Guilbert LJ, Mori T, Wegmann TG (1991) The *in situ* expression of granulocyte-macrophage colony-stimulating factor (GM-CSF) mRNA at the maternal-fetal interface. Growth Factors 5:69–74.
142. Armstrong DT, Chaouat G (1989) Effects of lymphokines and immune complexes on murine placental cell growth in vitro. Biol Reprod 40:466–474.
143. Drake BL, Head JR (1994) GM-CSF and CSF-1 stimulate DNA synthesis but not cell proliferation in short-term cultures of mid-gestation murine trophoblast. J Immunol 26:41–56.

144. Nishinakamura R, Miyajima A, Mee PJ, Tybulewicz LJ, Murray R (1996) Hematopoiesis in mice lacking the entire granulocyte-macrophage colony-stimulating factor/interleukin-3/interleukin-5 functions. Blood 88:2458–2464.
145. Motro B, Van Der Kooy D, Rossant J, Reith A, Bernstein A (1991) Contiguous patterns of c-*kit* and *steel* expression: analysis of mutations at the W and Sl loci. Development 113:1207–1221.
146. Hoire K, Kujita J, Takakura K, Kanzaki H, Kaneko Y, Iwai M, Nakayama H, Mori T (1992) Expression of c-kit protein during placental development. Biol Reprod 47:614–620.
147. Pampfer S, Arceci RJ, Pollard JW (1993) Role of two growth factors, colony stimulating factor-1 and stem cell factor, and their receptors in murine pre-implantation development, In: Implantation in Mammals, Serono Symposium Series, vol. 91 (Gianaroli L, Campana A, Trounson AD, eds.), Raven, New York, pp. 289–300.
148. Sharkey A, Jones DSC, Brown KD, Smith SK (1992) Expression of messenger RNA for kit-ligand in human placenta: Localization by *in situ* hybridization and identification of alternatively spliced variants. Mol Endocrinol 6:1235–1241.
149. Russell ES (1979) Hereditary anemias of the mouse: a review for geneticists. Adv Genetics 20: 357–459.
150. Ware CB, Horowitz MC, Renshaw BR, Hunt JS, Liggitt D, Koblar SA, Gliniak BC, McKenna HJ, Papayannopoulou T, Thoma B, Cheng L, Donovan PJ, Peschon JJ, Bartlett PF, Willis CR, Wright BD, Carpenter MK, Davison BL, Gearing DP. Targeted disruption of the low-affinity leukemia inhibitory factor receptor gene causes placental, skeletal, neural, and metabolic defects and results in perinatal death. Development 121:1283–1299.
151. King A, Jokhi PP, Smith S, Sharkey A, Loke YW (1995) Screening for cytokine mRNA expression in purified human villous and extravillous trophoblast populations using the reverse-transcriptase polymerase chain reaction (RT-PCR). Cytokine 7:364–371.
152. Sawai K, Matsuzaki N, Kameda T, Hashimoto K, Okada T, Shimoya K, Nobunaga T, Taga T, Kishimoto T, Saji F (1995) Leukemia inhibitory factor produced at the fetomaternal interface stimulates chorionic gonadotropin production: Its possible implication during pregnancy, including implantation period. J Clin Endocrinol Metab 80:1449–1456.
153. Stephanou A, Handwerger S (1994) Interleukin-6 stimulates placental lactogen expression by human trophoblast cells. Endocrinology 135:719–723.
154. Morrish DW, Bhardwaj D, Dabbagh LK, Marusyk H, Siy O (1987) Epidermal growth factor induces differentiation and secretion of human chorionic gonadotropin and placental lactogen in normal human placenta. J Clin Endocrinol Metab 65:1282–1290.
155. Oberbauer AM, Strong DD, Linkhart TA, Mohan S, Longo LD (1993) Fibroblast growth factor enhances the transcription and stability of human chorionic gonadotropin β-subunit messenger ribonucleic acid in Jar choriocarcinoma cells. Endocrinology 132:757–762.
156. Bhaumick B, Dawson EP, Bala RM (1987) The effects of insulin-like growth factor-I and insulin on placental lactogen production by human term placental explants. Biochem and Biophys Res Commun 144:674–682.
157. Nestler JE (1993) Interleukin-1 stimulates the aromatase activity of human placental cytotrophoblasts. Endocrinology 132:566–570.
158. Morrish DW, Bhardwaj D, Paras MT (1991) Transforming growth factor $\beta 1$ inhibits placental differentiation and human chorionic gonadotropin and human placental lactogen secretion. Endocrinology 129:22–26.
159. Graham CH, Lysiak JJ, McCrae K, LaLa PK (1992) Localization of transforming growth factor-β at the human fetal-maternal interface: Role in trophoblast growth and differentiation. Biol Reprod 46:561–572.
160. Saito S, Saito M, Enomoto M, Ito A, Motoyoshi K, Nakagawa T, Ichijo M (1993) Human macrophage colony-stimulating factor induces the differentiation of trophoblast. Growth Factors 9:11–19.
161. Poli V, Balena R, Fattori El, Markatos A, Yamamoto M, Tanaka H, Cilliberto G, Rodan GA, Costantini F (1994) Interleukin-6 deficient mice are protected from bone loss caused by estrogen depletion. EMBO J 13:1189–1196.
162. Pollard JW, Henninghausen L (1994) Colony stimulating factor 1 is required for mammary gland development during pregnancy. Proc Natl Acad Sci USA 91:9312–9316.
163. Pollard JW (1997) Role of colony-stimulating factor-1 in reproduction and development. Mol Reprod Dev 46:54–61.
164. Nagy A Gocza E, Merentes Diaz E, Prideaux VR, Ivanyi E, Markkula M, Rossant J (1990) Embryonic stem cells alone are able to support fetal development in the mouse. Development 110:815–821.

165. Guillemot F, Nagy A, Auerbach A, Rossant J, Joyner AL (1994) Essential role of Mash-2 in extra-embryonic development. Nature 371:333–336.
166. Damsky CH, Fitzgerald ML, Fisher SJ (1992) Distribution pattern of extracellular matrix components and adhesion receptors are intricately modulated during first trimester cytotrophoblast differentiation along the invasive pathway, *in vivo*. J Clin Invest 89:210–222.
167. Damsky C, Sutherland A, Fisher S (1993) Extracellular matrix 5: adhesive interactions in early mammalian embryogenesis, implantation, and placentation. FASEB J 7:1320–1329.
168. Librach CL, Feigenbaum SL, Bass KE, Cui TY, Nerastas N, Sadovsky Y, Quigley JP, French DL, Fisher SJ (1994) Interleukin-1β regulates human cytotrophoblast metalloproteinase activity and invasion *in vitro*. J Biol Chem 269:17,125–17,131.
169. Bass KE, Morrish D, Roth I, Bhardwaj D, Taylor R, Shou Y, Fisher SJ (1994) Human cytotrophoblast invasion is up-regulated by epidermal growth factor: evidence that paracrine factors modify this process. Dev Biol 164:550–561.
170. Librach CL, Werb Z, Fitzgerald ML, Chiu K, Corwin N, Esteves RA, Grobelny D, Galardy R, Damsky CH (1991) 92-kD type IV collagenase mediates invasion of human cytotrophoblasts. J Cell Biol 113:437–449.
171. Haining REB, Schofield JP, Jones DSC, Rajput-Williams J, Smith SK (1991) Identification of mRNA for epidermal growth factor and transforming growth factor-α present in low copy number in human endometrium and decidua using reverse transcriptase-polymerase chain reaction. J Mol Endocrinol 6:207–214.
172. Graham CH, Hawley TS, Hawley RG, MacDougall JR, Kerbel RS, Khoo N, LaLa PK (1993) Establishment and characterization of first trimester human trophoblast cells with extended lifespan. Exp Cell Res 206:204–211.
173. Bulmer JN (1996) Cellular constituents of human endometrium in the menstrual cycle and early pregnancy, In: Reproductive Immunology (Bronson RA, Alexander NJ, Anderson D, Branch DW, Kutteh WH, eds.), Blackwell Sciences, Cambridge, pp. 212–239.
174. Hunt JS, Pollard JW (1992) Macrophages in the uterus and placenta. Curr Prog Microbiol Immunol 181:39–63.
175. Heyborne K, Silver RM (1996) Immunology of postimplantation pregnancy, In: Reproductive Immunology (Bronson RA, Alexander NJ, Anderson D, Branch DW, Kutteh WH, eds.), Blackwell Science, Cambridge, pp. 383–417.
176. Wegmann TG, Lin H, Guilbert L, Mosmann TR (1993) Bidirectional cytokine interactions in the maternal-fetal relationship: is successful pregnancy a $T_{H}2$ phenomenon? Immunol Today 14: 353–356.
177. Lin H, Mosmann TR, Guilbert L, Tuntipopipat S, Wegmann TG (1993) Synthesis of T helper 2-type cytokines at the maternal-fetal interface. J Immunol 151:4562–4573.
178. Roth I, Corry DB, Locksley RM, Abrams JS, Litton MJ, Fisher SJ (1996) Human placental cytotrophoblasts produce the immunosuppressive cytokine interleukin 10. J Exp Med 184:539–548.
179. Hunt JS (1989) Cytokine networks in the uteroplacental unit: macrophages as pivotal regulatory cells. J Reprod Immunol 16:1–17.
180. De M, Sanford T, Wood GW (1993) Relationship between macrophage colony-stimulating factor production by uterine epithelial cells and accumulation and distribution of macrophages in the uterus of pregnant mice. J Leukocyte Biol 53:240–248.
181. Hunt JS, Robertson SA (1996) Uterine macrophages and environmental programming for pregnancy success. J Reprod Immunol 32:1–25.
182. Robertson SA, Mau VJ, Hudson SN, Tremellen KP (1997) Cytokine-leukocyte networks and the establishment of pregnancy. Am J Reprod Immunol 37:438–442.
183. Cecchini MG, Dominguez MG, Mocci S, Wetterwald A, Feliz R, Fleisch H, Chisholm O, Hofstetter W, Pollard JW, Stanley ER (1994) Role of colony stimulating factor-1 in the establishment and regulation of tissue macrophages during postnatal development of the mouse. Development 120: 1357–1372.
184. Pollard JW, Stanley ER (1996) Pleiotropic roles for CSF-1 in development defined by the mouse mutation osteopetrotic (op). Adv Dev Biochem 4:153–193.
185. Webb SE, Pollard JW, Jones GE (1996) Direct observation and quantification of macrophage chemoattraction to the growth factor CSF-1. J Cell Sci 109:793–803.
186. Hunt JS, Chen H-L, Hu X-L, Pollard JW (1993) Normal distribution of tumor necrosis factor-α messenger ribonucleic acid and protein in the uteri, placentas and embryos of osteopetrotic (*op/op*) mice lacking colony-stimulating factor-1. Biol Reprod 49:441–452.

187. Robertson SA, Seamark AC, Seamark RF (1994) Uterine epithelial GM-CSF and its primary interlocutory role during early pregnancy in the mouse, In: Immunobiology of Reproduction (Hunt JS, ed.), Springer-Verlag, New York, pp. 83–98.
188. Willman CL, Stewart CC, Miller V, Yi T-L, Tomasi TB (1989) Regulation of MHC class II gene expression in macrophages by hematopoietic colony-stimulating factors (CSF). J Exp Med 170:1559.
189. Bilyk N, Holt PG (1995) Cytokine modulation of the immunosuppressive phenotype of pulmonary alevolar macrophage populations. Immunology 86:231–237.
190. Hunt JS, Manning LS, Wood GW (1984) Macrophages in murine uterus are immunosuppressive. Cell Immunol 85:499–510.
191. Hunt JS (1992) Immunobiology of pregnancy. Curr Opinion Immunol 4:591–596.
192. Chang MY, Pollard JW, Khalili H, Goyet SM, Diamond B (1993) Mouse placental macrophages have a decreased ability to present antigen. Proc Natl Acad Sci USA 90:462–466.
193. Clark DA, Chaouat G (1989) What do we know about spontaneous abortion mechanisms? Am J Reprod Immunol 19:28–37.
194. Chaouat G, Menu E, Clark DA, Dy M, Minkowski M, Wegmann TG (1996) Control of fetal survival in CBA × DBA/2 mice by lymphokine therapy. J Reprod Fertil 89:447–458.
195. Brandon JM, Bibby MC (1979) A study of changes in uterine mast cells during early pregnancy in the rat. Biol Reprod 20:977–980.
196. Kiso Y, Croy BA (1993) Granulated metrial gland cells: a natural killer cell subset of the pregnant mouse uterus. Microscpy Research and Technique 25:189–200.
197. Bulmer JN, Morrison L, Longfellow M, Ritson A, Pace D (1991) Granulated lymphocytes in human endometrium: histochemical and immunohistochemical studies. Hum Reprod 6:791–798.
198. Guimond M-J, Luross JA, Wang B, Terhorst C, Danial S, Croy BA (1997) Absence of natural killer cells during murine pregnancy is associated with reproductive compromise in TgE26 mice. Biol Reprod 56:168–179.
199. Roberts RM, Cross JC, Leaman DW (1992) Interferons as hormones of pregnancy. Endocr Rev 13:432–452.
200. Whaley AE, Meka CSR, Harbision LA, Hunt JS, Imakawa K (1994) Identification and cellular localization of unique interferon mRNA from human placenta. J Biol Chem 269:10,864–10,868.
201. Bulmer JN, Morrison L, Johnson PM, Meager A (1990) Immunohistochemical localization of interferons in human placental tissues in normal, ectopic, and molar pregnancy. Am J Reprod Immunol 22:109–116.
202. Paulseu L, Romagnoli R, Cintorino M, Ricci MG, Garotta G (1994) First trimester human trophoblast expresses both interferon-γ and interferon-γ-receptor. J Reprod Immunol 27:37–48.
203. Delassus S, Coutinho GC, Saucier C, Darche S, Kourilsky P (1994) Differential cytokine expression in maternal blood and placenta during murine gestation. J Immunol 152:2411–2420.
204. Peyman JA, Hammond GL (1992) Localization of IFN-γ receptor in first trimester placenta to trophoblasts but lack of stimulation of HLA-DRA, -DRB, or invariant chain mRNA expression by IFN-γ. J Immunol 149:2675–2680.
205. Chen HL, Kamath R, Pace JL, Russell SW, Hunt JS (1994) Expression of the interferon-γ receptor gene is mouse placentas is related to stage of gestation and is restricted to specific subpopulations of trophoblast cells. Placenta 15:109–121.
206. Garcia-Lloret MI, Yui J, Windler-Lowen B, Guilbert LJ (1996) Epidermal growth factor inhibits cytokine-induced apoptosis of primary human trophoblasts. J Cell Physiol 167:324–332.
207. Mattsson R, Holmdahl R, Scheynius A, Bernadotte F, Mattsson A, Van der Meide PH (1991) Placental MHC class I antigen expression is induced in mice following *in vivo* treatment with recombinant interferon-gamma. J Reprod Immunol 19:115–129.
208. Feinman MA, Kliman HJ, Main EK (1987) HLA antigen expression and induction by γ-interferon in cultured human trophoblasts. Am J Obstet Gynecol 157:1429–1434.
209. Hunt JS, Atherton RA, Pace JL (1990) Differential responses of rat trophoblast cells and embryonic fibroblasts to cytokines that regulate proliferation and class I MHC antigen expression. J Immunol 145:184–189.
210. Stewart CJR, Maura A, Farquharson A, Foulis AK (1992) The distribution and possible function of gamma-interferon immunoreactive cells in normal endometrium and myometrium. Virchows Arch A Pathol Anat 420:419–424.
211. Baccarini M, Sbarba PD, Buscher D, Bartocci A, Stanley ER (1992) IFN-γ/lipopolysaccharide activation of macrophages is associated with protein kinase C-dependent down-modulation of the colony-stimulating factor-1 receptor. J Immunol 149:2656–2661.

212. Tabibzadeh AA, Satyaswaroop PG, Rao PN (1988) Antiproliferative effect of interferon gamma in human endometrial epithelial cells *in vitro*: potential local growth modulatory role in endometrium. Endocrinol Metab 67:131–138.
213. Tabibzadeh S, Satyaswaroop PG, Rao PN (1988) Antiproliferative effect of interferon-γ in human endometrial epithelial cells *in vitro*: potential local growth modulatory role in endometrium. J Clin Endocrinol Metab 67:131–138.
214. Ebbesen P, Hager H, Norskov-Lauritsen N, Aboagye-Mathiesen G, Zdravkovic M, Villadsen J, Liu X, Petersen PM, Bambra C, Nyongo A (1995) Concurrence of high levels of interferons alpha and beta in cord and maternal blood and simultaneous presence of interferon in trophoblast in an African population. J Interferon Cytokine Res 15:123–128.
215. Schrader JW, Clark-Lewis I, Leslie KB, Ziltener HJ (1992) Interleukin-3, In: Human Cytokines: Handbook for Basic and Clinical Research (Aggarwal BB, Gutterman JU, eds.), Blackwell Scientific, Cambridge, MA, pp. 97–122.
216. Wegmann TG (1988) Maternal T cells promote placental growth and prevent spontaneous abortion. Immunol Lett 17:297–302.
217. Kover K, Liang L, Andrews GK, Dey SK (1995) Differential expression and regulation of cytokine genes in the mouse uterus. Endocrinology 136:1666–1673.
218. Tabibzadeh SS, Santhanam U, Sehgal PB, May LT (1989) Cytokine-induced production of IFN-$\beta_{2/IL-6}$ by freshly explanted human endometrial stromal cells. J Immunol 142:3134–3139.

4 Role of Growth Factors of Uterine and Fetal–Placental Origin During Pregnancy

Virginia Rider, PHD *and Marta Piva,* PHD

CONTENTS

INTRODUCTION

Embryo–Maternal Interactions

Implantation of the mammalian embryo and development of the placenta are interactive processes that depend on two-way communication between genetically distinct individuals. On the maternal side, the hormonal status of the uterus is crucial to change the uterus from a hostile environment to one that is receptive to the blastocyst *(1)*. On the embryonic side, development must proceed from the fertilized ovum to the blastocyst stage before an implantation reaction can be initiated. The importance of the synchrony between the uterus and embryo was originally suggested by the pioneering embryo transfer experiments of Chang *(2)*. Although the strictness of this relationship varies somewhat among species, the requirement for developmental synchrony has now been demonstrated to some extent for all species studied *(1,3,4)*. The establishment and maintenance of pregnancy are complicated processes that can be more easily conceptualized by subdividing prenatal life into three distinct phases. In the first phase, the embryo is free-living in the maternal reproductive tract. However, luminal fluids provide a rich source of growth factors and nutrients during this phase, particularly in ungulates *(5)*. Preimplantation development is remarkably similar among species even though there is exceptional diversity in placental types occurring later in pregnancy *(6)*. The second phase of prenatal life spans the period of attachment of the blastocyst to the uterus and subsequent development of the placenta and fetal organs. Embryonic loss at this stage is high *(7,8)* often because of inadequate development of the placental vascular connections *(9)*. Failure to produce bidirectional signals in the appropriate temporal sequence or amount may be largely responsible for embryo losses at this time (reviewed in *10*). The latter half of pregnancy is considered to be the third and final phase of prenatal development. During this time, the major changes involve growth of the fetus and the placenta (reviewed in *11*).

Considerable diversity exists in the placental types formed among domestic animals, rodents, and humans (reviewed in *12*). Placental types can be categorized by the number of tissue layers separating the maternal and fetal blood *(13)*. In this scheme of classification, the simplest form of placenta is an epitheliochorial attachment exemplified by the mare and sow. There is no intimate fusion of the tissues, and at birth, no maternal tissue is removed (nondeciduate). The deciduate type of placenta, formed in rodents and humans, involves intimate connection of the fetal and maternal tissues, and maternal tissue is shed with the placenta at birth *(12)*. Although such distinct differences in placental architecture suggest that no universal mechanisms exist regarding placental development, it is useful to remember that the placenta provides the means for two distinct organisms to coexist. Thus, in spite of distinct anatomical differences in placental types among species, placental functions are universally conserved. These functions include placental transport of nutrients from the mother to fetus, excretion of fetal wastes into the maternal circulation (reviewed in *14*), production of hormones that affect the physiology of both the mother and the fetus (reviewed in *15*), the protection of the fetus from the maternal immune system (reviewed in *16*), and the secretion of a variety of growth factors and cytokines that are absolutely required for the maintenance of pregnancy and embryonic development *(11,17)*.

Growth Factors as Modulators of Cell Function

Growth factors have been implicated in the control of a variety of cellular functions during prenatal development and pregnancy, including decidual formation, placental development, neovascularization, chemotaxis, differentiation of fetal organs, and fetal growth (reviewed in *18–21*). Recent attention to the temporal and spatial distribution of growth factors and their receptors in the embryo and uterus has provided a more complete picture of the potential mechanisms that regulate placental formation and function. However, growth and differentiation of female sex organs are primarily controlled by a balance of the sex steroids, estrogen and progesterone (reviewed in *22*), in part by controlling the production of growth factors and their receptors. Moreover, the placenta functions as an endocrine organ *(see 15)*. Therefore, a comprehensive understanding of the molecular mechanisms underlying embryo–maternal communication must take into account the effects of both hormones and growth factors in the establishment and maintenance of pregnancy.

Growth factors are polypeptides that belong to large gene families. Many growth factors, including epidermal growth factor (EGF), insulin-like growth factors (IGFs), transforming growth factor-α (TGF-α), platelet-derived growth factors (PDGFs), and fibroblast growth factors (FGFs) bind to high-affinity cell-surface receptors with tyrosine kinase activity *(23–25)*. Tyrosine kinase receptors comprise a large gene family of receptor proteins that have been divided into four (I–IV) subclasses based on their sequence similarity and structural characteristics *(23)*. Growth factor binding to high-affinity receptors results in receptor dimerization that catalyzes the phosphorylation of target substrates as well as tyrosine residues within their own polypeptide chains. Receptor dimerization is a conserved mechanism for growth factor receptor activation that increases the potential assortment of receptor–ligand interactions *(24)*. In addition, differential splicing of a single receptor gene generates a number of receptor variants capable of forming heterodimers and increasing receptor–ligand diversity *(see 25)*.

The biological action of individual growth factors within gene families often overlaps, thus causing confusion regarding individual function. Additional complexities in assessing the effects of individual growth factors arise from differential responses that depend on the cell's lineage or phenotype. Thus, pleiotropic actions in conjunction with overlapping function complicate assignment of a specific purpose to any given growth factor. In spite of these difficulties, considerable information has emerged about the molecular mechanisms involved in growth factor action. The development of tissue-culture methods has increased knowledge about individual cell function and how cells interact with each other and their environments. In early studies, cells were grown in media containing serum, since in its absence they arrested in G_0 of the cell cycle (reviewed in *26*). Subsequent purification of these "factors" from the serum revealed that mitogenic stimulants are largely growth factors. Some serum growth factors are able to stimulate the proliferation of cells from a wide variety of tissue origins, whereas others, such as erythropoietin, affect only a single cell type. Purification of most growth factors from serum and the subsequent analysis of their function have established the importance of these proteins in cell-cycle regulation.

Growth Factor Control of the Mammalian Cell Cycle

The best-characterized role of growth factors is their ability to regulate cell proliferation. When growth factors bind to high-affinity receptors on target cells, signal transduction cascades are activated that eventually lead to altered cell function. These changes in signal transduction pathways are mediated by the stimulation of second messengers, and by the activation of protein kinases and phosphatases (reviewed in *26–28*). The immediate result of growth factor receptor activation is increased protein phosphorylation of target substrates that stimulate the transcription of genes called the "early response genes." Early response genes primarily encode transcription factors necessary for regulating the delayed response genes. The synthesis and degradation of the delayed response gene products, including the G_1 cyclin-dependent kinases and their regulatory cyclin partners, drive cells through the restriction point of G_1 of the cell cycle (Fig. 1). The nature of the cdk–cyclin complexes present at a given time in a cell determines whether it will enter S phase or M phase, and these phases normally occur in a sequential fashion *(29)*.

Growth Factor Control of Angiogenesis

Another process controlled by growth factors that is crucial for placental function is development of the vascular connections between embryo and mother. Angiogenesis (new blood vessel formation) is a complex process requiring local degradation of the basement membrane from the parental vessel, migration of endothelial cells to form a sprout, proliferation, and differentiation of the endothelial cells into tube-like structures *(30–32)*. Fetal vascular growth, termed vasculogenesis, entails a process by which the development of blood vessels arise from the differentiation of endothelial cells *in situ (33)*. Although

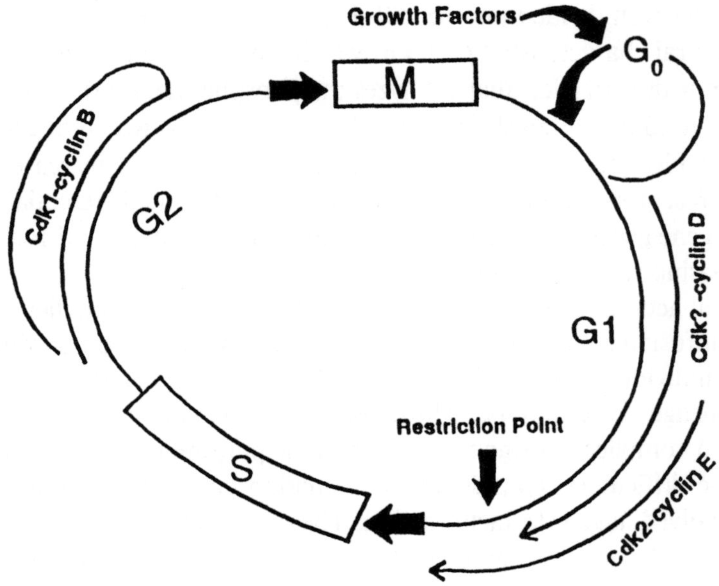

Fig. 1. Growth factors regulate the mammalian cell cycle. Mammalian cells use a small family of related cyclin-dependent kinases (cdks) to regulate progression through the cell cycle. Some of these (cyclins D and E) function during G_1 of the cell cycle, whereas others, such as cyclin B, function during the G_2 to M transition. The current model for the action of growth factors during G_1 of the cell cycle predicts that cyclin D and cyclin E levels increase resulting in formation of different cdk complexes that drive cells through the restriction point of G_1 into DNA replication. (Modified from *26*.)

angiogenesis occurs throughout the life of an organism, vasculogenesis may be limited to developmental stages. The importance of the vascular connections between mother and fetus has been well established *(see 20)*, and inadequate development of these connections contributes to embryonic loss and/or reduced birthweights *(see 14,20,34)*. A large number of growth factors have been shown to stimulate angiogenesis *(34,35)*; however, their mechanism of action is still not well defined.

Angiogenic factors have been mapped to the placenta in many species, but little evidence has emerged to support postulates regarding mechanisms by which vascular connections are established. The acquisition of the angiogenic phenotype is a complex process that is controlled by a balance of positive and negative factors *(30)*. This idea has obtained support from experiments in domestic animals, such as the cow *(36)* and ewe *(37)*, where angiogenic factors are produced primarily by the maternal placenta. The fetal tissues in these species produce factors that are proposed to inhibit maternal endothelial cell proliferation and migration throughout most of gestation (reviewed in *14*). These putative inhibitors are not expected to affect adversely fetal placental development, because vasculogenesis may be controlled independently from angiogenesis *(14)*. Additional difficulties in understanding the angiogenic process exist owing to variability in growth factor preparations, and to dissimilarities in the response of large and small endothelial cell vessels, smooth muscle cells, and pericytes to the same growth factor *(38)*.

Growth Factor Control of Cell Survival and Apoptosis

Growth factor action is not limited to cell-cycle control and angiogenesis. A variety of other proposed biological functions ranging from cellular differentiation, chemotaxis, immune regulation, and tissue regeneration to modulation of specific gene transcription have been advanced (Tables 1 and 2). Growth factors and steroid hormones regulate programmed cell death and cell survival by suppressing and stimulating apoptosis (reviewed in *39,40*). Direct evidence for the function of these factors in placental and fetal development in vivo is weak compared with evidence obtained from isolated cells in culture. However, it is likely that the molecular mechanisms involved in regulating cell function will be similar in reproductive processes as has been reported for other systems.

EGF FAMILY

Epidermal Growth Factor

EGF and several related polypeptides, including TGF-α, amphiregulin (AR), and heparin binding EGF (HB-EGF) are structurally related proteins that bind to the EGF receptor (EGFR), and promote cell proliferation and differentiation *(see 41,42)*. The action of these ligands is mediated through a 170-kDa transmembrane glycoprotein, which belongs to the type I tyrosine kinase family of receptors *(23)*. EGF is a 53 amino acid, single-chain polypeptide that exhibits potent mitogenic activity for a variety of cell types both in vivo and in vitro, including fibroblasts, epithelial cells, and keratinocytes *(43)*. It is generated from a larger 128-kDa glycosylated integral membrane protein called preproEGF by proteolytic cleavage *(44,45)*. Evidence suggests that EGF is a key modulator of embryo implantation, placental and fetal growth, and cellular differentiation *(46–48)*.

Immunoreactive EGF has been reported in the stromal cells of pregnant women and in association with the surface epithelium *(49)*. EGF has been immunolocalized to cytotrophoblast cells in human placenta at 4–5 wk, whereas at 6–12 wk EGF was detected in syncytiotrophoblast *(50)*. Cultured human trophoblast cells at all stages of functional differentiation, isolated from placental tissues of 6–9 wk of gestation *(51)*, contained both protein and mRNA for EGF and its receptor. EGFR colocalized with the ligand in the first trimester placenta *(50)*. In the second and third trimester pregnancy, EGF mainly localized to the cytotrophoblast, but EGFR was predominantly expressed in the syncytium *(50,52)*. The colocalization of EGF and its receptor to the same cell types in the first trimester of pregnancy suggested that EGF functions in an autocrine manner. However, localization of receptor and ligand to different cell types later in pregnancy suggested that EGF functions by paracrine mechanisms during the latter half of pregnancy *(50)*. In contrast to the above studies, third trimester placentae have been reported to show little to no immunoreactivity in either trophoblastic layer using two different monoclonal antibodies (MAb) to EGF *(53)*.

Recent evidence suggests that reinterpretation of the earlier immunolocalization studies may be required *(47)*. Experiments from Bass and colleagues *(47)* indicate that cytotrophoblasts do not express EGF or TGF-α. These ligands were not detected in conditioned culture medium containing cytotrophoblast from first term pregnancy. Furthermore, the mRNAs for these growth factors were absent from cultured cytotrophoblast cells after reverse transcription-polymerase chain reaction (RT-PCR) analysis. A panel of growth factors (TGF-β1, PDGF-AA, PDGF-BB, EGF, and TNF-α) were used to test growth factor effects on cytotrophoblast migration. Of those factors tested, only EGF increased the invasive capacity (migration distance) of first trimester cytotrophoblast cells. EGF had less effect on cytotrophoblast cells isolated from later times in gestation when their invasive capacity is normally diminished *(47)*. Since EGF is not expressed in first term cytotrophoblast, maternally derived EGF from the endometrium or placenta may be the agent responsible for cell division and invasion in the first trimester cytotrophoblast *(47)*. EGF

Table 1
Postulated Functions of Maternally Produced Growth Factors

	EGF	*TGF-α*	*HB-EGF*	*AR*	*FGFs*	*IFG-1*	*IGF-II*	*PDGF*	*VEGF/PlGF*	*TGF-β*	*TFN-α*
Endometrial cell proliferation/differentiation	+	+	+	+	+	+	+	+			+
Decidualization	+	+				+	+			+	
Extracellular matrix modification										+	+
Angiogenesis					+			+	+	+	+
Implantation	+	+	+	+							+
Placental growth					+	+	+	+			
Regulation of steroidogenesis	+	+				+					
Maternal immune function										+	

Table 2
Postulated Functions of Fetally Produced Growth Factors

	EGF	*TGF-α*	*HB-EGF*	*AR*	*FGFs*	*IFG-1*	*IGF-II*	*PDGF*	*VEGF/PlGF*	*TGF-β*	*TFN-α*
Implanatation attachment/migration	+		+								+
Cell proliferation or differentiation	+	+	+	+	+	+	+		+	+	+
Vasculogenesis/angiogenesis					+			+	+		+
Early fetal growth/ organogenesis		+			+	+	+			+	
Fetal/placental growth	+	+			+	+	+			+	
Regulation of steroidogenesis	+	+			+	+	+				
Immune modulation										+	

mRNA has been shown to be synthesized in human endometrium and decidua *(54)*. This apparent discrepancy between the results of Bass and colleagues *(47)* with the earlier immunolocalization analysis *(49,50,55,56)* is suggested to be owing to the use of whole antibodies that bind nonspecifically to the trophoblast Fc receptors *(47)*. An alternative interpretation is that EGF produced by the mother is detected in cytotrophoblast, because it is bound to cytotrophoblast EGF receptors *in situ*. Identification of the site of EGF synthesis using *in situ* hybridization will resolve this issue.

In nonhuman primates, there is a marked increase in EGF and EGFR immunoreactivity in decidualizing stromal cells during early pregnancy *(57,58)*. Later in pregnancy, EGF and EGFR immunolocalized to the syncytiotrophoblast, whereas TGF-α localized to the villous cytotrophoblast and endovascular cytotrophoblast within the maternal blood vessels *(58)*. The spatial distribution of EGF during early pregnancy in baboons suggested that this growth factor influences uterine decidualization and events associated with implantation of the embryo *(58)*. This interpretation is supported by data from rodents where EGF induces blastocyst implantation during embryonic delay *(59,60)* and augments the decidual cell response in a dose-dependent manner as measured by increased uterine weight wet in pseudopregnant rats *(59)*. A recent study by Harvey and colleagues *(48)* provides hints regarding a possible implantation mechanism. Proteinase activity produced by the early embryo is reported to be regulated by EGF and leukemia inhibitory factor (LIF). Transcripts for the proteinases were detected in the trophoblast giant cells in embryos at 7.5 d of development. The decidua immediately adjacent to the implanting blastocyst expressed the tissue inhibitor of metalloproteinase activity, TIMP-3. Both LIF and EGF stimulated matrix metalloproteinase gelatinase B (MMP-9) and urokinase-type plasminogen activator (uPA) expression when blastocysts were cultured in defined media containing the cytokine and growth factor, respectively. Since blastocysts express EGFRs, maternally produced EGF may stimulate the synthesis of proteinases facilitating blastocyst migration into the uterine stroma. The identification of TIMP-3 in the decidual cells adjacent to the blastocyst suggests endogenous uterine control of the invasive process.

EGF can influence placental function, since specific EGF binding sites are detected on rat, rabbit, and human placental homogenates *(61)*, and maternally administered EGF leads to a dramatic increase in placental permeability *(62)*. The levels of EGF in submandibular glands and plasma increased in pregnant and aged female mice *(63)*. Increased uterine wet weight during aging paralleled the increased concentration of EGF in both the submandibular glands and circulation *(63)*. Surgical removal (sialoadenectomy) prevented increased EGF in the circulation, increased abortions *(63)*, and significantly decreased live fetal weight and number *(64)*. These effects were reversed by the administration of EGF and augmented further by the administration of an antibody to EGF to the sialoadenectomized mice. Most interestingly, administration of TGF-α restored the litter size, but not the birthweight. The amino acid concentration in the maternal circulation is modified after sialoadenectomy, suggesting that the nutritional status of the mother is altered and that this affects the growth and development of the fetus *(65)*. In addition, maternal EGF effects may depend on gestational age *(66)*, since recombinant human EGF does not change the growth of 10-d-old rat embryos transplanted to the kidney capsule *(67)*.

Direct functions of EGF in placentation of domestic animals have yet to be demonstrated, but the spatial distribution and temporal expression of this growth factor and its receptor suggest its importance in a large number of species. In the fetal membranes of the sheep placenta, high- and low-affinity binding sites for ^{125}I-EGF have been reported *(68)*. The number of high-affinity binding sites peaked between d 90 and 100 of gestation, the time of rapid cotyledonary growth and increased placental hormonal secretion, suggesting that EGF functions in fetal aspects of ovine placental development *(68,69)*. EGF mRNA was first detected at approximately d 15 in the porcine conceptus, and its accumulation increased continuously up to d 22, whereas the protein immunolocalized in the d 22 fetus to the developing lung bud, gut loop, and the amnion *(70)*. At later stages of development, EGF mRNA was expressed primarily in the amnion *(70)*. Porcine embryos at all stages studied (d 7–22 of gestation) expressed EGFR mRNA. ^{125}I-EGF binds with high affinity to both glandular epithelial and stromal cells isolated from porcine endometrium *(71)*. However, the lack of notable changes of EGF and EGFR in the porcine endometrium during early pregnancy suggests that EGF functions in this species are related to embryo development *(72)*. Unlike pigs, EGF was absent from equine fetal membranes and was detected only in maternal tissues of mares *(73)*. In addition, the amount of EGF mRNA in the endometrium increased during early pregnancy in the mare, reaching a peak between d 35 and 45 coincident with the beginning of implantation and placentation *(73)*. Immunoreactive EGF is present in many fetal organs of the mouse, including liver, brain, lung, intestine, and placenta *(74)*. EGF has been implicated particularly in fetal lung development in several species *(75,76)*. The offspring of rats with autoantibodies against EGF have lower birthweights, and delayed lung maturation with decreased amounts of surfactant-protein A and increased perinatal mortality *(76)*. Sex-specific EGF effects on lung development in rabbits have been reported *(75)*. Female rabbit lung explants treated with EGF at 21 and 24 d of gestation (term 31 d) increased incorporation of glycerol into lamellar body diesaturated phosphatidylcholine, a principal surface-active component of surfactant *(77)*. Explants of lung from male rabbit fetuses at the same age were unresponsive to EGF in culture *(75)*, and were unable to synthesize diesaturated phosphatidylcholine.

The most direct evidence for EGF function in reproduction and development comes from recent analyses of mice lacking the EGFR owing to gene targeting mutagenesis *(78–80)*. Mice with the null allele for EGFR provide a range of phenotypes depending on the genetic background of the mice. Abnormalities can occur in the peri-implantation period because of defects in the ICM of the blastocyst, in the midgestation period owing to placental abnormalities, and during the perinatal period. In the latter case, the pups have normal birthweights, but reduced growth and wasting after birth *(78)*.

Transforming Growth Factor-α

TGF-α is a polypeptide that influences a variety of biological activities, including cellular transformation, mitosis, DNA synthesis, and neovascularization *(see 81)*. The protein is structurally related to EGF (30% homology), including conservation of all six cysteines *(see 42,81,82)*. Secreted TGF-α, like all secreted growth factors, is translocated across the membrane via a hydrophobic signal sequence in the amino-terminus of the protein *(81)*. Mature TGF-α exists in multiple forms owing to separate cleavage sites in the external precursor domain and to differential glycosylation *(81)*.

This growth factor has been identified in the uterus of rodents *(83–85)*, humans *(54)*, and pigs *(72)*. Human endometrial TGF-α immunoreactivity localized primarily to the epithelial cells and in the intermediate trophoblast cells within the decidua in the first trimester of pregnancy *(86)*. By the second and third trimesters, TGF-α expression declined. Villous trophoblast cells showed cytoplasmic and plasma membrane immunoreactivity *(86–88)*, whereas expression was variable in chorionic trophoblast *(87)*. Human placenta from early, mid- and late gestation contained more TGF-α mRNA and protein than EGF, suggesting that TGF-α could be more influential on human placental cell function than

EGF *(89)*. The origin of TGF-α mRNA in human endometrium was questionable. Since TGF-α is expressed in leukocytes, confirmation of uterine synthesis is difficult *(54)*. TGF-α has been proposed to function in decidualization of uterine stromal cells in the human *(86)*, baboon *(58)*, and rat *(83)*. Its spatial distribution in the placenta and the increased synthesis of 17β-hydroxysteroid dehydrogenase type 1 enzyme in response to TGF-α suggests that this growth factor may stimulate estrogen production in placental tissues *(90)*.

The distribution and temporal expression of TGF-α has not been extensively mapped in domestic animals. In the porcine endometrium beginning at d 10 and ending at d 22 of pregnancy, TGF-α transcripts were detected using RT-PCR *(72)*. Subsequent immunolocalization revealed that the protein was limited to the glandular epithelial cells at each day of pregnancy examined. Since the mRNA for TGF-α in the endometrium did not change qualitatively during pregnancy, it was suggested that TGF-α functions in this species may relate to development of the embryo *(72)*. Transcripts for TGF-α have been reported in sheep conceptuses (d 15–30) and in uterine tissues at this same time period *(91)*. Since EGF transcripts were not detected, TGF-α may serve as the natural ligand for EGFR activation in sheep *(91)*.

Consistent with a developmental role at later stages of pregnancy, TGF-α is expressed in a variety of fetal tissues. Human fetuses contain TGF-α mRNA *(92)* and protein *(93)* in the gastrointestinal tract. It is widely distributed in mesenchymal tissues of the gastrointestinal, genitourinary, and respiratory tracts in mid- to late gestation rats *(94)*. Development of the rat *(95)* and human lung *(96)* may be particularly influenced by TGF-α. Both TGF-α mRNA and protein were detected in rat lung during late gestation, reaching a peak when the respiratory acinus was formed and vascularized *(95)*.

Mice homozygous for a null mutation of the TGF-α gene are healthy and fertile, although they have hair follicle abnormalities and often develop corneal inflammation *(97,98)*. Thus, although TGF-α is widely expressed in both maternal and fetal tissues, its function does not appear to be required for survival of the embryo or for normal placental function. However, since EGF, AR, and HB-EGF bind and activate the EGFR, it is possible that these ligands can substitute for the normal function of TGF-α during pregnancy.

Heparin Binding EGF-Like Growth Factor

HB-EGF is a heparin binding mitogen for smooth muscle cells and fibroblasts that belongs to the EGF family of growth factors *(99)*. HB-EGF is initially synthesized as a large precursor of 208 amino acids that contains a highly hydrophobic sequence similar to the transmembrane domain of the TGF-α, AR, and EGF precursors *(100,101)*. The precursor protein from primates and humans has been identified as a cell-surface receptor for the internalization of the diphtheria toxin into eukaryotic cells *(102)*. Proteolytic cleavage of the precursor yields the mature protein. The carboxy-terminus of the protein shares 40% sequence identity with human EGF *(100,101)*. HB-EGF binds to the EGFR and stimulates its tyrosine kinase activity and receptor autophosphorylation *(101)*. HB-EGF and AR bind strongly to heparin, whereas EGF and TGF-α do not *(103,104)*.

In species like the pig that exhibit noninvasive epitheliochorial placentation, the composition of the uterine secretions is important in the establishment and early maintenance of pregnancy *(105)*. Biologically active HB-EGF has been isolated from uterine luminal flushings and uterine tissues of nonpregnant pigs *(106)*. Immunohistochemical analysis of uterine sections from pregnant animals revealed that HB-EGF was primarily located in cells of the endometrium *(106)*. The failure of an earlier study *(72)* to identify HB-EGF mRNA in porcine uterus is probably owing to differences in the PCR methodology *(106)*.

In the uterus of rats *(107,108)* and mice *(109)*, HB-EGF is expressed in epithelial and stromal cells. During implantation delay in mice, HB-EGF is not expressed in luminal epithelial cells at the site of blastocyst apposition. However, when blastocysts are stimulated to implant by injection of estradiol to the mother, HB-EGF transcripts are detected in the epithelium *(109)*.

Amphiregulin

AR is a polypeptide growth factor with significant amino acid similarity to the EGF family, and its biological effects are mediated via the EGFR *(110)*. The mature protein is generated by processing of a larger transmembrane precursor. AR is a bifunctional growth modulator, because it can promote the growth of normal epithelial cells and inhibit the proliferation of certain aggressive carcinoma cell lines. Significant amounts of a 1.4-kb AR transcript have been found in human placenta and ovaries *(110)*. Immunoreactive AR is localized to the nucleus and cytoplasm of the syncytiotrophoblast cell layer of the human chorionic villi from the 11th until the 18th wk of gestation *(111)*. Villous and extravillous cytotrophoblast cells, as well as decidual tissue, were negative for AR at all gestational ages examined. In mice, AR is expressed in uterine epithelial cells coincident with the timing of implantation *(112)*.

FIBROBLAST GROWTH FACTORS

FGFs were originally identified as mitogens for mouse 3T3 cells (reviewed in *113*). This growth factor family is now comprised of at least nine different members *(114,115)* based on varying degrees of shared protein sequence homology. FGFs promote proliferation of a wide variety of mesodermal and neuroectodermal cells, and they are angiogenic. The levels of FGFs are low in most adult tissues; however, basic FGF (bFGF) is stored in the basement membrane and extracellular matrix, where it is stably bound to heparan sulfate proteoglycans *(116–118)*. Extracellular residence of bFGF in the uterus where extensive remodeling can occur in preparation for implantation and placentation is a critical consideration for the bioactivity of bFGF and other growth factors that are sequestered and protected from proteolytic cleavage in extracellular stores *(119)*.

FGFs have been localized in the endometrium of human *(120–124)*, rhesus monkey *(125)*, mouse *(126,127)*, rat *(128,129)*, and pig *(130)*. FGF mRNAs for acidic (aFGF) and bFGF have been detected using RT-PCR amplification *(123)* and *in situ* hybridization *(131)*. The distribution of FGF-7 (KGF) mRNA has been mapped in the primate endometrium *(125)*. The proteins (bFGF and aFGF) localized to the basement membrane, extracellular matrix *(126,128)*, in smooth muscle cells surrounding the uterine and placental *(127)* blood vessels, and in endometrial stromal and decidual cells *(128)*. bFGF mRNA has been detected in syncytiotrophoblast, villous mesenchyme, amnion, and chorion in human placenta at term *(131)*. Uterine epithelial cells in mouse *(127)* and rat *(128)* contain granules at the apical surface that react with bFGF. Moreover, bFGF has been detected in the luminal flushings of pregnant pigs *(130)* and rats *(128)*. Since bFGF lacks a classical signal sequence *(132)*, it is not clear if the protein is exported from cells or released on damage. Several interesting proposals have been advanced for alternative export of bFGF *(133)*, but it remains to be shown how it arrives in the luminal fluid.

The widespread distribution of FGFs in fetal and maternal tissues suggests that these growth factors function in the establishment and maintenance of pregnancy. bFGF is a potent mitogen for cultured uterine stromal cells in both human *(134)* and rat *(135)*, providing that progesterone is in the culture medium. bFGF is expressed in the syncytiotrophoblast of first term human placenta *(131)*, and it stimulates mitosis of JEG-3 choriocarcinoma cells *(136)*. Cell division of JEG-3 cells and bFGF immunoreactivity are reduced after methotrexate treatment, a chemotherapeutic agent used to treat placental tumors *(122)*. Immunoreactive bFGF is lost from rat uterine stromal cells in early pregnancy if proliferation and implantation are blocked by administration of the progesterone receptor antagonist RU 486 *(129)*. bFGF increased the accumulation of human chorionic gonadotropin (hCG) in JAR choriocarcinoma cells *(137)*, and bFGF mRNA *(131)* and protein *(136)* are expressed in the syncytiotrophoblast, consistent with the view that bFGF may regulate placental production of hCG. bFGF immunoreactivity is found in the mesometrial sinusoids at d 9 of pregnancy in the mouse *(127)*, suggesting that it may be important in endothelial proliferation or migration. Endothelial cell migration is specifically stimulated by bFGF in the developing rat heart *(138)*. Both aFGF and bFGF stimulated proliferation of uterine endometrial epithelial cells from pseudopregnant rabbits *(139)*.

KGF (FGF-7) differs from other FGF growth factors because it is mitogenic for epithelial cells rather than fibroblast and endothelial cells *(140)*. The KGF receptor (KGFR) is an alternatively spliced form generated from the FGF receptor 2 (FGFR2) gene *(141)*. This receptor binds KGF and aFGF, but not bFGF, whereas FGFR2 binds aFGF and bFGF with high affinity (reviewed in *25*). KGF mRNA is expressed during the proliferative and secretory phases in human endometrium *(124)*. Enrichment of stromal and epithelial cells showed that KGF was expressed predominantly in stroma, whereas KGFR and FGFR2 expression was greatest in epithelium. These results were supported by the lack of KGF expression, but detectable KGFR and FGFR2 expression in epithelial cancer cell lines from endometrium *(124)*. In the primate endometrium, KGF is produced in the stromal cells *(125)*. Since KGF mRNA accumulated in response to progesterone whereas glandular epithelial cells proliferated, Koji and coworkers *(125)* speculated that KGF produced in stromal cells stimulates proliferation of glandular epithelial cells.

FGFs are also detected in a variety of fetal tissues during mammalian development *(142)*. FGFs stimulate proliferation of embryonic cells and clonal expansion of embryonic cell lines *(143,144)*, suggesting effects on cell lineage and organogenesis. F9 teratocarcinoma stem cells have certain features shared with the ICM cells of the mouse blastocyst *(145)*. F9 cells induced to differentiate into analogous cells of the embryonic parietal endoderm synthesize bFGF, but undifferentiated cells do not *(146)*. Only the differentiated cells export bFGF into the extracellular matrix, and this matrix-associated bFGF can stimulate the proliferation of endothelial cells. These results suggest that bFGF synthesized in one cell type can influence the proliferation of other cell types, indicating possible paracrine actions for FGFs in early development.

In order to exert biological function, FGFs must bind to their high-affinity tyrosine kinase receptors located on the surface of target cells. FGF receptors (FGFRs) are type IV tyrosine kinases *(23)*, including at least four (1–4) distinct members. Additional complexity exists, since numerous FGFR variants are produced by alternative splicing *(see 25)*. Target cells also express a large number of low-affinity binding sites for FGFs consisting of heparan sulfate proteoglycans, which bind FGFs both on the cell surface and within the extracellular matrix. Evidence suggests that FGF interaction with these low-affinity receptors is required for subsequent binding to high-affinity receptors *(147)*. FGFRs have been localized in a variety of tissues, but information on their distribution in the reproductive tract of most species is lacking. Multiple transcripts of FGFR1 have been reported for human fetal ovaries and uterus *(148)*. Differential distribution and alternative splicing of FGFRs have been reported for the endometrium of the pregnant rat, suggesting functions for bFGF in stromal cell proliferation and/or differentiation *(149)*. Most interestingly, proliferating stromal cells in culture express predominantly FGFRα *(135)*, whereas in whole uterus, both FGFRα and FGFRβ are present at approximately equal amounts *(149)*.

The proof of FGF function in cellular differentiation and pattern specification during early development continues to accumulate *(150,151)*. Because FGFs operate in mesoderm generation and pattern formation in amphibians *(151)*, recent work in mammalian embryos has focused on mapping FGFRs to different cell types in the embryo, and eliminating FGF function by targeted mutagenesis (reviewed in *152*). FGFR1, R2, and R3 are expressed in undifferentiated embryonal carcinoma (EC) and embryonic stem (ES) cells from the mouse *(153)*. Changes in expression of these three receptors occurred during differentiation of ES cells, whereas expression of FGFR4 correlated with formation of parietal endoderm. FGFR1 and FGFR2 are expressed during gastrulation *(154,155)*, and these receptors become differentially expressed in epithelial and mesenchymal tissues later in development *(156)*. FGFR1-deficient embryos show defects in their axial organization *(157)* and in the pattern of mesoderm formation during embryogenesis *(158)*. The FGFR1 defect is associated with growth retardation, and it is suggested that the FGFR1 defect results in reduced cell proliferation and perhaps mesodermal cell migration out of the primitive streak *(157,158)*. FGFR4 is detected by the late blastocyst stage of development and in the primitive streak during gastrulation *(159)*. Embryos homozygous for the null allele of FGFR4 implant and induce uterine decidualization, but development does not proceed owing to reduced proliferation of the inner cell mass *(160)*.

Taken together, the evidence indicates that bFGF promotes mitosis in placental cells, and its expression patterns suggest it participates in angiogenesis. Furthermore, expression of bFGF in the syncytiotrophoblast and amnion at term is consistent with an important role in placental function, including transport of nutrients across the fetal membrane *(131)*. Additional experiments to verify these proposed functions are necessary, since fetal growth retardation is expected from inadequate blood supply or nutrient transport. Mapping studies of the temporal and spatial distribution of FGFs and their receptors, and loss of function studies using targeted mutagenesis provide conclusive evidence that FGFs are major modulators of embryo development. It is clear that FGFs are important mitogens for a variety of embryonic cells, and that these growth factors play a role in pattern formation during development.

IGFs, IGF RECEPTORS (IGFRs) AND IGF BINDING PROTEINS (IGFBPs)

Insulin-like growth factor-I (IGF-I) and insulin-like growth factor II (IGF-II) are peptide growth factors with structural similarity to insulin *(161,162)*. IGF action occurs after ligand binding to type I (IGF1R) and type II (IGFR2) IGFRs. IGF1R is a transmembrane tyrosine kinase structurally related to the insulin receptor and, therefore, classified as a type II tyrosine kinase. IGF2R is identical to the cation-independent mannose 6-phosphate receptor, which functions in lysosomal enzyme trafficking *(see 162–164)*. The IGF1R is a tetrameric glycoprotein comprised of α-and β-subunits linked by disulfide bonds. Two half ($\alpha\beta$) receptors are joined by disulfide linkage between the α-chains to form the mature tetrameric ($\alpha\beta\alpha\beta$) holoreceptor *(165,166)*. The ligand binding domain is located at the amino-terminus of the protein in a cysteine-rich region of the extracellular α-subunit.

The receptor binds IGF-I with high affinity, IGF-II with similar or slightly lower affinity depending on the cell type, and insulin with 500 to 1000 times lower affinity *(167)*. On ligand binding, intracellular signaling is triggered through activation of the tyrosine kinase activity located in the transmembrane β-subunit. The IGF1R signal transduction pathway has not been well characterized compared to the insulin receptor pathway. However, similar to insulin receptor signaling, activation of IGF1R results in receptor autophosphorylation and activation of insulin receptor substrate-1 (IRS-1), an early substrate phosphorylated by insulin receptor activation. IRS-1 binds to the enzyme phosphatidylinositol 3-kinase and acts as a multivalent docking site for SH2 domains of other proteins involved in cellular signaling *(see 162,168)*.

IGF Binding Proteins

The biological actions of the IGFs are regulated further by a family of at least six specific binding proteins (IGFBPs) *(169)*. The affinity of IGFBPs for IGFs is partially dependent on the phosphorylation status of the binding protein, since the more extensively phosphorylated forms have a higher affinity for IGFs *(170,171)*. Most of the circulating IGFs are bound to IGFBP-3 as a 150-kDa complex *(172)*. Smaller amounts of IGFs circulate as complex of 40 kDa bound to IGFBP-1 and IGFBP-2. The larger 150-kDa complexes serve as a reservoir of circulating IGFs, whereas the smaller complexes function in the transfer of IGFs from the circulation into the extracellular space. These six IGFBPs are clearly distinct, but they share regions of homology, including the hydrophobic cysteine-rich N-terminal region and to a lesser extent the C-terminal domain *(173)*. All IGFBPs specifically bind IGF-I and IGF-II, having negligible affinity for insulin. IGFBPs have been proposed to play a key role in IGF bioavailability to the target tissues *(see 168)*, since these binding proteins transport IGFs in the circulation and are important for movement of IGFs out of the vascular compartment into target tissues. The IGFBPs provide a means of controlling the tissue-specific localization of the ligand, its accessibility to receptors, and protein turnover.

IGFBP-3, in solution, has a significantly higher affinity for IGF-I and IGF-II than IGF1R; therefore, the binding protein prevents ligand–receptor interaction *(168)*. IGFBP-3 functions are regulated during pregnancy by a maternal serum protease, which degrades the binding protein, reduces its affinity for IGFs *(174,175)*, and increases the growth factor availability and biological activity *(176)*. The main degradation product of IGFBP-3 does not bind IGFs. In the rat, there is a switch from IGFBP-3 to 2 in maternal serum and reproductive tissues as pregnancy progresses *(177)*. The decline in IGFBP-3 levels relates temporally to the appearance of IGFBP-3 protease activity that enhances the clearance of IGF-I from the maternal circulation toward the tissues *(178)*. This regulatory mechanism functions during human pregnancy, since the free form of IGF-I is significantly higher in pregnant than nonpregnant women owing to the endogenous pregnancy-related IGFBP-3 proteolytic activity *(179,180)*. However, Hills and collaborators *(181)* did not find a correlation between maternal serum total IGF-I, placental weight, and fetal birthweight, perhaps because they did not distinguish between free and bound IGF-I. In that study, however, maternal IGFBP-1 in serum was higher in small-for-gestational-age babies than in babies of average-for-gestational-weight, and lower in large-for-gestational-weight babies.

Growth hormone is absolutely required for growth in the infant. However, no such essential factor has been identified for fetal and placental growth in mammals (reviewed in *182*). Since growth factors stimulate cell division and growth in a variety of cell types, they became attractive candidates for promoting fetal and placental growth *(see 66,164,168, 182,183)*. In particular, attention has been focused on the IGFs, since IGF-I has anabolic effects in vivo and in vitro. IGF-I stimulates glucose and amino acid uptake, and decreases protein breakdown in adult animals of different species *(184–186)*. Human cytotrophoblast from first trimester chorionic villi showed increased glucose uptake in a dose-dependent manner in response to IGF-I and IGF-II *(187)*. IGF-I also stimulated amino acid uptake by these first trimester cells *(187)*. IGF-I and to a lesser extent IGF-II enhanced amino acid uptake by human cytotrophoblast cells isolated from term placenta *(188)*.

Localization

In the reproductive tissues, IGF-I is primarily detected in proliferative and early secretory human endometrium *(189)*. The level of IGF-I expression in the human placenta is low and restricted to the differentiated trophoblast cells *(190)*. Increased IGF-I binding capacity develops during differentiation of cytotrophoblast to syncytiotrophoblast in vitro *(191)*. IGF-I has been implicated in placental cell differentiation, since it potentiates the EGF-induced secretion of human placental lactogen by cultured trophoblast cells *(192)*. In contrast, IGF-II *(193,194)* and IGFBP-3 *(189)* genes are expressed at high levels in the proliferative cytotrophoblast of early human placenta *(195)*, and IGF-II has been shown to stimulate DNA synthesis in primary cultures of first trimester human cytotrophoblasts *(193)*. IGF1R and IGF2R are expressed during the secretory phase and in early pregnancy in the endometrium of the human *(189)*. Both receptors are detected later in cytotrophoblast and the mesenchymal stroma of the placental villi *(189)*.

IGF1R localizes to the decidualized stromal cells and the placental villi during early and late pregnancy in the baboon *(196)*. The decidua also expressed IGF-II, IGFBP-1, 2, and 3 genes *(195)*. IGFBP-1 and 2 were expressed predominantly in the endometrium and decidua, whereas IGFBP-3 was found in the placenta during early pregnancy *(197)*. At d 25 of pregnancy in primates, immunoreactivity for IGFBP-1 was limited to the endometrial trophoblastic junction *(197,198)*, but later it extended deeper into the stromal cells and the perivascular regions *(197)*. IGFBP-1 is the major secretory product of human *(199)* and nonhuman primate decidua during early pregnancy *(200,201)*.

Several different sizes of IGF-II transcripts have been detected in the invasive chorionic girdle that gives rise to the endometrial cups and in the noninvasive allantochorion that forms the diffuse, microcotyledonary placenta of the mare *(202)*. IGF-II was expressed in the equine fetus at all stages examined, particularly in tissues of mesodermal origin, in the extraembryonic mesoderm, invasive chorionic girdle, and mature endometrial cups. There was no evidence for IGF-II expression in maternal tissues at the times examined (d 14–150 gestation). In contrast to results reported for the mare, IGF-II mRNA is expressed in the bovine uterus. Moreover, the steady-state levels of IGF-II mRNA increased in the presence of the bovine conceptus *(203)*. IGF-II and IGFBP-2 mRNAs increased with the progression of pregnancy in the endometrium of the pig, but IGF-I mRNA levels declined *(204)*. On d 12 of pregnancy, the ratio of IGF-II:IGF-I mRNA levels in endometrium from Large White pigs (a breed with high conceptus mortality) was significantly higher than in Meishan pigs (a breed with low conceptus mortality). This difference was explained in terms of the conceptus P450 aromatase activity, a major source of estradiol, which was shown to be stimulated by IGF-I in pig conceptus *(205)* and strongly inhibited by IGF-II in cultured human cytotrophoblasts *(see 206)*. Addition of IGF-I to d 12 porcine conceptuses of filamentous morphology increased amounts of P450 aromatase mRNA *(207)*. The IGF2R is detectable by immunohistochemistry on trophectoderm cells in pig embryos from early pregnancy (d 4–10) and on fetal and maternal compartments of the placenta at d 20 *(208)*. In these very early stages, IGF2R is seen only in the endometrial cells of the placenta and not other placental structures or on embryonic tissue.

Biological Functions

Changes in the IGF axis are associated with metabolic changes in the mother to meet the increased nutritional requirements of the growing fetus. Maternal IGF-I promotes fetal growth in part by stimulating nutrient transfer across the placenta to the fetus in a variety of species. The nutritional requirements for the human fetus increase dramatically in the second half of gestation *(209)*. IGF-I specifically inhibits the release of the vasoconstrictors, such as thromboxane B_2 and prostaglandin $F_{2\alpha}$, in perfused human placenta *(210)*, thus affecting the supply of nutrients to the fetus by stimulating increased blood flow. At the end of the first trimester of pregnancy, the levels of IGF-I in human maternal serum are between 24 and 34 times higher than in fetal fluids *(180)*.

IGFs and IGFBPs in pregnant rabbits are correlated with maternal weight *(211)*. IGF-I, IGF-II, and IGFBPs levels in maternal serum peaked between d 21 and 23 of pregnancy and then decreased toward term (term 30–31 d). Maternal concentrations of IGF-II in circulation were higher in the rabbit than have been reported for other species. Although radiolabeled IGF-II does not cross the placenta in the ewe *(212)*, the hemochorial placenta of the rabbit could be permeable to proteins with a greater molecular mass. The increased amount of IGF-II and IGFBPs in the maternal serum of rabbits correlated temporally with inversion of the yolk sac and the initiation of functional activity of the true placenta.

Uteroplacental insufficiency (UPI) causes small-for-gestational-age fetuses because of nutritional deprivation. In this pathological situation, maternal serum levels of total IGF-I and IGFBP-3 were normal *(213)*, but fetal IGF-I, IGF-II, and IGFBP-3 levels were significantly lower than for the appropriate-for-gestation-age controls *(213,214)*. Furthermore, maternal serum IGFBP-3 protease activity was increased in UPI, probably as a compensatory mechanism to increase the bioavailable IGF-I.

Mice with high levels of maternal serum IGF-I do not exhibit the typical negative relationship between fetal mass and litter size *(215,216)*. Moreover, administration of IGF-I to mice throughout pregnancy resulted in large litters and increased fetal weight *(216)*. Generally speaking, IGF1R levels are regulated by the nutritional status of the mother *(217)*, circulating IGF-I concentrations *(218)*, and glycemia *(219)*. In addition, IGF1R is regulated both at the binding and at the transcription levels by several growth factors in different cell lines *(see 163)*. IGF-II receptors are developmentally regulated in the rat *(220)*, sheep *(221)*, and pig *(222)*. Receptor mRNA and protein levels were high in fetal tissues, and declined dramatically in late gestation and/or in the early postnatal period.

In the sheep placenta, IGF-I and IGF-II binding sites were detected at d 50, 75, 100, and 140 of pregnancy *(223)*. The highest concentrations of IGF-I occurred in the periepithelial endometrial stroma, whereas IGF-II mRNA was detected exclusively in the caruncular and endometrial stroma *(224)*. IGF1R transcripts localized mainly to the epithelium and stromal cells. Restriction of placental size in sheep retarded fetal growth by reducing the supply of nutrients and oxygen to the fetus *(225,226)* and significantly reducing fetal blood glucose, pO_2 and plasma IGF-I and IGFBP-3 levels in late pregnancy *(227,228)*. Furthermore, the quantity of IGF-I mRNA decreased in fetal muscle, liver, and kidney *(227)*, and correlated positively with fetal weight. Taken together, the findings suggest that IGF-I and not IGF-II contributes to late fetal growth in sheep.

Developmental Analysis of Mutant Mice

Detailed developmental analyses of mouse embryos carrying mutations in the IGFs and IGFRs have provided direct experimental evidence for IGF function in fetal growth *(229–231)*. Mice embryos homozygous (−/−) for the disrupted IGF-I gene (Igf1) weigh 90% of their wild-type counterparts at embryonic d 13.5 (E13.5), and slower growth continues until birth when mutants weigh 60% of their normal counterparts *(230)*. Depending on their genetic background, some Igf1 (−/−) mutants died shortly after birth, but others survived and reached adulthood. Surviving Igf1 (−/−) mutants were infertile and had retarded bone development, but continued to grow after birth, reaching 30% of the normal adult weight *(231)*. Mutation in either of the IGF genes (Igf1 [−/−] and Igf2 [p−]) produce similar phenotypes, but mice lacking both IGFs were more severely growth-retarded. Interestingly, Igf2 (p−) was the only mutation that decreased placental growth. IGF1R transcripts are expressed in the rat placenta throughout development *(232)*. Thus, it was surprising that receptor mutants (Igf1r, −/−) did not affect placental growth. To explain their findings, Baker and coworkers *(230)* postulated that IGF-II actions on the placenta were mediated by a third unknown receptor.

In contrast, all null mutants for the Igf1r gene died at birth of respiratory failure and were more severely growth-retarded, although morphogenesis appeared normal. Mouse mutant embryos homozygous (−/−) for the IRS-1 gene survived through gestation, but showed growth deficiencies at pre- and postnatal stages. Moreover, the null mutants were resistant to the hypoglycemic effects of insulin and IGFs *(233)*. Evidence that IGF1R is essential for cell growth has also been obtained from experiments in vitro. Mouse embryo-derived fibroblasts transfected with a selectively targeted disrupted Igf1r gene did not proliferate in a supplemented serum-free medium that stimulated the proliferation of normal fibroblasts *(234)*. Furthermore, this lack of proliferation was reversed when the transfections were carried out with the wild-type gene.

In contrast to the IGF1R, the IFG2R is a monomer with a short cytoplasmic tail and no tyrosine kinase activity *(163)*. This receptor targets lysosomal enzymes from the Golgi apparatus or the plasma membrane to the lysosomes, and mediates the rapid internalization and degradation of IGF-II (reviewed in *162,235*). The T hairpin (T^{hp}) chromosomal deletion, which leads to a dominant lethal maternal phenotype (Tme), encompasses the Igf2r locus *(236)*. Mice that inherit the T^{hp} chromosomal deletion from their mothers developed edema and died *in utero* at about d 15 of gestation *(237–239)*. Transmission through the paternal germline resulted in viable heterozygous offspring. The maternal lethal effect is attributed to a maternally imprinted locus called T-associated maternal effect. The heterozygote $T^{hp/+}$ embryos can be rescued to birth if they also lack IGF-II *(240)*.

Targeted Mutagenesis

The elimination of IGF2R function by targeted mutagenesis is lethal when maternally inherited *(241)*. Heterozygous Igf2r (−/+) and homozygous Igf2r (−/−) mutants die at birth and are approx 30% heavier in dry wt than their wild-type counterparts, depending on the genetic background of the mice *(241)*. They also show lung, heart, and skeletal abnormalities, and varying degrees of abnormal sorting of mannose-6-phosphate tagged proteins. The abnormal development was owing to an accumulation of IGF-II, because the introduction of a Igf2 null allele rescued the Igf2r phenotype. Some heterozygotes reactivated their paternal allele in various tissues and survived to adults, but no homozygotes survived. Taken together, these results indicate that IGF-II is essential for late fetal growth and development in mice, whereas the reactivated paternal allele IGF-II performs important functions in postnatal survival *(241)*.

PLATELET-DERIVED GROWTH FACTORS

PDGFs are mitogenic principally on mesenchymal connective-forming cells like fibroblasts, glial cells, and smooth muscle cells *(242)*. In addition to their mitogenic effects, PDGFs are chemotactic *(243–246)*, immunomodulatory *(247)*, and they affect specialized tissue function *(248)*. These growth factors stimulate tissue remodeling, and therefore, PDGFs have been implicated in the regenerative events that occur after injury (reviewed in *249*). Biologically active PDGF is a homo- or heterodimeric molecule comprised of two polypeptides designated PDFG-A and PDGF-B. The dimers share approx 60% amino acid homology *(250)*. Three possible isoforms (PDGF-AA, PDGF-AB, and PDGF-BB) can be generated, and the polypeptide chains are linked via disulfide bonds.

Similarly, PDGF receptor may be a homo- or heterodimeric molecule. The two subunits form three types of high-affinity type III tyrosine kinase PDGF receptors ($\alpha\alpha$ receptor, $\alpha\beta$ receptor, and $\beta\beta$ receptor) that interact with different specificities and affinities to the ligand isoforms, and may elicit different biological responses *(see 23,251)*. PDGF binding to its receptor induces receptor dimerization, autophosphorylation, as well as phosphorylation of a number of intracellular proteins that induces specific cellular responses.

PDGF has been implicated in the maintenance of pregnancy and fetal development during murine gestation *(252,253)*. Furthermore, Northern blot and immunocytochemical analyses reveal that mRNAs and protein for the PDGF-A, PDGF-B, PDGFα receptor, and PDGFβ receptor are time-dependent, and tissue specifically expressed in the placenta and uterus being progressively and coordinately upregulated as the pregnancy proceeds in the second half of murine gestation *(253)*. Ligand and receptors are present in multiple cell types of the placenta, gravid uterus, extraembryonic membranes, and in the nucleated fetal erythroid progenitor cells.

Early postimplantation embryos express PDGF-A mRNA in both embryonic ectoderm and in ectoderm lining the ectoplacental cavity, whereas PDGFα receptor mRNA is detected in the mesoderm layers of both embryonic and extraembryonic membranes *(254)*. These results suggest that after implantation, early mesoderm development depends on stimulation by ectodermally produced PDGF-A. Orr-Urtreger and Lonai *(255)* have expanded these findings to later stages of murine development. By *in situ* hybridization, they localized PDGF-A and PDGFα in separate, but adjacent germ layers of primitive streak embryos, early axial structures, the skin, the developing forelimb, the branchial arches, and various sense organs *(256)*. Homozygous Patch embryos, where PDGFα is deleted, mostly die before the 11th d of gestation. The embryos that survive until early organogenesis are very small, have hypertrophic yolk sacs, small and undifferentiated somites, convoluted neural tubes, large heart and pericardium, rudimentary limb buds, and branchial arches. In addition, the skin is missing the dermis, and connective tissue is reduced in many organs *(251)*.

PDGF plays a major role in platelet formation and kidney development. PDGFβ receptor-deficient mice are hemorrhagic, thrombocytopenic, and severely anemic *(257, 258)* with profound defects in kidney glomeruli, and die at or shortly before birth. However, many cell types and tissues that expressed the receptor, like major blood vessels and the heart, appear normal. In the latter case, a compensatory mechanism by the α-subunit has been proposed. PDGF-BB may act as a trophic factor for mesencephalic dopaminergic neurons in both humans and rats *(259)*. In addition, PDGF is an important mitogen and growth regulator for glial cells, and all three isoforms of PDGF and PDGFβ receptor are present in neural structures during development in mouse *(260)*. In cultured osteoblasts isolated from fetal rats, all three PDGF isoforms stimulated DNA, and collagen synthesis and alkaline phosphatase activity *(261)*.

PDGF receptors have been detected in the pig endometrium, and the protein has been mainly located in stromal and endothelial cells, the wall of endometrial blood vessels, and the nonvascular smooth muscle cells of the myometrium *(262)*. The smooth muscle cells of the tunica media of major uterine vessels also showed some immunoreactivity. PDGF receptors have been found in trophoblasts and adjoining blood capillaries. Immunoreactivity was intense in early pregnancy and at term, two periods under major estrogenic influence, in both fetal and maternal tissues. PDGF-AB and PDGFβ receptors have been detected in human endometrial tissue by immunocytochemistry *(263)*. The receptor localized in luminal and glandular epithelium and stromal cells. The ligand was present only in stromal cells. PDGF stimulates stromal cell proliferation in vitro, but only in the presence of progesterone *(134)*. PDGF is mitogenic for human cytotrophoblast cells in an autocrine manner and may play a role in successful implantation, since PDGF ligands and receptors are expressed in the invasive cytotrophoblastic portion of the first trimester human placenta *(264,265)*. Extravillous placental cytotrophoblast cells express the PDGFα and β receptors, both in vivo and in vitro, and produce PDGF-B protein. Immunocytochemical analysis shows that PDGFα receptors are located in the cell surface, but PDGFβ receptors are detected only intracellularly. The two types of receptors are expressed in different cytotrophoblast subpopulations. Furthermore, the addition of PDGF-AA and PDGF-BB to cytotrophoblast primary cultures induced a significant increase in DNA synthesis.

PDGF ligands and receptors are proposed to contribute to angiogenesis of the developing placenta *(266)*. Analysis of first trimester human placenta showed that most microcapillary endothelial cells coexpress the PDGF-B and PDGFβ receptor mRNAs. In contrast, endothelial cells of macroblood vessels have high levels of PDGF-B mRNA, whereas PDGFβ receptor mRNA was not detectable. However, the receptor could be found in the stromal and smooth muscle cells of the surrounding intima as the PDGF-B signaling pathway switched from an autocrine to a paracrine mechanism. Similarly, PDGF-B is induced in the vasculature after acute mechanical injury. In rat aorta, the activated expression of this gene is preceded by a marked increase in the amount of the early-growth-response gene product Egr-1 at the endothelial wound edge *(267)*.

Vascular Endothelial Growth Factor (VEGF)

VEGF was isolated from conditioned medium of folliculostellate cells by heparin-Sepharose affinity chromatography *(268)*. This growth factor is a potent mitogen for endothelial cells and increases vascular permeability *(see 269)*. Purification of vascular permeability factor (VPF) revealed that these two factors (VEGF and VPF) are in fact coded for by a single gene, and the protein variants are generated by alternative mRNA splicing *(270,271)*. VEGF has been considered a member of the PDGF gene family, because it contains eight conserved cysteines *(272)*, although it only shares 18% overall identity with PDGF-B. A gene related to VEGF termed placental growth factor (PlGF), has been isolated from a human placental cDNA library *(273)*, and it has at least two alternative spliced mRNAs *(273,274)*. Expression of PlGF has not been observed in tissues other than the placenta *(275)*, but it has been detected in a variety of endothelial cells *(276)*. PlGF, like VEGF isoforms, are homodimeric glycoproteins *(277)*. The purified isoforms of PlGF do not stimulate vascular proliferation or permeability, but they potentiate these actions of VEGF both in culture and in vivo *(277)*.

VEGF mRNA has been localized in first trimester and term placenta of humans *(278)*, and during vasculogenesis and embryonic angiogenesis in the mouse *(279,280)* and rat *(281)*. VEGF localized to the human maternal glandular epithelial cells and macrophages in first trimester pregnancy *(278)*. In the human fetal cells, VEGF mRNA localized primarily to cells within the placental villi adjacent to the fetal capillaries. This distribution suggests VEGF involvement in angiogenesis *(278)*. VEGF expression in term placenta suggests that this growth factor regulates vascular permeability at later stages of pregnancy *(278)*. Two transcripts for VEGF have been reported in ovine placenta *(282)*. A major transcript of 3.7 kb was found in the cotyledon, chorion, and amnion. The minor transcript of 1.7 kb was present only in cotyledon and chorion. The presence of VEGF mRNA between 100 and 140 d of pregnancy suggested that it is one factor promoting angiogenesis and vascular perfusion of the placental and fetal membranes in the sheep *(282)*.

Products corresponding to four of the predicted isoforms have been identified using RT-PCR in cycling human endometrium, first trimester trophoblast, first trimester decidua, and term placenta *(278)*. Western blot analysis of human placentae *(283)* verified expression of four VEGF isoforms. The form corresponding to the full-length translation product coding for the 206-kDa isoform was also found on immunoblots, although the mRNA was absent in previous studies *(278)*. The mRNA for this form of the protein could also be detected in placental villi following two rounds of PCR *(284)*. Immunolocalization studies identified VEGF in the villous cytotrophoblast in human first trimester placenta and in syncytiotrophoblast thereafter *(283)*. Diffuse VEGF was present in the villous stroma at term, suggesting matrix-bound VEGF could be utilized for capillary remodeling, repair, or maintenance throughout gestation *(283)*.

VEGF mRNA localized by in situ hybridization in the giant trophoblast cells of early postimplantation rat embryos, and to the mesometrium of the uterus at this same time *(281)*. ^{125}I-labeled VEGF bound to the hemangioblasts (blood islands) within the yolk sac and along the lumina of blood vessels of both embryonic and maternal origin. VEGF mRNA accumulates at the mesometrial and antimesometrial decidual beds in pregnant mice between d 6 and 8 of pregnancy *(280)*. VEGF is expressed in many human fetal tissues at midgestation *(285)*. Interestingly, at this time of pregnancy, the mRNA is found in epithelial cells and myocytes, and not in endothelial cells. This suggests that VEGF may act by paracrine mechanisms, since VEGF has been shown to be specifically mitogenic for endothelial cells *(286,287)*, and it supports cord-like blood vessel structure formation in E14 stage rat embryonic hearts cultured on collagen gels *(138)*.

The deduced amino acid sequence of the three VEGF receptors has revealed structural similarity to the fms family. These receptors constitute a gene family coding for type III tyrosine kinase receptors containing five immunoglobulin-like loops in their extracellular domains *(288–290)*. Related receptors in this family include the colony-stimulating factor-1 (CSF-1) gene receptor *(288)* and the PDGF receptor genes *(291)*. Three tyrosine kinase receptors Flt-1, Flt-4, and KDR/Flk-1 have been shown to bind VEGF with high affinity. Distinct patterns of expression have been reported in the human fetus *(292)* and mouse embryo *(293,294)*.

In the human fetus, distinct but overlapping patterns of expression for the three receptors have been reported *(292)*. The authors propose that differential expression of these receptors suggests they may have distinct functions in blood vessel growth or formation. This interpretation is supported by impaired vessel formation in embryos deficient in

KDR/Flk-1 *(295)* and Flt-1 *(296)*. In the human placenta at 9 wk, VEGF is produced by maternal macrophages found in the Nitabuch's layer *(297)*. Localization of flt-1 showed silver grains visible on the extravillous trophoblast cells and the cytotrophoblast shell around a villus. These results suggest that ligand is produced by the maternal side, and that receptors are expressed on the fetal side. Addition of VEGF to BeWo cells, a human trophoblast cell line, stimulated phosphorylation of MAP kinase in a time-dependent fashion. KDR/Flk-1 associates with endothelial cells at all stages of development in the mouse, including the blood islands in the yolk sac *(293)*. Colocalization of VEGF at these same developmental stages indicated expression of ligand and receptor in endothelial cells *(293)*. VEGF bound the KDR/Flk-1 receptor with high affinity, and receptor activation stimulated autophosphorylation as expected. Flt-1 expression is limited to endothelial cells in adult tissues, whereas the mRNA was expressed in early yolk sac mesenchyme *(294)*. On d 5–8 of pregnancy in the mouse, VEGF receptors accumulate primarily in cells of the decidualizing stromal bed *(280)*. The distribution of this growth factor and its receptors suggests that VEGF participates in angiogenesis at the mesometrial aspect of the endometrium, whereas its expression at the antimesometrial region is associated more with vascular permeability changes *(280)*.

High-affinity binding of VEGF to Flt-1 has been reported *(298)*, but this binding can fail to activate VEGF-dependent tyrosine phosphorylation *(288)*. Since BeWo cells express both Flt-1 and KDR/Flk-1 *(297)*, it is not clear which receptor is responsible for MAP kinase phosphorylation. KDR is expressed in endothelial cells from human, porcine, and rat *(276)*. It is also expressed in bovine and human placental tissues, but only in endothelial cells. PlGF does not bind with high affinity to KDR/Flk-1 receptor *(298)*, and KDR/Flk-1 antiserum does not precipitate ^{125}I-PlGF bound to human umbilical vein endothelial (HUVE) cells *(277)*. PlGF binds to FLT-1 with high affinity *(299)*; however, this binding is not sufficient to induce permeability changes or endothelial cell proliferation *(277)*, suggesting that receptor activation does not occur. Purified VEGF and PlGF are potent mitogens as heterodimers VEGF.PlGF for vascular endothelial cells, as are VEGF homodimers *(300)*. It will be of interest to identify the mechanisms involved in heterodimerization, and if this interaction between VEGF and PlGF is a mechanism for fine-tuning the regulation of vascular growth and permeability changes in the placenta.

The spatial and temporal expression of VEGF and PlGF suggests that these two factors are essential for angiogenesis and vasculogenesis, and as such, are closely involved with the efficiency of vascular exchanges between mother and fetus. These ligands alter cell function by binding and activating at least three tyrosine kinase receptors. Receptor activation is expected to promote endothelial cell proliferation and changes in vascular permeability. Since both of these growth factors interact with the same receptors, targeted disruption of the receptors did not precisely define unique roles for each of these ligands. However, recent evidence from VEGF knockout mice reveals abnormal blood vessel development and embryo lethality in mice lacking a single VEGF allele *(301,302)*. Thus, of the many growth factors that function in embryo–maternal interactions, VEGF has now been shown to be absolutely essential for establishment of the vascular system during placentation.

TRANSFORMING GROWTH FACTOR BETAs (TGFβs)

This large gene family of structurally related proteins includes TGF-βs, activins, inhibins, bone morphogenetic proteins, and Müllerian inhibiting substance *(303–305)*. Polypeptides in this growth factor family affect many cellular processes, such as angiogenesis, inflammation, osteogenesis, tissue repair and remodeling, and steroidogenesis. In this chapter, we focus on TGF-β as the prototype, since this growth factor has been implicated specificially in maternal–fetal interactions during pregnancy. There are three isoforms of TGF-β in mammals, and they are expressed in specific patterns during embryonic development and in many cell types in adult tissues *(306,307)*. One of the important functions of TGF-βs is to stimulate production of extracellular matrix molecules and their receptors, which is often accompanied by increased synthesis of protease inhibitors and repression of proteases that degrade the extracellular matrix *(see 304)*. TGF-βs have also been localized to the basement membrane and extracellular matrix providing a reservoir of TGF-β activity for surrounding cells.

TGF-β mRNAs have been localized throughout the uterine decidua at d 5–8 of pregnancy in the mouse *(308)*, and in decidual cells of rat uterus *(309)*. Using two different antibodies, it was shown that intracellular TGF-β was limited to cells in the primary decidual zone, but in the secondary decidual zone, immunoreactivity was found in the extracellular matrix *(308)*. The primary sites for extracellular accumulation of secreted TGF-βs were the decidualizing stroma, the secondary decidual zone, the decidual capsularis, and placental trophoblast cells *(308,309)*. TGF-β2 transcripts were present in the endometrium of the pregnant mare, and between d 38 and 42 of pregnancy, maternal leukocytes in the region of the developing endometrial cups were positive *(310)*. Moreover, TGF-β was localized within the leukocytes at the periphery of the degenerating endometrial cups *(310)*. TGF-β expression increased during conceptus elongation in the ewe, and variation in the spatial distribution and temporal expression of two distinct isoforms suggested an important role in early ovine development and placentation *(311,312)*. TGF-βs were more abundantly expressed in the allantoic membrane than in the chorion of the ovine placenta *(311)*. Two of the isoforms (TGF-β1 and β2) were present in chorion, allantois, placental endothelium, trophectoderm, and yolk sac of the sheep *(311)*. Mice homozygous for TGF-β1 null allele have defective yolk sac vasculogenesis and hematopoiesis *(313,314)*. Consistent with a possible role in angiogenesis, the number of erythroid cells within the yolk sac was reduced, and inadequate capillary tube formation was also observed in those mice *(314)*.

In the human endometrium, TGF-βs have been localized in decidua and placenta during the first trimester *(315,316)*. This growth factor was present in the extracellular matrix and chorionic villi during midgestation, and it also localized within decidual cells at term *(315)*. TGF-βs are proposed to regulate programmed cell death in uterine decidual cells *(317)*, a process that is necessary in early pregnancy to accommodate placental growth. The immunolocalization of TGF-βs at the implantation site suggested two possible functions *(318,319)*. First, TGF-βs may limit embryo migration *(318)*, since cell migration assays have shown that exogenous TGF-β stimulates integrin expression in trophoblast cells. Increased intergin receptor expression reduced embryo migration *(320)*. Second, expression of TGF-βs at the implantation site suggested possible functions in immunoprotection of the embryo, since TGF-βs are known immunomodulators in other cell types *(319)*.

Localization of TGF-βs at the maternal–fetal interface *(315)* suggests its importance in trophoblast differentiation. For example, there is induction of multinucleated cells in first trimester and term trophoblast cells in vitro *(315)*, a reduction in the amount of hCG and human placental lactogen secreted by cultured trophoblast, and an increase in production of oncofetal fibronectin in response to TGF-β *(321,322)*.

Recent evidence indicates that TGF-βs stimulate the production of oncofetal fibronectin deposition into the extracellular matrix connecting extravillous trophoblast and trophoblastic cell columns to the uterine decidua *(321)*. Enhanced spreading of cultured trophoblast cells on fibronectin substrates in response to TGF-β was also observed *(321)*. Maternally produced fibronectin may also promote trophoblast adhesion and spreading *(323,324)*. On d 6 of pregnancy in the rat, fibronectin mRNAs encoding the V95 and A regions were preferentially localized to the antimesometrial zone in the primary decidual cells. Accumulation of these mRNA splicing variants was dependent on decidualization, but the embryo was not required *(324)*. Taken together, these studies suggest that fibronectin deposition into the extracellular matrix promotes adhesion between embryonic and maternal tissues. An alternative interpretation of these observations is suggested by studies of mice lacking functional TGFβ-1, which have increased mononuclear leukocyte infiltration into multiple organs. Infiltration of leukocytes and increased adhesion to extracellular matrix proteins and endothelial cells may be explained by changes in the adhesive properties of leukocytic cells *(325)*. The increased cell adhesiveness was reduced by administration of polypeptides containing the cell and heparin binding sequences of fibronectin. Administration of the same fibronectin peptides to the knockout mice blocked leukocyte infiltration and moderated the lethal wasting syndrome. This suggests that newly synthesized fibronectin at the maternal–fetal interface may discourage maternal leukocyte infiltration.

The availability and efficacy of TGF-βs are controlled by a large group of binding proteins. Although the interaction of these proteins in TGF-β signaling is not understood, further clarification of their interactions with ligands will be important for understanding the biological action of TGF-βs. At least nine different proteins have been shown to bind TGF-β with binding constants in the nanomolar range (reviewed in *326,327*). Analysis of mutant cells suggests that two of the receptors, the type I and type II receptors, are required for intracellular signaling. Lung epithelial cell mutants that do not express TGF-β-dependent genes have lost type I and type II receptors. Since these cells do not express the genes normally induced by TGF-β, it suggests that the type I and type II receptors are key to intracellular signaling. Furthermore, type I and type II receptors have conserved regions, including nine cysteines and an intracellular serine/threonine kinase domain similar to the type II activin receptors *(328,329)*. Interaction between the type I and type II receptors is thought to be necessary for signal transduction.

The function of the other high-affinity binding proteins is not clear. Recent characterization of two of these proteins suggests their possible importance in pregnancy. TGF-β is present in a latent form in serum where it is bound to α_2-macroglobulin *(330,331)*. Pregnancy zone protein (PZP) is an abundant plasma protein in maternal circulation during pregnancy. Sequence identity between α_2-macroglobulin and PZP is approx 70%, and both are inhibitors of protease activity *(332)*. Comparison of the binding characteristics of PZP and α_2-macroglobulin showed that both inhibit the binding of TGF-β to high-affinity cell-surface receptors. Moreover, the affinity of TGF-β1 and TGF-β2 suggests that the availability of TGF-βs during pregnancy may be regulated by their binding to PZP *(332)*. Endoglin is a membrane glycoprotein that has been localized to vascular endothelial cells, hematopoietic cells, syncytiotrophoblast of first trimester and term placenta, and uterine stromal cells *(333–336)*. Crosslinking of TGF-β with its high-affinity receptors and subsequent immunoprecipitation with endoglin suggest that endoglin facilitates binding of TGF-βs to its high-affinity receptors *(335)*.

TGF-β1 and TGF-β2 were detected in postimplantation mouse embryos *(337,338)*. Transcripts were present prior to gastrulation only in the embryonic visceral endoderm. At 7.5 d after conception, the mRNAs for both transcripts were detected in all of the germ layers *(338)*. However, the signaling receptors were restricted to extraembryonic tissues at the time of gastrulation. The receptors were only found in the embryo proper during organogenesis. Mice lacking TGF-β3 exhibited delayed pulmonary development and defective palatogenesis, abnormalities consistent with defective epithelial-mesenchymal interactions, whereas the disruption of TGF-β1 receptors by targeted mutagenesis revealed mice with apparently normal phenotypes at birth, but approx 2 wk later, these mice began wasting and died *(339)*. In a subsequent set of experiments *(340)*, results indicated that the pups received TGF-β from the mother via the placenta and milk. A homozygous null female, and therefore lacking maternal TGF-β, was treated with dexamethasone to suppress wasting and death. She survived to reproduce a litter of seven pups. These pups died within 24 h of birth, and each exhibited cardiac abnormalities *(340)*. Taken together, these studies demonstrate that a gene "knockout" is not equivalent to a protein knockout, since the mother can serve as a protein source for the fetus as long as the protein is soluble.

One of the best supported functions for TGF-β1 is its immunosuppressive action on a variety of leukocytes. Disruption of the TGF-β1 gene by targeted mutagenesis leads to inflammatory disease after the pups are weaned *(341,342)*, whereas a protein with structural similarities to TGF-β2 called decidual suppressor factor (DSF) is released by small non-T-lymphocytes in murine decidua *(343,344)*. Lack of this latter factor or related proteins has been associated with recurrent abortion in humans *(345)*. Dore and coworkers *(312)* have suggested that the ovine embryo suppresses maternal TGF-β expression at the time of implantation. At later stages of pregnancy, there was stage-specific expression of the three TGF-β isoforms, suggesting that they play distinct roles during ovine placental development. Uterine luminal flushings from pregnant pigs contain a protein related to TGF-βs *(346)*. Partially purified luminal flushing fractions containing this protein suppressed thymidine incorporation into phytohemagglutinin-treated peripheral blood lymphocytes.

TUMOR NECROSIS FACTOR ALPHA (TNF-α)

TNF is a homotrimeric protein comprised of subunits with molecular masses of 17 kDa. TNF has traditionally been associated with activated macrophages and T-cells *(347)*. Accumulated evidence indicates that this growth factor/cytokine is a major modulator of the immune system. However, more recent results suggest that TNF also functions in pregnancy and early fetal development. Since the distribution, hormonal control, and postulated functions of TNF in reproduction have been thoroughly reviewed recently *(348,349)*, only the more salient points will be touched on here. The reader is referred to those excellent earlier reviews for more details.

Our chapter has primarily focused on growth factors that bind to high-affinity tyrosine kinase receptors and alter cell function. Compared with the tyrosine kinase receptors, little is known about cellular signal transduction pathways utilized by the TNF receptors. TNF receptors are comprised of a super gene family of related protein molecules. The family is comprised of type I and type II receptor proteins with amino acid similarities only in the extracellular domain *(350)*. The distribution and temporal expression of TNF receptors have not been extensively mapped in reproductive tissues. However, early reports indicated differences in the temporal expression patterns of TNF between the type I and type II receptors during pregnancy *(349)*. These findings suggest the potential for multiple TNF functions, perhaps via alternative signaling pathways, within the same tissue.

TNF mRNA and protein have been localized in the placentae of a wide variety of animals and humans (reviewed in *349*, refs. therein). The distribution of TNF is similar

Table 3
Hormonal Control of Growth Factors and Receptors

Ligand/receptor	*Hormone*	*Cell types*	*Species*	*References*
EGF	Estrogen	Epithelium/stroma	Mouse	*351,352*
EGF	Testosterone	Uterus	Mouse	*353*
EGFR	Estrogen/progesterone	Stroma	Mouse	*354,355*
TGF-α	Estrogen	Epithelium	Mouse	*85*
HB-EGF	Estrogen/progesterone	Epithelium/stroma	Rat	*107,108*
AR	Estrogen	Uterus	Mouse	*112*
bFGF	Estrogen	Adenocarcinoma	Human	*356*
	Estrogen/progesterone	Endometrial	Rat	*357*
IGF-1	Estrogen/progesterone	Uterus/stroma	Rodent	*358,369*
IGF-1	Estrogen	Uterus	Pig	*360*
IGF-1	Estrogen	Ishikawa cells	Human	*361*
IGFBP-1	Estrogen/progesterone	Uterus	Rodent	*362*
PDFG-A, PDGF-B	Estrogen	Epithelium/stroma	Mouse	*363*
PDFG-α, PDGF-β	Estrogen	Epithelium/stroma	Mouse	*363*
VEGF	Estrogen	Endometrial Adenocarcinoma	Human	*364*
VEGF	Estrogen/progesterone	Uterus	Rat	*364*
TGF-β2	Estrogen	Uterine epithelium	Mouse	*365*
TNF-α	Estrogen/progesterone	Uterus	Mouse	*349*
TNF-α-RI	Progesterone/estrogen	Uterus	Mouse	*349*

between the uterus and placenta of humans and rodents. Trophoblast cells from rodents and horse express TNF, and in humans, the trophoblast is the first lineage to express the TNF ligand *(349)*. Changes in the temporal and spatial distribution of TNF suggest it functions by both autocrine and paracrine mechanisms in the female reproductive tract. The well-characterized role of TNF in immunological cells, coupled with its interesting distribution in the uterus and placenta during early pregnancy, ensures continuing interest in the role of this growth factor in pregnancy and placental development.

HORMONAL CONTROL OF GROWTH FACTORS AND GROWTH FACTOR RECEPTORS

The uterus provides a unique example of a situation where tissue turnover is cyclical. Evidence has been emerging over the last five years to suggest that restructuring of uterine tissues is regulated in part by steroid hormones via their control of growth factor and growth factor receptor synthesis *(17–19)*. Estrogens in particular have been shown to stimulate a variety of growth factors and growth factor receptor mRNAs. The results from numerous studies are listed in Table 3, and readers are referred to the original references for details.

SUMMARY AND FUTURE DIRECTIONS

This chapter summarizes the spatial distribution and temporal expression of several growth factors and their receptors in maternal and conceptus tissues during pregnancy. The experimental evidence suggests that growth factors are important molecules whose biological activity participates in the complex cellular processes required for the establishment and maintenance of pregnancy in mammals. Variations in the temporal and spatial patterns of expression exist among species; however, our interpretation of the accumulating evidence is that the underlying mechanisms controlling placental and fetal growth appear more similar than different.

Clearly more research is required to delineate how growth factors and their receptors are regulated. This includes further understanding of hormonal control of the ligands and their receptors. However, transcriptional and posttranscriptional regulatory mechanisms known to regulate some factors are likely to represent but one facet of growth factor control. Additional mechanisms to consider include regulation of bioavailability via sequestration in the extracellular matrix and production of latent forms that become biologically active in response to specific signals.

Understanding the structural interactions of growth factors with their receptors has progressed rapidly in the last five yr. Ligand binding to receptor results in dimerization of the receptor followed by phosphorylation of tyrosine residues on a variety of substrate proteins. Activated receptors induce the production of second messengers, such as phospholipase C-γ, and trigger the *ras* signal transduction pathway. Key steps in these pathways have been identified, but many details remain obscure. Many growth factors and cytokines do not manifest intrinsic kinase activity, and defining their signal transduction pathway is a major challenge (*see* Chapter 3 of this vol.). Thus, more complete analysis of signal transduction cascades in reproductive tissues is an important area for future research. The biological importance of potential "fine-tuning" regulatory mechanisms, including receptor dimerization and alternative splicing, also needs to be clarified.

Insight into the function of particular growth factors has emerged from targeted mutagenesis studies. This approach will continue to provide important information about the developmental consequences of eliminating individual molecules. The evidence that the genetic background of an individual can affect the mutant phenotype *(78,79)* suggests the existence of complex developmental signal transduction pathways that are probably influenced by multiple gene products. Interpretation regarding the function of a given growth factor from mutant phenotypes, therefore, may require consideration of both the genetic background and the gender of the individual mutants. Scientists often support the importance of their favorite growth factor in biological processes. The lack of lethal effects from the gene knockout experiments (excepting VEGF) is very surprising, because growth factors regulate essential cellular processes. The lack of definable phenotypes from many knockout experiments suggests potential overlapping and redundant functions among growth factors. Although redundancy may complicate our understanding, it seems a fail-safe method to insure developmental success. The alternative viewpoint suggesting that expression of many proteins is superfluous *(366)* must also be considered. Considerable progress regarding the role of growth factors and their receptors has been accomplished in the last five yr. These proteins play essential roles in the establishment of pregnancy and in placental formation and fetal development. Increased understanding about the cellular consequences of growth factor action and the molecular mechanisms involved in their control in female reproduction seems a prudent strategy to enhance knowledge about bidirectional communication between the conceptus and mother. This knowledge may be used to plan effective methods to reduce infertility and to prevent fetal–placental growth retardation.

ACKNOWLEDGMENTS

The authors are deeply grateful to Joan Hunt (University of Kansas Medical Center), Rosalia Simmen (University of Florida), David Brigstock (Wexner Institute), and Lindsey

Hutt-Fletcher (UMKC) for their critical reading of this chapter and their helpful suggestions and comments. We thank our many colleagues, including Larry Reynolds (North Dakota State), Asgi Fazleabas (University of Illinois), Bob Bigsby (Indiana University), and Bob Wordinger (University of North Texas Health Science Center) for sharing their thoughts and reprints. The authors thank Jim Swafford (UMKC) for computer graphic assistance. We thank Theresa Parks and Rhonda Ploeger for help in the manuscript preparation. This work was supported by a grant from the University of Missouri Research Board.

REFERENCES

1. Psychoyos A (1986) Uterine receptivity for nidation. Ann NY Acad Sci 476:36–42.
2. Chang MC (1950) Development and fate of transferred rabbit ova or blastocyst in relation to the ovulation time of recipients. J Exp Zool 114:197–225.
3. Betteridge KJ, Eaglesome MD, Randall GCB, Mitchell D (1980) Collection, description, and transfer of embryos from cattle 10–16 days after oestrus. J Reprod Fertil 59:205–216.
4. Bergh PA, Navot D (1992) The impact of embryonic development and endometrial maturity on the timing of implantation. Fertil Steril 58:537–542.
5. Simmen FA, Simmen RCM, Bazer FW (1989) Maternal growth factors as mediators of embryonic and neonatal growth. Biochem Soc Trans 17:587–589.
6. Papaioannou VE, Ebert KM (1988) The preimplantation pig embryo: cell number and allocation to trophectoderm and inner cell mass of the blastocyst in vivo and in vitro. Development 102: 793–803.
7. Zavy MT (1994) Embryonic mortality in cattle, In: Embryonic Mortality in Domestic Species (Zavy MT, Geisert RD, eds.), CRC, Boca Raton, FL, pp. 99–140.
8. Nancarrow CD (1994) Embryonic mortality in the ewe and doe, In: Embryonic Mortality in Domestic Species (Zavy MT, Geisert RD, eds.), CRC, Boca Raton, FL, pp. 79–97.
9. Roberts JM, Redman CWG (1993) Pre-eclampsia: more than pregnancy-induced hypertension. Lancet 341:1447–1451.
10. Heap RB, Rider V, Wooding FBP, Flint APF (1986) Molecular and cellular signalling and embryo survival, In: Embryonic Mortality in Farm Animals (Sreenan JM, Diskin MG, eds.), Martinus Nijhoff, Dordrecht, 46–73.
11. Anthony RV, Pratt SL, Liang R, Holland MD (1995) Placental-fetal hormonal interactions: impact on fetal growth. J Anim Sci 73:1861–1871.
12. Amoroso EC (1952) Placentation, In: Marshall's Physiology of Reproduction (Parks AS, ed.), Longmans, London, pp. 127–311.
13. Mossman HW (1937) Comparative morphogenesis of the fetal membranes and accessory uterine structures. Contributions Embryology Carnegie Institution 26:129–246.
14. Reynolds LP, Redmer DA (1995) Utero-placental vascular development and placental function. J Anim Sci 73:1839–1851.
15. Strauss JF III, Martinez F, Kiriakidou M (1996) Placental steroid hormone synthesis: unique features and unanswered questions. Biol Reprod 54:303–311.
16. Roberts RM, Xie S, Mathialugan N (1996) Maternal recognition of pregnancy. Biol Reprod 54: 294–302.
17. Simmen FA, Simmen RCM (1991) Peptide growth factors and proto-oncogenes in mammalian conceptus development. Biol Reprod 44:1–5.
18. Pollard JW (1990) Regulation of polypeptide growth factor synthesis and growth factor-related gene expression in the rat and mouse uterus before and after implantation. J Reprod Fertil 88: 721–731.
19. Brigstock DR (1991) Growth factors in the uterus: steroidal regulation and biological actions. Baillière's Clin Endocrinol Metab 5:791–808.
20. Cross JC, Werb Z, Fisher SJ (1994) Implantation and the placenta: key pieces of the development puzzle. Science 266:1508–1518.
21. Giudice LC (1994) Growth factors and growth modulators in human uterine endometrium: their potential relevance to reproductive medicine. Fertil Steril 61:1–17.

22. Clarke CL, Sutherland RL (1990) Progestin regulation of cellular proliferation. Endocr Rev 11: 266–301.
23. Ullrich A, Schlessinger J (1990) Signal transduction by receptors with tyrosine kinase activity. Cell 61:203–212.
24. Schlessinger J, Ullrich A (1992) Growth factor signaling by receptor tyrosine kinases. Neuron 9: 383–391.
25. Johnson DE, Williams LT (1993) Structural and functional diversity in the FGF receptor multigene family. Adv Cancer Res 60:1–41.
26. Murray A, Hunt T (1993) The Cell Cycle. Oxford University Press.
27. Pendergast AM (1996) Nuclear tyrosine kinases: from Abl to WEE1. Curr Opinion Cell Biol 8: 174–181.
28. Streuli M (1996) Protein tyrosine phosphatases in signaling. Curr Opinion Cell Biol 8:182–188.
29. Nurse P (1994) Ordering S phase and M phase in the cell cycle. Cell 79:547–550.
30. Folkman J, Shing Y (1992) Angiogenesis. J Biol Chem 267:10,931–10,934.
31. D'Amore PA, Thompson RW (1987) Mechanisms of angiogenesis. Ann Rev Physiol 49:453–464.
32. Klagsbrun M, D'Amore PA (1991) Regulators of angiogenesis. Annu Rev Physiol 53:217–239.
33. Risau W (1991) Vasculogenesis, angiogenesis and endothelial cell differentiation during embryonic development, In: The Development of the Vascular System (Feinberg RN, Sherer GK, Auerbach R, eds.), Krager, Basel, pp. 58–68.
34. Reynolds LP, Killilea SD, Redmer DA (1992) Angiogenesis in the female reproductive system. FASEB J 6:886–892.
35. Folkman J, Klagsbrun M (1987) Angiogenic factors. Science 235:442–447.
36. Reynolds LP, Redmer DA (1988) Secretion of angiogenic activity by placental tissues of cows at several stages of gestation. J Reprod Fertil 83:497–502.
37. Millaway DS, Redmer DA, Kirsch JD, Anthony RV, Reynolds LP (1989) Angiogenic activity of maternal and fetal placental tissues of ewes throughout gestation. J Reprod Fertil 86:689–696.
38. D'Amore PA, Smith SR (1993) Growth factor effects on cells of the vascular wall: a survey. Growth Factors 8:61–75.
39. Schwartzman RA, Cidlowski JA (1993) Apoptosis: The biochemistry and molecular biology of programmed cell death. Endocr Rev 14:133–151.
40. Collins MKL, Rivas AL (1993) The control of apoptosis in mammalian cells. Trends Biochem Sci 18:307–309.
41. Browne CA (1991) Epidermal growth factor and transforming growth factor α. Baillière's Clin Endocrinol Metab 5:553–569.
42. Prigent SA, Lemoine NR (1992) The type I (EGFR-related) family of growth factor receptors and their ligands. Prog Growth Factor Res 4:1–24.
43. Carpenter G, Cohen S (1979) Epidermal growth factor. Annu Rev Biochem 48:193–216.
44. Heidaran MA, Fleming TP, Bottaro DP, Bell GI, Di Fiore PP, Aaronson SA (1990) Transformation of NIH3T3 fibroblasts by an expression vector for the human epidermal growth factor precursor. Oncogene 5:1265–1270.
45. Breyer JA, Cohen S (1990) The epidermal growth factor precursor isolated from murine kidney membranes. Chemical characterization and biological properties. J Biol Chem 265:16,564–16,570.
46. Evain-Brion D, Alsat E (1994) Epidermal growth factor receptor and human fetoplacental development. J Pediatr Endocrinol 7:295–302.
47. Bass KE, Morrish D, Roth I, Bhardwaj D, Taylor R, Zhou Y, Fisher SJ (1994) Human cytotrophoblast invasion is up-regulated by epidermal growth factor: evidence that paracrine factors modify this process. Dev Biol 164:550–561.
48. Harvey MB, Leco KJ, Arcellana-Panlilio MY, Zhang X, Edwards DR, Schultz GA (1995) Proteinase expression in early mouse embryos is regulated by leukaemia inhibitory factor and epidermal growth factor. Development 121:1005–1014.
49. Hofmann GE, Scott RT Jr, Bergh PA, Deligdisch L (1991)Immunohistochemical localization of epidermal growth factor in human endometrium, decidua, and placenta. J Clin Endocrinol Metab 73:882–887.
50. Ladines-Llave CA, Maruo T, Manalo AS, Mochizuki M (1991) Cytologic localization of epidermal growth factor and its receptor in developing human placenta varies over the course of pregnancy. Am J Obstet Gynecol 165:1377–1382.
51. Amemiya K, Kurachi H, Adachi H, Morishige K-I, Adachi K, Imai T, Miyake A (1994) Involvement of epidermal growth factor (EGF)/EGF receptor autocrine and paracrine mechanism in human trophoblast cells: functional differentiation *in vitro*. J Endocrinol 143:291–301.

52. Mühlhauser J, Crescimanno C, Kaufmann P, Höfler H, Zaccheo D, Castellucci M (1993) Differentiation and proliferation patterns in human trophoblast revealed by c-erbB-2 oncogene product and EGF-R. J Histochem Cytochem 41:165–173.
53. Duello TM, Bertics PJ, Fulgham DL, Van Ess PJ (1994) Localization of epidermal growth factor receptors in first- and third-trimester human placentas. J Histochem Cytochem 42:907–915.
54. Haining RE, Schofield JP, Jones DS, Rajput-Williams J, Smith SK (1991) Identification of mRNA for epidermal growth factor and transforming growth factor-alpha present in low copy number in human endometrium and decidua using reverse transcriptase-polymerase chain reaction. J Mol Endocrinol 6:207–214.
55. Hofmann GE, Drews MR, Scott RTJ, Navot D, Heller D, Deligdisch L (1992) Epidermal growth factor and its receptor in human implantation trophoblast: immunohistochemical evidence for autocrine/paracrine function. J Clin Endocrinol Metab 74:981–988.
56. Hofmann GE, Horowitz GM, Scott RT Jr, Navot D (1993) Transforming growth factor-α in human implantation trophoblast: immunohistochemical evidence for autocrine/paracrine function. J Clin Endocrinol Metab 76:781–785.
57. Fazleabas AT, Hild-Petito S, Verhage HG (1994) Secretory proteins and growth factors of the baboon (*papio anubis*) uterus: potential roles in pregnancy. Cell Biol Int 18:1145–1153.
58. Slowey MJ, Verhage HG, Fazleabas AT (1994) Epidermal growth factor, transforming growth factor-α, and epidermal growth factor receptor localization in the baboon (*papio anubis*) uterus during the menstrual cycle and early pregnancy. J Soc Gynecol Invest 1:277–284.
59. Tamada H, Kai Y, Mori J (1994) Epidermal growth factor-induced implantation and decidualization in the rat. Prostaglandins 47:467–475.
60. Johnson DC, Chatterjee S (1993) Epidermal growth factor (EGF) replaces estradiol for the initiation of embryo implantation in the hypophysectomized rat. Placenta 14:429–438.
61. Bramley TA, Menzies GS (1992) Specific binding sites for ^{125}I-labelled epidermal growth factor in the ovine corpus luteum and human placenta. J Endocrinol 135:5–16.
62. Mimouni F, Hoath SB, Hammond G (1991) Effects of maternally administered epidermal growth factor on placental permeability. Am J Obstet Gynecol 165:173–176.
63. Tsutsumi O, Taketani Y, Oka T (1993) The uterine growth-promoting action of epidermal growth factor and its function in the fertility of mice. J Endocrinol 138:437–443.
64. Kamei Y, Tsutsumi O, Kuwabara Y, Taketani Y (1993) Intrauterine growth retardation and fetal losses are caused by epidermal growth factor deficiency in mice. Am J Physiol 264:497–600.
65. Odaka K, Hiramatsu Y, Eguchi K, Kudo T (1993) Effects of epidermal growth factor on mouse fetal growth. Asia Oceania J Obstet Gynaecol 19:213–216.
66. Price WA, Stiles AD (1994) Determinants of fetal and neonatal growth. Curr Opinion Pediatr 6:135–141.
67. Alarid ET, Chen P, Schaudies RP, Nicoll CS (1993)Differential effects of an antiserum to epidermal growth factor on the development of transplanted rat embryos and fetal structures in vivo. Growth Factors 8:235–243.
68. Lacroix MC, Kann G (1993) Ontogeny and characterization of epidermal growth factor receptors on the fetal area of the sheep placenta. J Endocrinol 136:43–50.
69. Gharib-Hamrouche N, Chene N, Guillomot M, Martal J (1993) Localization and characterization of EGF/TGF-α receptors on peri-implantation trophoblast in sheep. J Reprod Fertil 98: 385–392.
70. Vaughan TJ, James PS, Pascall JC, Brown KD (1992) Expression of the genes for TGF alpha, EGF and the EGF receptor during early pig development. Development 116:663–669.
71. Zhang Z, Krause M, Davis DL (1992) Epidermal growth factor receptors in porcine endometrium: binding characteristics and the regulation of prostaglandin E and F2 alpha production. Biol Reprod 46:932–936.
72. Kennedy TG, Brown KD, Vaughan TJ (1994) Expression of the genes for the epidermal growth factor receptor and its ligands in porcine oviduct and endometrium. Biol Reprod 50:751–756.
73. Stewart F, Power CA, Lennard SN, Allen WR, Amet L, Edwards RM (1994) Identification of the horse epidermal growth factor (EGF) coding sequence and its use in monitoring EGF gene expression in the endometrium of the pregnant mare. J Mol Endocrinol 12:341–50.
74. Shigeta H, Taga M, Katoh A, Minaguchi H (1993) Ontogenesis and distribution of epidermal growth factor immunoreactivity and binding activity in the mouse fetal and neonatal tissues. Endocr J 40:641–647.
75. Klein JM, Nielsen HC (1992) Sex-specific differences in rabbit fetal lung maturation in response to epidermal growth factor. Biochim Biophys Acta 1133:121–126.

76. Raaberg L, Nexo E, Jorgensen PE, Poulsen SS, Jakab M (1995) Fetal effects of epidermal growth factor deficiency induced in rats by autoantibodies against epidermal growth factor. Pediatr Res 37:175–181.
77. Mendelson CR, Boggaram V (1990) Hormonal and developmental regulation of pulmonary surfactant synthesis in fetal lung. Baillières Clin Endocrinol Metab 4:351–378.
78. Threadgill DW, Dlugosz AA, Hansen LA, Tennenbaum T, Lichti U, Yee D, LaMantia C, Mourton T, Herrup K, Harris RC, Barnard JA, Yuspa SH, Coffey RJ, Magnuson T (1995) Targeted disruption of mouse EGF receptor: effect of genetic background on mutant phenotype. Science 269: 230–233.
79. Sibilia M, Wagner EF (1995) Strain-dependent epithelial defects in mice lacking the EGF receptor. Science 269:234–238.
80. Miettinen PJ, Berger JE, Meneses J, Phung Y, Pedersen RA, Werb Z, Derynck R (1995) Epithelial immaturity and multiorgan failure in mice lacking epidermal growth factor receptor. Nature 376:337–341.
81. Derynck R (1988) Transforming growth factor α. Cell 54:593–595.
82. Massagu J (1990) Transforming growth factor-α. A model for membrane-anchored growth factors. J Biol Chem 265:21,393–21,396.
83. Han VKM, Hunter ES III, Pratt RM, Zendengui JG, Lee DC (1987) Expression of rat transforming growth factor alpha mRNA during development occurs predominantly in the maternal decidua. Mol Cell Biol 7:2335–2343.
84. Tamada H, Das SK, Andrews GK, Dey SK (1991) Cell-type-specific expression of transforming growth factor-alpha in the mouse uterus during the peri-implantation period. Biol Reprod 45: 365–372.
85. Nelson KG, Takahashi T, Lee DC, Luetteke NC, Bossert NL, Ross K, Eitzman BE, McLachlan JA (1992) Transforming growth factor-α is a potential mediator of estrogen action in the mouse uterus. Endocrinology 131:1657–1664.
86. Horowitz GM, Scott RT Jr, Drews MR, Navot D, Hofmann GE (1993) Immunohistochemical localization of transforming growth factor-α in human endometrium, decidua, and trophoblast. J Clin Endocrinol Metab 76:786–792.
87. Lysiak JJ, Han VK, Lala PK (1993) Localization of transforming growth factor alpha in the human placenta and decidua: role in trophoblast growth. Biol Reprod 49:885–894.
88. Filla MS, Zhang CX, Kaul KL (1993) A potential transforming growth factor α/epidermal growth factor receptor autocrine circuit in placental cytotrophoblasts. Cell Growth Differ 4:387–393.
89. Bissonnette F, Cook C, Geoghegan T, Steffen M, Henry J, Yussman MA, Schultz G (1992) Transforming growth factor-alpha and epidermal growth factor messenger ribonucleic acid and protein levels in human placentas from early, mid, and late gestation. Am J Obstet Gynecol 166:192–199.
90. Lewintre EJ, Orava M, Vihko R (1994) Regulation of 17β-hydroxysteroid dehydrogenase type 1 by epidermal growth factor and transforming growth factor-α in choriocarcinoma cells. Endocrinology 135:2629–2634.
91. Gharib-Hamrouche N, Chene N, Martal J (1995) Comparative expression of TGF-alpha and EGF genes in the ovine conceptus and uterine endomterium in the peri-implantation period. Reprod Nutr Dev 35:291–303.
92. Miettinen PJ (1993) Transforming growth factor-alpha and epidermal growth factor expression in human fetal gastrointestinal tract. Pediatr Res 33:481–486.
93. Hormi K, Lehy T (1994) Developmental expression of transforming growth factor-alpha and epidermal growth factor receptor proteins in the human pancreas and digestive tract. Cell Tissue Res 278:439–450.
94. Burton PBJ, Quirke P, Sorensen CM, Nehlsen-Cannarella SL, Bailey LL, Knight DE (1993) Growth factor expression during rat development: a comparison of TGF-β_3, TGF-α, bFGF, PDGF and PDGF-R. Int J Exp Pathol 74:87–96.
95. Kubiak J, Mitra MM, Steve AR, Hunt JD, Davies P, Pitt BR (1992) Transforming growth factor-alpha gene expression in late-gestation fetal rat lung. Pediatr Res 31:286–290.
96. Strandjord TP, Clark JG, Hodson WA, Schmidt RA, Madtes DK (1993) Expression of transforming growth factor-alpha in mid-gestation human fetal lung. Am J Respir Cell Mol Biol 8: 266–272.
97. Mann GB, Fowler KJ, Gabriel A, Nice EC, Williams RI, Dunn AR (1993) Mice with a null mutation of the TGFα gene have abnormal skin architecture, wavy hair, and curly whiskers and often develop corneal inflammation. Cell 73:249–261.

98. Luetteke NC, Qui TH, Peiffer RL, Oliver P, Smithies O, Lee DC (1993) TGFα deficiency results in hair follicle and eye abnormalities in targeted and waved-1 mice. Cell 73:263–278.
99. Besner GE, Whelton D, Crissman-Combs MA, Steffen CL, Kim GY, Brigstock DR (1992) Interaction of heparin-binding EGF-like growth factor (HB-EGF) with the epidermal growth factor receptor: modulation by heparin, heparinase, or synthetic heparin-binding HB-EGF fragments. Growth Factors 7:289–296.
100. Higashiyama S, Abraham JA, Miller J, Fiddes JC, Klagsbrun M (1991) A heparin-binding growth factor secreted by macrophage-like cells that is related to EGF. Science 251:936–939.
101. Higashiyama S, Lau K, Besner GE, Abraham JA, Klagsbrun M (1992) Structure of heparin-binding EGF-like growth factor. Multiple forms, primary structure, and glycosylation of the mature protein. J Biol Chem 267:6205–6512.
102. Naglich JG, Metherall JE, Russell DW, Eidels L (1992) Expression cloning of a diphtheria toxin receptor: identity with a heparin-binding EGF-like growth factor precursor. Cell 69:1051–1061.
103. Besner GE, Higashiyama S, Klagsbrun M (1990) Isolation and characterization of a macrophage-derived heparin-binding growth factor. Cell Regul 1:811–819.
104. Cook PW, Mattox PA, Keeble WW, Pittelkow MR, Plowman GD, Shoyab M, Adelman JP, Shipley GD (1991) A heparin sulfate-regulated human keratinocyte autocrine factor is similar or identical to amphiregulin. Mol Cell Biol 11:2547–2557.
105. Roberts RM, Bazer FW (1988) The functions of uterine secretions. J Reprod Fertil 82:875–892.
106. Kim GY, Besner GE, Steffen CL, McCarthy DW, Downing MT, Luquette MH, Abad MS, Brigstock DR (1995) Purification of heparin-binding epidermal growth factor-like growth factor from pig uterine luminal flushings, and its production by endometrial tissues. Biol Reprod 52: 561–571.
107. Zhang Z, Funk C, Roy D, Glasser S, Mulholland J (1994) Heparin-binding epidermal growth factor-like growth factor is differentially regulated by progesterone and estradiol in rat uterine epithelial and stromal cells. Endocrinology 134:1089–1094.
108. Zhang Z, Funk C, Glasser SR, Mulholland J (1994) Progesterone regulation of heparin-binding epidermal growth factor-like growth factor gene expression during sensitization and decidualization in the rat uterus: effects of the antiprogestin, ZK 98.299. Endocrinology 135:1256–1263.
109. Das SK, Wang X-N, Paria BC, Damm D, Abraham JA, Klagsbrun M, Andrews GK, Dey SK (1994) Heparin-binding EGF-like growth factor gene is induced in the mouse uterus temporally by the blastocyst solely at the site of its apposition: a possible ligand for interaction with blastocyst EGF-receptor in implantation. Development 120:1071–1083.
110. Plowman GD, Green JM, McDonald VL, Neubauer MG, Disteche CM, Todaro GJ, Shoyab M (1990) The amphiregulin gene encodes a novel epidermal growth factor-related protein with tumor-inhibitory activity. Mol Cell Biol 10:1969–1981.
111. Lysiak JJ, Johnson GR, Lala PK (1995) Localization of amphiregulin in the human placenta and decidua throughout gestation: role in trophoblast growth. Placenta 16:359–366.
112. Das SK, Chakraborty I, Paria BC, Wang X-N, Plowman G, Dey SK (1995) Amphiregulin is an implantation-specific and progesterone-regulated gene in the mouse uterus. Mol Endocrinol 9: 691–705.
113. Gospodarowicz D, Ferrara N, Schweigerer L, Neufeld G (1987) Structural characterization and biological functions of fibroblast growth factors. Endocr Reviews 8:95–114.
114. Basilico C, Moscatelli D (1992) The FGF family of growth factors and oncogenes. Adv Cancer Res 59:115–165.
115. Miyamoto M, Naruo KI, Seko C, Matsumoto S, Kondo T, Kurokawa T (1993) Molecular cloning of a novel cytokine cDNA encoding the ninth member of the fibroblast growth factor family, which has a unique secretion property. Mol Cell Biol 13:4251–4259.
116. Folkman J, Klagsbrun M, Sasse J, Wadzinski M, Ingber D, Vladovsky I (1988) A heparin-binding angiogenic protein-basic fibroblast growth factor is stored within basement membrane. Am J Pathol 130:393–400.
117. Aviezer D, Hecht D, Saftan M, Eisinger M, David G, Yayon A (1994) Perlecan, basal lamina proteoglycan, promotes basic fibroblast growth factor-receptor binding, mitogenesis, and angiogenesis. Cell 79:1005–1013.
118. Spivak-Kroizman T, Lemmon MA, Dikic I, Ladbury JE, Pinchasi DM, Huang J, Jaye M, Crumley G, Schlessinger J, Lax I (1994) Heparin-induced oligomerization of FGF molecules is responsible for FGF receptor dimerization, activation, and cell proliferation. Cell 79:1015–1024.
119. Logan A, Hill DJ (1992) Bioavailability: is this a key event in regulating the action of peptide growth factors? J Endocrinol 134:157–161.

120. Cordon-Cardo C, Vlodavsky I, Haimovitz-Friedman A, Hicklin D, Fuks Z (1990) Expression of basic fibroblast growth factor in normal human tissues. Lab Invest 63:832–840.
121. Rusnati M, Casarotti G, Pecorelli S, Ragnotti G, Presta M (1990) Basic fibroblast growth factor in ovulatory cycle and postmenopausal human endometrium. Growth Factors 3:299–307.
122. Cattini PA, Nichel B, Bock M, Kardami E (1991) Immunolocalization of basic fibroblast growth factor (bFGF) in growing and growth-inhibited placental cells: a possible role for bFGF in placental cell development. Placenta 12:341–352.
123. Ferriani RA, Charnock-Jones DS, Prentice A, Thomas EJ, Smith SK (1993) Immunohistochemical localization of acidic and basic fibroblast growth factors in normal human endometrium and endometriosis and the detection of their mRNA by polymerase chain reaction. Hum Reprod 8: 11–16.
124. Pekonen F, Nyman T, Rutanene E-M (1993) Differential expression of keratinocyte growth factor and its receptor in the human uterus. Mol Cell Endocrinol 95:43–49.
125. Koji T, Chedid M, Rubin JS, Slayden OD, Csaky KG, Aaronson SA, Brenner RM (1994) Progesterone-dependent expression of keratinocyte growth factor mRNA in stromal cells of the primate endometrium: keratinocyte growth factor as a progestomedin. J Cell Biol 125:393–401.
126. Wordinger RJ, Moss AE, Lockard T, Gray D, Chang I-FC, Jackson TL (1992) Immunohistochemical localization of basic fibroblast growth factor within the mouse uterus. J Reprod Fertil 96:141–152.
127. Wordinger RJ, Smith KJ, Bell C, Chang I-FC (1994) The immunolocalization of basic fibroblast growth factor in the mouse uterus during the initial stages of embryo implantation. Growth Factors 11:175–186.
128. Carlone DL, Rider V (1993) Embryonic modulation of basic fibroblast growth factor in the rat uterus. Biol Reprod 49:653–665.
129. Rider V, Psychoyos A (1994) Inhibition of progesterone receptor function results in loss of basic fibroblast growth factor expression and stromal cell proliferation during uterine remodelling in the pregnant rat. J Endocrinol 140:239–249.
130. Brigstock DR, Heap RB, Barker PJ, Brown KD (1990) Purification of heparin-binding growth factors from porcine uterus. Biochem J 266:273–282.
131. Shams M, Ahmed A (1994) Localization of mRNA for basic fibroblast growth factor in human placenta. Growth Factors 11:105–111.
132. Abraham JA, Whang J-L, Tumulo A, Mergia A, Friedman J, Gospodarowicz D, Fiddes JC (1986) Human basic fibroblast: nucleotide sequence and genomic organization. EMBO J 5: 2523–2528.
133. Mignatti P, Morimoto T, Rifkin DB (1992) Basic fibroblast growth factor, a protein devoid of secretory signal sequence, is released by cells via a pathway independent of the endoplasmic reticulum-golgi complex. J Cell Physiol 151:81–93.
134. Irwin JC, Utian WH, Eckert RL (1991) Sex steroids and growth factors differentially regulate the growth and differentiation of cultured human endometrial stromal cells. Endocrinology 129: 2385–2392.
135. Piva M, Flieger O, Rider V (1996) Growth factor control of cultured rat uterine stromal cell proliferation is progesterone dependent. Biol Reprod 55:1333–1342.
136. Ferriani RA, Ahmed A, Sharkey A, Smith SK (1994) Colocalization of acidic and basic fibroblast growth factor (FGF) in human placenta and the cellular effects of bFGF in trophoblast cell line JEG-3. Growth Factors 10:259–268.
137. Oberbauer AM, Strong DD, Linkhart TA, Mohan S, Longo LD (1993) Fibroblast growth factor enhances the transcription and stability of human chorionic gonadotropin β-subunit messenger ribonucleic acid in jar choriocarcinoma cells. Endocrinology 132:757–762.
138. Ratajska A, Torry RJ, Kitten GT, Kolker SJ, Tomanek RJ (1995) Modulation of cell migration and vessel formation by vascular endothelial growth factor and basic fibroblast growth factor in cultured embryonic heart. Developmental Dynamics 203:399–407.
139. Simmen RCM, Ko Y, Simmen FA (1993) Insulin-like growth factors and blastocyst development. Theriogenology 39:163–175.
140. Finch PW, Rubin JS, Miki T, Ron N, Aaronson SA (1989) Human KGF is FGF-related with properties of a paracrine effector of epithelial cell growth. Science 245:752–755.
141. Yayon A, Zimmer Y, Guo-Hong S, Avivi A, Yarden Y, Givol D (1992) A confined variable region confers ligand specificity on fibroblast growth factor receptors: implications for the origin of the immunoglobulin fold. EMBO J 11:1885–1890.

142. Gonzalez A-M, Buscaglia M, Ong, M, Baird A (1990) Distribution of basic fibroblast growth factor in the 18-day rat fetus: localization in the basement membranes of diverse tissues. J Cell Biol 110:753–765.
143. Matsui Y, Zsebo K, Hogan BLM (1992) Derivation of pluripotential embryonic stem cells from murine primordial germ cells in culture. Cell 70:841–847.
144. Resnick JL, Bixler LS, Cheng I, Donavan PJ (1992) Long term proliferation of mouse primordial germ cells in culture. Nature 359:550–551.
145. Martin GR (1980) Teratocarcinomas and mammalian embryogenesis. Science 290:768–776.
146. Braunhut SJ, D'Amore PA, Gudas LJ (1992) The location and expression of fibroblast growth factor (FGF) in F9 visceral and parietal embryonic cells after retinoic acid-induced differentiation. Differentiation 50:141–152.
147. Klagsbrun M, Baird A (1991) A dual receptor system is required for basic fibroblast growth factor activity. Cell 67:229–231.
148. Yeh, J, Osathanondh R (1993) Expression of messenger ribonucleic acids encoding for basic fibroblast growth factor (FGF) and alternatively spliced FGF receptor in human fetal ovary and uterus. J Clin Endocrinol Metab 77:1367–1371.
149. Rider V, Piva M, Cohen ME, Carlone DL (1995) Alternative splicing and differential targeting of fibroblast growth factor receptor 1 in the pregnant rat uterus. Endocrinology 136:3137–3145.
150. Hrabe De Angelis M, Kirchner C (1993) Fibroblast growth factor induces primitive streak formation in rabbit pre-implantation embryos in vitro. Anat Embryol 187:269–273.
151. Slack J (1994) Role of fibroblast growth factors as inducing agents in early embryonic development. Mol Reprod Develop 39:118–125.
152. Yamaguchi TP, Rossant J (1995) Fibroblast growth factors in mammalian development. Curr Opinion Genet Dev 5:485–491.
153. Mummery CL, Van Rooyen M, Bracke M, Van den Eijnden-van Raaij J, Van Zoelin EJ, Alitalo K (1993) Fibroblast growth factor-mediated growth regulation and receptor expression in embryonal carcinoma and embryonic stem cells and human germ cell tumours. Biochem Biophys Res Commun 191:188–195.
154. Orr-Urtreger A, Givol D, Yagan A, Yarden Y, Lonai P (1991) Developmental expression of two murine fibroblast growth factor receptors, flg and bek. Development 109:911–923.
155. Yamaguchi TP, Conlon RA, Rossant J (1992) Expression of the fibroblast growth factor receptor FGFR-1/flg during gastrulation and segmentation in the mouse embryo. Dev Biol 152:75–88.
156. Peters KG, Werner S, Chen G, Williams LT (1992) Two FGF receptor genes are differentially expressed in epithelial and mesenchymal tissues during limb formation and organogenesis in the mouse. Development 114:233–243.
157. Deng C-X, Wynshaw-Boris A, Shen MM, Daugherty C, Ornitz DM, Leder P (1994) Murine FGFR-1 is required for early postimplantation growth and axial organization. Genes Dev 8: 3045–3057.
158. Yamaguchi TP, Harpal K, Henkemeyer M, Rossant J (1994) *Fgfr-1* is required for embryonic growth and mesodermal patterning during mouse gastrulation. Genes Dev 15:3032–3044.
159. Niswander L, Martin GR (1992) *Fgf-4* expression during gastrulation, myogenesis, limb and tooth development in the mouse. Development 114:755–768.
160. Feldman B, Poueymirou W, Papaioannou VE, Dechiara TM, Goldfarb M (1995) Requirement of FGF-4 for post implantation mouse development. Science 267:246–249.
161. Sussenbach JS (1989) The gene structure of the insulin-like growth factor family. Prog Growth Factor Res 1:33–48.
162. Nielsen FC (1992) The molecular and cellular biology of insulin-like growth factor II. Prog Growth Factor Res 4:257–290.
163. LeRoith D, Werner H, Beitner-Johnson D, Roberts CT Jr (1995) Molecular and cellular aspects of the insulin-like growth factor I receptor. Endocr Rev 16(2):143–163.
164. LeRoith D, Kavsan VM, Koval AP, Roberts CT Jr (1993) Phylogeny of the insulin-like growth factors (IGFs) and receptors: a molecular approach. Mol Reprod Dev 35:332–336.
165. Ullrich A, Gray A, Tam AW, Yang-Feng T, Tsubokawa M, Collins C, Henzel W, Le Bon T, Kathuria S, Chen E (1986) Insulin-like growth factor I receptor primary structure: comparison with insulin receptor suggests structural determinants that define functional specificity. EMBO J 5:2503–2512.
166. Siddle K (1992) The insulin receptor and type I IGF receptor: comparison of structure and function. Prog Growth Factor Res 4:301–320.

167. De Meyts P, Christoffersenrso B, Wallach B, Gronskov K, Yakushiji F, Symko RM (1995) Role of the time factor in signaling specificity: application to mitogenic and metabolic signaling by the insulin and insulin-like growth factor-I receptor tyrosine kinases. Metabolism 44:2–11.
168. Jones JI, Clemmons DR (1995) Insulin-like growth factors and their binding proteins: biological actions. Endocr Rev 16:3–34.
169. Rechler MM, Brown AL (1992) Insulin-like growth factor binding proteins: gene structure and expression. Growth Regul 2:55–68.
170. Frost RA, Mazella J, Tseng L (1993) Insulin-like growth factor binding protein-1 inhibits the mitogenic effect of insulin-like growth factors and progestins in human endometrial stromal cells. Biol Reprod 49:104–111.
171. Jones JI, D'Ercole AJ, Camacho-Hubner C, Clemmons DR (1991) Phosphorylation of insulin-like growth factor (IGF)-binding protein 1 in cell culture and in vivo: effects on affinity for IGF-I. Proc Natl Acad Sci USA 88:7481–7485.
172. Martin JL, Baxter RC (1992) Insulin-like growth factor binding protein-3: biochemistry and physiology. Growth Regul 2:88–99.
173. Drop SL, Schuller AG, Lindenbergh-Kortleve DJ, Groffen C, Brinkman A, Zwarthoff EC (1992) Structural aspects of the IGFBP family. Growth Regul 2:69–79.
174. Lamson G, Giudice LC, Cohen P, Liu F, Gargosky S, Muller HL, Oh Y, Wilson KF, Hintz RL, Rosenfeld RG (1993) Proteolysis of IGFBP-3 may be a common regulatory mechanism of IGF action in vivo. Growth Regul 3:91–95.
175. Lassarre C, Binoux M (1994) Insulin-like growth factor binding protein-3 is functionally altered in pregnancy plasma. Endocrinology 134:1254–1262.
176. Blat C, Villaudy J, Binoux M (1994) In vivo proteolysis of serum insulin-like growth factor (IGF) binding protein-3 results in increased availability of IGF to target cells. J Clin Invest 93:2286–2290.
177. Davenport ML, Pucilowska J, Clemmons DR, Lundblad R, Spencer JA, Underwood LE (1992) Tissue-specific expression of insulin-like growth factor binding protein-3 protease activity during rat pregnancy. Endocrinology 130:2505–2512.
178. Bastian SE, Walton PE, Wallace JC, Ballard FJ (1993) Plasma clearance and tissue distribution of labelled insulin-like growth factor-I (IGF-I) and an analogue LR3IGF-I in pregnant rats. J Endocrinol 138:327–336.
179. Hasegawa T, Hasegawa Y, Takada M, Tsuchiya Y (1995) The free form of insulin-like growth factor I increases in circulation during normal human pregnancy. J Clin Endocrinol Metab 80:3284–3286.
180. Nonoshita LD, Wathen NC, Dsupin BA, Chard T, Giudice LC (1994) Insulin-like growth factors (IGFs), IGF-binding proteins (IGFBPs), and proteolyzed IGFBP-3 in embryonic cavities in early human pregnancy: their potential relevance to maternal-embryonic and fetal interactions. J Clin Endocrinol Metab 79:1249–1255.
181. Hills FA, English J, Chard T (1996) Circulating levels of IGF-I and IGF-binding protein-1 throughout pregnancy: relation to birthweight and maternal weight. J Endocrinol 148:303–309.
182. Chard T (1994) Insulin-like growth factors and their binding proteins in normal and abnormal human fetal growth. Growth Regul 4:91–100.
183. Simmen RA, Green ML, Simmen FA (1995) IGF system in periimplantation uterus and embryonic development, In: Molecular and Cellular Aspects of Periimplantation Processes (Dey SK, ed.), Serono Symposia, Norwell, MA, pp. 185–204.
184. Jacob R, Barret E, Plewe G, Fagin KD, Sherwin RJ (1989) Acute effects of insulin-like growth factor-I on glucose and amino acid metabolism in the awake fasted rat. J Clin Invest 83:1717–1723.
185. Turkalj I, Keller U, Ninnis R, Vosmeer S, Stauffacher W (1992) Effect of increasing doses of recombinant human insulin-like growth factor-I on glucose, lipid, and leucine metabolism in man. J Clin Endocrinol Metab 75:1186–1191.
186. Douglas RG, Gluckman PD, Ball K, Breier B, Shaw JH (1991) The effects of infusion of insulin-like growth factor (IGF) I, IGF-II, and insulin on glucose and protein metabolism in fasted lambs. J Clin Invest 88:614–622.
187. Kniss DA, Shubert PJ, Zimmerman PD, Landon MB, Gabbe SG (1994) Insulinlike growth factors: their regulation of glucose and amino acid transport in placental trophoblasts isolated from first-trimester chorionic villi. J Reprod Med 39:240–256.
188. Karl PI (1995) Insulin-like growth factor-1 stimulates amino acid uptake by the cultured human placental trophoblast. J Cell Physiol 165:83–88.

189. Giudice LC, Dsupin BA, Jin IH, Vu TH, Hoffman AR (1993) Differential expression of messenger ribonucleic acids encoding insulin-like growth factors and their receptors in human uterine endometrium and decidua. J Clin Endocrinol Metab 76:1115–1122.
190. Wang C-Y, Diamon M, Shen S-J, Engelmann GL, Ilan J (1988) Insulin-like growth factor-I messenger ribonucleic acid in the developing human placenta and in term placenta of diabetics. Mol Endocrinol 2:217–229.
191. Milio LA, Hu J, Douglas GC (1994) Binding of insulin-like growth factor I to human trophoblast cells during differentiation in vitro. Placenta 15:641–651.
192. Bhaumick B, George D, Bala RM (1992) Potentiation of epidermal growth factor-induced differentiation of cultured human placental cells by insulin-like growth factor-I. J Clin Endocrinol Metab 74:1005–1011.
193. Ohlsson R, Holmgren L, Glaser A, Szpecht A, Pfeifer-Ohlsson S (1989) Insulin-like growth factor 2 and short-range stimulatory loops in control of human placental growth. EMBO J 8:1993–1999.
194. Ohlsson R, Larsson E, Nilsson O, Wahlstrom T, Sundstrom P (1989) Blastocyst implantation precedes induction of insulin-like growth factor II gene expression in human trophoblasts. Development 106:555–559.
195. Glaser A, Luthman H, Stern I, Ohlsson R (1992) Spatial distribution of active genes implicated in the regulation of insulin-like growth factor stimulatory loops in human decidual and placental tissue of first-trimester pregnancy. Mol Reprod Dev 33:7–15.
196. Hild-Petito S, Verhage HG, Fazleabas AT (1994) Characterization, localization, and regulation of receptors for insulin-like growth factor I in the baboon uterus during the cycle and pregnancy. Biol Reprod 50:791–801.
197. Tarantino S, Verhage HG, Fazleabas AT (1992) Regulation of insulin-like growth factor-binding proteins in the baboon (*papio anubis*) uterus during early pregnancy. Endocrinology 130: 2354–2362.
198. Hustin J, Philippe E, Teisner B, Grudzinskas JG (1994) Immunohistochemical localization of two endometrial proteins in the early days of human pregnancy. Placenta 15:701–708.
199. Bell SC, Hales MW, Patel S, Kirwan PH, Drife JO (1985) Protein synthesis and secretion by the human endometrium and decidua during early pregnancy. Br J Obstet Gynaecol 92:793–803.
200. Fazleabas AT, Verhage HG, Waites G, Bell SC (1989) Characterization of an insulin-like growth factor binding protein, analogous to human pregnancy-associated secreted endometrial alpha 1-globulin, in decidua of the baboon (*papio anubis*) placenta. Biol Reprod 40:873–885.
201. Fazleabas AT, Verhage HG, Bell SC (1990) Insulin-like growth factor binding protein and pregnancy: regulation and function in the primate, In: Early Embryo Development and Paracrine Relationships (Heyner S, Wiley LM, eds.), Wiley and Liss, New York, 137–152.
202. Lennard SN, Stewart F, Allen WR (1995) Insulin-like growth factor II gene expression in the fetus and placenta of the horse during the first half of gestation. J Reprod Fertil 103:169–179.
203. Geisert RD, Lee CY, Simmen FA, Zavy MT, Fliss AE, Bazer FW, Simmen RC (1991) Expression of messenger RNAs encoding insulin-like growth factor-I, -II, and insulin-like growth factor binding protein-2 in bovine endometrium during the estrous cycle and early pregnancy. Biol Reprod 45:975–983.
204. Simmen FA, Simmen RCM, Geisert RD, Martinat-Botte F, Bazer FW, Terqui M (1992) Differential expression, during the estrous cycle and pre- and postimplantation conceptus development, of messenger ribonucleic acids encoding components of the pig uterine insulin-like growth factor system. Endocrinology 130:1547–1556.
205. Hofig A, Simmen FA, Bazer FW, Simmen RC (1991) Effects of insulin-like growth factor-I on aromatase cytochrome P450 activity and oestradiol biosynthesis in preimplantation porcine conceptuses in vitro. J Endocrinol 130:245–250.
206. Nestler JE (1993) Regulation of the aromatase activity of human placental cytotrophoblasts by insulin, insulin-like growth factor-I, and -II. J Steroid Biochem Mol Biol 44:449–457.
207. Green ML, Simmen RC, Simmen FA (1995) Developmental regulation of steroidogenic enzyme gene expression in the periimplantation porcine conceptus: a paracrine role for insulin-like growth factor-I. Endocrinology 136:3961–3970.
208. Chastant S, Monget P, Terqui M (1994) Localization and quantification of insulin-like growth factor-I (IGF-I) and IGF-II/mannose-6-phosphate (IGF-II/M6P) receptors in pig embryos during early pregnancy. Biol Reprod 51:588–596.
209. Chard T (1989) Hormonal control of growth in the human fetus. J Endocrinol 123:3–9.

210. Siler-Khodr TM, Forman J, Sorem KA (1995) Dose-related effect of IGF-I on placental prostanoid release. Prostaglandins 49:1–14.
211. Nason KS, Binder ND, Labarta JI, Rosenfeld RG, Gargosky SE (1996) IGF-II and IGF-binding proteins increase dramatically during rabbit pregnancy. J Endocrinol 148:121–130.
212. Bassett NS, Breier BH, Moore L, Gluckman PD (1990) Disappearance of labeled IGF-2 from plasma of the ovine fetus in late gestation. J Dev Physiol 13:295–301.
213. Langford KS, Nicolaides KH, Jones J, Abbas A, McGregor AM, Miell JP (1995) Serum insulin-like growth factor-binding protein-3 (IGFBP-3) levels and IGFBP-3 protease activity in normal, abnormal, and multiple human pregnancy. J Clin Endocrinol Metab 80:21–27.
214. Giudice LC, De Zegher F, Gargosky SE, Dsupin BA, De Las Fuentes L, Crystal RA, Hintz RL, Rosenfeld RG (1995) Insulin-like growth factors and their binding proteins in the term and preterm human fetus and neonate with normal and extremes of intrauterine growth. J Clin Endocrinol Metab 80:1548–1555.
215. Morel PC, Blair HT, Ormsby JE, Breier BH, McCutcheon SN, Gluckman PD (1994) Influence of fetal and maternal genotype for circulating insulin-like growth factor I on fetal growth in mice. J Reprod Fertil 101:9–14.
216. Gluckman PD, Morel PC, Ambler GR, Breier BH, Blair HT, McCutcheon SN (1992) Elevating maternal insulin-like growth factor-I in mice and rats alters the pattern of fetal growth by removing maternal constraint. J Endocrinol 134:R1–3.
217. Thissen JP, Ketelslegers JM, Underwood LE (1994) Nutritional regulation of the insulin-like growth factors. Endocr Rev 15:80–163.
218. Eshet R, Werner H, Klinger B, Silbergeld A, Laron Z, LeRoith D, Roberts CT Jr (1993) Up-regulation of insulin-like growth factor-I (IGF-I) receptor gene expression in patients with reduced serum IGF-I levels. J Mol Endocrinol 10:115–120.
219. Werner H, Shen-Orr Z, Stannard B, Burguera B, Roberts CJ Jr, LeRoith D (1990) Experimental diabetes increases insulin-like growth factor I and II receptor concentration and gene expression in the kidney. Diabetes 39:1490–1497.
220. Nissley P, Kiess W, Sklar M (1993) Developmental expression of the IGF-II/mannose 6-phosphate receptor. Mol Reprod Dev 35:408–413.
221. O'Mahoney JV, Brandon MR, Adams TE (1991) Developmental and tissue-specific regulation of ovine insulin-like growth factor II (IGF-II) mRNA expression. Mol Cell Endocrinol 78:87–96.
222. Lee CY, Chung CS, Simmen FA (1993) Ontogeny of the porcine insulin-like growth factor system. Mol Cell Endocrinol 93:71–80.
223. Lacroix MC, Servely JL, Kann G (1995) IGF-I and IGF-II receptors in the sheep placenta: evolution during the course of pregnancy. J Endocrinol 144:179–191.
224. Stevenson KR, Gilmour RS, Wathes DC (1994) Localization of insulin-like growth factor-I (IGF-I) and -II messenger ribonucleic acid and type 1 IGF receptors in the ovine uterus during the estrous cycle and early pregnancy. Endocrinology 134:1655–1664.
225. Owens JA, Falconer JF, Robinson JS (1987) The effect of restriction of placental growth on oxygen delivery to and consumption by the gravid uterus and fetus. J Dev Physiol 9:137–150.
226. Owens JA, Falconer JF, Robinson JS (1987) The effect of restriction of placental growth on fetal and utero-placental metabolism. J Dev Physiol 9:225–238.
227. Kind KL, Owens JA, Robinson JS, Quinn KJ, Grant PA, Walton PE, Gilmour RS, Owens PC (1995) Effect of restriction of placental growth on expression of IGFs in fetal sheep: relationship to fetal growth, circulating IGFs and binding proteins. J Endocrinol 146:23–34.
228. Owens JA, Kind KL, Carbone F, Robinson JS, Owens PC (1994) Circulating insulin-like growth factors-I and -II and substrates in fetal sheep following restriction of placental growth. J Endocrinol 140:5–13.
229. DeChiara TM, Efstratiadis A, Robertson EJ (1990) A growth-deficiency phenotype in heterozygous mice carrying an insulin-like growth factor II gene disrupted by targeting. Nature 345:78–80.
230. Baker J, Liv J-P, Robertson EJ, Efstratiadis A (1993) Role of insulin-like growth factors in embryonic and postnatal growth. Cell 75:73–82.
231. Liu J-P, Baker J, Perkins AS, Robertson EJ, Efstratiadis A (1993) Mice carrying null mutations of the genes encoding insulin-like growth factor I (lgf-1) and type 1 IGF receptor (lgf1r). Cell 75: 59–72.
232. Zhou J, Bondy C (1992) Insulin-like growth factor-II and its binding proteins in placental development. Endocrinology 131:1230–1240.

233. Tamemoto H, Kadowaki T, Tobe K, Yagi T, Sakura H, Hayakawa T, Terauchi Y, Ueki K,Kaburagi Y, Satoh S (1994) Insulin resistance and growth retardation in mice lacking insulin receptor substrate-1. Nature 372:182–186.
234. Li S, Ferber A, Miura M, Baserga R (1994) Mitogenicity and transforming activity of the insulin-like growth factor-I receptor with mutations in the tyrosine kinase domain. J Biol Chem 269: 32,558–32,564.
235. Kornfeld S (1992) Structure and function of the mannose 6-phosphate/insulinlike growth factor II receptors. Annu Rev Biochem 61:307–330.
236. Barlow DP, Stoger R, Harrmann BG, Saito K, Schweifer N (1991) The mouse insulin-like growth factor type-2 receptor is imprinted and closely linked to the Tme locus. Nature 349:84–87.
237. Johnson DR (1974) Hairpin-tail: a case of post-reductional gene action in the mouse eggs? Genetics 76:795–805.
238. Johnson DR (1975) Further observations on the hairpin tail (Thp) mutation in the mouse. Genet Res 24:207–213.
239. Winklin H, Silver LM (1984) Characterization of a recombinant mouse T haplotype that expresses a dominant lethal maternal effect. Genetics 108:1013–1020.
240. Filson AJ, Louvi A, Efstratiadis A, Robertson EJ (1993) Rescue of the T-associated maternal effect in mice carrying null mutations in *Igf-2* and *Igf2r*, two reciprocally imprinted genes. Development 118:731–736.
241. Wang Z-Q, Fund MR, Barlow DP, Wagner EF (1994) Regulation of embryonic growth and lysosomal targeting by the imprinted *Igf2/Mpr* gene. Nature 372:464–467.
242. Westermark B, Heldin C-H (1993) Platelet-derived growth factor. Acta Oncol 32(2):101–105.
243. Grotendorst GR, Seppa HEJ, Kleinman MK, Martin GR (1981) Attachment of smooth muscle cells to collagen and their migration toward platelet-derived growth factor is chemotactic for fibroblasts. Proc Natl Acad Sci USA 78:3669–3673.
244. Grotendorst GR, Chang T, Seppa HE, Kleinman HK, Martin GR (1982) Platelet-derived growth factor is a chemoattractant for vascular smooth muscle cells. J Cell Physiol 113:261–266.
245. Seppa HEJ, Grotendorst GR, Seppa S, Schiffmann E, Martin GR (1982) Platelet-derived growth factor is chemotactic for fibroblasts. J Cell Biol 92:584–588.
246. Hosang M, Rouge M, Wipf B, Eggimann B, Kaufmann F, Hunziker W (1989) Both homodimeric isoforms of PDGF (AA and BB) have mitogenic and chemotactic activity and stimulate phosphoinositol turnover. J Cell Physiol 140:558–564.
247. Pierce GF (1990) Macrophages: important physiologic and pathologic sources of polypeptide growth factors. Am J Respir Cell Mol Biol 2:233–234.
248. Hosgood G (1993) Wound healing. The role of platelet-derived growth factor and transforming growth factor beta. Vet Surg 22:490–495.
249. Antoniades HN (1991) PDGF: a multifunctional growth factor. Baillère's Clin Endocrinol Metab 5:595–613.
250. Johnsson A, Heldin C-H, Westermark B, Wasteson A (1982) Platelet growth factor: identification of constituent polypeptide chains. Biochem Biophys Res Commun 104:66–74.
251. Schatteman GC, Morrison-Graham K, Van Koppen A, Weston JA, Bowen-Pope DF (1992) Regulation and role of PDGF receptor α-subunit expression during embryogenesis. Development 115: 123–131.
252. Mercola M, Wang C, Kelly J, Brownlee C, Jackson-Grusby L, Stiles C, Bowen-Pope D (1990) Selective expression of PDGF A and its receptor during early mouse embryogenesis. Dev Biol 138:114–122.
253. Bidwell MC, Eitzman BA, Walmer DK, McLachlan JA, Gray KD (1995) Analysis of messenger ribonucleic acid and protein for the ligands and receptors of the platelet-derived growth factor signaling pathway in the placenta, extraembryonic membranes, and uterus during the latter half of murine gestation. Endocrinology 136:5189–5201.
254. Palmieri SL, Payne J, Stiles CD, Biggers JD, Mercola M (1992) Expression of mouse PDGF-A and PDGF alpha-receptor genes during pre- and postimplantation development: evidence for a developmental shift from an autocrine to a paracrine mode of action. Mech Dev 39:181–191.
255. Orr-Urtreger A, Lonai P (1992) Platelet-derived growth factor-A and its receptor are expressed in separate, but adjacent cell layers of the mouse embryo. Development 115:1045–1058.
256. Orr-Urtreger A, Bedford MT, Do MS, Eisenbach L, Lonai P (1992) Developmental expression of the alpha receptor for platelet-derived growth factor, which is deleted in the embryonic lethal patch mutation. Development 115:289–303.

257. Soriano P (1994) Abnormal kidney development and hematological disorders in PDGF beta-receptor mutant mice. Genes Dev 8:1888–1896.
258. Leveen P, Pekny M, Gebre-Medhin S, Swolin B, Larsson E, Betsholtz C (1994) Mice deficient for PDGF B show renal, cardiovascular, and hematological abnormalities. Genes Dev 8:1875–1887.
259. Nikkhah G, Odin P, Smits A, Tingstrom A, Othberg A, Brundin P, Funa K, Lindvall O (1993) Platelet-derived growth factor promotes survival of rat and human mesencephalic dopaminergic neurons in culture. Exp Brain Res 92:516–523.
260. Hutchins JB, Jefferson VE (1992) Developmental distribution of platelet-derived growth factor in the mouse central nervous system. Brain Res Dev Brain Res 67:121–135.
261. Pfeilschifter J, Krempien R, Naumann A, Gronwald RG, Hoppe J, Ziegler R (1992) Differential effects of platelet-derived growth factor isoforms on plasminogen activator activity in fetal rat osteoblasts owing to isoform-specific receptor functions. Endocrinology 130:2059–2066.
262. Rodríguez-Martinez H, Persson E, Hurst M, Stanchev P (1992) Immunohistochemical localization of platelet-derived growth factor receptors in the porcine uterus during the oestrous cycle and pregnancy. Zentralbl Veterinarmed A 39:1–10.
263. Chegini N, Rossi MJ, Masterson BJ (1992) Platelet-derived growth factor (PDGF), epidermal growth factor (EGF), and EGF and PDGF beta-receptors in human endometrial tissue: localization and in vitro action. Endocrinology 130:2373–2385.
264. Holmgren L, Claesson-Welsh L, Heldin CH, Ohlsson R (1992) The expression of PDGF alpha- and beta-receptors in subpopulations of PDGF-producing cells implicates autocrine stimulatory loops in the control of proliferation in cytotrophoblasts that have invaded the maternal endometrium. Growth Factors 6:219–231.
265. Guilbert L, Robertson SA, Wegmann TG (1993) The trophoblast as an integral component of a macrophage-cytokine network. Immunol Cell Biol 71:49–57.
266. Holmgren L, Glaser A, Pfeifer-Ohlsson S, Ohlsson R (1991) Angiogenesis during human extra-embryonic development involves the spatiotemporal control of PDGF ligand and receptor gene expression. Development 113:749–754.
267. Khachigian LM, Lindner V, Williams AJ, Collins T (1996) Egr-1-induced endothelial gene expression: a common theme in vascular injury. Science 271:1427–1432.
268. Gospodarowicz D, Abraham D (1989) Isolation and characterization of a vascular endothelial cell mitogen produced by pituitary-derived folliculo stellate cells. Proc Natl Acad Sci USA 86:7311–7315.
269. Neufeld G, Tessler S, Gitay-Goren H, Cohen T, Levi B-Z (1994) Vascular endothelial growth factor and its receptors. Prog Growth Factor Res 5:89–97.
270. Tischer E, Gospodarowicz D, Mitchell R, Silva M, Schilling J, Lau K, Crisp T, Fiddes JC, Abraham JA (1989) Vascular endothelial growth factor: a new member of the platelet-derived growth factor gene family. Biochem Biophys Res Commun 165:1198–1206.
271. Houk KA, Ferrara N, Winer J, Cachianes G, Li B, Leung DW (1991) The vascular endothelial growth factor family-identification of a fourth molecular species and characterization of alternative exon splicing. Mol Endocrinol 5:1806–1814.
272. Keck PJ, Hauser SD, Krivi G, Sanzo K, Warren T, Feder J, Connolly DT (1989) Vascular permeability factor, an endothelial cell mitogen related to PDGF. Science 246:1309–1312.
273. Maglione D, Guerriero V, Viglietto G, Delli-Bovi P, Persico MG (1991) Isolation of a human placenta cDNA coding for a protein related to the vascular permeability factor. Proc Natl Acad Sci USA 88:9267–9271.
274. Hauser S, Weich HA (1993) A heparin-binding form of placenta growth factor (PIGF-2) is expressed in human umbilical vein endothelial cells and in placenta. Growth Factors 9:259–268.
275. Hatva E, Kaipainen A, Mentula P, Jääskeläinen J, Paetau A, Haltia M, Alitalo K (1995) Expression of endothelial cell-specific receptor tyrosine kinases and growth factors in human brain tumors. Amer J Pathol 146:368–378.
276. Barleon B, Hauser S, Schöllman C, Weindel K, Marmé D, Yayon A, Weich HA (1994) Differential expression of the two VEGF receptors flt and KDR in placenta and vascular endothelial cells. J Cell Biochem 54:56–66.
277. Park JE, Chen HH, Winer J, Houck KA, Ferrara N (1994) Placenta growth factor. J Biol Chem 269:25,646–25,654.
278. Sharkey AM, Charnock-Jones DS, Boocock CA, Brown KD, Smith SK (1993) Expression of mRNA for vascular endothelial growth factor in human placenta. J Reprod Fertil 99:609–615.
279. Brier G, Albrecht U, Sterrer S, Risau W (1992) Expression of vascular endothelial growth factor during embryonic angiogenesis and endothelial cell differentiation. Development 114:521–532.

280. Chakraborty I, Das SK, Dey SK (1995) Differential expression of vascular endothelial growth factor and its receptor mRNAs in the mouse uterus around the time of implantation. J Endocrinol 147:339–352.
281. Jakeman LB, Armanini M, Philips HS, Ferrara N (1993) Developmental expression of binding sites and messenger ribonucleic acid for vascular endothelial growth factor suggests a role for this protein in vasculogenesis and angiogenesis. Endocrinology 133:848–859.
282. Cheung CY, Serigh M, Ebaugh MJ, Brace RA (1995) Vascular endothelial growth factor gene expression in ovine placenta and fetal membranes. Am J Obstet Gynecol 173:753–759.
283. Jackson MR, Carney EW, Lye SJ, Knox Ritchie JW (1994) Localization of two angiogenic growth factors (PDECGF and VEGF) in human placentae throughout gestation. Placenta 15:341–353.
284. Anthony FW, Wheeler T, Elcock CL, Pickett M, Thomas EJ (1994) Short report: identification of a specific pattern of vascular endothelial growth factor mRNA expression in human placenta and cultured placental fibroblasts. Placenta 15:557–561.
285. Shifren JL, Doldi N, Ferrara N, Mesiano S, Jaffe RB (1994) In the human fetus, vascular endothelial growth factor is expressed in epithelial cells and myocytes, but not vascular endothelium: implications for mode of action. J Clin Endocrinol Metabol 79:316–322.
286. Ferrara N, Henzel WJ (1989) Pituitary follicular cells secrete a novel heparin-binding growth factor specific for vascular endothelial cells. Biochem Biophys Res Commun 161:851–858.
287. Leung DW, Cachianes G, Kuang WJ, Goeddel DV, Ferrara N (1989) Vascular endothelial growth factor is a secreted angiogenic mitogen. Science 246:1306–1309.
288. De Vries C, Escobedo JA, Ueno H, Houck K, Ferrara N, Williams LT (1992) The *fms*-like tyrosine kinase, a receptor for vascular endothelial growth factor. Science 255:989–991.
289. Terman BI, Carrion ME, Kovacs E, Rasmussen BA, Eddy RL, Shows TB (1991) Identification of a new endothelial growth factor receptor tyrosine kinase. Oncogene 6:1677–1683.
290. Terman BI, Dougher-Vermazen M, Carrion ME, Dimitrov D, Armeilino DC, Gospodarowicz D (1992) Identification of the KDR tyrosine kinase as a receptor for vascular endothelial cell growth factor. Biochem Biophys Res Commun 187:1579–1586.
291. Matsui T, Heideman M, Miki T, Popeseu N, La Rochelle W, Kraus M, Pierce J, Aaronson S (1989) Isolation of a novel receptor cDNA establishes the existence of two PDGF receptor genes. Science 243:800–804.
292. Kaipainen A, Korhonen J, Pajusola K, Aprelikova O, Persico MG, Terman BI, Alitalo K (1993) The related FLT4, FLT1, and KDR receptor tyrosine kinases show distinct expression patterns in human fetal endothelial cells. J Exp Med 178:2077–2088.
293. Millauer B, Wizigmann-Voos S, Schnürch H, Martinez R, Moller NPH, Risau W, Ullrich A (1993) High affinity VEGF binding and developmental expression suggest flk-1 as a major regulator of vasculogenesis and angiogenesis. Cell 72:835–846.
294. Peters KG, De Vries C, Williams LT (1993) Vascular endothelial growth factor receptor expression during embryogenesis and tissue repair suggests a role in endothelial differentiation and blood vessel growth. Proc Natl Acad Sci USA 90:8915–8919.
295. Shalaby F, Rossant J, Yamaguchi TP, Gertsenstein M, Wu X-F, Breltman ML, Schuh AC (1995) Failure of blood-island formation and vasculogenesis in flk-1-deficient mice. Nature 376:62–65.
296. Fong G-H, Rossant J, Gertsenstein M, Breitman ML (1995) Role of the flt-1 receptor tyrosine kinase in regulating the assembly of vascular endothelium. Nature 376:66–70.
297. Charnock-Jones DS, Sharkey AM, Boocock CA, Ahmed A, Plevin R, Ferrara N, Smith SK (1994) Vascular endothelial growth factor receptor localization and activation in human trophoblast and choriocarcinoma cells. Biol Reprod 51:524–530.
298. Kendall RL, Wang G, DiSalvo J, Thomas KA (1994) Specificity of vascular endothelial cell growth factor receptor ligand binding domains. Biochem Biophys Res Commun 201:326–330.
299. Terman BI, Khandke L, Dougher-Vermazan M, Maglione D, Lassam NJ, Gospodarowicz D, Persico MG, Böhlen P, Eisinger M (1994) VEGF receptor subtypes KDR and FLT1 show different sensitivities to heparin and placenta growth factor. Growth Factors 11:187–195.
300. Di Salvo J, Bayne ML, Conn G, Dwok PW, Trivedi PG, Sondermann DD, Palisi TM, Sullivan KA, Thomas KA (1995) Purification and characterization of a naturally occurring vascular endothelial growth factor, placenta growth factor heterodimer. J Biol Chem 270:7717–7723.
301. Carmeliet P, Ferreira Valérie, Breier G, Pollefeyt S, Kieckens L, Gertsenstein M, Fahrig M, Vandenhoeck A, Harpal K, Eberhardt C, Declercq C, Pawling J, Moons L, Collen D, Risau W, Nagy A (1996) Abnormal blood vessel development and lethality in embryos lacking a single VEGF allele. Nature 380:435–438.

302. Ferrara N, Carver-Moore K, Chen H, Dowd M, Lu L, O'Shea KS, Powell-Braxton L, Hillan KJ, Moore MW (1996) Heterozygous embryonic lethality induced by targeted inactivation of the VEGF gene. Nature 380:439–442.
303. Massagué J (1990) The transforming growth factor-β family. Annu Rev Cell Biol 6:597–641.
304. Roberts AB, Sporn MB (1990) The transforming growth factor-βs, In: Peptide Growth Factors and Their Receptors (Sporn MB, Roberts AB, eds.), Springer Verlag, New York, pp. 419–472.
305. Flanders KC, Marascalco BA, Roberts AB, Sporn MB (1990) Transforming growth factor β: a multifunctional regulatory peptide with actions in the reproductive system, In: Growth Factors in Reproduction (Schomberg DW, ed.), Springer Verlag, New York, pp. 23–37.
306. Milan FA, Denhez F, Kondaiah P, Akhurst RJ (1991) Embryonic gene expression patterns of TGFβ1, β2 and β3 suggest different developmental functions in vivo. Development 111:131–144.
307. Pelton RW, Saxena B, Jones M, Moses HL, Gold LI (1991) Immunohistochemical localizations of TGFβ1, TGFβ2 and TGFβ3 in the mouse embryo. Expression patterns suggest multiple roles during embryonic development. J Cell Biol 115:1091–1105.
308. Tamada H, McMaster MT, Flanders KC, Andrews GK, Dey SK (1990) Cell type-specific expression of transforming growth factor-β1 in the mouse uterus during the periimplantation period. Mol Endocrinol 4:965–972.
309. Chen H, Yelavarthi KK, Hunt JS (1993) Identification of transforming growth factor-β1 mRNA in virgin and pregnant rat uteri by in situ hybridization. J Reprod Immunol 25:221–233.
310. Lea RG, Stewart F, Allen WR, Ohno I, Clark DA (1995) Accumulation of chromotrope 2R positive cells in equine endometrium during early pregnancy and expression of transforming growth factor-β2 (TGF-β2). J Reprod Fertil 103:339–347.
311. Doré JJE Jr, Wilkinson JE, Godkin JD (1995) Early gestational expression of transforming growth factor beta isoforms by the ovine placenta. Biol Reprod 53:143–152.
312. Doré JJE, Wilkinson JE, Godkin JD (1996) Ovine endometrial expression of transforming growth factor β isoforms during the peri-implantation period. Biol Reprod 54:1080–1087.
313. Martin JS, Dickson MC, Cousins FM, Kulkarni AB, Karlsson S, Akhurst RJ (1995) Analysis of homozygous TGF beta 1 null mouse embryos demonstrates defects in yolk sac vasculogenesis and hematopoiesis. Ann NY Acad Sci 752:300–308.
314. Dickson MC, Martin JS, Cousins FM, Dulkarnia AB (1995) Defective haematopoiesis and vasculogenesis in transforming growth factor-β knock out mice. Development 121:1845–1854.
315. Graham CH, Lysiak JJ, McCrae KR, Lala PK (1992) Localization of transforming growth factor-β at the human fetal-maternal interface: role in trophoblast growth and differentiation. Biol Reprod 46:561–572.
316. Dungy LJ, Siddiqi TA, Khan S (1991) Transforming growth factor-β1 expression during placental development. Am J Obstet Gynecol 165:853–857.
317. Moulton BC (1994) Transforming growth factor-β stimulates endometrial stromal apoptosis *in vitro*. Endocrinology 134:1055–1060.
318. Selik CE, Horowitz GM, Gratch M, Scott RT Jr, Navot D, Hofmann GE (1994) Immunohistochemical localization of transforming growth factor-β in human implantation sites. J Clin Endocrinol Metab 78:592–596.
319. Kauma S, Matt D, Strom S, Eierman D, Turner R (1990) Interleukin-β1, human leukocyte antigen HLA-DRα, and transforming growth factor-β expression in endometrium, placenta, and placental membranes. Am J Obstet Gynecol 163:1430–1437.
320. Irving JA, Lala PK (1995) Functional role of cell surface integrins on human trophoblast cell migration: regulation by TGF-β, IGF-II, and IGFBP-1. Exp Cell Res 217:419–427.
321. Feinberg, RF, Kliman HJ, Wang C-L (1994) Transforming growth factor-β stimulates trophoblast oncofetal fibronectin synthesis *in vitro*: implications for trophoblast implantation *in vivo*. J Clin Endocrinol Metab 78:1241–1248.
322. Morrish DW, Bhardwaj D, Paras MT (1991) Transforming growth factor β1 inhibits placental differentiation and human chorionic and human placental lactogen secretion. Endocrinology 129: 22–26.
323. Kaartinen V, Voncken JW, Shuler C, Warburton D, Bu D, Heisterkamp N, Groffen J (1995) Abnormal lung development and cleft palate in mice lacking TGF-beta 3 indicates defects of epithelial-mesenchymal interaction. Nat Genet 11:415–421.
324. Rider V, Carlone DL, Witrock D, Cai C, Oliver O (1992) Uterine fibronectin mRNA content and localization are modulated during implantation. Developmental Dynamics 195:1–14.

325. Hines KL, Kulkarni AB, McCarthy JB, Tian H, Ward JM, Christ M, McCartney-Francis NL, Furcht LT, Karlsson S, Wahl SM (1994) Synthetic fibronectin peptides interrupt inflammatory cell infiltration in transforming growth factor beta 1 knockout mice. Proc Natl Acad Sci USA 91:5187–5191.
326. Massagué J (1992) Receptors for the TGF-β family. Cell 69:1067–1070.
327. Lin HY, Lodish HF (1993) Receptors for the TGF-β super family: multiple polypeptides and serine/threonine kinases. Trends Cell Biol 3:14–19.
328. Bassing CH, Yingling JM, Howe DJ, Wang T, He WW, Gustafson ML, Shah P, Danahoe PK, Wang XF (1994) A transforming growth factor-β type I receptor that signals to activate gene expression. Science 263:87–89.
329. Franzn P, Ten Dijke P, Ichijo H, Yamashita H, Schultz P, Heldin C, Miyazonok (1993) Cloning of a TGFβ type I receptor that forms a heteromeric complex with the TGFβ type II receptor. Cell 75:681–692.
330. O'Connor-McCourt MD, Wakefield LM (1987) Latent transforming growth factor-β in serum. A specific complex with α_2 macroglobulin. J Biol Chem 262:14,090–14,099.
331. Danielpour D, Sporn MB (1990) Differential inhibition of transforming growth factor $\beta 1$ and $\beta 2$ activity by α_2 macroglobulin. J Biol Chem 265:6973–6977.
332. Philip A, Bostedt L, Stigbrand T, O'Connor-McCourt MD (1994) Binding of transforming growth factor-β (TGF-β) to pregnancy zone protein (PZP). Comparison to the TGF-β-α_2-macroglobulin interaction. J Biochem 221:687–693.
333. Gougos A, Letarte M (1988) Identification of a human endothelial cell antigen with monoclonal antibody 44G4 against a pre-B leukemic cell line. J Immunol 141:1925–1933.
334. Gougos A, St-Jacques S, Greaves A, O'Connell PJ, d'Apice AJF, Buhring H-J, Bernabeu C, Van Mourik JA, Letarte M (1992) Identification of distinct epitopes of endoglin, an RGD containing glycoprotein of endothelial cells, leukemic cells and syncytiotrophoblasts. Int Immunol 4:83–92.
335. Yamashita H, Ichijo H, Grimsby S, Morén A, Ten Dijke P, Miyazono K (1994) Endoglin forms a heteromeric complex with the signaling receptors for transforming growth factor-β. J Biol Chem 269:1995–2001.
336. St-Jacques S, Cymerman U, Pece N, Letarte M (1994) Molecular characterization and *in situ* localization of murine endoglin reveal that it is a transforming growth factor-β binding protein of endothelial and stromal cells. Endocrinology 134:2645–2657.
337. Slager HG, Lawson KA, Van Den Eijnden-Van Raaij AJM, De Laat SW, Mummery CL (1991) Differential localization of TGF-β_2 in mouse preimplantation and early postimplantation development. Dev Biol 145:205–218.
338. Roelen BAJ, Lin HY, Knežević, Freund E, Mummery CL (1994) Expression of TGF-βs and their receptors during implantation and organogenesis of the mouse embryo. Dev Biol 166:716–728.
339. Kulkarni AB, Karlsson S (1993) Transforming growth factor-$\beta 1$ knockout mice. A mutation in one cytokine gene causes a dramatic inflammatory disease. Am J Pathol 143:3–9.
340. Letterio JJ, Geiser AG, Kulkarni AB, Roche NS, Sporn MB, Roberts AB (1994) Maternal rescue of transforming growth factor-$\beta 1$ null mice. Science 264:1936–1938.
341. Christ M, McCartney-Francis NL, Kulkarni AB, Ward JM, Mizel DE, Mackall CL, Gress RE, Hines KL, Tian H, Karlsson S (1994) Immune dysregulation in TGF-beta 1-deficient mice. J Immunol 153:1936–1946.
342. Boivin GP, O'Toole BA, Orsmby IE, Diebold RJ, Eis MJ, Doetschman T, Kier AB (1995) Onset and progression of pathological lesions in transforming growth factor-beta 1-deficient mice. Am J Pathol 146:276–288.
343. Clark DA, Flanders KC, Hirte H, Dasch JR, Coker R, McAnulty RJ, Laurent J (1995) Characterization of murine pregnancy decidua transforming growth factor β-1. Transforming growth factor β-2 like molecules of unusual molecular size released in bioactive form. Biol Reprod 52:1380–1388.
344. Clark DA, Flanders KC, Banwatt D, Millar-Brook W, Manuel J, Stedronska-Clark J, Rowley B (1990) Murine pregnancy produces a unique immunosuppressive molecule related to transforming growth factor $\beta 2$. J Immunol 144:3008–3014.
345. Lea RG, Underwood J, Flanders KC, Hirte H, Banwatt D, Finotto S, Ohno I, Da S, Harley C, Michel M (1995) A subset of patients with recurrent spontaneous abortion is deficient in transforming growth factor beta-2-producing "suppressor cells" in uterine tissue near the placental attachment site. Am J Reprod Immunol 34:52–64.

346. Segerson EC (1995) Immunosuppressive activity of a porcine high-molecular weight uterine macromolecule is associated with transforming growth factor-beta. J Reprod Immunol 29:47–60.
347. Robertson SA, Seamark RF, Guilbert LJ, Wegmann TG (1994) The role of cytokines in gestation. Crit Rev Immunol 14:239–292.
348. Hunt JS (1993) Expression and regulation of the tumour necrosis factor-α gene expression in the tissues of normal mice. Reprod Fertil Dev 5:141–153.
349. Hunt JS, Chen H-L, Miller L (1996) Tumor necrosis factors: pivotal components of pregnancy? Biol Reprod 54:554–562.
350. Smith CA, Farrah T, Goodwin RG (1994) The TNF receptor superfamily of cellular and viral proteins: activation, costimulation, and death. Cell 76:959–962.
351. Gardner RM, Verner G, Kirkland JL, Stancell GM (1989) Regulation of uterine growth factor (EGF) receptors by estrogen in the mature rat and during the estrous cycle. J Steroid Biochem 32:339–343.
352. Huett-Hudson YM, Chakraborty C, De SK, Suzuki Y, Andrews GK, Dey SK (1990) Estrogen regulates the synthesis of epidermal growth factor in mouse uterine epithelial cells. Mol Endocrinol 4:510–523.
353. Gupta C, Singh M (1996) Stimulation of epidermal growth factor gene expression during the fetal mouse repoductive tract differentiation: Role of androgen and its receptor. Endocrinology 137:705–711.
354. Das SK, Tsukamura H, Paria BC, Andrews GK, Dey SK (1994) Differential expression of epidermal growth factor receptor (EGF-R) gene and regulation of EGF-R bioactivity by progesterone and estrogen in the adult mouse uterus. Endocrinology 134:971–981.
355. Kleinstein J, Westermann W, Mennenga K, Gustmann C, Gips H (1993) Estrogen induces expression of endometrial epidermal growth factor receptors before implantation. Am J Reprod Immunol 30:58–62.
356. Presta M (1988) Sex hormones modulate the synthesis of basic fibroblast growth factor in human endometrial adenocarcinoma cells: implications for the neovascularization of normal and neoplastic endometrium. J Cell Physiol 137:593–597.
357. Rider V, Carlone DL, Foster RT (1997) Oestrogen and progesterone control basic fibroblast growth factor messenger RNA in the rat uterus. J Endocrinol 154:75–84.
358. Rajkumar K, Dheen T, Krsek M, Murphy LJ (1996) Impaired estrogen action in the uterus of insulin-like growth factor binding protein-1 transgenic mice. Endocrinology 137:1258–1264.
359. Kapur S, Tamada H, Dey SK Andrews GK (1992) Expression of insulin-like growth factor-I (IGFI) and its receptor in the peri-implantation mouse uterus, and cell-specific regulation of IGF-I gene expression by estradiol and progesterone. Biol Reprod 46:208–219.
360. Simmen RCM, Simmen FA, Hofig A, Farmer SJ, Bazer, FW (1990) Hormonal regulation of insulin-like growth factor gene expression in pig uterus. Endocrinology 127:2166–2174.
361. Hana V, Murphy LJ (1994) Expression of insulin-like growth factors and their binding proteins in the estrogen responsive Ishikawa human endometrial cancer cell line. Endocrinology 135:2511–1516.
362. Sadek S, Unterman TG, Bell SC (1994) Epithelial localization of insulin-like growth factor binding protein 1 in the uterus of the rat during pregnancy, deciduoma-bearing pseudopregnancy and hormone treatment. J Reprod Fertil 101:67–75.
363. Gray K, Eitzman B, Raszmann, K, Steed T, Geboff A, McLachlan J, Bidwell M (1995) Coordinate regulation by diethylstilbesterol of the platelet-derived growth factor-A (PDGF-A) and -B chains and the PDGF receptor α- and β-subunits in the mouse uterus and vagina: potential mediators of estrogen action. Endocrinology 136:2325–2340.
364. Cullinan-Bove K, Koos RD (1993) Vascular endothelial growth factor/vascular permeability factor expression in the rat uterus: rapid stimulation by estrogen correlates with estrogen-induced increases in uterine capillary permeability and growth. Endocrinology 133:829–837.
365. Das SK, Flanders KC, Andreqws GK, Dey SK (1992) Expression of transforming growth factor-β isoforms (β2 and β3) in the mouse uterus: analysis of the periimplantation period and effects of ovarian steroids. Endocrinology 130:3459–3466.
366. Erickson HP (1993) Gene knockouts of c-scr, transforming growth factor β1, and tenascin suggest superfluous, nonfunction expression of proteins. J Cell Biol 120:1079–1081.

5 Novel Concepts in Neuroendocrine Regulation of Reproductive Tract Functions

Ch. V. Rao, PHD

CONTENTS

INTRODUCTION

The female reproductive tract transports gametes and provides an optimal environment for fertilization of the oocyte, growth, development, and implantation of early embryo, and continuation of pregnancy until labor begins. Regulatory agents that arrive by general or local blood circulation or those produced by embryos and the reproductive tract itself can influence its functions. It has long been believed that the reproductive tract is primarily regulated by ovarian steroid hormones synthesized in response to stimulatory actions of pituitary gonadotropins, luteinizing hormone (LH), follicle-stimulating hormone (FSH), and placental gonadotropin, i.e., chorionic gonadotropin (CG), in primates. Until recently, it had never been thought that the reproductive tract could directly respond to pituitary or placental gonadotropins. Since it is now known that it does, the whole perspective has changed, and a completely new area of reproductive biology has begun. The purpose of this chapter is to review these advances, and present novel concepts in the physiologic and pathologic regulation of the reproductive tract.

Most of these advances came from human studies. However, the functional implications may also apply to animals with exceptions for species having unique reproductive functions. In the animals that lack CG, LH may fulfill the same functions. Human chorionic gonadotropin (hCG) is commonly used in LH receptor binding and functional studies in all species simply because of its availability and purity.

LH and hCG are heterodimeric glycoprotein hormones consisting of dissimilar α- and β-subunits noncovalently bound to each other *(1)*. The β-subunits of LH and hCG are similar to one another, but not to the other members of this glycoprotein hormone family (FSH and thyroid-stimulating hormone). hCG and LH also belong to the family of cystine knot growth factors, which includes platelet-derived growth factor, nerve growth factor, and transforming growth factor-β *(2)*. As growth factors in this family, hCG and LH have diverse mitogenic and nonmitogenic effects in the gonadal and nongonadal tissues of the body *(3–6)*. In fact, it now appears that there are very few differences between traditional growth factors and hCG and LH.

LH and hCG bind to the same receptors, which belong to a family of G-protein-coupled receptors *(7,8)*. The members of this family are single-chain transmembrane glycoproteins, consisting of variable lengths of extracellular hormone binding domain, seven transmembrane-spanning regions, and a relatively short cytoplasmic tail.

LH/hCG RECEPTORS IN THE UTERUS

The first direct evidence for the presence of LH/hCG receptors in uterus came from pig *(9)*. These authors have shown, by traditional ligand binding techniques, that all myometrial specimens and some endometrial specimens contain high-affinity and low-capacity receptors. Subsequently, uterine LH/hCG receptors have been identified in rabbit *(10,11)*, rat *(11–14)*, human *(15–24)*, mouse *(25)*, and cow *(26)*. The techniques used to detect these receptors and the effects of exogenous LH and hCG on uterine functions are summarized in Table 1. Although the affinity of uterine receptors generally appears to be similar to that for ovarian receptors, i.e., $K_d \sim 10^{-10} M$, the number of available receptors per mg protein is considerably lower in uterus than in the gonads *(9–12,25,26,37)*. The in vivo uptake of ^{125}I-hCG is also lower in the uterus than in the gonads *(37)*. However, the reproductive tract should be considered a significant source of LH/hCG receptors in the body simply because of its greater weight as compared to ovaries and the increase in its size during pregnancy.

The uterine LH/hCG receptors are tissue- and hormone-specific. Thus, liver, kidney, heart, skeletal smooth muscle, and so forth, do not contain these receptors, and uterine LH/hCG receptors do not bind any other hormones except hCG and LH *(9–12,25,26,37)*.

Traditional ligand binding studies have not been very useful in studying human uterine LH/hCG receptors, the reason being that human uterus contains too few specific binding sites and too many nonspecific binding sites. The problem of receptor detection by ligand binding techniques was overcome by ligand blotting and covalent receptor crosslinking techniques *(17,20,22,24)*. They probably worked because of the use of very high concentrations of ^{125}I-hCG in the binding reaction.

Human uterus contains a major 4.3-kb and several minor transcripts of LH/hCG receptors. Receptor proteins of 80, 50, and 35 kDa have been detected in whole uterine tissue and in isolated cells *(17,20–22, 24,35,36)*. All the receptor proteins can bind ^{125}I-hCG. Since human specimens cannot always be obtained under optimal conditions, it is possible that some of the lower-molecular-size receptor proteins are artifacts of proteolytic degradation that occurred before it could be prevented by protease inhibitors present in the

Table 1
Uterine LH/hCG Receptors from Various Species

Species	*Method(s) of receptor detection*	*Effects of exogenous hCG/LH*	*References*
Porcine	Ligand binding	Inhibits contractions Increases cyclic AMP and inositol phosphates	*9,27–29*
Rat	Ligand binding	Increases cyclic AMP and progesterone synthesis	*11,12–14,30*
Rabbit	Ligand binding	—	*10,11*
Human	Ligand binding	—	*19*
	Northern, Western, and ligand blotting; covalent Receptor crosslinking; Nested reverse transcription-polymerase chain reaction; *in situ* hybridization, and immunocytochemistry	Inhibits contractions Downregulates gap junctions Increases myometrial smooth muscle cell number and size Promotes the differentiation of endometrial stromal cells Downregulates LH/hCG receptor gene expression Upregulates COX-2 gene expression Increases vasodialatory and decreases vasoconstrictive eicosanoids Decreases vascular resistance index of uterine arteries	*15–18, 20–24, 31–36*
Mouse	Ligand binding	Increases the size of uterus Decreases ascorbic acid content Increases the synthesis of estradiol and progesterone	*25*
Cow	Ligand binding	Increases COX protein and $PGF_{2\alpha}$ synthesis	*26*

tissue collection buffers. At the same time, the possibility of smaller-size receptor proteins being real cannot be ignored.

In situ hybridization and immunocytochemistry have revealed that uterine receptors are present in longitudinal and circular smooth muscle layers of myometrium, glands and stroma of endometrium, and endothelium and smooth muscle of blood vessels *(15,16,18, 20,21,24)*. Among the cell types, endometrial glandular epithelium contains the highest receptor levels. It is not known whether circular and longitudinal myometrial smooth muscle layers differ in LH/hCG receptor levels. The uterine artery contains very few receptors before entering the uterus *(38)*. After it enters, the receptors begin to appear and then progressively increase from the parametrial and myometrial junction *(38)*. The smaller intramyometrial arteries contain more receptors than the larger intramyometrial arteries.

The uterine receptors are high during the progesterone-dominated phase of the cycle and low during postmenopause *(15)*. These findings suggest that either estrogens may downregulate and/or progesterone may upregulate LH/hCG receptors. In pigs, treatment with estradiol benzoate increases uterine LH/hCG receptors *(39)*. Treatment with progesterone alone or in combination with estradiol benzoate results in a greater increase as compared to treatment with estradiol benzoate alone *(39)*. These findings, plus the fact that estradiol and progesterone have a permissive role in hCG actions in human endometrial stromal cells *(22,33)*, suggest that estradiol may modestly increase uterine LH/hCG receptors during the proliferative phase and that progesterone in the luteal phase acts on the estrogen-primed uterus to cause a much greater increase.

Whether lower uterine LH/hCG receptors in postmenopausal women are owing to a decrease in estradiol and progesterone levels is not known. However, progesterone supplementation in hormone replacement therapy does not affect the uterine LH/hCG receptors *(23)*. This leads to the possibility that elevated LH levels may be responsible for decreased uterine receptors in postmenopausal women. In support of this possibility, treatment of human endometrial stromal cells with hCG results in a dose-dependent and hormone-specific downregulation of receptors by decreasing the stability of transcripts rather than decreasing the transcription rate of the LH/hCG receptor gene *(35)*. Hypophysectomy results in an increase of uterine LH/hCG receptors without affecting ovarian receptors in rats *(11)*.

Human myometrium from third trimester pregnancy also contains LH/hCG receptors *(24)*. The specimens from women in labor contain lower receptor levels than those from women not in labor at preterm or term pregnancies. The direct comparison of pregnant and nonpregnant myometria has not been made to determine whether one contains more receptors than the other.

The cyclicity and reproductive state dependence of uterine LH/hCG receptors have also been demonstrated in rat, pig, and cow, suggesting that similar hormonal control mechanisms may operate in these species *(9,12,14,26)*.

LH/hCG RECEPTORS IN THE OVIDUCT

Oviduct, which is a physical continuation of the uterus, is derived from the same embryological precursor as uterus and also contains LH/hCG receptors *(40)*. Human and bovine oviductal receptors have been identified by one or more of the following techniques: Northern, Western, and ligand blotting, covalent receptor crosslinking, *in situ* hybridization, and immunocytochemistry *(40,41)*. There are obvious segmental differences in human (ampulla > isthmus), but not in bovine (fimbria = ampulla = isthmus) oviduct (*40,* Sun et al., unpublished data). The hormone binding specificity of oviductal LH/hCG receptors is the same as in uterus and ovaries *(40)*. Although there are no quantitative data, it appears that oviduct contains similar receptor levels as the uterus.

The receptors are present in epithelial cells, smooth muscle, and blood vessels of oviduct with ciliated and nonciliated epithelial cells containing similar receptor levels *(40)*. Progesterone-dominated oviduct contains more receptors than estrogen-dominated uterus, suggesting a similar scenario of hormonal regulation as in uterus *(40)*. Postpartum oviduct contains similar receptor levels as proliferative phase oviduct, and both contain higher levels than postmenopausal oviduct *(40)*. The lower receptor levels in postpartum as compared with secretory phase may suggest that high hCG levels present during pregnancy may have downregulated the receptors. The very low LH/hCG receptor levels in the tubal tissues from postmenopausal women could be owing to a receptor downregulation by chronically elevated LH levels in the presence of very low levels of ovarian steroid hormones. In fact, as in uterus *(35)*, LH/hCG can downregulate their own receptor levels in oviductal epithelial cells in culture *(42)*.

Whole tubal tissue or isolated epithelial cells contain a major 4.3-kb and several minor transcripts and an 80-kDa protein of LH/hCG receptors *(40,43)*. There is a possibility that the size and relative abundance of receptor transcripts and protein may differ with oviductal cell type and reproductive state.

THE ROLE OF LH AND hCG IN UTERINE FUNCTIONS

The Effect of LH and hCG on Uterine Weight and Steroidogenesis

Ovariectomy results in a decrease of uterine weight in mice *(25)*. Treatment of these animals with LH results in a restoration of uterine weight, a decrease in uterine ascorbic acid content, and an increase in uterine synthesis of estradiol and progesterone *(25)*. The effect of LH on uterine weight appears to be mediated by increasing the synthesis of estrogens in the uterus *(25)*. Rat uterus also makes small amounts of progesterone, which increases following treatment with LH via a cyclic AMP-dependent mechanism *(30)*.

The Effect of hCG on Human Endometrial Cells

Glandular and luminal epithelial cells contain the highest LH/hCG receptor levels, suggesting that these cells are prime targets of regulation by these gonadotropins. In fact, treatment of human endometrial glandular epithelial cells in culture with highly purified hCG results in a time- and dose-dependent and hormone-specific increase in cyclooxygenase (COX) 2 protein levels *(44)*. Prostaglandins (PGs) have long been implicated in the regulation of numerous functions of uterine endometrium. The new findings suggest that LH and hCG, through increasing the formation of PGs via the upregulation of COX-2, may control all the endometrial functions that have been previously attributed to PGs.

The functional significance of LH/hCG receptors in stromal cells has been extensively investigated. Endometrial stromal cells resemble fibroblasts. They can differentiate under appropriate hormonal conditions into bigger and morphologically active protein hormone-secreting decidual cells. The differentiation takes place from the sequential actions of estradiol and progesterone during the menstrual cycle *(45,46)*. In vitro, progesterone alone can induce differentiation because the cells have already been primed in vivo with estradiol. In addition to the steroid hormones, numerous other agents, such as epidermal growth factor, insulin-like growth factor I and II, (IGF-I, IGF-II) androgens, relaxin, and even prolactin, have been shown to promote the differentiation of stromal cells *(47–54)*. Among these, prolactin action suggests that it is formed as a consequence of functional differentiation, and can act in an autocrine and paracrine manner to amplify the differentiation process. It also implies that stromal and/or decidual cells also contain prolactin receptors, which have not yet been identified in these cells.

Recently, exogenous hCG, LH, and FSH have been shown to promote the differentiation of stromal cells *(22,34)*. Of these gonadotropins, LH and hCG action has been investigated in detail *(22)*. These hormones have very little effect on their own on the morphologic or functional differentiation of stromal cells. However, in the presence of estradiol and progesterone, LH and hCG, can further enhance the differentiation, suggesting that the steroid hormones have a permissive role in the action of LH and hCG, and that steroid hormones and gonadotropins are required for a complete or a maximal differentiation of stromal cells. The mechanism of permissive action of steroid hormones has not been investigated. However, it is possible that progesterone may help maintain LH/hCG receptor levels. Such a role for progesterone is possible in view of the findings that uterine receptors are highest during the progesterone-dominated (secretory) phase of the menstrual cycle *(15)*.

The effect of hCG on promoting stromal cell differentiation is time- and dose-dependent with the maximal effect occurring at about 10 d of culture with about 10 ng/mL hCG *(22)*. The effect of hCG and LH is hormone-specific, requires the conformation of native hormone, and is probably mediated by cyclic AMP. In support of cyclic AMP mediation, hCG can stimulate cyclic AMP formation in the rat uterus *(30)*, and exogenous dibutyryl cyclic AMP or elevation of endogenous cyclic AMP by cholera toxin and relaxin can stimulate decidual reaction in animals or promote the differentiation of human endometrial stromal cells *(55–58)*. The effect of hCG on functional differentiation as determined by increased prolactin production appears at least partly to be owing to an increased transcription rate of the prolactin gene *(59)*.

The differentiation of endometrial stromal cells into decidua is an important fundamental event that is required for the implantation of blastocyst. Therefore, promoting this event, LH and hCG have a direct role in the implantation process itself. Moreover, LH is present when the process begins, and hCG is present as it continues. Interestingly, the administration of LH to hypophysectomized rats has been shown a long time ago to induce implantation *(60,61)*. This could have been a direct effect of LH on endometrium, but at that time, it was never suspected *(5)*.

During the LH and hCG action to promote in vitro decidualization, LH/hCG receptor mRNA and protein levels decrease in a dose-dependent and hormone-specific manner *(35)*. The decrease in steady-state LH/hCG receptor mRNA transcript levels was owing to a decrease in the stability of transcripts rather than a decrease in the transcription rate of LH/hCG receptor gene *(35)*.

Like LH and hCG, exogenous prostaglandin E_2 (PGE_2) can also promote the differentiation of stromal cells into decidua in the presence of estradiol and progesterone *(62)*. PGE_2 is formed by the catalytic action of COX-1 and 2 *(63)*. Since PGE_2 is produced locally and is not a primary regulator, the possibility that hCG can regulate the formation of PGE_2 during its action to promote stromal cell differentiation was investigated. The results showed that indeed hCG can increase the formation of PGE_2 by increasing the expression of COX-2 gene in a dose-dependent and hormone-specific manner *(33)*. The effect of hCG on COX-2 gene expression involves an increase in the stability of transcripts rather than increasing the transcription rate of the gene *(33)*. The treatment with LH also increases COX protein and prostaglandins $F_{1\alpha}$ ($PGF_{2\alpha}$) synthesis in the cow uterus, but the relevance of this change to a specific uterine function is not known *(26)*.

Once decidulization begins, it continues throughout pregnancy *(64)*. It is not known what hormone(s) is responsible for this continuation. Progesterone is important, but it alone may not be sufficient. hCG may play a vital role in the continuation of decidualization throughout pregnancy. Pregnancy decidua contains LH/hCG receptors, and these receptors are functional in regulating eicosanoid biosynthetic enzymes *(65)*. Again, through mediation by eicosanoids, hCG may influence decidual synthesis of various hormones, cytokines, and growth factors that are important for maternal and fetal communication throughout pregnancy *(66–68)*.

The Effect of LH and hCG on Uterine Blood Flow

As previously indicated, uterine arteries contain LH/hCG receptors in both endothelial cells and smooth muscle. The presence of LH/hCG receptors in uterine blood vessels suggests that these gonadotropins may directly affect uterine blood flow *(36,38)*. Also, it is logical to consider such an effect for gonadotropins because a commensurate increase in blood flow would increase the delivery of nutrients and removal of metabolic waste products from the cells that are functioning at increased levels under the influence of gonadotropins.

In vitro studies have shown that treatment with hCG increases prostacyclin and decreases thromboxane A_2 in both endothelial and smooth muscle layers of uterine arteries *(36)*. These findings suggest that LH and hCG may increase uterine blood flow by increasing the synthesis of vasodialatory eicosanoids and decreasing the synthesis of vasoconstrictive eicosanoids.

Doppler ultrasonography showed that administration of 10,000 IU hCG for ovulation induction in women resulted in a decrease of the resistence index of uterine arteries, indicating an increase in uterine blood flow *(36)*. The decreased vascular resistance correlated well with the appearance of hCG in the circulation from the im injection rather than an increase in estradiol or progesterone levels from the gonadotropin stimulation of the ovaries *(36)*.

In rats, a single injection of a superovulating dose of 50 IU hCG results in a decrease of uterine blood flow, as determined by a microspheres technique *(69)*. Removal of the ovaries, however, results in a loss of response, suggesting that hCG action on decreasing uterine blood flow is indirect. The decrease of uterine blood flow by hCG was unexpected, and it may be a pharmacologic response in which very high doses of hCG may have an opposite effect from that seen with physiologic doses. Superovulated rats are usually used for harvesting ovaries. It is not known whether superovulated rats can become pregnant in the face of decreased uterine blood flow. These findings may have clinical relevance to reproductive medicine, since the recommended hCG doses in some women could be too high causing an implantation failure owing to decreased uterine blood flow.

Direct application of hCG to rat uterine arterioles in microcirculatory preparations results in a dialation on diestrus-1 and 2 and constriction on proestrus *(70)*. Removal of ovaries had no significant effect, suggesting that hCG action is direct. Thus, the hCG effects on uterine blood flow in rats involve both indirect and direct mechanisms.

It has also been recently demonstrated that LH/hCG can directly increase lumen diameter of prearteriolar uterine and mesenteric vessels in nonpregnant and pregnant rats *(71)*. The uterine vessels are more sensitive in pregnant rats, and mesenteric vessels are more sensitive in nonpregnant animals. Nevertheless, blood vessels from both groups of animals responded to hCG treatment. Based on these findings, these authors have suggested that hCG is the main embryonic signal that not only regulates ovarian and uterine blood flow, but also triggers the cascade of adoptive cardiovascular processes seen in early pregnancy *(71)*.

Previous to the above studies, estradiol and/or progesterone was thought to be responsible for regulating uterine blood flow in women *(72–77)*. Consistent with such a possibility, uterine blood vessels contain estradiol and progesterone receptors *(78,79)*. Nevertheless, the presumptive effect of steroid hormones was based on circumstantial evidence such as:

1. Increased uterine blood flow during the preovulatory period when estrogen levels are high *(72,80–82)*;
2. Increased uterine blood flow during pregnancy when progesterone levels are high;
3. Increased uterine blood flow following treatment with estradiol *(74,83,84)*; and
4. Decreased uterine blood flow following treatment with GnRH analogs, which decrease estradiol levels *(85)*.

In all these cases, either LH levels increase or decrease or hCG is present. However, these gonadotropins have not been suspected of playing any role in uterine blood flow. The fact that LH and hCG may increase uterine blood flow does not necessarily rule out a role for estradiol and progesterone, since both of these groups of hormones may act in an overall control of uterine vascular function.

The effect of LH and hCG on increasing uterine blood flow may be physiologically relevant during the preovulatory period when LH levels reach a peak and during pregnancy when hCG is present. These are the two time periods during which increased uterine blood flow is required, and it may be fulfilled in part by gonadotropins. Aberrant uterine vascular responses to LH or hCG may cause infertility, pregnancy loss, or circulatory problems in pregnancy, including excessive obstetrical hemorrhage.

The increase of uterine blood flow by hCG may also result from relaxation of myometrial smooth muscle and growth of new blood vessels. Even though angiogenesis or neovascularization may not be a significant phenomenon in the myometrium, it could be very important in the endometrium, since it is shed and regrows in every nonfertile cycle. LH from the preovulatory surge and hCG from early pregnancy may stimulate angiogenesis in the endometrium. This action, coupled with a possible increase in vascular permeability by LH, may constitute a part of the tropic actions of hCG in the endometrium.

Tubal blood vessels also contain LH/hCG receptors *(40)*. However, whether LH and hCG can directly increase tubal blood flow has not been investigated.

The Effect of hCG on Myometrial Hyperplasia and Hypertrophy

The size of the uterus increases tremendously during pregnancy to accommodate the growing fetus. This increase includes both myometrial smooth muscle cell number and cell size. A role for hCG in this process was considered because myometrial smooth muscle cells contain LH/hCG receptors and either LH or hCG is present during pregnancy in all species. It turns out that hCG is a mild mitogen in human myometrial smooth muscle cells *(17)*. The hCG effect is hormone-specific, time- and dose-dependent, and mediated by protein kinase A signaling. Eicosanoids from the COX pathway of arachidonic acid metabolism are probably not involved in this hCG action. Estradiol, which is generally considered a uterotropic hormone, had very little effect on its own and it could not modify hCG action on the growth of myometrial smooth muscle cells. Progesterone also had no effect on myometrial cell growth. Epidermal growth factor (EGF) is also mitogenic in human myometrial smooth muscle cells, but its relationship with hCG is not known *(86)*.

In addition to mitogenesis, hCG can cause hypertrophy in a small subpopulation of myometrial smooth muscle cells *(17)*). These cells become very large while retaining normal chromosomal ploidy. How these cells are different from the other myometrial smooth muscle cells is not known.

The Role of hCG in Myometrial Contractions and Gap Junctions

Myometrial quiescence is very important for the implantation of blastocysts and also for the continuation of pregnancy to term. Even though the pregnant myometrium is relatively quiescent, there are low-frequency and low-amplitude contractions that increase tremendously with the onset of labor. Obviously, it is very important to understand better hormonal control of myometrial quiescence, since such knowledge could help formulate strategies for prevention of preterm labor in women.

It is generally believed that progesterone is responsible for maintaining myometrial quiescence during pregnancy. Consistent with such a possibility, pregnancy myometrium contains progesterone receptors, and progesterone can downregulate myometrial gap junctions and inhibit the contractions of myometrium *(31,87–89)*.

The presence of LH/hCG receptors in pregnant human myometria and lower receptor levels in specimens from women in labor compared to women not in labor at preterm and term pregnancies suggest that hCG may also play a role in maintaining myometrial quiescence *(23)*. In fact, hCG can directly inhibit myometrial contractions *(32)*. Priming with estradiol and stimulation with oxytocin are required for hCG to inhibit the amplitude of contractions; however, the frequency of contractions increases. The action of hCG on myometrial contractions is accompanied by a decrease in intracellular Ca^{2+} levels *(32)*. The effect of hCG on myometrial contractions is only detected in myometrial specimens from the proliferative, but not from the secretory phase of the cycle. The lack of effect is not owing to the absence of receptors, because secretory phase specimens contain even more LH/hCG receptors than proliferative phase specimens. If hCG is expected to maintain myometrial quiescence during pregnancy, then the lack of hCG effect in secretory phase specimens is a paradox. Although the reasons are not known, it is possible that hCG may only counteract the actions of myometrial-stimulating agents, such as oxytocin. If this is the case, then secretory phase specimens do not contain, whereas pregnancy specimens contain an oxytocin-response system.

The inhibitory action of hCG on myometrial contractions was probably owing to downregulation of gap junctions *(31)*. In fact, the treatment of pregnant human myometrial smooth muscle cells with hCG results in a dose- and time-dependent decrease in myometrial gap junctions *(31)*. The effect of hCG is hormone-specific and mediated by protein kinase A signaling. Oxytocin treatment increases myometrial smooth muscle cell gap junctions, and hCG blocks the oxytocin action *(31)*. The downregulating effect of hCG on myometrial gap junctions is similar to that of progesterone *(31)*. In fact, progesterone may be involved in the hCG actions because RU-486, a progesterone receptor antagonist, can block the downregulating effect of hCG on myometrial gap junctions *(31)*. The involvement of progesterone in the action of hCG could be in the form of hCG stimulating myometrial synthesis of progesterone and/or transactivation of progesterone receptors by activated LH/hCG receptors.

In porcine uterus, hCG is capable of inhibiting both frequency and amplitude of spontaneous contractions *(27)*. Interestingly, as in human uterus, estradiol priming is required for the effect of hCG, and the progesterone-dominated pig uterus in the luteal phase does not respond to hCG *(27)*.

THE ROLE OF hCG/LH IN OVIDUCTAL FUNCTIONS

There are at least two direct effects described for LH and hCG in oviducts or fallopian tubes. First, LH and hCG can upregulate the COX-2 mRNA and protein, and PGE_2 synthesis in epithelial cells in a dose- and time-dependent and hormone-specific manner *(43)*. The upregulation involves increasing the stability of transcripts rather than increasing the transcription rate of the COX-2 gene *(43)*. The importance of LH and hCG in regulating the COX-2 gene lies in the fact that PGE_2 formed by the catalytic action of this enzyme has been shown to inhibit tubal contractions and stimulate ciliary beat frequency *(90–95)*. Both are very important in early pregnancy. For example, inhibition of tubal contractions favors fertilization of the oocyte and prevents premature transport of the early embryo into the uterus for implantation. The stimulation of ciliary beat frequency, on the other hand, may allow timely transport of the early embryo out of the oviduct for implantation in the uterus.

The second effect found for LH and hCG in oviductal epithelial cells is that they increase the synthesis of oviductal glycoprotein (OGP) *(41)*. The effect is time- and dose-dependent, hormone-specific, and requires the conformation of native hCG. Generally, estradiol is considered to increase the synthesis of this protein simply because its levels increase in the late follicular phase and then disappear *(96)*. In the late follicular phase, LH also increases, but this was never suspected to play a role, because the presence of LH/hCG receptors in tubal epithelial cells was not known until recently. The importance of LH and hCG in increasing the OGP synthesis lies in the fact that this protein binds to the zona pellucida and perivitelline membranes of ovulated oocytes and also to spermatozoa, in some species, to increase the rate of fertilization of oocytes *(see 97)*. The OGP also binds two- to four-cell embryos, suggesting that it might promote early embryonic growth and development *(see 97)*. By increasing the synthesis of this protein, LH and hCG may play a direct role in enhancing the fertilization of oocytes and early embryonic growth and development. Thus, the sum of the total effects of LH and hCG in oviducts may be to create optimal conditions for fertilization of the oocyte, growth and development of the early embryo, and its timely transport into the uterus for implantation.

LH/hCG RECEPTORS IN UTERINE PATHOLOGIES

Endometriosis is a benign gynecologic disease in women. It is characterized by translocation of uterine endometrium to various peritoneal surfaces in the body. There are a number of theories on the cause of this disease, but none has been universally accepted.

Like eutopic endometrium, ectopic endometrial implants contain LH/hCG receptors *(16)*; however, there was no consistent difference between them. Although eutopic endometrial LH/hCG receptors are cyclic, the implants show no cyclic variation *(16)*. The relevance of these findings to the etiology of this disease is not known. The fact that endometriosis generally subsides during pregnancy and is not seen in postmenopausal women who have elevated gonadotropins levels, does not necessarily rule out a possible role for LH in endometriosis, since other hormonal and biophysical changes may explain the findings in these women.

Adenomyosis is another benign gynecologic disease in women. In this disease, endometrial glands and stroma invade myometrium. The invading glands contain more LH/hCG receptors than noninvading glands in the same uterus *(18)*. The overexpression of LH/hCG receptors is selective, as invading stroma does not overexpress this receptor and invading glands do not overexpress cell adhesion molecule, such as cadherin. The cause of adenomyosis and the significance of LH/hCG receptor overexpression in the invading uterine glands are not known.

Leiomyomas or fibroids are benign outgrowths of myometrial and vascular smooth muscle in women. They contain LH/hCG receptors, but at lower levels than in adjacent unaffected myometrium *(21)*. The lower receptor levels could be owing to lower smooth muscle content, a lower number of blood vessels, or higher amounts of extracellular matrix proteins present in leiomyomas as compared to adjacent normal myometria. As in unaffected normal adjacent myometrium, LH/hCG receptors in leiomyomas are functional in downregulating a gap junctional protein, connexin-43 *(21)*. Although the significance of LH/hCG receptors in leiomyomas is not known, the possibility that LH and hCG may influence the synthesis of extracellular matrix proteins, thus altering the growth control mechanisms, may be considered.

All of the above benign gynecologic conditions cause pelvic pain, abnormal uterine bleeding, and dysmenorrhea, pregnancy loss, and infertility. Surgical and/or medical treatment with GnRH analogs are the current options.

Endometrial carcinoma is the most common gynecological malignancy in Western countries *(98)*. It exceeds the incidence of ovarian and cervical cancers. Endometrial carcinomas overexpress LH/hCG receptors as compared with normal endometrium *(20)*. The receptor expression increases with increasing tumor grade. These findings may be relevant to understanding endometrial carcinomas better. For example, endometrial carcinoma is generally considered an estrogen-related disease *(99)*, but this disease frequently occurs in postmenopausal women who have very low estrogen levels. Even though it has been shown that endometrial cancer tissue can convert peripheral androgens into estrogens *(100)*, there are no clear data demonstrating that cancer tissue contains higher levels of estrogens than the adjacent normal uterine tissue. Also, there are no obvious differences in circulating estradiol and estrone levels between postmenopausal women with endometrial cancer as compared to those without cancer *(101)*. Contrary to these findings, LH levels are elevated in postmenopausal women. Moreover, bioactive, but not total (bioactive and immunoreactive), LH levels are higher in postmenopausal women with endometrial cancer than those without cancer *(102)*. These findings support a role for LH, but not for estrogens in endometrial carcinoma. However, this may be too simplistic and both hormones may somehow be involved in this disease. For example, LH may sensitize the endometrial cancer tissue to low levels of estrogens by upregulating its receptors and also by increasing local synthesis of estrogens. For such a case, both hormones will be important, but LH would have a primary role.

Treatment with GnRH analogs is one of the options in endometriosis, adenomyosis, leiomyomas, and endometrial cancer. This treatment is presumed to work by decreasing estrogen levels. The hypoestrogenism is a consequence of decreased LH levels. Since LH/hCG receptors are present in all these tissues, at least part of any therapeutic benefit may come from decreased LH levels. In the case of endometrial cancer, the theory of decreased estrogen levels causing therapeutic benefit may not apply because the estrogen levels are already low and treatment with GnRH analogs may not further reduce these levels.

Another possibility in these conditions is that gonadotropin-releasing hormone (GnRH) analogs act directly on the tissue. Consistent with such a possibility, GnRH receptors are present in some of these tissues *(103,104)*. In view of the new findings on LH/hCG receptors in endometrial cancer, it is possible that treatment with GnRH analogs may downregulate LH/hCG receptors in endometrial cancer tissue. As a consequence, LH may not be able to sensitize the tissue to estrogens, which would also lead to a therapeutic benefit.

THE ROLE OF LH/hCG RECEPTORS AND hCG IN OVIDUCTAL INFECTIONS

Pathogens that express either hCG or LH-like or LH/hCG receptor-like molecules may infect oviducts by a mechanism of molecular mimicry. In this mechanism, the pathogens mimic a ligand by binding to the epethelial cell surface, which already contains both hCG and LH/hCG receptor molecules. The binding results in endocytosis or transcytosis of pathogens into the cell interior and submucosal spaces, respectively. Once pathogens are in these sites, they may begin causing cellular damage and provoke inflammatory changes by increasing the formation of eicosanoids just as a normal ligand would do.

The experimental evidence for this possibility includes the fact that several pathogens that can potentially infect the reproductive tract contain LH or hCG or LH/hCG receptor-like molecules *(105–108)*. Infection of fallopian tubes by *Neisseria gonorrhea* can be inhibited by treatment with anti-hCG antibody, and prior treatment with hCG protects the tubal tissue from infection by enhancing the local mucosal cell immune response by increasing the secretion of IgA *(109)*. *Chlamydia trachomatis*, which invades fallopian tubes from the lower genital tract in women, causes subclinical or clinical salpingitis and infertility. The DNA extracted from elementary and reticular bodies of this organism contain LH/hCG receptor-like sequences as determined by Southern blotting under high-stringency conditions with rat and porcine LH/hCG receptor cDNAs (Li et al., unpublished data). These elementary and reticular bodies also contain a 46-kDa protein that is recognized by a polyclonal antibody raised against a synthetic N-terminus amino acid sequence of 15–38 of rat LH/hCG receptors (Li et al., unpublished data). McCoy cells and epithelial cells from human fallopian tubes do not contain a 46-kDa protein. However, when they are infected with *C. trachomatis*, a 46-kDa protein appears, suggesting that it is derived from the organism (Li et al., unpublished data). These findings suggest that this 46-kDa protein is probably encoded by a LH/hCG receptor-like gene sequence in *C. trachomatis* and that this protein may bind to hCG in epithelial cell membranes, resulting in invasion of the organism into the cells and the submucosal spaces.

INTERRELATIONSHIPS BETWEEN LH/hCG AND OTHER HORMONES IN CONTROL OF REPRODUCTIVE TRACT FUNCTIONS

LH, hCG, progesterone, and relaxin have similar actions in the reproductive tract. This raises a question concerning why we have all these hormones when only one may be adequate to do the job. The answer may partly lie in the following possibilities. First, all these hormones may not be present at the same time. Even if they were all present, they may not work in tandem. In other words, there may be a hierarchy that allows one hormone to regulate another and so on. Second, more than one hormone may be required for maximal effect, and finally, different hormones may be active in different reproductive states.

hCG can inhibit oxytocin-stimulated myometrial contractions, and can oppose the action of oxytocin on myometrial gap junctions and intracellular Ca^{2+} levels *(31,32)*. The downregulating action of hCG on myometrial gap junctions can be blocked by the progesterone receptor antagonist, RU-486 *(31)*. Estradiol and progesterone have a permissive role in LH and hCG actions in endometrial stromal cells and in oviductal epithelial cells *(22,33,43)*. Although molecular mechanisms of permissiveness of ovarian steroid hormones and the interaction of hCG with other hormones are not known, they underscore the importance of various groups of hormones of similar or opposing actions in the overall control and fine-tuning of reproductive tract functions.

THE SOURCE OF HORMONES THAT BIND TO REPRODUCTIVE TRACT LH/hCG RECEPTORS

The hormones that bind to reproductive tract LH/hCG receptors can come from peripheral and/or local sources. The peripheral source is the hormones present in blood circulation. This will be LH in the nonpregnant state, hCG in human pregnancy, and LH in pregnant animals. The local sources include LH or hCG or similar molecules produced by the reproductive tract itself or embryo, placenta, or even pathogens present in the reproductive tract *(40,105,107,109,110)*.

THE ROLE OF OTHER NEUROENDOCRINE FACTORS IN REPRODUCTIVE TRACT FUNCTIONS

Human uterus has recently been shown to contain FSH receptors *(111)*. These receptors seem to mediate the action of exogenous FSH in upregulating LH/hCG receptors and restoring the loss of mitogenic response of human myometrial smooth muscle cells to hCG.

Uterus and/or oviduct have been shown to contain receptors for growth hormone, prolactin, oxytocin, relaxin, vasopressin, and GnRH *(102,112–117)*. The hormones that bind to the corresponding receptors in the reproductive tract may not necessarily come from the central nervous system, since they may be produced locally. In fact, such local synthesis has been demonstrated for prolactin, oxytocin, and relaxin *(45,118–120)*. Growth hormone has a direct mitogenic effect in the uterus *(121)*. Prolactin, produced locally as a result of decidualization, can further promote the decidualization process. Oxytocin and vasopressin stimulate myometrial contractions via distinct receptors *(122)*. Relaxin inhibits the contractions of myometrial smooth muscle, and perhaps also oviductal smooth muscle, and may regulate numerous other functions of the reproductive tract *(119,123)*. GnRH has been shown to inhibit uterine contractions in humans and to stimulate them in rat *(124,125)*. Immunoneutralization experiments have revealed that GnRH may also affect endometrial functions *(126)*.

SUMMARY AND PERSPECTIVES

The reproductive tract, which was once considered only an indirect target of gonadotropins, has now been found to be directly regulated by LH and hCG. Recent advances have provided compelling evidence for the presence of LH/hCG receptors in uterus and oviduct, and for these gonadotropins to regulate numerous functions of the female reproductive tract (Fig. 1). These findings are seminal and are the seeds for a new area of reproductive biology that is certain to grow a great deal in the future.

hCG plays an important role in maternal recognition of pregnancy in women by supporting luteal synthesis of progesterone. The new findings suggest that the pregnancy recognition signal also includes numerous changes induced by hCG in the reproductive tract of a fertile cycle. These changes could be just as important as maintaining luteal function. In animals, there is no hCG, but there is LH and there are LH receptors in the uterus. The current data on maternal recognition of pregnancy in animals suggest that the trophoectoderm of the conceptus makes trophoblast interferon τ *(127)*. This protein blocks expression of genes for estradiol and oxytocin receptors and, therefore, uterine production of $PGF_{2\alpha}$, which causes luteal demise *(127)*. As a result, the corpus luteum is rescued and pregnancy is recognized. In view of the findings that the uterus of animals also contains LH receptors, it is possible that these receptors may also be involved in the maternal recognition of pregnancy. In support of such a possibility is the recent finding that LH can regulate COX enzymes in the cow uterus *(26)*. Thus, LH can potentially decrease $PGF_{2\alpha}$ and/or increase PGE_2 synthesis in the uterus, either of which can support rescue of the corpus luteum. In addition, as in women, LH may induce changes in the uterus of animals that could be just as important as maintaining luteal function. Concern-

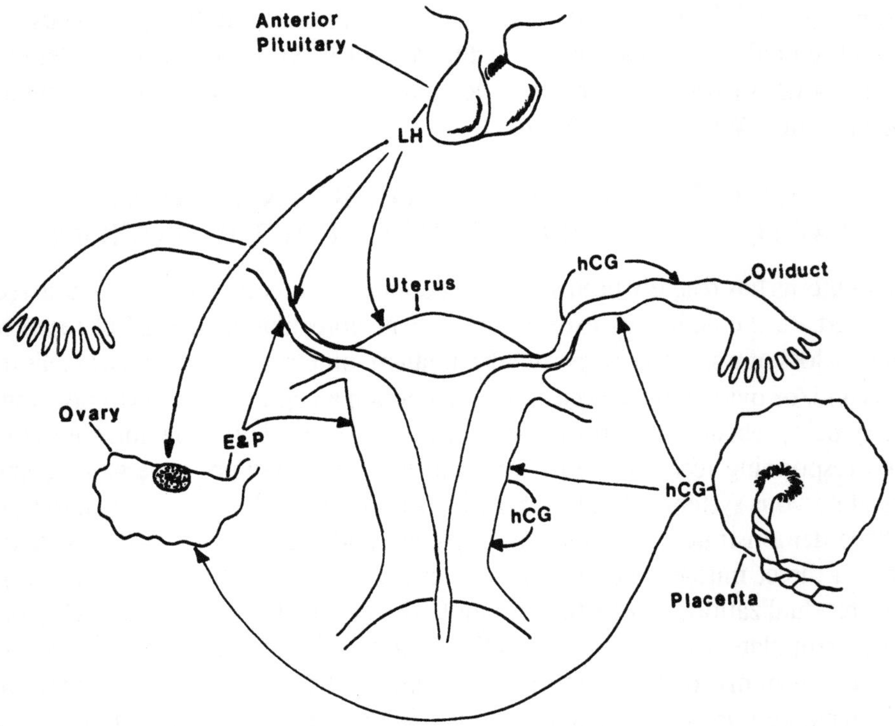

Fig. 1. Concepts in LH and hCG regulation of reproductive tract functions. Shown in this figure is an old concept in which LH from the anterior pituitary and hCG from human placenta act on ovaries to increase estradiol (E) and progesterone (P) synthesis, which would then regulate reproductive tract functions. Also shown is a new concept in which LH and hCG also directly regulate reproductive tract functions. Human fallopian tubes make small amounts of hCG, which may affect its functions in both an autocrine and paracrine manner. An implanting early embryo may make hCG or hCG-like molecules, which may affect uterine functions. Autocrine and paracrine actions of hCG in the reproductive tract may involve local synthesis of estradiol and progesterone.

ing the source of ligand for the uterine receptors, it will be interesting to determine whether the conceptus of animals can synthesize LH or LH-like molecules.

The new findings on LH and hCG actions in the reproductive tract may have potential clinical applications in reproductive medicine. For example, it is known that coculture of oviductal epithelial cells with embryos results in a greater embryonic development, presumably because the epithelial cells secrete stimulatory factors *(128,129)*. The knowledge that LH and hCG can increase the synthesis of oviductal glycoprotein *(41)* and perhaps other molecules by oviductal epithelial cells could be utilized to devise new strategies to enhance embryonic development further. The findings that LH and hCG actions in oviduct and uterus promote beneficial events for fertilization of the oocyte, as well as growth, development, and implantation of the early embryo *(22,33,36,41,43)* suggest that inclusion of hCG in the transfer media used for gamete intrafallopian tube transfers and in vitro fertilization, and embryo transfers may improve pregnancy rates. Either of these two possibilities would have tremendous relevance to assisted reproductive technologies. Another example of a potential clinical application has to do with treatment of preterm labor. Since we now know that hCG can downregulate myometrial gap junctions and inhibit contractions *(31,32)*, hCG and/or its analogs may be used for treatment of preterm labor in women. Even though these women will have hCG in their blood, it may not be present in adequate concentrations; therefore, administering exogenous hCG may suppress myometrial contractions. Since hCG is normally present anyway in the body and is frequently used in reproductive medicine, administering a dose of exogenous hCG should not cause any anaphylactic reaction.

hCG is widely used for ovulation induction in women. It must be realized that administration of hCG for these and any other therapeutic reasons can affect reproductive tract functions, and any final clinical outcome may represent a sum of all of the changes. Favorable or adverse effects may result depending on the dose, frequency, and time of hCG administration. The new findings may also impact the development of contraceptive or cancer vaccines using anti-hCG antibodies. These vaccines rely on the assumption that only the ovaries and cancer tissues produce and/or respond to hCG. Since LH/hCG receptors are present in the reproductive tract and other organs, the consequences of unintended alterations of their functions should be considered when planning vaccine strategies.

REFERENCES

1. Pierce JG, Parsons TF (1981) Glycoprotein hormones: structure and function. Annu Rev Biochem 50:466–495.
2. Lapthorn AJ, Harris DC, Littlejohn A, Lustbader JW, Canfield RE, Machin KJ, Morgan FJ, Isaacs NW (1994) Crystal structure of human chorionic gonadotropin. Nature 369:455–461.
3. Rodway MR, Rao ChV (1995) A novel perspective on the role of human chorionic gonadotropin during pregnancy and in gestational trophoblastic disease. Early Pregnancy: Biol Med 1:176–187.
4. Rao ChV (1996) The beginning of a new era in reproductive biology and medicine: Expression of low levels of functional luteinizing hormone/human chorionic gonadotropin receptors in nongonadal tissues. J Physiol Pharmacol 47:41–53.
5. Rao ChV, Sanfilippo JS (1997) New understanding in the biochemistry of implantation: potential direct roles of luteinizing hormone and chorionic gonadotropin. Endocrinologist 7:107–111.
6. Rao ChV (1997) Potential novel roles of luteinizing hormone and human chorionic gonadotropin during early pregnancy in women. Early Pregnancy: Biol Med 3:1–9.
7. McFarland KC, Sprengel R, Phillips HS, Köhler M, Rosemblit N, Nikolics K, Segaloff DL, Seeburg PH (1989) Lutropin-choriogonadotropin receptor; an unusual member of the G-protein-coupled receptor family. Science 245:494–499.
8. Loosfelt H, Misrahi M, Atger M, Salesse R, Vu MT, Thi HL, Jolivet A, Guiochon-Mantell A, Sar S, Jallal B, Garnier J, Milgrom E (1989) Cloning and sequencing of porcine LH-hCG receptor cDNA: variants lacking transmembrane domain. Science 245:525–528.
9. Ziecik AJ, Stanchev PD, Tilton JE (1986) Evidence for the presence of luteinizing hormone/human chorionic gonadotropin-binding sites in the porcine uterus. Endocrinology 119:1159–1163.
10. Jensen JD, Odell WD (1988) Identification of LH/hCG receptors in rabbit uterus (42775). Proc Soc Exp Biol Med 189:28–30.
11. Sawitzke AL, Odell WD (1991) Uterine binding sites for LH/hCG can be modulated by hormonal status in rabbits and rats. Acta Endocrinol (Copenh) 124:322–330.
12. Bonnamy PJ, Benhaim A, Leymarie P (1990) Estrous cycle-related changes of high affinity luteinizing hormone/human chorionic gonadotropin binding sites in the rat uterus. Endocrinology 126: 1264–1269.
13. Sen S, Bhattacharya S (1992) Binding of radiolabelled luteinizing hormone to intact and ovariectomized rat uterus. Indian J Exp Biol 30:972–976.
14. Bonnamy PJ, Benhaim A, Leymarie P (1993) Uterine luteinizing hormone/human chorionic gonadotropin-binding sites in the early pregnant rat uterus: Evidence for total occupancy in the periimplantation period. Endocrinology 132:1240–1246.
15. Reshef E, Lei ZM, Rao ChV, Pridham DD, Chegini N, Luborsky JL (1990) The presence of gonadotropin receptors in nonpregnant human uterus, human placenta, fetal membranes and decidua. J Clin Endocrinol Metab 70:421–430.

16. Lincoln S, Lei ZM, Rao ChV, Yussman MA (1992) The expression of human chorionic gonadotropin/human luteinizing hormone receptors in ectopic human endometrial implants. J Clin Endocrinol Metab 75:1140–1144.
17. Kornyei J, Lei ZM, Rao ChV (1993) Human myometrial smooth muscle cells are novel targets of direct regulation by human chorionic gonadotropin. Biol Reprod 49:1149–1157.
18. Lei ZM, Rao ChV, Lincoln S, Ackermann DM (1993) Increased expression of human chorionic gonadotropin/human luteinizing hormone receptors in adenomyosis. J Clin Endocrinol Metab 76:763–768.
19. Bhattacharya S, Banerjee J, Sen S, Manna PR (1993) Human chorionic gonadotropin binding sites in the human endometrium. Acta Endocrinol 129:15–19.
20. Lin J, Lei ZM, Lojun S, Rao ChV, Satyaswaroop PG, Day Jr TG (1994) Increased expression of luteinizing hormone/human chorionic gonadotropin receptor gene in human endometrial carcinomas. J Clin Endocrinol Metab 79:1483–1491.
21. Singh M, Zuo J, Li X, Ambrus G, Lei ZM, Yussman MA, Sanfilippo JS, Rao ChV (1995) The decreased expression of functional human chorionic gonadotropin/luteinizing hormone receptor gene in human uterine leiomyomas. Biol Reprod 53:899–904.
22. Han SW, Lei ZM, Sanfilippo JS, Rao ChV (1995) Human chorionic gonadotropin as a new regulator of human endometrial stromal cells differentiation into decidua, In: The Program of the Endocrine Society Annual Meeting, Abstract P2–84.
23. Zuo J, Lei ZM, Rao ChV (1994) Human myometrial chorionic gonadotropin/luteinizing hormone receptors in preterm and term deliveries. J Clin Endocrinol Metab 79:907–911.
24. Bernardini L, Moretti-Rojas I, Brush M, Rojas FJ, Balmaceda JP (1995) Status of hCG/LH receptor and G proteins in human endometrium during artificial cycles of hormone replacement therapy. J Soc Gynecol Invest 2:630–635.
25. Mukherjee D, Manna PR, Bhattacharya S (1994) Functional relevance of luteinizing hormone receptor in mouse uterus. Eur J Endocrinol 131:103–108.
26. Freidman S, Gurevich M, Shemesh M (1995) Bovine cyclic endometrium contains high-affinity luteinizing hormone/human chorionic gonadotropin binding sites. Biol Reprod 52:1020–1026.
27. Flowers B, Ziecik AJ, Caruolo EV (1991) Effects of human chorionic gonadotropin on contractile activity of steroid-primed pig myometrium in vitro. J Reprod Fertil 92:425–432.
28. Ziecik AJ, Gajewski Z, Jedruch J, Barcikowski B (1993) Effect of human chorionic gonadotropin on myometrial electrical activity in the pig. Anim Reprod Sci 31:131–139.
29. Kisielewska J, Flint APF, Ziecik AJ (1996) Phospholipase C and adenylate cyclase signalling systems in the action of hCG on porcine myometrial smooth muscle cells. J Endocrinol 148: 175–180.
30. Bonnamy PJ, Benhaim A, Leymarie P (1989) Human chorionic gonadotropin affects tissue levels of progesterone and cyclic adenosine 3′-5′-monophosphate in the metestrus rat uterus in vitro. Biol Reprod 40:511–516.
31. Ambrus G, Rao Ch.V (1994) Novel regulation of pregnant human myometrial smooth muscle cell gap junctions by human chorionic gonadotropin. Endocrinology 135:2772–2779.
32. Eta E, Ambrus G, Rao ChV (1994) Direct regulation of human myometrial contractions by human chorionic gonadotropin. J Clin Endocrinol Metab 79:1582–1586.
33. Han SW, Lei ZM, Rao ChV (1996) Upregulation of cyclooxygenase-2 gene expression by chorionic gonadotropin during the differentiation of human endometrial stromal cells into decidua. Endocrinology 137:1791–1797.
34. Tang B, Gurpide E (1993) Direct effect of gonadotropins on decidualization of human endometrial stromal cells. J Steroid Biochem Mol Biol 47:115–121.
35. Han SW, Lei ZM, Rao ChV (1997) Homologus downregulation of luteinizing hormone/ chorionic gonadotropin receptors by increasing the degradation of receptor transcripts in human endometrial stromal cells. Biol Reprod 57:158–164.
36. Toth P, Li X, Rao ChV, Lincoln SR, Sanfilippo JS, Spinnato JA, Yussman MA (1994) Expression of functional human chorionic gonadotropin/human luteinizing hormone receptor gene in human uterine arteries. J Clin Endocrinol Metab 79:307–315.
37. Ziecik AJ, Derecka-Reszka K, Rzucidlo SJ (1992) Extragonadal gonadotropin receptors, their distribution and function. J Physiol Pharmacol 43:33–49.
38. Lei ZM, Reshef E, Rao ChV (1992) The expression of human chorionic gonadotropin/ luteinizing hormone receptors in human endometrial and myometrial blood vessels. J Clin Endocrinol Metab 75:651–659.

39. Ziecik AJ, Jedlinska M, Rzucidlo SJ (1992) Effect of estradiol and progesterone on myometrial LH/hCG receptors in pigs. Acta Endocrinol 127:185–188.
40. Lei ZM, Toth P, Rao ChV, Pridham D (1993) Novel co-expression of human chorionic gonadotropin (hCG)/human luteinizing hormone receptors and their ligand, hCG, in human fallopian tubes. J Clin Endocrinol Metab 77:863–872.
41. Sun T, Lei ZM, Rao ChV (1997) A novel regulation of the oviductal glycoprotein gene expression by luteinizing hormone in bovine oviductal epithelial cells. Mol Cell Endocrinol 131:87–108.
42. Han SW, Lei ZM, Rao ChV (1997) Regulation of luteinizing hormone/human chorionic gonadotropin receptor levels in human fallopian tube epithelial cells by estradiol and human chorionic gonadotropin. J Soc Gynecol Invest 4:Suppl 1, Abstract #605.
43. Han SW, Lei ZM, Rao ChV (1996) Upregulation of cyclooxygenase-2 gene expression by chorionic gonadotropin in mucosal cells from human fallopian tubes. Endocrinology 137: 2929–2937.
44. Zhou XL, Lei ZM, Rao ChV (1997) Regulation of cyclooxygenase-2 in human endometrial glandular epithelial cells by human chorionic gonadotropin and luteinizing hormone. J Soc Gynecol Invest 4:Suppl 1, Abstract #633.
45. Noyes RW, Hertig AT, Rock J (1950) Dating the endometrial biopsy. Fertil Steril 1:3–25.
46. Maslar IA, Riddick DH (1979) Prolactin production by human endometrium during the normal menstrual cycle. Am J Obstet Gynecol 135:751–754.
47. Huang JR, Tseng L, Bischof P, Janne OA (1987) Regulation of prolactin production by progestin, estrogen, and relaxin in human endometrial stromal cells. Endocrinology 121:2011–2017.
48. Irwin JC, Utian WH, Eckert RL (1991) Sex steroids and growth factors differentially regulate the growth and differentiation of cultured human endometrial stromal cells. Endocrinology 129: 2385–2392.
49. Randolph JF Jr, Peegel H, Ansbacher R, Menon KMJ (1990) *In vitro* induction of prolactin production and aromatase activity by gonadal steroids exclusively in the stroma of separated proliferative endometrium. Am J Obstet Gynecol 162:1109–1114.
50. Zhu HH, Huang JR, Mazella J, Rosenberg M, Tseng L (1990) Synergistic effects of progestin and relaxin on the synthesis and production of prolactin in long term cultures of human endometrial stromal cells. J Clin Endocrinol Metab 71:889–899.
51. Bell SC, Jackson JA, Ashmore J, Zhu HH, Tseng L (1991) Regulation of insulin-like growth factor binding protein-1 (hIGFBP-1) synthesis and secretion by progestin and relaxin in long term cultures of human endometrial stromal cells. J Clin Endocrinol Metab 72:1014–1024.
52. Irwin JC, Fuentes LDL, Dsupin BA, Guidice LC (1993) Insulin-like growth factor regulation of human endometrial stromal cells function coordinate effects on insulin-like growth factor binding protein-1, cell proliferation and prolactin secretion. Regul Pept 48:165–177.
53. Irwin JC, Kirk D, King RJB, Quigley MM, Gwatkin RBL (1989) Hormonal regulation of human endometrial stromal cells in culture: an *in vitro* model for decidualization. Fertil Steril 52:761–768.
54. Naurkawa S, Kanzaki H, Inoue T, Imai K, Higuchi T, Hatayama H, Kariya M, Mori T (1994) Androgens induce prolactin production by human endometrial stromal cells *in vitro*. J Clin Endocrinol Metab 78:165–168.
55. Alleva JJ, Kenimer JG, Jordan AW, Lamanna C (1983) Induction of estrogen and progesterone receptors and decidualization in the hamster uterus by cholera toxin. Endocrinology 112: 2095–2100.
56. Ebert KM, Fox KA (1977) Induction of implantation in the rat by cyclic nucleotides. Contraception 16:149–154.
57. Holmes PV, Bergström S (1975) Induction of blastocyst implantation in mice by cyclic AMP. J Reprod Fertil 43:329–335.
58. Webb FTG (1975) Implantation in ovariectomized mice treated with dibutyryl adenosine 3′,5′-monophosphate (dibutyryl cyclic AMP). J Reprod Fertil 42:511–517.
59. Han SW, Lei ZM, Rao ChV (1996) Transcriptional regulation of prolactin gene by chorionic gonadotropin during the differentiation of human endometrial stromal cells into decidua. Biol Reprod 54:Suppl 1, Abstract #343.
60. McDonald GJ, Armstrong DT, Greep RO (1967) Initiation of blastocyst implantation by luteinizing hormone. Endocrinology 80:172–176.
61. Gidley-Baird AA, Emmens CW (1978) Pituitary hormone control of implantation in the mouse. Aust J Biol Sci 31:657–665.

62. Frank GR, Brar AK, Cedars MI, Handwerger S (1994) Prostaglandin E_2 enhances human endometrial stromal cell differentiation. Endocrinology 134:258–263.
63. Funk CD (1993) Molecular biology in the eicosanoid field. Prog Nucleic Acids Res Mol Biol 45:67–98.
64. Wu W-X, Brooks J, Glasier AF, McNeilly AS (1995) The relationship between decidualization and prolactin mRNA and production at different stages of human pregnancy. J Mol Endocrinol 14:255–261.
65. Toth P, Li X, Lei ZM, Rao ChV (1996) Expression of human chorionic gonadotropin (hCG)/luteinizing hormone receptors and regulation of cyclooxygenase-1 gene by exogenous hCG in human fetal membranes. J Clin Endocrinol Metab 81:1283–1288.
66. Petraglia F, Tabanelli S, Galassi MC, Garuti GC, Mancini AC, Genazzani AR, Gurpide E (1992) Human decidua and *in vitro* decidualized endometrial stromal cells at term contain immunoreactive corticotropin-releasing factor (CRF) and CRF messenger ribonucleic acid. J Clin Endocrinol Metab 74:1427–1431.
67. Sakakibara H, Taga M, Saji M, Kida H, Minaguchi H (1994) Gene expression of epidermal growth factor in human endometrium during decidualization. J Clin Endocrinol Metab 79: 223–226.
68. Hatayama H, Kanzaki H, Iwai M, Kariya M, Fujimoto M, Higuchi T, Kojima K, Nakayama H, Mori T, Fujita J (1995) Progesterone enhances macrophage colony-stimulating factor production in human endometrial stromal cells *in vitro*. Endocrinology 135:1921–1927.
69. Hill JB, Jiminez AL, Passmore JC, Rao ChV (1996) Effect of human chorionic gonadotropin on reproductive organ blood flow in cycling rats. Proc Soc Exp Biol Med 211:94–99.
70. Hill JB, Alsip NL, Rao ChV, Asher EF (1997) Human chorionic gonadotropin directly and indirectly alters uterine arteriolar diameters in cycling rats. Am J Obstet Gynecol 176:150–157.
71. Hermsteiner GJ, Zoltan DR, Clapp JF III (1977) Human chorionic gonadotropin is a potent vasodialator of pre-arteriolar uterine and mesenteric vessels in pregnant and nonpregnant rats. J Soc Gynecol Invest 4:Suppl 1, Abstract #123.
72. Goswamy RK, Steptoe PC (1988) Doppler ultrasound studies of the uterine artery in spontaneous ovarian cycles. Hum Reprod 3:721–726.
73. Thaler I, Manor D, Brandes J, Rottem S, Itskovitz J (1990) Basic principles and clinical applications of the transvaginal Doppler duplex system in reproductive medicine. J In Vitro Fertil Embryo Transfer 7:74–85.
74. deZiegler D, Bessis R, Frydman R (1991) Vascular resistance of uterine arteries: physiological effects of estradiol and progesterone. Fertil Steril 55:775–779.
75. Greiss Jr FC, Anderson SG (1970) Effect of ovarian hormones on the uterine vascular bed. Am J Obstet Gynecol 107:829–836.
76. Huckabee WE, Crenshaw C, Curet LB, Mann L, Barron DH (1970) The effect of exogenous oestrogen on the blood flow and oxygen consumption of the uterus of the nonpregnant ewe. Q J Exp Physiol 55:16–24.
77. Killam AP, Rosenfeld CR, Battaglia FC, Makowski EL, Meschia G (1973) Effect of estrogen on the uterine blood flow of oophorectomized ewes. Am J Obstet Gynecol 115:1045–1052.
78. Perrot-Applanat M, Groyer-Picart MT, Garcia E, Lorenzo F, Milgrom E (1988) Immunocytochemical demonstration of estrogen and progesterone receptors in muscle cells of uterine arteries in rabbits and humans. Endocrinology 123:1511–1519.
79. Perrot-Applanat M, Deng M, Fernandez H, Lelaidier C, Meduri G, Bouchard P (1994) Immunohistochemical localization of estradiol and progesterone receptors in human uterus throughout pregnancy: expression in endometrial blood vessels. J Clin Endocrinol Metab 78:216–224.
80. Battaglia C, Larocca E, Lanzani A, Valentini M, Genazzani AR (1990) Doppler ultrasound studies of the uterine arteries in spontaneous and IVF stimulated cycles. Gynecol Endocrinol 4: 245–250.
81. Kurjak A, Kupesic-Urek S, Schulman H, Zalud I (1991) Transvaginal color flow Doppler in the assessment of ovarian, uterine blood flow in infertile women. Fertil Steril 56:870–873.
82. Kupesic S, Kurjak A (1993) Uterine and ovarian perfusion during periovulatory period assessed by transvaginal color Doppler. Fertil Steril 60:439–443.
83. Hillard TC, Bourne TH, Whitehead MI, Crayford TB, Collins WP, Campbell S (1992) Differential effects of transdermal estradiol and sequential progestogens on impedence to flow within the uterine arteries of postmenopausal women. Fertil Steril 58:959–963.
84. Bourne T, Hillard TC, Whitehead MI, Crook D, Campbell S (1990) Oestrogens, arterial status and post menopausal women. Lancet 335:1470–1471.

85. Matta WHM, Stabile I, Shaw RW, Campbell S (1988) Doppler assessment of uterine blood changes in patients with fibroids receiving the gonadotropin-releasing hormone agonist buserelin. Fertil Steril 49:1083–1085.
86. Környei JL, Li X, Lei ZM, Rao ChV (1995) Analysis of epidermal growth factor action in human myometrial smooth muscle cells. J Endocrinol 146:261–270.
87. How H, Huang ZH, Zuo J, Lei ZM, Spinnato II JA, Rao ChV (1995) Myometrial estradiol and progesterone receptor changes in preterm and term pregnancies. Obstet Gynecol 86:936–940.
88. Csapo AI (1976) Effects of progesterone, prostaglandin $F_{2\alpha}$, and its analogue ICI 81008 on the excitability and threshold of the uterus. Am J Obstet Gynecol 124:367–378.
89. Beck P, Adler P, Szlachter N, Goldsmith LT, Steinetz BG, Weiss G (1982) Synergistic effect of human relaxin and progesterone on human myometrial contractions. Int J Gynecol 20:141–144.
90. Sandberg F, Ingelman-Sundberg A, Ryden G (1964) The effect of prostaglandin E_2 and E_3 on the human uterus and fallopian tubes in vitro. Acta Obstet Gynecol Scand 43:95–102.
91. Coutinho EM, Maia H (1971) The contractile response of the human uterus, fallopian tubes and ovary to prostaglandins in vivo. Fertil Steril 22:539–543.
92. Spilman CH, Harper MJK (1975) Effects of prostaglandins on oviductal motility and egg transport. Gynecol Invest 6:186–205.
93. Lindblom B, Hamberger L, Wiqvist N (1978) Differential contractile effect of prostaglandins E and F on the isolated circular and longitudinal smooth muscle of the human oviduct. Fertil Steril 30:553–559.
94. Nozaki M, Ito Y (1986) Menstrual cycle and sensitivity of human fallopian tube to prostaglandins. Am J Physiol 251:R1126–R1136.
95. Verdugo P, Rumery R, Tam PY (1980) Hormonal control of oviductal ciliary activity: effect of prostaglandins. Fertil Steril 33:193–196.
96. Nancarrow CD, Hill JL (1995) Oviduct proteins in fertilization and early embryo development. J Reprod Fertil Suppl 49:3–13.
97. O'Day-Bowman MB, Mavrogianis PA, Reuter LM, Johnson DE, Fazleabas AT, Verhage HG (1996) Association of oviduct-specific glycoproteins with human and baboon (*Papio anubis*) ovarian oocytes and enhancement of human sperm binding to human hemizonae following in vitro incubation. Biol Reprod 54:60–69.
98. Kurman RJ, Norris HI (1987) Endometrial carcinoma, In: Blausteins Pathology of the Female Genital Tract, 3rd ed. (Kuman RJ, ed.), Springer-Verlag, New York, pp. 338–372.
99. Lucas, WE (1974) Casual relationships between endocrine-metabolic variables in patients with endometrial carcinomas. Obstet Gynecol 29:507–528.
100. Tseng L, Mozella J, Mann WT, Chumas J (1982) Estrogen synthesis in normal and malignant human endometrium. J Clin Endocrinol Metab 55:1029–1031.
101. Nagamani M, Stuart CA, Doherty MG (1992) Increased steroid production by the ovarian stromal tissue of postmenopausal women with endometrial cancer. J Clin Endocrinol Metab 74:172–176.
102. Nagamani M, Doherty MG, Smith ER, Yallampalli C (1992) Increased bioactive luteinizing hormone levels in postmenopausal women with endometrial cancer. Am J Obstet Gynecol 167: 1825–1830.
103. Wiznitzer A, Marback M, Hazum E, Insler V, Sharoni Y, Levy J (1988) Gonadotropin-releasing hormone-specific binding sites in uterine leiomyomata. Biochem Biophys Res Commun 152: 1326–1331.
104. Emons G, Schroder B, Ortmann O, Westphalen S, Schulz K-D, Schally AV (1993) High affinity binding and direct antiproliferative effects of luteinizing hormone-releasing hormone analogs in human endometrial cancer cell lines. J Clin Endocrinol Metab 77:1458–1464.
105. Hussa RO (1980) Biosynthesis of human chorionic gonadotropin. Endocr Rev 1:268–294.
106. Acevedo HF, Pardo M, Campbell-Acevedo E, Domingue GJ (1987) Human choriogonadotropin-like material in bacteria of different species: electron microscopy and immunocytochemical studies with monoclonal and polyclonal antibodies. J Gen Microbiol 133:783–791.
107. Robinson Jr EN, McGee ZA (1988) Detection of human hormone-like molecules elaborated *in vitro* by *Neisseria gonorrhoeae*. J Cell Biochem 12B(Suppl):30.
108. Bramley TA, Menzies GS, Williams RJ, Adams RJ, Kinsman OS (1990) Specific high-affinity binding sites for human luteinizing hormone (hLH) and human chorionic gonadotropin (hCG) in *Candida* species. Biochem Biophys Res Commun 167:1050–1056.
109. Gorby GL, Clemens CM, Barley LR, McGee ZA (1991) Effect of human chorionic gonadotropin (hCG) on *Neisseria gonorrhoeae* invasion of and IgA secretion by human fallopian tube mucosa. Microbial Pathogen 10:373–384. .

110. Heap RB, Flint APF, Gadsby JE (1979) Role of embryonic signals in the establishment of pregnancy. Br Med Bull 35:129–134.
111. Kornyei JL, Li X, Lei ZM, Rao ChV (1996) Restoration of human chorionic gonadotropin response in human myometrial smooth muscle cells by treatment with follicle stimulating hormone (FSH): Evidence for the presence of FSH receptors in human myometrium. Eur J Endocrinol 134:225–231.
112. Soloff MS, Swartz TL, Steinberg AH (1974) Oxytocin receptors in human uterus. J Clin Endocrinol Metab 38:1052–1058.
113. Fuchs AR, Fuchs F, Soloff MS (1985) Oxytocin receptors in nonpregnant human uterus. J Clin Endocrinol Metab 60:37–41.
114. Maggi M, Genazzani AD, Giannini S, Torrisi C, Baldi E, Tomasso M, Munson PJ, Rodbard D, Serio M (1988) Vasopressin and oxytocin receptors in vagina, myometrium, and oviduct of rabbits. Endocrinology 122:2970–2980.
115. Jenner LJ, Parkinson TJ, Lamming GE (1991) Uterine oxytocin receptors in cyclic and pregnant cows. J Reprod Fert 91:49–58.
116. Yang S, Rembiesa B, Bullesbach EE, Schwabe C (1992) Relaxin receptors in mice: demonstration of ligand binding in symphyseal tissues and uterine membrane fragments. Endocrinology 130: 179–185.
117. Sharara FI, Nieman LK (1995) Growth hormone receptor messenger ribonucleic acid expresion in leiomyoma and surrounding myometrium. Am J Obstet Gynecol 172:814–819.
118. Lefebvre DL, Giaid A, Bennett H, Larivière R, Zingg HH (1992) Oxytocin gene expression in rat uterus. Science 256:1553–1555.
119. Tang XM, Chegini N (1995) Human fallopian tube as an extraovarian source of relaxin: messenger ribonucleic acid expression and cellular localization of immunoreactive protein and ^{125}I-relaxin binding sites. Biol Reprod 52:1343–1349.
120. Tashima L, Greenwood FC, Bryant-Greenwood GD, Peaker M (1988) Identification of mRNA for relaxin in the endometrium of the pregnant guinea-pig. J Endocrinol 188:R9–R11.
121. Grattarola R, Li CH (1959) Effect of growth hormone and its combination with estradiol-17β on the uterus of hypophysectomized-ovariectomized rats. Endocrinology 65:802–810.
122. Guillon G, Balestre MN, Roberts JM, Bottari SP (1987) Oxytocin and vasopressin:distinct receptors in myometrium. J Clin Endocrinol Metab 64:1129–1134.
123. MacLennan AH, Grant P, Ness D, Down A (1986) Effect of porcine relaxin and progesterone on rat, pig and human myometrial activity in vitro. J Reprod Med 1986;31:43–49.
124. Kendall JZ, Mathias JR, Van Hook JW (1991) Leuprolide acetate stimulates smooth muscle of the human reproductive tract. Fertil Steril 56:993–994.
125. Medeiros YS, Claixto JB, Ballejo G (1988) Inhibitory effect of GnRH on isolated rat uterine muscle contractility. Life Sci 42:2055–2062.
126. Asirvatham AL, Johnson GA, Belden EL, Van-Kirk EA, Moss GE, Murdoch WJ (1994) Immunization of mice against a synthetic N-terminal extracellular domain gonadotropin-releasing hormone receptor peptide: evidence for a direct uterine effect. Am J Reprod Immunol 32:95–100.
127. Bazer FW, Spencer TE, Ott TL (1996) Placental interferons. Am J Reprod Immunol 35:297–308.
128. Gandolfi F, Moor RM (1987) Stimulation of early embryonic development in the sheep by coculture with oviduct epithelial cells. J Reprod Fertil 81:23–28.
129. White KL, Hehnke K, Rickords LF, Southern LL, Thompson DL, Wood TC (1989) Early embryonic development in vitro by coculture with oviductal epithelial cells in pigs. Biol Reprod 41:425–430.

6 The Rodent Placental Prolactin Family and Pregnancy

Michael J. Soares, PHD, *Guoli Dai,* DVM, PHD, *Christopher B. Cohick,* MS, *Heiner Müller,* MD, *and Kyle E. Orwig,* PHD

CONTENTS

INTRODUCTION

Endocrine signals produced by the placenta have a pivotal role in the establishment and maintenance of pregnancy. These signals include hormones, cytokines, and growth factors that act to coordinate events in maternal, extraembryonic, and embryonic compartments. Among the various regulatory signals secreted by the placenta are a prominent family of proteins related to pituitary prolactin (PRL). These proteins have amassed a rich history of investigation in several species.

In this chapter, we will focus on the current state of knowledge of structural and functional PRL homologs produced by the rodent placenta. Several reviews related to the subject have appeared in recent years *(1–6)*.

THE PLACENTAL PRL FAMILY: HISTORICAL ASPECTS

The initial identification of placental hormones possessing characteristics similar to pituitary PRL grew out of classic studies in the rat and mouse on the control of corpus luteum and mammary gland function during pregnancy *(see 2)*. For several decades, it was known that the anterior pituitary synthesized and secreted a substance (PRL) responsible for controlling the development and function of the corpus luteum (luteotrophic) and mammary gland (mammotrophic/lactogenic; *see 7*). The continued development of these

PRL target tissues following removal of the anterior pituitary gland during the latter half of pregnancy suggested the existence of extrapituitary sources of substances with luteotrophic, mammotrophic, and lactogenic actions. Replacement paradigms further demonstrated that the placenta was the source of substances that stimulated corpus luteum and mammary gland function. The eventual isolation and characterization of rodent placental proteins possessing PRL-like actions were very much dependent on the establishment of two experimentally powerful in vitro assays for monitoring PRL-like biological activities *(8,9)*: (1) radioreceptor assay for lactogenic hormones, and (2) the rat Nb2 lymphoma cell proliferation assay. Additional members of the placental PRL family were discovered during attempts to characterize further the proteins responsible for the placental PRL-like biological activities. Research on the biology and biochemistry of the placental PRL family has benefited immeasureably from the efforts and leadership of Henry G. Friesen and Frank Talamantes.

THE PLACENTAL PRL FAMILY: NOMENCLATURE

The placental PRL family represents a collection of structurally related proteins expressed by trophoblast cells of the placenta. Some proteins are also expressed by non-placental tissues. Each member of the family bears similarity to the structure of pituitary PRL, especially regarding the positioning of four core cysteine residues and some other key amino acids *(10)*. Shared functional characteristics with pituitary PRL are not a prerequisite for inclusion in the PRL family. Nomenclature for members of the placental PRL family reflects biological activities (placental lactogens), structural relationships with PRL (PRL-like proteins, PRL-related proteins), or association with proliferation (proliferin). At present, the terminology for some of the PRL family members is not entirely optimal; however, it seems inappropriate to make significant changes until we have a better appreciation of the biological actions of each of the ligands.

THE RODENT PLACENTAL PRL FAMILY

Placental proteins sharing characteristics with pituitary PRL have been demonstrated in only a limited number of rodent species, including the rat, mouse, hamster, and guinea pig *(11,12)*.

Members of the PRL family can be subdivided into two groups based on their biological actions: (1) classical and (2) nonclassical (Table 1). Classical members of the PRL family are functional PRL homologs, whereas nonclassical members possess biological actions not normally attributed to PRL. Although it has not been shown, some members of the PRL family may utilize both classical and nonclassical modes of action. Subfamilies can also be identified based on structural relationships. To date, nine members of the rat placental PRL family have been identified. Two homologs have been described in the mouse and hamster. An additional two apparently novel members of the placental PRL family have been reported in the mouse. A number of features of the placental PRL family are summarized in Table 2 and Figs. 1 and 2.

Before proceeding into a discussion of the rodent placental PRL family, it is necessary to review briefly the organization of the tissues responsible for their expression. We will subsequently examine our present understanding of the structural features of each member of the PRL family and its expression pattern, distribution, and biological actions.

Table 1
Rodent Placental Prolactin Family

Hormone	*Species*
Classical members:	
Placental lactogen-I subfamily:	
Placental lactogen-I (PL-I)	Mouse, rat, hamster
Placental lactogen-I variant (PL-Iv)	Rat
Placental lactogen-II (PL-II)	Mouse, rat, hamster
Nonclassical members:	
Prolactin-like protein-A (PLP-A)	Rat
Prolactin-like protein-B (PLP-B)	Rat
Prolactin-like protein-C subfamily:	
Prolactin-like protein-C (PLP-C)	Rat
Prolactin-like protein-C variant (PLP-Cv)	Rat
Prolactin-like protein-D (PLP-D)	Rat
Prolactin-related protein (d/tPRP)	Rat
Proliferin (PLF)(SSP) (ESP)	Mouse
Proliferin-related protein (PRP)	Mouse, hamster

Table 2
Characteristics of Placental PRL Family Members[a]

Hormone	*Mol wt of reduced forms, kDa*	*Cysteine residues*	*Glycoprotein*	*Peak serum levels during pregnancy, ng/mL[b]*	*Functional characteristics*
Rat					
PRL	23	6	No	1500–200	PRL-R[d] activation
PL-I	36–42	5	Yes	2000–3000	PRL-R activation
PL-Iv	29 and 33	5	Yes	?	PRL-R activation
PL-II	25	4	No	600–800	PRL-R activation
PLP-A	29 and 33	5	Yes	?	Unknown
PLP-B	31	4	Yes	?	Unknown
PLP-C	29	6	Yes/no	?	Unknown
PLP-Cv	?	6	?	?	Unknown
PLP-D	?	6	?	?	Unknown
d/tPRP	29	6	Yes	?	Unknown[c]
Mouse					
PRL	23	6	No	200–300	PRL-R activation
PL-I	29–32 and 36.5–42	5	Yes	300–400	PRL-R activation
PL-II	25	4	No	300–500	PRL-R activation
PLF	27 and 35	6	Yes	3000–4000	Stimulates angiogenesis
PLF-RP[d]	36–44	5	Yes	3000–4000	Inhibits angiogenesis
Hamster					
PRL	23	6	No	600–1000	PRL-R activation
PL-II	25	6	No	10,000–12,000	PRL-R activation
PLF-RP	?	4	?	?	Unknown

[a] *See text* for discussion.
[b] Please note serum levels are only an approximation and vary depending on hormone standards used in the analyses.
[c] d/tPRP may increase tumor incidence and similarly the establishment of pregnancy.
[d] PRL-R, PRL receptor; PLF-RP, Proliferin-related protein.

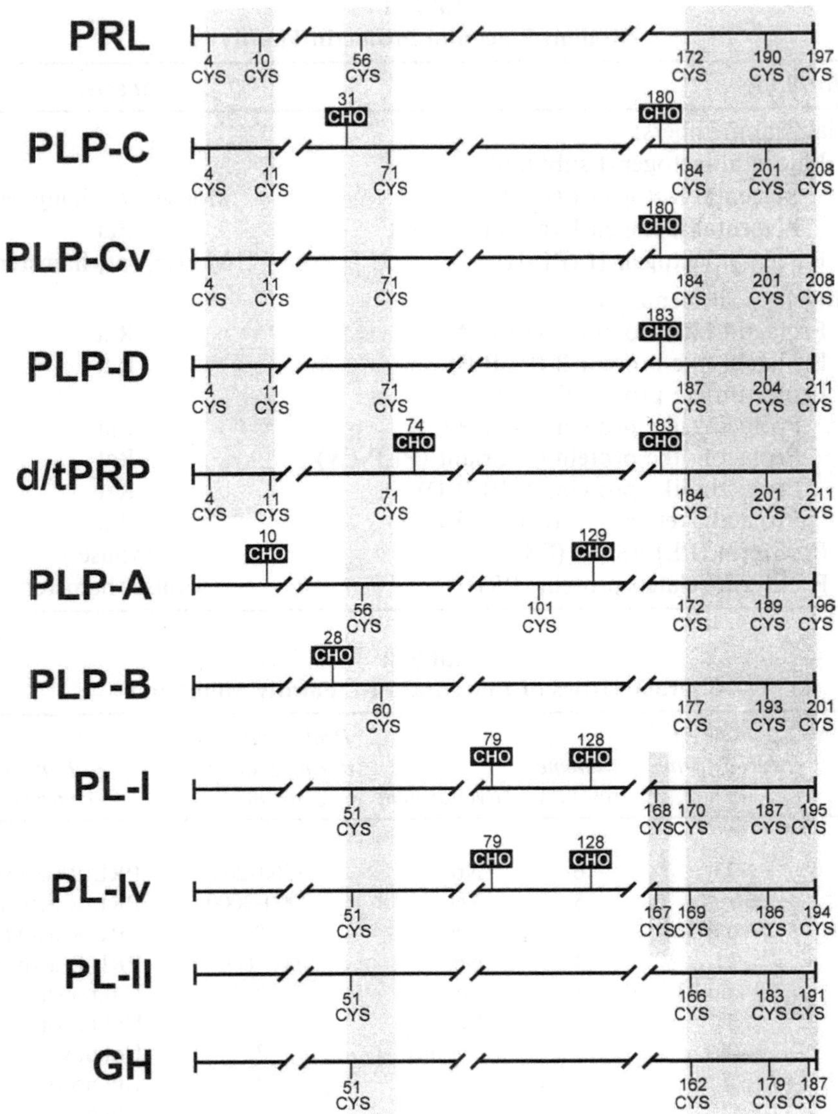

Fig. 1. Schematic comparisons of the current rat PRL family. Sites for N-linked glycosylation are shown above each line, and cysteine residues are shown below each line. Locations of homologous cysteine residues are shaded. Abbreviations: PRL, prolactin; PLP-C, prolactin-like protein C; PLP-Cv, prolactin-like protein C variant; PLP-D, prolactin-like protein D; d/tPRP, decidual/trophoblast prolactin-related protein; PLP-A, prolactin-like protein A; PLP-B, prolactin-like protein B; PL-I, placental lactogen-I; PL-Iv, placental lactogen-I variant; PL-II, placental lactogen-II; GH, growth hormone.

Organization of the Endocrine Placenta

The following overview relates to specific anatomical relationships associated with placental endocrinology in the rat and mouse *(see 3,4,13,14)*. Two prominent placental structures: (1) choriovitelline placenta and (2) chorioallantoic placenta, and two trophoblast cell types: (1) trophoblast giant cells and (2) spongiotrophoblast cells are responsible for the endocrine activities of the rodent placenta (Fig. 3). The choriovitelline placenta is important from postimplantation stages until midgestation, whereas the chorioallantoic placenta first develops at midgestation and continues until term.

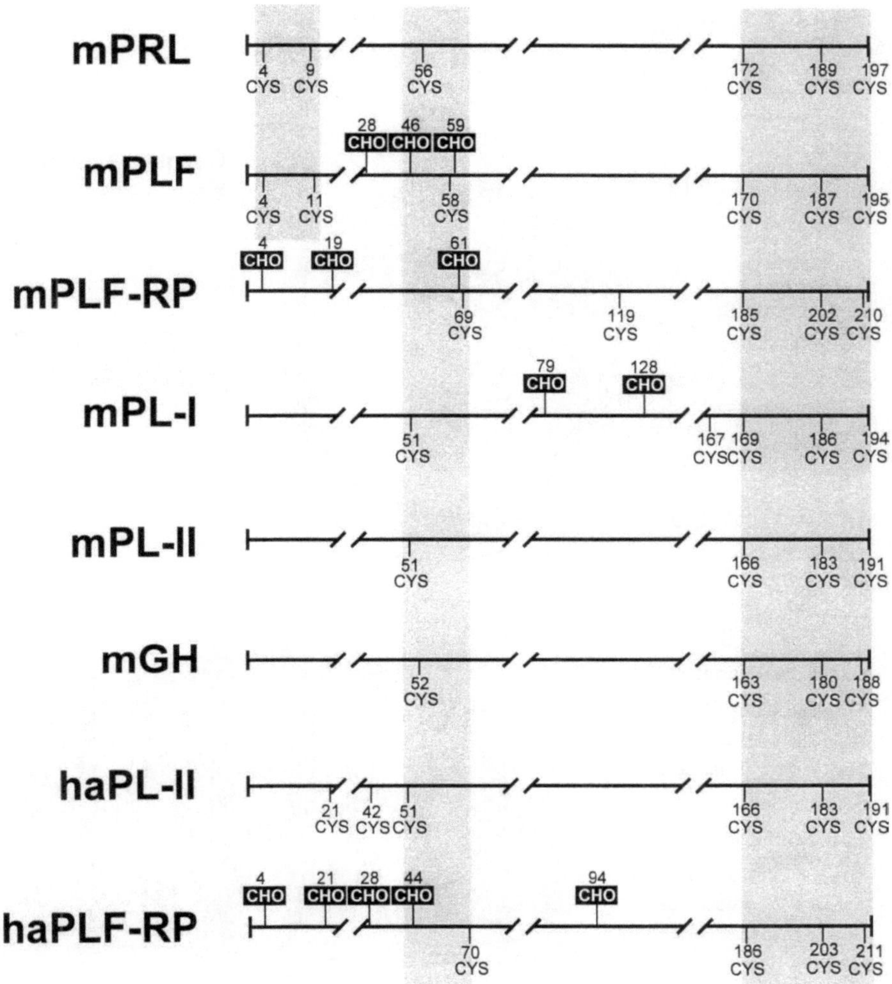

Fig. 2. Schematic comparisons of the mouse PRL family and hamster PL-II and PLF-RP. Sites for N-linked glycosylation are shown above each line, and cysteine residues are shown below each line. Locations of homologous cysteine residues are shaded. Abbreviations: mPRL, mouse prolactin; mPLF, mouse proliferin; mPLF-RP, mouse PLF-related protein; mPL-I, mouse placental lactogen-I; mPL-II, mouse placental lactogen-II; mGH, mouse growth hormone; haPL-II, hamster PL-II; haPLF-RP, hamster PLF-related protein.

Trophoblast giant cells are endocrinologically active from implantation until term. As gestation progresses, these important cells produce hormones attributed to the choriovitelline placenta, and subsequently they contribute to hormones produced by the chorioallantoic placenta. On their initial appearance and thereafter, trophoblast giant cells are positioned at the maternal–placental interface. During the final week of gestation, they also appear in a component of the chorioallantoic placenta located nearest the developing fetus and referred to as the labyrinth zone. The labyrinth zone is a site of bidirectional fetal–maternal transport *(15)*. A unique rat trophoblast cell line, referred to as Rcho-1, is a useful in vitro model for studying regulatory pathways controlling trophoblast giant cell differentiation *(16,17)*. In vitro, Rcho-1 trophoblast cells can be manipulated to recapitulate trophoblast giant cell development *(17–22)*.

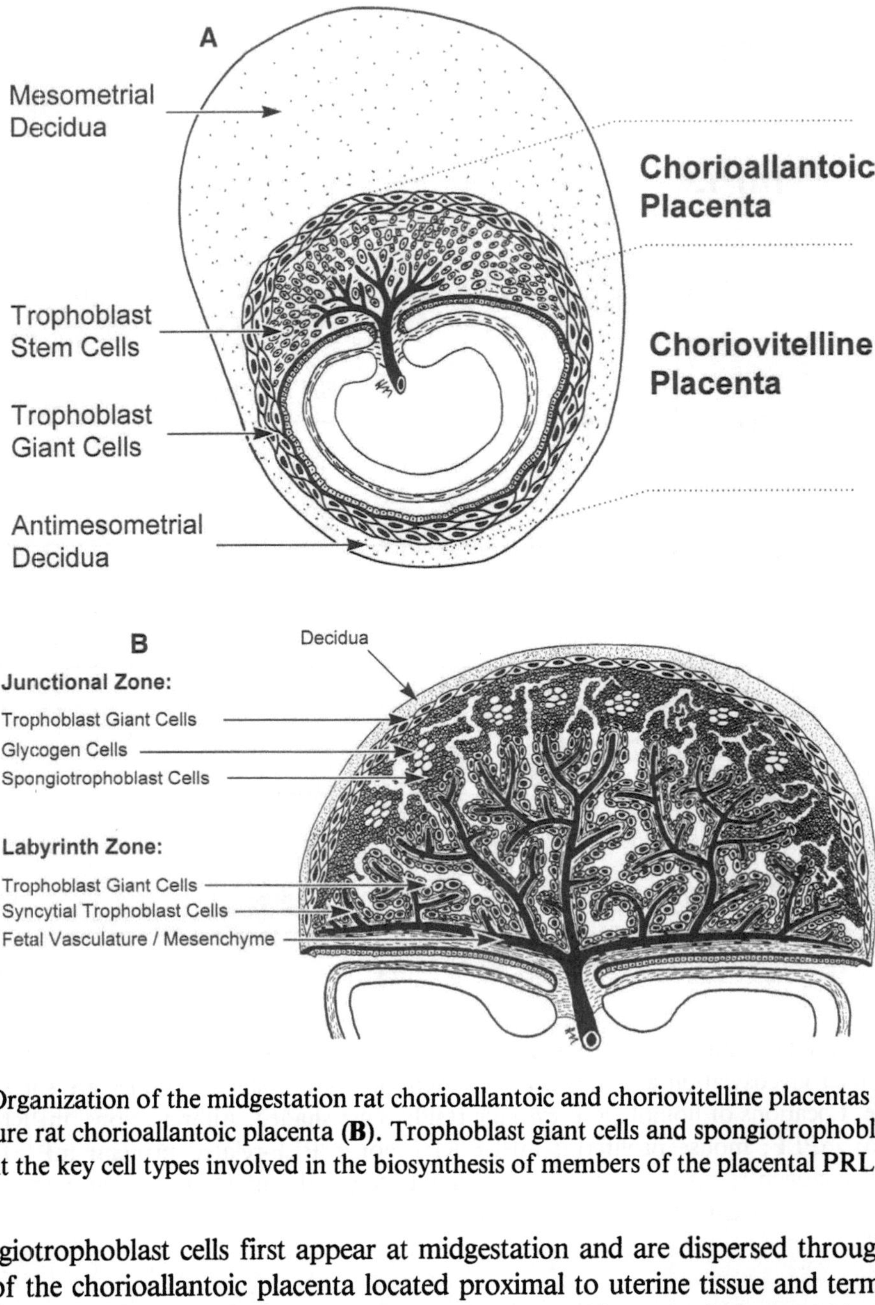

Fig. 3. Organization of the midgestation rat chorioallantoic and choriovitelline placentas (**A**) and the mature rat chorioallantoic placenta (**B**). Trophoblast giant cells and spongiotrophoblast cells represent the key cell types involved in the biosynthesis of members of the placental PRL family.

Spongiotrophoblast cells first appear at midgestation and are dispersed throughout a region of the chorioallantoic placenta located proximal to uterine tissue and termed the junctional zone. These cells are active sites of hormone biosynthesis from midgestation until term.

Classical Members of the Placental PRL Family

Classical members of the PRL family utilize the PRL receptor signaling pathway. Mouse, rat, and hamster homologs for two classical members of the PRL family have been investigated. The guinea pig placenta produces a classical member of the PRL family *(12)*; however, it has not been isolated or characterized, and will not be further discussed.

Placental Lactogen-I (PL-I) Subfamily. The PL-I subfamily consists of two members sharing considerable structural similarity and some functional overlap.

Placental Lactogen-I (PL-I). A prominent placental lactogen, PL-I, was identified in midpregnant placental tissues from the mouse, rat, and hamster *(23–29)*. PL-I was purified to homogeneity from midgestation mouse placental tissue *(30)*, and its corresponding cDNA isolated from both mouse and rat placental cDNA libraries *(31,32)*. A rat placental cDNA, closely related to the "original" rat PL-I cDNA *(32)*, termed PL-I mosaic (PL-Im), has been reported *(33)*. Similarly, we isolated a PL-I cDNA from a Rcho-1 trophoblast cell cDNA library that closely resembled PL-Im *(34)*. Using an assortment of polymerase chain reaction (PCR) strategies, we have not been successful in isolating the "original" PL-I transcript from midgestation rat placental tissue, from the PL-I expressing Rcho-1 trophoblast cell line, or the "original" PL-I gene from a rat genomic library *(34)*. Alternatively, the PL-Im sequence can be amplified from each of these sources *(34)*. Given these results, we re-examined the original PL-I cDNA by PCR and nucleotide sequence analyses. The sequence differed from the original report, and was found to be identical to the Rcho-1 PL-I and PL-Im cDNA clones *(34)*. Thus, PL-I, Rcho-1 PL-I, and PL-Im are equivalent and should be referred to as PL-I. Although, evidence for a hamster PL-I homolog also exists *(28)*, it has not been purified nor has its cDNA been isolated.

Structural Characteristics. PL-I is a heterogeneous high-mol-wt glycoprotein (36–42 kDa) possessing approx 30% sequence identity with pituitary PRL *(30–34)*. The PL-I cDNA encodes a 224 amino acid protein possessing a 30 amino acid signal peptide, 5 cysteine residues, and 2 putative N-linked glycosylation sites *(31,33,34)*. Carbohydrate constituents of PL-I fail to bind to Concanavalin A (Con A) *(35)*, which may be a characteristic of the cells that produce PL-I rather than the PL-I structure itself. Transcription from the PL-I gene is initiated 63 nucleotides upstream of the PL-I translation start site *(36)*.

Expression. Trophoblast giant cells are the exclusive source of PL-I *(32,37–40)*. PL-I expression is initiated shortly after implantation and terminates at midgestation *(32,38,39)*.

A limited amount of information is available on the control of trophoblast giant cell PL-I production. During the first half of gestation, PL-I expression is tightly coupled to trophoblast giant cell development. At midpregnancy, PL-I biosynthesis is abruptly terminated. Following midgestation, trophoblast giant cell formation continues, but is not associated with PL-I expression. Factors responsible for determining the ontogeny or cessation of PL-I production are largely unknown. The anterior pituitary is a possible source of regulators that are associated with decreased serum PL-I levels *(41,42)*. This may be through the production of factors that inhibit PL-I production or modulate PL-I clearance. Seemingly, contradictory in vitro data suggest that substances secreted by the anterior pituitary may actually stimulate PL-I biosynthesis *(43)*. A number of other factors potentially modulating PL-I production in vitro through direct or indirect mechanisms have been reported. Epidermal growth factor (EGF), leukemia inhibitory factor (LIF), oncostatin M (OM), and interleukin-11 (IL-11) stimulated, whereas progesterone and transforming growth factor α (TGF-α) inhibited PL-I production by mixed mouse placental cell cultures *(44–48)*. Cyclic adenosine-3′,5′-monophosphate (cAMP) can stimulate or inhibit PL-I production depending on the gestational age of the placental cells *(48,49)*. The nature of the in vitro model used in these experiments makes mechanistic interpretations difficult.

5′-Flanking DNA associated with the mouse PL-I gene has been isolated and studied in the Rcho-1 trophoblast cell line *(36)*. This cell line is particularly useful, because it consists of trophoblast stem cells that can be manipulated to differentiate into trophoblast giant cells *(17,19)*. A minimal 274-bp PL-I promoter effectively targets reporter expression to trophoblast giant cells in vitro *(36)*. Within this promoter region are important cis-regulatory elements that bind AP-1 and GATA factors *(36,50)*. Mutation of these elements is associated with significant reductions in in vitro PL-I promoter activity. Two GATA factors, GATA-2 and GATA-3, are expressed in trophoblast cells and have been shown to activate the PL-I promoter specifically in a nontrophoblast cell system *(50)*. Furthermore, GATA-2 and GATA-3 null mutant placentae show decreased PL-I expression *(51)*. Additionally, when members of the basic helix-loop-helix (bHLH) transcription factor family are cotransfected with PL-I promoter-reporter constructs into Rcho-1 trophoblast cells, PL-I promoter activity is influenced *(52)*. *Id-1* and *Hxt* (also known as Thing-1 and e-HAND; *53,54*) have modest inhibitory and stimulatory effects on PL-I promoter activity, respectively *(52)*. The expression of each of the bHLH factors in differentiating Rcho-1 trophoblast cells parallels its actions and the expression of PL-I. A putative bHLH DNA binding element (E-Box) is located within the PL-I minimal promoter. The collective importance of each of these assorted DNA regulatory regions and trans-acting factors to the in vivo regulation of PL-I expression has yet to be demonstrated.

Distribution. PL-I circulates in maternal blood *(55,56)*. Maternal serum PL-I levels peak at midgestation and decline precipitously accompanying the termination of trophoblast giant cell PL-I expression *(55)*. PL-I has a prolonged serum half-life relative to PL-II *(23)*. At midgestation, PL-I has also been detected in cerebrospinal fluid *(57)*.

Biological Actions. The actions of PL-I have been primarily studied via the generation of recombinant PL-I in Chinese hamster ovary (CHO) or HRP-1 cell lines *(34,56,58)*. PL-I binds to PRL receptors present in maternal and fetal tissues *(59–62)*, and possesses both stimulatory and inhibitory actions previously attributed to pituitary PRL. Rat Nb2 lymphoma cell proliferation *(31,34,56)*, mouse mammary gland epithelial cell proliferation, α-lactalbumin and insulin-like growth factor binding protein (29-kDa IGFBP) biosynthesis *(34,58,63)*, islet B-cell proliferation and insulin secretion *(64)*, luteal cell progesterone production *(65)*, and maternal behavior *(57,66)* are stimulated, whereas pituitary PRL secretion is inhibited *(67)*. PL-I is equipotent with pituitary PRL, and is the predominant lactogen in circulation between implantation and midgestation.

Placental Lactogen-I Variant (PL-Iv). A second member of the PL-I subfamily was identified as a result of two independent lines of investigation. During the purification of PRL-like protein A (PLP-A; *see below*) from late-gestation rat placental tissue, a major contaminating protein was purified and its N-terminal amino acid sequence determined *(35)*. The amino-terminus of the isolated protein exhibited approx 88% sequence identity with PL-I *(35)* and its cDNA subsequently isolated with a mouse PL-I cDNA from a late-gestation placental cDNA library *(68)*. A second strategy involved the detection of an mRNA from late-gestation placentas with a rat PL-I cDNA *(32)*. A rat PL-I cDNA was then used to isolate the late-gestation PL-I-related cDNA *(69)*. The cDNAs encoded for proteins closely related to PL-I and were referred to as PL-I variant (PL-Iv). Although, PL-Iv has only been definitively demonstrated in the rat, there is some evidence for existence of multiple PL-I genes and possibly additional PL-I immunoreactive proteins in the mouse *(31,55)*.

Structural Characteristics. PL-Iv is a close relative of PL-I. Both are glycoproteins, and possess considerable sequence (89% amino acid identity) and antigenic similarities *(35, 68,69)*. The PL-Iv cDNA encodes for a 223 amino acid protein containing a 28 amino acid signal peptide *(68)*. Five cysteine residues are present in PL-Iv and two putative N-linked glycosylation sites *(68,69)*. The nature of the glycosylated constitutents of PL-I and PL-Iv is different. In contrast to the 36–42 kDa PL-I species, PL-Iv avidly binds to Con A and is synthesized as 29- and 33-kDa mol-wt species *(35)*. As indicated above, PL-I and PL-Iv glycosylation patterns may reflect the cell types responsible for their synthesis.

Expression. PL-Iv is expressed during the second half of gestation primarily by spongiotrophoblast cells with minor contributions from trophoblast giant cells located at the maternal–placental interface *(35,69)*. Differentiating spongiotrophoblast cells spontaneously gain the capacity to produce PL-Iv in vitro *(70)*. The expression of PL-Iv by differentiating spongiotrophoblast cells can be specifically inhibited by treatment with retinoic acid *(70)*. Regulatory DNA associated with PL-Iv gene expression has not been defined. Because of the marked contrast in the cell- and temporal-specific patterns of PL-I vs PL-Iv gene expression, we would predict the existence of significant structural differences in their promoter sequences.

Distribution. PIv is present in maternal blood during the latter part of gestation as determined by a specific radioimmunoassay *(71)*.

Biological Actions. The biological activities of PL-Iv have been investigated with SDS-gel electrophoresis-purified PL-Iv and heterologously expressed recombinant PL-Iv *(35,68,71)*. Each of the preparations is capable of stimulating rat Nb2 lymphoma cell proliferation; however, none of the preparations are as potent as pituitary PRL *(35,68,71)*. Recombinant PL-Iv is also capable of competing with pituitary PRL for PRL receptors, again at a reduced potency *(68,71)*. PL-Iv also activates the Jak2 tyrosine kinase, a component of the intracellular PRL receptor signaling cascade *(68)*. Our current information suggests that PL-Iv is a functional homolog of pituitary PRL with somewhat reduced biological potency. The physiological significance of a limited PRL agonist is yet to be fully resolved. Additionally, it is not entirely clear that PL-Iv actions are restricted to the PRL receptor signal transduction system.

PLACENTAL LACTOGEN-II (PL-II). The protein responsible for the PRL-like biological activities of the second half of pregnancy is referred to as PL-II. PL-II was the first rodent PL discovered, purified to homogeneity, and its cDNA isolated from mouse, rat, and hamster placental cDNA libraries *(72–78)*.

Structural Characteristics. PL-II is a nonglycosylated protein with a mol wt approximating 25 kDa *(79,80)*. Each of the characterized rodent PL-II sequences possesses four cysteine residues in locations that are also conserved in all members of the PRL family and exhibit approx 35% amino acid sequence identity with PRL *(73,75,78)*. Hamster PL-II has two additional cysteines not present in mouse or rat PL-II that are proposed to influence its ability to interact with other proteins *(78)*. Rat PL-II is somewhat unique, in that it has been reported to exist in multiple forms *(74,81)*. The biochemical basis and physiological significance of these molecular isoforms are yet to be determined.

The mouse PL-II gene has a five-exon/four-intron organization identical to the well-conserved organization of the PRL gene *(82–85)*. A major transcription start site is situated 59 nucleotides upstream of the translation start site *(85)*.

Expression. PL-II is the exclusive product of trophoblast giant cells from midgestation until term *(38–40,86–89)*. At least some of the same trophoblast giant cells that are responsible for PL-I expression go on to express PL-II *(90,91)*. There are also positional effects related to PL-II gene expression. Around midgestation, PL-II is expressed in trophoblast giant cells associated with the maternal–placental interface of both the choriovitelline and chorioallantoic placentas *(38)*. During the latter part of pregnancy, trophoblast giant cells located in the labyrinth zone of the chorioallantoic placenta become a significant source of PL-II *(35,86,92)*.

In vivo experimental manipulations have yielded findings suggesting that the fetus produces substances that increase serum PL-II levels, whereas the anterior pituitary and ovaries produce substances that decrease circulating PL-II concentrations *(41,42,93–101)*. The positive fetal influences on circulating PL-II production seem to be indirect via effects on the development of the labyrinthine trophoblast giant cell population *(102)*. Negative modulatory influences of the anterior pituitary appear to be associated with growth hormone, and its mechanism of action appears to be through altering PL-II clearance rates *(95)*. In vivo studies have implicated estrogen and in vitro experiments have implicated progesterone as ovarian factors involved in the inhibitory control of PL-II *(98,100)*. Calcyclin, a calcium binding protein produced by decidual cells, has a positive stimulatory effect on PL-II biosynthesis *(103)*. An array of additional factors potentially modulating PL-II production in mixed placental cell cultures has been reported. Insulin, inhibin, and growth hormone-releasing hormone (GHRH) stimulate, but EGF, IL-6, IL-1, tumor necrosis factor-α (TNF-α), transforming growth factor-β_1, activin, LIF, OM, IL-11, and cAMP inhibit PL-II production *(45–49,104–111)*.

Progress in dissecting the molecular control of PL-II gene expression has been hindered by the apparent absence of suitable in vitro models. A 2.7-kb mouse PL-II promoter–reporter construct shows some limited activity in primary cultures of mouse placental cells *(112)*. Surprisingly, Rcho-1 trophoblast cells, which are capable of expressing the endogenous PL-II gene *(17)*, have thus far proven to be of limited value in studying the activities of either mouse or rat PL-II promoter–reporter constructs *(85,113)*. Whether additional DNA regulatory regions or more complex mechanisms are required for activity of these reporter constructs in Rcho-1 trophoblast cells remains to be determined. Some advances in identifying PL-II gene regulatory regions have been obtained utilizing transgenic approaches. The above-mentioned 2.7-kb mouse PL-II promoter directed expression of an SV40 large T-antigen reporter transgene in a pattern parallel to expression of the endogenous PL-II gene *(85)*. A shorter region of PL-II 5′-flanking DNA (569 bp) was ineffective in targeting expression of the transgene to the mouse placenta *(85)*. Thus, regulatory elements located within a rather broad region between 569 and 2700 bp upstream of the PL-II transcription start site direct trophoblast-specific PL-II gene expression.

Distribution. PL-II is present in maternal and fetal blood during the latter half of gestation *(1,24,26,59)*. Maternal serum PL-II increases gradually from low levels at midgestation to relatively high levels at term. In the rat and mouse, PL-II predominantly circulates in a monomeric form *(27,29)*, whereas in the hamster, PL-II circulates bound to α_2-macroglobulin *(114)*. During late gestation, PL-II has also been detected in cerebrospinal fluid *(57)*.

Biological Actions. The actions of PL-II have been primarily studied with native PL-II purified from either the mouse or rat placenta *(72,74,76)*. PL-II was originally characterized based on its ability to bind PRL receptors and mimic PRL biological activities *(59,61, 72,76,77,115)*. Among the spectrum of PL-II actions resembling pituitary PRL are stimulation of a variety of cellular processes, including rat Nb2 lymphoma cell proliferation *(25,34)*, mouse mammary gland epithelial cell proliferation, α-lactalbumin and IGFBP (29 kDa) biosynthesis *(34,63,77,116)*, islet B-cell proliferation and insulin secretion *(64,117)*, luteal cell progesterone production *(65)*, and maternal behavior *(57)*. Several amino acids within the PL-II structure critical to activation of PRL receptor signal transduction pathways have been identified *(118,119)*. Furthermore, structural requirements for PL-II binding to the PRL receptor have been dissociated from requirements for PRL receptor activation *(118,119)*. PL-II is equipotent with PRL and is the most prominent circulating lactogenic hormone of the latter half of pregnancy.

Nonclassical Members of the Placental PRL Family

Inclusion in this category of PRL family members reflects an inability of the ligand to activate the PRL receptor signal transduction system. This subgroup is comprised of six members from the rat and two members from the mouse. Mouse homologs for the rat members and rat homologs for the mouse members have not been reported. A possible hamster homolog for one of the mouse nonclassical members has recently been described *(see below)*.

PRL-Like Protein-A (PLP-A). PRL-like protein-A (PLP-A) is one of a group of structurally related proteins that are prominent secretory products of the rat placenta. A cDNA to PLP-A was one of three cDNAs structurally related to PRL originally identified during a search for the PL-II cDNA *(120)*.

Structural characteristics. The PLP-A cDNA encodes a 227 amino acid protein possessing a 31 amino acid signal peptide, five cysteine residues, two putative N-linked glycosylation sites, and overall a 30% amino acid sequence identity with pituitary PRL *(120)*. Four of the cysteines are located in regions homologous to the four core cysteine residues present in all members of the PRL family. The fifth cysteine is positioned toward the middle of its sequence. PLP-A protein species were first identified and partially characterized with antipeptide antibodies generated to three different regions of the predicted PLP-A amino acid sequence *(121)*. The antibodies recognized two placental protein species migrating at 29 and 33 kDa. Each species bound Con A and could be converted to species migrating at 25 kDa following treatment with *N*-glycanase *(121)*. The nature of the carbohydrate modification differs depending on the trophoblast cell type producing PLP-A *(122)*. The PLP-A gene has been partially characterized, and its transcription start site localized to 45 nucleotides upstream of the PLP-A translation start site *(113)*.

Expression. PLP-A protein and mRNA are specifically expressed in spongiotrophoblast cells and trophoblast giant cells of the junctional zone of the rat chorioallantoic placenta during the latter half of pregnancy *(86,87)*. Differentiating spongiotrophoblast cells express abundant amounts of PLP-A in vitro *(70)*. Some initial attempts to investigate the transcriptional regulation of PLP-A in the trophoblast giant cell lineage have been performed with the RCHO cell line (related to the Rcho-1 trophoblast cell line), which is capable of expressing the endogenous PLP-A gene *(113)*. PLP-A promoter–reporter constructs containing either 4.6 or 975 bp of 5′-flanking DNA are active in RCHO cells, but not in rat pituitary cells *(113)*. The 975-bp PLP-A promoter contains sequence motifs that correspond to cis-acting elements shown to be important in the developmental regulation of other genes. The relevance of these regulatory elements in directing trophoblast giant cell-specific expression of PLP-A has not been reported.

Distribution. PLP-A has been detected in fetal and maternal serum where it circulates as a high-mol wt complex (67–150 kDa; *121,123*). High-molecular-weight PLP-A complexes show decreased immunoreactivity that increases markedly following treatment with reducing agents, such as 2-mercaptoethanol *(123)*. An involvement of a free sulfhydral within the PLP-A structure has been postulated to be responsible for the formation of the circulating high-mol wt complexes *(123)*. Western blot analysis of PLP-A from pregnant serum with antibodies to recombinant PLP-A under nonreducing conditions results in the detection of immunoreactive species migrating at approx 110 and 230 kDa *(123)*. Cross-linking experiments with radiolabeled PLP-A and rat serum indicated the presence of complexes at approx 70, 110, 130, and 250 kDa *(124)*. Formation of the complexes could not be competed with PRL, growth hormone (GH), or human PL, but could be competed with excess PLP-A. The identity of the PLP-A binding proteins is yet to be determined. In addition to its secretion, some evidence exists for a nuclear targeting of PLP-A *(123)*. The significance of this latter observation is not readily apparent.

Biological Actions. Although, PLP-A has significant structural homologies to PRL and GH, it does not possess classic PRL or GH actions, as demonstrated by the Nb2 lymphoma cell proliferation assay or the adipocyte conversion assay, respectively *(124)*. The biological role of PLP-A during pregnancy is presently unknown.

PRL-LIKE PROTEIN-B (PLP-B). PRL-like protein-B (PLP-B) is characterized by its dual expression in the uterus and placenta. A cDNA to PLP-B was another one of the cDNAs, structurally related to PRL, originally identified during a search for the PL-II cDNA *(125)*.

Structural Characteristics. The PLP-B mRNA encodes for a 234 amino acid protein containing four cysteine residues, a single putative N-linked glycosylation site, a 33 amino acid signal peptide, and overall a 31% amino acid sequence identity with pituitary PRL *(125)*. The PLP-B protein is secreted as a 31-kDa glycoprotein by both uterine and placental tissues *(126)*. Both uterine and placental PLP-B mRNAs consist of two equally expressed transcripts estimated to be 0.9 and 1.2 kb in size and postulated to contain differing amounts of 5′-untranslated sequence *(125,127)*. Multiple transcription start sites have been identified in the PLP-B gene, possibly accounting for the two transcripts *(125)*. All other members of the PRL family are transcribed predominantly as a single transcript approx 0.9–1.0 kb in size.

Expression. As indicated above, PLP-B is dually expressed in uterine and trophoblast tissues. PLP-B is expressed at relatively low levels in the antimesometrial compartment of rat decidual tissue *(127)*. Temporally, decidual PLP-B production follows the growth, development, and regression of the antimesometrial deciduum *(127)*. After midgestation, PLP-B expression shifts to spongiotrophoblast cells of the rat chorioallantoic placenta where it is expressed at high levels until it declines during the final days of gestation *(70,87, 125,126,128)*. Unlike other members of the PRL family, PLP-B expression is rapidly activated by enzymatic dispersion of placental cells *(70)*. Another unique feature of the PLP-B placental expression pattern is its absence in trophoblast giant cells. Consistent with these observations PLP-B is also not expressed in the trophoblast giant cell lineage-restricted Rcho-1 trophoblast cell line *(17,129)*.

Distribution and Biological Actions. The existence of PLP-B in maternal or fetal circulation has not been reported. Identification of PLP-B in decidual tissue prompted Croze and coworkers to speculate that it may represent a decidual luteotrophin (dLTH) previously postulated by Gibori and coworkers *(127,130)*. In order to examine the actions of PLP-B, we expressed PLP-B in CHO cells *(126)*. Recombinant PLP-B exhibited similar immunoreactive and electrophoretic characteristics with PLP-B produced by the rat placenta and decidua; however, PLP-B did not effectively bind to PRL receptors or activate the PRL receptor signaling pathway *(126)*. Our observations to date have not supported a relationship between PLP-B and the dLTH. Although specific biological actions for PLP-B have not been elucidated, the sustained pattern of expression of PLP-B throughout much of gestation suggests that its presence is likely beneficial for pregnancy. Furthermore, the rapid response of PLP-B expression following trophoblast cell dispersion *(70)* may suggest that PLP-B participates in cellular responses to tissue injury. Furthermore, the fall in PLP-B expression prior to the end of pregnancy may be a necessary event that allows parturition to proceed without the counteracting influences of wound repair. PLP-B may represent a hormone/cytokine that has important modulatory actions on other hormones/cytokines responsible for the establishment of pregnancy and the initiation of parturition.

PRL-Like Protein C Subfamily. The PRL-like protein C subfamily represents a collection of four proteins possessing a close structural relationship. Additional members of this subfamily may exist *(131)*.

PRL-Like Protein-C (PLP-C). PRL-like protein-C (PLP-C) was originally identified via two approaches: (1) as a major placental secretory protein of late gestation *(123,131)*, and (2) as a major contaminant during the isolation of the 29-kDa isoform of the PLP-A protein *(123,132)*.

Structural Characteristics. PLP-C is secreted in glycosylated and nonglycosylated isoforms of 29 and 25 kDa, respectively *(132)*. The PLP-C cDNA encodes for a 238 amino acid protein, containing a 30 amino acid signal peptide, six cysteine residues, two putative N-linked glycosylation sites, and overall a 26% amino acid sequence identity with pituitary PRL *(133,134)*. Alignment of the six cysteine residues in PLP-C is homologous with PRL *(133,134)*. PLP-C also contains a 10-residue segment rich in aromatic amino acids that is uniquely present in PLP-C subfamily members and mouse proliferin-related protein *(see below; 133–138)*. The significance of this aromatic domain is unknown. Several putative transcription start sites located approx 43 and 61 nucleotides upstream of the PLP-C translation start site have been identified *(134)*. Evidence for an alternatively spliced form of PLP-C lacking a signal peptide has also been reported *(135)*.

Expression. PLP-C is expressed during the second half of gestation primarily by spongiotrophoblast cells with minor contributions from trophoblast giant cells located at the maternal–placental interface *(132,133)*. This pattern of expression is similar to the pattern observed for PL-Iv *(35,69)* and PLP-A *(86,87)*. PLP-C expression is spontaneously activated in differentiating spongiotrophoblast cells maintained in vitro and is inhibited by retinoic acid *(70)*.

Distribution and Biological Actions. The existence of PLP-C in maternal or fetal circulation has not been reported. Actions of PLP-C are currently unknown. Recombinant PLP-C generated from a bacterial expression system lacks the ability to interact with PRL receptors and fails to stimulate the proliferation of lactogen-dependent Nb2 lymphoma cells *(139)*.

Prolactin-Like Protein-C Variant (PLP-Cv). As a consequence of attempting to characterize the PLP-C gene, we identified a related gene that we have termed PLP-C variant (PLP-Cv; *134*).

Structural Characteristics. Screening of a rat genomic library with a PLP-C cDNA resulted in the isolation of a gene, PLP-Cv, closely related to, but distinct from PLP-C. The PLP-Cv gene possessed a six exon/five intron organization unique among members of the PRL family *(134)*. Primer extension analysis revealed multiple putative transcription start sites located approx 42 and 60 nucleotides upstream of the PLP-Cv translation start site. A PCR strategy involving primers based on the PLP-Cv gene was used to isolate a placental PLP-Cv cDNA. The predicted PLP-Cv protein contains 238 amino acids, including a 30 amino acid signal peptide and a single putative N-linked glycosylation site. PLP-Cv showed 90 and 78% sequence identity with PLP-C at nucleotide and amino acid levels, including the homologous alignment of the six cysteine residues, respectively. The PLP-Cv protein has not been directly identified.

Expression. Expression of PLP-Cv is restricted to the trophoblast lineage (spongiotrophoblast and trophoblast giant cells), and is coordinately activated with PLP-C beginning at d 11 of gestation and continuing until term *(134)*. 5′-Flanking DNA of the PLP-Cv gene exhibits homology with flanking DNA of other placental PRL genes and contains cis-elements implicated in controlling trophoblast-specific gene expression. PLP-Cv promoter-luciferase reporter constructs are specifically activated in differentiating trophoblast giant cells of the Rcho-1 cell line *(134)*.

Distribution and Biological Actions. The distribution and biological activities of the PLP-Cv protein have not been determined. Based on the homology of PLP-Cv to PLP-C, we anticipate that PLP-Cv will not utilize the PRL receptor signaling system, but may share biological actions with other members of the PLP-C subfamily.

Prolactin-Like Protein-D (PLP-D). A cDNA was isolated using a differential display strategy designed to find late-gestation placenta-specific cDNAs. On sequencing, the cDNA was found to possess significant similarity to PLP-C and was termed prolactin-like protein-D (PLP-D; *137*).

Structural Characteristics. The predicted PLP-D protein contains 240 amino acids, including a 29 amino acid signal peptide, and a single putative N-linked glycosylation site *(137)*. PLP-D showed 80 and 65% sequence identity with PLP-C at nucleotide and amino acid levels, including the homologous alignment of the six cysteine residues, respectively *(137)*. The PLP-D protein has not been directly identified.

Expression. Expression of PLP-D appears to be restricted to the trophoblast lineage (spongiotrophoblast and trophoblast giant cells), and is coordinately expressed during the second half of pregnancy with PLP-C and PLP-Cv *(134,137)*.

Distribution and Biological Actions. The distribution and biological activities of the PLP-D protein have not been determined. Based on the homology of PLP-D to PLP-C, we anticipate that PLP-D will not utilize the PRL receptor signaling system, but may share biological actions with other members of the PLP-C subfamily.

Decidual/Trophoblast Prolactin-Related Protein (d/tPRP). d/tPRP was originally identified during the attempts to characterize the PLP-B protein from decidual tissue *(138)*. It was subsequently shown to be expressed in both decidual and trophoblast cells *(140)*.

Structural Characteristics. A 29-kDa protein was isolated from medium conditioned by decidual explants. The protein possessed an affinity for Con A and crossreactivity with antibodies to amino acids 140–159 of PLP-B. N-terminal sequencing of the isolated decidual protein indicated it shared significant sequence identity with the N-terminus of PLP-C, and limited similarity with PLP-B. Consistent with these observations, antibodies to PLP-C were shown to recognize the decidual protein. The decidual protein was initially termed decidual PRL-related protein (dPRP), and following its discovery in trophoblast tissue, d/tPRP. A PLP-C cDNA was used to identify d/tPRP cDNAs from a rat decidual cDNA library *(133,138)*. Nucleotide sequence analyses of the d/tPRP cDNAs predicted a protein of 239 amino acids, including a 28 amino acid signal sequence, and overall a 29% amino acid sequence identity with pituitary PRL. The predicted d/tPRP amino acid sequence contains two putative N-linked glycosylation sites and six cysteine residues. The six cysteines are located in positions homologous to the cysteines of PLP-C and PRL. Overall, d/tPRP exhibits approx 70% amino acid homology with PLP-C. Additional sequence similarities with members of the PRL family are evident. Similar to the PLP-Cv gene, the d/tPRP gene possesses a six exon/five intron organization *(141)*.

Expression. Cell- and temporal-specific patterns of d/tPRP expression have been determined with cytochemical and biochemical procedures *(138,140,142)*. d/tPRP expression was first detected in decidual tissue at d 6 of pregnancy. Expression increased with the growth of the deciduum and declined with decidual regression. Throughout the first half of pregnancy, d/tPRP protein and mRNA were predominantly localized to the antimesometrial deciduum of the developing conceptus. During the second half of gestation, d/tPRP expression shifts to the chorioallantoic placenta. Both trophoblast giant cells and spongiotrophoblast cells within the junctional zone of the chorioallantoic placenta express d/tPRP. The decidua-trophoblast shift in d/tPRP expression closely resembles that reported for PLP-B *(see above)*. In contrast to PLP-B, d/tPRP is expressed at high levels in decidua and within trophoblast giant cells of the chorioallantoic placenta *(140)*. Factors and molecular mechanisms responsible for the control of d/tPRP expression in any tissue are yet to be elucidated.

Distribution. Analysis of serum from pseudopregnant rats indicated that unlike some other members of the PRL family, d/tPRP was not readily detectable in circulation *(143)*. d/tPRP associates with heparin-containing molecules and resides, at least in part, within the decidual extracellular matrix *(143)*. Modulatory factors present in the decidual extracellular matrix would be well situated to influence the behavior of decidual cells and other cell types traversing the decidual extracellular matrix, such as trophoblast, endothelial, and various immune cells. Most interestingly, d/tPRP is expressed in the junctional zone of the chorioallantoic placenta during the latter half of pregnancy *(140)*, a region conspicuously devoid of heparan sulfate proteoglycan *(144)*. The distribution of d/tPRP within placental and extraplacental tissues and in circulation during the latter part of gestation has not been reported.

Biological Actions. The coordinated pattern of d/tPRP expression from postimplantation until term involving both maternal and extraembryonic tissues implies some physiologic importance to d/tPRP. An approach similar to those described above regarding the generation of recombinant d/tPRP protein was employed *(143)*. Recombinant d/tPRP exhibited features that closely resembled native d/tPRP isolated from decidua and placenta, and was used to evaluate biological functions representing classical and nonclassical actions previously attributed to members of the PRL family. d/tPRP failed to bind to PRL receptors and lacked the ability to promote the proliferation of the PRL-dependent Nb2 lymphoma cell line. d/tPRP did not markedly influence the development of vascular structures as evaluated in both in vitro and in vivo assays *(143)*. Heterologous expression of d/tPRP in CHO cells did, however, significantly increase the ability of CHO cells to form tumors following transplantation into athymic mice *(143)*. We hypothesize that d/tPRP in some way alters the relationship between the tumor cells and the host, thereby increasing the success rate for establishing a tumor. d/tPRP may be mediating similar processes during the establishment of pregnancy.

Proliferin (PLF). Proliferin (PLF) is one of two nonclassical members of the PRL family expressed in the mouse placenta *(145)*. PLF was originally discovered as an mRNA and protein expressed in association with serum/growth factor-stimulated 3T3 cell proliferation *(146–150)*.

Structural Characteristics. Major PLF species expressed by trophoblast and nontrophoblast cell types are derived from at least five closely related genes *(151,152)*. Two of the PLF proteins PLF-1 and PLF-2 differ at only four residues along their 224 amino acid sequence *(145,149)*. The significance of multiple PLF genes has not been described. PLF contains a 29 amino acid signal peptide, six cysteines present in locations homologous to PRL, three putative N-linked glycosylation sites, and overall a 30% amino acid sequence identity with pituitary PRL *(149)*. Trophoblast cells secrete PLF as a heterogeneous glycoprotein with major molecular species approximating 27 and 35 kDa *(153,154)*. The PLF gene contains the prototypical PRL five exon/four intron organization *(152)*.

Expression. PLF expression in the placenta is restricted to trophoblast giant cells *(40, 91,155)*. Expression begins at least by d 6, peaks at d 10, and gradually declines during the remainder of gestation *(40,136,145,155,156)*. Some trophoblast giant cells capable of expressing PLF also express PL-I and/or PL-II *(91,155)*.

Limited research has been reported concerning the control of PLF expression in trophoblast giant cells. GATA-2 and GATA-3 transcription factors have been indirectly implicated in the control of placental PLF expression. Mutant placentas lacking GATA-2 or GATA-3 show decreased proliferin expression *(50)*. There is also some evidence that activators of the cAMP/protein kinase A pathway stimulate trophoblast cell PLF production *(157)*. In contrast, the regulation of PLF expression in nontrophoblast cell types by various growth modulators has been the focus of several reports *(152,158–160)*. PLF gene expression is stimulated by phorbol esters via an AP-1 site situated within the PLF promoter and inhibited by glucocorticoids through a glucocorticoid response element also present in the PLF promoter *(161,162)*. A range of chemical agents that transform cells also induce PLF expression *(163–165)*. Increases in PLF expression following immortalization appear to be related to changes in RNA processing or transcript stability *(158, 166–168)*. The overall significance of experimentation in nontrophoblast cells to the regulation of placental PLF expression remains to be determined.

Distribution. PLF is present in both maternal and fetal compartments *(42,154,155, 169)*. During pregnancy, PLF is first detectable in maternal serum on d 8, peaks between d 10–12, and gradually declines to low levels by the end of pregnancy *(42,155)*. PLF concentrations in amniotic fluid show a similar gestational profile *(155)*. PLF appears to be specifically transported through the yolk sac to fetal structures *(169)*. Unlike PL-I and PL-II, circulating PLF concentrations are not significantly influenced by the anterior pituitary *(42)*.

Biological Actions. PLF was the first nonclassical member of the PRL family to be identified and the first shown to exhibit distinct biological actions. PLF lacks the ability to interact with PRL receptors or influence the behavior of lactogen-dependent Nb2 lymphoma cells or the lactogen-dependent pigeon crop-sac (*170*; Horseman, personal communication). However, PLF can be converted into a lactogen through site-directed mutagenesis *(119)*. Progress in determining the biological role of PLF first appeared from investigations on the effects of PLF on the pigeon crop-sac and from studies on the 16-kDa proteolytic fragment of PRL (16-kDa PRL). Horseman observed prominent vascular changes at the injection site of the pigeon crop-sac (Horseman, personal communication). Clapp and Weiner *(171)* demonstrated that the 16-kDa PRL possessed antiangiogenic actions and interacted with a unique endothelial cell membrane receptor that also apparently possessed some affinity for PLF. Through an elegant series of experiments, Linzer and his coworkers demonstrated that PLF stimulated endothelial cell migration and blood vessel development *(170)*. These PLF actions do not appear to involve the 16-kDa PRL receptor, but instead are likely mediated by PLF interaction with mannose-6-phosphate/ IGF-II receptors present on endothelial cells and other PLF targets *(169,172–174)*. PLF binding is specifically competed by mannose-6-phosphate and dependent on its carbohydrate constituents *(169,173)*. Additional PLF actions independent of the mannose-6-phosphate/IGF-II receptor have also recently been described. PLF specifically binds to uterine membranes where it stimulates uterine cell proliferation *(175)*. PLF has also been shown to inhibit muscle cell-specific gene expression and muscle cell differentiation following transfection, but not following addition of the hormone to muscle cell cultures *(176,177)*. These latter actions may be dependent on some form of intracellular action of PLF.

The reported actions of PLF are beginning to expand. As they increase in number, it may be helpful that we appreciate PLFs are encoded by multiple genes, exist in multiple posttranslationally processed forms, and have access to maternal, extraembryonic, and embryonic tissues.

PLF-Related Protein (PLF-RP). PLF-RP cDNA was originally discovered during the identification of PLF cDNAs in a mouse placental cDNA library *(136)*. A possible hamster PLF-RP has also been recently characterized *(178)*.

Structural Characteristics. The cDNA for PLF-RP encodes a 244 amino acid protein containing a 30 amino acid signal peptide and three putative N-linked glycosylation sites *(136)*. PLF-RP possesses 30 and 32% amino acid sequence identity with pituitary PRL and PLF, respectively. Regions of extensive homology between PLF-RP and PLF exist, especially within the first 100 nucleotides of their cDNAs *(136)*. In addition to the four core cysteine residues present in all members of the PRL family, PLF-RP contains a fifth cysteine situated toward the middle of its sequence. PLF-RP also bears some limited homology, in the so-called "aromatic domain," with members of the PLP-C subfamily. The significance of this relationship is unknown. PLF-RP is secreted as a glycoprotein with molecular sizes ranging from 36–44 kDa *(154)*. A possible hamster PLF-RP homolog bears 75 and 58% identity with mouse PLF-RP at nucleotide and amino acid levels, respectively *(178)*.

Expression. PLF-RP is expressed primarily by mouse spongiotrophoblast cells with a lesser contribution from trophoblast giant cells *(40,154)*. Expression is initiated by d 8, peaks at d 12, and continues to be expressed throughout the remainder of gestation *(40, 136,154)*. In the hamster, the putative PLF-RP appears to be restricted to spongiotrophoblast cells *(178)*. Overall, the expression pattern for PLF-RP largely follows the growth and development of spongiotrophoblast cells.

Distribution. PLF-RP circulates at relatively high levels in the mother, but does not appear to enter fetal circulation *(42,154)*. Targets for PLF-RP action are likely confined to maternal and extraembryonic compartments.

Biological Actions. Our present understanding of PLF-RP action is coupled with the functions of PLF. As was true for PLF, PLF-RP also lacks the ability to interact with PRL receptors and influence lactogen-dependent Nb2 lymphoma cells *(170)*. Additionally, similar to PLF, PLF-RP has been reported to compete with 16-kDa PRL binding to endothelial cell membranes *(171)*. However, in contrast to the angiogenic actions of PLF, PLF-RP inhibits endothelial cell migration and blood vessel development stimulated by a variety of angiogenic factors, including PLF *(170)*. PLF-RP has been postulated to provide an important "gestational brake" on PLF-stimulated angiogenesis *(170)*. Most interestingly, the intraplacental location of PLF-RP expression (junctional zone) is conspicuously devoid of vasculature *(40,154)*. Thus, PLF-RP may also have a central role in the morphogenesis of the chorioallantoic placenta.

STRUCTURAL RELATIONSHIPS OF THE PLACENTAL PRL FAMILY

A few comments are provided regarding structural relationships for members of the placental PRL family. The design of each ligand is based on the specific assembly of smaller component parts or domains. Identification of these domains may provide considerable insight into functional attributes of the ligands.

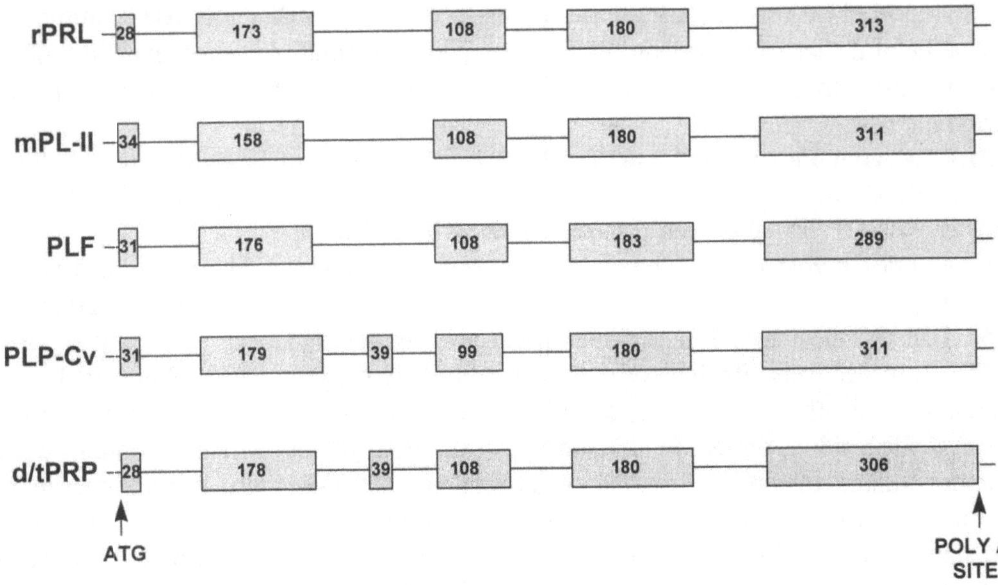

Fig. 4. Representations of the rat PRL (rPRL), mouse placental lactogen-II (mPL-II), mouse PLF (PLF), rat PLP-Cv (PLP-Cv), and rat d/tPRP genes. Exons are depicted by shaded boxes. Numbers within the boxes refer to the size of the exons. Please note that the PLP-Cv and d/tPRP genes contain an extra exon situated between the second and third exons of the prototypical PRL exonic organzation seen in PRL, PL-II, and PLF.

Genomic Organization

Two basic gene structures have been elucidated for members of the placental PRL family (Fig. 4): (1) the prototypical PRL structure of five exons and four introns shared among many members of the family, and (2) a six exon–five intron arrangement characteristic of at least two members of the PLP-C subfamily (PLP-Cv and d/tPRP). Major differences in these two gene structures correspond to the addition of a small exon in the PLP-C subfamily members situated between exons two and three of the prototypical PRL gene *(82,83,134,141)*. The significance of the additional small exon is yet to be fully appreciated *(see below)*.

Genes for each member of the rat PRL family have been localized to chromosome 17 of the rat genome *(6,34,68,133,134,138,179)*, whereas chromosome 13 of the mouse genome is the site of the mouse PRL family genes *(180)*. These chromosomal loci are homologous with the PRL gene locus on human chromosome 6 *(181)*. Specific linkage arrangements of the PRL family genes on their respective chromosomes have not been reported. Analysis of the genomic organization of the PRL family members may lead to the identification of additional members of the family and new insights regarding their regulation. The apparent absence of significant cross-species homologs for some members of the family is suggestive that the rodent PRL family is a result of more recent evolutionary events. The use of proteins with PRL-like biological activities (PRL/human GH) as a prototype for the derivation of families of proteins expressed during pregnancy, with seemingly novel actions, has independently occurred several times (human, bovine, mouse, and rat; *2,182,183)*. As these gene families have evolved, it is apparent that the biological actions of some members of each family center around the utilization of the PRL receptor. However, it is also apparent that the actions of other members are independent of PRL receptor activation. At present, evidence for signaling mechanisms independent of the PRL receptor is modest. It is not entirely clear whether specific and unique receptor signaling systems have coevolved with the PRL family members, whether PRL family members utilize signaling pathways for other known ligands, or whether PRL family members act through receptor-independent mechanisms (e.g., transport proteins, binding proteins, and so forth). As indicated above, the mechanism of action of PLF provides us with a glimpse of what we might expect for other PRL family members. PLF can influence cellular behavior through the mannose-6-phosphate receptor/IGF-II receptor *(173)* and also interacts with other presumably unique receptors *(175)*.

Are There Structural Motifs That May Give Us Clues Regarding Function?

There are likely several domains shared among subsets of PRL family members that potentially influence function. These structural motifs may influence ligand–receptor interactions, accessibility to biological compartments, and functional life-span. Several examples exist of structural relationships in primary sequence that likely affect conformation and hormone action *(184)*. The positioning of cysteine residues is one of the key elements used in ligand classification. All members have four core cysteines. Subgroups can be identified, at least in part, through the sharing of additional cysteine residues. Some members possess an odd number of cysteine residues, implicating the existence of putative reactive free sulfhydrals. Each of these attributes likely has a significant impact on protein folding, protein–protein interactions, and thus, the mode and spectrum of actions of a given PRL family member. Some amino acids critical to ligand interaction and activation of the PRL receptor are conserved in classical members of the PRL family *(10,118,119,184)*. A subgroup of PRL family members (PLP-C subfamily members and PLF-RP) contains an additional 10 amino acid region referred to as the "aromatic" domain. In at least some of the genes for this subgroup, the "aromatic" domain is encoded by a unique exon. The biological consequences of this exonic addition are not yet fully appreciated. Overall sequence identity with pituitary PRL is not necessarily an indication of functional characteristics.

Glycosylation is a prominent posttranslational event that can dramatically affect ligand function. PLF's utilization of the carbohydrate binding domain of the mannose-6-phosphate/IGF-II receptor *(173)* indicates the potential importance of glycosylation in placental PRL family function. Carbohydrate modifications on PRL family members are strikingly affected by their cellular source and structure *(122)*, thus creating the potential for additional modes of functional regulation via ligand-and cell type-specific selection.

COORDINATION AND INTEGRATION OF EXPRESSION AND ACTIONS OF THE PRL FAMILY DURING PREGNANCY

Over the past decade, we have gained an appreciation of specific regulatory networks involving members of the PRL family during pregnancy.

Classical PRL-PL Regulatory Network

The biosynthesis of classical members of the PRL family is exquisitely orchestrated through the activities of the anterior pituitary and placenta (Fig. 5). These tissues produce ligands that potentially activate PRL receptor signaling pathways in maternal, extraembryonic, and embryonic tissues.

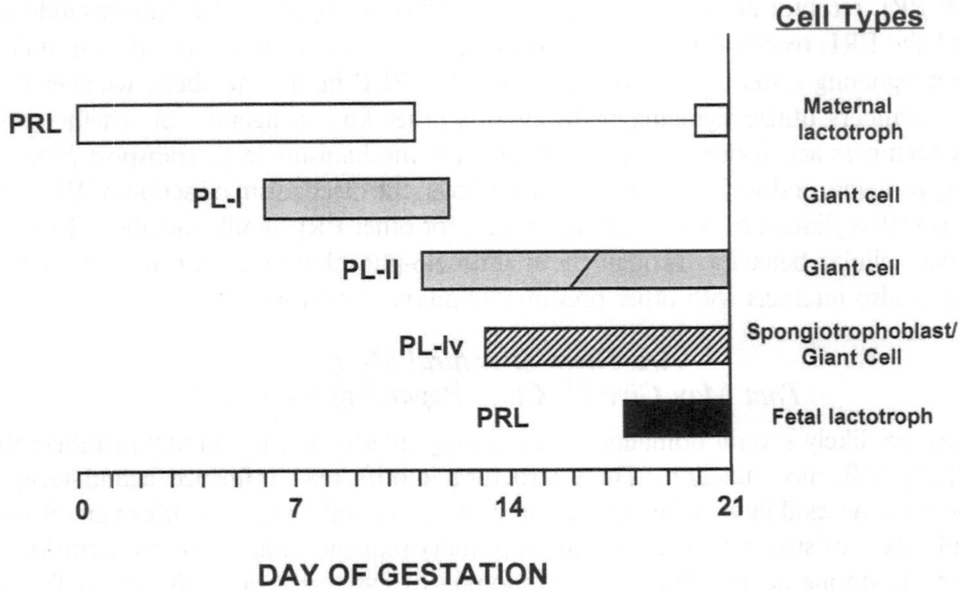

Fig. 5. Classical PRL-PL regulatory network. Schematic diagram of the temporal pattern of expression of components of the PRL-PL regulatory network. The scale on the bottom of the diagram refers to the duration of gestation in the rat. Positions of the horizontal bars represent the duration of expression. Expression patterns for PRL from the maternal lactotroph (open bar), PL-I and PL-II from trophoblast giant cells (gray bars), PL-Iv from both spongiotrophoblast cells and trophoblast giant cells (striped bar), and PRL from the fetal lactotroph (black bar) are shown. Please note the diagonal line in the PL-II bar depicts a shift in the primary source of PL-II from trophoblast giant cells associated with the junctional zone to trophoblast giant cells of the labyrinth zone. Abbreviations: PRL, prolactin; PL-I, placental lactogen-I; PL-II, placental lactogen-II; PL-Iv, placental lactogen-I variant. (d 0 = sperm positive; d 4 = implantation; d 21 = parturition.)

At the outset of pregnancy, the copulatory stimulus initiates a neuroendocrine reflex that culminates in the generation of a twice-daily secretory pattern of anterior pituitary PRL for the first half of gestation *(185–187)*. These PRL surges are critical for the maintenance of the corpus luteum *(188)*. At implantation, trophoblast giant cells arise, and uterine stromal cells decidualize. The development of trophoblast giant cells may be influenced by the expression and actions of a bHLH transcription factor, Thing-1/Hxt/e-HAND *(52)*. This limited number of early trophoblast giant cells is a significant source of a "potent" and "long-acting" PRL agonist, PL-I *(38)*. PL-I effectively mimics the actions of PRL on the corpus luteum, mammary glands, and other PRL targets, including the hypothalamus and anterior pituitary, where it inhibits the twice-daily secretion of PRL *(34,58,65,67)*. At midgestation, trophoblast giant cells have significantly increased in numbers and begin secreting another "potent," but "short-acting" PRL agonist, PL-II *(38)*. PL-I production subsequently terminates and a "weaker-acting" PRL agonist, PL-Iv, is expressed predominantly by the spongiotrophoblast population of cells of the chorioallantoic placenta *(35)*. Spongiotrophoblast cells arise at midgestation under the control of signaling pathways involving another bHLH transcription factor, Mash-2, and possibly a pathway involving the EGF receptor *(189–192)*. PL-II and PL-Iv continue to be produced through the remainder of gestation and activate PRL receptor signaling systems *(65,68, 116)*. During the last week of gestation, trophoblast giant cells of the labyrinthine region

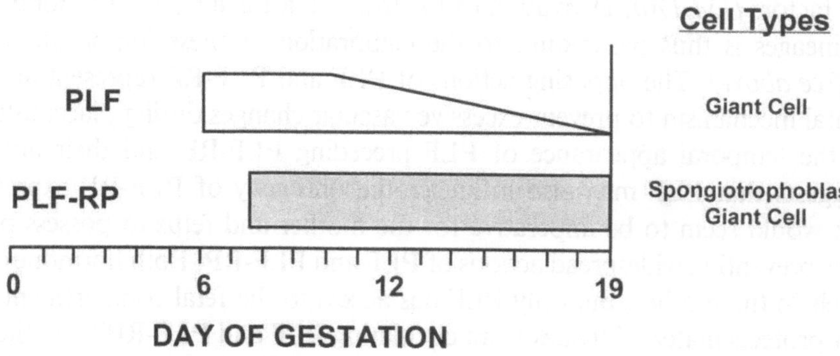

Fig. 6. PLF/PLF-RP angiogenesis regulatory network. Schematic diagram of the temporal pattern of expression of PLF and PLF-RP protein during mouse pregnancy. The scale on the bottom of the diagram refers to the duration of gestation in the mouse. Positions of the horizontal bars represent the duration of expression. Expression patterns for PLF from trophoblast giant cells (open bar) and PLF-RP from spongiotrophoblast cells and trophoblast giant cells (gray bar) are shown. The width of the bars corresponds to the magnitude of expression. (d 0 = sperm positive; d 4 = implantation; d 19 = parturition.)

are the major source of PL-II *(35,88,92)*. This shift may facilitate the entry of PL-II into the fetal compartment. The physiological importance of extrapituitary PRL receptor ligands is further illustrated by the broad tissue distribution of the PRL receptor in the fetus *(193)* and the developmental abnormalities associated with targeted disruption of the PRL receptor *(194)*. Immediately prior to parturition, fetal pituitary PRL expression is first detectable and maternal pituitary PRL secretion is reinitiated *(195–200)*. The coordination of these events in maternal, extraembryonic, and fetal tissues is striking.

Unanswered questions abound regarding this regulatory network. Why produce four different ligands for the PRL receptor? There are certainly differences regarding the sources of the ligands and aspects of their regulation; however, do they also possess unique attributes allowing them to access specific biological compartments or differentially activate PRL receptor signaling pathways? Redundancy is evident, but is there also specificity? What is responsible for the termination of PL-I expression? Is the shutoff intrinsic to trophoblast cells or dependent on extratrophoblast signals? What is the significance of the production of a "weak-acting" lactogen, PL-Iv? Does PL-Iv act as a lactogen antagonist? Does PL-Iv possess unique nonlactogen actions? We are at a very early stage in understanding how these ligands act on known PRL targets, such as the mammary gland, ovary, liver, uterus, and so on, and unfortunately do not have any clues regarding other possible targets tissues. The availability of biologically active recombinant ligands and various molecular and immunological tools will permit these important questions to be investigated.

PLF/PLF-RP Angiogenesis Regulatory Network

One of the chief roles of trophoblast cells is to establish the vascular connectivity required in providing nourishment for the developing embryo/fetus. PLF and PLF-RP represent an important regulatory network controlling angiogenesis in the mouse (Fig. 6). PLF is produced shortly after implantation at the maternal–placental interface by trophoblast giant cells and promotes blood vessel development *(155,170)*. PLF-RP is expressed later, primarily by spongiotrophoblast cells, and acts to counter the effects of PLF and other angiogenic factors *(154,170)*. Derivation of the trophoblast giant cell and spongiotrophoblast cell lineages is thus paramount to the elaboration of these important regulatory molecules *(see above)*. The opposing actions of PLF and PLF-RP represent an effective intraplacental mechanism to prevent excessive vascular changes during placentation. Furthermore, the temporal appearance of PLF preceding PLF-RP and their antagonistic actions suggests that PLF may also influence the ontogeny of PLF-RP expression. In addition, it would seem to be imperative for the mother and fetus to possess protective mechanisms preventing widespread actions of PLF and PLF-RP. Both hormones circulate at high levels in the mother, but only PLF has access to the fetal compartment *(42,154, 155)*. What protects maternal tissues from circulating PLF and PLF-RP? Are there transport proteins that limit the availability of these endothelial cell-acting hormones? Do specific amino acid sequence motifs or posttranslational modifications influence PLF's entry into and PLF-RP's exclusion from the fetus? These are important questions that when addressed will provide a more complete understanding of the PLF/PLF-RP angiogenesis regulatory network. The role of members of the PRL family in the regulation of placental and uterine angiogenesis in other species is not known.

Are There Other Regulatory Networks Involving the PRL Family?

The examples of regulatory networks illustrated above represent two distinct types of circuitry. One involves a series of ligands with redundant and overlapping biological actions (PRL/PL), whereas the other involves ligands of opposing actions (PLF/PLF-RP). Although we know little of the biology of other members of the PRL family, we may be able to formulate some predictions. The PLP-C subfamily and PLP-B have signature features that are suggestive of a regulatory network (Fig. 7). Components of this putative circuit are coordinately and/or sequentially expressed throughout gestation in both maternal and extraembryonic tissues. This proposed network includes a series of closely related ligands, the PLP-C subfamily, potentially exhibiting redundant and overlapping biological actions. PLP-B is only distantly related to the PLP-C subfamily, but is coordinately expressed with at least one of the PLP-C subfamily ligands during the course of pregnancy. This observation prompts us to suggest that PLP-C subfamily, actions may be functionally opposed by PLP-B. We currently hypothesize that PLP-C subfamily members promote utero–placental remodeling, but PLP-B prevents excessive alterations.

In the preceding brief discussions, we have placed each of the members of the rodent placental PRL family, except for PLP-A, into regulatory networks ("real" or "imagined"). PLP-A possesses many unique and intriguing features *(see above)*; however, its role in pregnancy and relationship with other members of the PRL family have been somewhat elusive.

FINAL COMMENTS

The PRL family represents an intriguing developmental paradigm with important implications for the establishment and maintenance of pregnancy, fetal development, hormone action, and cell differentiation. It is evident that each member of the PRL family contributes to the physiological adjustments of pregnancy. Although the nature of the actions of some members are yet to be fully appreciated, many of the experimental tools are now in place to elucidate the biological relevance of the placental PRL family. Genes comprising the PRL family can also be viewed as valuable indices of lactotroph, decidual cell, and trophoblast cell differentiation. Understanding the nature of how these genes are controlled will provide greater insights into how the respective cell lineages are regulated.

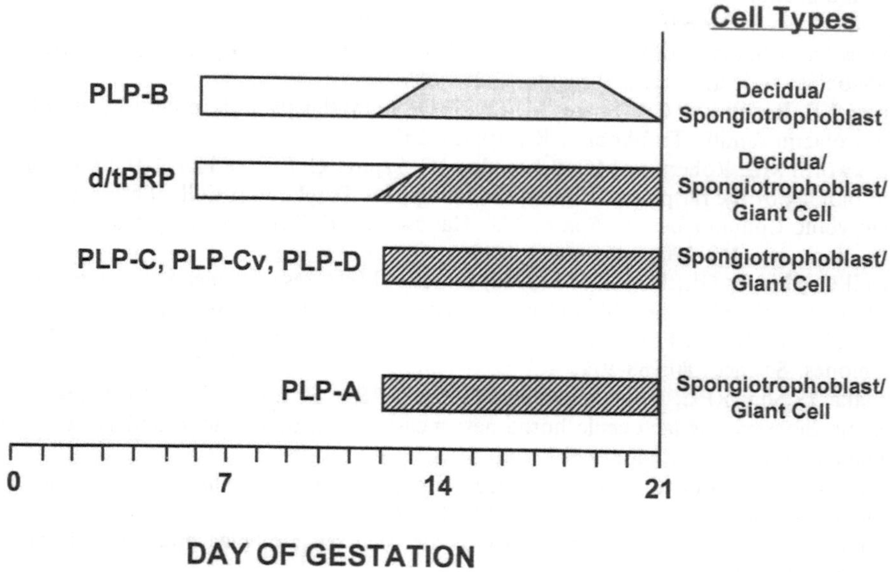

Fig. 7. Other possible PRL family regulatory networks. Schematic diagram of the temporal pattern of expression of prolactin-like protein B (PLP-B), the prolactin-like protein C subfamily (PLP-C, PLP-Cv, PLP-D, d/tPRP), and prolactin-like protein A (PLP-A) during pregnancy in the rat. The scale on the bottom of the diagram refers to the duration of gestation in the rat. Positions of the horizontal bars represent the duration of expression. Expression patterns for PLP-B in decidua (open bar) and in spongiotrophoblast cells (gray bar), d/tPRP in decidua (open bar) and in spongiotrophoblast cells and trophoblast giant cells (striped bar), and PLP-C, PLP-Cv, PLP-D, and PLP-A in spongiotrophoblast cells and trophoblast giant cells (striped bars) are shown. The width of the bars corresponds to the magnitude of expression. (d 0 = sperm positive; d 4 = implantation; d 21 = parturition.)

We are approaching a meaningful stage in the investigation of placental endocrinology. To date, a largely phenomenological approach has garnered information highlighting the diversities associated with placental structure and function. However, this will soon change. Scientific advancements at mechanistic levels are forthcoming utilizing several different species (primates, domestic animals, and rodents). Implementation of transgenic and gene targeting strategies for testing hypotheses derived from these advances will ensure a pivotal role of rodent models in future placental research. The cumulative progress from these endeavors will soon make it possible to identify the fundamental principles governing placental development and function.

ACKNOWLEDGMENT

We would like to acknowledge the National Institute of Child Health and Human Development for providing financial support for research conducted in our laboratory.

REFERENCES

1. Ogren L, Talamantes F (1988) Prolactins of pregnancy and their cellular source. Int Rev Cytol 112:1–65.
2. Soares MJ, Faria TN, Roby KF, Deb S (1991) Pregnancy and the prolactin family of hormones: coordination of anterior pituitary, uterine, and placental expression. Endocr Rev 12:402–423.
3. Soares MJ, Faria TN, Hamlin GP, Lu XJ, Deb S (1993) Trophoblast cell differentiation: expression of the placental prolactin family, In: Trophoblast Cells: Pathways for Maternal-Embryonic

Communication (Soares MJ, Handwerger S, Talamantes F, eds.), Springer-Verlag, New York, pp. 45–67.
4. Soares MJ, Chapman BM, Rasmussen CA, Dai G, Kamei T, Orwig KE (1996) Differentiation of trophoblast endocrine cells. Placenta 17:277–289.
5. Orwig KE, Rasmussen CA, Soares MJ (1997) Decidual signals in the establishment of pregnancy: the prolactin family. Trophoblast Res 10:329–343.
6. Duckworth ML, Robertson MC, Schroedter IC, Szpirer C, Friesen HG (1993) Molecular genetics and biology of the rat placental prolactin family, In: Trophoblast Cells: Pathways for Maternal-Embryonic Communication (Soares MJ, Handwerger S, Talamantes F, eds.), Springer-Verlag, New York, pp. 169–190.
7. Nicoll CS, Mayer GL, Russell SM (1986) Structural features of prolactins and growth hormones that can be related to their biological properties. Endocr Rev 7:169–203.
8. Shiu RPC, Kelly PA, Friesen HG (1973) Radioreceptor assay for prolactin and other lactogenic hormones. Science 180:968–971.
9. Tanaka T, Shiu RPC, Gout PW, Beer CT, Noble RL, Friesen HG (1980) A new sensitive and specific bioassay for lactogenic hormones: measurement of prolactin and growth hormone in human serum. J Clin Endocrinol Metab 51:1058–1062.
10. Southard JN, Talamantes F (1991) Placental prolactin-like proteins in rodents: variations on a structural theme. Mol Cell Endocrinol 79:C133–C140.
11. Talamantes F (1975) Comparative study of the occurrence of placental prolactin among mammals. Gen Comp Endocrinol 27:115–121.
12. Kelly PA, Tsushima T, Shiu RPC, Friesen HG (1976) Lactogenic and growth hormone-like activities in pregnancy determined by radioreceptor assays. Endocrinology 99:765–774.
13. Enders AC (1965) A comparative study of the fine structure of the trophoblast in several hemochorial placentas. Am J Anat 116:29–67.
14. Soares MJ, Chapman BM, Kamei T, Yamamoto T (1995) Control of trophoblast cell differentiation: lessons from the genetics of early pregnancy loss and trophoblast neoplasia. Dev Growth Differ 37:355–364.
15. Sibley CP (1994) Mechanisms of ion transfer by the rat placenta: a model for the human placenta? Placenta 15:675–691.
16. Teshima S, Shimosato Y, Koide T, Kuroki M, Kikuchi Y, Aizawa M (1983) Transplantable choriocarcinoma of rats induced by fetectomy and its biological activities. Gann 74:205–212.
17. Faria TN, Soares MJ (1991) Trophoblast cell differentiation: establishment, characterization, and modulation of a rat trophoblast cell line expressing members of the placental prolactin family. Endocrinology 129:2895–2906.
18. Hamlin GP, Soares MJ (1995) Regulation of DNA synthesis in proliferating and differentiating trophoblast cells: involvement of transferrin, transforming growth factor-beta, and tyrosine kinases. Endocrinology 136:322–331.
19. Hamlin GP, Lu X-J, Roby KF, Soares MJ (1994) Recapitulation of the pathway for trophoblast giant cell differentiation in vitro: stage-specific expression of members of the prolactin gene family. Endocrinology 134:2390–2396.
20. Yamamoto T, Roby KF, Kwok SCM, Soares MJ (1994) Transcriptional activation of cytochrome P450 side chain cleavage enzyme expression during trophoblast cell differentiation. J Biol Chem 269:6517–6523.
21. Yamamoto T, Chapman BM, Clemens JW, Richards JS, Soares MJ (1995) Analysis of cytochrome P450 side-chain cleavage gene promoter activation during trophoblast cell differentiation. Mol Cell Endocrinol 113:183–194.
22. Yamamoto T, Chapman BM, Johnson DC, Givens CR, Mellon SH, Soares MJ (1996) Cytochrome P450 17alpha-hydroxylase gene expression in differentiating rat trophoblast cells. J Endocrinol 150:161–168.
23. Kelly PA, Shiu RPC, Robertson MC, Friesen HG (1975) Characterization of rat chorionic mammotropin. Endocrinology 96:1187–1195.
24. Robertson MC, Friesen HG (1981) Two forms of rat placental lactogen revealed by radioimmunoassay. Endocrinology 108:2388–2390.
25. Robertson MC, Gillespie B, Friesen HG (1982) Characterization of the two forms of rat placental lactogen (rPL): rPL-I and rPL-II. Endocrinology 111:1862–1866.
26. Soares MJ, Colosi P, Talamantes F (1982) The development and characterization of a homologous radioimmunoassay for mouse placental lactogen. Endocrinology 110:668–670.
27. Soares MJ, Colosi P, Ogren L, Talamantes F (1983) Identification and partial characterization of a lactogen from the midpregnant mouse conceptus. Endocrinology 112:1313–1317.

28. Southard JN, Campbell GT, Talamantes F (1987) Hamster placental lactogens: gestational profiles and high mol-wt forms. Endocrinology 121:900–906.
29. Soares MJ, Julian JA, Glasser SR (1985) Trophoblast giant cell release of placental lactogens: temporal and regional characteristics. Dev Biol 107:520–526.
30. Colosi P, Ogren L, Thordarson G, Talamantes F (1987) Purification and partial characterization of two prolactin-like glycoprotein hormone complexes from the midpregnant mouse conceptus. Endocrinology 120:2500–2511.
31. Colosi P, Talamantes F, Linzer DIH (1987) Molecular cloning and expression of mouse placental lactogen I complementary deoxyribonucleic acid. Mol Endocrinol 1:767–776.
32. Robertson MC, Croze F, Schroedter IC, Friesen HG (1990) Molecular cloning and expression of rat placental lactogen-I complementary deoxyribonucleic acid. Endocrinology 127:702–710.
33. Hirosawa M, Miura R, Min KS, Hattori N, Shiota K, Ogawa T (1994) A cDNA encoding a new member of the rat placental lactogen family, PL-I mosaic (PL-Im). Endocr J 41:387–397.
34. Dai G, Imagawa W, Liu B, Szpirer C, Levan G, Kwok SCM, Soares MJ (1996) Rcho-1 trophoblast cell placental lactogens: complementary DNAs, heterologous expression, and biological activities. Endocrinology 137:5020–5027.
35. Deb S, Faria TN, Roby KF, Larsen D, Kwok SCM, Talamantes F, Soares MJ (1991) Identification and characterization of a new member of the prolactin family, placental lactogen-I variant. J Biol Chem 266:1605–1610.
36. Shida MM, Ng Y-K, Soares MJ, Linzer DIH (1993) Trophoblast-specific transcription from the mouse placental lactogen-I gene promoter. Mol Endocrinol 7:181–188.
37. Nieder GL, Jennes L (1990) Production of mouse placental lactogen-I by trophoblast giant cells in utero and in vitro. Endocrinology 126:2809–2814.
38. Faria TN, Deb S, Kwok SCM, Talamantes F, Soares MJ (1990) Ontogeny of placental lactogen-I and placental lactogen-II expression in the developing rat placenta. Dev Biol 141:279–291.
39. Faria TN, Ogren L, Talamantes F, Linzer DIH, Soares MJ (1991) Localization of placental lactogen-I in trophoblast giant cells of the mouse placenta. Biol Reprod 44:327–331.
40. Carney EW, Prideaux V, Lye SJ, Rossant J (1993) Progressive expression of trophoblast specific genes during formation of mouse trophoblast giant cells in vitro. Mol Reprod Dev 34:357–368.
41. Lopez MF, Carrion FA, Talamantes F (1992) Pituitary-placental interaction: hypophysectomy modulates the secretion of mouse placental lactogen-I. Endocrinology 129:2325–2328.
42. Lopez MF, Ogren L, Linzer DIH, Talamantes F (1993) Pituitary-placental interaction during pregnancy: regulation of prolactin-like proteins. Endocr J 1:513–518.
43. Yamaguchi M, Miyake A (1996) Regulation of mouse placental lactogen secretion by factors secreted from the pituitary in vitro. Eur J Endocrinol 134:123–127.
44. Yamaguchi M, Endo H, Thordarson G, Ogren L, Talamantes F (1992) Modulation of mouse placental lactogen-I secretion in vitro: effects of progesterone and mouse placental lactogen-II. Endocrinology 130:2897–2905.
45. Yamaguchi M, Ogren L, Endo H, Thordarson G, Kensinger R, Talamantes F (1992) Epidermal growth factor stimulates mouse placental lactogen I but inhibits mouse placental lactogen II secretion in vitro. Proc Natl Acad Sci USA 89:11,396–11,400.
46. Yamaguchi M, Taga T, Kishimoto T, Miyake A (1995) Cytokines that use gp130 as a signal transducer stimulate mouse placental lactogen-I (mPL-I) but inhibit mPL-II production in vitro. Biol Reprod 53:399–406.
47. Yamaguchi M, Ogren L, Kurachi H, Hirota K, Imai T, Talamantes F (1995) Opposite effects of transforming growth factor alpha and epidermal growth factor on mouse placental lactogen I secretion. Proc Natl Acad Sci USA 92:2830–2834.
48. Yamaguchi M, Imai T, Maeda T, Sakata M, Miyake A (1995) Cyclic adenosine-3′,5′-monophosphate stimulates mouse placental lactogen-I (mPL-I) secretion but inhibits mPL-II secretion at midpregnancy. Endocrinology 136:1388–1393.
49. Yamaguchi M, Miyake A (1996) Regulation of mouse placental lactogen secretion by G proteins before midpregnancy. J Endocrinol Invest 19:492–498.
50. Ng Y-K, George KM, Engel JD, Linzer DIH (1994) GATA factor activity is required for the trophoblast-specific transcriptional regulation of the mouse placental lactogen I gene. Development 120:3257–3266.
51. Ma G, Roth M, Groskopf JC, Tsai F-Y, Orkin SH, Grosveld F, Engel JD, Linzer DIH (1997) GATA-2 and GATA-3 regulate trophoblast-specific gene expression in vivo. Development 124:907–914.
52. Cross JC, Flannery ML, Blanar MA, Steingrimmission E, Jenkins NA, Copeland NG, Rutter WJ, Werb Z (1995) Hxt encodes a basic helix-loop-helix transcription factor that regulates trophoblast cell development. Development 121:2513–2523.

53. Cserjesi P, Brown D, Lyons GE, Olson EN (1995) Expression of the novel basic helix-loop-helix gene eHAND in neural crest derivatives and extraembryonic membranes during mouse development. Dev Biol 170:664–678.
54. Hollenberg SM, Sternglanz R, Cheng PF, Weintraub H (1995) Identification of a new family of tissue-specific basic helix-loop-helix proteins with a two-hybrid system. Mol Cell Biol 15:3813–3822.
55. Ogren L, Southard JN, Colosi P, Linzer DIH, Talamantes F (1989) Mouse placental lactogen-I: RIA and gestational profile in maternal serum. Endocrinology 125:2253–2257.
56. Robertson MC, Cosby H, Fresnoza A, Cattini PA, Shiu RPC, Friesen HG (1994) Expression, purification, and characterization of recombinant rat placental lactogen-I: a comparison with the native hormone. Endocrinology 134:393–400.
57. Bridges RS, Robertson MC, Shiu RPC, Friesen HG, Stuer AM, Mann PE (1996) Endocrine communication between conceptus and mother: placental lactogen stimulation of maternal behavior. Neuroendocrinology 64:57–64.
58. Colosi P, Ogren L, Southard JN, Thordarson G, Linzer DIH, Talamantes F (1988) Biological, immunological, and binding properties of recombinant mouse placental lactogen-I. Endocrinology 123:2662–2667.
59. Freemark M, Kirk K, Pihoker C, Robertson MC, Shiu RPC, Driscoll P (1993) Pregnancy lactogens in the rat conceptus and fetus: circulating levels, distribution of binding, and expression of receptor messenger ribonucleic acid. Endocrinology 133:1830–1842.
60. Freemark M, Kirk K, Robertson MC (1994) Cellular distribution of placental lactogen binding sites in the pregnant rat. Endocr J 2:199–205.
61. MacLeod KR, Smith WC, Ogren L, Talamantes F (1989) Recombinant mouse placental lactogen-I binds to lactogen receptors in mouse liver and ovary: partial characterization of the ovarian receptor. Endocrinology 125:2258–2266.
62. Pihoker C, Robertson MC, Freemark M (1993) Rat placental lactogen-I binds to the choroid plexus and hypothalamus of the pregnant rat. J Endocrinol 139:235–242.
63. Fielder PJ, Thordarson G, English A, Rosenfeld RG, Talamantes F (1992) Expression of a lactogen-dependent insulin-like growth factor-binding protein in cultured mouse mammary epithelial cells. Endocrinology 131:261–267.
64. Brelje TC, Scharp DW, Lacy PE, Ogren L, Talamantes F, Robertson M, Friesen HG, Sorenson RL (1993) Effect of homologous placental lactogens, prolactins, and growth hormones on islet B-cell division and insulin secretion in rat, mouse, and human islets: implication for placental lactogen regulation of islets function during pregnancy. Endocrinology 132:879–887.
65. Galosy SS, Talamantes F (1995) Luteotropic actions of placental lactogens at midpregnancy in the mouse. Endocrinology 136:3993–4003.
66. Bridges RS, Roberston MC, Shiu RPC, Sturgis JD, Henriquesz BM, Mann PE (1997) Central lactogenic regulation of maternal behavior in rats: steroid dependence, hormone specificity, and behavioral potencies of rat prolactin and rat placental lactogen I. Endocrinology 138:756–763.
67. Voogt JL, Soares MJ, Robertson MC, Arbogast LA (1996) Rat placental lactogen-I abolishes nocturnal prolactin surges in the pregnant rat. Endocrine 4:233–238.
68. Cohick CB, Dai G, Xu L, Deb S, Kamei T, Levan G, Szpirer C, Szpirer J, Kwok SCM, Soares MJ (1996) Placental lactogen-I variant utilizes the prolactin receptor signaling pathway. Mol Cell Endocrinol 116:49–58.
69. Robertson MC, Schroedter IC, Friesen HG (1991) Molecular cloning and expression of rat placental lactogen-Iv, a variant of rPL-I present in late pregnant rat placenta. Endocrinology 129: 2746–2756.
70. Lu X-J, Deb S, Soares MJ (1994) Spontaneous differentiation of trophoblast cells along the spongiotrophoblast pathway: expression of the placental prolactin gene family and modulation by retinoic acid. Dev Biol 163:86–97.
71. Robertson MC, Cosby H, Shiu RPC (1996) Rat placental lactogen-I variant (rPL-Iv), product of an unique gene, is biologically different from rPL-I. Endocrinology 137:5242–5249.
72. Colosi P, Marr G, Lopez J, Haro L, Ogren L, Talamantes F (1982) Isolation, purification, and characterization of mouse placental lactogen. Proc Natl Acad Sci USA 79:771–775.
73. Duckworth ML, Kirk KL, Friesen HG (1986) Isolation and identification of a cDNA clone of rat placental lactogen II. J Biol Chem 261:10,871–10,878.
74. Kishi K, Hirashiba M, Hasegawa Y (1992) Multiple forms of rat placental lactogen-II (rPL-II): purification and partial characterization of rPL-II. Placenta 13:63–79.
75. Jackson LL, Colosi P, Talamantes F, Linzer DIH (1986) Molecular cloning of mouse placental lactogen cDNA. Proc Natl Acad Sci USA 83:8496–8500.

76. Robertson MC, Friesen HG (1975) The purification and characterization of rat placental lactogen. Endocrinology 97:621–629.
77. Southard JN, Thordarson G, Talamantes F (1986) Purification and partial characterization of hamster placental lactogen. Endocrinology 119:508–514.
78. Southard JN, Do L, Smith WC, Talamantes F (1989) Hamster placental lactogen-II contains a structural feature unique among the growth hormone-prolactin-placental lactogen family. Mol Endocrinol 3:1710–1713.
79. Southard JN, Talamantes F (1987) Immunological studies of rodent placental lactogens. Mol Cell Endocrinol 50:29–36.
80. Deb S, Hashizume K, Boone K, et al. (1989) Antipeptide antibodies reveal structural and functional characteristics of rat placental lactogen-II. Mol Cell Endocrinol 63:45–56.
81. Soares MJ, De SK, Foster BA, Julian JA, Glasser SR (1988) Identification of multiple low mol-wt placental prolactin-like proteins produced by rat trophoblast cells. J Endocrinol 116:101–106.
82. Chien Y-H, Thompson EB (1980) Genomic organization of rat prolactin and growth hormone genes. Proc Natl Acad Sci USA 77:4583–4587.
83. Cooke NE, Baxter JD (1982) Structural analysis of the prolactin gene suggests a separate origin for its 5′ end (1982) Nature 297:603–606.
84. Maurer RA, Erwin CR, Donelson JD (1981) Analysis of 5′ flanking sequences and intron-exon boundaries of the rat prolactin gene. J Biol Chem 256:10,524–10,528.
85. Shida MM, Jackson-Grusby LL, Ross SR, Linzer DIH (1992) Placental-specific expression from the mouse placental lactogen II gene promoter. Proc Natl Acad Sci USA 89:3864–3868.
86. Campbell WJ, Deb S, Kwok SCM, Joslin JA, Soares MJ (1989) Differential expression of placental lactogen-II and prolactin-like protein-A in the rat chorioallantoic placenta. Endocrinology 125:1565–1574.
87. Duckworth ML, Schroedter IC, Friesen HG (1990) Cellular localization of rat placental lactogen II and rat prolactin-like proteins A and B by in situ hybridization. Placenta 11:143–155.
88. Hall J, Talamantes F (1984) Immunocytochemical localization of mouse placental lactogen in the mouse placenta. J Histochem Cytochem 32:379–382.
89. Jones MA, Renegar RH (1994) Temporal and regional expression of placental lactogen-II messenger ribonucleic acid and protein in the hamster placenta. Biol Reprod 50:581–592.
90. Yamaguchi M, Ogren L, Endo H, Thordarson G, Bigsby RM, Talamantes F (1992) Production of mouse placental lactogen-I and placental lactogen-II by the same giant cell. Endocrinology 131: 1595–1602.
91. Yamaguchi M, Ogren L, Endo H, Soares MJ, Talamantes F (1994) Co-localization of placental lactogen-I, placental lactogen-II, and proliferin in the mouse placenta at midpregnancy. Biol Reprod 51:1188–1192.
92. Soares MJ (1987) Developmental changes in the intraplacental distribution of placental lactogen and alkaline phosphatase in the rat. J Reprod Fertil 79:93–98.
93. Daughad WH, Trivedi B, Kapadia M (1979) The effect of hypophysectomy on rat chorionic somatomammotropin as measured by prolactin and growth hormone radioreceptor assays: possible significance in maintenance of somatomedin generation. Endocrinology 105:210–214.
94. D JR, Ogren L, Talamantes F (1986) The effect of hypophysectomy on serum placental lactogen and progesterone in the mouse. Endocrinology 119:898–903.
95. Kishi K, Ogren L, Southard JN, Talamantes F (1988) Pituitary factors regulating mouse placental lactogen-II (mPL-II) secretion during the last half of pregnancy in mice. Endocrinology 122: 2309–2317.
96. Pinon I, Kishi K, Talamantes F (1988) The kinetics of disappearance of endogenous mouse placental lactogen-II in intact and hypophysectomized pregnant mice. Mol Cell Endocrinol 55: 45–51.
97. Robertson MC, Owens RE, Klindt J, Friesen HG (1984) Ovariectomy leads to a rapid increase in rat placental lactogen secretion. Endocrinology 114:1805–1811.
98. Robertson MC, Owens RE, McCoshen JA, Friesen HG (1984) Ovarian factors inhibit and fetal factors stimulate the secretion of rat placental lactogen. Endocrinology 114:22–30.
99. Soares MJ, Bartke A, Colosi P, Talamantes F (1984) Identification of a placental lactogen in pregnant Snell and Ames dwarf mice. Proc Soc Exp Biol Med 175:106–108.
100. Soares MJ, Talamantes F (1985) Placental lactogen secretion in the mouse: in vitro responses and ovarian and hormonal influences. J Exp Zool 234:97–104.
101. Tonkowicz PA, Voogt JL (1984) Ovarian and fetal control of rat placental lactogen and prolactin secretion at midpregnancy. Endocrinology 114:254–259.

102. Roby KF, Soares MJ (1993) Trophoblast cell differentiation and organization: role of fetal and ovarian signals. Placenta 14:529–545.
103. Thordarson G, Southard JN, Talamantes F (1991) Purification and characterization of mouse decidual calcyclin: a novel stimulator of mouse placental lactogen-II secretion. Endocrinology 129:1257–1265.
104. Kishi K, Itoh M, Kanamori S, Hirashiba M, Kawai M (1993) Stimulation of rat placental lactogen-II (rPL-II) secretion by cultured trophoblasts by insulin: development of a rat placental cell culture system and effects of peptide hormones on rPL-II seceretion in vitro. J Reprod Fertil 99: 519–527.
105. Yamaguchi M, Ogren L, Southard JN, Kurachi H, Miyake A, Talamantes F (1993) Interleukin 6 inhibits mouse placental lactogen II but not mouse placental lactogen I secretion in vitro. Proc Natl Acad Sci USA 90:11,905–11.909.
106. Yamaguchi M, Kurachi H, Tadokoro C, Sakata M, Yoshimoto Y, Masumoto N, Tasaka K, Miyake A (1994) Tumor necrosis factor-alpha (TNFalpha) inhibits expression of mouse placental lactogen-II through TNF alpha type-I but not type-II receptor. Biochem Biophys Res Commun 202:1599–1605.
107. Yamaguchi M, Ogren L, Barnard R, Imai T, Sawada T, Miyake A, Talamantes F (1994) Selective inhibition of mouse placental lactogen II secretion by tumour necrosis factor-alpha. J Endocrinol 143:95–105.
108. Yamaguchi M, Maeda T, Yoneda M, Nishizaki T, Miyake A (1995) Posttranscriptional inhibition of mouse placental lactogen-II secretion by transforming growth factor beta1: synergistic effects with epidermal growth factor and interleukin-6. Biol Reprod 53:373–379.
109. Yamaguchi M, Tasaka K, Ogura K, Sakata M, Mizuki J, Miyake A (1995) Activin inhibits but inhibin activates mouse placental lactogen-II secretion. J Endocrinol 146:469–474.
110. Yamaguchi M, Sakata M, Ogura K, Adachi K, Mammoto A, Miyake A (1996) Inhibition of mouse placental lactogen-II release from placental cells by interleukin-1 after mid-pregnancy. J Endocrinol 147:423–429.
111. Yamaguchi M, Sawada K, Miyake A (1996) Lipopolysaccharides selectively inhibit mouse placental lactogen-II secretion through stimulation of interleukin-1α (IL-1α) and IL-6 production. J Endocrinol Invest 19:415–421.
112. Shida M, Ng Y-K, Linzer DIH (1993) Transcriptional regulation of the placental lactogen genes in mouse trophoblast giant cells, In: Trophoblast Cells. Pathways for maternal–Embryonic Communication (Soares MJ, Handwerger S, Talamantes F, eds.), Springer-Verlag, New York, pp. 243–252.
113. Vuille J-C, Cattini PA, Bock ME, Verstuyf A, Schroedter IC, Duckworth ML, Friesen HG (1993) Rat prolactin-like protein-A partial gene and promoter structure: promoter activity in placental and pituitary cells. Mol Cell Endocrinol 96:91–98.
114. Southard JN, Talamantes F (1989) High mol-wt forms of placental lactogen: evidence for lactogen-macroglobulin complexes in rodents and humans. Endocrinology 125:791–800.
115. Harigaya T, Smith WC, Talamantes F (1988) Hepatic placental lactogen receptors during pregnancy in the mouse. Endocrinology 122:1366–1372.
116. Thordarson G, Villalobos R, Colosi P, Southard J, Ogren L, Talamantes F (1986) Lactogenic response of cultured mouse mammary epithelial cells to mouse placental lactogen. J Endocrinol 109:263–274.
117. Kawai M, Kishi K (1997) In vitro studies on the stimulation of insulin secretion and B cell proliferation by rat placental lactogen II during pregnancy in rats. J Reprod Fertil 109:145–152.
118. Davis JA, Linzer DIH (1989) A mutant lactogenic hormone binds, but does not activate, the prolactin receptor. Mol Endocrinol 3:949–953.
119. Davis JA, Linzer DIH (1989) Mutational analysis of a lactogenic hormone reveals a role for lactogen-specific amino acid residues in receptor binding and mitogenic activity. Mol Endocrinol 3:1987–1995.
120. Duckworth ML, Peden LM, Friesen HG (1986) Isolation of a novel prolactin-like cDNA clone from developing rat placenta. J Biol Chem 261:10,879–10,884.
121. Deb S, Youngblood T, Rawitch AB, Soares MJ (1989) Placental prolactin-like protein A. Identification and characterization of two major glycoprotein species with antipeptide antibodies. J Biol Chem 264:14,348–14,353.
122. Manzella SM, Dharmesh SM, Cohick CB, Soares MJ, Baenziger JU (1997) Developmental regulation of a pregnancy-specific oligosaccharide structure, NeuAcα2,6GalNAcβ1,4GlcNAc on select members of the rat placental prolactin family. J Biol Chem 272:4775–4782.

123. Deb S, Soares MJ (1990) Characterization of placental prolactin-like protein-A in intracellular and extracellular compartments. Mol Cell Endocrinol 74:163–172.
124. Deb S, Hamlin GP, Roby KF, Kwok SCM, Soares MJ (1993) Heterologous expression and characterization of prolactin-like protein-A. Identification of serum binding proteins. J Biol Chem 268:3298–3305.
125. Duckworth ML, Peden LM, Friesen HG (1988) A third prolactin-like protein expressed by the developing rat placenta: complementary deoxyribonucleic acid sequence and partial structure of the gene. Mol Endocrinol 2:912–920.
126. Cohick CB, Xu L, Soares MJ (1997) Prolactin-like protein-B: heterologous expression and characterization of placental and decidual species. J Endocrinol 152:291–302.
127. Croze F, Kennedy TG, Schroedter IC, Friesen HG (1990) Expression of rat prolactin-like protein B in deciduoma of pseudopregnant rat and in decidua during early pregnancy. Endocrinology 127:2665–2672.
128. Ogilvie S, Duckworth ML, Larkin LH, Buhi WC, Shiverick KT (1990) De novo synthesis and secretion of prolactin-like protein-B by rat placental explants. Endocrinology 126:2561–2566.
129. Faria TN, Deb S, Vandeputte M, Talamantes F, Soares MJ (1990) Transplantable rat choriocarcinoma cells express placental lactogen: identification of placental lactogen-I immunoreactive protein and messenger ribonucleic acid. Endocrinology 127:3131–3137.
130. Gibori G, Jayatilak PG, Khan I, Rigby B, Puryear T, Nelson S, Herz Z (1987) Decidual luteotropin secretion and action: its role in pregnancy maintenance in the rat, In: Regulation of Ovarian and Testicular Function (Mahesh VB, Dhindsa DS, Anderson E, Kalra SP, eds.), Plenum, New York, pp. 379–397.
131. Ogilvie S, Buhi WC, Olson JA, Shiverick KT (1990) Identification of a novel family of growth hormone-related proteins secreted by rat placenta. Endocrinology 126:3271–3273.
132. Deb S, Roby KF, Faria TN, Larsen D, Soares MJ (1991) Identification and immunochemical characterization of a major placental secretory protein related to the prolactin-growth hormone family, prolactin-like protein-C. Endocrinology 128:3066–3072.
133. Deb S, Roby KF, Faria TN, Szpirer C, Levan G, Kwok SCM, Soares MJ (1991) Molecular cloning and characterization of prolactin-like protein-C complementary deoxyribonucleic acid. J Biol Chem 266:23,027–23,032.
134. Dai G, Liu B, Szpirer C, Levan G, Kwok SCM, Soares MJ (1996) Prolactin-like protein-C variant: complementary DNA, unique six exon gene structure, and trophoblast cell-specific expression. Endocrinology 137:5009–5019.
135. Conliffe PR, Simmen RCM, Buhi WC, Shiverick KT (1995) Cloning of a novel rat placental prolactin-like protein C-related cDNA. Mol Reprod Dev 41:167–176.
136. Linzer DIH, Nathans D (1985) A new member of the prolactin-growth hormone gene family expressed in mouse placenta. EMBO J 4:1419–1423.
137. Iwatsuki K, Shinozaki M, Hattori N, Hirasawa K, Itagaki S-I, Shiota K, Ogawa T (1996) Molecular cloning and characterization of a new member of the rat placental prolactin (PRL) family PRL-like protein D (PLP-D). Endocrinology 137:3849–3855.
138. Roby KF, Deb S, Gibori G, Szpirer C, Levan G, Kwok SCM, Soares MJ (1993) Decidual prolactin-related protein. Identification, molecular cloning, and characterization. J Biol Chem 268:3136–3142.
139. Conliffe PR, Farmerie WG, Charles GD, Buhi WC, Kelly PA, Simmen RCM, Shiverick KT (1994) Expression and characterization of recombinant rat placental prolactin-like protein C. Mol Cell Endocrinol 106:121–130.
140. Rasmussen CA, Orwig KE, Vellucci S, Soares MJ (1997) Dual expression of prolactin-related protein in decidua and trophoblast tissues during pregnancy. Biol Reprod 56:647–654.
141. Orwig KE, Dai G, Rasmussen CA, Soares MJ (1997) Decidual prolactin-related protein: characterization of gene structure and cell-specific expression. Endocrinology 138:2491–2500.
142. Gu Y, Soares MJ, Srivastava RK, Gibori G (1994) Expression of decidual prolactin-related protein in the rat decidua. Endocrinology 135:1422–1427.
143. Rasmussen CA, Hashizume K, Orwig KE, Vellucci S, Xu L, Soares MJ (1996) Decidual prolactin-related protein: heterologous expression and characterization. Endocrinology 137:5558–5566.
144. Laurie GW (1985) Lack of heparan sulfate proteoglycan in a discontinuous and irregular placental basement membrane. Dev Biol 108:299–309.
145. Linzer DIH, Lee S-J, Ogren L, Talamantes F, Nathans D (1985) Identification of proliferin mRNA and protein in mouse placenta. Proc Natl Acad Sci USA 82:4356–4359.

146. Nilsen-Hamilton M, Shapiro JM, Massoglia SL, Hamilton RT (1980) Selective stimulation by mitogens of incorporation of ^{35}S-methionine into a family of proteins released into the medium by 3T3 cells. Cell 20:19–28.
147. Nilsen-Hamilton M, Hamilton RT, Alvarez-Azaustre E (1987) Relationship between mitogen-regulated protein (MRP) and proliferin (PLF), a member of the prolactin/growth hormone family. Gene 51:163–170.
148. Linzer DIH, Nathans D (1983) Growth-related changes in specific mRNAs of cultured mouse cells. Proc Natl Acad Sci USA 80:4271–4275.
149. Linzer DIH, Nathans D (1984) Nucleotide sequence of a growth-related mRNA encoding a member of the prolactin-growth hormone family. Proc Natl Acad Sci USA 81:4255–4259.
150. Parfett CL, Hamilton RT, Howell BW, Edwards DR, Nilsen-Hamilton M, Denhardt DT (1985) Characterization of a cDNA clone encoding murine mitogen-regulated protein: regulation of mRNA levels in mortal and immortal cell lines. Mol Cell Biol 5:3289–3292.
151. Wilder EL, Linzer DIH (1986) Expression of multiple proliferin genes in mouse cells. Mol Cell Biol 6:3283–3286.
152. Connor AM, Waterhouse P, Khokha R, Denhardt DT (1989) Characterization of a mouse mitogen-regulated protein/proliferin gene and its promoter: a member of the growth hormone/prolactin gene superfamily. Biochim Biophys Acta 1009:75–82.
153. Lee S-J, Nathans D (1987) Secretion of proliferin. Endocrinology 120:208–213.
154. Colosi P, Swiergiel JJ, Wilder EL, Oviedo A, Linzer DIH (1988) Characterization of proliferin-related protein. Mol Endocrinol 2:579–586.
155. Lee S-J, Talamantes F, Wilder E, Linzer DIH, Nathans D (1988) Trophoblastic giant cells of the mouse placenta as the site of proliferin synthesis. Endocrinology 122:1761–1768.
156. Nilsen-Hamilton M, Jang YJ, Alvarez-Azaustre E, Hamilton RT (1988) Regulation of the production of a prolactin-like protein (MRP/PLF) in 3T3 cells and in the mouse placenta. Mol Cell Endocrinol 56:179–190.
157. Yamaguchi M, Imai T, Maeda T, Sakata M, Miyake A, Linzer DIH (1995) Cyclic adenosine 3′,5″-monophosphate stimulation of placental proliferin and proliferin-related protein secretion. Endocrinology 136:2040–2046.
158. Linzer DIH, Wilder EL (1987) Control of proliferin gene expression in serum-stimulated mouse cells. Mol Cell Biol 7:2080–2086.
159. Linzer DIH, Mordacq JC (1987) Transcriptional regulation of proliferin gene expression in response to serum in transfected mouse cells. EMBO J 6:2281–2288.
160. Nilsen-Hamilton M, Jang YJ, Delgado M, Shim JK, Bruns K, Chiang CP, Fang Y, Parfett CL, Denhardt DT, Hamilton RT (1991) Regulation of the expression of mitogen-regulated protein (MRP; proliferin) and cathepsin L in cultured cells and in the murine placenta. Mol Cell Endocrinol 77:115–122.
161. Mordacq JC, Linzer DIH (1989) Co-localization of elements required for phorbol ester stimulation and glucocorticoid repression of proliferin gene expression. Genes Dev 3:760–769.
162. Groskopf JC, Linzer DIH (1994) Characterization of a delayed early serum response region. Mol Cell Biol 14:6013–6020.
163. Parfett CLJ (1992) Induction of proliferin gene expression by diverse chemical agents that promote morphological transformation in C3H/10T1/2 cultures. Cancer Lett 64:1–9.
164. Parfett CL, Pilon R (1993) Tri-n-butyltin chloride promotes morphological transformation and induces proliferin expression in C3H10T1/2 cells. Cancer Lett 71:167–176.
165. Parfett CL, Pilon R (1995) Oxidative stress-regulated gene expression and promotion of morphological transformation induced in C3H/10T1/2 cells by ammonium metavanadate. Food Chem Toxicol 33:301–308.
166. Edwards DR, Parfett CL, Smith JH, Denhardt DT (1987) Evidence that post-transcriptional changes in the expression of mitogen regulated protein accompany immortalization of mouse cells. Biochem Biophys Res Commun 147:467–473.
167. Malyankar UM, Rittling SR, Connor A, Denhardt DT (1994) The mitogen-regulated protein/proliferin transcript is degraded in primary mouse embryo fibroblast but not 3T3 nuclei: altered RNA processing correlates with immortalization. Proc Natl Acad Sci USA 91:335–339.
168. Malyankar UM, Rittling SR, Denhardt DT (1996) Instability of endogenous MRP/proliferin transcripts in the nucleus of mouse embryo fibroblasts contrasts with their stability when produced during transient transfections. J Cell Biochem 60:198–210.
169. Jackson D, Linzer DIH (1997) Proliferin transport and binding in the mouse fetus. Endocrinology 138:149–155.

170. Jackson D, Volpert OV, Bouck N, Linzer DIH (1994) Stimulation and inhibition of angiogenesis by placental proliferin and proliferin-related protein. Science 266:1581–1584.
171. Clapp C, Weiner RI (1992) A specific, high affinity, saturable binding site for the 16-kilodalton fragment of prolactin on capillary endothelial cells. Endocrinology 130:1380–1386.
172. Volpert O, Jackson D, Bouck N, Linzer DIH (1996) The insulin-like growth factor II/mannose 6-phosphate receptor is required for proliferin-induced angiogenesis. Endocrinology 137:3871–3876.
173. Lee S-J, Nathans D (1988) Proliferin secreted by cultured cells binds to mannose 6-phosphate receptors. J Biol Chem 263:3521–3527.
174. Rogers SA, Purchio AF, Hammerman MR (1990) Mannose 6-phosphate-containing peptides activate phospholipase C in proximal tubular basolateral membranes from canine kidney. J Biol Chem 265:9722–9727.
175. Nelson JT, Rosenzweig N, Nilsen-Hamilton M (1995) Characterization of the mitogen-regulated protein (proliferin) receptor. Endocrinology 136:283–288.
176. Muscat GE, Gobius K, Emery J (1991) Proliferin, a prolactin/growth hormone-like peptide represses myogenic-specific transcription by the suppression of an essential serum response factor-like DNA-binding activity. Mol Endocrinol 5:802–814.
177. Wilder EL, Linzer DIH (1989) Participation of multiple factors, including proliferin, in the inhibition of myogenic differentiation. Mol Cell Biol 9:430–441.
178. Barnes SW, Renegar RH (1996) Identification, characterization, and expression of a new prolactin-like molecule in the hamster placenta. Biol Reprod 55:370–378.
179. Cooke NE, Szpirer C, Levan G (1986) The related genes encoding growth hormone and prolactin have been dispersed to chromosomes 10 and 17 in the rat. Endocrinology 119:2451–2454.
180. Jackson-Grusby LL, Pravtcheva D, Ruddle FH, Linzer DIH (1988) Chromosomal mapping of the prolactin/growth hormone gene family in the mouse. Endocrinology 122:2462–2466.
181. Owerbach D, Rutter WJ, Cooke NE, Martial JA, Shows TB (1981) The prolactin gene is located on chromosome 6 in humans. Science 212:815,816.
182. Schuler LA, Scott P, Kessler MA (1993) Molecular genetics and biology of the bovine placental prolactin family, In: Trophoblast Cells. Pathways for Maternal–Embryonic Communication (Soares MJ, Handwerger S, Talamantes F, eds.), Springer-Verlag, New York, pp. 191–205.
183. Cooke NE, Jones BK, Urbanek M, Misra-Press A, Lee AK, Russell JE, MacLeod JN, Liebhaber SA (1993) Placental expression and function of the human growth hormone gene cluster, In: Trophoblast Cells. Pathways for Maternal–Embryonic Communication (Soares MJ, Handwerger S, Talamantes F, eds.), Springer-Verlag, New York, pp. 222–239.
184. Goffin V, Shiverick KT, Kelly PA, Martial JA (1996) Sequence-function relationships within the expanding family of prolactin, growth hormone, placental lactogen, and related proteins in mammals. Endocr Rev 17:385–410.
185. Erskine MS (1995) Prolactin release after mating and genitosensory stimulation in females. Endocr Rev 16:508–528.
186. Gunnet JW, Freeman ME (1983) The mating-induced release of prolactin: a unique neuroendocrine response. Endocr Rev 4:44–61.
187. Neill JD (1980) Neuroendocrine regulation of prolactin secretion. Frontiers Neuroendocrinol 6: 129–155.
188. Morishige W, Rothchild I (1974) Temporal aspects of the regulation of corpus luteum function by luteinzing hormone, prolactin, and placental luteotrophin during the first half of pregnancy in the rat. Endocrinology 95:260–272.
189. Guillemot F, Nagy A, Auerbach A, Rossant J, Joyner A (1994) Essential role of Mash-2 in extraembryonic development. Nature 371:333–336.
190. Guillemot F, Caspary T, Tilghman SM, Copeland, NG, Gilbert DJ, Jenkins NA, Anderson DJ, Joyner AL, Rossant J, Nagy A (1995) Genomic imprinting of Mash2, a mouse gene required for trophoblast development. Nature Genetics 9:235–241.
191. Sibilia M, Wagner EF (1995) Strain-dependent epithelial defects in mice lacking the EGF receptor. Science 269:234–238.
192. Threadgill DW, Dlugosz AA, Hansen J, Tennenbaum T, Lichti U, Yee D, LaMantia C, Mourton T, Herrup K, Harris RC, Barnard JA, Yuspa SH, Coffey RJ, Magnuson T (1995) Targeted disruption of mouse EGF receptor: effect of genetic background on phenotype. Science 269:230–234.
193. Royster M, Driscoll P, Kelly PA, Freemark M (1995) The prolactin receptor in the fetal rat: cellular localization of messenger ribonucleic acid, immunoreactive protein, and ligand-binding activity and induction of expression in late gestation. Endocrinology 136:3892–3900.

194. Ormandy CJ, Binart N, Camus A, Barra J, Damotte D, Lucas B, Buteau H, Edery M, Brousse N, Babinet C, Binart N, Kelly PA (1997) Null mutation of the prolactin receptor gene produces multiple reproductive defects in the mouse. Genes Dev 11:167–178.
195. Bridges RS, Goldman BD (1975) Ovarian control of prolactin secretion during late pregnancy in the rat. Endocrinology 97:496–498.
196. Chatelain A, Dupuoy JP, Dubois MP (1979) Ontogenesis of cells producing polypeptide hormones (ACTH, MSH, LPH, GH, Prolactin) in the fetal hypophysis of the rat: influence of the hypothalamus. Cell Tissue Res 196:409–427.
197. Grattan D, Averill RLW (1990) Effect of ovarian steroids on a nocturnal surge of prolactin secretion that precedes parturition in the rat. Endocrinology 126:1119–1205.
198. Simmons DM, Voss JW, Ingraham HA, Holloway JM, Broide RS, Rosenfeld MG, Swanson LW (1990) Pituitary cell phenotypes involve cell-specific Pit-1 mRNA translation and synergistic interactions with other classes of transcription factors. Genes Dev 4:695–711.
199. Tong Y, Zhao H, Labrie F, Pelletier G (1989) Ontogeny of prolactin mRNA in the rat pituitary gland as evaluated by in situ hybridization. Mol Cell Endocrinol 67:11–16.
200. Watanabe YG, Daikoku S (1979) An immunohistochemical study of the cytogenesis of adenohypophysial cells in fetal rats. Dev Biol 68:557–567.

7 Expression of Steroid Hormone Receptors in the Pregnant Uterus

William C. Okulicz, PHD*, Sheri Hild-Petito,* PHD*, and Beverly Chilton,* PHD

CONTENTS

INTRODUCTION

The uterus of mammalian species plays the central role in providing the appropriate environment for the establishment and maintenance of pregnancy. The coordinated actions of estradiol (E) and progesterone (P) are essential for all stages of pregnancy from implantation to parturition. These steroid hormones exert their effects on gene expression primarily through specific receptors (R) present in uterine tissue and compartmentalized within different cell types. Because of their central importance in female reproductive functions, the presence and regulation of these ligand-inducible transcription factors have been the focus of numerous studies. Although many other regulatory molecules are believed to be part of the hormonal cascade of action triggered by E and P, these factors and their roles in pregnancy are discussed elsewhere in this volume.

The focus of this chapter is the expression and regulation of steroid hormone receptors in the pregnant uterus. Our particular emphasis will be on ER and PR because of their importance and the extensive literature available. A brief overview of current concepts on the mechanism of action and hormonal regulation of these receptors will be followed by a

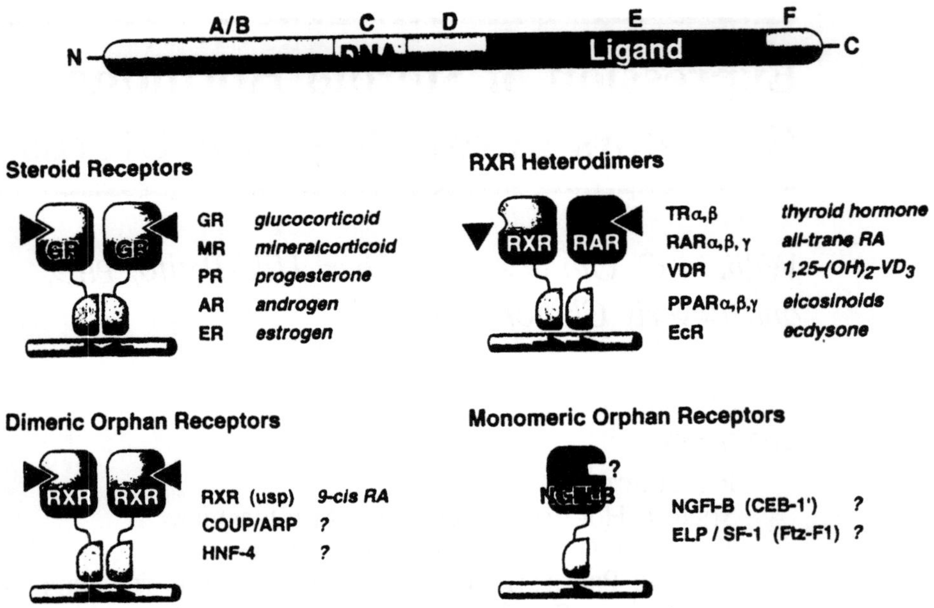

Fig. 1. Nuclear receptors share common structure/function domains. Reprinted with permission *(1)*.

description of the changes in uterine receptor binding activity during pregnancy in several mammalian systems. The recent availability of specific antibodies and nucleic acid probes for steroid hormone receptors has allowed their identification and localization by both immunohistochemical and *in situ* hybridization techniques, respectively. With these tools, specific morphological compartments and cell types within target tissues that contain these receptors can be identified. Because of the increased recognition of the importance of cell type-specific regulation, we have chosen to separate a discussion of receptor ligand binding studies of the pregnant uterus from cell type-specific studies. Finally, we conclude with discussion of other members of the steroid receptor superfamily that may potentially play a role in uterine function during pregnancy.

STEROID HORMONE RECEPTORS: AN OVERVIEW

The nuclear receptor superfamily can be divided into the steroid receptor family and the thyroid/retinoid/vitamin D (or nonsteroid) receptor family. The glucocorticoid (GR) and estrogen receptors, the first cellular transcription factors identified, were cloned in the mid-1980s. Then came the discovery of the receptor for retinoic acid, and ecdysone, the first insect receptor. By 1990, the development of radiolabeled ligands, purified hormones, and antibodies had facilitated the identification of 15 receptors, one for each of the known lipophilic hormones. Since that time, molecular cloning techniques have led to the identification of numerous unliganded (orphan) receptors, resulting in a family of more than 150 members in species as diverse as mammals and arthropods *(1)*.

Based on structure and function, a typical member of the nuclear receptor superfamily can be divided into five regions denoted A/B,C,D,E, and F *(1,2)* (Fig. 1). Region A/B is the hypervariable N-terminal region that contains a transactivation domain (AF1). The suggestion that the function of this domain is not conserved by family members is based on the variable length of the region, i.e., 20 amino acids in the vitamin D_3 receptor compared to 600 amino acids in the mineralcorticoid receptor *(3)*. Region C is centrally located and contains the highly conserved DBD with an invariant pattern of cysteine residues and a dimerization domain. Many receptor-encoding genes were cloned as a result of screening cDNA libraries with probes to this highly conserved region. The DBD, which directs the receptor to specific DNA sequences called hormone response elements (HREs), is characterized by two highly conserved zinc-finger motifs that are folded together to form a single structural domain. Structural stability requires the presence of both zinc fingers *(4)*. This structural affiliation distinguishes the zinc-finger motif of the nuclear receptors from the classical modular zinc fingers of other DNA binding proteins *(5)*. Mutations in the DBD can result in receptor dysfunction and a disease state. For example, six independent mutations have been mapped to the DBD of the vitamin D receptor in patients with hereditary rickets. In two different families, the single nucleotide change in either zinc finger resulted in a loss of DNA binding activity *(6,7)*. Immediately adjacent to the C-terminal zinc-finger motif is a short, ligand-dependent, nuclear localization domain (NLD), which encroaches on the variable hinge region (D). Region E is the ligand binding domain (LBD), which contains a dimerization region and two transactivation domains (AF-2 and AF-2a). The LBD functions as the molecular on/off switch, selectively binding hormone and converting the receptor from an inactive state to a transcriptionally active state. Mutations in the LBD can also result in a disease state, i.e., several mutations have been reported in the LBD of the androgen receptor in patients with testosterone insensitivity syndrome *(6,7)*. Regions C and E contain the DBD and the LBD, which are the signature motifs of the nuclear receptor superfamily. In contrast, no function has been assigned to region F at the C-terminus.

Nuclear receptors can be subdivided into four classes according to their ligand binding, DNA binding, and dimerization properties *(1,8–11)* (Fig. 1). Nuclear receptors associate directly with specific DNA sequences or HREs, which are composed of direct repeats, inverted repeats, or everted repeats of a hexad core sequence. Specificity of the hormone response is determined by the number of nucleotides placed between the two core elements, differences in the sequence of the hexad half-site, and differences in the 5′-extensions of the HREs. Class I or steroid receptors are ligand-induced homodimers that bind to palindromic HREs. Receptors for glucocorticoids, mineralcorticoids, P, and androgens recognize the same AGAACA half-site. The ER recognizes AGGTCA, the same half-site recognized by the class II, nonsteroid nuclear receptors (called RXR heterodimers in Fig. 1). All the nonsteroid, ligand-dependent receptors, such as the thyroid and ecdysone receptors, heterodimerize with the retinoid X receptor (RXR) and typically bind to direct repeats. Known ligands for this group include vitamin D, thyroid hormone, retinoids, and prostanoids. However, some RXR heterodimer partner receptors have no known ligands (or activators) and are therefore called orphan receptors. Homodimeric orphan receptors (chick ovalbumin upstream promotor [COUP]/apolipoprotein regulatory protein [ARP] and hepatocyte nuclear factor [HNF-4] receptors) and monomeric orphan receptors (nerve growth factor inducible [NGF1-B] and embryonal long-terminal repeat binding protein [EL]P/steroidogenic factor [SF-1] receptors) comprise classes III and IV, respectively.

The steroid hormone receptors (SHRs) exhibit the modular structure typical of the nuclear receptor superfamily. Moreover, they are known to interact with a diverse group of proteins *(12)*. The SHRs are unique in that their unliganded forms are maintained in an inactive, ligand-ready conformation through their affiliation with a large multiprotein complex of chaperones. This heterocomplex, which includes heat shock protein (Hsp) 90 and the immunophilin Hsp56, binds to the LBD and maintains the receptor in a transcriptionally inactive state. Dissociation of this heterocomplex results in the conversion of the receptor to the DNA binding state *(13)*. Immunolocalization of Hsps in human endometrium suggests that Hsp70 expression is related to cell proliferation and/or down-regulation of SHRs *(14)*.

Liganded SHRs bind to DNA and communicate with the transcription initiation complex, which consists of RNA polymerase II and relevant basal transcription factors *(15–17)*. More poorly defined SHR-protein interactions include evidence that the AF-2 site of the C-terminus of the ER contacts intermediary factors, such as receptor interacting protein (RIP140). TIF1 interacts with ER and PR, and suppressor for galactose (SUG1), a component of the RNA polymerase II holoenzyme, has been identified as another AF-2 binding protein. It is increasingly apparent that the classical model for ligand–receptor interaction in which the effect of the ligand was determined directly by its interaction with the receptor is being replaced with a tripartite model that involves ligand, receptor, and effector interactions *(18)*.

The ER and PR are two members of the SHR family that directly transduce signals from their hormone effectors into uterine-specific gene expression. Because PR synthesis is positively regulated by the ER, its presence indicates a functionally active ER response pathway *(19)*. Prolactin has also been shown to increase PR expression in the uterus *(20)*. In fact, a servomechanism (feedback) exists between PRL and P, in which PRL binds to its receptor and increases PR concentration. This in turn enhances the cellular response to P, including an increase in PRL receptor number *(21)*. The PR from most species exists as subtypes A and B. One exception is the rabbit, where the functional PR is a single 110-kDa protein (B form). The A form is missing the N-terminal 127 (chick) or 164 (human) amino acids present in the B form. Proposed mechanisms for the generation of these two subtypes include alternate initiation of transcription from the same message or transcription from two different estrogen-regulated promoters in the same gene. It is well documented that PR expression is decreased in response to P. Recent evidence *(22,23)* indicates the A form of the receptor can act as a transcriptional activator or as a dominant repressor of B activity. Phosphorylation might also differentially alter the two isoforms *(24)*.

The PR has been implicated in the regulation of some early events of pregnancy. P and to a lesser extent E regulate the preimplantation uterine expression of uteroglobin (UG), a protein with potent anti-inflammatory activity *(25)*. The highest levels of UG expression in the rabbit and in the human endometrium coincide with the events of embryo implantation. The recent localization of a high-affinity UG binding protein on human trophoblast cells *(26)* suggests that UG may play a pivotal role in regulating cellular invasiveness. PR has also been implicated in the induction of apoptosis in uterine endometrium. Apoptosis, the genetically governed process that is complementary to mitosis, is the usual form of cell death *(27)*. The most completely described group of cell death-modulating proteins is the Bcl-2 family *(28)*. The ratio of Bcl-2 to its partner, Bax, is thought to be regulatory, i.e., Bcl-2 is death-inhibitory, whereas Bax facilitates death. In the uterus, P may regulate apoptosis during blastocyst implantation and decidualization by controlling the balance between Bcl-2 and Bax expression *(29)*.

The interaction between SHRs and DNA likely involves chromatin structure. Transcriptional activation by GR and ER in yeast requires switch (SWI)/sucrose nonfermenting (SNF) proteins *(30)*. The SWI/SNF complex of proteins is believed to participate in the unwinding of chromatin in the region of the promoter *(31,32)*, thereby reorganizing chromatin to facilitate the binding of transcription factors. A human homolog to the yeast SWI/SNF, human homolog of *Drosophila brahma* (hBrm), potentiates transcriptional activation by the GR and the retinoic acid receptor *(33)*. Another human SWI/SNF homology, BRM/SWI2-related gene (BRG1), restored transcriptional activation by the GR in yeast strains lacking SWI2. New evidence for P-dependent posttranscriptional processing of two SWI/SNF-related proteins that bind to the UG promoter *(34)* provides evidence for PR-mediated recruitment of chromatin remodeling factors.

SHRs were thought to be essential for neonatal survival, sexual differentiation, and fertility. However, the development of mice with mutations in ER *(35)* and PR *(36)*, i.e., knockouts for the sex steroid receptors, did not lead to embryonic lethality. The balanced sex ratio suggests that their ablation does not alter the process of sex determination. Homozygous female mice without ER were, however, infertile. They developed ovaries with cystic and hemorrhagic follicles, but no corpora lutea. Uteri were hypoplastic and unable to respond to an estrogen challenge. Female mice without PR (homozygous) were also infertile. They failed to ovulate, displayed uterine hyperplasia and inflammation, and they failed to display any P-facilitated sexual behavior (lordosis response). Collectively, these studies confirm the critical role of ER and PR in normal reproductive function, and emphasize the need for additional studies to determine the relative contribution of each receptor.

TEMPORAL CHANGES IN ESTROGEN RECEPTOR AND PROGESTERONE RECEPTOR BINDING IN THE PREGNANT UTERUS: PERI-IMPLANTATION THROUGH PARTURITION

Rodent/Rabbit Models

The rat is the most commonly used rodent model for reproductive studies, and much of the early work on the hormonal regulation and establishment of pregnancy has used this species. The importance of P and E in the development of uterine receptivity for blastocyst implantation has been well documented in the rat *(37)*. Between d 1 and 4 of pregnancy, there is a transitory increase in serum E *(38)* that is associated with an increase in uterine nuclear ER binding on d 2–3, which subsequently declines by d 4 *(39)*. During this period there appears to be little difference in uterine PR binding compared to the nonpregnant luteal phase uterus *(40,41)*. A transitory increase in nuclear PR during this period has also been reported in the myometrium and may reflect increased serum P *(41)*. After implantation occurs (d 5–6), studies have shown significant differences between implantation and nonimplantation sites *(42)*. Nuclear ER and PR binding at implantation sites was approximately twofold higher than at nonimplantation sites. Furthermore, these differences were not observed in decidualized vs nondecidualized endometrium in the absence of a blastocyst. These results are consistent with secretion of a local steroid or other factor from the blastocyst during implantation. These results have, however, been disputed by the work of Martel and Psychoyos *(43)*. In contrast to the striking changes noted above, these authors observed no differences in cytosolic or nuclear ER binding between implantation and noninplantation sites. Although a number of studies in other species have shown that signals from the blastocyst are recognized by the uterus *(44)*, further studies will be needed to determine their role in the regulation of uterine ER and PR in the rat.

Although a gradual increase in both uterine cytosolic and nuclear PR binding has been reported during pregnancy and until just before parturition *(40)*, other studies have shown a gradual decline in nuclear PR binding that is associated with decreases in serum P *(45)*. In contrast, nuclear ER binding gradually increased to peak levels on d 21 (the day before parturition) *(45,46)*. The elevated level of nuclear ER binding at this time was associated with elevated levels of serum E during the last few days of pregnancy. It has been suggested that this elevated level of nuclear ER binding is a sign of increased E action that leads to increased myometrial contractility necessary for parturition. The observed decreases in nuclear PR concomitant with increases in ER binding are consistent with the known effects of P on ER levels, i.e., decreases in P action reverse the inhibitory effect of P on ER levels. The most dramatic change in uterine ER binding occurred just prior to and during parturition *(45)*. Nuclear ER binding fell rapidly from its peak level on d 21 through d 22 and during the postpartum period. This decrease in ER binding was associated with a rise in serum P at this time and may reflect a transitory return of P inhibition of ER binding.

McCormack and Glasser *(47)* were the first to show the presence of ER binding sites in the basal region of the placenta. Subsequently, the maternal decidua basalis has also been shown to contain both ER and PR *(48,49)*. ER binding sites declined approx 70% from d 9 through d 17 to almost undetectable levels. The high levels of ER binding between d 8 and 10 were associated with the differentiation and growth of the decidua basalis. In contrast to the classical action of P inhibition of ER binding, studies have shown that P may serve to increase and maintain the expression of ER in this tissue perhaps by a posttranslational mechanism *(50)*. PR binding in the decidua basalis declined to undetectable levels during the last week of gestation in the rat coincident with the regression of this tissue during the last week of pregnancy. Although P has been shown to decrease PR binding, this may not be the case for all target tissues, since placental PR binding can be maintained during pregnancy by exogenous P *(51)*.

The female hamster, like the rat, has been used extensively to study the hormonal control mechanisms that are operative during pregnancy and parturition. In the pregnant hamster, myometrial cytosolic and nuclear receptors for ER and PR remained relatively steady from d 6 of pregnancy through d 14 *(52)*. Prior to parturition on d 16, there were striking changes in ER binding. Both cytosolic and nuclear ER binding increased sharply between d 14 and 16. The increase in nuclear ER binding during this period of pregnancy has been subsequently shown to be primarily owing to an increase in the occupied form (ligand-bound form) of nuclear ER *(53)*. In contrast to the rat, there was no prepartum increase in serum E associated with this increase in ER binding. The most likely explanation for this increase in ER binding is the sharp decrease in serum P that occurred during this period that removed the inhibitory influence of P on ER binding. Myometrial cytosolic PR binding also increased sharply at this time and probably reflects an increase in E action (E-dependent PR induction) as well as a decrease of P downregulation of its own receptor. A similar pattern of ER and PR expression was observed in the myometrium of the pseudopregnant hamster *(54)*.

Changes in ER and PR binding have also been studied in the developing deciduoma in pseudopregnant hamsters *(52,55)*. The deciduoma of the pseudopregnant hamster typically remains viable until approximately d 8 of pseudopregnancy and involutes on d 9. During d 6–9 of pseudopregnancy, the levels of serum P and E remain relatively steady. Cytosolic PR binding increased from d 6 to a peak level on d 8, whereas nuclear PR binding showed little or no change during this period. Cytosolic and nuclear ER binding showed a striking decrease between d 7 and 8. Although the concentrations of ER and PR in the hamster deciduoma differ somewhat from the levels in the myometrium, the changes observed follow a similar temporal pattern.

Uterine ER and PR binding have been measured during pregnancy in other species, such as the mouse *(56)*, guinea pig *(57)*, and rabbit *(58)*. Although there are some differences during pregnancy, there are also differences between species. Because of the few detailed studies, it is difficult to interpret and reconcile these differences.

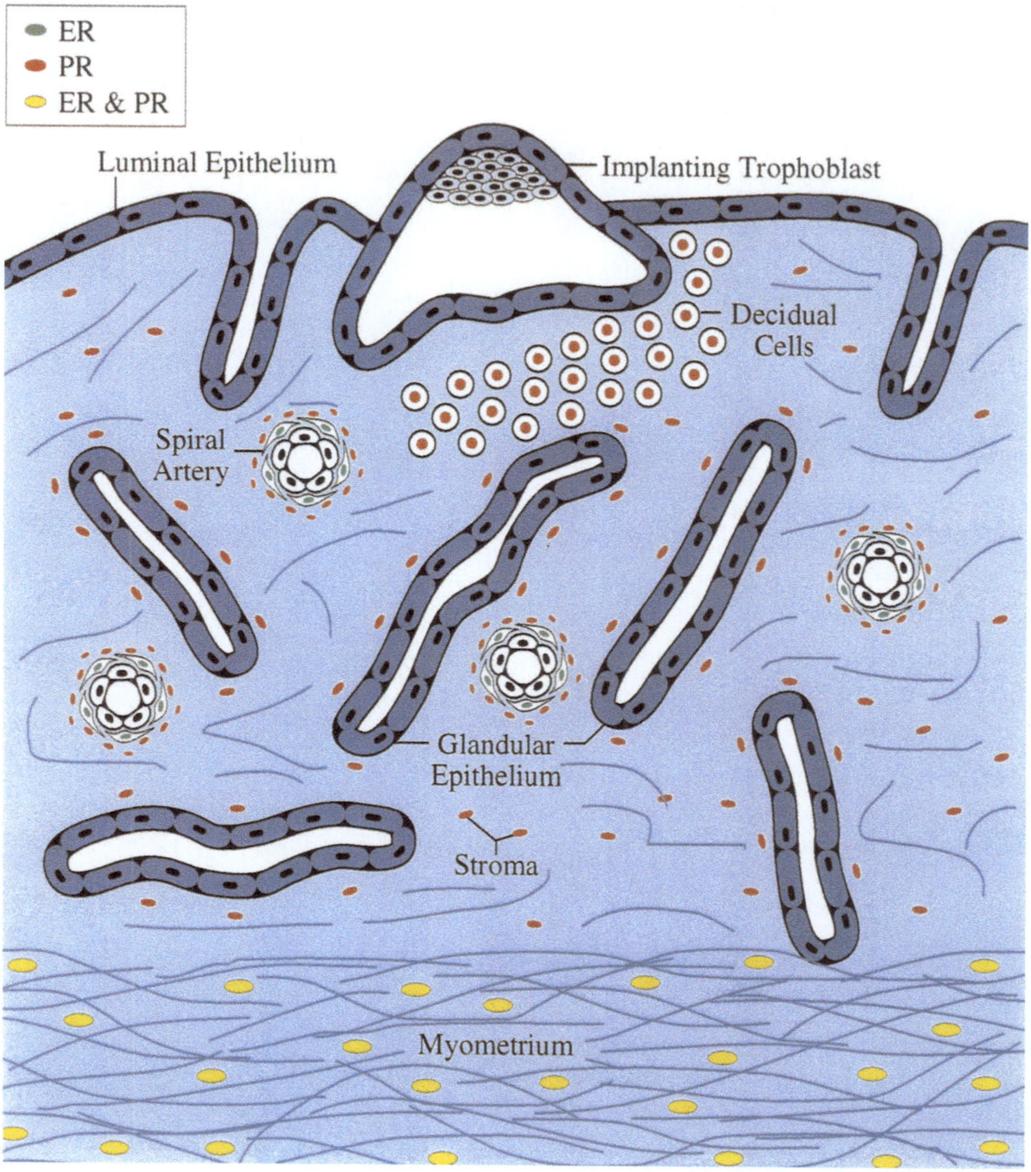
ER
PR
ER & PR
Luminal Epithelium
Implanting Trophoblast
Decidual Cells
Spiral Artery
Glandular Epithelium
Stroma
Myometrium

Domestic Animal Models

The pregnant ewe has historically been one of the most studied domestic animal models in reproductive biology. The day of estrus (mating) is defined as d 0 of pregnancy, and distinct morphological changes in the uterus are not apparent until d 15, the day of implantation. Cytosolic ER binding between d 9 and 15 in pregnant ewes was lower in caruncular and intercaruncular tissue than ER binding in the nonpregnant uterus *(59)*. Although uterine ER binding decreased in both pregnant and nonpregnant ewes from d 9 to d 13, nonpregnant ewes showed a sharp increase in cytosolic ER on d 15, whereas no change was observed in pregnant ewes. This increase in cytosolic ER binding in cyclic ewes occurred at the time of luteolysis, and most likely reflects decreasing P levels and the subsequent loss of P-induced inhibition of ER binding. Similar results in total endometrial ER binding have been reported between d 10 and 16 in pregnant ewes with a concomitant 80% decrease in ER mRNA by d 16 *(60,61)*. In contrast, there was little difference in endometrial PR binding during this period of pregnancy despite a 50% decrease in the steady-state mRNA level *(61)*.

Local signals from the blastocyst have been shown to play a role in the maternal recognition of pregnancy in the ewe *(44,62,63)*. It has recently been demonstrated that interferon τ originating from the blastocyst can regulate ER expression in the ovine uterus *(64,65)*. The secretion of interferon τ by the conceptus is believed to prevent normal luteolytic mechanisms by suppressing uterine ER expression and therefore preventing the upregulation of uterine oxytocin receptors that mediate luteolysis in the ewe *(66)*. The suppressed levels of ER expression in the pregnant uterus compared to the nonpregnant uterus reflect this mechanism. The role and potential mechanism of action of signals from the conceptus that regulate the maternal recognition of pregnancy are covered in detail elsewhere in this volume.

Both cytosolic ER and PR binding remained suppressed between d 56 and 112 of gestation in caruncular and intercaruncular tissue of ewes *(67)*. Decreased endometrial ER mRNA levels are consistent with the suppressed protein expression pattern during this period *(67)*. Although nuclear ER binding remained low in these endometrial tissue compartments during this period, nuclear PR binding showed a significant increase on d 84 and d 112. This observation may be owing to increased levels of serum E during this period and was similar to the increase in myometrial PR binding during the latter half of gestation *(see below)*.

The regulation of myometrial ER and PR during the peri-implantation period in the ewe is somewhat different from that described above for the endometrium. Myometrial cytosolic ER and PR binding decreased between d 5 and 14 in cyclic and pregnant ewes compared to the day of estrus *(68)* similar to that described above for the endometrium. These changes in cytosolic ER and PR protein expression parallel the changes in the steady-state levels of ER and PR mRNA through d 13 *(61)*. Subsequently, between d 13 and 25 there was an increase in PR mRNA expression in the endometrium, whereas myometrial levels remained suppressed. The decrease in ER and PR binding during this period most likely reflects the increasing levels of serum P in pregnant ewes *(60)*, resulting in an inhibition of ER binding and an autologous downregulation of PR similar to that shown for the endometrium. Myometrial ER and PR binding showed little change throughout most of the pregnancy, except for a tendency of cytosolic PR to increase from d 65 to d 130 *(68)*. This latter increase in myometrial PR binding may be a result of increased levels of serum E *(69)*, which would potentially lead to an increase in PR.

There are few studies on uterine ER and PR levels in the ewe just before and during parturition. The dramatic changes in steroid hormone levels that accompany labor would be expected to cause significant changes in the levels of ER and PR binding similar to those described above for rodent models. These changes would be expected to manifest themselves in the tissue compartment that is most intimately involved in labor, the myometrium. A recent study has, however, shown that both ER protein and ER mRNA level were significantly elevated in myometrial, endometrial, and cervical tissue during glucocorticoid-induced parturition *(70)*. The authors suggested that during spontaneous labor glucocorticoids originating from the fetus may play a role in the upregulation of ER during parturition. As noted above for other species, the upregulation of uterine ER expression just before and during parturition was associated with rising serum E levels and declining P levels during spontaneous parturition *(69)*.

The role of E during early pregnancy in the pig is quite different from sheep and would be expected to alter the pattern of uterine expression of ER and PR binding. The secretion of E from the conceptus in the pig has been shown to be important in the maintenance of the corpus luteum in early pregnancy *(44)*. This luteotrophic action of E in the pig is in contrast to the ewe where elevated E and E action promotes luteolysis *(63)*. These differences were evident during the early stages of pregnancy (d 10–19) in the pig. Uterine ER binding and ER mRNA levels were elevated and were not suppressed by increased serum P during the luteal phase as observed in the ewe *(71)*. Indeed, nuclear ER binding in the endometrium has been shown to increase between d 16 and 19 of pregnancy in the pig *(72)*.

The levels of myometrial ER and PR binding during pregnancy in the pig have been documented and correlated with serum E and P levels *(73)*. Similar to observations in several other species, there were no remarkable changes in myometrial ER and PR binding levels throughout most of pregnancy. Cytosolic and nuclear PR binding remained elevated during most of pregnancy, whereas cytosolic and nuclear ER showed an opposite pattern, i.e., increased levels as parturition approached. Just before and during parturition, the levels of serum E increased and the levels of P decreased similar to observations in the ewe. These changes were associated with increased myometrial ER binding, and most likely reflect a decline in P action, i.e., loss of P inhibition of ER binding. As reported for other species, these changes have been interpreted as a reflection of increased E action and subsequent changes in myometrial contractility, which is a prerequisite for labor and the expulsion of the fetus.

Human and Nonhuman Primates

During the midluteal phase of the human menstrual cycle (peri-implantation period), ER and PR binding were significantly lower than during the late proliferative phase *(74–76)*. These differences were similar to that described above for several other species and are a result of the known effects of elevated P levels during the luteal phase, i.e., P inhibition of ER and PR binding. Although ethical considerations clearly prohibit studies on human implantation sites, there are several studies that have been done during early pregnancy (8–10 wk, elective abortion) and during late pregnancy (38–40 wk, cesarean section). Endometrial ER (cytosolic and nuclear) remained low during early and late pregnancy, and were comparable to levels during the midsecretory period of the menstrual cycle *(74,75)*. Although total (cytosolic and nuclear) endometrial PR was also similar to that of a secretory endometrium, a larger fraction of PR binding was found in the nuclear compartment *(75)*. This may be related to the very high levels of serum P during this stage of pregnancy. No significant differences in endometrial PR binding were observed during late pregnancy (38–40 wk).

ER binding (cytosolic and nuclear) in term myometrium has been shown to be comparable to that observed during the proliferative phase of the menstrual cycle *(77,78)*. Interestingly, occupied nuclear ER were elevated compared to normal secretory phase myometrium, despite the very high levels of serum P at this time. Changes in steroid hormone levels during parturition in several species *(see above)* often correlate with the expected regulation of ER and PR by these hormones. However, in the human, serum P levels do not fall during parturition, and the initiation of labor occurs despite high serum and local uterine tissue P levels *(79,80)*. Indeed, PR binding in the myometrium was higher in the nuclear compartment than in the cytosolic fraction and was typical of a progestational tissue *(76,78)*. The changes in ER and PR binding during pregnancy in the human and their role, if any, in the initiation of labor remain unclear.

Similar to that observed for many species, ER and PR binding in nonhuman primates were considerably lower in the midsecretory phase compared to the follicular phase *(81–84)*. These binding data correspond with the decrease observed in the mRNAs for both ER and PR in baboon endometrium during the luteal phase (Hild-Petito and Fazleabas, unpublished observations). A study of the rhesus monkey during early gestation (d 2–6), prior to implantation, showed changes in endometrial ER and PR binding compared to nonfertile endometria *(85)*. This study showed that cytosolic and nuclear ER and nuclear PR binding increased during d 3–6 in subsequently fertile endometria. Other studies have also shown an increase in endometrial nuclear ER binding during the peri-implantation period (cycle d 24, midsecretory phase) and during rescue of the corpus luteum during normal pregnancy *(86)*. Cytosolic PR binding remained similar to that observed in nonfertile endometria during this period of early gestation. The above changes in nuclear ER and PR binding lend further support to the concept that blastocyst-derived factors may affect biochemical parameters in the endometrium prior to potential implantation and represent an early sign of maternal recognition of pregnancy. Following implantation in the baboon (d 18–32 postovulation), the mRNAs for both ER and PR were reduced more than that observed during the luteal phase of nonpregnant baboons (Hild-Petito and Fazleabas, unpublished observations). Taken together, these data suggest that there are changes in ER and PR occurring during the implantation period.

In the pregnant rhesus monkey, there was little difference in uterine nuclear and cytosolic ER binding during late pregnancy vs parturition *(87)*. The absence of any difference was observed for both decidual and myometrial tissues. As in women, serum P levels are elevated prior to and during parturition in the rhesus monkey, and the "withdrawal" of P that leads to increased myometrial contractility must occur by a mechanism(s) that remains to be defined. These data suggest that similar to the human, striking changes (increases) in ER binding associated with initiation of parturition in other species do not appear to play a role in the initiation of parturition in the rhesus monkey.

CELL TYPE-SPECIFIC EXPRESSION AND REGULATION DURING PREGNANCY

The pregnant uterus in mammalian species is distinctly different from the nonpregnant uterus. Specific uterine cell types undergo differentiation, regression, or demonstrate increased growth and development. The morphological changes that occur in the uterus during pregnancy have been described elsewhere in this volume. Briefly, the endometrium of the nonpregnant uterus consists of luminal and glandular epithelium, stromal cells, vascular cells of arteries, arterioles, capillaries, veins, and occasional infiltration of immune cells, such as leukocytes, eosinophiles, and macrophages. During early pregnancy, the stromal cells differentiate into decidual cells, which are considered to be a marker of pregnancy. Decidualization of the endometrium can also occur in some species under experimental conditions. The glandular epithelium undergoes varying degrees of regression depending on the species. For example, the glandular endometrium completely converts to a decidulized endometrium of pregnancy in primates. Throughout pregnancy the endometrial and myometrial vasculature undergoes increased growth and development. Likewise the smooth muscle cells of the myometrium demonstrate increased growth during pregnancy.

Since the actions of estrogen and progestin are essential to the development of the pregnant uterus, localization of ER and PR to specific uterine cell types has been investigated in various species. Immunocytochemistry, utilizing specific monoclonal or polyclonal antibodies against ER and PR, has demonstrated that these receptors are differentially regulated in specific uterine cell types of the nonpregnant uterus *(88–93)*. Recent *in situ* hybridization studies using labeled complementary DNA probes have shown that localization of the ER mRNA corresponds with the localization of ER receptor protein *(94)*. This section will concentrate on the localization and regulation of ER and PR in uterine cell types during pregnancy or during hormonal treatments that mimic pregnancy.

Rodent/Rabbit Models

The distribution of both ER and PR to specific uterine cell types has been determined during early pregnancy in the rat *(95–97)*. On d 10 of pregnancy (d 1 = d vaginal sperm detected), ER were localized in stromal cells of the decidua basalis, but not the junctional or labyrinth zones *(95)*. The chorioallantoic placenta also did not demonstrate staining for ER. The intensity of ER staining and the number of positive cells located in the decidua basalis decreased on d 13 and 14 of pregnancy. This corresponded to decreases in ER protein as detected by immunoblot analysis and binding assays *(95)*. The number of epithelial and stromal cells staining positive for PR and the intensity of the nuclear staining for PR increased during the first 4 d of pregnancy. There was a decrease in PR staining in both cell types after d 4 postcoitum. In contrast, the PR staining of myometrial smooth muscle cells remained constant throughout early pregnancy. The downregulation of both ER and PR by d 4 correlates with decreased nuclear and cytosolic binding of radiolabeled progestin *(42)*. In addition, the decrease in PR staining in epithelial and stromal cells occurred in the nonpregnant uterus of rats treated with E and P, which mimics the hormonal environment of early pregnancy *(96)*. These data support the hypothesis that the distribution of ER and PR in the uterus is primarily regulated by the steroid hormones.

Immunocytochemical studies in the pregnant guinea pig and rabbit have focused on the localization of ER and PR in the vasculature of the uterus *(98,99)*. ER were localized to the endothelial, smooth muscle, and adventitia layers of uterine arteries in pregnant guinea pigs. The number of ER-staining cells was higher in nonpregnant and term pregnant uteri as compared to midpregnancy *(98)*. In pregnant rabbit uterus, ER and PR were detected in smooth muscle cells of the tunica media of blood vessels and perivascular cells of the capillaries *(99)*. No ER or PR staining was detected in the endothelial cells of the rabbit vasculature.

Domestic Animal Models

The localization of ER in the endometrium of the pregnant ewe on d 14 and 21 was similar to staining observed at midcycle in the nonpregnant ewe *(100,101)*. ER were present in the deep glandular epithelium, but the luminal epithelium and superficial glands did not contain ER. Some stromal cells contained ER, and ER staining was present in the smooth muscle cells of the myometrium. In addition, cells adjacent to the caruncles were ER-positive, whereas cells further from the caruncles were not. This agrees with the binding data that demonstrated higher ER binding in caruncular vs intercaruncular tissues *(59)*. ER staining was also detected in some trophoblast cells on d 21 of pregnancy. The staining pattern for PR in the uterus of the pregnant ewe on d 14 and 21 was similar to the staining observed on d 14 of the estrous cycle *(101)*. PR was absent in the luminal epithelium, deep glands, and stroma. The smooth muscle cells of the myometrium stained positive for PR, but only light staining for PR was detected in some superficial glands.

In the pig, the localization of ER during d 5–12 of pregnancy (d 0 = estrus) was similar to that observed during the estrous cycle *(71)*. Intense ER staining was present in the surface and glandular epithelium and some underlying stromal cells, particularly on d 10–12 of pregnancy. However, there was a considerable reduction in ER staining in the glandular epithelium by d 15 of pregnancy, and ER were not detectable in the stromal cells. Immunocytochemical localization of PR during pregnancy in the pig demonstrated a pattern similar to that observed during the estrous cycle *(102)*. PR staining was absent from the luminal epithelium, but detectable in the glandular epithelium and stroma on d 10 of pregnancy. The intensity of staining was much lower than that observed during estrus. By d 15 of pregnancy, PR were only detectable in stromal cells. On d 18 of pregnancy, an increase in PR staining was observed in stromal cells closely associated with endometrial capillaries. The smooth muscle cells of the myometrium stained positive for PR, and the staining intensity for PR did not change throughout early pregnancy. These results support the hypothesis that P downregulates the expression of both ER and PR. However, the degree of downregulation for each receptor appears to differ between the specific cell types. Stromal cells appear to be more sensitive to P-induced downregulation of ER, whereas epithelial cells may be more sensitive to P downregulation of PR. In contrast, PR expression in smooth muscle cells appears to be independent of P regulation.

The distribution of ER and PR has also been examined in the uterus of the pregnant domestic house cat *(103)*. In this study, the downregulation of ER and PR was apparent by d 7 postcoitum. Luminal epithelium lost both ER and PR staining by d 5 postcoitum, whereas the glandular epithelium maintained ER staining from d 7 postcoitum through d 28 of pregnancy. Tissues were not examined after d 28 of pregnancy. Some of the stromal cells maintained staining for both ER and PR prior to implantation (d 12). Throughout trophoblast invasion and placental development in this species (d 14–28), most of the stromal cells contained PR, whereas staining for ER was similar to the preimplantation endometrium. Myometrial smooth muscle cells contained both ER and PR, and staining remained consistent throughout early pregnancy (d 28). The tissues were examined closely for differences in ER and PR staining between the implantation and nonimplantation sites, but no differences were detected. In addition, E and P treatment of ovariectomized nonpregnant cats resulted in staining similar to that observed during pregnancy. These data further support the hypothesis that estrogen and progestins regulate these receptors.

Human and Nonhuman Primates

In humans, the distribution of ER and PR staining in the uterus has been examined during early (wk 5–10 of gestation) pregnancy *(104–106)*. Both ER and PR were detected in the smooth muscle cells of the myometrium throughout early pregnancy *(105)*. In contrast, neither ER nor PR was detected in the developing placenta *(106)*. During early pregnancy, both ER and PR were detected in the stromal or decidual cells of the endometrium. However, the staining intensity for ER was weak in stromal cells. Increased staining for ER was observed in the decidual capsularis compared to the decidual parietalis *(105)*. In contrast, the glandular epithelium did not demonstrate staining for ER, and glandular staining for PR was considered negative in two studies *(104,105)* and variable in the other *(104)*. Both ER and PR were associated with arterioles *(104–106)*. Two studies localized PR in the smooth muscle cells and pericytes of spiral arteries *(104,106)*. The localization of PR in smooth muscle cells was confirmed by colocalization of PR with either desmin or smooth muscle actin *(106)*. One study *(104)* detected PR in endothelial cells based on colocalization of PR and Factor VIII, an endothelial cell-specific protein. However, the other study *(106)* did not detect either ER or PR in endothelial cells that stained positive for a specific endothelial cell antigen (BNH9). These discrepancies may be related to different binding affinities of the respective PR antibodies. Another possibility may be related to difficulty in distinguishing specific cell types based on only one marker. The study by Perrot-Applanat et al. *(106)* used two marker proteins for smooth muscle cells (desmin and α-smooth muscle actin) and one marker for endothelial cells (BNH9). The other study utilized one marker protein for endothelial cells (Factor VIII), but did not attempt to distinguish smooth muscle cells.

The distribution of ER and PR in the baboon uterus during early pregnancy has also been reported *(92)*. A diagrammatic representation of the localization of ER and PR in the baboon uterus is depicted in Fig. 2. The distribution of PR was similar to that reported for humans (present in stromal and decidual cells, absent in glandular and luminal epithelia, and associated with the vasculature). In contrast, ER was not detected in stromal or decidual cells of the baboon during early pregnancy (d 18–32 postovulation). ER were localized in the blood vessels, including spiral arteries of the pregnant baboon uterus. The location of the ER- and PR-positive cells indicated that there were no steroid hormone receptors in the endothelial cells. Instead, ER appeared to be localized in smooth muscle cells, and PR was associated with pericytes. The PR-positive cells may also have been smooth muscle cells, since the walls of spiral arteries in the endometrium of pregnancy are thicker *(106)*. However, the distribution of ER- and PR-positive cells within the wall of blood vessels was not determined by colocalization of cell-specific markers. The smooth muscle cells of the baboon myometrium contained both ER and PR throughout early pregnancy (d 18–32). However, the staining for ER was weak. A study performed with intact baboons treated with hormones to mimic early pregnancy (chorionic gonadotropin + E and P or E and P only) demonstrated a similar distribution of ER and PR in the endometrium *(107)*. These data support the hypothesis that steroid hormones primarily regulate ER and PR during pregnancy as opposed to a conceptus/trophoblastic factor(s).

In addition, the localization of ER and PR in primates was determined during late pregnancy in baboons or at term in rhesus monkeys and women *(87,92,106)*. Tissues obtained during late pregnancy in the baboon (d 150 of pregnancy) also demonstrated PR staining of the decidua, but no ER staining in the decidua *(92)*. In contrast, ER were detected in the decidua of pregnant and parturient rhesus monkeys *(87)*, and some faint staining for ER was detectable in the decidua of women undergoing cesarian sections near term (35–38 wk of gestation) *(106)*. This difference in ER staining of decidua may reflect species differences or may be related to the stage at which the tissues were obtained, late pregnancy vs term. During late pregnancy, the smooth muscle cells of the myometrium demonstrated strong staining for PR, but weak staining for ER in the baboon *(92)*. A similar staining pattern was observed in the myometrium from women near term *(106)*.

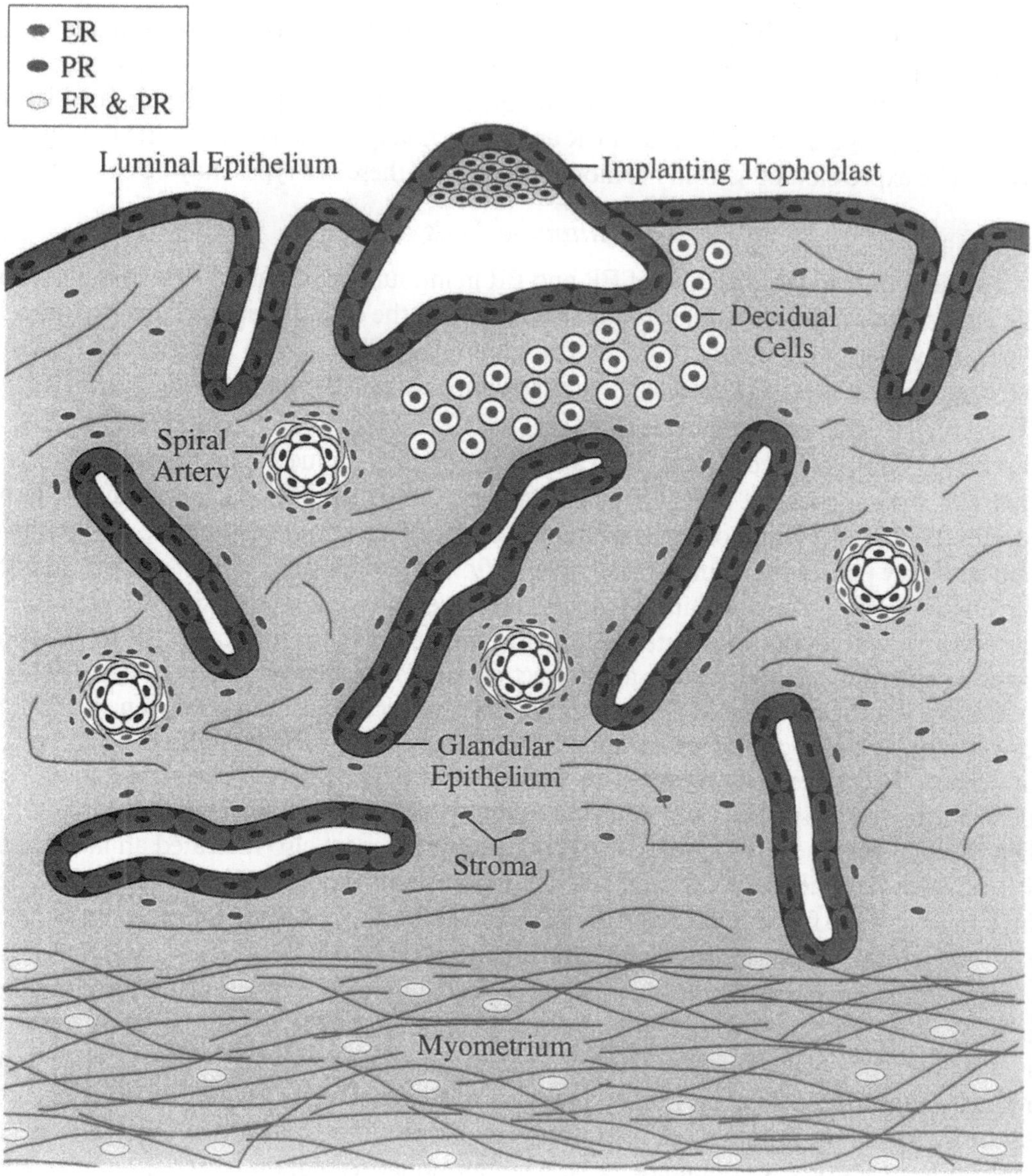

Fig. 2. Diagrammatic representation of the baboon uterus during early pregnancy demonstrating the distribution of ER and PR in the nuclei of specific cell types. The cell types are labeled with the exception of the various cell types within the spiral arteries. The inner layers represent ER-positive smooth muscle cells, whereas the pericytes surrounding the arteries contain PR. ER, Green; PR, Red; and cells containing both ER and PR, yellow.

However, the authors reported only a few smooth muscle cells (< 1%) staining faintly for ER in the myometrium. These differences may be species- or stage-related. In addition, placental tissues from either early or late pregnancy in the baboon or amnion and chorion from late pregnancy in the baboon or at term in the rhesus monkey did not stain positive for ER or PR *(87,92)*.

Overall, both ER and PR are downregulated during pregnancy in the uterus of all species. The decrease in both ER and PR occurs preferentially in the luminal and glandular epithelium. Stromal, decidual, and smooth muscle cells of the myometrium and blood vessels continue to express PR throughout pregnancy in most species. The results of studies in which nonpregnant animals have been treated with hormones to mimic pregnancy support the hypothesis that ER and PR are primarily regulated by estrogen and progestin. However, ER and PR persist in particular cell types despite the elevated levels of progestin, suggesting that ER and PR are differentially regulated in specific uterine cell types. The expression of steroid hormone receptors in these cell types may be constitutive.

Immune Cells

The detection and localization of ER and PR in immune cells, particularly cells invading the uterus, have not been studied to the same extent as the endometrial and myometrial cell types. However, the presence of ER or PR in immune cells has been investigated. Specific estrogen binding sites were detected in human lymphoid and thymic cells (K_d = 0.18–2.4 × 10^{-9} *M [108]*) and T-lymphocytes (K_d = 2.5 × 10^{-10} *M [109]*). Colocalization of CD8, a marker of cytotoxic T-cells, and CD4, a marker of helper/inducer lymphocytes, indicated that ER were associated with CD8-positive cells *(109)*. Monoclonal antibodies (MAb) localized ER in the lymphoid cells of human endometrial stroma during the proliferative and secretory phases of the menstrual cycle *(110)*. These data suggest that estrogen can act directly on immune cells within the uterus. However, a recent study using dual immunohistochemistry to detect ER in uterine mucosal leukocytes failed to localize ER to lymphocytes or macrophages, suggesting an indirect effect of estrogen on these cell types *(111)*.

Reports on the presence of PR in immune cells, particularly during pregnancy, are also conflicting. P binding to lymphocytes *(112)* and detection of PR by indirect immunofluorescence *(113)* have been reported in women who have recurrent pregnancy loss. The percentage of PR-staining lymphocytes during pregnancy was increased compared to lymphocytes obtained during the cycle *(114)*. Another report also indicated an increase in PR-positive peripheral blood lymphocytes in pregnant women *(115)*. However, other investigators have failed to detect PR in peripheral blood lymphocytes of pregnant women *(116)* or uterine lymphocytes obtained during the cycle *(110,111)*.

These data are currently inconclusive regarding the presence of ER and PR in immune cells. Overall, the data suggest that under certain conditions, ER and PR may be expressed in specific types of leukocytes. Further studies are required to determine whether hormonally dependent effects on immune cells are mediated directly via a receptor-dependent pathway within the immune cells or through an indirect mechanism that involves a signal from other ER- or PR-containing cells. The hormonal regulation of these putative ER- and/or PR-positive leukocytes and their relevance to a successful pregnancy also remain to be determined.

POTENTIAL ROLE OF OTHER UTERINE STEROID HORMONE RECEPTORS DURING PREGNANCY

Glucocorticoid Receptor

Glucocorticoid binding sites have been shown to be present in endometrium, myometrium, and decidua *(117)*. Glucocorticoids have been implicated in the initiation of labor in several species *(68)*, and the presence of these receptors in the uterus suggests that the uterus is a target tissue for glucocorticoids. A recent study has described the localization of GR and GR mRNA by immunohistochemical and *in situ* hybridization techniques, respectively, in the sheep uterus during pregnancy and parturition *(69)*. The data from this study suggest that glucocorticoids from the fetus may interact with myometrial GR to upregulate

ER and E action. These changes may serve as a mechanism for increases in myometrial contractility necessary for parturition. Although the above study suggests that glucocorticoids may act on the pregnant uterus through its cognate receptor, P can also interact with and bind to the GR. Interestingly, corticosteroid binding globulin (CBG) and its mRNA have been shown to be present in uterine tissue *(118)*. CBG possesses high affinity for glucocorticoids and P, and may serve as a local reservoir for these hormones. It is presently unknown whether the high levels of P during gestation are capable of mediating glucocorticoid action in the uterus. Future research may lead to a better understanding of the role and potential importance of GR and CBG in the pregnant uterus.

Androgen Receptor

Several studies have documented the presence of the androgen receptor in the rodent and human uterus *(119–121)*. The presence of the androgen receptor suggests that androgens may also play a role in the regulation of uterine function. In vitro studies have shown that androgens can inhibit endometrial cell proliferation *(122)*. In addition, androgens were shown to decrease ER binding in human breast cancer cells *(123)*. Both ligand binding assays and immunohistochemical techniques have shown the presence of the androgen receptor in the decidua of early pregnancy in the human *(119)*. Although androgen receptors have been localized in decidual cells of early pregnancy in the human, their potential role in modulating and/or regulating function in the nonpregnant or pregnant uterus has yet to be elucidated.

Orphan Receptors

Orphan receptors are a group of potential ligand-dependent transcription factors that possess nucleotide sequence homology to the superfamily of nuclear steroid hormone receptors *(124)*. DNA sequence homology has shown that this growing family of receptors possesses zinc-finger DBDs similar to those of other steroid hormone receptors. Although their presence in mammalian uterine tissue has yet to be determined, they may potentially serve some role in the nonpregnant and pregnant uterus. Despite the fact that these receptors are in search of a ligand, there are many possible candidates, such as metabolites of E, P, glucocorticoids, or androgens. Indeed, during pregnancy, there are very high concentrations of the P metabolite 5-dihydroxyprogesterone (5-DHP) *(125)*. These data suggest that this metabolite and other steroid hormone metabolites may play a role in uterine function and response. Only future research will determine the ligands for this class of receptors and their potential roles in the pregnant and nonpregnant uterus.

SUMMARY

It is clear from results presented in this chapter that the regulation of uterine steroid hormone receptors during pregnancy, specifically ER and PR, does not necessary follow a similar pattern in all species. Species differences in the circulating concentrations of E and P during pregnancy most likely are the basis for many of these differences. Overall, the well-documented heterologus and homologous regulation of ER and PR by their respective ligands appears to dominate. That is, E increases its receptor level and promotes nuclear localization, whereas P decreases cellular levels of its receptor and promotes nuclear localization. P also decreases the level of cellular ER and as a result, redirects the response of the uterus to a progestational tissue. The above effects of these hormones are expected to result in the tissue and cell type-specific action characteristic of each hormone. Although the actions of these hormones on their own receptors and each other's receptors are generally consistent, there are notable species, tissue, and cell type-specific differences *(see above)*. In addition, the regulation of these receptors, which is expected in most cases to be an indication of tissue response, can also be regulated by newly identified extrauterine factors e.g., signals emanating from the conceptus. A resolution of these differences in cell type- and tissue-specific regulation will require continued research efforts with modern cellular and molecular biological methods.

The evolving model of steroid hormone action has clearly provided, and will continue to provide, multiple avenues for investigation of the mechanisms that regulate uterine response during pregnancy. It is clear that steroid hormone action, which is essential for pregnancy, involves a cascade of signals that stem from the initial interaction of the hormone with its cognate receptor. Although ER and PR are the primary receptors that mediate uterine response, other steroid hormone receptors, such as those for glucocorticoids, androgens, orphan ligands, as well as other members of the nuclear receptor superfamily, may play a role in the regulation of uterine responses during pregnancy. A wide variety of steroid hormone-regulated transcription factors, cofactors necessary for transscriptional activation, autocrine/paracrine factors, as well as yet undiscovered cellular entities will undoubtedly provide fertile areas of research in the future. The important phenomenon of tissue-specific gene expression has been appreciated in the past and is widely appreciated now. With the advent of cellular probes for identification of specific antigens and their corresponding mRNAs has come, however, a deeper appreciation of the importance of steroid hormone regulation of spatial (cell type-specific) and temporal responses. The future holds much promise with regard to our understanding of the regulation of steroid hormone receptors and the vast array of regulatory molecules triggered by these ligand-dependent transcription factors that are essential for a successful pregnancy.

NOTE ADDED IN PROOF

The recent discovery of a second estrogen receptor (ERβ) and its presence in the rat uterus may have important implications on the regulation of the pleiotropic effects of estrogens (Kuiper GGJM, Carlsson B, Grandien K, Enmark E, Haggblad J, Nilsson S, Gustafsson J-A (1977) Comparison of the ligand binding specificity and transcript tissue distribution of estrogen receptors α and β. Endocrinology 138:863–870). Future studies will certainly determine its role and importance in the peri-implantation and pregnant uterus.

ACKNOWLEDGMENTS

This publication was supported in part by grants from the NIH (HD-31620, William C. Okulicz and HD-29457, Beverly S. Chilton). Its contents are solely the responsibility of the authors and do not necessarily represent the official views of the NIH.

REFERENCES

1. Mangelsdorf DJ, Thummel C, Beato M, Herrlich P, Schütz G, Umesono K, Blumberg B, Kastner P, Mark M, Chambon P, Evans RM (1995) The nuclear receptor superfamily: The second decade. Cell 83:835–839.
2. Gronemeyer H (1991) Transcriptional activation by estrogen and progesterone receptors. Ann Rev Genetics 25:89–123.
3. Parker MG (1993) Structure and function of the oestrogen receptor. J Neuroendocrinol 5:223–228.
4. Freedman LP (1992) Anatomy of the steroid receptor zinc finger region. Endocr Rev 13:129–145.
5. Klug A, Schwabe JWR (1995) Zinc fingers. FASEB J 9:597–604.

6. Freedman LP, Luisi BF (1993) On the mechanism of DNA binding by nuclear hormone receptors: A structural and functional perspective. J Cell Biochem 51:140–150.
7. Carson-Jurica MA, Schrader WT, O'Malley BW (1990) Steroid receptor family: Structure and functions. Endocr Rev 11:201–220.
8. Giguere V (1994) Retinoic acid receptors and cellular retinoid binding proteins: complex interplay in retinoid signaling. Endocr Rev 15:61–79.
9. Kastner P, Mark M, Chambon P (1995) Nonsteroid nuclear receptors: What are genetic studies telling us about their role in real life? Cell 83:859–869.
10. Mangelsdorf DJ, Evans RM (1995) The RXR heterodimers and orphan receptors. Cell 83:841–850.
11. Thummel CS (1995) From embryogenesis to metamorphosis: the regulation and function of drosophila nuclear receptor superfamily members. Cell 83:871–877.
12. Beato M, Herrlich P, Schutz G (1995) Steroid hormone receptors: many actors in search of a plot. Cell 83:851–857.
13. Pratt WB, Welsh MJ (1994) Chaperone functions of the heat shock proteins associated with steroid receptors. Sem Cell Biol 5:83–93.
14. Koshiyama M, Konishi I, Nanbu K, Nanbu Y, Mandai M, Komatsu T, Yamamoto S, Mori T, Fujii S (1995) Immunohistochemical localization of heat shock proteins HSP70 and HSP90 in the human endometrium: Correlation with sex steroid receptors and Ki-67 antigen expression. J Clin Endocrinol Metab 80:1106–1112.
15. Gronemeyer H (1991) Transcription activation by estrogen and progesterone receptors. Annu Rev Genet 25:89–123.
16. Knight DC, Eden JA (1995) Phytoestrogens—a short review. Maturitas 22:167–175.
17. Truss M, Beato M (1993) Steroid hormone receptors: interaction with deoxyribonucleic acid and transcription factors. Endocr Rev 14:459–479.
18. Katzenellenbogen JA, O'Malley BW, Katzenellenbogan BS (1996) Tripartite steroid hormone receptor pharmacology: interaction with multiple effector sites as a basis for the cell- and promoter-specific action of these hormones. Mol Endocrinol 10:119–131.
19. Osbourne CK, Elledge RM, Fuqua SAW (1996) Estrogen receptors in breast cancer therapy. Sci Am Sci Med 3:32–41.
20. Daniel JC Jr, Jetton AE, Chilton BS (1984) Prolactin as a factor in the uterine response to progesterone in rabbits. J Reprod Fertil 72:443–452.
21. Chilton BS, Mani SK, Bullock DW (1988) A servomechanism of prolactin and progesterone in regulating uterine gene expression. Mol Endocrinol 2:1169–1175.
22. Vegeto E, Shahbaz MM, Wen DX, Goldman ME, O'Malley BW, McDonnell DP (1993) Human progesterone receptor A form is a cell- and promoter-specific repressor of human progesterone receptor B function. Mol Endocrinol 7:1244–1255.
23. Tung L, Kamel Mohamed M, Hoeffler JP, Takimoto GS, Horwitz KB (1993) Antagonist-occupied human progesterone B-receptors activate transcription without binding to progesterone response elements and are dominantly inhibited by A-receptors. Mol Endocrinol 7:1256–1265.
24. Orti E, Bodwell JE, Munck A (1992) Phosphorylation of steroid hormone receptors. Endocr Rev 13:105–128.
25. Miele L, Cordella-Miele E, Mukherjee AB (1987) Uteroglobin: structure, molecular biology, and new perspectives on its function as a phospholipase A2 inhibitor. Endocr Rev 8:474–490.
26. Kundu GC, Mantile G, Miele L, Cordella-Miele E, Mukherjee AB (1996) Recombinant human uteroglobin suppresses cellular invasiveness via a novel class of high affinity cell surface binding site. Proc Natl Acad Sci USA 93:2915–2929.
27. Welsh AO (1993) Uterine cell death during implantation and early placentation. Microsc Res Tech 25:223–245.
28. Wyllie AH (1995) The genetic regulation of apoptosis. Curr Opinion Genet Dev 5:97–104.
29. Akcali KC, Khan SA, Moulton BC (1996) Effect of decidualization on the expression of regulators of apoptosis, BAX and BCL-2, in the rat endometrium. Endocrinology 137:3123–3130.
30. Yoshinaga SK, Petersen CL, Herskowitz I, Yamamoto KR (1992) Roles of SWI1, SWI2, and SWI3 proteins for transcriptional enhancement by steroid receptors. Science 258:1598–1604.
31. Winston F, Carlson M (1992) Yeast SNF/SWI transcriptional activators and the SPT/SIN chromatin connection. Trends Genet 8:387–391.
32. Carlson M, Laurent BC (1994) The SNF/SWI family of global transcriptional activators. Curr Opinion Cell Biol 6:396–402.
33. Muchardt C, Yaniv M (1993) A human homologue of Saccharomyses cerevisiae SNF2/SWI2 and drosophila brm genes potentiates transcriptional activation by the glucocorticoid receptor. EMBO J 12:4279–4290.

34. Hayward-Lester A, Hewetson A, Beale EG, Oefner PJ, Doris PA, Chilton BS (1996) Cloning, characterization and steroid-dependent posttrranscriptional processing of RUSH-1α and β, two uteroglobin promoter-binding proteins. Mol Endocrinol 10:1335–1349.
35. Lubahn DB, Mgyer JS, Golding TS, Couse JF, Korach KS, Smithies O (1993) Alteration of reproductive function but not prenatal sexual development after insertional disruption of the mouse estrogen receptor gene. Proc Natl Acad Sci USA 90:11,162–11,166.
36. Lydon JP, DeMayo FJ, Funk CR, Mani SK, Hughes AR, Montgomery CA, Jr., Shyamala G, Conneely OM, O'Malley BW (1995) Mice lacking progesterone receptor exhibit pleiotropic reproductive abnormalities. Genes Dev 9:2266–2278.
37. Shelesnyak MC (1986) A history of research on nidation. Ann NY Acad Sci 476:5–24.
38. Yoshinaga K, Hawkins RA, Stocker JF (1969) Estrogen secretion by the rat ovary in vivo during the estrous cycle and pregnancy. Endocrinology 85:103–112.
39. Glasser SR, Clark JH (1975) A determinant role for progesterone in the development of uterine sensitivity to decidualization and ovo-implantation. Symp Soc Dev Biol 33:311–345.
40. Vu Hai MT, Warembourg M, Milgrom E (1977) Hormonal control of progesterone receptors. Ann NY Acad Sci 286:199–209.
41. Chikusu PMA, McConnell N, Green B (1982) Progesterone nuclear receptors in the rat uterine myometrium during pregnancy. J Steroid Biochem 16:489–492.
42. Logeat F, Sartor P, VuHai MT, Milgrom E (1980) Local effect of the blastocyst on estrogen and progesterone receptors in the rat endometrium. Science 207:1083–1085.
43. Martel D, Psychoyos A (1981) Estrogen receptors in the nidatory sites of the rat endometrium [Abstract]. Science 211:1454–1455.
44. Bazer FW, Vallet JL, Roberts RM, Sharp DC, Thatcher WW (1986) Role of conceptus secretory products in establishment of pregnancy. J Reprod Fertil 43:39–47.
45. Sakamoto H, MacLusky N, Naftolin F (1986) Steroid receptors in the pregnant uterus, In: The Physiology and Biochemistry of the Uterus in Pregnancy and Labor (Huszar G, ed.), CRC, Boca Raton, FL, pp. 35–51.
46. Yu WCY, Leung BS (1982) Variations of cytoplasmic content of estrogen and progesterone receptors in the mammary gland and uterus of rats at time of parturition. Biol Reprod 27:658–664.
47. McCormack SA, Glasser SR (1978) Ontogeny and regulation of a rat placental estrogen receptor. Endocrinology 102:273–280.
48. Ogle TF, Mills TM, Soares MJ (1989) Changes in cytosolic and nuclear progesterone receptors during pregnancy in rat placenta. Biol Reprod 40:1012–1019.
49. Ogle TF, Soares MJ, Zhou Y, Chorich L, Mahesh VB (1993) Regulation of the estrogen receptor and estrogen receptor messenger ribonucleic acid in rat decidua basalis and placenta during pregnancy. J Steroid Biochem 12:1–12.
50. Ogle TF, Mills TM, Soares MJ (1986) Evidence for nuclear processing of progesterone receptors in rat placenta. J Steroid Biochem 25:183–190.
51. Ogle TF, Mills TM, Costoff A (1990) Progesterone maintenance of the placental progesterone receptor and placental growth in ovariectomized rats. Biol Reprod 43:276–284.
52. Leavitt WW, MacDonald RG, Okulicz WC (1983) Hormonal regulation of estrogen and progesterone receptor systems, In: Biochemical Actions of Hormones (Litwack G, ed.), Academic, New York, pp. 324–356.
53. Leavitt WW, Okulicz WC (1985) Occupied and unoccupied estrogen receptor during estrous cycle and pregnancy. Am J Physiol 249:E589–594.
54. Leavitt WW (1985) Hormonal regulation of myometrial estrogen, progesterone, and oxytocin receptors in the pregnant and pseudopregnant hamster. Endocrinology 116:1079–1084.
55. Leavitt WW, Chen TJ, Evans RW (1979) Regulation and function of estrogen and progesterone receptor systems, In: Steroid Hormone Receptor Systems (Leavitt WW and Clark JH, eds.), Plenum, New York, pp. 197–222.
56. Philibert D, Raynaud JP (1977) Cytoplasmic progestin receptors in mouse uterus, In: Progesterone Receptors in Normal and Neoplastic Tissue (McQuire WL, Raynaud JP, Baulieu EE, eds.), Raven, New York, pp. 227–243.
57. Milgrom E, Perrot M, Atger M, Baulieu EE (1972) Progesterone in uterus and plasma. V. An assay of the progesterone cytosol receptor of the guinea pig uterus. Endocrinology 90:1064–1070.
58. Gutierrez-Sagal R, Perez-Palacios G, Langley E, Pasapera AM (1993) Endometrial expression of progesterone receptor and uteroglobin genes during early pregnancy in the rabbit. Mol Reprod Dev 34:244–249.

59. Findlay JK, Clarke IJ, Swaney J, Colvin N, Doughton B (1982) Oestrogen receptors and protein synthesis in caruncular and intercaruncular endometrium of sheep before implantation. J Reprod Fertil 64:329–339.
60. Ott TL, Zhou Y, Mirando MA, Stevens C, Harney JP, Ogle TF, Bazer FW (1993) Changes in progesterone and oestrogen receptor mRNA and protein during maternal recognition of pregnancy and luteolysis in ewes. J Mol Endocrinol 10:171–183.
61. Spencer TE, Bazer FW (1995) Temporal and spatial alterations in uterine estrogen receptor and progesterone receptor gene expression during the estrous cycle and early pregnancy in the ewe. Biol Reprod 53:1527–1543.
62. Bazer FW, Ott TL, Spencer TE (1994) Pregnancy recognition in ruminants, pigs and horses: Signals from the trophoblast. Theriogenology 41:79–94.
63. Bazer FW, Thatcher WW, Haansen DJ, Mirando MA, Ott TL, Plante C (1986) Physiological mechanism of pregancy recognition in ruminants. J Reprod Fertil 43:39–47.
64. Mirando MA, Harney JP, Zhou Y, Ogle TF, Ott TL, Moffatt RJ, Bazer FW (1993) Changes in progesterone and oestrogen receptor mRNA and protein and oxytocin receptors in endometrium of ewes after intrauterine injection of ovine trophoblast interferon. J Mol Endocrinol 10:185–192.
65. Spencer TE, Bazer FW (1996) Ovine interferon tau suppresses transcription of the estrogen receptor and oxytocin receptor genes in the ovine endometrium. Endocrinology 137:1144–1147.
66. Spencer TE, Becker WC, George P, Mirando MA, Ogle TF, Bazer FW (1995) Ovine interferron-tau regulates endometrial expression of receptor for estrogen and oxytocin, but not progesterone. Biol Reprod 53:732–745.
67. Miller BG, Tassell R, Stone GM (1983) Growth of the endometrium and cotyledons during pregancy in the ewe: rates of protein secretion and synthesis and nuclear and cytosol steroid hormone receptor levels. J Endocrinol 96:137–146.
68. Rexroad CE, Jr (1984) Steroid receptors in the myometrium during pregnancy in the ewe. J Anim Sci 58:1278–1284.
69. Thorburn GD, Challis JRG, Robinson JS (1977) Endocrine control of parturition, In: Biology of the Uterus (Wynn RM, ed.), Plenum, New York, pp. 653–732.
70. Wu WX, Derks JB, Nathanielsz PW (1996) Effects of glucocorticoids on estrogen receptor messenger ribonucleic acid in the pregnant ovine myometrium in vivo and in vitro. Biol Reprod 54:230–241.
71. Geisert RD, Brenner RM, Moffatt RJ, Harney JP, Yellin T, Bazer FW (1993) Changes in oestrogen receptor protein, mRNA expression and localization in the endometrium of cyclic and pregnant gilts. Reprod Fertil Dev 5:247–260.
72. Rexroad CE Jr, Guthrie HD (1984) Cytoplasmic and nuclear estrogen receptors and leucine incorporation in endometrium of cyclic and pregnant pigs to d 19 postestrus. J Anim Sci 59:1286–1294.
73. Thilander G, Eriksson H, Edqvist LE, Rodriguez-Martinez H (1990) Variations in oestradiol and progesterone receptor levels in the porcine myometrium and cervix during pregnancy and parturition. J Vet Med 37:329–338.
74. Limpaphayom K, Lee C, Jacobson HI, King TM (1971) Estrogen receptor in human endometrium during the menstrual cycle and early pregnancy. Am J Obstet Gynecol 111:1064–1068.
75. Levy C, Robel P, Gautray JP, De Brux J, Verma U, Descomps B (1980) Estradiol and progesterone receptors in human endometrium: normal and abnormal menstrual cycles and early pregnancy. Am J Obstet Gynecol 136:646–651.
76. Giannopoulos G, Goldberb P, Shea TB Tulchinsky D (1979) Cytoplasmic and nuclear progestin receptors in human myometrium during the menstrual cycle and in pregnancy at term. J Clin Endocr Metab 49:100–106.
77. Giannopoulos G, Goldberg P, Shea TB, Tulchinsky D (1980) Unoccupied and occupied estrogen receptors in myometrial cytosol and nuclei from nonpregnant and pregnant women. J Clin Endocrinol Metab 51:702–710.
78. Khan-Dawood FS, Dawood MY (1984) Estrogen and progesterone receptor and hormone levels in human myometrium and placenta in term pregnancy. Am J Obstet Gynecol 150:501–505.
79. Bedford CA, Challis JRG, Harrison FA (1972) The role of oestrogens and progesterone in the onset of parturition in various species. J Reprod Fertil 16:1–23.
80. Batra S, Bengtsson LP (1978) 17β-Estradiol and progesterone concentrations in myometrium of pregnancy and their relationship to concentrations in peripheral plasma. J Clin Endocrinol Metab 46:622–626.
81. West NB, Brenner RM (1983) Estrogen receptor levels in the oviduct and endometria of cynomolgus macaques during the menstrual cycle. Biol Reprod 29:1–303.

82. Kreitmann-Gimbal B, Goodman AL, Bayard F, Hodgen DG (1979) Characterization of estrogen and progesterone receptors in monkey endometrium: methodology and effects of estradiol and/or progesterone on endometrium of castrate monkeys. Steroids 34:749–770.
83. Okulicz WC, Savasta AM, Hoberg LM, Longcope C (1990) Biochemical and immunohistochemical analyses of estrogen and progesterone receptors in the rhesus monkey uterus during the proliferative and secretory phases of artificial menstrual cycles. Fertil Steril 53:913–920.
84. Okulicz WC, Balsamo M, Tast J (1993) Progesterone regulation of endometrial estrogen receptor and cell proliferation during the late proliferative and secretory phase in artificial menstrual cycles in the rhesus monkey. Biol Reprod 49:24–32.
85. Ghosh D, Sengupta J (1988) Patterns of estrogen and progesterone receptors in rhesus monkey endometrium during secretory phase of normal menstrual cycle and preimplantation stages of gestation. J Steroid Biochem 31:223–229.
86. Kreitmann-Gimbal B, Bayard F, Hodgen GD (1981) Changing ratios of nuclear estrone to estradiol binding in endometrium at implantation: regulation by chorionic gonadotropin and progesterone during rescue of the primate corpus luteum. J Clin Endocrinol Metab 52:133–137.
87. Haluska GJ, West NB, Novy MJ, Brenner RM (1990) Uterine estrogen receptors are increased by RU486 in late pregnant rhesus macaques but not after spontaneous labor. J Clin Endocrinol Metab 70:181–186.
88. Press MF, Nousek-Goebl N, King WJ, Herbst AL, Greene GL (1984) Immunohistochemical assessment of estrogen receptor distribution in the human endometrium throughout the menstrual cycle. Lab Invest 51:495–503.
89. Press MF, Greene GL (1988) Localization of progesterone receptor with monoclonal antibodies to the human progestin receptor. Endocrinology 122:1165–1175.
90. Okulicz WC, Padykula HA, Kaiserman-Abramof IR, Longcope C (1987) Immunohistochemical localization and biochemical analysis of estrogen and progesterone receptors in the rhesus monkey endometrium. J Cell Biol 105:9A.
91. Lessey BA, Killam AP, Metzger DA, Haney AF, Greene GL, McCarty KS Jr (1988) Immunohistochemical analysis of human uterine estrogen and progesterone receptors throughout the menstrual cycle. J Clin Endocrinol Metab 67:334–340.
92. Hild-Petito S, Verhage HG, Fazleabas AT (1992) Immunocytochemical localization of estrogen and progestin receptors in the baboon (*Papio anubis*) uterus during implantation and pregnancy. Endocrinology 130:2343–2353.
93. Brenner RM, Slayden OD (1994) Cyclic changes in primate oviduct and endometrium, In: The Physiology of Reproduction (Knobil E, Neill JD, eds.), Raven, New York, pp. 541–569.
94. Koji T, Brenner RM (1993) Localization of estrogen receptor messenger ribonucleic acid in rhesus monkey uterus by nonradioactive *in situ* hybridization with digoxigenin-labeled oligodeoxynucleotides. Endocrinology 132:382–392.
95. Ogle TF, George P (1995) Regulation of the estrogen receptor in the decidua basalis of the pregnant rat. Biol Reprod 53:65–77.
96. Ohta Y, Sato T, Iguchi T (1993) Immunocytochemical localization of progesterone receptor in the reproductive tract of adult female rats. Biol Reprod 48:205–213.
97. Rider V, Psychoyos A (1994) Inhibition of progesterone receptor function results in loss of basic fibroblast growth factor expression and stromal cell proliferation during uterine remodelling in the pregnant rat. J Endocrinol 140:239–249.
98. Leiberman JR, Van Vroonhoven CCJ, Beckmann I, Van der Kwast TH, Wallenburg HCS (1990) Uterine artery estrogen receptors in the nonpregnant and pregnant guinea pig. Am J Obstet Gynecol 163:1685–1688.
99. Perrot-Applanat M, Groyer-Picard MT, Garcia E, Lorenzo F, Milgrom E (1988) Immunocytochemical demonstration of estrogen and progesterone receptors in muscle cells of uterine arteries in rabbits and humans. Endocrinology 123:1511–1519.
100. Cherny RA, Salamonsen LA, Findlay JK (1991) Immunocytochemical localization of oestrogen receptors in the endometrium of the ewe. Reprod Fertil Dev 3:321–331.
101. Wathes DC, Hamon M (1993) Localization of oestradiol, progesterone and oxytocin receptors in the uterus during the oestrous cycle and early pregnancy of the ewe. J Endocr 138:479–492.
102. Geisert RD, Pratt TN, Bazer FW, Mayes JS, Watson GH (1994) Immunocytochemical localization and changes in endometrial progestin receptor protein during the porcine oestrous cycle and early pregnancy. Reprod Fertil Dev 6:749–760.
103. Li W, Boomsma RA, Verhage HG (1992) Immunocytochemical analysis of estrogen and progestin receptors in uteri of steroid-treated and pregnant cats. Biol Reprod 47:1073–1081.

104. Wang J-D, Fu Y, Shi WL, Zhu PD, Cheng J, Qiao GM, Wang YQ, Greene GL (1992) Immunohistochemical localization of progesterone receptor in human decidua of early pregnancy. Hum Reprod 7:123–127.
105. Wu W-X, Brooks J, Millar MR, Ledger WL, Glasier AF, McNeilly AS (1993) Immunolocalization of oestrogen and progesterone receptors in the human decidua in relation to prolactin production. Hum Reprod 8:1129–1135.
106. Perrot-Applanat M, Deng M, Fernandez H, Lelaidier C, Meduri G, Bouchard P (1994) Immunohistochemical localization of estradiol and progesterone receptors in human uterus throughout pregnancy: Expression in endometrial blood vessels. J Clin Endocrinol Metab 78:216–224.
107. Hild-Petito S, Donnelly KM, Miller JB, Verhage HG, Fazleabas AT (1995) A Baboon (*Papio anubis*) simulated-pregnant model: Cell specific expression of insulin-like growth factor binding protein-1 (IGFBP-1), type I IGF receptor (IGF-1 R) and retinol binding protein (RBP) in the uterus. Endocrine 3:639–651.
108. Danel D, Souweine G, Monier JC, Saez S (1983) Specific estrogen binding sites in human lymphoid cells and thymic cells. J Steroid Biochem 18:559–563.
109. Stimson WH (1988) Oestrogen and human T lymphocytes: presence of specific receptors in the T-suppressor/cytotoxic subset. Scand J Immunol 28:345–350.
110. Tabibzadehk SS, Satyaswaroop PG (1989) Sex steroid receptors in lymphoid cells of the human endometrium. Am J Clin Pathol 91:656–663.
111. King A, Gardner L, Loke YW (1996) Evaluation of oestrogen and progesterone receptor expression in uterine mucosal lymphocytes. Hum Reprod 11:1079–1082.
112. Szekeres-Bartho J, Csernus V, Hadnagy J, Pacsa AS (1983) Immunosuppressive effect of serum progesterone during pregnancy depends on the progesterone binding capacity of the lymphocytes. J Reprod Immunol 5:81–88.
113. Chiu L, Nishimura M, Ishii Y, Nieda M, Maeshima M, Takedani Y, Shibata Y, Tadokora K, Juji T (1996) Enhancement of the expression of progesterone receptor on progesterone-treated lymphocytes after immunotherapy in unexplained recurrent spontaneous abortion. Am J Reprod Immunol 35:552–557.
114. Szekeres-Bartho J, Szekeres G, Debre P, Autran B, Chaouat G, (1990) Reactivity of lymphocytes to a progesterone receptor-specific monoclonal antibody. Cell Immunol 125:273–283.
115. Szekeres-Bartho J, Reznikoff-Etievant MF, Varga P, Pichon MF, Varga Z, Chaouat G (1989) Lymphocytic progesterone receptors in normal and pathological human pregnancy. J Reprod Immunol 16:239–247.
116. Mansour I, Reznikoff-Etievant MF, Netter A (1994) No evidence for the expression of progesterone receptor on peripheral blood lymphocytes during pregnancy. Hum Reprod 9:1546–1549.
117. Giannopoulos G, Jackson K, Tulchinsky D (1982) Specific glucocorticoid binding in human uterine tissues. J Steroid Biochem 17:371–375.
118. Misao R, Hori M, Ichigo S, Fujimoto J, Tamaya T (1994) Corticosteroid-binding globulin mRNA levels in human uterine endometrium. Steroids 59:603–607.
119. Horie K, Takakura K, Imai K, Liao S, Mori T (1992) Immunohistochemical localization of androgen receptor in the human endometrium, decidua, placenta and pathological conditions of the endometrium. Hum Reprod 7:1461–1466.
120. Muechler EK (1987) The androgen receptor of the human endometrium. Endocr Res 13:69–84.
121. Sar M, Lubahn DB, French FS, Wilson ME (1990) Immunohistochemical localization of the androgen receptor in rat and human tissues. Endocrinology 127:3180–3186.
122. Rose GL, White JO, Dowsett M, Jeffcoate SL, Mudge JE (1988) The inhibitory effects of danazol, danazol metabolites, gestrinone, and testosterone on the growth of human endometrial cells in vitro. Fertil Steril 49:224–228.
123. Poulin R, Simard J, Labrie C, Petitclerc L, Dumont M, Lagac L, Labrie F (1990) Down-regulation of estrogen receptors by androgens in the ZR-75-1 human breast cancer cell line. Endocrinology 127:392–399.
124. O'Malley BW, Conneely OM (1992) Orphan receptors: In search of a unifying hypothesis for activation. Mol Endocrinol 6:1359–1361.
125. Eley RM, Thatcher WW, Bazer FW, Fields MJ (1983) Steroid metabolism by the bovine uterine endometrium and conceptus. Biol Reprod 28:804–816.

8 Endocrine Control of Trophoblast–Uterine Epithelial Cell Interactions

Robert C. Burghardt, PHD, *Jeffery A. Bowen,* PHD,
and Fuller W. Bazer, PHD

CONTENTS

INTRODUCTION

Implantation in mammals refers to a series of highly orchestrated interactions that begin with an intimate association of the conceptus and uterine endometrium and end with the formation of a placenta as a means to support embryonic/fetal development to the end of pregnancy. Before any cell–cell contacts are established, the embryo and uterine histotrophe exert a mutual influence to support further development of the conceptus and its secretion of the signal that sustains the function of the corpus luteum during the early stages of pregnancy, a process referred to as "maternal recognition of pregnancy" *(see 1–3)*. Implantation is then initiated with an uncommon union between apical plasma membranes of the genetically distinct endometrial epithelium and embryonic trophectoderm subsequent to hatching from the zona pellucida *(see 4)*. In some species, the blastocyst is gradually implanted in the endometrial stroma following trophoblast penetration of uterine epithelium (invasive hemochorial and endotheliochorial implantation), but in others, stromal invasion does not occur, and the intimate association between uterine epithelium and conceptus tissues is retained (noninvasive epitheliochorial implantation). In the latter situation, which is seen, for example, in the pig, horse, and all ruminants, the trophoblast and its supporting layer of extraembryonic mesoderm is simply apposed to the uterine epithelium. There is no displacement or invasion of the maternal tissues, and the conceptus remains within the uterine lumen throughout gestation *(5)*. However, species, such as rodents and primates, in which implantation is invasive, penetration of the uterine epithelium triggers a series of stromal responses collectively identified as decidualization. During decidualization, the endometrium is transformed into a specialized tissue by hyperplasia and hypertrophy of stromal cells, secretion of prolactin and the extracellular matrix (ECM) proteins laminin and fibronectin, the invasion by large numbers of immune system cells, and the formation of extensive cell–cell contacts *(6)*. This specialized tissue is believed to provide an important element of control of trophoblast invasion during implantation *(7)* in addition to a number of other endocrine and paracrine functions.

The development of techniques for assisted reproduction in infertile couples has highlighted our ignorance of the details of implantation, a process that is regarded as the most relevant limiting factor for successful pregnancy (cf *8)*. Ethical considerations and the limited accessibility of the uterine lumen for extensive evaluation proscribe experimental manipulation of the events of implantation in humans. Comparative investigations employing animal models and in vitro culture systems have contributed greatly to our understanding of implantation, although the diversity of placentation strategies and the complexity of the maternal–fetal dialog highlight the differences and limitations of these model systems. The implantation process remains a frontier in reproductive endocrinology owing to our incomplete understanding of the cell biology, immunology, and endocrinology of implantation. At the present time, there is considerable interest in markers that identify or predict uterine receptivity to implantation as well as in the development of noninvasive approaches to detect these markers.

This chapter highlights some comparative aspects of structural and functional changes that take place in the uterine endometrial epithelium during the peri-implantation period and are under endocrine control. Included are studies that involve the search for markers of uterine receptivity in domestic farm animals, which may provide additional perspectives on the utility of these animal models and culture systems derived from endometrial tissues for this purpose. Comparative studies in mammals and the use of in vitro model systems have led to the common division of the process of implantation into phases of apposition, attachment or adhesion, and in those species where it occurs, invasion. The use of domestic farm animals to study apposition and attachment, that are necessary stages in all species, may be advantageous owing to the absence of invasiveness, which could obscure or erase the events of the previous phases. The role of the decidua during implantation is covered elsewhere in this volume.

UTERINE RECEPTIVITY

The uterine epithelium is remarkable in that it is the only tissue to which blastocysts cannot attach ubiquitously *(9)* without suitable hormonal priming. However, the conceptus will implant in the uterine wall independently of reproductive status or hormonal priming if the integrity of the epithelium is compromised *(10)*. Blastocysts, which are inherently invasive, can attach and invade a diverse array of artificial ectopic sites (including male tissue; *11)*, and biological matrices in vivo and in vitro without discrimination and without the need for prior ovarian hormonal conditioning *(12)*. Even the pig blastocyst, which does not invade the uterine endometrial epithelium during implantation, will invade and undergo syncytium formation when transplanted to an ectopic site *(13)*. Although the type of implantation differs among species, the barrier to implantation is a maternal property resident in the uterine epithelium until it is cyclically transformed to respond to embryonic signals and permit adhesive contact with conceptus epithelial tissues. This condition of the uterus is referred to as the receptive state.

The expression of nonreceptive (i.e., prereceptive and refractory) and receptive states to blastocyst implantation are a consequence of the exceptional structural and physiological plasticity of the uterus in its responses to ovarian cues with orderly cycles of tissue differentiation, glandular secretion, and regional turnover of terminally differentiated cells. Uterine receptivity is programmed to be synchronous with blastocyst development. Arrival of a blastocyst in the prereceptive uterus is therefore compatible with further embryonic development prior to interaction of blastocyst trophectoderm with uterine epithelial cells during the "window of receptivity," and results in the progressive phases of implantation. In the absence of pregnancy or failure of maternal recognition of pregnancy, this transient state is replaced by a refractory stage, which is incompatible with embryonic attachment and becomes hostile to further embryonic development *(3,14)*.

Although it is evident that estrogen and progesterone induce essential proliferative and differentiative changes in the endometrium that lead to a temporary state of uterine receptivity *(15)*, a number of other factors are required to establish the necessary dialog between the blastocyst and endometrium. For example, even though luteal function has been maintained, a large number of embryos in domestic farm animals are lost at the stage of pregnancy when embryonic and uterine epithelial cells are closely apposed and cellular attachment is achieved between trophoblastic and endometrial epithelium *(16,17)*. This emphasizes the importance of additional signals, which must be sent and received, because as implantation progresses, the maternal–conceptus interactions shift from long-range molecular dialogue employing secreted factors involved in maintenance of the corpus luteum to more intimate and local exchanges involved in nidation. This interaction is, at least in part, under the control of the growth factors and cytokines, that are the subject of other chapters in this volume.

Although the following discussion focuses primarily on the epithelial cell component of the endometrial compartment during the peri-implantation period, the potential contributions of other cells to the generation of the nonreceptive and receptive status of the epithelium must be mentioned. Despite the fact that the principal cells of the endometrium are separated by a basal lamina, the classic experiments of Cunha et al. *(18)* define the importance of epithelial–stomal cell interactions in the production of stage-specific responses of the epithelium to endocrine signals. In a number of species, when the uterus enters the receptive phase, circulating progesterone levels are high, and these conditions result in a marked decrease in immunologically detectable steroid receptors in the luminal epithelium *(19–22)*. Other cells, including stroma, myometrium, and/or vascular cells, are likely to mediate the action of steroid hormones (e.g., estromedins, progestomedins) on the surface epithelium. For example, keratinocyte growth factor (KGF, also known as FGF-7) has been shown to be a stromally derived, progesterone-induced growth factor that may function as a progestomedin on uterine epithelial cell proliferation in primates *(23)*. The selective expression of KGF in stroma and the KGF receptor in uterine epithelial cells *(24)* support the paracrine function of this growth factor in uterine epithelial cells. Similarly, insulin-like growth factor-I (IGF-I) *(25,26)* and epidermal growth factor (EGF) *(26)* have been implicated as mediators of estrogen action in the uterus. Additional interactions may also be mediated by cell–cell contacts that will be described in more detail.

STRUCTURAL MARKERS OF UTERINE RECEPTIVITY

The restricted adhesive properties of a blastocyst to a uterine epithelium that is appropriately prepared by ovarian steroid hormones suggest that under certain conditions, the apical surface of uterine epithelial cells express molecules that do not permit (or prevent) blastocyst attachment. Experimental evidence is accumulating that the uterine epithelium responds to a variety of regulatory agents (growth factors, cytokines) in addition to the action of nidatory estrogen on the progesterone-dominated uterus that modulates structural and functional properties of the uterine epithelium during the transformation from the nonreceptive to receptive state. Insight into the specialized characteristics of uterine epithelial and stromal cells and their interactions has also provided improvements in culture systems, which permit the discrimination of functions that are under direct hormonal control from those that are controlled through hormonal effects on other uterine cell types or more distant tissues. Procedures for culturing uterine epithelium in a polarized fashion *(27)* have stimulated renewed analysis of epithelial receptivity in vitro. Because polarized epithelial cells regain their nonreceptive state in vitro and mimic attributes of these cells in vivo *(28–30)*, the utility of these model systems to support the search for, and analysis of potential markers of uterine receptivity is increasing.

Structural Modification of Uterine Epithelium at the Apical Plasma Membrane

As noted previously, the initial interaction between trophoblastic cells and the receptive uterine epithelium constitutes an unusual apical–apical contact between genetically distinct simple epithelia. In order for this contact to be established, dramatic changes in uterine luminal epithelial cell morphology and molecular organization of apical and basolateral plasma membrane domains take place regardless of the mode of placentation (Fig. 1). Details of the transformation involving reduction of epithelial cell polarity and cytoskeletal alterations, changing patterns of adhesion molecule expression, activation of various classes of enzymes, and changing profiles of protein and glycoprotein secretion are the subject of a number of recent reviews *(4,9,31,32)*. As a consequence of this epithelial cell reorganization, the apical uterine epithelial cell plasma membrane is capable of forming stable attachment with the blastocyst. Considerable effort is being devoted to the identification of adhesion molecules involved in this attachment and the mechanisms by which the expression of adhesive properties of heterologous apical plasma membranes are integrated.

Prior to the receptive phase in the rat and human uterus, the surface epithelium is characterized by a dense distribution of long, thin microvilli with a uniformly thick glycocalyx. In response to the action of nidatory estrogen on the progesterone-dominated uterus, there is a thinning of the glycocalyx as the microvilli become shorter and develop blunt projections referred to as pinopodes, that develop over a 1–2 d interval in humans *(33)*. The pinopodes appear to be a useful marker for the period of uterine receptivity during a precise interval of the secretory phase of the menstrual cycle, since these structures appear to be strictly controlled by progesterone and can be observed in artificially induced and stimulated cycles *(34,35)* as well as in postmenopausal uteri functionally restored by hormone replacement *(9)*. Although identified as a morphological marker of uterine receptivity more than 25 yr ago *(36)*, their function has not yet been defined.

Modifications in the actin cytoskeleton contribute to changes in the polarized properties of uterine epithelial cells at the time of uterine receptivity in rats. Loss of the terminal web at the subapical region of the cell is under maternal ovarian hormonal control and does not depend on the presence of the blastocyst. In rats, this is accompanied by the appearance of an extensive actin network in pinopodes *(37)*. An increase in the density of intramembrane protein particles in the apical plasma membrane during the period of uterine receptivity revealed by freeze-fracture techniques *(38–40)* could be a consequence of these cytoskeletal changes as could the observed changes in tight junctions (zonula

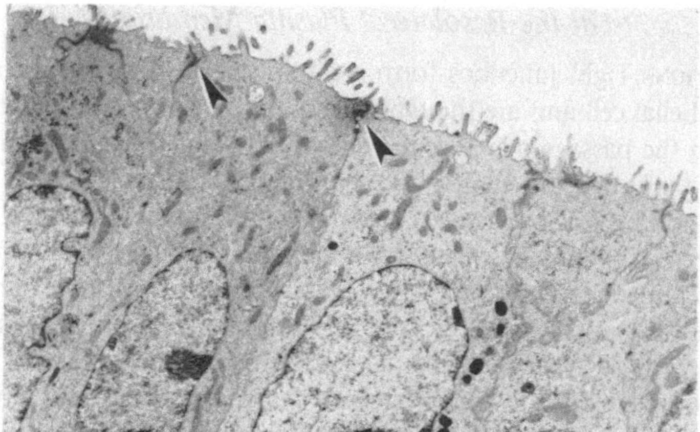

Fig. 1. Reorganization of the apical plasma membrane in porcine uterine epithelial cells during the conversion from the prereceptive period **(A)** to the receptive period **(B)**. **(A)** The prereceptive luminal uterine epithelium (d 1 of the estrous cycle) appears as a simple columnar epithelium. The flat apical surface exhibits numerous microvilli and the Pico-lateral location of the tight junctional complex is visible (arrowheads). **(B)** The apical surface of uterine epithelial cells in the receptive uterus (d 15 of pregnancy) in close contact with the trophectoderm (T) exhibit a dome-like appearance and loss of microvilli. The tight junctional complex (arrowheads) appears to be located in a more baso-lateral region of the epithelial cell (×4250).

occludens), which are located in the subapical plasma membrane. Freeze-fracture techniques have also led to the identification of unusual cell-surface contacts along projections of the apical plasma membrane of uterine epithelial cells in rats only at the time of blastocyst implantation or artificially induced hormonal states compatible with implantation *(41)*. These structures, that appear identical to gap junctions, are termed "reflexive" gap junctions to identify such junctions formed by the plasma membrane of the same cell *(42)*. Although gap junctions are normally restricted to the lateral plasma membrane, their expression in the apical plasma membrane may be linked to changes in the polarized functions of receptive uterine cells, including modifications occurring in the basolateral plasma membrane.

Structural Modification of Uterine Epithelium at the Basolateral Plasma Membrane

TIGHT JUNCTIONS. Tight junctions form a continuous belt around the apical region of the uterine epithelial cell and are thought to play a role as an intercellular barrier, selectively regulating the passage of molecules across the paracellular pathway to control the fluid content of the lumen and, thereby, the environment of the blastocyst. These structures also play an important role in passively separating molecules in the apical and basolateral plasma membrane domains to create and maintain cell polarity *(see 43)*. Considerable progress has been made recently in defining protein constituents of the tight junction. One transmembrane component, occludin *(44)*, and several peripheral proteins, such as ZO-1 *(45)*, ZO-2 *(46)*, 7H6 *(47)*, and cingulin *(48,49)*, have been characterized. In addition, the actin-based cytoskeleton located in the vicinity of tight junctions is involved in the maintenance of junctional tightness as indicated by the organization of junctional strands *(50)*.

Changes in both organization and numbers of junctional strands occur in uterine epithelial tight junctions in rodents as a function of steroid hormone treatment *(51)*, during pseudopregnancy *(40)*, and in early pregnancy *(38)*. Similar kinds of structural alterations occur in tight junctions of human tissues during the menstrual cycle *(39)*. Proliferation of the tight junctional belt requires both progesterone and estrogen in ovariectomized animals *(51)*, and is consistent with the increase in tight junctional complexity occurring in rodents during the preimplantation phase of pregnancy associated with uterine receptivity and during pseudopregnancy *(38,40)*. The proliferation of tight junctional strands and their extension toward the basal pole of the cell during progesterone dominance is interpreted to be indicative of a reduction of polar organization along the apico–basal axis *(4)*.

This general pattern of tight junction modulation does not appear to be unique to species in which blastocysts invade the uterine epithelial cell layer during implantation. A similar tight junction reorganization also accompanies an increase in circulating progesterone concentration in species exhibiting noninvasive implantation, such as the pig *(52)*. The consequence of amplification of tight junctions during reduction of apico–basal polarity, which correlates with alterations in the actin-based cytoskeleton *(9)*, is a decrease in epithelial cell paracellular permeability. This is thought to reflect an important change in the uterine milieu in preparation for pregnancy. In this context, the finding that uterine luminal epithelial cells acquire the ability to form reflexive gap junctions at the apical membrane during the receptive phase or in progesterone- and estrogen-primed rats *(38)* takes on significance. Although reflexive gap junctions in apical processes probably do not confer any unique function within the uterine luminal epithelial cell, they may reflect changes in the ability of tight junctions to separate apical and basolateral plasma membrane domains of epithelial cells.

GAP JUNCTIONS. Gap junction expression in the lateral plasma membranes of uterine endometrial epithelial cells, like their expression in other tissue-level compartments of the uterus, is extraordinary. Although gap junctions are constitutively expressed in most adult tissues, their expression in different tissue-level compartments of the uterus exhibits unique tissue-specific spatial and temporal patterns that correlate with the changing functional activities of uterine compartments. For example, the endocrine control of the brief expression of large numbers of gap junctions in uterine smooth muscle at the end of pregnancy and their role in the birth process are best understood *(53)*. However, prior to the discovery that reflexive gap junctions appear in apical epithelium of the artificially induced or naturally occurring receptive uterus, gap junction expression in uterine epithelium was thought to be modest. Advances in the biology of gap junctions and their complex regulation in uterine tissues have suggested that gap junctions exhibit a distinct spatial and temporal pattern of expression in uterine epithelium and stroma, and thus cell–cell communication mediated by these structures may constitute an important element of the regulatory mechanisms involved in the integration of implantation *(54–56)*.

Proteins comprising these structures are members of an evolutionarily conserved multigene family of channel-forming proteins called connexins (Cx), which assemble as hexameric hemichannels (connexons) in cell membranes to form an aqueous channel of about 1.5-nm diameter on alignment in adjacent cells *(see 57)*. Consequently, gap junctions are thought to facilitate diffusion of ions (electrical coupling) and small metabolites (metabolic coupling) between channel-bearing cells. The diffusible metabolites include regulatory and informational molecules, such as second messengers (Ca^{2+}, cAMP, cGMP, IP_3, cADP-ribose), which govern the activity of protein kinases *(58)* as well as molecules involved in cellular homeostasis. Analysis of cloned family members has revealed diversity in gap junction phenotypes, which may be functionally specialized owing to differences in unitary conductances and permeability properties. Further, properties of these channels may be differentially modulated by voltage gradients, intracellular pH, or changes in cyclic nucleotide concentration *(59)*. Certain connexins are phosphoproteins whose properties are modulated by protein kinases, and thus, gap junction channels may have specific functions in certain tissues *(60)*.

The 13 known members of the Cx multigene family in rodents (and presumably all mammals) share sequence homology and a predicted membrane topology *(see 61)*. Commonly used nomenclature identifies Cx with the predicted molecular mass in kDa of the protein deduced from the cDNA sequence. For example, the cDNA for Cx43 isolated from rat heart contained a single 1146-bp open reading frame coding for a predicted protein of 382 amino acids with a molecular mass of 43,036 Dalton, which corresponds to a 44–47 kDa peptide in SDS gels *(62)*. An alternative classification currently assigns known connexins into two classes, α and β, based on their primary sequence and evolutionary relationships *(61)*. Although there is divergence among the different connexin isoforms, there is significant sequence conservation across species for comparable connexin isoforms (e.g., in human and rat Cx32 differ by only 4 amino acid changes, but human and rat Cx43 differ by 9 of 382 amino acids) *(62)*.

The connexin family members identified in the uterine endometrium to date include Cx26, Cx32, Cx37, and Cx43; however, only Cx26, Cx32, and Cx43 appear to be expressed in a temporal and spatial pattern, which is under steroid hormone control *(54,56)*. Comparison of the membrane topology of Cx26, Cx32, and Cx43 indicates that a major difference between these three connexin species is the length of the C-terminal domain of 18 amino acids in Cx26, 76 amino acids in Cx32, and 156 in Cx43. The larger two connexins are phosphoproteins whose permeability may be modulated by the action of protein kinases, whereas Cx26 does not appear to be phosphorylated *(63)*.

The preimplantation uterine endometrium in the rabbit and rat is characterized by the suppression of cell–cell communication *(54,55,64)*, which appears to be regulated by an increase in maternal progesterone *(65)*, whereas epithelial gap junction expression in the rat can be strongly enhanced by estrogen treatment. However, the progesterone-induced suppression in both rats and rabbits appears to be abolished in response to the implanting blastocyst *(55,64)*, and dramatic gap junction expression is initiated locally in the vicinity of the blastocyst and spreads outward to the blastocystfree segments of the uterus. In response to the invading trophoblast in rodents, gap junction expression also increases dramatically in the developing decidua.

Interestingly, Cx26 and/or Cx32 appear to be the only connexin family members present in endometrial epithelial cells in animals exhibiting invasive implantation. In the rabbit, Cx32 is the predominant connexin expressed; induction of Cx32 expression requires physical contact with the blastocyst *(64)*. In the rat, Cx26 is the predominant connexin, although low-level expression of Cx32 has been reported *(56)*. Recent studies of human endometrial epithelial cells have indicated that gap junctions cannot be detected during the early proliferative phase of the cycle, whereas Cx26 expression increases in luminal and glandular epithelium from d 11–15 of the cycle, but disappears in the late secretory phase. Furthermore, weak Cx32 staining in the basal membrane region of glandular cells was detected in the late proliferative and early secretory phases, suggesting that these two connexins could represent markers for the proliferation and differentiation of human endometrium during the menstrual cycle *(66)*.

As noted above, steroid hormones have been implicated in the regulation of endometrial epithelial cell gap junction expression. Grümmer et al. *(65)* have shown that Cx26 mRNA levels in ovariectomized steroid-treated rats were enhanced by estradiol and suppressed by progesterone treatment. Administration of a progesterone antagonist during the first 3 d of pregnancy reversed the normal decline in Cx26 transcript levels that occurs during the preimplantation phase. These data are consistent with a positive estrogen and negative progesterone modulation of endometrial Cx26 expression. In a subsequent report by Risek et al. *(67)*, there was no detectable effect of estrogen on steady-state levels of Cx26 in uteri treated with estrogen and progesterone, suggesting a synergistic rather than antagonistic interaction of the two steroids. The synergistic action of these steroids on luminal epithelium was supported by immunohistochemical data.

Studies of endometrial gap junction expression in animal models characterized by non-invasive implantation have been limited; however, gap junctions appear to be absent in uterine luminal epithelial populations of domestic farm animals (horse, pig, sheep, goat). Immunocytochemical analysis using antibodies to Cx26, Cx32, and Cx43 have identified Cx43 expression colocalized with the tight junction-associated protein ZO-1 exclusively in the glandular epithelium, but not luminal epithelium of the horse, sheep, and goat *(68,69)*. The uterine glandular expression of Cx43 in the mare is restricted to a period beginning d 3 postovulation though d 14 of diestrus and until d 23 of pregnancy, whereas Cx43 is absent within uterine glands during anestrus, estrus, and after d 25 of pregnancy (Day and Burghardt, unpublished observations). Surprisingly, no evidence for Cx26, Cx32, and Cx43 in porcine luminal or glandular epithelium has been detected at any stage of the estrous cycle or pregnancy. Further, no evidence for gap junction expression or immunostaining for the three junctional proteins was detected at implantation sites (although trophectoderm staining of Cx43 was detected) *(70)*.

The significance of differences in gap junction expression during invasive and non-invasive implantation is not yet clear. It has been suggested that gap junction-mediated intercellular communication may play a role in regulating trophoblast invasion *(55)* and that metabolic coupling of endometrial gland cells may coordinate their secretory activity. The regional gap junctional response to an embryo in rodents might also be associated with the mechanism for message transmission through luminal epithelial cells to underlying tissues to initiate decidualization. The absence of a gap junctional response and decidualization in the endometrial stroma in domestic farm animal species may, therefore, be involved in limiting trophoblast invasiveness. The necessity of a highly integrated uterine luminal epithelial cell layer in these species may not be as great as in animals with small blastocysts and a relatively large luminal surface, such as rodents and humans.

FUNCTIONAL MODIFICATIONS OF UTERINE EPITHELIUM

The embryos of most species enter the uterine lumen at the four- to eight-cell stage surrounded by a nonadhesive glycoprotein coat, the zona pellucida *(71)*, which is typically shed in the uterus within 4–8 d postovulation. The interval between conceptus arrival and initial apposition/attachment (i.e., the prereceptive stage) is variable. For instance, in rodents and primates, the conceptus implants within 10 h following blastocyst hatching from the zona pellucida, whereas in domestic farm animals, there is an extended prereceptive stage where the apical surface of the uterine epithelium remains nonadhesive and the embryo is free within the uterus. The equine conceptus secretes a nonadhesive mucin-like glycoprotein "capsule," which allows the conceptus to remain free within the uterus for an additional 10 d following hatching *(72)*. During this prereceptive stage, the conceptus is dependent on the uterine secretory products (histotrophe) prior to the development of receptivity.

Of the molecular changes in the composition of the apical luminal uterine epithelium that accompany the reduction of glycocalyx and decreased surface charge with the development of receptivity, the changing patterns of cell-surface glycoconjugates have attracted considerable interest as important events that define the transition from prereceptive to receptive status. Patterns of glycoconjugate expression (including extrinsic and intrinsic plasma membrane proteins, glycoproteins and glycolipids, and ECM constituents) involve the upregulation of some glycoconjugates and the downregulation of others superimposed on the constitutive expression of still others. Molecules that have been evaluated relative to their potential contribution to the antiadhesive character of prereceptive uterine epithelium and the development of adhesive properties in uterine epithelium and trophectoderm are summarized in Table 1. The following section provides an overview of glycoconjugates listed in Table 1 that are thought to contribute to the functional characteristics of the peri-implantation uterus in a number of animal models. Changes in the molecular composition at the surface of the trophoblast and uterus, which result in mutually adhesive interactions, are a necessary preliminary event for implantation in all species, and the search for markers of receptivity and the prereceptive period has been an important impetus for these studies.

Muc-1

Apically disposed surface glyconjugates expressed by uterine epithelial cells under most conditions are nonadhesive; however, there is recent experimental evidence that the removal of mucin-like glycoproteins from the cell surface may contribute to generation of the receptive state. One of the few candidate glycoprotein markers for the prereceptive stage is an integral mucin-type glycoprotein (Muc-1), which appears to be modulated during the estrous cycle and early pregnancy. Another potential marker of the prereceptive phase, cellCAM-105 or C-CAM, is described under the Immunoglobulin (Ig) Superfamily section.

Studies in the mouse, baboon, and pig indicate that Muc-1 is present at the apical surface of both luminal and glandular uterine epithelium during the prereceptive stage, and disappears during the implantation window *(30,73,75,76,82,111)*. This large (200–1000 kDa), heavily glycosylated, proline-rich, transmembrane protein is a major constituent of the apically expressed glycocalyx of many epithelial cell types *(111)*. Its antiadhesive properties have been demonstrated in transfection studies in which cell–cell and cell–matrix interactions are inhibited on cell-surface expression of Muc-1 at high levels *(112,113)*.

Table 1
Molecules Examined in Relation to Uterine Receptivity

Group	*Specific molecule*	*Species*	*Notes*
Mucins	Muc-1	Mouse	Regulated—present during estrus and downregulated during receptive phase *(30,73)*
		Human	Regulated—highest level d 7 after LH surge, which coincides with the time of implantation *(74)*
		Pig	Regulated—high levels during estrous and non-detectable by receptive phase; downregulated by progesterone *(75)*
		Baboon	Regulated—loss from surface epithelium correlates with receptive phase *(76)*
		Horse	Expressed on apical surface of the luminal epithelium; regulation is unknown (Day et al., unpublished data); equine capsule contains a mucin-like substance *(72)*
Integrins	LFA-1 or αLβ2	Human	Regulated—seen throughout the menstrual cycle in stroma and epithelium—increased around time of menstruation *(77)*
	Mac-1 or αMβ2	Human	Regulated—seen in stroma only and increased around time of menstruation *(77)*
	α1	Human	Regulated—seen in uterine glands and stroma; high in all secretory phases *(78)*
		Porcine	Not regulated—low-intensity expression on uterine epithelium *(75)*
	α2	Human	Regulated—decreased expression on luminal epithelium during secretory, continuous expression in glandular epithelium *(32,78)*
	α3	Human	Not regulated—present on uterine epithelium; regulated in stroma *(78)*
		Porcine	Not regulated—present in basal and lateral aspects of uterine epithelium *(75)*
	α4	Human	Regulated—expressed in glands, high in early and midsecretory phases *(78)*
		Porcine	Regulated—highest expression on luminal uterine epithelium during window of implantation *(75)*
	α5	Human	Not regulated—expressed in stroma only *(78)*
		Porcine	Regulated—luminal epithelium expression is highest during window of implantation *(75)*
		Bovine	Found in preimplantation trophoblast *(79)*
		Rats	Regulated—high during proestrus and low throughout the rest of the cycle *(80)*
	α6β4	Human	Not regulated—present in uterine epithelium *(78)*
	α9	Human	Not regulated—strongly expressed in luminal epithelium; regulated in glands *(78)*
	αvβ3	Human	Regulated throughout uterus; highest expression during window of implantation *(78)*
	αv	Porcine	Not regulated—constitutively expressed at a high intensity throughout estrous cycle *(75)*
	αvβ5	Human	Regulated—detected in stroma only *(78)*
	β1	Human	Not regulated—constitutively expressed at a high level *(81)*
		Porcine	Regulated—highest expression on luminal epithelium during window of implantation *(75)*

Table 1 (Continued)

Group	*Specific molecule*	*Species*	*Notes*
		Bovine	Found in pre- and peri-implantation trophoblast *(79)*
	β3	Porcine	Not regulated—constitutively expressed at a high intensity *(75)*
	β5	Human	Present on the apical surface of uterine epithelium; regulation unknown *(82)*
	β6	Human	Regulated—decreased expression on luminal epithelium during midsecretory phase *(78)*
Specific carbohydrate residues	LNF-1	Mouse	Regulated—present on the apical surface of uterine epithelium; exogenous LNF-1 can inhibit attachment *(83,84)*
	LNF-II	Mouse	Not regulated on uterine epithelium *(83,84)*
	LNF-III	Mouse	Not regulated on uterine epithelium *(83,84)*
	LND-I	Mouse	Not regulated on uterine epithelium *(83,84)*
	Galactose	Mouse	Regulated—glycoconjugates with a terminal galactose are positively correlated with uterine receptivity *(85)*
	Lactosamino-glycans	Mouse	Regulated—present on uterine epithelial cells—questionable at implantation *(86)*
		Human	Regulated—changes observed throughout the menstrual cycle—questionable at implantation *(87)*
HSPG	Syndecan	Mouse	Present on external surface of preimplantation trophectoderm, but switches to internal surface when attachment competent *(88)*
	Perlecan	Mouse	Present at implantation sites on trophectoderm only *(89)*
HSPG binding sites		Human	Regulated—found on the surface of uterine epithelium during receptive phase *(90)*
		Mouse	Regulated—found on the surface of uterine epithelium during the receptive phase *(91)*
	HIP	Human	Regulated—found on the apical surface of uterine epithelium during receptive phase *(92)*
Trophinin		Human/ monkey	Regulated—present on uterine epithelium and trophectoderm only during peri-implantation phase *(93)*
CD44		Human	Regulated—present on uterine epithelium at low levels in proliferative phase and high levels during secretory phase *(94,95)*
		Rabbit	Regulated—present on uterine epithelium during peri-implantation phase, may be triggered by embryonic signal—only a weak stromal reaction *(96)*
Cadherins	E-cadherin	Rabbit	Regulated—moves from subapical region of uterine epithelium during the prereceptive phase to a more evenly dispersion throughout the lateral membrane *(4)*
		Mouse	Present and coexpressed at the interface of uterine epithelium and trophectoderm *(97)*
		Mouse	Not found on the interface between maternal and fetal tissues *(98)*
		Mouse	Antibodies against E-cadherin did not inhibit embryo attachment to various substrates included UE *(99)*

Table 1 (Continued)

Group	Specific molecule	Species	Notes
	P-cadherin	Mouse/human	Present on mouse trophoblast and decidua, but not human *(100)*
Selectins	E-Selectin	Human	Present, only detected within the vascular in decidual tissue *(101)*
	L-Selectin	Human	Present on lymphocytes within the decidua *(101)*
Ig superfamily	C-CAM	Rat	Regulated—found on the apical surface of uterine epithelium—downregulated during early pregnancy *(102)*
	ICAM-1	Human	Regulated—present in stroma throughout the menstrual cycle; high just prior to menstruation and found in the decidua *(77,101)*
	PECAM	Human	Regulated—present in stroma throughout the menstrual cycle; high just prior to menstruation *(77)*
	VCAM-1	Human	Present on stroma cells within the decidua *(101)*
	NCAM	Mouse	A heparin binding protein not expressed in the uterus *(92)*
Extracellular matrix components	Osteopontin	Human	Present on apical surface of uterine epithelium; ligand for $\alpha v\beta 3$ *(103)*
	Oncofetal fibronectin	Human	Present on peri-implantation embryos *(104,105)*
		Porcine	Present on uterine epithelium and embryonic trophectoderm *(129)*
	Fibronectin	Human	Present on preimplantation embryos
		Porcine	Present on peri-implantation embryos *(75)*
	Laminin	Human	Present on peri-implantation embryos *(106)*
		Mouse	Present on peri-implantation embryos *(107)*
	Vitronectin	Porcine	Present on peri-implantation embryos and uterine epithelium *(75)*
	Entactin nidogen	Mouse	Present on peri-implantation embryos *(107)*
	Bone	Human	Present on trophoblast cells in human placenta; ligand for $\alpha v\beta 3$ (108)
	Sialoprotein tenascin	Mouse	Regulated—induced in uterine epithelium at implantation sites and interferes with UE adhesion *(109)*
		Human	Regulated—found in proliferative phase surrounding glandular uterine epithelium and in subepithelial regions of uterine epithelium *(78,110)*

LNF, lacto-*N*-fucopentaose; LND, lacto-*N*-difucohexaose; C-CAM, CellCAM105; ICAM, intercellular adhesion molecule; PECAM, platelet endothelial cell adhesion molecule; VCAM, vascular adhesion molecule; NCAM, neural cell adhesion molecule; LFA-1, lymphocyte-associated antigen-1; Mac-1, macrophage antigen-1; HIP, heparin/heparan sulfate-interacting protein.

Muc-1 mRNA and protein are constitutively expressed in ovariectomized mice, but are significantly downregulated following administration of progesterone *(73)*. Modulation of Muc-1 expression was also observed in ovariectomized gilts *(75)*, suggesting a comparable pattern of expression regardless of implantation strategy. These observations support suggestions that Muc-1 can function as an antiadhesive molecule and that its expression on surface epithelium serves as a marker for the prereceptive phase. Further reduction or loss

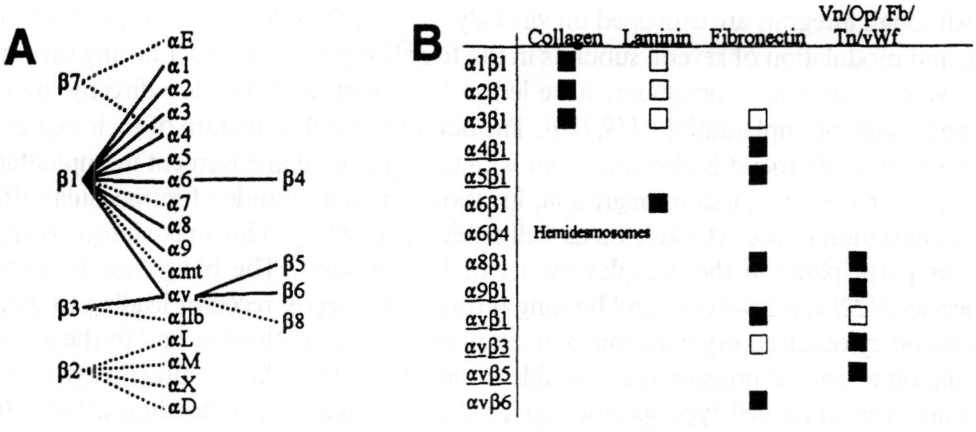

Fig. 2. The integrin family of receptors. **(A)** The 23 known integrin heterodimer combinations that can be formed from the 17α- and 8β-subunits are shown. Heterodimer combinations with thick lines have been identified in uterine tissue from a variety of species. Broken lines are heterodimer combinations that have not been found within the uterus. **(B)** Binding specificity of possible heterodimer combinations from integrin subunits detected within the uterus from different species. Integrin subunits that are potential candidates for trophectoderm–epithelial interactions are underlined. All of these heterodimers are members of the vitronectin and fibronectin family of adhesion molecules. Solid box indicates strong affinity between receptor and ligand; open box indicates weak affinity. Vn, vitronectin; Op, osteopontin; Fb, fibrinogen; Tn, tenascin; vWF, vonWillebrand's Factor.

of Muc-1 could contribute to the acquisition of endometrial receptivity by exposing constitutively expressed or hormone-induced adhesion molecules and/or their ligands.

Studies of Muc-1 in humans have provided paradoxical findings. Although the expression of Muc-1 mRNA and protein is hormonally regulated during the estrous cycle, maximal expression occurs 1 wk after ovulation, the time when implantation would be expected if conception were to occur *(114)*. Several forms of Muc-1 have been reported to arise by alternative splicing of its mRNA, including the common cell-surface form and two variants of the larger cell-surface form. One of the variants (identified as MUC1/Y) has a smaller extracellular domain, and the second splice variant (MUC1/S) is secreted owing to the absence of transmembrane and intracellular regions. All three isoforms have been detected by mRNA analyses in the endometrium of women throughout the menstrual cycle *(114)*, and the balance between cell-surface-associated and secreted forms is considered to be critical if the function of Muc-1 in humans is comparable to the other species examined to date *(115)*. Further, it remains a possibility that Muc-1 could play a role in human implantation if it carries binding sites specific for the conceptus *(115)*, similar to the selectin–carbohydrate interactions, which will be discussed further.

Integrins

The integrins are another family of glycoconjugates containing members that are expressed on the uterine luminal epithelium, and have spatial and temporal relationships with blastocyst development and implantation. These cation-dependent heterodimeric intrinsic membrane glycoproteins, comprised of noncovalently bound α- and β-subunits, participate in cell–cell and cell–substratum adhesion by virtue of their large extracellular domains *(116)*. At least 23 heterodimer combinations are known to be formed from the currently identified 17 α- and 8 β-subunits *(117,118)* with ligand specificity determined by the α- and β-subunit combinations (*see* Fig. 2).

Although integrins are expressed on virtually all cells, the spatial and temporal distribution and modulation of several subunits in the female reproductive tract during the reproductive cycle and early pregnancy have led to the notion that they are directly involved in the process of implantation *(119,120)*. The developmental regulation of their expression on the mouse blastocyst is also consistent with their potential involvement in implantation *(121)*. Their role in adhesion, migration, invasion, and a multitude of intracellular effects on organization of the cytoskeleton as well as bidirectional signaling make integrins attractive as participants in the complex events of implantation. The bidirectional signaling processes *(122)* can involve ligand binding through an integrin receptor leading to specific effects on cytoskeletal organization, activation of signaling pathways, and to the eventual regulation of gene expression (i.e., outside-in signaling). In addition, integrin cytoplasmic domains transduce cell type-specific signals that modulate ligand binding affinity (i.e., inside-out signaling). The likely involvement of these central functions of integrin receptors in trophectoderm-uterine epithelial cell interactions have been discussed *(123)*.

Much of the data on uterine integrin receptors have come from clinical studies and experiments in rodents, although recent experiments have been reported using a porcine model *(75)*. Therefore, comparative information relative to invasive and noninvasive modes of implantation is emerging.

At least 14 different integrin subunits (9 α and 5 β integrin subunits) have been identified in human endometrium *(78)* and 7 subunits (5 α and 2 β integrin subunits) have been reported for the pig uterine endometrium *(75)*. The uterine epithelial cell expression of several integrin subunits in both species is temporally and spatially regulated during the reproductive (estrus or menstrual) cycle, whereas others are constitutively expressed. At the present time, the species-specific differences are thought to reflect the major differences in the mode of implantation, although several common subunits have been identified.

In humans, subunits $\alpha 2$, $\alpha 3$, $\alpha 6$, $\alpha 9$, αv, $\beta 1$, $\beta 3$, $\beta 4$, $\beta 5$, and $\beta 6$, have been identified on uterine luminal epithelium, whereas $\alpha 1$ and $\alpha 4$, but not $\beta 5$ and $\beta 6$, are expressed in glandular epithelium *(32,78,82,119,120)*. Subunits $\alpha 5$ and $\alpha 8$ have not been found in human uterine epithelium *(78,120,124)*. Therefore, the following discussion summarizes experimental evidence for the possible known heterodimers available at the uterine luminal epithelial surface, including $\alpha 2\beta 1$, $\alpha 3\beta 1$, $\alpha 6\beta 1$, $\alpha 6\beta 4$, $\alpha 9\beta 1$, $\alpha v\beta 1$ $\alpha v\beta 3$, $\alpha v\beta 5$, and $\alpha v\beta 6$.

The expression of three of these integrin receptors appears to be particularly well suited for an early role in the implantation process; $\alpha 9\beta 1$, $\alpha v\beta 1$, and $\alpha v\beta 3$ are all members of the fibronectin and vitronectin family of integrin receptors (*see* Fig. 2). The $\alpha 9\beta 1$ receptor (which can bind to the fibronectin type III repeat in the ECM component, tenascin) is strongly expressed on the luminal epithelium throughout the menstrual cycle, whereas it is regulated on the glandular epithelium and only expressed during the mid- to late-secretory phase *(78)*. $\alpha 9\beta 1$ is a potential participant in the early attachment phase of implantation. The expression of $\alpha v\beta 1$ on the apical surface of uterine epithelium has been postulated *(82)*. This integrin receptor binds fibronectin with high affinity and vitronectin with weak affinity through the common RGD amino acid (Arg-Gly-Asp) sequence. However, analysis of this particular receptor is complicated, since each subunit of the dimer is capable of forming heterodimer combinations with other subunits, which could mask subtle changes in expression by either subunit. Most attention has been given to $\alpha v\beta 3$ owing to its potential use as a marker of uterine receptivity *(78,81,120,124)*. Expression of $\alpha v\beta 3$ is regulated during the menstrual cycle with maximal expression coincident with the rise in progesterone during the period of maternal recognition of pregnancy; aberrant expression of $\alpha v\beta 3$ is associated with infertility *(78,120)*. This heterodimer, which was localized at along apical microvilli and secretory granules of endometrial epithelial cells *(78)*, is the most versatile integrin receptor capable of binding to a variety of ECM components, including vitronectin, fibronectin, oncofetal fibronectin, and osteopontin. It is noteworthy that $\alpha4\beta1$ has also been detected during the putative implantation window in human endometrium *(32,81,120,124)*; however, its expression in the glandular epithelium reduces the likelihood that it is directly involved in the early events of implantation.

Two integrin receptors that are constitutively expressed during the menstrual cycle ($\alpha3\beta1$ and $\alpha6\beta4$) are members of the collagen/laminin family of receptors and hemidesmosomes, respectively *(78)*. The $\alpha6\beta1$ receptor is not thought to be present in uterine epithelium (since immunostaining of the $\alpha6$ subunit colocalized only with $\beta4$ staining in the basal aspect of the cell). The pattern of expression of $\alpha3\beta1$ and $\alpha6\beta4$ in the uterine epithelium does not suggest a direct involvement in early implantation owing to their localization on the basolateral aspect of epithelial cells. However, a role in early implantation cannot be excluded, because these integrins could be exposed during the reduction of polar organization of the uterine luminal epithelial cells that occurs during the peri-implantation period *(38,39)*.

Another pair of integrin receptors, $\alpha2\beta1$ and $\alpha v\beta6$, a collagen/laminin and a fibronectin receptor, respectively, are regulated during the menstrual cycle, but appear to be downregulated during the midsecretory phase *(78)*. Both of these integrins are thought to be involved in cell–cell and cell–substratum interactions and their downregulation may further contribute to the changes in epithelial cell polarity occurring during the window of implantation.

The final heterodimer of the integrin receptors considered here, which are potentially present on the apical surface of human uterine luminal epithelial cells, is the $\alpha v\beta5$ receptor. Apical staining of the $\beta5$-subunit has been reported *(82)*; however, use of an antibody raised against the $\alpha v\beta5$ heterodimer failed to reveal epithelial cell expression of this integrin *(78)*. This vitronectin receptor remains a potential, but controversial candidate for involvement in the implantation process.

Recent analyses of integrin and ECM expression in the baboon endometrium during the menstrual cycle and early pregnancy revealed a remarkably similar pattern to that seen in humans, including the changing integrin patterns in the decidua of pregnancy *(125)*. However, the expression of $\alpha v\beta3$, which appears on apical uterine endometrial epithelial cells during the implantation window in humans appeared well after the time of initial blastocyst attachment in the baboon, but correlates with enhanced glandular secretion in both species.

The significance of the integrin receptors and their modulation must be considered in the context of the available receptors and ligands present on both conceptus and uterine epithelial cells. In humans, oncofetal fibronectin, referred to as "trophoblast glue," is present on the invading human trophoblast *(104)*, and osteopontin is present on the apical surface of uterine epithelium *(103)*. Both oncofetal fibronectin and osteopontin are ligands for the integrin receptors present on the uterine epithelium during the implantation period in humans. Coexpression of both osteopontin and $\alpha v\beta3$ was recently reported in both glandular epithelium and decidualizing stomal cells as well as cytotrophoblast cells in baboon *(125)*. In addition, other integrin binding ligands, fibronectin and vitronectin, have been implicated in murine trophoblast outgrowth and attachment *(see 4,99)*, and this process can be blocked with RGD-containing peptides in vitro *(126)*.

The preimplantation human embryo exhibits constitutive expression of $\alpha3$, $\alpha5$, αv, $\beta1$, $\beta3$, $\beta4$, and $\beta5$ integrin subunits from the oocyte to the blastocyst stage *(127)*. With the exception of the $\beta4$-subunit (which presumably binds with $\alpha6$ in hemidesmosomes), all of the possible integrin heterodimers are capable of binding either fibronectin with low affinity ($\alpha3\beta1$), or are members of the family of fibronectin and vitronectin receptors, and are similar to those expressed on human uterine epithelium.

In the mouse, $\alpha5\beta1$ and $\alpha v\beta3$ are expressed on trophectoderm during initial stages of apposition and adhesion *(123)*. However, once the trophoblast becomes invasive, $\alpha1\beta1$, $\alpha6\beta1$, and $\alpha7\beta1$ appear; these receptors are capable of binding laminin and collagen, and presumably support invasion of epithelium and stroma. Only the invasive cells of the mouse trophoblast express both $\alpha5\beta1$ and $\alpha1\beta1$. In experiments where the function of the fibronectin receptor, $\alpha5\beta1$, was blocked with antibodies, invasion was inhibited, suggesting that the interaction of this integrin receptor and its ligand regulate the invasion of the mouse trophoblast cells *(128)*.

As noted above, comparative studies of integrin expression are limited; the only noninvasive implantation animal model studied to date is the pig. Uterine luminal epithelial cell expression of integrin subunits $\alpha1$, $\alpha3$, $\alpha4$, $\alpha5$, αv, $\beta1$, and $\beta3$ were monitored using immunofluorescence microscopy during the estrous cycle and early pregnancy (including sites of conceptus attachment) *(75)*. These subunits exhibited three distinct patterns of expression classified as:

1. Low or no expression ($\alpha1$ and $\alpha3$);
2. High-intensity constitutive expression (αv and $\beta3$); and
3. High-intensity, modulated expression ($\alpha4$, $\alpha5$, $\beta1$).

Modulation of $\alpha4$, $\alpha5$, $\beta1$ resulted in maximal expression during the period corresponding to maternal recognition of pregnancy (i.e., d 10–15). In the same study, experimental evidence for steroid modulation of integrin subunits was obtained in ovariectomized gilts. Integrin subunits classified as the high-intensity, modulated subunits ($\alpha4$, $\alpha5$, $\beta1$) were expressed at a higher intensity in gilts that were treated with progesterone (or progesterone in combination with estrogen) than in estrogen-treated animals.

Analysis of implantation sites indicated that integrin subunits $\alpha4$, $\alpha5$, αv, $\beta1$, and $\beta3$ were expressed at sites of trophectoderm contact with the uterine epithelium (e.g., Fig. 3). The integrin receptors potentially formed from the heterodimers identified in this study included $\alpha4\beta1$, $\alpha5\beta1$, $\alpha v\beta1$, and $\alpha v\beta3$. These receptors, like those identified above from human studies (during the initial events of attachment), are all members of the fibronectin/vitronectin family of integrin receptors.

The porcine conceptus was also found to express the same integrin subunits ($\alpha4$, $\alpha5$, αv, $\beta1$, and $\beta3$) as the uterine epithelium. In addition, the ECM constituents, fibronectin, oncofetal fibronectin, and vitronectin, are all expressed by the conceptus during the time of implantation (the porcine uterine epithelium expressed vitronectin and oncofetal fibronectin) *(75,129)*. The distribution and type of ECM components correspond with the integrin subunits expressed on uterine epithelial cells during implantation in the pig.

Integrins $\alpha1\beta1$ and $\alpha3\beta1$ are members of the collagen/laminin receptor family. The restricted expression of these integrins at the basal aspect of porcine uterine epithelium is consistent with cellular attachment to the basement membrane. Integrins $\alpha4\beta1$, $\alpha5\beta1$, and $\alpha v\beta1$ are members of the large family of fibronectin receptors, which makes them possible candidates for trophectoderm/uterine epithelium attachment based on the finding that fibronectin and vitronectin are present on the contacting surfaces between the conceptus and the uterine epithelium. In addition, $\alpha v\beta3$ can also bind to fibronectin with weak affinity. The expression of several different fibronectin receptors on the uterine epithelium and

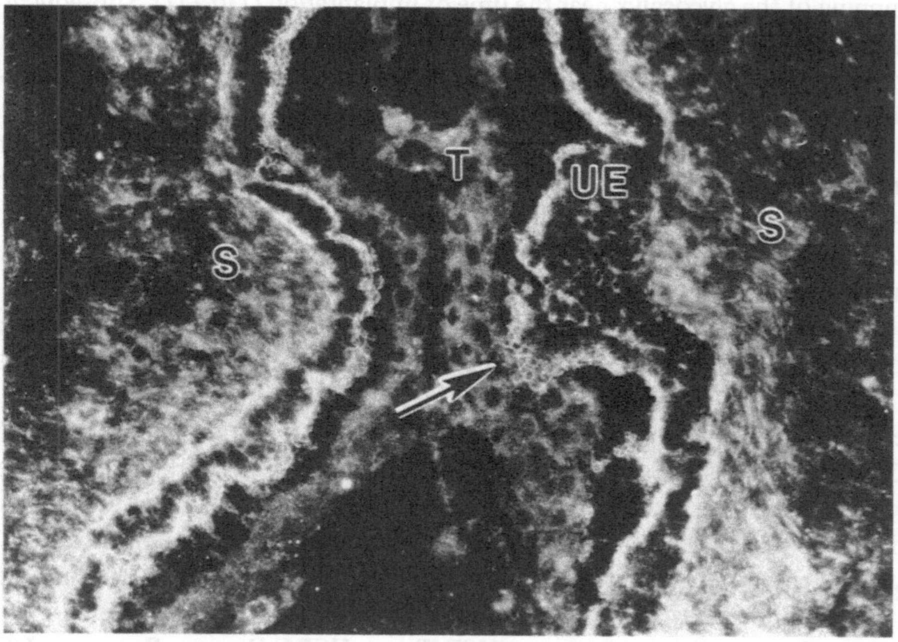

Fig. 3. The expression of the fibronectin receptor α5-subunit during implantation in the pig. Immunofluorescence microscopy of α5-labeled endometrium and conceptus (d 15) revealed staining of the trophectoderm (T), the apical aspect of uterine epithelium (UE), and the underlying stroma (S). The presence of the α5-subunit on both the uterine epithelium and trophectoderm, and at sites of attachment (arrow) suggests the presence of the fibronectin receptor at the implantation site (×235).

the trophectoderm allows for the integrins to bind to fibronectin at two different locations, α4β1 integrin binds to the amino acid sequence, EILDV (Glu-Ile-Leu-Asp-Val), within the IIICS region of fibronectin, whereas the remaining integrins will bind to the RGD sequence of fibronectin *(116)*. The αvβ3 (vitronectin receptor) and αvβ1 (weak affinity vitronectin receptor) can also bind to the RGD sequence found in fibronectin. Thus, two ECM proteins (fibronectin and vitronectin) and the four integrin heterodimers are available for participation in implantation events of the porcine conceptus. This redundancy in integrin receptors may ensure the ability of the conceptus to attach to the uterine epithelium.

In summary, regardless of the mode of implantation, it appears that the expression of integrin receptors and their ligands are important elements of attachment and adhesion of the conceptus to uterine epithelium. Integrin receptors expressed on the conceptus appear to be largely conserved between species examined to date, and consist of integrins that are also expressed on uterine epithelium. This strategy may represent a conserved mechanism of conceptus attachment. The induction of new integrin receptor populations (specific for collagen and laminin) occurs later in conceptuses from species that exhibit invasive implantation.

Molecules Expressing Specific Carbohydrate Residues

LNF-I and Related Determinants. Changes in carbohydrate expression on the epithelium lining the uterine lumen were initially suggested by the reduction in surface charge and thinning of the glycocalyx near the time of implantation *(130,131)*. Subsequent studies have identified specific carbohydrate determinants that may play a role in the implantation process. Monoclonal antibodies (MAb) developed against a blood group-related oligosaccharide determinant, lacto-*N*-fucopentaose-1 (LNF-I), have shown that the expression of this epitope on the surface of mouse uterine epithelial cells changes during the preimplantation period *(83,84,132)*. LNF-I (but not polysaccharides with similar structures, such as LNF-II, LNF-III, lacto-*N*-difucohexaose, lacto-*N*-tetraose, and lactodifucotetraose) *(133)* and an anti-LNF-I MAb have also been shown to significantly inhibit embryo attachment using an in vitro model for implantation *(84)*.

In ovariectomized mice, estrogen administration stimulated LNF-I, but progesterone did not alter LNF expression, whereas the combination of the two hormones was synergistic and resulted in maximal expression *(132)*. In pregnant mice, the maximal LNF-I epithelial surface expression occurred on d 1–4 and decreased dramatically by d 5 and 6 *(83)*. Since the expression of LNF-I does not span the entire duration of the receptive phase, it is thought that the potential role for LNF-I may be limited to initial steps of adhesion. Mouse conceptuses are believed to contain specific binding sites for LNF-I, although specific receptors have not been identified. Comparative studies in humans or other animal models have not yet been reported.

Heparan Sulfate Proteoglycans (HSPG) and HSPG Binding Proteins. HSPG are expressed on the mouse trophectoderm, and it has been suggested that HSPG "receptors" become distributed on the apical plasma membrane of uterine epithelium during the receptive phase in the mouse *(134)*. Perlecan is an HSPG detected on mouse conceptuses and uterine epithelial cells and is also found at sites of attachment, suggesting its role in adhesion during early implantation *(89)*. Another HSPG, syndecan, is also expressed at the exterior surface of trophectoderm in preimplantation mouse conceptuses. Since syndecan is redistributed to the interior surface just prior to attachment competence *(88)*, its role in attachment seems unlikely.

A novel cell-surface heparin/heparan sulfate binding protein expressed by a variety of human epithelia, heparin/heparan sulfate-interacting protein (referred to as HIP), has recently been isolated and cloned from a human uterine epithelial cell line *(135)*. This putative HSPG receptor has been localized at the apical and basal surfaces of human luminal and glandular uterine epithelium. Intense HIP expression during the first 7 d postovulation and detection of stromal expression on d 13 postovulation are consistent with a role in conceptus attachment *(92)*.

HSPG are also capable of complexing with a number of growth factors and modulate cellular functions *(99)*. A heparin-binding epidermal growth factor-like growth factor (HB-EGF) is synthesized as a transmembrane form in mouse uterine epithelium; HB-EGF mRNA is expressed in uterine luminal epithelium just prior to implantation and only at the site of blastocyst apposition *(136)*. Recent experimental evidence indicates that HB-EGF can function as a juxtacrine adhesion factor that could be one of the mediators of blastocyst adhesion during early implantation *(137)*. Uterine expression of colony-stimulating factor-1 (CSF-1) in the pig exhibits an interesting similarities to HB-EGF *(138)*. CSF-1 was detected on the apical side of porcine trophectoderm and immunocytochemical analysis suggests that this may be a membrane-bound form of CSF-1 *(138)*. CSF-1 may interact with CSF-1 receptor expressed on both trophectoderm and endometrial cells by a juxtacrine mechanism, since the CSF-1 receptor is expressed by both porcine conceptus and endometrium (Tuo and Bazer, unpublished data).

Trophinin

Trophinin was first identified on transformed epithelial cell lines (a trophoblastic teratocarcinoma, HT-H, and endometrial adenocarcinoma, SNG-M, cell lines) and named for the cell type in which it was originally cloned *(93)*. This intrinsic transmembrane, divalent cation-independent protein with a predicted mol wt of 69 kDa, is found on the apical surface of these cells and appears to bind to a trophinin counterpart on the neighboring cell. Trophinins are not present in the endometrium of women during the proliferative and ovulatory phases, but are expressed only by the surface of uterine epithelium during the implantation window *(93)*. In the same study, it was also reported that trophinins are present at the surface of both uterine epithelium and monkey blastocysts at the implantation site.

Trophinin has an associated cytoplasmic protein necessary for trophinin function. The protein, tastin, named for its action as a trophinin-assisting protein, has a predicted mol wt of 83 kDa, but no significant amino acid sequence homology to any known protein. Tastin interacts with the cytoskeleton and participates in the clustering of trophinin on the cell surface. Tastin also contains numerous phosphorylation sites (including 2 that are cAMP/cGMP-dependent, 11 potential casein kinase II, and 16 potential protein kinase C phosphorylation sites), which may allow for subtle regulation of tastin and/or tastin-trophinin complexes. The relationship of trophinin and tastin to other members of the classes of adhesion molecules discussed thus far is unknown, since sequence homology to other known nucleotide or peptide sequences has not been established.

CD44

The integral membrane protein, CD44, is a highly glycosylated adhesion molecule that exists in a variety of mol wt isoforms in mammals (85–160 kDa) and has a large extracellular domain with a short carboxy-terminal cytoplasmic domain *(139)*. CD44 is expressed by leukocytes, where it acts as a homing molecule during the adhesion cascade, and on epithelial and mesenchymal cells, where it appears to function as a receptor for hyaluronic acid.

Uterine epithelia of both humans and rabbits express CD44 with maximal expression coinciding with uterine receptivity, although they have not been examined *in uteri* from other mammals *(94–96)*. The dual functions of CD44 for both cell–cell and cell–matrix interactions along with the modulation of these proteins make them candidates for involvement in the implantation process. Further study is needed to identify potential interactions between CD44 and the trophectoderm, and expression relative to differences in implantation strategies.

Cadherins

Cadherins are transmembrane calcium-dependent cell–cell adhesion molecules that bind to one another by means of homophilic interactions and are involved in establishing and maintaining intercellular connections between neighboring epithelial cells *(100)*. Many members of the cadherin family have been identified based on their immunological differences. Cadherins were originally found in epithelial, nervous, and placental tissues (E-, N-, and P-cadherin, respectively). E-cadherin has been found on both uterine epithelial cells and the developing conceptus, suggesting that cadherin adhesion between the embryonic trophectoderm and epithelium may exist. In rabbit uterine epithelium, cadherin expression moves from a subapical region of the uterine epithelium during the prereceptive phase and becomes more evenly dispersed throughout the lateral membrane *(4)*. The change in cadherin localization is consistent with the changes that occur when the polarized uterine epithelial cell organization is reduced during the receptive phase. In the mouse, immunocytochemical studies reveal cadherin expression at points where trophectoderm and uterine epithelial cells interact *(97)*. However, earlier work *(98)* showed staining of cadherins in uterine epithelium and trophoblast, but not at the site of contact. Although it is unclear exactly what role cadherins play in implantation and the maintenance of pregnancy, E-cadherin is not required for the implantation cascade, since antibodies against E-cadherin do not inhibit embryo attachment to various substrates, including uterine epithelial cells *(99)*.

Selectins

There are three known family members of the selectin family of adhesion molecules, including E-selectin (originally detected on endothelium), P-selectin (identified on platelets), and L-selectin (identified on leukocytes). Selectin is a term proposed to highlight the common amino-terminal lectin domain, and to indicate the selective function and expression of these molecules. All members of the selectin family contain the unique extracellular region composed of an amino-terminal calcium-dependent lectin domain, which is central to the carbohydrate binding properties of all three selectins. Additionally, this family contains epidermal growth factor-like domain, and two to nine short consensus repeat units, which are highly conserved between species *(140,141)*.

There have been few reports of selectin expression within the uterus during normal cycling or during implantation. E-selectin was detected in the vascular endothelium within the decidual tissue, and L-selectin was only detected on decidual lymphocytes *(101)*. Although uterine epithelial expression of selectins has not yet been reported, the logic for a selectin-like molecule exists. All selectins studied to date bind to the sialylated-fucosylated structures (sialyl Lewis X). The sialyl Lewis X motifs are found in Muc-1, which is expressed at the time of implantation in humans *(74)*. Fucosylated carbohydrates are also expressed on the uterine epithelium during the implantation process in the form of LNF-I *(142)*.

Immunoglobulin (Ig) Superfamily

The Ig superfamily includes a variety of proteins that share an Ig-like structure consisting of 70–110 amino acids arranged into seven to nine β-pleated sheets stabilized by disulfide bridges between two β-sheets *(139)*. Most of these membrane-bound proteins are involved in cell–cell recognition and include molecules that function in cellular immunity (e.g., major histocompatibility antigen, CD4, CD8, and so on), neural development (N-CAM), leukocyte trafficking (ICAM-1, VCAM-1, PECAM, and so forth), and signal transduction (e.g., CSF-1 and PDGF receptors), and thus, are very responsive to cytokines *(143)*.

One member of the Ig superfamily, cellCAM-105 (or C-CAM), which contains four extracellular immunoglobulin domains, a transmembrane domain, and a cytoplasmic domain is involved in intercellular adhesion by the homophilic interaction of C-CAMs on neighboring cells *(144)*. C-CAM may serve as a marker for the prereceptive phase of the rat uterine epithelium, and since it is expressed on the apical surface of luminal epithelium during estrus, it is downregulated in the presence of progesterone, and is absent during implantation *(102)*. Additionally, expression of C-CAM was also detected on rat d 4 blastocysts, but disappeared as blastocysts developed to the adhesive stage.

To date, the role of other Ig superfamily members in the implantation process has not been reported. However, several members of this superfamily function as cell–cell adhesion molecules and most cells express at least one Ig superfamily member. ICAMs and VCAM-1 are ligands for integrins LFA-1 and $\alpha4\beta1$, respectively. Both $\alpha4\beta1$ and LFA-1 have also been found in human endometrium *(77)*, and $\alpha4\beta1$ has been detected on the uterine epithelium of both women and gilts *(75,78,81,120,124)*. The role of ICAMs and VCAM-1 in conceptus attachment requires further study.

Uterine expression of other members of the Ig superfamily have indicated that N-CAM does not appear in mouse uterus *(92)*. PECAM-1 was detected on endothelial cells and focal areas of stroma throughout the menstrual cycle, and may be related to the influx of leukocytes into the uterus during menstruation *(77)*. Similarly, ICAM-1 was found in endothelium and in focal areas of the stroma, and the staining increases around the time of menstruation in humans *(77)*. Unlike PECAM-1, ICAM-1 was determined to be extensively distributed throughout the decidua *(101)*. VCAM-1, the ligand for the integrin $\alpha4\beta1$, was localized to endothelium and stromal cells within the decidua of humans *(101)*.

Implantation as an Adhesion Cascade

The adhesion events that occur during implantation are likely to involve a highly coordinated set of sequential interactions that include many different adhesion molecules with distinct, but interrelated functions. The molecular interactions involved in apposition and attachment of the conceptus and apical uterine luminal epithelial cell surface may constitute an implantation adhesion cascade with core events that are comparable to other adhesion cascades. Examples include the cytokine-mediated activation of granulocyte-endothelial interactions, activation and migration of distinct maturational stages of lymphocyte populations to different lymphoid organs, and metastasis of malignant cells *(see 145,146)*. Similarities of early implantation events to the leukocyte-endothelial adhesion cascade *(123,133)* and metastatic process *(99)* have been recognized.

Shweighoffer and Shaw *(145)* have highlighted three core elements of adhesion cascades including:

1. A triggering molecule on the cell surface capable of interacting with an extracellular ligand;
2. A biochemical signal (or series of signals) generated by physical association of the trigger molecule to the adhesion molecule; and
3. An adhesion molecule whose adhesive nature is altered by the biochemical signal.

The molecules that function to trigger the adhesion cascade are diverse and represented by many families of molecules that could include cytokine receptors, carbohydrate–selectin interactions, and membrane lipid metabolites, which are linked to a variety of signal transduction pathways *(147,148)*. Although there is considerable diversity among triggering molecules, integrins are the dominant adhesion systems in each of the adhesion cascades, and their capacity to mediate adhesion is linked to their activation by engaging another surface molecule *(145)*. However, selectins and members of the Ig superfamily can also undergo activation-dependent changes in binding capacity.

The conditions that control the developmental expression of adhesion receptors and ligands in the uterus are precisely regulated through the action of ovarian steroids, growth factors, and cytokines (*see* Fig. 4). During the prereceptive phase, the blastocyst is free to move within the uterus, a condition that appears to be supported in a number of species by the nonadhesive nature of the large glycoprotein Muc-1. Muc-1 may extend outward from the apical cell surface further than receptors or triggering molecules, and thereby

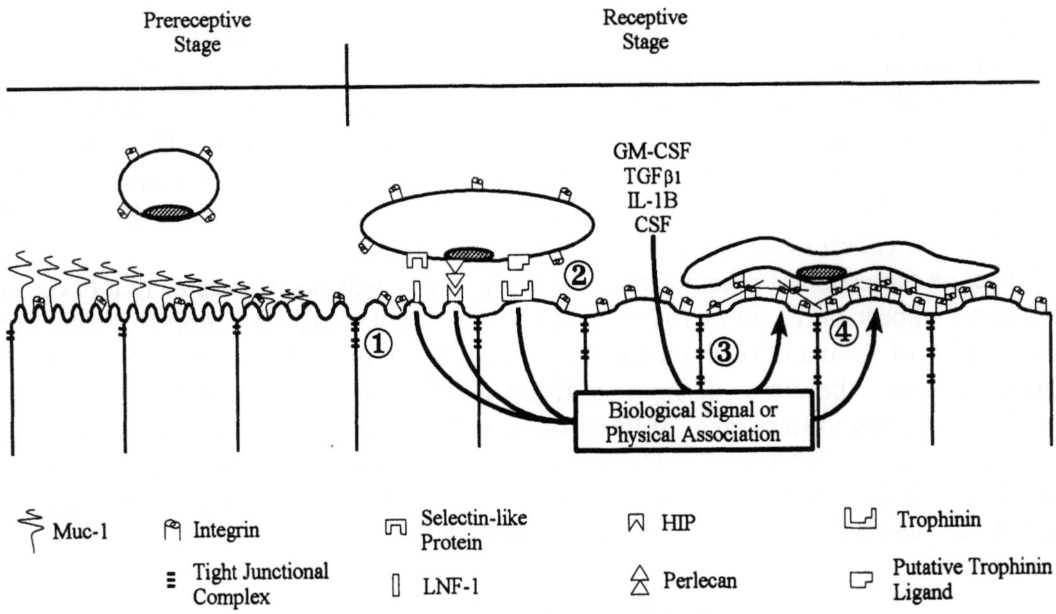

Fig. 4. A schematic representation of implantation as an adhesion cascade. Transition of uterine luminal epithelium from prereceptive to receptive requires downregulation of the antiadhesive mucin, Muc1, thought to inhibit sterically the interaction of the conceptus with adhesion molecules at the trophectoderm/uterine epithelium interface. The sequential events of implantation resemble the events of other adhesion cascades *(140)* and consist of four steps, which are numbered 1–4 on the illustration. 1. The progesterone-induced structural changes that result in reduction of epithelial polarity are indicated by loss of apical microvilli, alteration of tight junction organization, the formation of pinopodes, and a dome-like apical surface, which allows close apposition of conceptus and apical uterine epithelium. 2. Initial interaction between the two genetically distinct cell types occurs with triggering and/or tethering molecules, which are either induced or constitutively expressed, but unavailable until loss of Muc-1. The triggering molecules that initiate the implantation cascade are involved in low-affinity and weak molecular interactions. 3. Transduction of signals from the triggering molecules can include a diverse array of biochemical and/or physical interactions, including calcium fluxes, protein phosphorylation, or cytoskeletal alterations. 4. The final adhesion event between the conceptus and uterine epithelium is mediated by the strong, high-affinity integrin–ligand interactions. The potential heterodimer combinations that are strong candidates for the implantation cascade identified to date are all members of the fibronectin and vitronectin family of receptors. LNF-1, lacto-*N*-fucopentaose; HIP, heparin/heparan sulfate-interacting protein; GM-CSF, granulocyte macrophage-colony-stimulating factor; TGFβ1, transforming growth factor β1; IL-1β, interleukin 1β; CSF, colony-stimulating factor.

have the capacity to inhibit sterically the interaction of the embryo with adhesion molecules at the maternal/fetal interface *(115)*.

Entry into the receptive phase in synchrony with conceptus development and the expression and/or unmasking of adhesion molecules permit the primary interactions involving low-affinity bonds with triggering molecules *(149)*. Several candidates for this role have been described in this chapter. The appearance of LNF-I and LNF-I-containing fucosylated lactosaminoglycans in the rodent uterine epithelium is suggestive of a carbohydrate–selectin interaction, although no selectin-type molecule has as yet been described in uterine epithelium or trophectoderm during implantation *(133)*.

Two recently identified molecules, trophinin and HIP, may function in this capacity. Although no ligand has yet been found for trophinin, expression of trophinin by transfection of cells causes them to become adhesive *(93)*. The formation of trophinin complexes with the cytoskeletal-associated protein, tastin, which has many potential phosphorylation sites could potentially result in the downstream biochemical regulation of integrins. HIP is expressed on the apical surface of uterine epithelium during the receptive phase and can bind heparin/heparan sulfate proteoglycans, such as perlecan *(92)*. If HIP is involved in the adhesion cascade, it is likely to occur through early physical association providing low-affinity tethering or docking of the conceptus prior to the high-affinity adhesion associated with integrin binding.

Although not discussed in this chapter, cytokines, growth factors, and paracrine hormones may act as triggering mechanisms or signals involved in the implantation cascade. Potential participants in this process include, but are not limited to, transforming growth factor (TGF-β_1), interferon gamma (IFNγ), granulocyte macrophage-colony-stimulating factor (GM-CSF), and interleukin-1β (IL-1β) *(150)*. These and other cytokines discussed in previous chapters are present in the uterus during the window of implantation and could initiate integrin activation during signaling events.

It should also be noted that changes in the polarized functions that occur during the receptive phase result in cytoskeletal alterations and changes in the distribution of plasma membrane proteins and lipids partitioned by tight junctions. These changes may contribute to conformational alterations in the integrins, which could lead to activation *(151,152)*.

As discussed previously, the involvement of integrins in adhesion, migration, and invasion, their numerous effects on organization of the cytoskeleton, and bidirectional signaling are consistent with these adhesion molecules as dominant participants in the implantation cascade. The upregulation of several integrin subunits and exposure of others on loss of Muc-1 during the receptive period provide a number of heterodimer combinations that are members of the fibronectin and vitronectin family of integrin receptors. The redundancy in the potential integrin receptors present and the variety of potential triggering molecules and ligands highlight the physiological complexity of the implantation cascade. Recent studies in which aggregation of integrin receptors has been demonstrated as sufficient to induce transmembrane accumulation of at least 20 signal transduction molecules *(153,154)* are indicative of both the complexity of the process and our limited understanding of the details of the implantation cascade.

Culture systems that can be regulated in vitro to study uterine epithelial cell–conceptus interactions would be of great value to explore the molecular aspects of uterine receptivity and the implantation cascade. Improvements in endometrial culture systems that accommodate the polarized functions of uterine epithelial cells *(27)* and coculture of segregated endometrial stromal and epithelial cells for use in implantation studies have been reported *(155)*. These culture systems should facilitate a better appreciation of uterine epithelial and stromal cell interactions and identification of functions that are under endocrine or paracrine control. Because polarized epithelial cells regain many in vivo characteristics *(28–30,156–158)*, there is considerable utility of these model systems to investigate in detail the events occurring at the conceptus-uterine epithelial interface.

Recent studies in our laboratory that capitalize on porcine uterine epithelial cells *(75)* and conceptus-derived trophoblastic vesicles offer encouragement in this area *(75,157,158)*. Modulation of Muc-1 and integrin expression have been detected in polarized porcine uterine epithelial cells in vitro if conditions for development and maintenance of epithelial cell polarity are provided *(158)*. The modulation of both Muc-1 and integrin expression in vitro resembled that detected in uterine epithelium in vivo *(75)*. Similarly, the expression of integrin subunits on trophoblastic vesicles was identical to their expression on trophectoderm of intact conceptuses in vivo.

CONCLUSIONS

During the peri-implantation period, coordination of a variety of signals arising from the ovary, the endometrium, and the conceptus are necessary to overcome the uterine epithelial cell barrier to implantation. The structural and functional alterations of uterine epithelial cells that permit the apical-apical union of conceptus and uterine epithelium surveyed here are complex and account for the fact that in the 20 years of assisted human reproduction, 85% of the transferred human embryos resulting from in vitro fertilization fail to implant *(159)*. In contrast, improved implantation rates in domestic and laboratory animals suggest that the identification of markers that identify or predict uterine receptivity to implantation and the development of noninvasive approaches to detect these markers may facilitate attempts to improve pregnancy rates in women who have difficulty in conceiving because of implantation failure. Although new insights into human blastocyst implantation will depend on studies in experimental animals, improved endometrial culture systems that faithfully reproduce events occurring in vivo will be of great value to explore the molecular aspects of uterine receptivity and the implantation cascade.

ACKNOWLEDGMENTS

This work was supported by USDA grant 92-37203-7952. We thank Stanley R. Glasser and Gary R. Newton for helpful discussions, and William E. Day for providing unpublished data.

REFERENCES

1. Bazer FW, First NL (1983) Pregnancy and parturition. J Anim Sci 57(Suppl 2):425–460.
2. Bazer FW (1992) Mediators of maternal recognition of pregnancy in mammals. Proc Soc Expt Biol Med 199:373–384.
3. Psychoyos A (1986) Uterine receptivity for nidation. Ann NY Acad Sci 476:36–42.
4. Denker H-W (1993) Implantation: a cell biological paradox. J Exp Zool 266:541–558.
5. Burton GJ (1992) Human and animal models: limitations and comparisons, In: The First Twelve Weeks of Gestation (Barnea ER, Hustin J, Janiaux E, eds.), Springer-Verlag, Berlin, pp. 469–485.
6. Loke YW, King A, Burrows TD (1995) Decidua in human implantation. Human Reprod 10(Suppl 2):14–21.
7. Loke YW, King A (1995) Human Implantation: Cell Biology and Immunology. Cambridge University Press, Cambridge, UK.
8. Simón C, Francés A, Pellicier A, Polan ML (1995) Cytokines in implantation. Semin Reprod Endocrinol 13:142–151.
9. Murphy CR (1995) The cytoskeleton of uterine epithelial cells: a new player in uterine receptivity and the plasma membrane transformation. Human Reprod Update 1:567–580.
10. Cowell TP (1969) Implantation and development of mouse eggs transferred to the uterus of non-progestational mice. J Reprod Fertil 19:239–245.
11. Kirby DRS (1963) The development of mouse blastocysts transplanted to the cryptorchid and scrotal testis. J Anat 97:119–130.
12. Glasser SR, Mullholland J, Mani SJ, Julian J, Munir MI, Lampelo S, Soares MJ (1991) Blastocyst-endometrial relationships: reciprocal interactions between uterine epithelial and stromal cells and blastocysts. Trophoblast Res 5:229–280.
13. Samuel CA, Perry JS (1972) The ultrastructure of pig trophoblast transplanted to an ectopic site in the uterine wall. J Anat 113:139–149.

14. Dickman Z, Noyes RW (1960) The fate of ova transferred into the uterus of the rat. J Reprod Fertil 12:197–206.
15. Finn CA, Martin L (1974) The control of implantation. J Reprod Fertil 39:195–206.
16. Ayalon W (1978) A review of early embryonic mortality in cattle. J Reprod Fertil 54:483–493.
17. Pope WF (1994) Embryonic mortality in swine, In: Embryonic mortality in Domestic Species (Zavy MT, Geisert RD, eds.), CRC, Baton Rouge, pp. 53–78.
18. Cunha GR, Hhung LWK, Shannon JM, Tagichi O, Fujii H (1983) Hormone-induced morphogenesis and growth: role of mesenchymal-epithelial interactions. Rec Prog Horm Res 39:559–598.
19. Hild-Petito S, Verhage HG, Fazleabas A (1992) Immunocytochemical localization of estrogen and progestin receptors in baboon (*Papio anubis*) uterus during implantation and pregnancy. Endocrinology 130:2343–2353.
20. Lessey BA, Killam AP, Metzger DA, Haney AF, Greene GL, McCarty KS, Jr (1988) Immunohistochemical analysis of human uterine estrogen and progesterone receptors throughout the menstrual cycle. J Clin Endocrinol Metab 67:334–340.
21. Geisert RD, Short EC, Morgan GL (1994) Establishment of pregnancy in domestic farm species, In: Embryonic Mortality in Domestic Species (Zavy MT, Geisert RD, eds.), CRC, Boca Raton, pp. 23–51.
22. Spencer TE, Bazer FW (1995) Temporal and spatial alterations in uterine estrogen receptor and progesterone receptor gene expression during the estrous cycle and early pregnancy in the ewe. Biol Reprod 53:1527–1543.
23. Koji T, Chedid M, Rubin JS, Slayden Ov D, Csaky KG, Aaronson SA, Brenner RM (1994) Progesterone-dependent expression of keratinocyte growth factor mRNA in Stromal cells of the primate endometrium: keratinocyte growth factor as a progestomedin. J Cell Biol 125:393–401.
24. Pekonen F, Nyman T, Rutanen EM (1993) Differential expression of keratinocyte growth factor and its receptor in the human uterus. Mol Cell Endocrinol 95:43–49.
25. Guidice LC, Dsupin BA, Jin IH, Vu TH, Hoffman AR (1993) Differential expression of messenger ribonucleic acids encoding insulin-like growth factors and their receptors in human uterine endometrium and decidua. J Clin Endocrinol Metab 76:1115–1122.
26. Hana V, Murphy LJ (1994) Interdependence of epidermal growth factor and insulin-like growth factor-I expression in the mouse uterus. Endocrinology 135:107–112.
27. Glasser SR, Julian J, Decker GL, Tang J-P, Carson DD (1988) Development of morphological and functional polarity in primary cultures of immature rat uterine epithelial cells. J Cell Biol 107:2409–2423.
28. Julian J, Carson DD, Glasser SR (1992) Polarized rat uterine epithelium in vitro: responses to estrogen in defined medium. Endocrinology 130:68–78.
29. Julian JA, Carson DD, Glasser SR (1992) Polarized rat uterine epithelium in vitro: Constitutive expression of estrogen "induced" proteins. Endocrinology 130:79–87.
30. Valdizan MC, Julian J, Carson DD (1992) WGA-binding, mucin glycoproteins protect the apical cell surface of mouse uterine epithelium. J Cell Physiol 151:451–465.
31. Glasser SR, Mullholland J (1993) Receptivity is a polarity dependent special function of hormonally regulated uterine epithelial cells. Micros Res Tech 25:106–120.
32. Tabibzadeh S, Babaknia A (1995) The signals and molecular pathways involved in implantation, symbiotic interaction between blastocyst and endometrium involving adhesion and tissue invasion. Hum Reprod 10:1579–1602.
33. Nikas G, Drakakis P, Loutradis D, Mara-Skoufari C, Koumantakis E, Michalas S, Psychoyos A (1995) Uterine pinopodes as markers of the "nidation window" in cycling women receiving exogenous oestradiol and progesterone. Hum Reprod 10:1208–1213.
34. Martel D, Frydman R, Glissant M, Maggioni C, Roche D, Psychoyos A (1987) Scanning electron microscopy of postovulatory human endometrium in spontaneous cycles and cycles stimulated by hormone treatment. J Endocrinol 114:319–324.
35. Massai MR, Bergeron C, Martel D, de Ziegler D, Meduri G, Psychoyos A, Frydman R, Bouchard P (1993) Physiological estradiol and progesterone replacement cycles in women with ovarian failure, a model to study endometrial maturation and sex steroid receptor regulation by exogenous hormones. Hum Reprod 8:1828–1834.
36. Psychoyos A, Mandon P (1971) Etude de la surface de l'épithélium utérin au microscope électronique à balayage. Observations chez la ratte au 4ème et 5ème jours de la gestation. CR Acad Sci Paris 272:2723–2729.
37. Luxford KA, Murphy CR (1992) Reorganization of the apical cytoskeleton of uterine epithelial cells during early pregnancy in the rat: a study with myosin subfragment 1. Biol Cell 74:195–202.

38. Murphy CR, Swift JG, Mukherjee TM, Rogers AW (1982) The structure of tight junctions between uterine luminal epithelial cells at different stages of pregnancy in the rat. Cell Tissue Res 223: 281–286.
39. Murphy CR, Swift JG, Need JA, Mukherjee TM, Rogers AW (1982) A freeze-fracture electron microscopic study of tight junctions of epithelial cells in the human uterus. Anat Embryol 163: 367–370.
40. Winterhager E, Kuhnel W (1982) Alterations in intercellular junctions of the uterine epithelium during preimplantation phase in the rabbit. Cell Tissue Res 224:517–526.
41. Murphy CR, Swift JG, Mukherjee TM, Rogers AW (1982) Reflexive gap junctions on uterine luminal epithelial cells. Acta Anat 112:92–96.
42. Herr JC (1976) Reflexive gap junctions. Gap junctions between processes arising from the same ovarian decidual cell. J Cell Biol 69:495–501.
43. Citi S (1993) The molecular organization of tight junctions. J Cell Biol 121:485–489.
44. Furuse M, Itoh M, Hirase T, Nagafuchi A, Yonemura S, Tsukita S, Tsukita (1994) Direct association of occludin with ZO-1 and its possible involvement in the localization of occludin at tight junctions. J Cell Biol 127:1617–1626.
45. Stevenson BR, Siliciano JD, Mooseker MS, Goodenough DA (1986) Identification of ZO-1: a high mol-wt polypeptide associated with the tight junction (zonula occludens) in a variety of epithelia. J Cell Biol 103:755–766.
46. Gumbiner B, Lowenkopf T, Apatira D (1991) Identification of a 160-kDa polypeptide that binds to the tight junction protein ZO-1. Proc Natl Acad Sci USA 88:3460–3464.
47. Zhong Y, Saitoh T, Minase T, Sawada N, Enomoto K, Mori M (1993) Monoclonal antibody 7H6 reacts with a novel tight junction-associated protein distinct from ZO-1, cingulin, and ZO-2. J Cell Biol 120:477–483.
48. Citi S, Sabanay H, Jakes R, Geiger B, Kendrick-Jones J (1988) Cingulin, a new peripheral component of tight junctions. Nature (Lond) 333:272–276.
49. Stevenson BR, Heintzelman MB, Anderson JM, Citi S, Mooseker MS (1989) ZO-1 and cingulin: tight junction proteins with distinct identities and localizations. Am J Physiol 257:C621–C628.
50. Madara J (1987) Intestinal absorptive cell tight junctions are linked to cytoskeleton. Am J Physiol 253:C171–C175.
51. Murphy CR, Swift JG, Mukherjee TM, Rogers AW (1981) Effects of ovarian hormones on cell membranes in the rat uterus. II. Freeze-fracture studies on tight junctions of the lateral plasma membrane of the luminal epithelium. Cell Biophys 3:57–69.
52. Johnson SA, Morgan G, Wooding FBP (1988) Alterations in uterine epithelial tight junction structure during the oestrous cycle and implantation in the pig. J Reprod Fertil 83:915–922.
53. Garfield RE, Ali M, Yallampalli C, Izumi H (1995) Role of gap junctions and nitric oxide in control of myometrial contractility. Sem Perinatol (19:41–51.
54. Winterhager E, Stutenkemper R, Traub O, Beyer E, Willecke K (1991) Expression of different connexin genes in rat uterus during decidualization and at term. Eur J Cell Biol 55:133–142.
55. Winterhager E, Grümmer R, Janh E, Willecke K, Traub O (1993) Spatial and temporal expression of connexin26 and connexin43 in rat endometrium during trophoblast invasion. Dev Biol 157: 399–409.
56. Risek B, Guthrie S, Kumar N, Gilula NB (1990) Modulation of gap junction transcript and protein expression during pregnancy in the rat. J Cell Biol 110:269–282.
57. Goodenough DA, Goliger JA, Paul DL (1996) Connexins, connexons, and intercellular communication. Ann Rev Biochem 65:475–502.
58. Stagg RB, Fletcher WH (1990) The hormone-induced regulation of contact-dependent cell-cell communication by phosphorylation. Endocr Rev 11:302–325.
59. Bennett MVL, Barrio LC, Bargiello TA, Spray DC, Hertzberg E, Saez JC (1991) Gap junctions: new tools, new answers, new questions. Neuron 6:305–320.
60. Willecke K, Hennemann H, Dahl E, Jungbluth S, Heynkes R (1991) The diversity of connexin genes encoding gap junctional proteins. Eur J Cell Biol 56:1–7.
61. Kumar NM, Gilula NB (1996) The gap junction communication channel. Cell 84:381–388.
62. Beyer EC, Paul DL, Goodenough DA (1987) Connexin43: a protein from rat heart homologous to a gap junction protein from liver. J Cell Biol 105:2621–2629.
63. Traub O, Look J, Dermietzel R, Brümmer F, Hülser D, Willecke K (1989) Comparative characterization of the 21-kD and 26-kD gap junction proteins in murine liver and cultured hepatocytes. J Cell Biol 108:1039–1051.

64. Winterhager E, Brümmer F, Dermietzel R, Hulser DF, Denker HW (1988) Gap junction formation in rabbit uterine epithelium in response to embryo recognition. Dev Biol 126:203–211.
65. Grümmer R, Chwalisz K, Mullholland J, Traub O, Winterhager E (1994) Regulation of connexin26 and connexin43 expression in rat endometrium by ovarian steroid hormones. Biol Reprod 51: 1109–1116.
66. Jahn E, Classen-Linke I, Kusche M, Beier HM, Traub O, Grümmer R, Winterhager E (1995) Expression of gap junction connexins in the human endometrium throughout the menstrual cycle. Hum Reprod 10:2666–2670.
67. Risek B, Klier G, Phillips A, Hahn DW, Gilula NB (1995) Gap junction regulation in the uterus and ovaries of immature rats by estrogen and progesterone. J Cell Sci 108:1017–1032.
68. Brady HA, Blanchard TL, Evans JW, Varner DD, D WE, Schwab CA, Risek B, Gilula NB, Burghardt RC (1995) Gap junction expression in equine endometrium. Biol Reprod Monogr 1:507–514.
69. Burghardt RC, Bowen JA, Day WE, Barhoumi R, Bazer FW, Glasser SR, Newton GR (1996) Comparative analysis of gap junction protein expression in porcine, equine, and caprine endometrium. Biol Reprod 54(Suppl 1):174a.
70. Bowen JA (1996) The development and characterization of a polarized in vitro model of porcine uterine epithelial cells. PhD thesis, Texas A&M University, College Station, TX.
71. Wassarman PM (1987) Early events in mammalian fertilization. Ann Rev Cell Biol 3:109–142.
72. Oriol JG, Betteridge KJ, Clarke AJ, Sharom FJ (1993) Mucin-like glycoproteins in the equine embryonic capsule. Mol Reprod Dev 34:255–265.
73. Braga VM, Gendler SJ (1993) Modulation of Muc-1 mucin expression in the mouse uterus during the estrus cycle and early pregnancy. J Cell Sci 105:397–405.
74. Aplin JD, Hey NA (1995) MUC1, endometrium and embryo implantation. Biochem Soc Trans 23:826–831.
75. Bowen JA, Bazer FW, Burghardt RC (1996) Spatial and temporal analyses of integrin and Muc-1 expression in porcine uterine epithelium and trophectoderm in vivo. Biol Reprod 55:1098–1106.
76. Hild-Petito S, Fazleabas A, Julian J, Carson DD (1996) Mucin (Muc-1) expression is differentially regulated in uterine luminal and glandular epithelia of the baboon (*Papio anubis*). Biol Reprod 54:939–947.
77. Tawia SA, Beaton LA, Rogers PAW (1993) Immunolocalization of the cellular adhesion molecules, intercellular adhesion molecule-1 (ICAM-1) and platelet endothelial cell adhesion molecule (PECAM-1), in human endometrium throughout the menstrual cycle. Hum Reprod 8:175–181.
78. Lessey BA, Ilesanmi AO, Lessey MA, Riben M, Harris JE, Chwalisz K (1996) Luminal and glandular endometrial epithelium express integrins differentially throughout the menstrual cycle: Implications for implantation, contraception, and infertility. Am J Reprod Immunol 35:195–204.
79. MacLaren LA, Wildeman AG (1995) Fibronectin receptors in preimplantation development: cloning, expression, and localization of the $\alpha5$ and $\beta1$ integrin subunits in bovine trophoblast. Biol Reprod 53:153–165.
80. Nishida T, Murakami J, Otori T (1991) Expression of fibronectin receptor (integrin) in the uterus of rats in relation to the estrous cycle. Histochemistry 96:279–283.
81. Lessey BA, Castelbaum AJ (1995) Integrins in the endometrium. Reprod Med Rev 4:43–58.
82. Aplin JD, Seif MW, Graham RA, Hey NA, Behzad F, Campbell S (1994) The endometrial cell surface and implantation. Expression of the polymorphic mucin MUC-1 and adhesion molecules during the endometrial cycle. Ann NY Acad Sci 734:103–121.
83. Kimber SJ, Lindenberg S, Lundblad A (1988) Distribution of some Gal β1-24 GlcNAc related carbohydrate antigens on the mouse uterine epithelium in relation to the peri-implantation period. J Reprod Immunol 12:297–313.
84. Lindenberg S, Sundberg K, Kimber SJ, Lundblad A (1988) The milk oligosaccharide, lacto-*N*-fucopentaose I, inhibits attachment of mouse blastocysts on endometrial monolayers. J Reprod Fertil 83:149–158.
85. Chavez DJ, Anderson TL (1985) The glycocalyx of the mouse uterine luminal epithelium during estrus, early pregnancy, the peri-implantation period, and delayed implantation. I. Acquisition of *Ricinus communis* I binding sites during pregnancy. Biol Reprod 32:1135–1142.
86. Dutt A, Carson DD (1990) Lactosaminoglycan assembly, cell surface expression, and release by mouse uterine epithelial cells. J Biol Chem 265:430–438.
87. Hadley MA, Weeks BS, Kleinman HK, Dym M (1990) Laminin promotes formation of cord-like structures by Sertoli cells in vitro. Dev Biol 140:318–327.

88. Sutherland AE, Anderson RD, M Mayes, Seiberg, M, Calarco PG, Bernfield M, Damsky CH (1991) Expression of syndecan, a putative low affinity fibroblast growth factor receptor, in the early mouse embryo. Development 113:339–351.
89. Carson DD, Tang JP, Julian J (1993) Heparin sulfate proteoglycan (perlecan) expression by mouse embryos during acquisition of attachment competence. Dev Biol 155:97–106.
90. Rohde LH, Carson DD (1993) Heparin-like glycosaminoglycans participate in binding of human trophoblastic cell line (JAR) to a human uterine epithelial cell line (RL95). J Cell Physiol 155: 185–196.
91. Tang J-P, Julian J, Glasser SR, Carson DD (1987) Heparan sulfate proteoglycan syntheses and metabolism by mouse uterine epithelial cells in vitro. J Biol Chem 262:12,832–12,842.
92. Rohde LH, Julian J, Babaknia A, Carson DD (1996) Cell surface expression of HIP, a novel Heparin/heparan sulfate-binding protein, of human uterine epithelial cells and cell lines. J Biol Chem 271:11,824–11,830.
93. Fukuda MN, Sato T, Nakayama J, Klier G, Mikami M, Aoki D, Nozawa S (1995) Trophinin and tastin, a novel cell adhesion molecule complex with potential involvement in embryo implantation. Genes Dev 9:1199–1210.
94. Albers A, Thie M, Hohn H-P, Denker H-W (1995) Differential expression and localization of integrins and CD44 in the membrane domains of human uterine epithelial cells during the menstrual cycle. Acta Anat 153:12–19.
95. Yaegashi N, Fujita N, Yajima A, Nakamura M (1995) Menstrual cycle dependent expression of CD44 in normal human endometrium. Hum Pathol 26:862–865.
96. Hohn H-P, Huch G, Tlolka U, Denker H-W (1995) Differential expression of CD44 in rabbit uterine epithelium during early pregnancy. Acta Anat 152:185–194.
97. Kadokawa Y, Fuketa I, Nose A, Takeichi M, Nadatsuji N (1989) Expression pattern of E- and P-cadherin in mouse embryos during the peri-implantation period. Dev Growth Differ 31:23–30.
98. Vestweber D, Gossler A, Boller K, Kemler R (1987) Expression and distribution of cell adhesion molecule uvomorulin in mouse preimplantation embryos. Dev Biol 124:451–456.
99. Wegner CC, Carson DD (1994) Cell adhesion processes in implantation. Oxford Rev Reprod Biol 16:87–137.
100. Takeichi M (1991) Cadherin cell adhesion receptors as a morphogenetic regulator. Science 251: 1451–1455.
101. Ruck P, Marzusch K, Kaiserling E, Horny HP, Dietl J, Geiselhart A, Handgretinger R, Redman CW (1994) Distribution of cell adhesion molecules in decidua of early human pregnancy. An immunohistochemical study. Lab Invest 71:94–101.
102. Svalander PC, Odin P, Nilsson BO, Obrink B (1990) Expression of cellCAM-105 in the apical surface of rat uterine epithelium is controlled by ovarian steroid hormones. J Reprod Fertil 88: 213–221.
103. Brown LF, Bers B, Van Dewater L (1992) Expression and distribution of oesteopontin in human tissues: Widespread association with luminal epithelial surfaces. Mol Biol Cell 3:1169–1180.
104. Feinberg RF, Kliman HJ, Lockwood CJ (1991) Is oncofetal fibronectin a trophoblast glue for human implantation? Am J Pathol 138:537:543.
105. Turpeenniemi-Hujanen T, Feinberg RF, Kauppila A, Puistola U (1995) Extracellular matrix interactions in early humanembryos: implications for normal implantation events. Fertil Steril 64: 132–138.
106. Turpeenniemi-Hujanen T, Thorgeirsson UP, Rao CN, Liotta LA (1992) Laminin in the human embryo implantation: analogy to the invasion of malignant cells. Fertil Steril 58:105–113.
107. Wu T-C, Wan Y-J, Chung AE, Damjanov I (1983) Immunohistochemical localization of entactin and laminin in mouse embryos and fetuses. Dev Biol 100:496–505.
108. Bianco P Fisher LW, Young MF, Termine JD, Gehron Robey P (1991) Expression of bone sialoprotein (BSP) in developing human tissues. Calcif Tissue Int 49:421–426.
109. Julian J, Chiquet-Ehrismann R, Erikson HP, Carson DD (1994) Tenascin is induced at the implantation sites in the mouse uterus and interferes with epithelial cell adhesion. Development 120: 661–671.
110. Vollmer G, Siegal GP, Chiquet-Ehrismann R, Lightner VA, Arnholdt H, Knuppen R (1990) Tenascin expression in the human endometrium and in endometrial adenocarcinomas. Lab Invest 62:725–730.
111. Pemberton L, Taylor-Papadimitrou J, Gendler SJ (1992) Antibodies to the cytoplasmic domain of Muc-1 mucin show conservation throughout mammals. Biochem Biophys Res Commun 185: 167–175.

112. Hilkens J, Ligtenberg MJL, Vos HL, Litvinov SV (1992) Cell membrane-associated mucins and their adhesion-modulating properties. TIBS 17:359-363.
113. Wesseling J, van der Valk SE, Vos HL, Sonnenberg A, Hilkens J (1995) Episialin (MUC1) over-expression inhibits integrin-mediated cell adhesion to extracellular matrix components. J Cell Biol 129:255-265.
114. Hey NA, Graham RA, Seif MW, and Aplin JD (1994) The polymorphic epithelial mucin Muc1 in human endometrium is regulated with maximal expression in the implantation phase. J Clin Endocrinol Metab 78:337-342.
115. Aplin JD, Hey NA, Li TC (1996) MUC1 as a cell surface and secretory component of endometrial epithelium: reduced levels in recurrent miscarriage. Am J Reprod Immunol 35:261-266.
116. Hynes RO (1992) Integrins: Versatility, modulation, and signaling in cell adhesion. Cell 69:11-25.
117. Luscinskas FW, Lawler J (1994) Integrins as dynamic regulators of vascular function. FASEB J 8:929-938.
118. Gullberg D, Velling T, Sjoberg G, Sejersen T (1995) Up-regulation of a novel integrin α-chain (α_{mt}) on human fetal myotubes. Dev Dynamics 204:57-65.
119. Tabibzadeh S (1990) Immunoreactivity of human endometrium: correlation with endometrial dating. Fertil Steril 54:624-631.
120. Lessey BA, Damjanovich L, Coutifaris C, Castelbaum A, Albelda SM, Buck CA (1992) Integrin adhesion molecules in the human endometrium. Correlation with the normal and abnormal menstrual cycle. J Clin Invest 90:188-195.
121. Sutherland AE, Calarco PG, Damsky CH (1993) Developmental regulation of integrin expression at the time of implantation in the mouse embryo. Development 119:1175-86.
122. Humphries MJ (1993) Mechanisms of ligand binding by integrins. Biochem Soc Trans 22:275-282.
123. Damsky C, Sutherland A, Fisher S (1993) Extracellular matrix 5: Adhesive interactions in early mammalian embryogenesis, implantation and placentation. FASEB J 7:1320-1329.
124. Lessey BA, Lei Y, Castlebaum AJ, Yowell CW, Buck CA, Sun J (1994) Further characterization of endometrial integrins during the menstural cycle and in pregnancy. Fertil Steril 62:497-506.
125. Fazleabas AT, Bell SC, Flemming A, Sun J, Lessey B (1997) Distribution of integrins and the extracellular matrix proteins in the baboon endometrium during the menstrual cycle and early pregnancy. Biol Reprod 56:348-356.
126. Kao LC, Caltabiano S, Wu S, Strauss JF III, Kliman HJ (1988) The human villous cytotrophoblast: interactions with extracellular matrix proteins, endocrine function, and cytoplasmic differentiation in the absence of syncytium formation. Dev Biol 130:693-702.
127. Campbell S, Swann HR, Seif MW, Kimber SJ, Aplin JD (1995) Cell adhesion molecules on the oocyte and preimplantation human embryo. Hum Reprod 10:1571-1578.
128. Cross JC, Werb Z, Fisher SJ (1994) Implantation and the placenta: Key pieces of the development puzzle. Science 266:1508-1518.
129. Tuo W, Bazer FW (1996) Expression of oncofetal fibronectin by porcine conceptuses and uterus throughout gestation. Reprod Fertil Dev 8:1207-1214.
130. Enders AC, Schlafke S (1974) Surface coats of the mouse blastocyst and uterus during the preimplantation period. Anat Rec 180:31-45.
131. Hewitt K, Beer AE, Grinnell F (1979) Disappearance of anionic sites from the surface of the rat endometrial epithelium at the time of blastocyst implantation. Biol Reprod 21:691-707.
132. Kimber SJ, Lindenberg S (1990) Hormonal control of a carbohydrate epitope involved in implantation in mice. J Reprod Fertil 89:13-21.
133. Kimber SJ, White S, Cook A, Illingworth I (1994) The initiation of implantation: parallels between attachment of the embryo and neutrophil-endothelial interaction, In: Gamete and Embryo Quality (Mastroianni L, Jr, Coelingh Bennink HJT, Suzuki S, Vemer HM, eds.), Parthenon, London, pp. 171-198.
134. Carson DD, Wilson OF, Dutt A (1990) Glycoconjugate expression and interactions at the cell surface of mouse uterine epithelial cells and peri-implantation stage embryos. Trophoblast Res 4:211-241.
135. Liu S, Smith SE, Julian J, Rohde LH, Karin NJ, Carson DD (1996) cDNA cloning and expression of HIP, a novel cell surface heparan sulfate/heparin-binding protein of human uterine epithelial cells and cell lines. J Biol Chem 271:11,817-11,823.
136. Das SK, Wang XN, Paria BC, Damm D, Abraham JA, Klagsbrun M, Andrews GK, Dey SK (1994) Heparin-binding EGF-like growth factor gene is induced in the mouse uterus temporally by the blastocyst solely at the site of its opposition: a possible ligand for interaction with blastocyst EGF-receptor in implantation. Development 120:1071-1083.

137. Raab G, Kover K, Paria B, Dey SK, Ezzell RM (1996) Mouse preimplantation blastocysts adhere to cells expressing the transmembrane form of heparin-binding EGF-like growth factor. Development 122:637–645.
138. Tuo W, Harney JP, Bazer FW (1995) Colony-stimulating factor-1 in conceptus and uterine tissues in pigs. Biol Reprod 53:133–142.
139. Albelda SM (1993) Biology of disease. Role of integrins and other cell adhesion molecules in tumor progression and metastasis. Lab Invest 68:4–17.
140. Tedder TF, Steeber DA, Chen A, Engel P (1995) The selectins: vascular adhesion molecules. FASEB J 9:866–873.
141. Etzioni A (1996) Adhesion molecules—their role in health and disease. Pediatr Res 39:191–198.
142. Kimber SJ, Brown DG, Pahlsson P, Nilsson B (1993) Carbohydrate antigen expression in murine embryonic stem cells and embryos. II. Sialylated antigens and glycolipid analysis. Histochem J 25:628–641.
143. Williams AF, Barclay AN (1988) The immunoglobulin superfamily. Domains for cell surface recognition. Ann Rev Immunol 6:381–405.
144. Obrink B (1991) C-CAM (cell-CAM 105) a member of the growing immunoglobulin superfamily of cell adhesion proteins. Bioessays 13:227–234.
145. Schweighoffer T, Shaw S (1992) Adhesion cascades: Diversity through combinatorial strategies. Curr Opinion Cell Biol 4:824–829.
146. Giancotti FG, Mainiero F (1994) Integrin-mediated adhesion and signaling in tumorigenesis. Biochim Biophys Acta 1198:47–64.
147. Stewart M, Thiel M, Hogg N (1995) Leukocyte integrins. Curr Opinion Cell Biol 7:690–696.
148. Schwartz MA, Schaller MD, Ginsberg MH (1995) Integrins: Emerging paradigms of signal transduction. Annu Rev Cell Dev Biol 11:549–599.
149. Skierczynski BA, Skalak R, Chien S (1995) Modeling of molecular mechanisms of cell adhesion. Biochem Cell Biol 73:399–409.
150. Roberson SA, Seamark RF, Guilbert LJ, Wegmann TG (1994) The role of cytokines in gestation. Crit Rev Immunol 14:239–292.
151. Conforti G, Zanetti A, Paxquali-Ronchetti I, Quaglino D, Neyroz P, Dejana E (1990) Modulation of vitronectin receptor binding by membrane lipid composition. J Biol Chem 265:4011–4019.
152. Hermanowski-Vosatka A, Van Strijp JAG, Swiggard WJ, Wright SD (1992) Integrin modulating factor-1: A lipid that alters the function of leukocyte integrins. Cell 68:341–352.
153. Clark RA, Brugge JS (1995) Integrins and signal transduction pathways: The road taken. Science 268:233–239.
154. Miyamoto S, Teramoto H, Coso OA, Gutkind S, Burbelo PD, Akiyama SK, Yamada KM (1995) Integrin function: molecular hierarchies of cytoskeletal and signaling molecules. J Cell Biol 131: 791–805.
155. Bentin-Ley U, Pedersen B, Lindenberg S, Falck Larsen J, Hamberger L, Horn T (1994) Isolation and culture of human endometrial cells in a three-dimensional culture system. J Reprod Fertil 101:327–332.
156. Jacobs AL, Decker GL, Glasser SR, Julian J, Carson DD (1990) Vectorial secretion of prostaglandins by polarized rodent uterine epithelial cells. Endocrinology 126:2125–2136.
157. Bowen JA, Newton GR, Weiss DW, Bazer F, Burghardt RC (1996) Characterization of a polarized porcine uterine epithelial cell model system. Biol Reprod 55:613–619.
158. Bowen JA, Bazer FW, Burghardt RC (1997) Spatial and temporal analyses of integrin and Muc-1 expression in porcine uterine epithelium and trophectoderm in vitro. Biol Reprod 56:409–415.
159. Edwards RG (1995) Clinical approaches to increasing uterine receptivity during human implantation. Hum Reprod 10 (Suppl 2):60–66.

9 The Influences of Immune Cells on the Success of Pregnancy

B. A. Croy, DVM, PHD, *P. F. Whitelaw*, BSC, PHD, *and H. Engelhardt*, BSC, MSC, PHD

INTRODUCTION

It is widely held that the immune system evolved for maintaining the health of an individual. Health promotion is achieved through the ability of immune competent T-cells to recognize pathogens and respond to them, in a manner causing elimination of the pathogens. However, since immune responses are triggered by a far broader range of peptides than those presented by pathogenic organisms, the concept evolved that the purpose of the immune system is discrimination between antigens representing self and nonself. Many of the ideas associated with self/nonself discrimination have been defined by organ and bone marrow transplantation. The development of tumors and the successful gestation of a fetus are two medical conditions thought to represent an overwhelming or failure of the mechanisms for self/nonself discrimination.

The immune system is a dynamic system of highly integrated subcomponents. Immune responses can be either antigen-specific or innate. The latter responses are also called natural immunity or nonspecific immunity. For antigen-specific immune responses, gene rearrangements in thymus-derived (T) and/or bone marrow-derived (B) lymphocytes provide unique antigen recognition elements, and responses develop over an interval of several days. Innate immune responses require no gene rearrangements, and the response is immediate in the prototype cells natural killer lymphocytes (NK cells), macrophages, and neutrophils.

A different classification of the immune system is systemic vs mucosal *(1)*. Linked together in the systemic immune system are liver, bone marrow, thymus, spleen, peripheral blood, lymph nodes, and thoracic duct. In many textbooks, the mucosal immune system is presented as the gastrointestinal tract, with its specialized lymphoid Peyer's patches and the respiratory system *(2,3)*. The reproductive tracts of both the female and male must be considered important components of the mucosal immune system. Since the female reproductive tract is under cyclic endocrine regulation during the reproductive phase of life, it is worth considering that there are unique immunological events and important neuroendocrine–immune relationships awaiting definition.

Evidence supporting sexual differences in immune responses has been obtained from both clinical reports and experimental studies. In females, puberty, pregnancy, lactation, and menopause induce changes in the immune system. Hormonally correlated differences in the immune system have been particularly well documented in autoimmune disease states *(4)*. The mechanisms by which the endocrine and nervous systems influence the immune system are not fully understood.

Pregnancy is an interval of special physiology in female mammals. Immunologically, the conceptus is a "nonself" or "foreign" component that over the course of gestation, will express developmentally regulated, unique embryonic antigens and paternally inherited antigens that stimulate the mothers immune system. Tissues expressing foreign antigens are grafts. Presentation of graft antigens, particularly a major histocompatibility complex (MHC) antigen haplotype, usually leads to acute (7–10 d) graft rejection. The conceptus, however, is not rejected. By analogy to organ transplantation, the mother is therefore considered to be immunologically tolerant of her developing offspring. The idea of maternal immune tolerance of the fetus has several implications. First, it implies that the immune participates in the promotion of pregnancy in ways beyond the simple maintenance of maternal systemic and uterine health. Second, it suggests that breakdown of tolerance will interrupt a pregnancy and result in active immune rejection of the fetus. Thus, fetal death and abortion or resorption could be interpreted as immunological events.

The fetal allograft hypothesis has dominated the thinking and experimental design of reproductive immunologists for almost 50 yr *(5)*. Recently, a strong challenge was raised against this hypothesis *(6)*, and investigators were urged to reappraise this central paradigm of reproductive immunology. The basis for this recommendation was that the fetal allograft hypothesis is steeped in the thinking of antigen-specific immunity, whereas over the past decade, most studies have suggested that the innate or nonspecific immune system dominates in the pregnant uterus *(6–8)*. Loke and King *(6)* suggest that invertebrates, particularly marine sponges, offer a model where, following recognition by natural immune mechanisms, interacting individuals secrete a collagen barrier between themselves to maintain independence. Although this is an extremely attractive position, it is not fully supported by the literature, since it implies too rigidly that the maternal–fetal interface is impervious to cell trafficking. Trafficking of immune-competent cells from the mother into the fetus and from the fetus into the mother, across the hemochorial placenta is well documented. This bidirectional movement of cells during gestation may be the basis for fetal allograft success or may be a random event of little significance *(9)*. Lymphoid microchimerism has been associated with successful organ engraftment. Long-term (25 yr+) survivors of human liver transplants who are removed from immunosuppressive drug therapy fall into two groups. One group undergoes acute rejection; the other sustains the transplant without drug therapy. Patients in the latter group have been found to have very low levels of lymphohematopoietic cells of the genotype of the original organ donor in their blood, marrow, and/or skin *(10)* which is postulated as the major mechanism providing clinical organ allograft success.

The hypothesis that cells of the innate immune system found in the pregnant uterus may be specialized or unique subsets with important functions in pregnancy promotion can be assessed whether or not one adheres to the notion that the fetus is an allograft. In mice, genetic depletion of lymphocytes from the NK cell lineage, but not from the T- or B-cell lineages, has been shown to reduce the success of pregnancy. This suggests that at least in mice, the only lymphocytes having truly critical functions associated with normal pregnancy are NK cells. The influences of the NK cell population were postimplantation and linked to placental growth, vascular relaxation, and fetal survival *(11,12)*. It is expected that this pregnancy-promoting function of the murine, innate immune system will have immunological parallels, although perhaps with variant mechanistic details *(13)*, in humans and livestock species.

This chapter will address briefly the major components of the immune system and tolerance. Definitions for abbreviated terms are found on p. 272. Influences of pregnancy and the endocrine system on the immune system will be discussed at both the systemic level and the local uterine level in several species. The suspected importance of the innate immune system, particularly NK cells, on fetal development will be emphasized.

THE LYMPHOHEMATOPOIETIC SYSTEM

Immune Competent Cells and Their Functions

The lymphohematopoietic system includes all cells found in blood, related cells found in tissues, and their progenitors and stem cells. Stem cells have the potential to generate all of the lymphohematopoietic cells. Progenitor cells are more restricted in the families of descendent cells they produce. The immune system is considered to have two or three lineages: lymphocytes, monocytes/macrophages, and usually neutrophils. Differentiation of immune competent cells from stem cells and progenitor cells is a unidirectional process, and the cells produced have finite-life spans that are well defined in many species. Antigen-specific lymphocytes (B-cells and T-cells) are thought to develop clonally, from individual, unique cells. In adults, bone marrow is considered the major source of both stem cells and progenitor cells.

Lymphocytes are divided into three classes. These are B-cells, derived from the bone marrow in mammals or the Bursa of Fabricius in birds, T-cells, which are lymphocytes that undergo a process of maturation within the thymus, and NK cells. The differentiation pathway of NK cells is less well defined than that of B-cells or T-cells. Deletion of the zinc-finger DNA binding transcription factor Ikaros results in transgenic mice without lymphocytes. This suggests that all lymphocytes are derived from a common progenitor *(14)*. B-cells differentiate to become antibody-producing cells and memory cells by the process of immunoglobulin (Ig) gene rearrangement. B-cells are subdivided into five subtypes by the Ig heavy chains they express.

T-cells are mature, postthymic, antigen-specific cells that have undergone rearrangement of three gene families to produce four antigen-specific T-cell receptor (TCR) chains. These are expressed in dimer pairs as $\alpha\beta$ or $\gamma\delta$. T-cells are stimulated by the presentation of short peptides processed from larger molecules, pathogens, or cells by antigen-presenting cells (APCs), which include macrophages, dendritic cells, which may be macrophage-related *(15)*, or memory B-cells *(16)*. B-cell antigen presentation occurs only in interactions with antigen-experienced, but not naive T-cells *(16)*. T-cells are subdivided by their antigen-induced responses into T-helper cells and T-cytotoxic/suppressor cells. Surface antisera distinguish between these as $CD4^+$ and $CD8^+$ cells, respectively. $CD4^+$ cells are further subclassified by the pattern of cytokines they produce: Th1 and Th2 cells are the most widely recognized, although there are others *(17)*. Th1 cells emphasize production of interleukin-2 (IL-2) and interferon gamma (IFNγ), whereas Th2 cells are characterized by their production of IL-4, IL-5, and IL-10. Other cytokines are produced by both of these Th subsets. Peptides are presented to $\alpha\beta$ T-cells in association with a receptor for MHC. Self-MHC is required for stimulation. $CD4^+$ T-cells respond to class II MHC engagement, and $CD8^+$ T-cells respond to class I MHC binding. T-cells expressing the $\gamma\delta$ TCR can respond to peptides in the context of MHC class I or II, but most $\gamma\delta$ T-cells appear to be MHC-independent and recognize larger peptides and nonproteinaceous ligands *(18)*.

Table 1 briefly lists antigens commonly used to discriminate immune competent cells from other cell types and to distinguish the various immune cells from each other. Protors of the T-cell lineage enter the thymus throughout life, and are "educated" in discrimination between self and nonself by thymic epithelial or dendritic cells *(19)*. The thymus is anatomically arranged into three zones. The subcapsular zone contains the most immature T-cell precursors recently arrived from marrow, which are called $CD4^-$ $CD8^-$ or double-negative cells. As the immature cells migrate more deeply into the organ, they enter the cortex, encounter high levels of class I and II MHC antigens, and begin to express both CD4 and CD8. Rearrangement of TCR genes is also initiated in the cortex. Positive selection for self-antigens will permit some of these cells to journey toward the medulla as mature single positive T-cells, either $CD4^+$ $CD8^-$ or $CD4^-$ $CD8^+$, which can exit into the blood and seed organs. Unselected thymocytes will undergo apoptosis in the thymus *(20)*. Most thymocytes (>90%) never emigrate to peripheral sites and die intrathymically. Many $\gamma\delta$ T-cells develop extrathymically and preferentially localize at mucosal surfaces rather than in lymphoid organs *(1,21)*.

The third lymphocyte lineage, the NK cell, is best defined in humans and rodents, but remains less well defined than either the B- or T-cell lineages. Transgenic mice, which have B-cells, but lack both T-cells and NK cells *(22)*, support earlier suggestions that NK cells are more related to T-cells than to B-cells *(23,24)*. NK cells are discriminated from the other lymphocytes by the absence of rearrangements in the genes encoding both the TCR and Igs, and the fact that they are not required to undergo a thymic education. Thus, NK cells and their progenitors are normal in immune-deficient mice, such as the *scid/scid* mouse *(25,26)*, because the mutation alters the recombination of TCR and Igs. Features shared by NK cells and T-cells include several common surface markers (i.e., Thy-1 in mice), common cytolytic machinery (i.e., perforin and serine esterases), and expression of components of CD3. In T-cells, CD3 is a complex of invariant peptides expressed in the cell membrane as a component that stabilizes the TCR and transmits signals to the cytosol following engagement of the TCR *(27,28)*. In NK cells and in their fetal liver or thymic progenitors, the γ, δ, ϵ, and ζ-chains of the CD3 complex can be found cytoplasmically, but the chains are never assembled into the CD3 complex *(24,29)*. NK cells kill target cells without prior activation, demonstrating that their mode of lytic activation differs from that of $CD8^+$ T-cells. T-cells require a longer time to respond and, thus, must be responding to different signals although employing similar killing mechanisms *(30,31)*.

NK cells can be identified by the surface phenotype $CD3^-$, $CD16^+$, and $CD56^+$ in humans and $CD3^-$ $NK1.1^+$ in mice *(32,33)*. Endogenous lytic function against specific targets was originally used to characterize NK cells, and it was also found that on activation with IL-2, NK cells rapidly became lymphokine-activated killer (LAK) cells capable

Table 1
Definitions of Cluster Determinants (CD)

Name	*Cell type for surface expression*	*Functions, where known*[a]
CD2	Thymocytes, T-cells, NK cells	Adhesion, activation, signal transduction
CD3	Thymocytes, T-cells, NK cells[b]	TCR-associated signal transduction
CD4	Thymocytes, class II MHC-restricted T-cells	Signal transduction
CD8	Thymocytes, class I MHC restricted T-cells	Signal transduction
CD11a	Leukocytes	Adhesion
CD11b	NK cells, granulocytes, monocytes	Adhesion
CD14	Monocytes, macrophages	Receptor for lipopolysaccharide
CD16	NK cells, granulocytes, macrophages	Receptor for IgG
CD18	Leukocytes	Adhesion
CD25	Activated lymphocytes and macrophages	IL-2Rα chain
CD34	Immature hemotopoietic cells	—
CD38	Immature lymphocytes, T- and B-cells	—
CD44	Leukocytes, erythrocytes	Homing receptor
CD45	Leukocytes	Signal transduction
CD56	NK cells	Isoform of NCAM
CD69	Activated lymphocytes	Early activation
CD95	Multiple cell types (Fas antigen)	Role in apoptosis

[a] *See* ref. *(2)*.
[b] Expression in NK cells is as unassembled cytoplasmic components.

of killing a wide range of virally infected, malignant, or normal cells. Killing by NK cells and LAK cells is associated with the release of the cytolytic proteins perforin, and serine esterases, which induce apoptotic death in the target cell and probably in the effector cell. IL-2 stimulation also induces the expression of the cytokines, including IFNγ, granulocyte macrophage-colony-stimulating factor (GM-CSF) and tumor necrosis factor-(TNF)α. The lytic activity of NK cells was thought to be "natural," since it did not appear to involve the recognition of antibodies or MHC class II, and was perceived as "non-MHC-restricted." However, this idea has been modified with the identification of specific receptors for MHC class I on the surface of NK cells.

Unlike T-cells, which require self-MHC presentation for target cell lysis, NK cells are inhibited from killing when they recognize target cells expressing MHC class I. Since MHC class I molecules are expressed on all healthy nucleated cells, the "missing self" hypothesis was proposed, *(34,35)* whereby NK cells scrutinize tissues for aberrantly expressed or absent MHC class I molecules, which might be found during tumorigenesis or infection. NK cells would then be freed from inhibitory signals and lyse the affected cell *(30,31,33,36–38)*. Human killer inhibitory receptors (KIR) have been identified (Table 2) which recognize distinct polymorphic determinants of HLA class I molecules (reviewed in *31*), including HLA-A, B, and C *(39,40)*.

In rodents, two families of receptors responsible for NK cell activation have been identified (Table 2). Both are type II transmembrane proteins with extracellular domains that resemble calcium-dependent (C-type) lectins *(38)*, and include NKR-P1 in the rat and NK1.1 in the mouse. In the mouse, most members of the LY-49(A-H) family of receptors inhibit NK killing by recognition of MHC class I molecules *(37)*. The ligands for these receptors are multiple cell-surface oligosaccharides *(52)*. The human NK receptors that have been identified and are sensitive to MHC represent a superfamily of Igs rather than lectins. Unlike the Igs of B-cells, these genes do not appear to undergo any form of somatic rearrangement *(39)*.

Table 2
Terms Currently Related to NK Cell Receptors and Activation Molecules

Species	*Term*	*Multiple genes*	*Dominant signal*	*Reference*
Human	CD16	No	Stimulation	*(41)*
	p58	Yes	Inhibition[b]	*(42)*
	NKB1	Yes	Inhibition[b]	*(43)*
	NKG2[a]	Yes	Inhibition[b]	*(44)*
	CD69	No	Activation	*(45)*
	CD94 (Kp43)[a]	No	Ambivalent	*(46)*
	NKR-P1A	No	Inhibition[b]	*(47)*
	NKAT4	Yes	Inhibition[b]	*(40)*
	NKLAM	No	Inhibition[b]	*(48)*
	p40	No	Inhibition[b]	*(49)*
Rodents	NKR-P1[a]	Yes	Activation	*(37)*
	Ly-49[a]	Yes	Inhibition	*(50)*
	Ly-49G2[a]	No	Activation	*(51)*

[a]Structures possessing C-type lectin domains; others belong to the immunoglobulin superfamily. The murine C-lectin families are located on chromosome 6, but in humans, an NK complex is located on chromosome 12 *(47)*.

[b]KIR: a term applied to groups of receptors associated with inhibition of lytic activity on NK cells. It appears that signaling is required to stimulate KIR, suggesting that the primary default response of NK cells is lysis of the target cell.

Defining the mechanisms for NK cell target recognition is currently an area of vigorous investigation. There is a consensus that NK cells do not recognize a single target MHC structure, but rather multiple target molecules are independently recognized by the effector cell. The density of the multiple recognition structures may play a major role in determining whether a signal for activation or inhibition of lysis is sent to the effector cell *(31)*. Table 2 outlines some of the receptor families found on human and rodent NK cells. Thus, NK cells have a complex receptor pattern that provides specificity without gene rearrangement, whereas T- and B-cells have a complex gene system that provides specificity through a unique receptor molecule. It is important to emphasize that not all NK cells are lytic, despite their name *(53)*, and that their activation results in cytokine production, particularly IFNγ *(32)*.

Neutrophils are cells of the myeloid lineage critical in inflammation. They are usually considered components of innate immunity. They are active phagocytes that kill microorganisms more rapidly than macrophages. Neutrophils are exquisitively sensitive to chemotactic signals (i.e., IL-8) *(54)*, and are generally the first cells recruited to sites of acute inflammation *(2)*. The mechanisms for diapedesis (i.e., the movement of cells from blood vessels into tissues) were initially defined through studies of neutrophils, but are also applicable to lymphocytes *(55,56)*.

Monocytes and macrophages are usually considered together as circulating and tissue forms in a common lineage. They are phagocytic cells that play important roles in processing of antigen and its presentation to lymphocytes. Differentiation of promonocytes in marrow is followed by egress of the cells to blood, and after a brief period of circulation, migration into tissues and final maturation. Kupffer cells of liver, alveolar macrophages, and brain microglia are all members of the monocyte/macrophage cell lineage. Macrophages are readily identified in the female reproductive tract *(57,58)*, but uterine macrophages have not been characterized as unique or specialized forms of the lineage.

Macrophages are microbicidal, cytotoxic cells whose functions are greatly enhanced in the presence of IFNγ. Macrophages are early participants in the acute inflammatory response. Their recruitment is followed by release of IL-1, IL-6, and TNF-α *(59)*. These cytokines act locally on fibroblasts and endothelial cells to increase vascular permeability and alter expression of adhesion molecules *(3)*. A parallel is often drawn between implantation of the conceptus and acute inflammatory events.

Dendritic cells are the final cell population associated with the immune system. They are bone marrow-derived cells found at sites commonly exposed to foreign antigens, such as skin, gastrointestinal tract, and lung. Dendritic cells have extensive stellate cytoplasmic processes, and are so central to antigen processing and presentation that they are often distinguished as "professional" APCs *(16)*. Dendritic cells have not yet been carefully distinguished from macrophages and subjected to extensive study in the uterus, but they have been mapped within the vagina and cervix *(58)*, sites routinely exposed to microbial agents and the components of seminal ejaculate.

Differentiation of the Lymphohematopoietic Lineages During Fetal Development

Since the fertilized zygote develops into a fetus, all cells in an individual have a common origin. During development, commitment to the various tissue lineages is usually not reversible. Many investigators, including those with interests in developmental biology and in cytokine, cell, and gene therapies, have sought to define mechanisms for commitment by studying relationships between committed progenitor cells both prenatally and postnatally *(60,61)*. The central dogma held for differentiation of lymphohematopoietic cells is that the progenitors first appear in embryos within blood islands of the yolk sac, migrate to fetal liver and the thymus, and, near term, become localized within bone marrow. In adults, the marrow alone remains as the progenitor tissue *(62–65)*. Many cytokines were first characterized by their capacity to direct lineage commitment during lymphohematopoietic cell differentiation.

Clinical interest in therapeutic human bone marrow transplantation has spurred extensive work on lymphohematopoietic progenitors, cytokines, and cytokine receptors using animal models. This has resulted in recent modifications of the lymphoid differentiation paradigm. It is now thought that an embryo-wide, multisite initiation of lymphohematopoiesis occurs in undifferentiated mesenchyme. This occurs on d 8.0 of gestation in the mouse, prior to development of the liver anlage. In concert with the development of blood islands in the fetal yolk sac, the paraortic splanchnopleure differentiates multipotential cells called colony-forming units, which include the progenitors of B-cells. The subsequent development of the fetal liver incorporates these cells, giving them the ability to circulate in the embryo *(66–69)*. It had also been thought that the peripheral blood and liver of adults did not contain pluripotent stem cells. However, this has been discounted in both humans and experimental animals, since adult liver, when grafted, can establish multiple, donor-derived hematopoietic lineages in recipients *(10,70)*. Flow cytometric studies of normal adult human blood has identified circulating lymphoid stem cells, characterized by their expression of the phenotypic markers CD34 and CD38 *(71)*. These cells are at a low frequency in peripheral blood, making human placental cord blood a more commonly sought source for CD34$^+$ stem cells for gene therapy-associated transplantation than adult peripheral blood *(72)*. Adult bone marrow and fetal liver are the most frequently used sources of CD34$^+$ cells for conventional transplantation *(73)*.

The T-lymphocyte lineage appears to be the earliest pathway to which lymphocytes can become committed. In mice (term = 19–20 d), pro-T-cells migrate in blood from both the yolk sac and liver to the thymic anlage as it develops between d 10 and 11 of gestation *(74)*. Pro-B-cells also circulate before entering the developing marrow as mature pro-B-cells (B220 antigen-positive) at d 17 of gestation *(69)*.

Less is known regarding establishment of the NK cell lineage during development. One reason for this may be the continuing difficulties in cloning murine NK cells. Tissue-culture techniques, including organ culture, clonal assays, and limiting dilution cloning, have been of major importance in defining the pathways of differentiation for both T-cells and B-cells. These approaches have defined the cytokines critical for the viability of the progenitor cells and for their commitment to maturation. Cloning has provided large numbers of identical, stable cells as lines that facilitated the understanding of the receptors on T- and B-cells and the responses of individual cells (i.e., signal transduction and regulation of genes, lysis and antibody or cytokine secretion) to stimuli. Clones were also vital for isolation of many cytokine receptor genes, understanding mechanisms of cytokine actions *(75)*, and quantification of cytokine levels by bioassay. Although long-term NK cell clones have been developed from human blood *(42,76)* and short-term human NK cell clones have been obtained from uterine decidua *(77,78)*, clones of murine NK cells have been difficult to obtain. In rodents, only a single rat tumor, NKR-1, has been widely available as a cell line to represent the NK cell lineage *(79)*.

In mice, transgenic manipulations have been more successful than cloning for gaining insight into the NK cell differentiation pathway. There are no spontaneous mutations deleting murine NK cells. The widely known *beige* mutation reduces lytic function in NK cells, but does not reduce NK cell frequency *(80)*. In 1995, DiSanto and his colleagues reported the first mouse with an immune deficiency that was almost exclusively an NK cell deficiency *(81)*. This mouse was produced by knockout of the IL-2Rγ chain gene, a situation that parallels a group of the human immune deficiency diseases *(82)*. Wang et al. *(22)* had previously reported several strains of transgenic mice deficient in both NK cells and T-cells, whereas Georgopoulos et al. *(14)* had obtained mice deficient in NK, T-, and B-cells by knockout of the Ikaros gene. The Wang mice overexpress a human transgene for CD3E under control of an endogenous promoter, resulting in death of the cells transcribing the transgene in the thymus at d 13 of gestation *(22)*. Renard and colleagues *(83)* knocked out the endogenous murine gene for CD3E, but did not observe the same phenotype, leaving open the basis for the NK cell lineage deficit in the human CD3E transgenic mice. Work with 6-wk-old human fetuses has also suggested that at least some NK progenitor cells are present in thymus *(24,33)*. It is uncertain, however, whether decidual blood cell contamination of this abortus-derived preparation may have contributed to the detection of NK progenitor cells *(84)*.

Postnatally, precursors of all of the lymphohematopoietic lineages are present in marrow. A life history proposed for NK cells from studies in mature mice is that most NK cells have a short life-span (2–4 d). They are continuously transported from marrow to spleen where they reside in a quiescent state awaiting signals for activation and recruitment to sites of need *(85–90)*. Some NK cells (10%) have a life-span of at least 2 mo. By comparison to the systemic immune system or the local immune system in the gastrointestinal tract, there are few studies on the development of the lymphocyte lineages within the fetal or juvenile uterus *(91–93)*.

Influences of the Endocrine System on the Normal Systemic Immune System

There is mounting experimental evidence for bidirectional regulation between the immune/inflammatory system and the neuroendocrine system. Regulatory molecules originally described in one system are known to affect cells in the other system. These molecules include steroids, cytokines, and neuropeptides. Systemic effects of pregnancy on the immune systems of normal females have been documented. These include increases in plasma concentrations of the cytokine IL-1 following ovulation *(94)* and of colony-stimulating factor-1 (CSF-1) in early gestation *(95)*, a decrease in the proportion of B-cells in marrow and blood *(96,97)*, and transient shifts in the numbers of circulating NK cells *(98,99)*. DNA repair in peripheral blood leukocytes (PBL) from women was found to be less successful during pregnancy than when cells from the same individuals were reassessed 6 wk postpartum *(100)*.

The mother's thymus experiences a dramatic depletion in lymphocytes during gestation *(101)*. Since the thymus produces multiple neuroendocrine mediators, including adrenocorticotropin, endorphins, gonadotropin-releasing hormone, norepinephrine, thyroid-stimulating hormone, and prolactin *(4)*, the lymphocyte depletion could be under neuroendocrine control. Loss of thymocytes during pregnancy could represent enhanced apoptosis or an enhanced exodus to peripheral tissues. However recent experiments support another mechanism. Ruhsinghani and colleagues *(102)* suggest, from the surface phenotyping patterns they obtained on murine thymocytes, that during pregnancy, T-cell development is blocked in the mother's thymus at the precursor level. They further suggest that this block in thymopoiesis may represent a mechanism for induction of maternal tolerance to the fetus. A gradual recovery of all of the thymocyte subsets occurs postpartum, but recovery is delayed by lactation. Thymocyte depletion was also achieved by administration of estradiol to nonpregnant mice *(102)*. This is consistent with an increase in "intermediate" T-cells (i.e., having the surface phenotype $CD4^-/CD8^-$, but TCR $\alpha\beta^+$ or TCR $\gamma\delta^+$) reported by Kimura and colleagues *(103)* in the liver and uterus of pregnant mice. The surface phenotype of the expanded T-cells is typical of extrathymic T-cell differentiation, which may be stimulated to compensate for pregnancy-induced thymic atrophy.

Only limited data support direct, receptor-mediated actions by progesterone or estrogen on immune competent cells in blood. Using a polyclonal antibody reagent to the human progesterone receptor (PR), Szekeres-Bartho *(104)* has found PR expression among PBL of pregnant women with impending abortion. Others have contradictory data *(105)*. In culture, progesterone favors development of human $CD4^+$ T-cells producing Th2-type cytokines *(106)*.

There are more data to support expression of estrogen receptor (ER) on immune competent cells, including thymocytes and macrophages. Expression of ER by endothelial cells could also contribute to the shifts among immune competent cells observed in various organs during pregnancy *(107)*. Estrogens have been shown to enhance human NK cell proliferation and lytic activity, which is blocked by the antiestrogen tamoxifen and not - induced by testosterone or progesterone *(108,109)*. The cloned human NK cell line YT-NI7 was shown to express 11.8 fmol/mg protein of ER, which was estimated at 5- to 10-fold greater than ER expression by other types of lymphohematopoietic cell lines *(108)*. Further, antiestrogens structurally related to tamoxifen, such as raloxifene and idoxifene, have been used with success in the treatment of autoimmune diseases. It is postulated that the therapeutic effect may be indirect and mediated through induction of immunosuppressive molecules *(110)*.

The expression of human chorionic gonadotropin/luteinizing hormone (hCG/LH) receptors by human lymphocytes has been inferred from functional studies, but it is relatively recently that proof of receptor expression was presented using nested reverse transcriptase polymerase chain reaction (RT-PCR) *(111)*. Gene expression was shown in a blood leukocyte subset prepared by Ficoll-Paque density gradient centrifugation and in blood T-cells recovered from a T-cell-enrichment column. The data were confirmed by immunoblotting. This study by Lin et al. *(111)* did not include analyses of the depleted blood or leukocyte fractions or samples from nonpregnant women, which limits the interpretations that can be made. Substance P, a neuropeptide, alters the cytokine release pattern from rat uterine mast cells, but direct binding to these leukocytes or others was not shown *(112)*.

There is a significant body of literature on the functions of immune cells in ovarian regulation. Readers are referred to recent reviews for further information on this topic *(113,114)*.

Immunological Tolerance and Autoimmunity

Tolerance is an extensively studied aspect of immunology that is still not fully understood *(16,115–120)*. Transgenic mice have been particularly valuable in defining many mechanistic aspects regarding tolerance *(121–123)*. Derived from observations that antigen-specific lymphocytes undergo clonal expansion in response to antigen, two major paths for tolerance induction were sought and demonstrated in both T-cells and B-cells. These are clonal deletion (i.e., death or passive tolerance) and clonal anergy (unresponsiveness or active tolerance). The latter has been thought to have antigen dosage and age restrictions, since tolerance can be induced in neonates or fetuses far more readily than in adults by either very low or very high doses of antigen. Intermediate antigen doses trigger an immune response in those cells reactive to the antigen.

The balance point between tolerance and immunity is not fixed, and it can be shifted toward autoimmunity or susceptibility to infection by genetic differences, or by the way in which an antigen is presented *(118,124)*. The balance point is normally set to evoke a robust response against pathogens, but not against one's own cells and tissues. Elimination of self-reactive immature B- and T-cells has been documented within the bone marrow and thymus *(125–128)*. Once B- and T- lymphocytes have been exported from the sites of primary lymphocyte production to peripheral tissues, their repertoire continues to be refined and reduced. Either lymphocyte type can be clonally eliminated in the periphery before or after an encounter with its specific antigen. In antigen-activated lymphocytes, signals involving Fas ligand and its receptor CD95 (also called Fas/APO-1) have been implicated in clonal elimination *(124)*.

B-cell and T-cell anergy is induced in peripheral sites. The nature of the antigen contributes to anergy; for example, T-cells presented with superantigens become difficult to expand as clones. In addition, blocks to effector functions leading to cytokine production and/or differentiation and the nature of costimuli presented with antigens can reduce or eliminate specific immune responses. Figure 1, adapted from Goodnow *(124)*, illustrates the sequential reduction in availability of the lymphocyte repertoire for antigen-specific immune responses. The stippled regions represent the zones of tolerance. For further information, interested readers are encouraged to consult Goodnow's recent excellent, yet concise review *(124)* on the balance between immunity and tolerance.

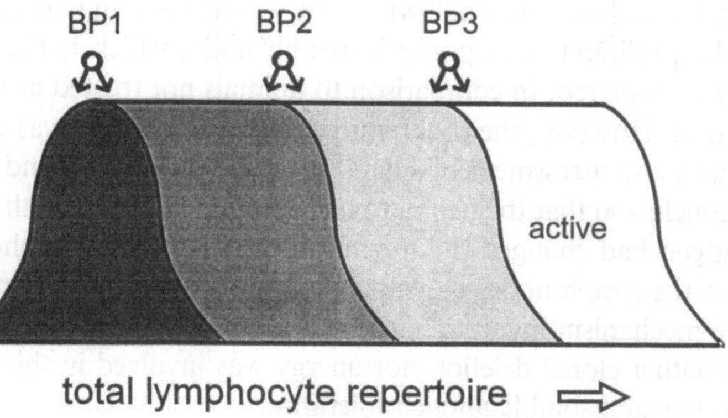

Fig. 1. Diagram of tolerance establishment adopted from Goodnow *(124)*. The *x*-axis represents the distribution of clones plotted from highest to lowest autoreactivity. The *y*-axis is an arbitrary frequency of clones. BPs represent the balance points for the different mechanisms that induce clonal deletion (BP1) or clonal anergy in naive (BP2) or antigen educated (BP3) lymphocytes. These balance points between tolerance and immunity are not fixed, but depend on such factors as amount of antigen presented, avidity of antigen binding, timing of antigen presentation, and costimulatory factors. The lymphocyte clones in the darkest stipple would be deleted, whereas those lighest stippling are anergic. The clones in the unstippled area provide active immunity.

Mate selection in a random-bred population is not controlled. Thus, peripheral tolerance promoting clonal anergy is a more probable explanation for tolerance toward the fetal allograft than is clonal deletion or thymic antigen presentation, which would be unlikely to occur in a perinatal female. Soluble antigens in the absence of adjuvant, low-dose antigens, chronic high-dose antigen stimulation, lack of costimulatory signals or of cytokines for B- or T-cell proliferation could each explain the absence of an antifetal rejection response. Experiments addressing the low levels and nature of MHC antigen expression on trophoblast and the immunosuppressive cytokine milieu in the pregnant uterus can be considered a partial evaluation of tolerance toward the fetus. Studies on clonal deletion, repertoire expression by uterine lymphocytes, or repertoire refinement to set new balance points during gestation are uncommon.

Recent investigations in transgenic mice have challenged the aspect of tolerance induction that relates to the fetal and neonatal period, and evaluated whether immunological tolerance is a component of pregnancy success. Data from three different model systems support rejection of the hypothesis that neonatal lymphocytes differ from those of adults and are susceptible to tolerance induction. Ridge and his colleagues *(118)* focused on the ratio between T-cells and APCs, which is quantitatively much greater in neonates than in adults, owing to the infrequency of APCs. Spleen cell suspensions, which are commonly used in experiments to induce alloantigen tolerance, contain many B-cells, but few dendritic APCs. The authors reasoned that T-cells in inoculated neonates would thus be presented with antigen in the context of a B-cell rather than a dendritic cell. Since the T-cells in the neonates are naive (not antigen-educated), they would not be expected to respond to B-cell presented antigens and would become tolerized. Inclusion of additional APCs with the spleen cell inoculum led to priming in neonates and a subsequent resistance to tolerance induction to the specific priming antigen. These studies show that neonatal T-cells are fully immune-competent and do not require a postnatal interval for functional maturation. Forsthuber et al. *(117)* examined the response of neonates to a soluble protein antigen given intraperitoneally in incomplete Freund's adjuvant. The response of these mice to an antigen recall challenge at 8 wk of age was assessed in lymph nodes and spleen. The fact that the proliferative response in lymph node, which is the traditional site of measurement, was impaired, in comparison to animals not treated as neonates, was suggestive of tolerance. However, the proliferative response in spleen was enhanced over that in control animals, and assessment of splenic cytokine production and systemic antibody supported the conclusion that the neonates had responded. These authors postulated that exposure to antigen had changed the migration pattern of the lymphocytes, so they no longer homed to the lymph node. Downregulation of L-selectin, a homing receptor, was suggested as the mechanism involved, since it is required for homing to lymph node, but not to spleen. Neither clonal deletion nor anergy was involved in this model, previously documented as neonatal soluble antigen tolerance.

Sarzotti and her colleagues *(120)* studied a mouse retrovirus challenge model. A protective cytotoxic T-cell response is induced by the virus challenge in weaning age and older mice, but not in neonates. By reducing the antigen dose by the difference in splenic T-cell frequency between the resistant weaning age and susceptible neonatal mice (3.5- to 5-fold), an immune response was induced in the neonates. The basis for the failure of neonates to respond to the higher dose of antigen was found to be the induction of a Th2-like cytokine pattern, as indicated by high IL-4 production. The immune response induced by the lower dose of viral antigen did not lead to production of IL-4, but rather IFNγ, a Th1 cytokine with protective antiviral activity. Together, these studies appear to refute the idea that a brief window of time exists in the newborn, which makes important contributions in the establishment of tolerance.

Tafuri and her colleagues began their investigations from the premise that neither tolerance nor ignorance of paternal alloantigens in maternal T-cells had been convincingly demonstrated *(129)*. Female mice with the MHC haplotype H-2^k, in which a transgene had been introduced to skew the T-cell repertoire toward the MHC class I-specific alloantigen H-$2K^b$, were mated to H-2^b males. As controls, genetically identical females were mated to syngeneic H-2^k males or MHC-unrelated third-party males. Only females mated to H-2^b males had reduced numbers of T-cells in the spleen capable of recognizing H-$2K^b$, demonstrating that the cells had become antigen-aware and removed from the periphery in response to the paternal transplantation antigens. Since no sequestration of the antigen-specific T-cells could be found in the placenta and placental cells do not express classical MHC class I antigen, the authors suggested that a leakage of fetal cells into the maternal circulation accounted for this deletion or anergic response in the mother to the paternal antigen. The H-$2K^b$-reactive cell population was restored in the spleen after the litter was born. Both depletion and reappearance of these T-cells occurred in intact as well as thymectomized pregnant transgenic mice. Further, the maternal immune "awareness" of the H-$2K^b$ fetal genotype induced a transient pregnancy-limited susceptibility to H-2^b-expressing tumor cells that was not seen in pregnancies involving the other mating combinations and was interpreted as pregnancy-associated tolerance.

Specific humoral or cell-mediated immune responses to constituents of ones own body tissues define autoimmunity. Mechanisms underlying the initiation of autoimmune disease remain elusive, although contributions from polygenic traits *(4)* and microbial infections *(130)* are leading postulates. The onset of an autoimmune disease implies that autoreactive lymphocytes were not clonally deleted or that peripheral anergy was not maintained *(131)*. Autoimmune diseases are a heterogeneous group of clinical diseases caused by different types of responses to different antigenic peptides, some of which are well defined *(132)*. Autoimmune diseases can be organ-restricted (i.e., rheumatoid arthritis or insulin-dependent diabetes mellitus or systemic (i.e., systemic lupus erythematosis [SLE]). Some of the autoimmune diseases seen in humans and other species occur predominantly in females. For example 9/10 cases of SLE and 10/11 cases of biliary cirrhosis occur in women *(132–134)*, and 4/5 mice in the spontaneously diabetic line NOD that become diabetic are females, although the prodromal stage of insulinitis occurs equally in NOD females and males *(135)*.

Data beyond sex ratio incidence also suggest an endocrine link in autoimmune disease. In both men and women with SLE, increased estrogen production has been measured *(136)* and SLE can become exacerbated during pregnancy. Rheumatoid arthritis typically remits during gestation and flares postpartum, particularly if the mother is lactating. Autoimmune thyroiditis is often first diagnosed postpartum *(4)*. In mutant mice with lupus-like pathology, ovariectomy decreases disease manifestations, whereas orchiectomy of males increases disease severity. The course of disease can also be manipulated in mice by administration of testosterone or estrogen. The former suppresses, but the latter accelerates pathogenesis *(133)*.

RELATIONSHIPS BETWEEN THE SYSTEMIC MATERNAL IMMUNE SYSTEM AND THE FETUS

Passively Acquired Maternal Antibody

Maternal-fetal communication is determined in a large part by the anatomy of the materno–fetal interface. In species having hemochorial placentation, maternal antibodies of some of the Ig subtypes cross freely into fetuses. Women with autoimmune diseases and autoantibodies are a high-risk group for antibody-mediated complications of pregnancy. Autoantibodies, particularly those directed against cell membrane phospholipids, are implicated in early pregnancy loss and recurrent early pregnancy failures *(137)*. Antibody-mediated thrombosis in placental vessels followed by placental ischemia and necrosis is believed to underlie the pregnancy failures *(138)*.

Live offspring can be born to women with autoimmunity. The effects of their disease on their developing fetuses and neonatal offspring vary according to the nature of the disease, whether systemic or tissue-restricted. Pregnant women with active SLE, a systemic disease, have about 65% probability of a live birth. In SLE, maternal renal failure is the most common complication associated with fetal loss. The overall outcome for SLE on the fetus is poor growth, although treatment of the mother to sustain the pregnancy can also contribute to intrauterine growth retardation. Elevated risk for neurologic and cardiac problems is also seen, including congenital heart block associated with passively transferred antiribonucleoprotein antibodies known as anti-SS-A (Ro) *(136)*.

Babies born to women with autoimmunity directed against a target tissue are at risk from more restricted complications involving the same target tissue. Fetal platelet destruction is observed and can be monitored in patients with autoimmune thrombocytopenic purpura *(138)*. Passively transferred maternal antibody destroys the circulating platelets in a manner analogous to the more familiar syndrome of hemolytic disease of the newborn that envolves by anti-Rh antibody-mediated destruction of erythrocytes. In thrombocytopenic purpura, the major complication for the fetus or neonate is hemorrhage, particularly intracerebral hemorrhage, which can be fatal. For this reason, vaginal deliveries are discouraged. Another example, neonatal thyrotoxicosis, has been recognized as a complication for fetuses exposed during gestation to passively acquired antibodies against thyrotropin receptors. These antibodies stimulate fetal thyroid activity *(139)*.

Maternal disease is not essential for the transfer of circulating autoantibodies to the fetus. Wellik and her colleagues *(140)* examined the hypothesis that naturally occurring insulin autoantibodies are intrinsic to the normal fetal immune system. Their study of 70 patients found that cord blood insulin autoantibody levels were more than double the levels present in maternal blood. Fetal autoantibody levels did not correlate to those in the mother, although the levels of insulin in the paired blood samples did correlate. The birthweight of the infants correlated to the insulin levels. A lack of glycemic control results in macrosomy of the fetus. Approximately 12% of macrosomic fetuses are born to diabetic women who would be expected to have higher levels of autoantibodies available for passive transfer to the fetus than the normal women examined in Wellik et al.'s study.

Generally, maternally derived Igs are thought to provide passive protection to the offspring during the perinatal period. However, because antibodies are proteins, it is possible for any animal (i.e., adult or fetus/neonate) receiving passive antibody to induce a response against the primary antibody, i.e., an anti-idiotype response or an anergic response. In this way, the mother and her inventory of antigen-induced responses can shape the immune repertoire selected by her developing offspring. The idiotypic interactions have been called a "molecular attention hypothesis" *(141)* and are based on the immunological network theory *(142,143)*. The network theory was proposed as a mechanism for homeostatic regulation of lymphocyte numbers and natural immune activities that are independent of external antigens, i.e., physiological.

The Hemochorial Placenta Is Porous to Both Maternal and Fetal Cell Passage

Fetal Cell Passage and Engraftment in Women. Bidirectional trafficking of fetal and maternal cells occurs in human pregnancy *(144)* and probably in mice (*129; discussed above*). Technical advances have now made it possible to isolate fetal cells from human maternal peripheral blood for prenatal diagnoses. Because venipuncture is a minimally invasive approach compared to amniocentesis or chorionic villus sampling, and presents no risk to the fetus, tremendous efforts are being made to validate maternal blood for prenatal diagnosis *(144–146)*. Although most approaches are based on enrichment or isolation of nucleated fetal erythrocytes, fetal leukocyte trafficking has also been documented *(71)*. Indeed, Bianchi and colleagues *(71)* reported that 13/19 patients carrying male fetuses had detectable male cells (PCR for a Y chromosome-specific sequence). More remarkable, however, was that 4 of 13 women carrying female fetuses and 6 of 8 nonpregnant women had detectable male cells from previously completed or terminated pregnancies. The male cells were lymphoid progenitors ($CD34^+$ $CD38^+$) and were found 1–27 yr after the gestation of a male conceptus. Thus, it is possible that low-dose shedding of fetal cells into the maternal circulation is a mechanism for peripheral tolerance of the maternal immune system during, and perhaps beyond pregnancy.

Maternal Cell Chimerism of Human Infants. Leukocyte trafficking is not unidirectional. Human clinical literature demonstrates unequivocally that maternal cells also pass into fetuses. Early studies showed that maternal blood collected near term, labeled, and autotransfused led to the appearance of labeled cells in fetal cord blood at birth *(147, 148)*. Questions remained concerning whether transfer of the label had occurred between cells postinfusion and if the phenomenon occurred only peripartum.

Investigations of immune-deficient children have provided stronger support for trafficking, since engrafted maternal cells have been found, isolated, and characterized *(149–152)*. In some children engrafted with maternal T-cells, graft vs host disease is evident, but in others it is not. The graft, however, can be an impediment to subsequent therapeutic bone marrow transplantation *(153–155)*. There is no evidence to suggest that the placenta of an immune-deficient baby differs from normal. Indeed, several children in the cited papers were reported as normal birthweight, full-term infants. Thus, it is reasonable to assume that maternal cells pass into all human fetuses, but are not harmful, and therefore, not sought out and characterized in normal infants.

Confirmation of Porosity of the Hemochorial Placenta in Experimental Animals. A thorough investigation of maternal-to-fetal cell trafficking is not possible in humans because of the sporadic availability of patients for study and ethical considerations. Rodents have a hemochorial placenta and short gestation period, and are the model animals of choice. Despite the genetic and immunological tools available, particularly in mice, there has not been a consensus on the frequency of maternal immune cells trafficking into fetuses. Early studies by Tuffrey and her colleagues *(156)* using a karyotypic marker indicated maternal cell passage into the offspring with subsequent engraftment. This was not confirmed by Hunziker et al. in 1984 *(157)* or by Shimamura et al. in 1994 *(158)*. The former investigators documented erythrocyte trafficking, but only rarely leukocyte passage (2/172 mice); the latter group found very low signals of maternal origin in PCR analysis of liver and spleen from pooled organs of neonates. In all three of these investigations, only immune-competent offspring were studied, and only the earliest work *(156)* examined the bone marrow compartment of the offspring.

The first suggestion that maternal-to-fetal cell trafficking could occur extensively in mice came from studies of xenogeneically engrafted mice. Ladel et al. *(159)* mated immune-deficient mothers of the genotype *scid/scid* (T-cell$^-$ B-cell$^-$) to syngeneic males. Prior to mating, however, the females had received an ip inoculation of human PBL to create mouse–human chimeras. At 16 wk of age, the animals born to and suckled by the chimeras were also human cell chimeras. The only source of human cells the offspring had been exposed to was their mother. The chimeric offspring spontaneously produced human Ig.

In a follow-up study, Greenwood and colleagues *(160)* examined *scid/scid* offspring from bovine PBL-reconstituted *scid/scid* dams. Not only did bovine cells cross the mouse placenta (this is in itself interesting because bovine cells do not cross the bovine placenta, which indicates placental structure is a crucial element in modeling), but the bovine cells remained competent to induction of a primary immune response, i.e., peripheral tolerance had not been established.

These two reports indicated that a reassessment of maternal-to-fetal cell trafficking in mice was necessary, using immune-deficient offspring to mimic the human clinical situation. Our laboratory has begun to explore a new model system that appears to have tremendous potential for analysis of materno–fetal chimerism. The model is based on embryo transfer of normal or genetically immune-deficient blastocysts to pseudopregnant females of the strain ROSA26. All nucleated cells in ROSA26 express the transgene *LacZ*, which transcribes the enzyme β-galactosidase. The enzyme can be readily detected by either flow cytometry or histochemistry *(161)*.

The result of initial studies of 51 embryos recovered on d 18.5 of gestation was that most (46/51) exhibited a degree of maternal cell chimerism. Among the immune-deficient fetuses, multiorgan engraftment was present with 86% of the positive thymic samples, and found mostly in livers and/or spleens. Less frequently, low levels of maternal cells were found in bone marrow, lung, and heart. In immune-competent fetuses, maternal cells were frequently found, but only in the bone marrow. Time-course analysis has been undertaken using immune-deficient fetuses. In these, maternal cell passage could not be demonstrated

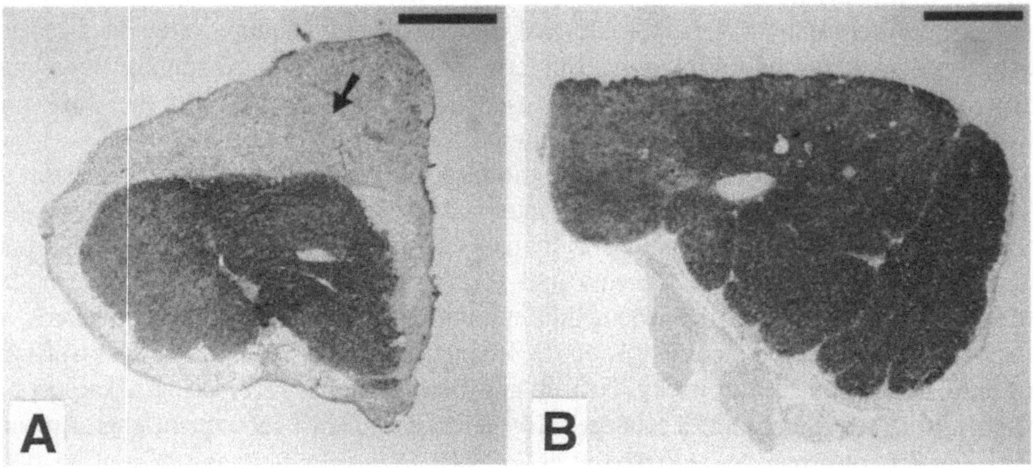

Fig. 2. Photomicrographs of sections of thymus biopsies from 3-wk-old *scid/scid* mice (**A**) gestated in an immune-deficient ICR *scid/scid* female or (**B**) gestated in a ROSA26 immune-competent female. The thymus depicted in B was much larger, the cortex was better developed, and the lymphoid cellularity was more dense. No LacZ + ROSA26 maternal cells were present in B or A (negative control). Stained with hematoxylin and eosin. Bar = 600 μm.

on d 6, 7, or 8 of gestation, but maternal cells restricted to the fetal thymus were present on d 12 of gestation *(161)*. The changes occurring between d 9 and 11 of gestation include establishment of placental circulation, and migration of fetal lymphoid progenitor cells. The nature of the maternal cells is as yet undefined, except for exclusion of erythrocytes, and it is not known whether the maternal cells are sustained as postnatal grafts. However, this study demonstrated that trafficking of maternal cells across the hemochorial placenta is a normal gestational event involving both immune-competent and immune-deficient fetuses. Further, for both immune-competent and immune-deficient fetuses, the major sites of engraftment are the primary lymphoid organs, those organs in which the mechanisms for repertoire development and central immune tolerance are becoming established. It is interesting that the level of immune competency determines the primary site of maternal cell chimerism. Does chimerism of the immune-deficient thymus, but not marrow indicate more readily availabile space, or does it reflect the developmental time-course of lymphoid tissue, thymic development preceding that of marrow? The numerous maternal cells in the marrow of immune-competent fetuses suggest that marrow is a growth-promoting environment or that there may be specific homing of the maternal cells. Could the role of maternal cells be to ensure the developing fetal immune system is tolerant of its mother as a safety measure? Could fetal cells in the mother be important for prevention of antifetal autoimmune disease when abortion is followed by a new conception, or when death from any underlying cause occurs in several members of a litter but littermates are spared *(162)*?

Implications of Maternal Lymphocyte Trafficking into Fetuses. Only three *scid/scid* mice gestated in ROSA26 females have been available for analysis after birth. Maternal cells were present in the thymus, liver, and spleen at 1 d of age, but were not found at wk 3 or 4 using flow cytometric analysis. Bone marrow was not assessed. It was observed that the lymphoid organs in these three mice were much larger than those in age-matched *scid/scid* mice gestated in *scid/scid* mothers. This was confirmed histologically *(163)* (Fig. 2). An increased cellularity and improvement in splenic and thymic architecture were observed. The simplest explanation for this is that growth factors and cytokines from the immune-competent mother cross freely into the fetus, and promote lymphopoiesis and lymphoid organ development. An alternate explanation is that the maternal T-cell microchimerism found in the fetus from d 12 of gestation until at least 24 h after birth produces cytokines at levels sufficient to stimulate lymphopoiesis in the thymus with enhanced seeding to the peripheral lymphoid organs.

It is not yet clear whether any circulating maternal cell has an equal, but random chance of crossing the placenta into the fetus, or whether lineage markers, proliferation markers, or other receptor properties endow some cells with a higher probability for transmission. Indeed, it is possible that the fetus may release chemotactic signals to recruit specific cells. If any cell has an equal probability of entering a fetus, then any cell containing a pathogen could also reach the fetus and potentially infect it. It would likely be necessary for some number of infected cells to reach the fetus to establish disease. This very direct mechanism could be involved in vertical transmission of the Epstein-Barr virus through B-cells or HIV-1 and related agents in T-cells. One of the major pathways for HIV-1 infection and the development of AIDS is to be born to an HIV-1$^+$ mother. Although many infants born to women seropositive for HIV-1 are not virally infected, a significant number are infected before birth *(164,165)*. Understanding the vertical transmission of this disease is an expanding area in reproductive immunology *(166)*.

The reciprocal migration of cells between the mother and fetus could also parallel a clinical organ grafting situation. Migration of donor cells from the organ graft into various tissues of the recipient has been demonstrated *(10)*. This allogeneic donor-type microchimerism has been associated with stable, long-term graft success, the absence of graft vs host disease, and donor-specific nonreactivity, which has permitted reductions or cessation in immunosuppressive drug therapy *(167–171)*. The ratios of lymphocytes to dendritic cells may be important for establishing donor-specific tolerance in these patients as was demonstrated in the neonatal tolerance induction experiments discussed earlier *(118)*. A failure to demonstrate microchimerism in the maternal–fetal situation *(9)* or in the attempts to establish its importance in prognosis for organ graft patients does not discredit the idea that allogeneic microchimerism is essential for fetal and organ graft success. The negative position is always very difficult to prove, since microchimerism may be present in tissues that were not sampled, such as marrow, may be at levels below the sensitivity of detection, or may be dynamic and fluctuate in its detectability *(168,170)*. It is clear that the issue of microchimerism needs further exploration in both pregnancy and organ grafting. It will also be of interest to know whether fetal cell microchimerism of the mother occurs in those livestock species in which the placenta is currently considered impervious to cell trafficking.

THE IMMUNE SYSTEM IN SPECIES WITH HEMOCHORIAL PLACENTATION

Leukocytes in the Rodent and Human Uterus

The hemochorial placenta characteristic of rodents and most primates represents the most invasive form of placentation. Blastocysts in these species attach to the uterine surface almost immediately and begin to invade. Although there are differences in the way trophoblasts breach the uterine epithelium and reorganize the endometrial stroma, there is direct contact between circulating maternal blood and trophoblast in both humans and rodents. Hemochorial placentae are further classified as either labyrinthine or villous, according to the structures containing maternal blood. In the labyrinthine placenta of rodents, trophoblast does not contact unmodified maternal connective tissue. The presence of a blastocyst in the uterus induces a "decidual response," which refers to modifications in the shape, organization, and metabolism of endometrial stromal cells. The decidual response is extensive by d 5–6, before the trophoblast reaches the basal lamina of the uterine epithelium. Under natural conditions, the decidual transformation is confined to areas adjacent to blastocysts, leaving areas of undecidualized endometrium between embryos. A generalized decidual response can be artifically induced by a wide variety of stimuli (pseudopregnancy).

In the villous hemochorial placenta of the human, predecidual changes take place in stromal cells throughout the uterus late in the luteal phase of the menstrual cycle whether or not a blastocyst is present. Initial implantation occurs in an undecidualized endometrium such that the trophoblast resides in unmodified endometrial stroma for 3–5 d. During the implantation process, the human trophoblast differentiates into an irregular cytotrophoblast surrounded at the point of invasion by an extensive outer syncytium, the syncytiotrophoblast. Trophoblast differentiates along villous and extravillous pathways. Villous trophoblast covers the chorionic villi and is concerned with metabolic exchange between mother and fetus. The villi are bathed in blood and hence contact is limited to maternal cells in the circulation. In contrast, extravillous trophoblast migrates deeply into the uterine mucosa as far as the myometrium and actually invades the spiral arteries of the decidua. Differential expression of MHC antigens occurs on villous syncytiotrophoblast, villous cytotrophoblast, and extravillous trophoblast *(6)*.

Leukocyte populations and their distribution have been studied extensively in both the human and rodent uterus. In the nonpregnant human endometrium, there are very few B-cells, and during normal pregnancy B-cells are almost totally absent from the implantation site *(6)*. T-cells are present in both nonpregnant endometrium and decidua with the numbers of CD3+ T-cells remaining constant (10% of total lymphocytes) throughout the menstrual cycle and early pregnancy *(172)*. In the pregnant human uterus, a population of large granulated lymphocytes (LGL) is distributed throughout the decidua and makes up 70% of the total leukocyte population. Human LGLs have been identified as a subset of NK cells because of their cell-surface markers. In the nonpregnant rodent uterus, B-cells make approx 2–3%, T-cells 30%, and NK cells 40% of the total number of leukocytes *(90)*.

Distribution and Function of T-Cells Within the Pregnant Uterus. The role of T-cells in the pregnant uterus is controversial. Studies in mice have tended to focus on the second half of gestation *(92,93,173,174)*, but in humans, the first trimester has been extensively studied *(175–177)*. Saito and colleagues *(175)* found by flow cytometry that in early human decidua, 84.8% of lymphocytes were CD16− CD56^{bright} NK cells, a subset found predominantly in the uterus, and 12.2% of lymphocytes were CD3+ T-cells with the percentages of CD4+ and CD8+ being 5.6 and 4.7%, respectively. In both humans and mice, effort has been invested into the characterization of the $\gamma\delta$ TCR+ cells, which have been reported to make up approx 5% of the CD3+ cells in human decidua *(178)*. In the nonpregnant mouse, $\gamma\delta$ T-cells account for 6.7% of intraepithelial lymphocytes (IELs), which, during allogeneic pregnancy, increase to 14.5% *(174)*. Heyborne and colleagues *(93)* found that relative to other CD3+ cells in the murine uterus, $\gamma\delta$ T-cells increased twofold during pregnancy. It should be pointed out, however, that $\gamma\delta$ T-cells make up < 1% of the total number of lymphocytes in the decidua. Interest in $\gamma\delta$ T-cells comes from their association with epithelial surfaces in other mucosal organs, particularly intestine.

Suzuki and colleagues *(174)* performed a series of experiments to determine the role of $\gamma\delta$ T-cells in successful murine pregnancy (d 12–20). The frequency of $\gamma\delta$ T-cells in uterine suspensions expressing the activation markers CD69 and IL-2Rα was asessed using flow cytometry. They found that a higher proportion of uterine $\gamma\delta$ T-cells displayed the activated phenotype in allogeneic pregnancy than in syngeneic pregnancies or nonpregnant animals. Despite their activated phenotype, the $\gamma\delta$ T-cells did not respond to stimulation in culture in a mixed-lymphocyte reaction (MLR). The authors concluded these T-cells may have been tolerant. However, in further MLR investigations involving uterine $\gamma\delta$ or $\alpha\beta$ T-cell-enriched and depleted culture conditions, they found that the $\gamma\delta$ T-cells suppressed the proliferative response observed in $\alpha\beta$ T-cells by secretion of TGF-β. The authors, therefore, suggest that uterine IEL $\gamma\delta$ T-cells play a physiological rather than a defensive role in the maternal recognition response to the fetus. It is important to note that in these experiments, the $\gamma\delta$ T-cells were isolated from the uterus after the placenta and trophoblast were removed (although uterine epithelium is no longer present at these hemochorial placentation sites). Therefore, the Suzuki et al. results should be viewed separately from information obtained from cell suspensions that include decidua and/or trophoblast.

In the human, Saito and colleagues *(175)* also found that the T-cell subsets of the pregnant uterus had an activated phenotype. Using flow cytometry, they identified CD4$^+$ and CD8$^+$ subsets in decidual lymphocytes, which expressed the HLA-DR, CD69, IL-2Rα, and IL-2Rβ activation markers. Mincheva-Nilsson and colleagues examined decidual lymphocytes with immunoelectron microscopy, and classified the leukocytes in terms of $\gamma\delta$ TCR and CD56 expression *(177)*. They found that approx 50% of $\gamma\delta$ TCR$^+$ were also CD56$^+$, despite evidence from other laboratories indicating that CD56$^+$ cells are NK cells *(172)*. In addition, the numbers of $\gamma\delta$ TCR$^+$ cells detected did not correlate with that of CD3$^+$ cells. This study is disputed *(6)*, and it is generally accepted that the predominant leukocytes in the pregnant human uterus are of the NK cell lineage.

Macrophages in the Uterus. Macrophages are abundant in the mesenchyme and stroma of the cycling and pregnant rodent uterus and constitute a significant proportion (7–10%) of the total cellular content in the nonpregnant uterus, rising to 20% during pregnancy *(179)*. Macrophages are recruited to target tissues through chemotactic products and cytokines, such as CSF-1, which is expressed by uterine epithelial cells in response to estrogen and progesterone *(180)*. De and Wood *(181)* pursued the concept of hormonal regulation of uterine macrophages in the mouse. Using the well-characterized antimouse macrophage antibody F4/80, they showed by immunohistochemistry that macrophages were evenly distributed throughout the endometrium in the intact mouse uterus during diestrus. However, during proestrus and estrus, macrophages became more concentrated in the subepithelial stroma and luminal epithelium. Ovariectomy resulted in a progressive decrease in macrophage numbers, a situation that was fully reversed by treatment with exogenous estradiol and progesterone. Thus, it appears that estrogen and progesterone have significant effects on the distribution of macrophages during the estrous cycle, which effectively position phagocytic cells close to the uterine lumen at a time when foreign antigens may enter the uterus during insemination.

During pregnancy, the distribution of macrophages in the rodent uterus is altered according to the extent of decidualization, which occurs adjacent to the blastocyst. In early stages of gestation, macrophages are scarce at implantation sites *(182)*, and when decidualization occurs, macrophages appear to be excluded from the decidua, so that there are virtually no cells bearing macrophage markers in the rat or mouse primary

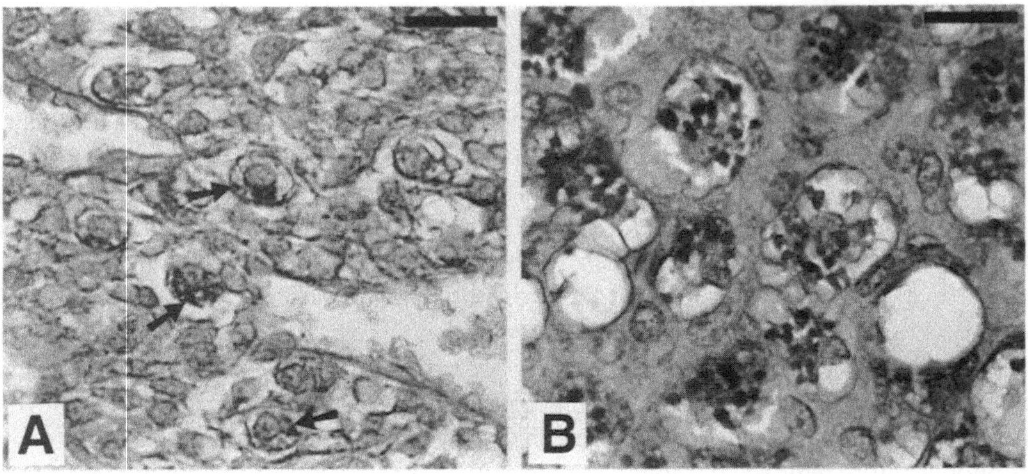

Fig. 3. Photomicrographs of **(A)** a young granulated murine uNK cell (arrowed) from d 8 of gestation and **(B)** a fully mature heavily granulated murine uNK cell from d 12 of gestation. Stained with PAS reagent. Bar, 20 μm.

decidual zone *(183,184)*. Redline et al. *(185)* suggested that mouse decidual tissue was not favorable for macrophage migration. The local production of cytokines, such as CSF-1, GM-CSF, TNF-α, and TGF-β, may be involved in the exclusion of macrophages from decidual tissue.

In the human, macrophages do not appear to be under hormonal control, because their numbers are relatively constant throughout the menstrual cycle (reviewed in *6,179,186*). Human macrophages are frequently identified by their expression of CD14. Uterine macrophages display phagocytic behavior typical of macrophages in other tissues and are thought to be involved in degradative activities associated with menstruation. Unlike the situation in the rodent, macrophages are in association with the decidua and are found near the implantation site in close contact with invading trophoblast *(179)*.

NK Cells in the Pregnant Uterus. In the young rodent, immature NK cells are distributed throughout the uterus *(187)* and can be identified by the NK cell marker LGL-1 *(188,189)*. This surface marker has since been identified as Ly49G2 *(51)*. In pregnant animals, the distribution and phenotype of these cells appear to change; first, the cells become localized at the sites of implantation and disappear from other parts of the decidualizing uterus. As gestation proceeds, proliferation of uterine NK (uNK) cells is only observed in their preferred location, a developing area mesometrial to the decidua known as the metrial gland *(190,191)*. Concurrently, the cells differentiate, increase dramatically in size (to as much as 50 μm in diameter), and gain a distinctive granular appearance owing to the synthesis of numerous lytic glycoprotein granules in the cytoplasm, which are detected histologically by periodic acid-Schiff reagent (PAS) (Fig. 3). It is thought that the marker LGL-1 is lost during this differentiation process, and the marker asialoGM-1 is acquired *(189,191)*, although there is no formal proof that a single cell makes these transitions.

The migration of uNK cells from bone marrow to the uterus is likely to be regulated by surface antigens expressed by the immature precursor cells and may involve stimulation by estrogen. Some progenitor cells are found in the virgin uterus *(192)*, but further studies are required to examine fully the development and trafficking of uNK cells. The development of the uNK cell population is hormone-dependent (reviewed in *190*). Progesterone prolongs the life-span of induced deciduomata, which contains uNK cells *(190)*. Other experiments, which involved the ovariectomy of pregnant mice and rats, may not be valid, since the ovary is the only source of progesterone throughout the pregnancy in the rodent (reviewed in *193*). Thus, the reported changes in uNK cell numbers and distribution following ovariectomy may have been owing to the imminently failing pregnancy, rather than simply the removal of hormonal support.

To characterize further the effects of estrogen and progesterone on uNK cells, the expression of the ER and PR was determined using RT-PCR and immunohistochemistry (*194* and Van den Heuvel et al., unpublished). At early stages of gestation (d 8), ER was expressed by a higher proportion (>90%) of uNK cells than PR (28%). Although PR expression was low early in gestation, it appeared to increase so that 80% of uNK cells expressed PR by d 16. The expression of steroid transcriptional regulators by uNK cells opens new areas of investigation, which will be important in understanding the biology of uNK cells and may distinguish the uNK subset as distinct from NK cells in lymphoid tissues.

The placenta and metrial gland have fully formed by d 10 and, as gestation progresses, uNK cells become larger, more granular, and often (>10%) binucleate *(190,195)*. Examination of DNA fragmentation in uNK cells in tissue sections indicates that not at d 11, but by d 12 of gestation, many uNKs are dying. Interestingly, it was somewhat common for one nucleus to be undergoing DNA fragmentation in a binucleate cell while the other had apparently intact DNA *(195,196)*. By parturition at d 19, the majority of uNK cells had ruptured in the mesometrial triangle area or had aligned along the basal aspect of the placenta. The latter were shed from the uterus with the placenta at parturition. It has been proposed that the increased granularity of the mature uNK cell and its subsequent death may be part of a mechanism to facilitate separation of the placenta from the uterine wall at parturition *(197,198)*.

The classification of uNK cells includes an evaluation of their ability to lyse traditional NK target cells in vitro. Lytic activity is relatively high in murine decidual cell suspensions early in gestation (d 6.5), but has decreased in decidual preparations on d 10 or 12 of pregnancy *(199)*. As uNK cells differentiate, they appear histologically to resemble highly activated cells *(188,191)*, and it has been thought for many years that uNK cells are lytic cells present to actively limit the invasion of trophoblast *(188,189,200)*. However, there is little evidence for this in vivo *(201,202)*. Even in vitro, uNK freshly isolated from the metrial gland region are unable to lyse of traditional NK target cells (YAC-1) or trophoblast *(199,203,204)*. Indeed it is only after incubation with IL-2, when uNK cells are transformed into LAK cells, that they become more efficient at lysis *(205)*. Some laboratories have noted the requirement for IL-2 in vitro for uNK migration and short-term viability *(204)*, whereas other laboratories find IL-2 unable to support or prolong the growth of uNK in vitro *(196,205)*. The confusion regarding the necessity for IL-2 in culture is probably indicative of a suboptimal culture system for murine uNKs rather than a requirement for IL-2 in vivo *(7)*.

Human decidual LGLs have been identified as a subset of NK cells because of their $CD56^{bright}$ $CD16^-$ $CD2^+$ $CD3^-$ surface phenotype *(175,206)*. King and her colleagues *(69, 207,208)* have investigated $CD3^-$ decidual uNK in detail using flow cytometry and immunohistochemistry. The majority of NK cells in peripheral blood are $CD16^+$ $CD56^{dim}$, and lack cytoplasmic granules *(209)*. The subset of blood NK cells displaying a phenotype matching that of uNK cells is a very small proportion estimated variously at <10–<1% *(6)*. Uterine NK cells are also present in the nonpregnant uterus where they proliferate and are greatest in number during the secretory phase of the menstrual cycle *(172,210)*. If pregnancy does not occur, the cells become pyknotic and die. However, the population of uNK cells is maintained in pregnancy, suggesting that these cells are progesterone-dependent *(176,208,210)*.

The cytolytic capacity of human uNK cells has been characterized both in the presence and absence of IL-2 *(6,211,212)*. Freshly isolated human decidual uNK cells were unable to kill first trimester human trophoblast, despite being able to lyse the human NK-target cell line K562. However, incubation of uNK cells with IL-2 promoted uNK differentiation into LAK cells, which, after an extended period of incubation (4–6 d), were able to kill normal trophoblast and JEG choriocarcinoma cells, a trophoblast-derived cell line. King and Loke *(208)* point out that the preference for killing malignant cells rather than trophoblast after IL-2 activation may indicate an in vivo role for uNK in the containment of exceptionally invasive or malignant trophoblast, as might be associated with hydatidiform mole pregnancy.

The receptor for IL-2 consists of α, β, and γ chains, each with different affinities for, and responses to, the cytokine. The high-affinity receptor found on activated NK and T-cells consists of all three subunits. When activated, this trimeric receptor induces the expression of immediate early genes involved in proliferation such as c-*myc* and c-*fos (213)*. The α-chain of the IL-2R has a molecular weight (mol wt) of 55 kDa (also referred to as p55 or CD25), and alone binds IL-2 with low affinity and little biological response. The β-chain has a mol wt of 75 kDa and intermediate affinity for IL-2, while the 64-kDa γ-chain has 70% homology between mice and humans and has been demonstrated to be important for intracellular signaling *(214)*. Circulating blood NK cells express IL-2R$\beta\gamma$ and can be stimulated by high levels of IL-2. The IL-2Rγ chain is an important molecule common to several cytokine receptors (IL-4, IL-7, and IL-15, an NK cell growth factor) *(215)*.

Clearly, uNK cells from both rodents and humans are responsive to IL-2 in vitro. However, it is important to assess the levels of both cytokine and receptor present in the decidua. Starkey *(210)* and King et al. *(212)* used immunohistology and flow cytometry to examine first trimester human decidua and found expression of the p75 β-chain on CD56$^{bright+}$ cells, but no expression of the p55 α-chain. Incubation with IL-2 in vitro did not induce expression of p55, but did stimulate cell proliferation and downregulation of p75 IL-2Rβ. A monoclonal antibody (MAb) to IL-2Rβ blocked IL-2-induced proliferation, indicating that the activation of decidual NK cells was occurring through the IL-2Rβ alone. Van den Heuvel et al. *(194)*, employing RT-PCR and immunocytochemistry techniques, found that at d 8 of gestation in mice, all three IL-2R chains were detectable on uNK cells, but by d 12, only the γ-chain was expressed and by d 16 this chain had also disappeared. Further, in the IL-2-depleted environment of IL-2$^{-/-}$ mice *(216)*, uNK morphology and placental development are normal *(11)*, suggesting that IL-2 is not required to maintain the viability of uNK precursor cells or to induce their differentiation, activation, or maturation.

Insights into Uterine NK Cell Functions from Studies in Immune-Deficient Mice

Previous work from this laboratory has used genetically immune-deficient mice to address questions in reproductive immunology *(7,11,12)*. The genetics, immunology, and short reproductive interval of this species are strengths of the approach. The *scid/scid* mouse lacks both B- and T-cells, but appears to have normal fertility. This indicates that neither B-cells nor T-cells are essential for successful pregnancy in this species. In double-mutant mice of genotype *scid/scid.bg/bg,* the lytic ability of NK cells is disabled. These double-mutant mice bred successfully for seven generations of study and continue to breed well as a commercially available stock *(217)*. Histological analysis of midgestational implantation sites from *scid/scid.bg/bg* mice revealed normal development with differentiation of both uNK cells and the metrial gland. This finding suggests that cytolytic ability is not an important function of uNK cells in vivo. This conclusion has recently been supported by studies of implantation sites in the perforin knockout mouse. Perforin is a component of the lytic machinery of NK and T-lymphocytes, and lymphocytes from these mice have severely restricted killing ability in culture *(218)*. Differentiation of uNK cells and of the metrial gland region occurs in the perforin knockout mice, and there is no reduction in fertility in comparison to the parental C57Bl/6 strain *(219)*.

Transgenic mice lacking NK cells have been developed *(14,22,81)*. We have established a breeding colony of the strain TgE26, which has a transgenic insert of > 30 copies of the human CD3E gene. The transgene leads to an almost absolute block in T-cell and NK cell development in the murine fetus at d 13 of gestation. Homozygous TgE26 females appear to ovulate, mate, and progress through early pregnancy in a manner identical to random-bred, inbred or transgenically related heterozygous females. At d 8 of gestation, the typical litters contain nine viable implantation sites that are histologically normal. When these females are mated by a homozygous TgE26 male, fetal resorption begins at d 10 of gestation, affecting about half of the fetuses in every litter *(11,12)*. Histological examination of the implantation sites of viable fetuses between d 10 and 14 of gestation revealed the absence of the metrial gland region and far fewer uNK cells than in immune-competent controls (3% of control). The placentae are much smaller than those in control mice (range 50–60% of control in area). However, differentiation of the fetal trophoblast into giant cells, spongiotrophoblast, and labyrinthine trophoblast occurs and the reduction in placental size appears to involve reductions in each trophoblast layer. Changes are also seen in the arterial blood vessels in regions of decidualization. The decidua itself is relatively acellular.

The earliest time-point at which vascular pathology is observed, using light microscopy, is d 10 of gestation (Fig. 4). The media of uterine arterial walls is thick and the endothelial cells appear swollen in every implantation site in the uterus. The vascular pathology is progressive. By d 12 of gestation, the arteriole walls appear to contain lipid deposits and macrophage foam cells, and the endothelium has flattened. By d 14 of gestation, the integrity of the endothelium is compromised, and erythrocyte leakage into tissue appears (Fig. 4). These progressive changes are highly suggestive of hypertension *(220–223)*. Pregnancy-induced hypertension (PIH) is a recognized condition in women and, when combined with pre-eclampsia, is a leading cause of pregnancy complication. The sequelae of PIH and pre-eclampsia include intrauterine growth retardation and small birthweight or fetal death *(224,225)*. To explore further a possible relationship between the pregnancy losses and vascular pathology seen in syngeneically mated TgE26 females and PIH/pre-eclampsia, blood vessels in other tissues of virgin and primiparous TgE26 were examined by light microscopy. Arterioles in the kidney, lung, spleen, liver, and virgin uterus were judged to be normal, as were the carotid arteries and aorta when compared to equivalent structures in immune-competent females. Arterioles in the postpartum TgE26 uterus also demonstrated normal morphology. Thus, the hypertensive-like vascular changes found in pregnant TgE26 mice are localized to the uterus, are only present during mid-to late gestation, and are reversible in the postpartum period *(11)*. This is quite similar to the PIH/pre-eclampsia syndrome, except that hypertensive pregnant women usually have vascular pathology within the kidney *(223)*.

Proteinuria, another feature of pre-eclampsia *(223,226)*, has been observed in two syngeneically mated TgE26 females studied to date. Peripartum urinary protein was > 500 mg/dL. These values fell to normal (trace to 30 mg/dL) 24 h after the litters were born. Daily blood pressure recordings on pregnant TgE26 females are in progress to determine whether systemic blood pressure elevation can be detected above the levels found in

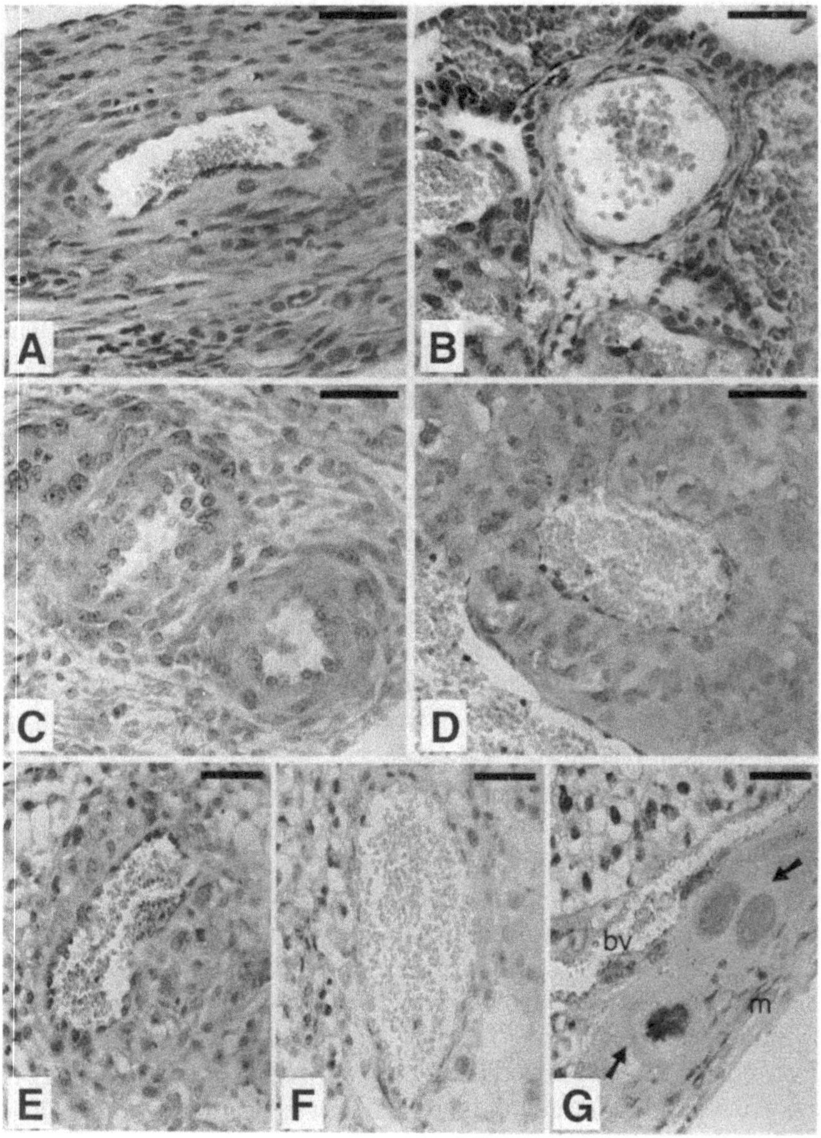

Fig. 4. Photomicrographs comparing features of implantation sites from d 10 (**A,C,E**) and 14 of gestation (**B,D,F,G**) in immune-competent CBA mice (A,B), NK^- and T^- TgE26 females carrying homozygous TgE26 fetuses (**C,D**) and NK^- and T^- TgE26 females carrying more immune competent (CD1 × TgE26) F_1 fetuses (**E,F,G**). In G, arrows show trophoblast giant cells in close association with a blood vessel (bv) wall and myometrium (m). Stained with hematoxylin and eosin. Bar, 50 μm.

pregnant immune-competent mice. It is our current thinking that the small placentae and fetal losses observed in the TgE26 model result from poor placental perfusion. Poor perfusion would limit metabolic exchange during an interval of rapid fetal growth. We feel that the critical role of uNK cells is in promoting uterine vessel relaxation, and thus, that the absence of uNK cells indirectly leads to fetal demise. Some TgE26 fetuses were examined during early resorption. Placental vessel thrombosis with neutrophil infiltration was observed. We think it unlikely that the resorbing fetuses are in any way abnormal; rather, we anticipate that normal fetuses are terminated because of the nutritional deficit and/or toxin elevation, in order to preserve some of the litter for a continued healthy gestation.

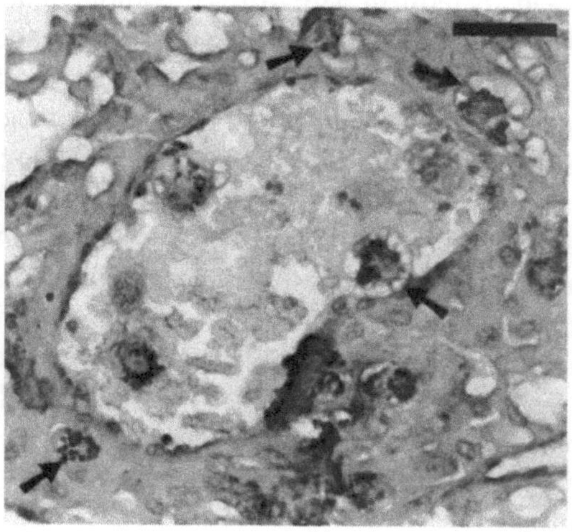

Fig. 5. Photomicrograph from an immune-competent mouse on d 12 of gestation showing normal localization of uNK cells (arrowed) within decidual arteriole walls. Other uNK cells appear to adhere to the endothelium suggesting initiation of extravasation. Bar, 20 μm.

Blood pressure is regulated at a number of levels. In the placenta, vascular relaxation is normal and a hypotensive state is promoted. This is thought to accommodate the large increase in uterine blood flow during the second half of gestation *(227–230)*. One of the major factors associated with vascular relaxation is nitric oxide (NO), which was formerly known as endothelium-derived relaxing factor. One of the vasoconstrictors found in the pregnant uterus is endothelin-1 *(231–234)*. Possible mechanisms that might be postulated for uNK cell promotion of arteriole relaxation in normal pregnancies include the production of NO, the induction of NO production in a target cell population, the production of enkephalinases, which would limit the activity of the endothelin converting enzymes *(235)*, or blocking of endothelin receptors *(231)*. Prostacyclin (PGI_2) and thromboxane A_2 are antagonistic molecules affecting vascular smooth muscle whose balance might also be sustained at least in part by uNK cells. It is of particular interest, and yet an enigma, that in normal pregnant mice, uNK cells are found within arteriole walls (Fig. 5). The movement of neutrophils and lymphocytes from the bloodstream into tissues (i.e., diapedesis) is usually described as occurring through venule walls, which are deficient in the smooth muscle media characteristic of arteries and arterioles *(56)*. Is it possible that vascular smooth muscle is a major target for lytic and/or other activities of uNK cells?

Peel, in her comprehensive monograph on rodent uNK cells *(190)*, described previous work in which an association was made between uNK cells and the relief of hypertension. Moore and colleagues, *(236)* studied deciduomata induction in ovariectomized, hypertensive rats. They detected a transient lowering of blood pressure over 8–14 d that was coincident with the appearance of uNK cells within the deciduomata. Both responses required progesterone, and it was not established whether uNK cells could act independently. Interestingly, hypertension returned while progesterone treatment was still being received, and late uNK cells were present, leading the authors to suggest that changes in uNK cell functions occur late in gestation. This idea has been advanced in current literature from entirely different types of data *(191,195,196,237–239)*. Today, estrogen is thought to be more important than progesterone in placental vessel relaxation *(228)*. Many investigators postulate that there is an immunological component in pre-eclampsia *(223,239)*; however, a possible role for uNK cells has not yet been explored in women with hypertension during pregnancy.

Pregnancy can proceed to term in TgE26 mice without fetal loss. This requires the gestation of an immune-competent fetus *(11)*. In these pregnancies, created by embryo transfer or mating to an immune-competent male, d 10 implantation sites could not be distinguished histologically from those in TgE26 females carrying TgE26 fetuses. That is, there was neither a metrial gland nor uNK cells. Vascular pathology was present, including thickening of the media and swelling of the endothelium (Fig. 4). As pregnancy continued, however, the implantation sites became noticeably different from those in syngeneically mated females. The same changes were not seen in every implantation site, but all fetuses remained viable. Most noticeably, the media of the decidual arterioles did not continue to thicken in a progressive manner, and foam cells did not invade. Rather, there was an unusual movement of trophoblast giant cells into the vascular walls (Fig. 4) and the development of fine branching, which suggested collateral recruitment of blood vessels into the decidual regions. The decidual region itself enlarged, but was relatively acellular and appeared to be edematous.

At least three possible explanations can be offered for the differences in pregnancy success between TgE26 females gestating immune-competent and immune-deficient fetuses. First, since the immune-competent fetuses studied were randombred CD1, the MHC haplotype, if expressed by trophoblast cells, was potentially different and may have triggered an immune response that led to an attempt to compensate for the pregnancy-induced hypertension. Alternately, the immune-competent fetus produces cytokines during the differentiation of its NK and T-cell lineages that are absent from immune-deficient fetuses. These cytokines may cross from the fetuses into the mother and facilitate a compensatory response that can carry the full litter to term. Cytokine production is not identical to that provided by normal uNK cells, since normal placental structure is not achieved in the presence of an immune-competent fetus (Fig 4). This may reflect production of different molecules by normal uNK cells than by normal fetuses or asynchrony in the production of the same molecules, which are provided earlier by uNK cells and not until d 13 of gestation by normal fetuses. This time-point can be established since the block to fetal T- and NK cell development in TgE26 mice is known to occur at d 13 of fetal age *(22)*. It is of interest to consider whether the corrective, fetally derived soluble mediators are simply molecules normally released during NK cell and T-cell development, or whether they are released as a response to fetal hypertension. Finally, but much less likely, one might postulate that the metabolic demands of an immune-competent fetus are much lower than those of an immune-deficient fetus, permitting the compromised placental circulation to support an entire litter of immune-competent fetuses, but only half of a litter of immune-deficient fetuses.

During our search for an animal model of uNK cell depletion, another line of mice was identified that also lacked uNK cells and metrial gland development *(11)*. These double-null mice lack both the IL-2Rβ and the p56^{lck} tyrosine kinase signal transduction pathway *(65)*. There is no fetal resorption in these mice, and they do not have vascular pathology similar to that seen in syngeneically mated TgE26. Rather, at d 14 of gestation, the decidua is replaced by an undefined, acellular mass that appears to be edema, but is weakly reactive with Masson's trichrome stain, suggesting the presence of some collagen. Owing to infertility in each of the foundation lines, experiments have not yet been undertaken to determine if either, both, or neither of the single null genotypes presents the pathology noted at this maternal–fetal interface.

Caution must be applied to the interpretation of the results from these two strains of transgenic mice. It appears to be a solid conclusion that the cells formerly called granulated metrial gland (GMG) cells are indeed of the NK cell lineage, since they are absent in both of the NK and T-cell-depleted strains. GMG cells have been found in all T-cell-deficient, but NK cell-sufficient mice studied to date. Both strains support the idea that the critical functions of uNK cells are provided after rather than before or during implantation, and they both seem to indicate that structures associated with decidua are those normally regulated by murine uNK cells *(239)*. The lack of concordant histopathology in the implantation sites from the two strains suggests there may be influences from insertional site mutagenesis or genetic background. Lymphocyte lineage reconstitution experiments using transplantation of marrow, fetal liver, and /or fetal thymus will be needed *(240)* to determine whether NK cells alone, T-cells alone, or the two lineages combined can "cure" the problems observed at TgE26 implantation sites. Further, the differences in placental architecture between mice and humans mean that the TgE26 cannot fully replicate the preeclampsia syndrome. In particular, the invasion of the spiral arteries by endovascular trophoblast in humans plays a major hypotensive role that cannot be addressed. However, having stated these reservations, it does appear that the TgE26 mouse has the potential to provide very important conceptual advances concerning the functions of uNK cells. This may represent the most important new information to emerge since surface phenotyping studies suggested that the large granulated lymphocytes found in the pregnant uteri of both women and rodents were lymphocytes of the NK lineage *(6,200,241–243)*.

Extracellular Matrices and uNK Cells

Murine uNK cells do not proliferate in culture and have reduced viability compared to in vivo *(196)*. However, culture on extracellular matrix (ECM) prolongs their life-span beyond what would be expected in vivo *(7,196)*. Both trophoblast cells and the stromal cells of the decidua produce ECM in large amounts. These substances are believed to be important in directing the behavior and shaping the environment of cells within the feto-maternal unit *(6)*. Both NK and uNK cells in rodents and humans have been shown to express receptors for ECM, and the distribution and specificity of the receptors are altered according to the degree of cell differentiation or activation *(244–247)*. For example, in mice at early stages of gestation (d 3–6), uterine LGL-1$^+$ cells expressed the integrin chains $\beta 1$, and $\alpha 1$, $\alpha 3$, $\alpha 4$, $\alpha 5$, and $\alpha 6$, which are binding receptors for collagen, fibronectin and laminin. However during midpregnancy (d 8–15), uNK cells expressed only $\beta 1$, $\alpha 4$, and $\alpha 5$, demonstrating that major changes had occurred between d 6 and 8 *(246)*. The integrin proteins still expressed at later stages are involved in binding to fibronectin, and are believed to be important in target cell recognition and regulation of the migration and extravasation of NK cells. In mutant mice that overproduce collagen, uNK cells do not colonize the mesometrial triangle efficiently, further supporting the importance of ECM in establishing the architecture of the maternal–fetal interface *(248)*.

Human decidual CD56^{bright} cells sorted by flow cytometry strongly express the fibronectin receptors $\alpha 4\beta 1$, $\alpha 5\beta 1$, and $\alpha 4\beta 7$ *(245)*. They also express the antigen HML-1, which is known to be important for the homing of lymphocytes to mucosal surfaces. Expression of the integrin $\alpha 4$-subunit, HML-1, and CD11b was decreased after IL-2 stimulation of uNK cells in culture, whereas that of CD18 increased. CD18 and CD11a are known to be correlated with increased cytolytic activity *(245)*. The identifying surface antigen for human uNK, CD56, corresponds to an embryonic form of the neural cell adhesion molecule (NCAM), although the specific isoform has not been identified. The function of this molecule on uNK cells is unknown. NCAM is involved in limiting proliferation of rat astrocytes in culture through an autocrine mechanism *(249)* and, by analogy, may restrict uNK proliferation in the pregnant uterus.

Cytokines and Uterine Lymphocytes

Cytokines are proteins secreted by cells as intercellular mediators. They influence growth, differentiation, and activation of the secreting cell or other cells, and are important nonantigen-specific effector molecules in the lymphohematopoietic system. Lymphocytes are an important source of cytokines, which are often secreted in response to antigen presentation or other activation signals. The study of cytokine functions in the pregnant uterus is an extremely active area with important potential diagnostic and therapeutic applications *(250)*. Information concerning cytokines in the pregnant uterus is somewhat confusing to read and interpret. The reasons for this are the pleiotrophic effects of individual cytokines, the shared chains in the cytokine receptor families *(251)*, and the redundancy in cell types contributing any one cytokine to this uterine milieu. An influential concept introduced by the late T. Wegmann and his colleagues is that the pregnant uterus represents a Th2-dominated environment, which would suppress maternal antifetal immune responses *(17,117,252,253)*. IL-10 is the molecule of major importance in this model. It might be recalled that among the lymphocytes present in the human and murine uterus, T-cells are not in the majority *(6)*. Although other lymphocytes, such as NK cells, may also contribute lymphocyte-derived cytokines, the maternal–fetal interface has many intimately related cytokine producing cell types. These include trophoblast and placental cells, decidual cells, and the vascular endothelium *(56,183,254–269)*. To this must also be added cytokines produced by lymphocytes in the developing fetus, based on the findings in TgE26 female mice carrying immune-competent fetuses (Fig. 4) *(11)*. Thus, suggesting which target cell is regulated by which cytokine-producing cell is a challenge. Another aspect for concern is that pregnancy can alter cytokine levels in blood. Therefore, the ovary, adrenal gland, or another distant site could be the responding tissue. The wisest approaches for studies of cytokine influences on pregnancy appear to employ null mice that lack an individual cytokine or receptor *(269)* or *in situ* procedures in which cell and tissue relationships are maintained. The latter can provide positional and semiquantitative information, and is free from artifacts induced by tissue dissociation. An extensive review of uterine cytokines can be found in Robertson et al. *(270)*.

UTERINE LEUKOCYTES IN SPECIES WITH EPITHELIOCHORIAL PLACENTATION

The Uterus Is a Component of the Mucosal Immune System

Mucosal surfaces are comprised of an epithelium resting on a basement membrane supported by a layer of connective tissue. Placentation in conventional livestock species (e.g., pig, cow, sheep, horse) is classified as epitheliochorial: all six components separating maternal and fetal blood supplies are retained (endothelium of maternal capillaries, uterine stroma, uterine epithelium, chorionic epithelium, fetal connective tissue or mesenchyme and fetal capillary endothelium). The maternal and fetal layers in direct apposition are the maternal epithelium and fetal chorion. Because the uterine epithelium is maintained throughout gestation, the pregnant uterus in these species more closely resembles nonreproductive mucosal surfaces than that in species with hemochorial placentation.

Mucosal surfaces typically contain lymphocytes within the epithelial layer and lymphocytes, neutrophils, macrophages, eosinophils, and mast cells in the stromal compartment.

IELs, usually T-cells, have unique functional and phenotypic characteristics. Although only a few IELs are found at a given site, their total number exceeds that of all lymphocytes in blood and lymphoid organs because of the extraordinarily large surface area of mucosa. In mice, intravenously injected cells from mesenteric lymph node migrate to several mucosal surfaces, including the female reproductive tract, whereas cells from peripheral lymph nodes return to peripheral lymph nodes *(271)*. This evidence supports the concept of a common mucosal immune system. In a subsequent report, McDermott and colleagues showed that migration of mesenteric lymph node cells to the female reproductive tract was greater at proestrus and estrus than at met- and diestrus, whereas migration to small intestine was unchanged *(272)*. Estradiol treatment stimulates the appearance of IgA-positive cells in the rat uterus *(273)*, and increases the tissue and intraepithelial content of IgA *(273,274)*. This response can be blocked by progesterone or dexamethasone when admininstered along with estradiol. These findings underscore the fact that although the female reproductive tract may have many features in common with other mucosal surfaces, it is likely influenced, either directly or indirectly, by fluctuations in circulating hormones, even in nonpregnant animals.

Within the gut, a protective local response against viruses, bacteria, and other hazardous agents is necessary, but local and systemic antigen-specific tolerance to nutritional components is also required. Similarly, the uterus must be able to eliminate infectious agents while coping with infusion of potentially antigenic male factors at mating and intimate contact with the genetically disparate conceptus throughout pregnancy. The following addresses current information on uterine immune cell populations in livestock species and pregnancy-induced changes.

The Maternal Immune Response to Mating

Exposure to semen at mating is the first immunological challenge to the maternal immune system in pregnancy. Semen consists of mature spermatozoa suspended in seminal plasma, which is composed of the combined secretions of the male accessory sex glands. Seminal plasma contains many factors with well-established immunological effects, such as prostaglandins, proteases, immunoglobulins, α2-macroglobulin, and β2-microglobulin (reviewed in *275*). When added to in vitro tests of immune function, seminal plasma has been shown to inhibit activities of most immune cell types *(275)*. However, in vitro systems do not necessarily reflect leukocyte responses within the uterus.

The pig provides an excellent model in which to investigate the immunological effects of semen on the uterus, because mating involves the deposition of up to 500 mL of semen directly into the uterine lumen. Most of this is absorbed by the uterine mucosa within 5 h *(276)*. Lovell and Getty *(277)* showed that 30 min after natural mating, numerous sperm were adhered to the uterine luminal surface, and leukocytes were present in both the endometrium (within and immediately below the epithelium) and the uterine lumen. By 1.75 h, luminal leukocytes contained phagocytosed sperm; by 27 h, only degenerating leukocytes were found in the lumen. Seminal plasma alone has been shown to cause a similar influx of leukocytes into the uterine lumen *(278)*, suggesting that seminal plasma factors rather than spermatozoa mediate the leukocytic response to mating in the pig. The luminal infiltrate in pigs has been reported to consist of primarily neutrophils (various times after mating; *277*) and macrophages (9–10 h after mating; *278*). Our studies, based on morphology in smears and flow cytometry (binding to a granulocyte/macrophage marker and scatter characteristics), found neutrophils to be the predominant cell type in luminal flushings collected approx 18 h after exposure to seminal plasma *(279)*. Similarly, in cows and goats, 95% of the leukocytes in the uterine lumen after mating were neutrophils, with the remainder being macrophages *(280)*.

In investigating maternal immune responses to mating, one must be careful to distinguish between responses resulting from exposure to semen components and those resulting from the endocrine milieu at estrus. The most striking change in uterine leukocyte distribution during the estrous cycle of the pig is the infiltration of large numbers of neutrophils at estrus *(281,282)*. This response occurs in unmated as well as mated animals and is detectable as early as d 18 (*282*; cycle length = 21 d, estrus = d 0) and is probably mediated, directly or indirectly, by the elevated concentrations of circulating estrogens. Estradiol has been shown to increase uterine blood flow *(283)* and endometrial vascular permeability in the pig *(284)*. To address the effect of circulating steroid concentrations on the leukocytic response to seminal plasma, we compared the number and distribution of endometrial leukocytes in pigs after intrauterine infusion of seminal plasma at either estrus or during the luteal phase of the cycle (d 10–12). Controls at each stage were infused with the same volume of a semen extender (diluent used in artificial insemination). Leukocytes were identified in paraffin-embedded tissue using a CD44 antibody, which binds to 100% of porcine peripheral blood leukocytes *(285)*. Regardless of treatment, most leukocytes tended to cluster at the epithelial/stromal interface in estrous animals, but were found deeper within the stroma in luteal-phase animals (Fig. 6A,B; *279*). In addition to differences in distribution, estrous animals had significantly greater numbers of $CD44^+$ cells both within the stroma and at the stromal/epithelial interface than did luteal-phase animals.

A similar leukocytic response to mating has been reported in cattle and goats. Neutrophils are numerous in uterine stroma 24 h after the onset of estrus; 90% are within 150 μm of the epithelial surface and some are within the epithelial layer itself, in the subepithelial stroma around and within uterine glands *(280)*. Although the distribution was similar in mated vs unmated animals, there were more luminal leukocytes in mated vs unmated goats. Together, this evidence suggests that the endocrine status of the animal determines the leukocyte distribution, but direct exposure of the uterine mucosa to seminal plasma is required to trigger an influx of leukocytes into the lumen.

The mechanism by which seminal plasma elicits the leukocytic response to mating has not been elucidated in the pig. Porcine seminal plasma has been reported to contain factors that stimulate proliferation and agglutination of leukocytes from peripheral blood *(286,287)*. Human seminal plasma has been shown to contain leukocyte chemotactic factors *(288)*. A leukocytic response to mating also occurs in rodents *(289,290)*. There is compelling evidence that the factor initiating the rodent response originates from seminal vesicles, and upregulates the synthesis of GM-CSF and IL-6 by estrogen-primed luminal epithelial cells *(291,292)*. GM-CSF is chemotactic in vitro for macrophages and neutrophils *(293,294)* and in vivo recruits monocytes and granulocytes into inflammatory sites in the skin *(295)*.

Both the hormonally mediated migration of leukocytes into the endometrium prior to estrus and the seminal plasma-mediated influx of leukocytes into the uterine lumen may be important in containing the inevitable microbial contamination introduced into the uterus by mating or insemination. Circulating steroid hormones are known to influence the susceptibility of the uterus to infection. Resistance to infection is highest at estrus when circulating estrogen levels are high and progesterone levels low, and conversely, susceptibility to infection is greatest during diestrus when progesterone levels are elevated. For example, insemination of luteal-phase or ovariectomized, progesterone-treated cows almost invariably results in pyometritis. Estrous or ovariectomized, estrogen-treated cows

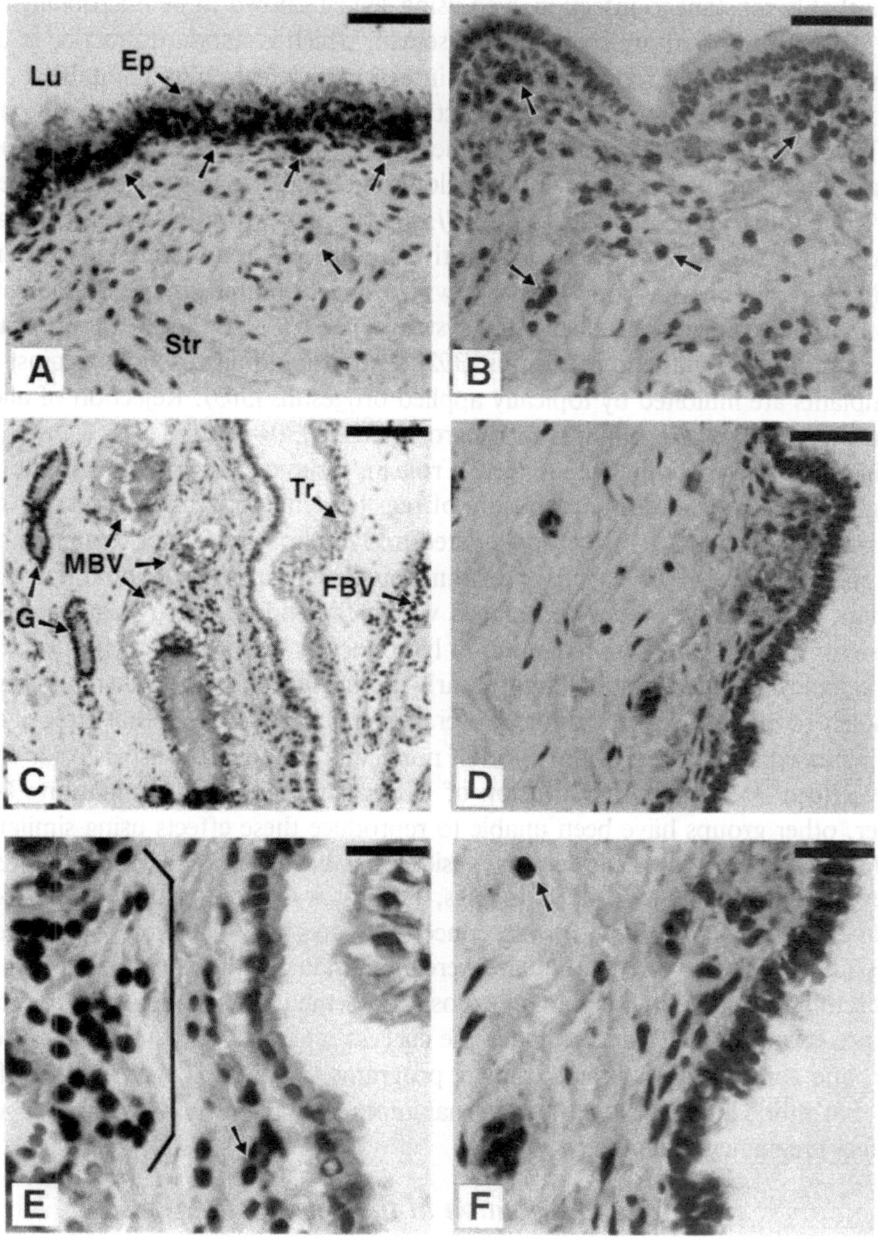

Fig. 6. Porcine endometrium obtained during the estrous cycle (**A**, estrus; **B**, diestrus) and early pregnancy (**C–F**, d 21–22), either at (C, E) or 'between' (D, F) conceptus attachment sites. Sections were stained by the streptavidin-biotin peroxidase technique with anti-CD44 (pan leukocyte marker). A, B: At estrus (A), $CD44^+$ leukocytes (arrows) were densely packed at the interface of luminal epithelium (Ep) and stroma (Str), whereas at diestrus (B), leukocytes were predominantly stromal in location. C: Note the trophoblast (Tr) that has been pulled away from the luminal epithelium during processing, fetal and maternal blood vessels (FBV, MBV) and uterine glands (G). At higher magnification (E), $CD44^+$ lymphocytes can be observed in a cluster between two blood vessels (bracket) and beneath the luminal epithelium (arrow). D, F: Between attachment sites, $CD44^+$ cell (arrow) are far fewer in number. (paraffin; hematoxylin counterstain). Bar, 150 μm (C), 75 μm (A, B, D), 37 μm (E, F).

are remarkably resistant to infection even using semen known to be microbially contaminated *(296)*. Addition of antibiotics to the semen, which is standard practice in artificial insemination of livestock today, prevented infection in luteal-phase animals.

Estrogen may increase resistance to infection indirectly by increasing uterine motility, blood flow, and vascular permeability. In the pig, the number of plasma cells is increased at estrus, although there are few immunoglobulin-containing plasma cells in the uterus compared to other mucosal surfaces *(297)*. In the rat, estradiol treatment has been reported to increase the number of IgA-positive uterine cells and uterine IgA content *(273, 274,298)*. Progesterone has long been known to have immunosuppressive activity. The rejection of allografts is curtailed after systemic *(299–301)* or local administration of various natural and synthetic progestins *(302)*, and granuloma reactions against foreign body implants are inhibited by topically applied progestins *(303)*. Rejection of allogeneic grafts in the uterus is also diminished by progesterone *(304–306)*.

Seminal plasma is hypothesized to have a role in "priming" the preimplantation uterus for pregnancy. Two to 4 d after exposure of pigs to seminal plasma, activation markers (IL-2Rα and MHC class II) were upregulated on lymphocytes from the uterine-draining lymph nodes *(307)*. MHC class II$^+$ cells increased beneath the endometrial glandular epithelium, and lymphocytes were reduced within the endometrium relative to levels in unmated control animals. The reduction in lymphocytes was similar to that occurring in early pregnancy *(308)*, suggesting that the early uterine response to fertile mating might be owing solely to seminal plasma factors. Several groups have reported that litter size in pigs can be increased by intrauterine infusion of nonviable semen at the estrus prior to breeding *(309,310)* or by intrauterine infusion of PBL at the time of insemination *(311,312)*. However, other groups have been unable to reproduce these effects using similar protocols *(313–315)*. Removal of the seminal vesicles has been reported to reduce pregnancy rates severely in rodents *(316,317)*. In pigs, fertility was reported to be unaffected by seminal vesicle removal *(318)*. However, conception rates (50%) and litter sizes (average of 7 piglets/litter) were low whether females were inseminated with semen from boars with or without seminal vesicles. In the human, exposure to semen has been reported to reduce the risk of pre-eclampsia *(319)* and enhance the success rate in in vitro fertilization, embryo transfer, and gamete intrafallopian transfer programs *(320,321)*. Together, these findings suggest that subtle influences on the maternal immune system even very early in gestation may affect pregnancy outcome.

Leukocyte Distribution in the Ruminant Uterus

Ovine and bovine blastocysts escape from their zonae early in the second week of gestation and begin rapid elongation after d 10. The chorionic vesicle(s) proliferates to fill almost the entire length of the uterus by d 14–15 in ewes *(322)* and d 21–22 in cows *(323)*, with developing embryos located just distal to the middle of the ipsilateral horn. The ruminant uterus possesses specialized caruncular regions composed of dense, aglandular stroma covered by a simple columnar epithelium. Caruncles are separated from each other by glandular intercaruncular regions. Caruncles interact with the adjacent "cotyledonary" areas of the chorioallantoic membrane to form placentomes. Contact between chorion and maternal epithelium is maintained by microvillous interdigitation, which is consolidated at the placentomes through penetration of chorionic villi into maternal crypts. As the placentomes mature, villi lengthen and branch, and the maternal crypts deepen *(324)*.

As attachment progresses, chorionic binucleate cells migrate across the placental interface and fuse with uterine epithelial cells, resulting in chimeric cells, or other binucleate cells *(325)*. In contrast to implantation in rodents and primates, chorionic cells in ruminants never penetrate beyond the basement membrane of the uterine epithelium. The multinucleate complexes subsequently spread or flatten to produce an extensive syncytium on the maternal side. In the ewe, syncytium formation is associated with degeneration of maternal cells such that migrant chorionic tissue replaces portions of the uterine epithelium *(326)*. In the cow, the uterine epithelium persists, resulting in small segments of syncytial tissue and clusters of multinucleated cells interspersed with maternal epithelial cells *(324)*.

Although the chorion attaches to all apposed surfaces of the uterus, the contact is clearly more intimate at placentomes. Interestingly, differentiation of endometrium into caruncular and intercaruncular components occurs during the development of the fetal uterus in both cattle *(327)* and sheep *(328)*. Thus, during pregnancy, it appears that the adjacent endometrium determines which areas of the chorion differentiate into cotyledons. One would predict that this communication would be bidirectional, and that the number and distribution of maternal immune cells in caruncular vs intercaruncular endometrium would be influenced by the proximity of trophoblast.

In early pregnancy in the cow (d 19–27; term = 278–290 d), a progressive decline in numbers of uterine IELs throughout both ipsilateral and contralateral horns was reported, which was associated with invasion of chorionic multinucleate cells and syncytium formation *(329)*. Using an antibody that recognized a monomorphic determinant of MHC class I molecules, Low and colleagues found that in mid- to late pregnancy, MHC class I antigens were expressed by limited areas of the chorionic epithelium in interplacentomal regions, but not on fetal cotyledonary villi at placentomes *(330)*. There was a corresponding difference in the distribution of maternal leukocytes: in intercaruncular endometrium, numerous cells expressing CD45 (leukocyte common antigen) were found in the epithelium and stroma, and a band of MHC class II^+ cells was present immediately under the epithelium. At placentomes, in contrast, there were only a few isolated class II^+ cells around blood vessels and some $CD45^+$ cells randomly distributed in the maternal caruncular septa.

In sheep, MHC class I expression was not detected on fetally derived placental tissues at any stage *(331)*. In interplacentomal regions, stroma and epithelium were positive throughout the period studied (d 9–125). At placentomes, the epithelium was positive up to d 19. However, the syncytial layer of the placentomes was consistently negative at later stages.

In early ovine pregnancy (d 21; term = 150 d), lymphocytes are present in similar numbers in caruncular and intercaruncular epithelium, but are never associated with continuous syncytium *(332)*. In intercaruncular regions, lymphocyte distribution is similar to that found in nonpregnant ewes: numerous lymphocytes are present within and beneath both luminal and glandular epithelia *(331)*. At placentomes, lymphocytes are commonly found within and just beneath the luminal epithelium and in the stroma before the establishment of chorionic villi. By the time chorionic villi form (d 30–35), lymphocytes are rare in the stroma and completely absent from the syncytial layer covering the caruncular septa *(331)*.

In both cycling and early pregnant sheep (d 18–46), the predominant leukocyte in caruncular, intercaruncular and glandular epithelia is a $CD8^+$ lymphocyte, which does not express the $\gamma\delta$ TCR *(333,334)*. Although no reagents are available to identify CD3 or the $\alpha\beta$ TCR on sheep lymphocytes, by analogy with other species, it is reasonable to assume that the cells, which comprise approx 50% of the IELs, are $\alpha\beta$ TCR^+. The remainder of the IELs express the CD45R antigen, which in peripheral blood recognizes a restricted epitope of CD45 present on B-cells and a small subset (5–6%) of T-lymphocytes *(335)*. Of these $CD8^+CD45R^+$ IELs, approximately half express the $\gamma\delta$ TCR and contain prominent granules. These cells are IgM and MHC class II negative, suggesting that they are not B-cells.

Pregnancy Associated $\gamma\delta$ T-Lymphocytes in the Ruminant Uterus. During pregnancy in sheep (d 18–46), there is a reduction in numbers of IELs in interplacentomal regions, particularly in the nongranulated subpopulation *(333)*. However, this decrease is overshadowed by a dramatic increase in the frequency of granulated lymphocytes in the luminal epithelium during mid- to late gestation *(333)*. These cells have been characterized as an unusual subset of T-cells with the phenotype $CD8^+CD45R^+$ $\gamma\delta$ TCR^+. By d 127–134, these $\gamma\delta$ T-cells make up approx 10% of the cells in the epithelium *(333)*. These cells increase in granularity (both size and number of granules) during mid- to late pregnancy, suggesting that they are undergoing activation *(331,333,334)*.

In the sheep, granulated cells within the uterine epithelium were first described as "globule leukocytes" by Kent *(336)*. Kellas noted similar cells, which he referred to as "intraepithelial granular cells," in the uterine epithelium of eight different ruminant species, including sheep, cattle, and goats *(337)*. The distribution of IELs has recently been investigated in the pregnant uterus of the deer, a ruminant that characteristically has a less extensive area of syncytium than cattle or sheep *(338)*. Although there was no appreciable change in the frequency of IELs during pregnancy, there was a shift in the relative proportion of lymphocyte types, such that numbers of large granulated IELs markedly increased and agranular IELs decreased as gestation progressed *(339)*. In contrast to sheep, the frequency of these lymphocyte types was similar in caruncular and intercaruncular endometrium, and the large granular IELs formed a much larger proportion of the total population. Also, these granular IELs increased in number early in pregnancy in deer, compared to midpregnancy in sheep *(333)*.

The $\gamma\delta$ T-cells are of particular interest in cattle and sheep in which they constitute up to 75% of circulating mononuclear cells *(340)*. In contrast to humans and mice, in which peripheral $\gamma\delta$ TCR^+ cells have the phenotype $CD2^+CD8^-CD4^-$, circulating $\gamma\delta$ T-cells in sheep and cattle are $CD2^-CD8^-CD4^-$ (triple-negative; reviewed in *341*). The CD2 molecule in the human is a T-cell antigen initially characterized by its ability to mediate rosette formation with sheep erythrocytes. CD2 is a cell-adhesion molecule that promotes the adherence of T-cells to target cells or APCs. Even when compared to $\gamma\delta$ T-cells at other sites in the sheep, the $\gamma\delta$ TCR^+ IELs of the ovine uterus have phenotypic peculiarities. Although most circulating ruminant $\gamma\delta$ T-cells (97–99%) express an antigen known as T19, a surface glycoprotein, this molecule is not expressed by the $\gamma\delta$ T-cells in the sheep uterine epithelium *(334)*. The fact that the $CD45R^+T19^-$ phenotype typical of the granulated $\gamma\delta^+$ IELs in the uterus represents only a minor subset of circulating $\gamma\delta$ T-cells implies that the uterine $\gamma\delta$ T-cells are selectively recruited from a small subpopulation of circulating $\gamma\delta$ T-cells. Despite the absence of CD8 on circulating ruminant $\gamma\delta$ T-cells, CD8 expression is consistently detectable on uterine granulated $\gamma\delta$ TCR^+ IELs, although at lower levels than on nongranulated TCR^- IELs *(334)*. Differences in CD8 phenotype between PBLs and IELs have been reported in other species. In mice, the $CD8\alpha\beta$ form predominates on PBLs, whereas a homodimeric form ($CD8\alpha\alpha$) is expressed on intestinal IELs *(342)*. Considered from a lineage perspective, the ovine uterine $\gamma\delta$ T-cells may provide equivalent functions to uNK cells found in other species. However, the timing of their activation and their position within the uterus suggest that they play other roles during pregnancy.

Regulation of Uterine Lymphocytes in Ruminants. During the period of conceptus attachment, IFNτ is secreted by the ruminant conceptus (sheep: d 11–15; cow: d 15–21;

reviewed elsewhere in this vol.). Although the primary role of IFNτ in these species is believed to be in prevention of luteolysis, this cytokine has also been shown to inhibit activation of blood lymphocytes in response to mitogenic or allogeneic stimulation *(343,344)* and to stimulate NK lytic activity *(345)*. Evidence that IFNτ affects uterine lymphocytes in vitro, or that the activity or distribution of uterine lymphocyte subpopulations changes during the time of IFNτ secretion in vivo is required before an immunomodulatory role for this cytokine can be proposed.

Although cytokine production by endometrial leukocytes has not been reported in ruminants, there is evidence for synthesis of several cytokines by uterine epithelial cells and trophoblast (IL-1, IL-6, GM-CSF, leukemia inhibitory factor [LIF]; reviewed in *346*). GM-CSF has been shown to stimulate production of IFτ *(347)*. It is possible that cytokines from these tissues influence both the conceptus and endometrial leukocytes in vivo.

Based on inhibitory effects of uterine fluid on lymphocyte function in vitro, it is believed that the ruminant conceptus is bathed by immunosuppressive substances and that this lymphocyte-inhibitory activity is under the control of progesterone *(346)*. In ovariectomized ewes, long-term treatment with progesterone (60 d) decreases numbers of endometrial MHC class II$^+$ cells and CD45R$^+$ lymphocytes *(348)*. Progesterone added directly to ovine, and bovine PBLs has been shown to inhibit mitogen-induced proliferation *(349, 350)*. However, the concentrations required to elicit these effects (10^{-6}–10^{-5} *M*) are several orders of magnitude above the K_d of the progesterone receptor (10^{-10} *M*; *351*). Furthermore, steroid antagonists not only failed to block progesterone effects, but were themselves inhibitory *(350)*. The reported in vitro effects of progesterone and other steroids may actually be owing to perturbations of membrane structure by these high concentrations of lipophilic substances. Staples and colleagues *(352)* found that the potency of steroid action on sheep lymphocytes tended to increase with lipid solubility.

Effects of progesterone are likely mediated through induction of other immunoregulatory molecules. Progesterone treatment of ovariectomized ewes induces secretion of substances into the uterine fluid that inhibit lymphocyte proliferation in vitro *(346,353)*. Most of the nondialyzable lymphocyte-inhibitory activity in uterine fluid of pregnant sheep has been attributed to a pair of related glycoproteins known as uterine milk proteins (UTMP). UTMPs, which are members of the serpin superfamily of serine protease inhibitors, are the predominant endometrial secretory protein in uterine fluids of pregnant and progesterone-treated ewes *(346,354)*. Similar proteins have also been demonstrated in the bovine uterus *(355)*.

Dipeptidyl peptidase-IV (DPPIV), a serine protease, is secreted by the ovine and bovine endometrium under the influence of progesterone *(356)*. DPPIV is homologous to CD26, a human T-cell-surface marker that is strongly expressed on IL-2-dependent T-cell lines and on a substantial portion of activated T-cells *(357–359)*. DPPIV has also been identified in the uterus of the rabbit *(360)* and mouse *(361)*. The physiological relevance of this molecule is unclear: it causes limited enhancement of PHA-stimulated lymphocyte proliferation in vitro *(356)*, but crude uterine fluid strongly inhibits lymphocyte proliferation, presumably owing to the actions of uterine milk proteins *(353)*.

Leukocyte Distribution in the Uterus of the Horse

The equine blastocyst sheds its zona 8–9 d after mating, but remains enclosed in a second noncellular membrane formed between the zona and the vitelline membrane *(362)*. The conceptus moves rapidly and apparently randomly throughout the entire uterus from the time it is first detectable by ultrasound (d 9 or 10), until it assumes a fixed position on d 15–16 *(363)*. The capsule is lost by d 21–22, by which time the conceptus is a 6–7 cm sphere lodged near the junction of one horn with the uterine body *(364)*. Equine conceptuses remain spherical for a longer period than other livestock species, and never achieve the slender filamentous forms that develop in ruminants and pigs *(324)*.

A yolk sac and then an allantochorionic placenta form, although the latter rapidly outgrows the former *(365)*. At the junction between the advancing allantois and regressing yolk sac, the chorion becomes thickened and corrugated, forming a band that completely surrounds the spherical conceptus, the chorionic girdle. The girdle becomes visible by about d 28 of gestation and reaches full development by about d 35 at which time it is a band 6–8 mm wide *(364,366)*. Between d 28 and 35, girdle ridges project into folds of the uterine lining.

At d 36–38 of gestation, cells of the chorionic girdle begin to invade the endometrium *(367,368)*. Most of the invading cells are binucleate at the time of migration into the uterine epithelium *(369)*. After approx 24 h in the epithelium, some of the chorionic cells migrate into the endometrial stroma. Those that fail to make contact with the basal lamina of the uterine epithelium degenerate *(369)*. Migrant cells that reach the stroma cease dividing, hypertrophy in a relatively uniform fashion, and congregate into structures known as endometrial cups. The regions of epithelium destroyed by invading girdle cells quickly regenerate and cover the cup surfaces by d 45 *(369,370)*.

The only known function of endometrial cup cells is the production of equine chorionic gonadotropin (eCG), formerly known as pregnant mare serum gonadotropin (PMSG), which is detectable in maternal blood between d 40 and 120 of gestation (term = 40 d; *367,368*). Production of eCG starts before the invasive phase of endometrial cup formation, as shown by the positive staining of d 33 chorionic girdle cells with antibodies directed against eCG *(371)*. The role of this gonadotropin in equine pregnancy is unclear. Although in other species, eCG has both follicle-stimulating hormone (FSH) and LH activity and is often used as an FSH substitute, it has very little FSH activity in equids *(372)*. However, eCG has luteotropic activity in the horse and may be involved in the ovulation/luteinization of the secondary corpora lutea *(373,374)* or, as hCG in humans *(375)*, the resurgence of the primary corpus luteum *(373,376)*.

The life-span of the endometrial cups is 80–100 d. Beyond about d 70, the cells at the luminal surface of the cup begin to degenerate, and maternal leukocytes invade its peripheral regions. By 100–120 d, the entire necrotic cup is sloughed off the endometrial surface *(377)*. Thus, placentation in the mare is relatively invasive compared to ruminants and pigs for the first half of gestation while the endometrial cups persist, but completely noninvasive for the second half.

The Maternal Immune Response to Endometrial Cup Cells. The presence of the fetally derived endometrial cups has a remarkable effect on the distribution of maternal leukocytes in the endometrium. A detailed morphological study of events occurring during girdle cell migration and endometrial cup formation has been carried out by Enders and Liu *(369)*. LGLs are numerous in the uterine epithelium, even at sites of invasion. Small lymphocytes, plasma cells, and macrophages are present in the endometrial stroma. With the initiation of epithelial invasion, there is a burst of small lymphocyte migration into the stroma, such that girdle cells migrate into a stroma already rich in lymphocytes. By the time the girdle cells differentiate into cup cells, leukocytes are no longer present within the cup, but are abundant in the surrounding stroma. Throughout the life-span of the cups, increasing numbers of leukocytes, mostly small lymphocytes with occasional plasma cells and eosinophils, accumulate in the endometrium at the periphery of each cup. The lymphocytes express either CD4 or CD8 (CD4:CD8 = 4:1; *378*).

Another unusual feature of equine pregnancy is that during gestation, >90% of primiparous mares develop high titers of alloantibodies that are cytotoxic for lymphocytes of the sire of the conceptus *(370,379)*. These antibodies are detectable in maternal serum between d 44 and 70 *(380)*, which is soon after the invasion of the chorionic girdle cells. The cytotoxic antibodies are directed exclusively against paternally derived MHC class I *(381)* and do not occur in mares carrying histocompatible conceptuses *(382)*. By comparison, cytotoxic antibodies to paternal lymphocyte antigens are detectable in a minority of women, and only relatively late in gestation (reviewed in *383*).

The leukocytic reaction associated with development and regression of the endometrial cups was thought to be a maternal immune response to paternally inherited MHC antigens. However, leukocyte accumulation also takes place in mares carrying histocompatible conceptuses *(382)*. Although chorionic girdle cells strongly express MHC class I before invasion (d 33–35; *384*), expression is low to undetectable after the cells differentiate into mature cups (d 60; *384–386*). MHC class I expression by allantochorion (noninvasive trophoblast) is undetectable at all stages. Maternal epithelium near the cups is strongly MHC$^+$, but expression on epithelium away from cups is variable and often diminished. The high level of MHC class I expression by invasive trophoblast cells followed by the loss of this expression by the descendant endometrial cup cells is believed to be a novel example of MHC gene regulation.

The leukocyte response may be mediated by eCG produced by the cup, but chemotactic properties of this molecule have not been investigated. It has been suggested that the endometrial damage resulting from invasion of the chorionic girdle cells initiates inflammation. However, the predominance of lymphocytes rather than neutrophils or macrophages in the infiltrate suggests otherwise. An equine trophoblast-specific antigen has been identified *(387)*. However, presence of this antigen on both invasive and noninvasive trophoblast makes it an unlikely stimulus for the leukocyte accumulation around endometrial cups. A population of suppressor cells having activity analogous to uterine TGF-β_2 found during pregnancy in the mouse *(262)* may protect cup cells from maternal leukocyte attack before d 70 *(388)*. In the horse, TGF-β_2 expression was not found before invasion of the endometrial by girdle cells, but maternal leukocytes expressing TGF-β_2 mRNA were observed in the region of the developing cups between d 38 and 43 *(389)*. At later stages (d 78 and 81), clusters of cells hybridizing with the TGF-β_2 riboprobe were localized within the dense band of leukocytes at the periphery of the degenerating cups *(389)*. On d 78, 90% of the TGF-β_2-expressing cells also stained with chromotrope 2R, which identifies eosinophils *(389)*.

It is tempting to speculate that death of endometrial cup cells is mediated by a non-MHCrestricted NK cell subset. LGLs are present in the equine uterine epithelium, but these cells have not been characterized with respect to surface phenotype *(369)*. Lymphocytes expressing CD8 are present in the infiltrate surrounding the endometrial cups *(378)*. There is some evidence to suggest that in horses as in pigs, NK cells are CD8$^+$ *(390)*. Clearly, further investigation is required to determine whether NK cells are present in the vicinity of endometrial cups.

The fact that members of the genus *Equus* successfully interbreed has allowed the comparison of intra-, inter-, and extraspecific pregnancies with respect to endometrial cup development, eCG production, the leukocytic response to the presence of the cups, and cytotoxic antibody production (reviewed in *391*). The donkey-in-horse model of pregnancy failure *(392)* offers some insights into normal pregnancy. Donkey-in-horse pregnancies (created by embryo transfer) have complete failure of endometrial cup formation, no production of eCG, but a dense accumulation of lymphocytes in maternal endometrium in contact with allantochorion *(388)*. These trophoblast of the donkey conceptuses shows tremendous variation in MHC expression and in the extent of interdigitation with the horse endometrium, ranging from firmly attached, MHC-negative trophoblast with few associated maternal lymphocytes to completely unattached, intensely MHC+ trophoblast associated with an endometrium densely packed with lymphocytes *(387)*. Even in normal horse and donkey pregnancies, regions of trophoblast overlying endometrial cups are MHC class I+ and at these points, the trophoblast does not have close intervillous attachment to the uterine epithelium. This led Kydd and her colleagues to propose that the lack of physical attachment either triggers a mechanism initiating expression of polymorphic molecules, such as MHC, or neutralizes a mechanism that normally blocks MHC expression *(387)*. Expression of polymorphic MHC along a substantial portion of the fetal–maternal interface, as in the abnormal donkey-in-horse pregnancies, could result in attraction of lymphocytes and abortion. It must be noted that although most of the donkey-in-horse pregnancies result in abortion by d 70–90, 10–30% are carried to term in the complete absence of endometrial cups or eCG *(392)*. Taken together with the few reported cases in the literature in which mares are able to carry to term in the absence of endometrial cups and/or eCG *(376,393)*, neither of these features seem absolutely essential for pregnancy in the horse.

Leukocyte Distribution in the Uterus of the Pig

Porcine blastocysts "hatch" 7–9 d after mating and enlarge uniformly for several days, forming spherical vesicles 8–10 mm in diameter. During this period the embryos migrate, becoming evenly distributed throughout the uterus. This spacing occurs even if ovulation is entirely unilateral *(394)*. On d 12 after fertilization, very rapid elongation occurs such that each conceptus forms a convoluted thread over a meter in length *(395)*, although because of their folding and twisting, each filamentous blastocyst occupies only a 10–20 cm length of luminal surface *(324)*. In contrast to primates and rodents, porcine conceptuses lodge in the mesometrial aspect of the uterus. Adhesion and attachment commence late in the second week in regions of apposition immediately adjacent to the embryonic disk. As attachment progresses, both the chorionic and uterine epithelia develop interdigitating cytoplasmic processes and microvilli. Beginning at the fourth week, chorionic ridges and secondary folds form, greatly increasing the surface area for metabolic exchange between mother and fetus. The chorioallantois becomes corrugated over the gland mouths, forming "areolae," which facilitate absorption of glandular secretions. These areolae increase in size and number as gestation proceeds.

The pig exemplifies the least intimate relationship between maternal and fetal tissues, even among species with epitheliochorial placentation. Invasion is completely prevented, and it is possible, with careful dissection, to obtain piglets complete with intact fetal membranes right up to term (115 d). However, properties of the uterine epithelium rather than the chorionic cells seem to limit invasion, since transplantation of porcine trophoblast to a variety of ectopic sites (within the uterine wall or beneath the capsule of the spleen or kidney) results in invasion of surrounding tissue and syncytial transformation typical of species with invasive placentation *(396,397)*.

The distribution of leukocyte populations within the uterus of the nonpregnant pig has been investigated by Bischof and colleagues in an immunohistochemical study using antibodies specific for porcine cell-surface markers *(282)*. Neutrophils were the predominant cells in the prepubertal uterus (~ 175 d of age); MHC class II+ cells (macrophages and dendritic cells) and lymphocytes were also common. In the cycling uterus, the most numerous leukocytes were lymphocytes, followed by macrophages and neutrophils.

Table 3
Frequency of Cells Reactive with Antiporcine CD44 MAb, a Pan Leukocyte Marker, in Porcine Endometrium During Early Pregnancy[a]

	Frequency of CD44⁺ cells, mean ± SEM	
Uterine	*Epithelium, #/mm²*	*Stroma, #/mm²*
At attachment sites	0.7 ± 0.3	323 ± 35
Between attachment sites	0.9 ± 0.3	98 ± 10

[a]Uterine tissue was collected either at or between conceptus attachment sites from pigs at d 16–25 of gestation (n = 6). Tissue blocks were fixed overnight in 0.5% zinc chloride in 0.1 M Tris plus 0.5% calcium acetate, and then processed routinely for paraffin embedding and immunohistology.

Lymphocytes were located in the stroma and the luminal epithelium, both between epithelial cells and in basal positions.

As discussed previously, a massive influx of neutrophils into the the subepithelial stroma and epithelium occurs at estrus *(282)*. The second major cyclical effect was a dramatic drop at midcycle (d 10–12; cycle length = 21 d) in numbers of lymphocytes relative to earlier in the cycle (d 2–4), in both the epithelial and stromal compartments. This observation is in conflict with an earlier report by King *(398)*, who noted a modest, but statistically significant increase in lymphocytes within the uterine epithelium through d 10–19 of the cycle. King did not assess numbers of stromal lymphocytes.

During the period of conceptus attachment, King *(398)* found that numbers of IELs in pregnant animals were significantly lower those that at comparable stages of the cycle (d 10, 13, 16, and 19), and decreased as pregnancy progressed. In contrast, Bischof and colleagues found no progressive decrease in IELs over the first 3 wk of gestation, although numbers of IELs were significantly lower in pregnant animals at d 2–3 and d 18–21 relative to cycling controls *(308)*. One methodological difference between these two studies was that in the King report *(398)*, tissue was collected from the mesometrial aspect of the uterus at attachment sites when possible (d 13, 16, 19), whereas Bischof and colleagues collected their tissue from the antimesometrial side of the uterus *(308)*. As previously noted, conceptus attachment in the pig occurs on the mesometrial aspect of the uterus, and the extensive contact between trophoblast and the epithelium has already induced localized differentiation of the endometrium by d 13 *(399)*.

Using the CD44 MAb, a pan leukocyte marker, we have compared leukocyte numbers in uterine tissue collected from the mesometrial aspect of the uterus at vs between conceptus attachment sites during early pregnancy (d 16–25; *400*). The number of CD44⁺ cells was assessed in 10 sites/section using image analysis software (Mocha, Jandel Scientific), and data were expressed per unit length of epithelium. The density of CD44⁺ cells/mm² was determined in the underlying stroma to a depth of 100–150 μm. In contrast to cycling animals (Fig. 6A,B), CD44⁺ cells were abundant in the stromal compartment, but rare in the epithelium. Over the gestational interval studied, stromal CD44⁺ cells were consistently three- to fourfold more numerous at vs between attachment sites (Table 3). Morphologically, the vast majority of these cells appear to be lymphocytes. The tissues are currently being probed using other surface markers to determine whether proximity to the conceptus affects the distribution of lymphocyte subpopulations.

Little is known about porcine uterine leukocyte distributions later in pregnancy. Bischof and colleagues reported that at attachment sites on d 28–30 of gestation, lymphocytes were present in the stroma around blood vessels and glands, and MHC class II⁺ macrophages were prominent under the epithelium. By d 45–60, the main leukocyte types observed in the stroma were macrophages and dendritic cells; many eosinophils were present and some lymphocytes *(308)*.

As in the small intestine *(401)*, the majority of lymphocytes in the pig uterus are CD2+ *(282,308)*. The CD2 antigen, a cell-adhesion molecule present on both T-cells and NK cells in the pig *(402)*, is believed to play a role in lymphocyte homing *(403)*. In porcine intestinal epithelium, two different CD2+ lymphocyte subpopulations have been identified: CD8− CD4− (double-negative) cells located apically and CD8+CD4− cells concentrated around the basement membrane *(401)*. In both pregnant and nonpregnant uteri, the CD2+ lymphocytes were predominantly CD8+ (particularly in the epithelium), with smaller numbers of CD4+ cells *(308)*. Through cell separation and remixing experiments, functional porcine uterine T-cells (responsive to the T-cell mitogen phyotohemagglutinin) have been demonstrated, as well as two independent populations capable of suppressing this response. No response was induced in unseparated cell suspensions *(404)*. The suppressor cells were also found in the uteri of pseudopregnant pigs, indicating that the presence of a conceptus was not required for their recruitment; cycling animals were not assessed.

In contrast to humans and mice, in which $\gamma\delta$ T-cells are a very minor subset of circulating T-cells with the phenotype CD2+CD8−CD4−, $\gamma\delta$ T-cells in pigs *(405)* as in cattle and sheep *(341)*, constitute a major circulating T-cell subpopulation with the predominant phenotype CD2−CD8−CD4− (triple-negative). Failure to account for these triple-negative cells may account for discrepancies between studies examining pregnancy effects on uterine IELs that are based on surface markers *(308)* and those based on morphology *(398)*. The lack of surface markers for $\gamma\delta$ TCR+ lymphocytes has limited investigations of these cells in the pig. The antibody "86D" recognizes an external epitope of the $\gamma\delta$ T-cell receptor, which is expressed by all CD2− T-lymphocytes of sheep and nearly all those of cattle *(341,406)*, but only a minor subset of $\gamma\delta$ T-cells in pigs *(405)*. An antibody recognizing a determinant of the δ-chain of the porcine $\gamma\delta$ TCR has recently become available (PGBL22A; VMRD Inc., Pullman, WA). In preliminary investigations using enzymatically dispersed, gradient-purified endometrial cells from d 21–22 of gestation, we have found that this anti-δ-chain antibody binds to similar proportions of CD44+ cells harvested either at or between attachment sites (~7%) and to a somewhat higher proportion of peripheral blood mononuclear cells (~23%).

Pregnancy-Associated NK Cells in the Porcine Uterus. The phenotype CD2+CD8+ predominant in lymphocytes of the pregnant and nonpregnant porcine uterus *(282,308)* is consistent with both the T-cell and NK cell lineages of the pig *(407)*. Dispersed porcine endometrial cells lyse conventional NK target cells in vitro *(408,409)*, suggesting that NK cells are present in the porcine endometrium. However, an antibody specific for porcine NK cells was not available at the time of these studies to confirm the identity of the endometrial effector cells. Endometrial cell lytic activity was elevated at d 10 and 20 of pregnancy and undetectable in cycling animals *(409)*. The fact that this increase in lytic activity was not detected at comparable stages of estrogen-induced pseudopregnancy *(409)* suggests that it was a response to the presence of conceptuses rather than the endocrine milieu of pregnancy.

The presence of potentially lytic cells in close proximity to the developing conceptus raised the question of whether porcine trophoblast cells were susceptible to lysis by uterine NK-like cells. In contrast to uNK cells in the human and mouse *(203,410,411)*, porcine endometrial cells obtained at early postattachment times (d 17–20) recognize and kill porcine trophoblast cells in culture without prior activation by IL-2 *(8)*. That the same endometrial population killed both K562 targets and trophoblast cells was supported by evidence that: (1) both targets were observed to bind to effector cells of similar morphology, and (2) killing of labeled K562 cells was inhibited in a parallel, dose-dependent manner by addition of unlabeled trophoblast or unlabeled K562 cells. Although IL-2 activation was not required for lysis, activity was increased by prior incubation of endometrial effectors with IL-2.

Investigations into the identity of these lytic cells have continued using the MAb "G7." This antibody was raised in mice immunized with a porcine peripheral blood fraction enriched for NK cells. G7 (generously provided by Y. B. Kim, The Chicago Medical School) is one of the best reagents available, but it also binds to granulocytes and 70% of monocytes/macrophages *(412)*. Using flow cytometry, we have compared numbers of $G7^+$ cells as a proportion of total leukocytes ($CD44^+$ cells) in endometrium obtained both at and between attachment sites during early pregnancy. Cell suspensions were prepared from endometrial tissue that was mechanically separated, minced, enzymatically dispersed, and purified by gradient centrifugation (Lympholyte-Mammal, CedarLane Laboratories, Hornby, ON, Canada) to remove granulocytes, erythrocytes, and nonleukocytic endometrial cells. The proportion of $CD44^+$ cells in samples collected at attachment sites was similar to that in preparations from cycling animals and was relatively constant over the stages of gestation studied (d 15–17: 81.4 ± 2.1%; d 21–22: 73.0 ± 5.0%; d 24–28: 69.8 ± 3.5%). However, CD44 binding progressively decreased in samples obtained between attachment sites (d 15–17: 81.1 ± 3.7%; d 21–22: 59.9 ± 5.3%; d 24–28: 31.4 ± 7.4%). Our interpretation of this effect is that in samples obtained between attachment sites, an increasing proportion of nonlymphoid, and therefore $CD44^-$ cells migrate to the mononuclear cell band during the gradient centrifugation step. To control for this artifact of the cell isolation procedure, G7 binding was expressed relative to $CD44^+$ leukocytes.

The frequency of $G7^+$ cells, as a proportion of the entire population of $CD44^+$ cells, was consistently higher in endometrial cells than in similarly prepared cells from peripheral blood of the same animals. However, there was no significant difference between numbers of $G7^+$ cells at vs between attachment sites. In both blood and endometrial cells, two distinct populations recognized by G7 were identified by their scatter characteristics: LGLs and monocytes/macrophages. LGLs were the more frequent $G7^+$ cell type in both endometrial samples (LGL:macrophages = 9.5 ± 1.7) and blood (LGL:macrophages = 6.7 ± 2.0). The frequency of $G7^+$ cells with LGL morphology was greater at attachment sites at d 21–22 (at: 36.3 ± 3.3%; between: 24.2 ± 1.5%) and at d 24–28 of gestation (at: 29.3 ± 8.0%; between: 12.4 ± 3.7%).

The distribution of uterine NK cells relative to the maternal–fetal interface during porcine pregnancy is not currently known. The granulated $CD2^+CD8^+$ lymphocytes found in the uterine epithelium of cycling and pregnant pigs *(307,308)* could be NK cells. However, phenotypically and morphologically similar lymphocytes in the porcine intestine appear to be T-cells because they display cytotoxic and helper T-cell functions and they do not lyse NK cell targets *(413)*. Thus, it is possible that the IELs in the porcine uterus are T-cells. Furthermore, porcine uterine IELs decrease in number through early pregnancy *(398)*, and are very rare (Table 3) when endometrial lytic activity is known to be elevated *(409)*. In the endometrial stroma $CD44^+$ lymphocytes are three- to fourfold more frequent in regions of stroma adjacent to trophoblast (Fig. 6C–F; Table 3). Together, this evidence suggests that in pigs, in common with humans and rodents, uterine NK cells localize to stromal, but not to epithelial tissue closely associated with conceptuses.

Interferon Production by Porcine Trophoblast. Porcine trophoblast has been shown to secrete high levels of antiviral activity between d 12 and 20 of pregnancy *(414,*

415). Subsequent characterization of this activity revealed that that it was owing to two distinct IFNs *(416)*, one of which was identified as IFNγ *(417)*; the other was a type II IFN resembling that produced by activated T- and NK cells. A novel type I IFN gene has been cloned from a d 14–15 porcine conceptus cDNA library that has been provisionally designated spI (short porcine type I) IFN *(418)*. This gene encodes the type I component of the antiviral activity secreted by the porcine conceptus. Pregnancy in the pig requires the conceptus to prevent luteal regression between d 11 and 15 after mating *(419)*. Since porcine IFNs are secreted during this interval, the possibility that these molecules have antiluteolytic activity, as in ruminants, has been addressed. However, intrauterine infusion of porcine conceptus-secretory proteins had no effect on luteal life-span when administered during d 12–15 of the cycle *(420)*. Prevention of luteal regression in pigs is believed to be mediated by conceptus-derived estrogen, which is also secreted at this time *(421)*.

IFNs are best known as a first line defense against viral diseases. D'Andrea and colleagues assessed porcine trophoblast and endometrial cells infected with vesicular stomatitis or transmissable gastroenteritis virus as possible targets for the antiviral activity of spI IFN and rIFNγ *(422)*. Endometrial cells were sensitive to the antiviral effects of these IFNs: stromal cells were highly sensitive to spI IFN and weakly sensitive to IFNγ; epithelial cells were sensitive to both IFNs. However, neither spI IFN nor rIFNγ had antiviral effects on trophoblast. Similarly, in the mouse, virally-induced IFN had no antiviral effect on preimplantation embryos *(423)*. In contrast to the pig, however, no significant IFN synthesis is detectable in the mouse uterus around the time of implantation *(424)*. Major intracellular effects of IFNs usually involve induction of 2′,5′-oligo(A) synthetase *(425)*. In contrast to D'Andrea et al. *(422)*, Short and colleagues found that porcine conceptus secretory proteins induced 2′,5′-oligo(A) synthetase in MDBK cells (a cell line used to assay antiviral activity) and in bovine endometrial explants, but had no effect in endometrial explants of pigs *(426)*. However, the use of whole endometrial explants rather than monolayers of isolated cell types in the latter study may have masked changes in enzyme activity.

Possible effects of porcine conceptus-derived IFNs on maternal leukocytes have not been addressed. IFNs are produced by activated T-cells and NK cells, and are major regulators of NK cell function *(427,428)*. These cytokines exert many immunoregulatory effects, such as enhancement of T- and NK cell-mediated cytotoxicity, B-cell differentiation, MHC antigen expression, and macrophage activation *(429)*. Evidence for coordinated IFN secretion by the porcine conceptus, elevation of endometrial NK-like activity, and an increase in lymphocyte density in endometrial stroma in the vicinity of conceptuses during early placentation raises the intriguing possibility that spI IFN is a messenger by which the porcine trophoblast activates the maternal immune system and directs its functions to the advantage of the fetus.

PREGNANCY-ASSOCIATED UTERINE LYMPHOCYTES: IS THERE A UNIFYING HYPOTHESIS?

The placenta is central to the evolutionary success of eutherian mammals, but as emphasized by Roberts and his colleagues *(13)*, its structure is disconcertingly variable. This variability has profound implication in all aspects of maternal–fetal communication, and there is no reason to assume that the mechanisms for immunological communication or its importance would be constant across species. Several principles appear to be universally applicable across the species and placental types. These are:

1. The female reproductive organs of all species are components of the immune system, because all classes of immune-competent cells are present.
2. Circulating hormones and paracrine regulatory factors influence cells of the immune system, altering their distribution and/or activity though the course of the menstrual/estrous cycle and pregnancy. This occurs at both the systemic and local uterine levels.
3. Both the innate and the antigen-specific arms of the immune system are affected by changes in reproductive status. In the uterus, however, changes in the innate immune system predominate.
4. Uterine NK cells and $\gamma\delta$ T-cells may be specialized subsets within their lineages with novel, pregnancy-associated functions.
5. Trophoblast has evolved unique patterns of regulated MHC expression in different species that may be obligatory for pregnancy success.

The major apparent differences in immunological communication at the maternal–fetal interface can be attributed to the anatomy of the interface as well as to the design, frequency, and depth of studies conducted among various species. In animals with hemochorial placentation, direct exchange of both maternal and fetal lymphocytes, antigen-specific antibodies, and other soluble immune mediators occurs across the placenta. In these pregnancies, microchimerism as a mechanism for inducing tolerance through clonal anergy in the mother and clonal deletion in the fetus needs to be more thoroughly addressed.

In immune-deficient mice raised under germ-free conditions, the only lymphocytes found to play a critical, pregnancy-associated role are NK cells. Their functions are necessary for normal, postimplantation development of decidua-associated structures, possibly including a role in modification of uterine arteries to promote adequate placental perfusion. Immune-deficient mice cannot be used to assess the roles of lymphocytes in an environment with normal microbial flora or in tolerance promotion when antigen-specific immune effector cells can be induced. For T-cells and B-cells, it can only be concluded that normal placental and fetal development can occur without their input.

In species with epitheliochorial placentation, immunological communication techniques between the mother and her conceptus(es) appear to be highly variable. Direct, two-way exchange of cells, antibodies, or other immune mediators across the placenta has not been demonstrated, although systemic effects of trophoblast-derived interferons are known.

In ruminants, unusual $\gamma\delta$ T-cells may become activated during mid- to late gestation. Morphologically, these cells resemble the mature granulated uterine NK cells found in the pregnant uterus of the human and mouse. However, ruminant $\gamma\delta$ T-cells are epithelial rather than stromal in location and are absent from the placentomes, the areas most closely associated with trophoblast.

Large granular intraepithelial lymphocytes have been reported in the pregnant horse uterus, but their lineage is unknown. Cells with similar morphology have not been reported in the uterus of the pig, but later stages of pregnancy remain unstudied. Evidence that $\gamma\delta$ T-cells constitute a major circulating T-cell population in pigs as in well as ruminants suggests that this T-cell subset may also be predominant in the uteri of other members of the order Artiodactyla (cloven-hoofed ungulates). The horse challenges immunological concepts usually associated with the idea of fetal allograft tolerance. In spite of high levels of MHC expression on the invading fetal trophoblast cells, the resulting high titers of cytotoxic alloantibodies early in pregnancy, and a vigorous cell-mediated reaction resulting in the death of the fetally derived endometrial cup cells, horses reproduce successfully! The pig is perhaps most similar to the human and rodent in that NK cells are present in the uterine stroma and seem to play a role in pregnancy. These cells are activated during early placental development and may be important in early interactions between the conceptus and the maternal immune system. Production of IFNγ by the porcine conceptus during this time directly contradicts the hypothesis based on human and rodent data that pregnancy is a Th2 phenomenon, and that IFNγ, a Th1 cytokine, is generally harmful to the maintenance of pregnancy.

Although immunological strategies for successful pregnancy vary enormously across species, the presence of the genetically foreign conceptus seems to activate maternal immune cells within the uterus and to redirect their activities toward promotion of fetal survival.

ABBREVIATIONS

APC(s), antigen-presenting cell(s); B-cell, bone marrow-derived lymphocyte or cell; CD3, a complex of invariant peptides originally described as T-cell surface proteins associated with TCR; subsequently some chains of CD3 were characterized as cytoplasmic proteins in NK cells—the CD3 peptides are γ, δ, ϵ, ζ, and η; CSF-1, colony-stimulating factor 1, also known as macrophage-CSF; ER, estrogen receptor; H-2, murine histocompatibility complex antigen system; HLA, human leukocyte antigen; GM-CSF, granulocyte macrophage-colony-stimulating factor; GMG cells, granulated metrial gland cells (older terminology for granulated uterine; natural killer cells); IDDM, insulin-dependent diabetes mellitus; IEL; intraepithelial lymphocyte; Ig, immunoglobulin; IL, interleukin, such as IL-2, IL-4, IL-10; IL-2R, receptor for IL-2; IFNγ, interferon γ; KIR, killer inhibitory receptors—these are found on NK cells; LAK, lymphokine-activated killer lymphocytes or cells; LGL, large granulated lymphocytes—this term is often applied to NK cells; MHC, major histocompatibility antigen complex, subclassed as class I, class II, and so forth; NK cell, natural killer lymphocyte or cell; NO, nitric oxide; NOD, nonobese diabetic, a mutant mouse genotype; PBL, peripheral blood leukocytes; PIH, pregnancy-induced hypertension; PR, progesterone receptor; SLE, systemic lupus erythematosis; T-cell, thymus-derived lymphocyte or cell; TCR, antigen-specific T-cell receptor, found as dimers of $\alpha\beta$ or $\gamma\delta$; TGF-β, transforming growth factor-β; Th as Th1, Th2, and so on, T-cell subsets, classified as helper cells but discriminated by patterns of cytokine production; NF-α, tumor necrosis factor-α; uNK cells, natural killer lymphocytes found in the uterus.

ACKNOWLEDGMENTS

This work was supported by the Ontario Ministry of Agriculture, Food and Rural Affairs, and the Natural Sciences and Engineering Council of Canada. P. W. is an NSERC Canada International Fellow, and H. E. is an OVC Postdoctoral Fellow. We thank Jeffrey Luross and John Swatman for preparation of the histological figure plates, the OVC Isolation Unit for their dedicated care of our immune-deficient mice, and the many students and colleagues whose work and discussions have made major contributions to our thinking.

REFERENCES

1. Poussier P, Julius M (1994) Thymus independent T cell development and selection in the intestinal epithelium. Ann Rev Immunol 12:521–553.
2. Abbas AK, Lichtman AH, Pober JS (1994) Cellular and Molecular Immunology, 2nd ed. WB Saunders, Philadelphia, PA.
3. Kuby J (1994) Immunology, 2nd ed. WH Freeman, New York, NY.
4. Wilder RL (1995) Neuroendocrine-immune system interactions and autoimmunity. Ann Rev Immunol 13:307–338.
5. Medawar PB (1953) Some immunological and endocrinological problems raised by the evolution of viviparity in vertebrates. Symp Soc Exp Biol 7:320–338.
6. Loke YW, King A (1995) Human Implantation: Cell Biology and Immunology. Cambridge University Press, Cambridge, UK.

7. Croy B, Kiso Y (1993) Granulated metrial gland cells: a natural killer cell subset of the pregnant murine uterus. Microsc Res Tech 25:189–200.
8. Yu Z-M, Croy BA, King GJ (1994) Lysis of porcine trophoblast cells by endometrial natural killer-like effector cells in vitro does not require interleukin-2. Biol Reprod 51:1279–1284.
9. Bonney EA, Matzinger P (1996) Beyond fetal cell migration into the maternal circulation. FASEB J, 10 Abstract #2104, A1364.
10. Starzl TE, Demetris AJ, Trucco M, Murase N, Ricordi C, Ildstad S, Ramoss H, Todo S, Tzakis A, Fung JJ, Nalesik M, Zeevi A, Rudert WA, Kocova M (1993) Cell migration and chimerism after whole organ transplantation: the basis of graft acceptance. Hepatology 17:1127–1152.
11. Guimond MJ, Luross JA, Wang B, Suzuki H, Mak TW, Terhorst C, Danial S, Croy BA (1996) Absence of natural killer cells during murine pregnancy is associated with reproductive compromise. Biol Reprod 56:169–179.
12. Guimond MJ, Wang B, Fujita J, Terhorst C, Croy BA (1996) Pregnancy-associated uterine granulated metrial gland cells in mutant and transgenic mice. Am J Reprod Immunol 35:501–509.
13. Roberts R, Xie S, Mathialaga M (1996) Maternal recognition of pregnancy. Biol Reprod 54: 294–302.
14. Georgopoulos K, Bigby M, Wang J-H, Molnar A, Wu P, Winandy S, Sharpe A (1994) The Ikaros gene is required for the development of all lymphoid lineages. Cell 79:143–156.
15. Zhou L-J, Tedder TF (1996) $CD14^+$ blood monocytes can differentiate into functionally mature CD83 dendritic cells. Proc Natl Acad Sci USA 93:2588–2592.
16. Matzinger P (1994) Tolerance, danger and the extended family. Ann Rev Immunol 12: 991–1045.
17. Mosmann TR, Sad S (1996) The expanding universe of T-cell subsets: Th1, Th2 and more. Immunol Today 17:138–146.
18. Kaufmann SHE (1996) γ/δ and other unconventional lymphocytes: what do they see and what do they do? Proc Natl Acad Sci USA 93:2272–2279.
19. Salaun J, Bandeira A, Khazaal I, Calman F, Coltey M, Coutinho A, Le Douarin NM (1990) Thymic epithelium tolerizes for histocompatibility antigens. Science 247: 1471–1474.
20. Shortman K, Wu L (1996) Early T lymphocyte progenitors. Ann Rev Immunol 14:29–48.
21. Goodman T, Lefrancois L (1989) Intraepithelial lymphocytes: anatomical site, not T cell receptor form, dictates phenotype and function. J Exp Med 170:1569–1581.
22. Wang B, Biron C, She J, Higgins K, Sunshine M-J, Lacy E, Lonberg N, Terhorst C (1994) A block in both early T lymphocyte and natural killer cell development in transgenic mice with high-copy numbers of the human CD3E gene. Proc Natl Acad Sci 91:9402–9406.
23. Gami-Wagner BA, Witte PL, Tutt MM, Kuziel WA, Tucker PW, Bennett M, Kumar V (1990) Natural killer cells in the thymus. Studies in mice with severe combined immune deficiency. J Immunol 144:796–803.
24. Phillips JH, Hori T, Nagler A, Bhat N, Spits H, Lanier LL (1992) Ontogeny of human natural killer (NK) cells: fetal NK cells mediate cytolytic function and express cytoplasmic CD3 epsilon, delta proteins. J Exp Med 175:1055–1066.
25. Kumar V, Hackett J Jr, Tutt MM, Gami-Wagner BA, Kuziel WA, Tucker PW, Bennett M (1989) Natural killer cells and their precursors in mice with severe combined immunodeficiency. Curr Top Microbiol Immunol 152:47–52.
26. Moore T, Bennett M, Kumar V (1995) Transplantable NK cell progenitors in murine bone marrow. J Immunol 154:1653–1663.
27. Klausner RD, Samelson LE (1991) T cell antigen receptor activation pathway: the tyrosine kinase connection. Cell 64:875–878.
28. Love PE, Shores EW, Johnson MD, Tremblay ML, Lee EJ, Grinberg A, Huang SP, Singer A, Westphal H (1993) T cell development in mice that lack the zeta chain of the T cell antigen receptor complex. Science 261:918–921.
29. Beecher MS, Baiocchi RA, Linett ML, Krajewski CA, Caligiuri MA (1994) Expression of the zeta protein subunit in CD3(−) NK effectors derived from human thymus. Cell Immunol 155:508–516.
30. Yokoyama WM (1995) Natural killer cell receptors specific for major histocompatibility complex class I molecules. Proc Natl Acad Sci USA 92:3081–3085.
31. Moretta A, Bottino C, Vitale M, Pende D, Biassoni R, Mingari MC, Moretta L (1996) Receptors for HLA-Class-1 molecules in human natural killer cells. Ann Rev Immunol 14:619–648.
32. Trinchieri G (1989) Biology of natural killer cells. Adv Immunol 47:187–376.
33. Lanier LL, Spits H, Phillips JH (1992) The developmental relationship between NK cells and T cells. Immunol Today 13:392–395.
34. Karre K, Ljunggren H-G, Piontek G, Kiessling R (1986) Selective rejection of H-2 deficient lymphoma variants suggests alternative immune defense strategy. Nature 319:675–678.

35. Karre K (1995) Express yourself or die: peptides, MHC molecules, and NK cells. Science 267: 978–979.
36. Moretta L, Ciccone E, Moretta A, Höglund P, Öhlén, Kärre K (1992) Allorecognition by NK cells: nonself or no self? Immunol Today 13:300–306.
37. Yokoyama WM (1993) The LY-49 and NKR-P1 gene families encoding lectin-like receptors on natural killer cells: The NK gene complex. Ann Rev Immunol 11:613–635.
38. Gumperz JE, Parham P (1995) The enigma of the natural killer cell. Nature 378:245–248.
39. Colonna M, Samaridis J (1995) Cloning of immunoglobulin-superfamily members associated with HLA-C and HLA-B recognition by human natural killer cells. Science 268:405–408.
40. Dohring C, Scheidegger D, Samaridis J, Cella M, Colonna M (1996) A human killer inhibitory receptor specific for HLA-A. J Immunol 156:3098–3101.
41. Anegon I, Cuturi MC, Trinchieri G, Perussia B (1988) Interaction of the Fcγ receptor (CD16) ligand induces transcription of interleukin-2 receptor (CD25) and lymphokine genes and expression of its products in natural killer cells. J Exp Med 167:452–472.
42. Moretta A, Vitale M, Bottino C, Orengo AM, Morelli L, Augugliaro R, Barbaresi M, Ciccone E, Moretta L (1993) P58 molecules as putative receptors for major histocompatability complex MHC class I molecules in human natural killer NK cells: anti-p58 antibodies reconstitute lysis of MHC class I-protected cells in NK clones displaying different specificities. J Exp Med 178:597–604.
43. Litwin V, Gumperz J, Parham P, Phillips JH, Lanier LL (1994) NKB1: an NK cell receptor involved in the recognition of polymorphic HLA-B molecules. J Exp Med 180:537–543.
44. Houchins JP, Yabe T, McSherry C, Bach FH (1991) DNA sequence analysis of NKG2, a family of related cDNA clones encoding type II integral membrane proteins on human natural killer cells. J Exp Med 173:1017–1020.
45. Schnittger S, Hamann J, Dannenberg C, Fiebig H, Strauss M, Fonatsch C (1993) Regional sublocalization of the human CD69 gene to chromosome bands 12p12.3-p13.2, the predicted region of the human natural killer cell gene complex. Eur J Immunol 23:27112713.
46. Perez-Villar JJ, Melero I, Rodriguez A, Carretero M, Aramburu J, Sivori S, Orengo AM, Moretta A, Lopez-Botet M (1995) Functional ambivalence of the Kp43 CD94 NK cell-associated surface antigen. J Immunol 154:5779–5788.
47. Lanier LL, Chang C, Phillips JH (1994) Human NKR-P1A. A disulfide linked homodimer of the C-type lectin superfamily expressed by a subset of NK and T lymphocytes. J Immunol 153: 2417–2428.
48. Kornbluth J, Kozlowski M, Portis T (1995) Identification of a novel cytokine-inducible gene associated with NK cytolytic activity [Abstract]. Nat Immun 14:72.
49. Poggi A, Pella N, Morelli L, Spada F, Revello V, Sivori S, Augugliaro R, Moretta L, Moretta A (1995) p40, a novel surface molecule involved in the regulation of the non-major histocompatibility complex-restricted cytolytic activity in humans. Eur J Immunol 25:369–376.
50. Smith HRC, Karlhofer FM, Yokoyama WM (1994) Ly-49 multigene family expressed by IL-2 activated NK cells. J Immunol 153:1068–1079.
51. Mason LH, Ortaldo JR, Young HA, Kumar V, Bennett M, Anderson SK (1995) Cloning and functional characteristics of murine large granular lymphocyte-1: a member of the Ly-49 gene family (Ly49G2). J Exp Med 182:293–303.
52. Bezouska K, Yuen C-T, O'Brien J, Childs RA, Chai W, Lawson AM, Drbal K, Fiserova A, Pospisil M, Feizi T (1994) Oligosaccharide ligands for NKR-P1 protein activate NK cells and cytotoxicity. Nature 372:150–157.
53. Jewett A, Bonavida B (1995) Target-induced anergy of natural killer cytotoxic function is restricted to the NK-target conjugate subset. Cell Immunol 160:91–97.
54. Baggiolini M, Dewald B, Moser B (1994) Interleukin 8 and related chemotactic cytokines-CXC and CC chemokines. Adv Immunol 55:97–179.
55. Lewinson DM, Bargatze RF, Butcher EC (1987) Leukocyte-endothelial cell recognition: evidence of a common molecular mechanism shared by neutrophils, lymphocytes and other leukocytes. J Immunol 138:4313–4327.
56. Springer TA (1995) Traffic signals on endothelium for lymphocyte recirculation and leukocyte emigration. Ann Rev Physiol 57:827–872.
57. Hunt JS (1989) Cytokine networks in the uetroplacental unit: macrophages as pivotal regulatory cells. J Reprod Immunol 16:1–17.
58. Parr MB, Parr EL (1996) Immunoglobulins in the female genital tract, In: Reproductive Immunology (Bronson R, Alexander NJ, Anderson D, Branch WK, Kutteh WH, eds.), Blackwell Scientific, Oxford, pp. 275–308.
59. Dinarello CA (1992) Role of interleukin-1 in infectious diseases. Immunol Rev 127:119– 146.

60. Lecuit T, Brook WJ, Ng M, Calleja M, Sun H, Cohen SM (1996) Two distinct mechanisms for long range patterning by Decapentaplegic in the *Drosophila* wing. Nature 381:387–393.
61. Averbock MR, Brinster CJ, Brinster R (1996) Reconstitution of spermatogenesis from frozen spermatogonial stem cells. Nature Med 2:693–696.
62. Snodgrass HR, Dembic Z, Steinmetz M, von Boehmer H (1985) Expression of T cell antigen receptor genes during fetal development in the thymus. Nature 315:232,233.
63. Hardy RR, Carmack CE, Shinton SA, Kemp JD, Hayakawa K (1991) Resolution and characterization of pro-B and pre-pro-B-cell stages in normal mouse bone marrow. J Exp Med 173:1213–1225.
64. Cumano A, Paige CJ, Iscove NN, Brady G (1992) Bipotential precursors of B cells and macrophages in murine fetal liver. Nature 356:612–615.
65. Pfeffer K, Mak TW (1994) Lymphocyte ontogeny and activation in gene targeted mutant mice. Ann Rev Immunol 12:367–411.
66. Godin IE, Garcia-Porrero JA, Coutinho A, Dieterlen-Lievre F, Marcos MAR (1993) Para-aortic splanchnopleura from early mouse embryos contains B1a cell progenitors. Nature 364:67–70.
67. Godin I, Dieterlen-Lievre F, Cumano A (1995) Emergence of multipotent hematopoietic cells in the yolk sac and paraortic splanchnopleura in mouse embryos beginning at 8.5 d post coitus. Proc Natl Acad Sci USA 92:773–777.
68. Cumano A, Furlonger C, Paige C (1993) Differentiation and characterization of B-cell precursors detected in the yolk sac and embryo body of embryos beginning at the 10- to 12-somite stage. Proc Natl Acad Sci USA 90:6429–6433.
69. Delassus S, Cumano A (1996) Circulation of hematopoietic progenitors in the mouse embryos. Immunity 4:97–106.
70. Taniguchi H, Toyoshima T, Fukao K, Nakauchi H (1996) Presence of hematopoietic stem cells in adult liver. Nature Med 2:198–203.
71. Bianchi DW, Ziekwolf GK, Weil GJ, Sylvester S, DeMaria MA (1996) Male fetal progenitor cells persist in maternal blood for as long as 27 years post partum. Proc Natl Acad Sci USA 93:705–708.
72. Kohn DB, Weinberg KI, Nolta JA, Heiss LN, Lenarsky C, Crooks GM, Hanley ME, Annett G, Brooks JS, El-Khoureiy A, Lawrence K, Wells S, Moen RC, Bastian J, Williams-Herman DE, Elder M, Wara D, Bowen T, Hershfield MS, Mullen CA, Blaese RM, Parkman R (1995) Engraftment of gene-modified umbilical cord blood cells in neonates with adenosine deaminase deficiency. Nature Med 1:1017–1023.
73. Johnson FL, Pochedly C (eds.) (1990) Bone Marrow Transplantation in Children. Raven, New York.
74. Rodewald HR, Kretzschmar K, Takeda S, Hohl C, Dessing M (1994) Identification of prothymocytes in murine fetal blood: T lineage committment can precede thymus colonization. EMBO J 13:4229–4240.
75. Ihle JN, Witthuhn BA, Quelle FW, Yamamoto K, Silvennoinen O (1995) Signalling through the hematopoietic cytokine receptors. Ann Rev Immunol 13:369–398.
76. Vitale M, Sivori S, Pende D, Moretta L, Moretta A (1995) Co-expression of two functionally independent p58 inhibitory receptors in human natural killer cell clones results in the inability to kill all normal allogeneic target cells. Proc Natl Acad Sci USA 92:3536–3540.
77. Christmas SE, Bulmer JN, Meager A, Johnson PM (1990) Phenotypic and functional analysis of human CD3- decidual leukocyte clones. Immunology 71:182–189.
78. Christmas SE, Brew R, Thorton SM, Deniz G, Flanagan BF (1995) Extensive TCR junctional diversity of Vδ9/Vζ2 clones from human female reproductive tissues. J Immunol 155:2543–2458.
79. Winkler-Pickett RT, Young HA, Kuta A, Ortaldo JR (1991) Analysis of rat natural killer cytotoxic factor (NKCF): mechanism of action and relationships to other cytotoxic/cytostatic factors. Cell Immunol 135:42–54.
80. Roder JC, Duwe AK (1979) The beige mutation in the mouse selectively impairs natural killer cell function. Nature 278:451–453.
81. DiSanto JP, Muller W, Guy-Grand D, Fischer A, Rajewsky K (1995) Lymphoid development in mice with a targeted deletion of the interleukin 2 receptor gamma chain. Proc Natl Acad Sci USA 92:377–381.
82. Sugamura K, Asao H, Kondo M, Tanaka N, Ishii N, Ohbo K, Nakamura M, Takeshita T (1996) Interleukin-2 receptor gamma chain: its role in multiple cytokine receptor complexes and T cell development in XSCID. Ann Rev Immunol 14:179–205.
83. Renard V, Ardoulin L, Malissen M, Milon G, Lebastard M, Gillet A, Malissen B, Vivier E (1995) Normal development and function of natural killer cells in CD3E delta 5/delta 5 mutant mice. Proc Natl Acad Sci USA 92:7545–7549.
84. King, A, Burrows, T, Loke YW (1996) Human uterine natural killer cells. Natural Immunity 15:41–52.

85. Haller OR, Kiessling R, Orn A, Wigzell H (1977) Generation of natural killer cells: an autonomous function of the bone marrow. J Exp Med 145:1411–1416.
86. Miller SC (1982) Production and renewal of murine natural killer cells in the spleen and bone marrow. J Immunol 129:2282–2286.
87. Pollack SB, Rosse C (1987) The primary role of murine bone marrow in the production of natural killer cells. A cytokinetic study. J Immunol 139:2149–2156.
89. Miller SC (1994) The development of natural killer (NK) cells from Thy-1^{lo}Lin^{-}Sca-1^{+} stem cells: acquisition by NK cells in vivo of the homing receptor Mel-14 and the integrin Mac-1. Immunobiol 190:385–398.
90. Pollack SB, Linnemeyer PA (1996) NK cells in the nonpregnant murine uterus. Natural Immunity 15:34–40.
91. Itohara S, Farr AG, Lafaille JJ, Bonneville M, Takagaki Y, Haas W, Tonegawa S 1990 Homing of a gamma/delta thymocyte subset with homogeneous T-cell receptors to mucosal epithelia. Nature 343:754–757.
92. Heyborne KD, Cranfill RL, Carding SR, Born WK, O Brien RL (1992) Characterisation of $\gamma\delta$ T lymphocytes at the maternal-fetal interface. J Immunol 149:2872–2878.
93. Heyborne K, Fu Y-X, Nelson A, Farr A, O'Brien R, Born W (1994) Recognition of trophoblasts by $\gamma\delta$ T cells. J Immunol 153:2918–2926.
94. Cannon JG, Dinarello CA (1984) Increased plasma interleukin-1 in women after ovulation. Science 227:1247–1249.
95. Bartocci A, Pollard JW and Stanley ER (1986) Regulation of colony stimulating factor-during pregnancy. J Exp Med 164:954–961.
96. Kincade PW, Medina KL, Smithson G and Scott DC (1994) Pregnancy: a clue to normal regulation of B lymphopoiesis. Immunol Today 15:539–544.
97. Bhat NM, Mithal A, Bieber MM, Herzenberg LA, Teng NN (1995) Human CD5^{+} B cells (B-1 cells) decrease in peripheral blood during pregnancy. J Reprod Immunol 28:53–60.
98. Baines MG, Pross HF, Miller KG (1977) Spontaneous human lymphocyte-mediated cytotoxicity against tumor target cells. IV. The suppressive effect of normal pregnancy. Am J Obstet Gynecol 130:741–744.
99. Gregory CD, Lee H, Scott IV, Golding PR (1987) Phenotypic heterogeneity and recycling capacity of natural killer cells in normal human pregnancy. J Reprod Immunol 11:135–145.
100. Skoner JM, Sigmon J, Larcom LL (1995) Suppressed DNA repair capacity of peripheral lymphocytes in pregnant women. Mol Cell Endocrinol 108:179–183.
101. Clark AG, Kendall MD (1994) The thymus in pregnancy: the interplay of neural, endocrine and immune influences. Immunol Today 15:545–551.
102. Ruhsinghani AG, Bhatia S, Trgrett LT, Waldschmidt TJ (1996) Effect of pregnancy on thymic T cell development. Am J Reprod Immunol 35:523–528.
103. Kimura M, Hanawa H, Watanabe H, Ogawa M, Abo T (1995) Synchronous expansion of intermediate TCR cells in the liver and uterus during pregnancy. Cell Immunol 162:16–25.
104. Szekeres-Bartho J (1995) Progesterone receptors on lymphocytes. Hum Reprod 10:695,696.
105. Mansour I, Reznikoff-Etievant MF, Netter A (1994) No evidence for the expression of progesterone receptor on peripheral blood lymphocytes during pregnancy. Hum Reprod 9:1546–1549.
106. Piccinni MP, Giudizi MG, Biagiotti R, Beloni L, Giannarini L, Sampognaro S, Parronchi P, Manetti R, Annunziato F, Livi C, Romagnani S, Maggi E (1995) Progesterone favors development of human T helper cells producing Th2-type cytokines and promotes both IL-4 production and membrane CD30 expression in established Th1 cell clones. J Immunol 155:128–133.
107. Cutolo M, Sulli A, Seriolo B, Accardo S, Masi AT (1995) Estrogens, the immune response and autoimmunity. Clin Exp Rheumatol 13:217–226.
108. Sorachi K, Kumagai S, Sugita M, Yodoi J, Imura H (1993) Enhancing effect of 17 beta-estradiol on human NK cell activity. Immunol Lett 36:31–35.
109. Screpanti I, Felli MP, Toniato E, Meco D, Martinotti S, Frati L, Gulino A, Santoni A (1991) Enhancement of natural killer cell susceptibility of human breast-cancer cells by estradiol and v-Ha-ras oncogene. Int J Cancer 47:445–449.
110. Grainger DJ, Metacalfe JC (1996) Tamoxifen: teaching an old drug new tricks. Nature Med 2: 381–385.
111. Lin J, Lojun S, Lei ZM, Wu WX, Peiner SC, Rao CV (1995) Lymphocytes from pregnant women express human chorionic gonadotropin/luteinizing hormone receptor gene. Mol Cell Endocrinol 111:R13–R17.

112. Cocchiara R, Albeggiani G, Azzolina A, Bongiovanni A, Lampiasi N, Di Blasi F, Geraci D (1995) Effect of substance P on uterine mast cell cytokine release during the reproductive cycle. J. Neuroimmunol 60:107–115.
113. Pate JL (1995) Involvement of immune cells in regulation of ovarian function. J Reprod Fertil Suppl 49:365–377.
114. Bukovsky A, Caudle MR, Keenan JA, Wimalasena J, Upadhyaya NB, Van Meter SE (1995) Is corpus luteum regression an immune-mediated event? Localization of immune system components and luteinizing hormone receptor in human corpora lutea. Biol Reprod 53:1373–1384.
115. Nossal GJV (1992) Cellular and molecular mechanisms of B cell tolerance. Adv Immunol 52: 283–331.
116. Nossal GJV (1995) Choices following antigen entry: antibody formation or immunologic tolerance? Ann Rev Imm 13:1–27.
117. Forsthuber T, Yip HC, Lehmann PV (1996) Induction of Th1 and Th2 immunity in neonatal mice. Science 271:1728–1730.
118. Ridge JP, Fuchs EJ, Matzinger P (1996) Neonatal tolerance revisited: turning on newborn T cells with dendritic cells. Science 271:1723–1726.
119. Mondino A, Khoruts A, Jenkins MK (1996) The anatomy of T cell activation and tolerance. Proc Natl Acad Sci USA 93:2245–2252.
120. Sarzotti M, Robbins DS, Hoffman PM (1996) Induction of protective CTL responses in newborn mice by a murine retrovirus. Science 271:1726–1728.
121. Rocha B, von Boehmer H (1991) Peripheral selection of the T cell repetoire. Science 251:1225–1228.
122. Goodnow CC (1992) Transgenic mice and analysis of B cell tolerance. Ann Rev Immunol 10: 489–518.
123. Andre I, Gonzalez A, Wang B, Katz J, Benoist C, Mathis D (1996) Checkpoints in the progression of autoimmune disease: lessons from diabetes models. Proc Natl Acad Sci USA 93:2260–2263.
124. Goodnow CC (1996) Balancing immunity and tolerance: deleting and fine tuning. Proc Natl Acad Sci USA 93:2264–2271.
125. Kisielow P, Bluthmann H, Staerz U, Steinmetz M, von Boehmer H (1988) Tolerance in T-cell receptor transgenic mice involves deletion of nonmature CD4+8+thymocytes. Nature 333: 742–746.
126. MacDonald HR, Schneider R, Lees RK, Howe RC, Acha-Orbea H, Festenstein H, Zinkernagel RM, Hengartner H (1988) T cell receptor V beta use predicts reactivity and tolerance to MIsa-coded antigens. Nature 332:40–45.
127. Okamoto M, Murakami M, Shimizu A, Ozaki S, Tsubata T, Kumagi S, Honjo T 1992 A transgenic model of autoimmune hemolytic anemia. J Exp Med 175:71–79.
128. Vasquez NJ, Kaye J, Hedrick SM (1992) In vivo and in vitro clonal deletion of double-positive thymocytes. J Exp Med 175:1307–1316.
129. Tafuri A, Alferink J, Moller P, Hammerling GJ, Arnold B (1995) T cell awareness of paternal alloantigens during pregnancy. Science 270:630–633.
130. Gianani R, Sarvetnick N (1996) Viruses, cytokines, antigens and autoimmunity. Proc Natl Acad Sci USA 93:2257–2259.
131. Parish NM, Hutchings PR, O'Rielly L, Quartey-Papafro R, Healey D, Ozegbe P, Cooke A (1996) Tolerance induction as a therapeutic strategy for the control of autoimmune endocrine disease in mouse models. Immunol Rev 144:269–300.
132. Steinman L (1996) A few autoreactive cells in an autoimmune infiltrate control a vastpopulation of non-specific cells: a tale of smart bombs and the infantry. Proc Natl Acad Sci USA 93:2253–2256.
133. Homo-Delarche F, Fitzpatrick F, Christeff N, Numez EA, Bach JF, Dardenne M 1991 Sex steroids, glucocorticoids, stress and immunity. J Steroid Biochem Mol Biol 40:619–637.
134. Lahita RG (1992) The importance of estrogens in systemic lupus erythematosus. Clin Immunol Immunopathol 63:17,18.
135. Kikutani H, Makino S (1992) The murine autoimmune diabetes model: NOD and related strains. Adv Immunol 51:285–322.
136. Gimovsky ML, Montoro M (1991) Systemic lupus erythematosus and other connective tissue diseases in pregnancy. Clin Obstet Gynecol 34:35–50.
137. Lockwood CJ, Rand JH (1994) The immunobiology and obstetrical consequences of antiphospholipid antibodies. Obstet Gynecol Survey 49:432–441.
138. Moise KJ (1991) Autoimmune thrombocytopenic purpura in pregnancy. Clin Obstet Gynecol 34: 51–63.

139. Matsuura N, Fujieda K, Iida Y, Fujimoto S, Konishi J, Kasagi K, Hagisawa M, Fukushi M, Takasugi N (1988) TSH-receptor antibodies in mothers with Graves' disease and outcome in their offspring. Lancet 1:14–17.
140. Wellik SR, de Veciana M, Morgan MA, Berkowitz KM, Arquilla ER (1995) Naturally occurring insulin autoantibodies in neonates of normal pregnancies and their relationship to insulinemia and birth weight. Am J Obstet Gynecol 173:1878–1784.
141. Anderson RW (1995) On the maternal transmission of immunity: a "molecular attention" hypothesis. BioSystems 34:87–105.
142. Jerne NK (1974) Towards a network theory of the immune system. Ann Immunol (Inst Pasteur). 125C:373–389.
143. Coutinho A (1995) The network theory: 21 years later. Scand J Immunol 42:3–8.
144. Wachtel S, Elias S, Price J, Wachtel G, Phillips O, Shulman L, Meyers C, Simpson JL, Dockter M (1991) Fetal cells in the maternal circulation: isolation by multiparameter flow cytometry and confirmation by PCR. Hum Reprod 6:1466–1469.
145. Geifman-Holtzman O, Blatman RN, Bianchi DW (1994) Prenatal genetic diagnosis by isolation and analysis of fetal cells circulating in maternal blood. Semin Perinatol 18:366–375.
146. Simpson JL, Elias S (1994) Isolating fetal cells in maternal circulation for prenatal diagnosis. Prenat Diagn 14:1229–1242.
147. Desai RG, Creger WP (1963) Maternal passage of leukocytes and platelets in man. Blood 21: 665–673.
148. Zarou DM, Lichtman HC, Hellman LM (1964) The transmission of chromium-51 tagged maternal erythrocytes from mother to fetus. Am J Obstet Gynecol 88:565–571.
149. Pollack MS, Kirkpatrick D, Kapoor N, DuPont B, O'Reilly RJ (1982) Identification by HLA-typing of intrauterine-derived maternal T cells in four patients with severe combined immunodeficiency. N Engl J Med 307:662–666.
150. Geha RS, Reinherz E (1983) Identification of circulating T and B lymphocytes in uncomplicated severe combined immunodeficiency by HLA typing of subpopulations of T cells separated by fluorescence-activated cell sorter and of Epstein Barr virus-derived B cell lines. J Immunol 130: 2493–2495.
151. Thompson LF, O'Connor RD, Bastian JF (1984) Phenotype and function of engrafted maternal cells in patients with severe combined immunodeficiency. J Immunol 133:2513–2517.
152. Knobloch C, Goldman SF, Friedrich W (1991) Limited T cell receptor diversity of transplacentally acquired maternal T cells in severe combined immunodeficiency. J Immunol 146:4157–4164.
153. Fischer A, Griscelli C, Friedrich W, Kubanek B, Levinsky R, Morgan G, Vossen J, Wagemaker G, Landais P (1986) Bone marrow transplantation for immunodeficiencies and osteopetrosis. European Survey 1968–1985. Lancet 2:1080–1984.
154. Neudorf SML, Yanik GA, Pietryga (1990) Bone marrow transplantation for correction of primary immuno-deficiencies, In: Bone Marrow Transplantation in Children (Johnson FL, Pochedly C, eds.), Raven, New York, pp. 165–180.
155. Le Diest F, Raffoux C, Griscelli C, Fischer A (1987) Graft vs graft reaction resulting in the elimination of maternal cells in a SCID patient with maternofetal GVHD after one HLA identical marrow transplantation. J Immunol 138: 423–427.
156. Tuffrey M, Bishun NP, Barnes RD (1969) Porosity of mouse placenta to maternal cells. Nature 221:1029,1030.
157. Hunziker RD, Gambel P, Wegmann TG (1984) Placenta as a selective barrier to cellular traffic. J Immunol 133:667–671.
158. Shimamura M, Ohta S, Suzuk R, Yamazaki K (1994) Transmission of maternal blood cells to the fetus during pregnancy. Blood 83:926–930.
159. Ladel CH, Puschner H, Kaufman SH, Bamberger U (1992) Human peripheral blood leukocytes transferred on CB17 *scid/scid* mice are transferred to their offspring. Eur J Immunol 22:1735–1740.
160. Greenwood JD, Bos N, Croy BA (1996) Offspring of xenogeneically-reconstituted *scid/scid* mice are capable of a primary xenogenic immune response to DNP-KLH. Vet Immunol Immunopathol 50:145–155.
161. Piotrowski P, Croy BA (1996) Maternal cells are widely distributed in murine fetuses during normal pregnancy. Biol Reprod 54:1103–1110.
162. Copp A (1995) Death before birth: clues from gene knock-outs and mutants. Trends Genet 11:87–93.
163. Custer RP, Bosma GC, Bosma MJ (1985) Severe combined immunodeficiency (SCID) in the mouse: pathology, reconstitution, neoplasms. Am J Pathol 120:464–477.

164. Faden RR, Geller G, Powers M (eds.) (1991) AIDS, Women and the Next Generation. Towards a Morally Acceptable Public Policy for HIV Testing of Pregnant Women and Newborns. Oxford University Press, New York, NY.
165. Lapointe N, Michaud J, Pekovic D, Chasseau JP, Dupuy JM (1985) Transplacental transmission of HTLV-III virus. Lancet 312:132S.
166. David FJ, Tran HC, Serpente N, Autran B, Vaquero C, Djian V, Menu E, Barre-Sinoussi F, Chaouat G (1995) HIV infection of choriocarcinoma cell lines derived from human placenta: the role of membrane CD4 and Fc-Rg in HIV entry. Virology 208:784–788.
167. Burlingham WJ, Grailer AP, Fechner JH Jr, Kusaka S, Trucco M, Kocova M, Belzer FO, Sollinger HW (1995) Microchimerisms linked to cytotoxic T lymphocyte functional unresponsiveness (clonal anergy) in a tolerant renal transplant recipient. Transplantation 59:1147–1155.
168. Hisanaga M, Hundrieser J, Uthoff K, Wahlers T, Pichlmayr R, Schlitt JH (1995) Graft function and rejection patterns in heart-transplanted patients with and without systemic microchimerism. Transplant Proc 27:202–204.
169. Mazariegos GV, Ramos H, Shapiro R, Zeevi A, Fung JJ, Starzl TE (1995) Weaning of immunosuppression in long-term recipients of living renal transplants: a preliminary study. Transplant Proc 27:207–209.
170. Hundrieser J, Hisanaga M, Boker K, Raddatz G, Brederlau A, Nashan B, Pichlmayr R, Schlitt H-J (1995) Long term chimerism in liver transplantation: no evidence for immunological relevance but requirement for graft persistence. Transplant Proc 27:216–218.
171. Rao AS, Fontes P, Zeevi A, Trucco M, Dodson FS, Rybka WB, Shapiro R, Jordan M, Pham SM, Rito HL, Seskey T, Todo S, Scantlebury V, Vivas C, Demetrius AJ, Fung JJ, Starzl TE (1995) Augmentation of chimerism in whole organ recipients by simultaneous infusion of donor bone marrow cells. Transplant Proc 27: 210–212.
172. King A, Wellings V, Gardner L, Loke YW (1989) Immunocytochemical characterization of the unusual large granular lymphocytes in the human endometrium throughout the menstrual cycle. Hum Immunol 24:195–205.
173. Redline RW, Lu CY (1989) Localization of fetal major histocompatibility complex antigens and maternal leukocytes in murine placenta: Implications for maternal–fetal immunological relationship. Lab Invest 61:27–36.
174. Suzuki T, Hiromatsu K, Ando Y, Okamoto T, Tomada Y, Yoshikai Y (1995) Regulatory role of $\gamma\delta$ T cells in uterine intraepithelial lymphocytes in maternal antifetal immune response. J Immunol 154:4476–4484.
175. Saito N, Nishikawa K, Morii T, Narita N, Enomoto M, Ichijo M (1992) Expression of activation antigens CD69, HLA-DR, interleukin-2 receptor-alpha IL-2R-α and IL-2Rβ on T cells of human decidua at an early stage of pregnancy. Immunology 75:710–712.
176. Starkey PM, Clover LM, Rees MCP (1991) Variation during the menstrual cycle of immune cell populations in human endometrium. Eur J Obstet Gynecol Reprod Biol 39:203–207.
177. Mincheva-Nilsson L, Baranov V, Yeung MM-W, Hammarstrom S, Hammarstrom M-L (1994) Immunomorphologic studies of human decidua-associated lymphoid cells in normal early pregnancy. J Immunol 152:2020–2032.
178. Dietl J, Handgretinger R, Horny H-P, Marzusch K, Geiselhart A, Kaiserling E (1994) CD3+ cells in first trimester decidua. Am J Obstet Gynecol 171:577,578.
179. Hunt JS Pollard JW (1992) Macrophages in the uterus and placenta. Topics Microbiol 181:39–63.
180. Pollard JW, Bartocci A, Arceci R, Orlofsky A, Ladner MB, Stanley ER (1987) Apparent role of the macrophage growth factor CSF-1 in placental development. Nature 330:484–487.
181. De M, Wood GW (1990) Influence of oestrogen and progesterone on macrophage distribution in the mouse uterus. J. Endocrinol. 126:417–424.
182. Brandon JM (1993) Leucocyte distribution in the uterus during the preimplantation period of pregnancy and phagocyte recruitment to sites of blastocyst attachment in mice. J Reprod Fertil 98: 567–576.
183. Yelavarthi KK, Chen HL, Yang Y, Cowley BD Jr, Fishback JL, Hunt JS (1991) Tumor necrosis factor-alpha mRNA and protein in rat uterine and placental cells. J Immunol 146:3840–3848.
184. Pollard JW, Hunt JS, Wiktor-Jerdrzejczak W, Stanley ER (1991) A pregnancy defect in the osteopetrotic mouse (op/op) mouse demonstrates the requirement for CSF-1 in female fertility. Dev Biol 148:273–283.
185. Redline RW, McKay DB, Vazquez MA, Papaioannou VE, Lu CY (1990) Macrophage functions are regulated by the substratum of murine decidual stromal cells. J Clin Invest 85:1951–1958.

186. Hunt JS (1994) Immunologically relevant cells in the uterus Biol Reprod 50:461–466.
187. Kiso Y, McBey B-A, Mason L, Croy BA (1992) Histological assessment of the mouse uterus from birth to puberty for the appearance of LGL-1+ natural killer cells. Biol Reprod 47:227–232.
188. Parr EL, Young LHY, Parr MB, Young JD-E (1990) Granulated metrial gland cells of pregnant mouse uterus are natural killer-like cells that contain perforin and serine esterases. J Immunol 145:2365–2372.
189. Parr EL, Parr MB, Zheng LM, Young JD-E (1991) Mouse granulated metrial gland cell originate by local activation of uterine natural killer lymphocytes. Biol Reprod 44:834–841.
190. Peel S (1989) Granulated metrial gland cells. Adv Anat Embryol Cell Biol 115:1–112.
191. Head JR (1996) Uterine natural killer cells during pregnancy in rodents. Natural Immunity 15:7–12.
192. Kiso Y, Yamashiro S, McBey B-A, Croy BA (1992) Tissue-specific differentiation of a natural killer cell subset in ectopically grafted murine uterine tissue. Transplantation 54: 185–187.
193. Liggins GC, Thorburn GD (1994) Initiation of parturition, In: Marshalls Physiology of Reproduction, vol III (4th ed.), part 2 (Lamming GE, ed.), Chapman and Hall, NY, pp. 863–1003.
194. Van den Heuvel M, McBey B-A, Hahnel AC, Croy BA (1996) An analysis of the uterine lymphocyte-derived hybridoma cell line GWM 1-2 for expression of receptors for estrogen, progesterone and interleukin 2. J Reprod Immunol 31:37–50.
195. Delgado SR, McBey B-A, Yamashiro S, Kiso Y, Croy BA (1996) Accounting for the peripartum loss of natural killer cell-like, granulated metrial gland cells from the pregnant mouse uterus. J Leukocyte Biol 59:262–269.
196. Croy BA, McBey B-A, Villeneuve LA, Kiso Y, van den Heuvel M (1997) Characterization of the cells that migrate from metrial glands during explant culture. J Reprod Immunol 32:241–263.
197. Larkin LH (1972) Electron microscopy of granule release in metrial gland cells of the pregnant rat. Anat Rec 172:109–126.
198. Straatsburg IH, Gossrau R (1993) Enzyme histochemistry of the regressing rat decidua and metrial gland. Acta Histochem 94:202–219.
199. Gambel P, Croy BA, Moore WD, Hunziker RD, Wegmann TG, Rossant J (1985) Characterization of immune effector cells present in early murine decidua. Cell Immunol 93:303–314.
200. Mukhtar DDY, Stewart IJ, Croy BA (1989) Leucocyte membrane antigens on mouse granulated metrial gland cells. J Reprod Immunol 15:269–279.
201. Stewart IJ (1991) Granulated metrial gland cells: Pregnancy specific leukocytes? J Leuk Biol 50:198–207.
202. Stewart IJ (1994) Granulated metrial gland cells—not part of the natural killer cell lineage? J Reprod Immunol 26:1–15.
203. Drake BL, Head JR (1989) Murine trophoblast can be killed by lymphokine activated killer cells. J Immunol 143:9–14.
204. Linnemeyer PA, Pollack SB (1991) Murine granulated metrial gland cells at uterine implantation sites are natural killer lineage cells. J Immunol 147:2530–2535.
205. Croy BA, Reed N, Malashenko BA, Kwon BS (1991) Demonstration of YAC target cell lysis by murine granulated metrial gland cells. Cell Immunol 133:116–126.
206. King A, Wooding P, Gardner L, Loke YW (1993) Expression of perforin, granzyme A and TIA-1 by human uterine $CD56^+$ NK cells implies they are activated and capable of effector functions. Hum Reprod 8:2061–2067.
207. King A, Balendran N, Wooding P, Carter NP, Loke YW (1991) CD^{3-} leukocytes present in the human uterus during early placentation: phenotypic and morphologic characterization of the $CD56^{++}$ population. Dev Immunol 1:169–190.
208. King A, Loke YW (1991) On the nature and function of human uterine granular lymphocytes. Immunol Today 12:432–435.
209. Lanier LL, Le AM, Civin CI, Loken MR, Phillips JH (1986) The relationship of CD16 leu-11 and Leu-19 NKH-1 antigen expression on human peripheral blood NK cells and cytotoxic T lymphocytes. J Immunol 136:4480–4486.
210. Starkey PM (1991) Expression on cells of early human pregnancy decidua of the p75, IL-2 and p145, IL-4 receptor proteins. Immunology 73:64–70.
211. King A, Loke YW (1990) Uterine large granular lymphocytes: A possible role in embryonic implantation? Am J Obstet Gynecol 162:308–310.
212. King A, Wheeler R, Carter NP, Francis DP, Loke YW (1992) The response of human decidual leukocytes to IL-2. Cell Immunol 141:409–421.
213. Naume B, Johnseni A-C, Espevik T, Sundan A (1993) Gene expression and secretion of cytokines and cytokine receptors from highly purified $CD56^+$ stimulated with IL-2, interleukin 7 and interleukin 12. Eur J Immunol 23:1831–1838.

214. Nakamura Y, Russel SM, Mess SA, Friedmann M, Erdos M, Francois C, Jaques Y, Adelstein S, Leonard WJ (1994) Heterodimerization of the IL-2 receptor β- and γ chain cytoplasmic domains is required for signalling. Nature 369:330–336.
215. Giri JG, Ahdieh Eisenman J, Shanebeck K, Grabstein K, Kumaki S, Namen A, Cosman D, Anderson D (1994) Utilization of the beta and gamma chains of the IL-2 receptor by the novel cytokine IL-15. EMBO J 13:28–22.
216. Schorle H, Holtschke T, Hunig T, Schimpl A, Horak I (1991) Development and function of T cells in mice rendered interleukin-2 deficient by gene targeting. Nature 352:621–24.
217. Croy BA, Chapeau C (1990) Evaluation of the pregnancy immunotropism hypothesis by assessment of the reproductive performance of young adult mice of genotype *scid/scid.bg/bg*. J Reprod Fertil 88:231–239.
218. Kagi D, Ledermann B, Burki K, Seiler P, Odermatt B, Olsen KJ, Podack ER, Zinkernagel RM, Hengartner H (1994) Cytotoxicity mediated by T cells and natural killer cells is greatly impaired in perforin-deficient mice. Nature 369:31–37.
219. Stallmach T, Ehrenstein T, Isenmann S, Muller C, Hengartner H, Kagi D (1995) The role of perforin-expression by granular metrial gland cells in pregnancy. Eur J Immunol 25:3342–3348.
220. Tennant M, Dilley RJ, McGeachie JK, Prendergast FJ (1990) Histogenesis of arterial intimal hyperplasia and atherosclerosis. Aust NZ J Surg 60:79–85.
221. Bondjers G, Glukhova M, Hansson GK, Postnov YV, Reidy MA, Schwartz SM (1991) Hypertension and a therosclerosis. Cause and effect, or two effects with one unknown cause? Circulation 84 Suppl VI:VI 2-VI 16.
222. O'Brien WF (1992) The prediction of preeclampsia. Clin Obstet Gynecol 35:351–364.
223. Cummingham FG, MacDonald PC, Grant NF (1989) Hypertensive disorders in pregnancy, In: Williams Obstetrics, 18th ed., Appleton and Lange, Norwalk, CT, pp. 653–694.
224. Loudin I (1991) Some historical aspects of toxaemia of pregnancy. Br J Obstet Gynecol 98:853–858.
225. Singh GK, Yu SM (1995) Infant mortality in the United States: trends, differentials, and projections, 1950 through 2010. Am J Public Health 85:957–964.
226. Conrad KP (1990) Animal models of pre-eclampsia: do they exist? Fetal Med Rev 2:67–88.
227. Mastrogiannis DS, O'Brien WF, Krammer J, Benoit R (1991) Potential role of endothelin-1 in normal and hypertensive pregnancies. Am J Obstet Gynecol 165:1711–1716.
228. Van Buren GA, Yang DS, Clark KE (1992) Estrogen-induced uterine vasodilatation is antagonized by L-nitroarginine methyl ester, an inhibitor of nitric oxide synthesis. Am J Obstet Gynecol 167: 828–833.
229. Yallampalli C, Garfield RE (1993) Inhibition of nitric oxide synthesis in rats during pregnancy produces signs similar to those of preeclampsia. Am J Obstet Gyencol 169:1316–1320.
230. Weiner CP, Knowles RG, Moncada S (1994) Induction of nitric oxide synthases early in pregnancy. Am J Obstet Gynecol 171:838–843.
231. Wilkes BM, Mento PF, Hollander AM, Maita ME, Sung S, Girardi EP (1990) Endothelin receptors in human placenta: relations to vascular resistance and thromboxane release. Am J Physiol 258: E864–E870.
232. Robaut C, Mondon F, Bandet J, Ferre F, Cavero I (1991) Regional distribution and pharmacological characterization of [125I] endothelin-1 binding sites in human fetal placental vessels. Placenta 12:55–67.
233. Peri A, Vannelli GB, Fantoni G, Giannini S, Barni T, Orlando C, Serio M, Maggi M 1992) Endothelin in rabbit uterus during pregnancy. Am J Physiol 263:E158–E167.
234. Myatt L, Brewer AS, Langdon G, Brockman DE (1992) Attenuation of the vasoconstrictor effects of thromboxane and endothelin by nitric oxide in the human fetal-placental circulation. Am J Obstet Gynecol 166:224–230.
235. Opgenorth TJ, Wu-wong JR, Shiosaki K (1992) Endothelin-converting enzymes. FASEB J 6: 2653–2659.
236. Moore HC, Cserhati I, Wilson K (1970) The duration of the fall of blood pressure following the induction of deciduomata and the administration of progesterone in steroid hypersensitive rats. Acta Endocrinol 63:242–252.
237. Sargent IL, Smarason AK (1995) Immunology of pre-eclampsia; current views and hypothesis, In: Immunology of Human Reproduction (Kurpisz M, Fernandez N, eds.), Bios Scientific Publishers, Oxford, pp. 355–367.
238. Croy BA (1994) Granulated metrial gland cells: hypotheses concerning possible functions during murine gestation. J Reprod Immunol 27:85–94.
239. Welsh AO, Enders AC (1993) Chorioallantoic placenta formation in the rat III. Granulated cells invade the uterine luminal epithelium at the time of epithelial cell death. Biol Reprod 49:38–57.

240. Hollander GA, Wang B, Nichogiannopoulou A, Platenburg PP, van Ewijk W, Burakoff SJ, Gutierrez-Ramos J-C, Terhorst C (1995) Developmental control point in induction of thymic cortex regulated by a subpopulation of prothymocytes. Nature 373:350–353.
241. Parr EL, Parr MB, Young JD-E (1987) Localization of a pore-forming protein, (perforin) in granulated metrial gland cells. Biol Reprod 37:1327–1335.
242. Bulmer JN (1994) Human endometrial lymphocytes in normal pregnancy and pregnancy loss. Ann NY Acad Sci 734:185–192.
243. Braga VMM, Gendler SJ (1993) Modulation of muc-1 mucin expression in the mouse uterus during the estrous cycle, early pregnancy and placentation. J Cell Sci 105:397–405.
244. Somersalo K, Tarkkanen Patarroyo M, Saksela E (1992) Involvement of β integrins in the migration of human natural killer cells. J Immunol 149:590–598.
245. Burrows TD, King A, Loke YW (1993) Expression of cell adhesion molecules by human decidual large granular lymphocytes. Cell Immunol 147:81–94.
246. Kiso Y, Yoshizawa M, Wilson JA, McBey B-A, Croy BA (1994) Immunohistochemical analysis of β1-integrin receptors displayed by murine uterine natural killer cells over the course of successful pregnancy. J Reprod Immunol 27:213–25.
247. Sluvkin II, Chernyshov VP, Merkula AA, Vodyanik MA, Kalinovsky AK (1994) Differential expression of adhesion and homing molecules by human decidual and peripheral blood lymphocytes in early pregnancy. Cell Immunol 158:29–45.
248. Kiso Y, McBey B-A, Croy BA (1992) Granulated metrial gland cells in the pregnant uterus of mice expressing the collagen mutation tight-skin (Tsk/+). Cell Tissue Res 268:393–396.
249. Sporns O, Edelman GM, Crossin KL (1995) The neural cell adhesion molecule (N-CAM) inhibits proliferation in primary cultures of rat astrocytes. Proc Natl Acad Sci USA 92:542–546.
250. Hill JA, Polgar K, Anderson DJ (1995) T-helper-1 immunity to trophoblast in women with recurrent spontaneous abortion. J Am Med Assoc 273:1933–1936.
251. Miyajima A, Kitamura T, Harada N, Yokota T, Arai K (1992) Cytokine receptors and signal transduction. Ann Rev Immunol 10:295–331.
252. Lin H, Mosmann TR, Guilbert L, Tuntipopipat S, Wegmann TG (1993) Synthesis of T helper 2-type cytokines at the maternal-fetal interface. J Immunol 151:4562–4573.
253. Wegmann TG, Lin H, Guilbert L, Mosmann TR (1993) Bidirectional cytokine interactions in the maternal-fetal relationship: is successful pregnancy a Th2 phenomenon? Immunol Today 14: 353–356.
254. Arceci RJ, Shanahan F, Stanley ER, Pollard J (1989) Temporal expression and location of colony-stimulating factor 1 (CSF-1) and its receptor in the female reproductive tract are consistent with CSF-1 regulated placental development. Proc Natl Acad Sci USA 86:8818–8822.
255. Regenstreif LJ, Rossant J (1989) Expression of the c-fms proto-oncogene and of the cytokine, CSF-1, during mouse embryogenesis. Dev Biol 133:284–294.
256. Chen H-L, Kamath R, Pace JL, Russell SW, Hunt JS (1994) Gestation-related expression of the interferon-γ receptor gene in mouse uterine and embryonic hematopoietic cells. J Leukocyte Biol 55:617–625.
257. De los Santos M, Mercader A, Frances A, Portoloes E. Remohi J. Pellicer A, Simon C (1996) Role of endometrial factors in regulating secretion of components of the immunoreactive human embryonic interleukin-1 system during embryonic development. Biol Reprod 54:563–574.
258. Haynes MK, Jackson LG, Tuan RS, Shepley KS, Smith JB (1993) Cytokine production in first trimester chorionic villi: detection of mRNAs and protein products in situ. Cell Immunol 151:300–308.
259. Jokhi PP, King A, Sharkey AM, Smith SK, Loke YW (1994) Screening for cytokine messenger ribonucleic acids in purified human decidual lymphocyte populations by reverse-transcription polymerise chain reaction. J Immunol 153:4427–4435.
260. Kauma S, Matt D, Strom S, Eierman D, Turner T (1990) Interleukin-1 beta, human leukocyte antigen HLA-DR alpha, and transforming growth factor-beta expression in endometrium, placenta, and placental membranes. Am J Obstet Gynecol 163:1430–1437.
261. King A, Jokhi PP, Smith SK, Sharkey AM, Loke YW (1995) Screening for cytokine mRNA in human villous and extra villous trophoblast using reverse-transcriptase polymerise chain reaction. Cytokine 7:364–371.
262. Lea RG, Flanders KC, Harley CB, Mauel J, Banwatt D, Clark DA (1992) Release of a transforming growth factor (TGF)-β2-related suppressor factor from post-implantation murine decidual tissue can be correlated with the detection of a subpopulation of cells containing RNA for TGF-β2. J Immunol 148:778–787.

263. Masuhiro K, Masuzaki N, Nishino E, Taniguchi T, Kameda T, Li Y, Saji F, Tanizawa O (1991) Trophoblast-derived interleukin-1 (IL-1) stimulates the release of human chorionic gonadotropin by activating IL-6 and IL-6 receptor systems in first trimester human trophoblasts. J Clin Endocrinol Metab 72:594–601.
264. Parr EL, Chen HL, Parr MB, Hunt JS (1995) Synthesis and granular localization of tumor necrosis factor-alpha in activated NK cells in the pregnant mouse uterus. J Reprod Immunol 28:31–40.
265. Saito S, Nishikawa K, Morii T, Enomoto M, Narita N, Motoyoshi K, Ichijo M (1993) Cytokine production by CD16-CD56 bright natural killer cells in the human early pregnancy decidua. Int Immunol 5:559–563.
266. Yamaguchi M, Taga T, Kishimoto T, Miyake A (1995) Cytokines that use gp130 as a signal transducer stimulate mouse placental lactogen-I (mPL-I) but inhibit mPL-II production in vitro. Biol Reprod 53:399–406.
267. Shi C, Lee W-S, He Q, Zhang D, Fletcher DL, Jr, Newell JB, Haber E (1996) Immunological basis of transplant-associated arteriosclerosis. Proc Natl Acad Sci USA 93:4051–4056.
268. Gurtner GC, Davis V, Li H, McCoy MJ, Sharpe A, Cybulsky MI (1995) Targeted disruption of the murine VCAM-I gene: essential role of VCAM-1 in chorioallantoic fusion and placentation. Genes Dev 9:1–14.
269. Tabibzadeh S, Babaknia A (1995) The signals and molecular pathways involved in implantation, a symbiotic interaction between blastocyst and endometrium involving adhesion and tissue invasion. Hum Reprod 10:1579–1602.
270. Robertson SA, Seamark RF, Guilbert LJ, Wegmann TG (1994) The role of cytokines in gestation. Crit Rev Immunol 14:239–292.
271. McDermott MR, Bienenstock J (1979) Evidence for a common mucosal immunologic system: I. Migration of B immunoblasts into intestinal, respiratory, and genital tissues. J Immunol 122: 1892–1898.
272. McDermott MR, Clark DA, Bienenstock J (1980) Evidence for a common mucosal immunologic system: II. Influence of the estrous cycle on B immunoblast migration into genital and intestinal tissues. J Immunol 124: 2536–2539.
273. Wira CR, Hyde E, Sandoe CP, Sullivan D, Spencer S (1980) Cellular aspects of the rat uterine IgA response to estradiol and progesterone. J Steroid Biochem 12:451–459.
274. Wira CR, Sullivan DA, Sandoe CP (1983) Epithelial cell involvement in the estrogen-stimulated accumulation of IgA in the rat uterus. J Steroid Biochem 19:469–474.
275. Alexander NJ, Anderson DJ (1987) Immunology of semen. Fertil Steril 47:192–205.
276. du Mesnil du Buisson F, Dauzier L (1955) La remontée des spermatozoides du verrat dans le tractus génital de la truie en oestrus. Comptes Rendus des Société Biologie (Paris) 149:76–79.
277. Lovell JE, Getty R (1968) Fate of semen in the uterus of the sow: histologic study of endometrium during the 27 hours after natural service. Am J Vet Res 29:609–624.
278. Hadjisavas M, Armstrong DT, Seamark RF (1994) Purification of a cell-cell adhesion regulator from porcine seminal vesicle fluid. Biochem Biophys Res Commun 205:1206–1216.
279. Engelhardt H, Small MR, King GJ (1996) Exposure of pigs to seminal plasma at estrus recruits leukocytes to the uterine epithelium. Biol Reprod 54(Suppl 1):abstract 476.
280. Mattner PE (1968) The distribution of spermatozoa and leucocytes in the female genital tract in goats and cattle. J Reprod Fert 17:253–261.
281. Corner GW (1921) Cyclic changes in the ovaries and uterus of the sow, and their relation to the mechanism of implantation. Contrib Embryol 13:117–146.
282. Bischof RJ, Brandon MR, Lee C-S (1994) Studies on the distribution of immune cells in the uteri of prepubertal and cycling gilts. J Reprod Immunol 26:111–129.
283. Ford SP, Christenson RK (1979) Blood flow to uteri of sows during the estrous cycle and early pregnancy: local effect of the conceptus on the uterine blood supply. Biol Reprod 21:617–624.
284. Keys JL, King GJ (1988) Morphological evidence for increased uterine vascular permeability at the time of embryonic attachment in the pig. Biol Reprod 39:473–487.
285. Zuckerman FA, Binns RM, Husmann R, Yang H, Carr MM, Kim YB, Davis WC, Misfeldt M, Lunney JK (1994) Analyses of monoclonal antibodies reactive with porcine CD44 And CD45. Vet Immunol Immunopathol 43:293–305.
286. Kovacs PR, Tekpetey FR, Armstrong DT (1994) Response of peripheral blood leucocytes to mitogenic factor(s) in porcine seminal plasma. Immunol Cell Biol 72:129–135.
287. Hadjisavas M, Laurenz JC, Bazer FW (1994) Seminal plasma (SPL); a potential mediator of inflammation in the uterus following mating in the pig. Biol Reprod 50 (Suppl 1):abstract 76.

288. Pandya IJ, Cohen J (1985) The luekocytic reaction of the human uterine cervix to spermatozoa. Fertil Steril 43:417–421.
289. De M, Choudhuri R, Wood GW (1991) Determination of the number and distribution of macrophages, lymphocytes and granulocytes in the mouse uterus from mating through implantation. J Leuk Biol 50:252–262.
290. Kachkache M, Acker GM, Chaouat G, Noun A, Garabedian M (1991) Hormonal and local factors control the immunohistochemical distributions of immunocytes in the rat uterus before conceptus implantation: Effects of ovariectomy, fallopian tube section and injection. Biol Reprod 45:860–868.
291. Robertson SA, Seamark RF (1990) Granulocyte macrophage colony stimulating factor (GM-CSF) in the murine reproductive tract: Stimulation by seminal factors. Reprod Fertil Dev 2:359–368.
292. Robertson SA, Mayrhofer G, Seamark RF (1992) Uterine epithelial cells synthesize granulocyte-macrophage colony-stimulating factor and interleukin-6 in pregnant and nonpregnant mice. Biol Reprod 46:1069–1079.
293. Wang JM, Colella S, Allavena P, Mantovani A (1987) Chemotactic activity of human recombinant granulocyte-macrophage colony-stimulating factor. Immunol 60:439–444.
294. Gasson JC, Weisbart RH, Kaufman SE, Clark, SC, Hewick RM, Wong GG, Golde DW (1984) Purified human granulocyte-macrophage colony-stimulating factor: Direct action on neutrophils. Science 226:1339–1342.
295. Robertson FM, Oberyszyn TM, Sabourin CLK, Pellegrini AE, Bijur GN, Oberyszyn AS, Boros LG (1994) Granulocyte macrophage colony stimulating factor gene expression and function during tumor promotion. Carcinogenesis 15:1017–1029.
296. Rowson LEA, Lamming GE, Fry RM (1953) The relationship between ovarian hormones, and uterine infection. Vet Rec 65:335–340.
297. Hussein AM, Newby TJ, Stokes CR, Bourne FJ (1983) Quantitation and origin of immunoglobulin A, G and M in the secretions and fluids of the reproductive tract of the sow. J Reprod Immunol 5:17–26.
298. Sullivan DA, Wira CR (1983) Hormonal regulation of immunoglobulins in the rat uterus: uterine immunoglobulin response to a single estradiol treatment. Endocrinology 112:260–268.
299. Turcotte JG, Haines RF, Bordy GL, Meyer TJ, Schwartz SA (1968) Immunosuppression with medroxyprogesterone acetate. Transplantation 6:248–260.
300. Munroe JS (1971) Progesteroids as immunosuppressive agents. J Reticuloendothelial Soceity 9:361–375.
301. Kountz SL, Wechter WJ (1977) Immunosuppression with melengestrol. Transplant Proc 9:1447–1453.
302. Beer AE, Billingham RE (1979) Maternal immunological recognition mechanisms during pregnancy, In: Ciba Foundation Symposium 64 (Wjelan EJ, ed.), Oxford, Excerpta Medica, pp. 293–322.
303. Siiteri PK, Febres F, Clemens LE, Chang RJ, Gondos B, Stites D (1977) Progesterone and maintenance of pregnancy: is progesterone natures immunosuppressant? Ann NY Acad Sci 286:384–397.
304. Watnick AS, Russo RA (1968) Survival of skin homografts in uteri of pregnant and progesterone-estrogen treated rats. Proc Soc Exp Biol Med 128:1–4.
305. Moriyama I, Sugawa T (1972) Progesterone facilitates implantation of xenogeneic cultured cells in hamster uterus. Nature New Biol 236:150–152.
306. Hansen PH, Bazer, FW, Sergerson EC (1986) Skin graft survival in the uterine lumen or ewes treated with progesterone. Am J Reprod Immunol Microbiol 12:48–54.
307. Bischof RJ, Lee C-S, Brandon MR, Meeusen E (1994) Inflammatory response in the pig uterus induced by seminal plasma. J Reprod Immunol 26:131–146.
308. Bischof RJ, Brandon MR, Lee C-S (1995) Cellular immune responses in the pig uterus during pregnancy. J Reprod Immunol 29:161–178.
309. Murray FA, Grifo AP, Parker CF (1983) Increased litter size in gilts by intrauterine infusion of seminal plasma and sperm antigens before breeding J Anim Sci 56:895–900.
310. Murray FA, Grifo APJ (1986) Intrauterine infusion of killed semen to increased litter size in gilts. J Anim Sci 62:187–190.
311. Skjervoid H, Amlid T, Onstad O, Fossum K (1979) Evidence of immunological influence on the number of live embryos in pigs. A Tierzuchtg Zuchtgsbiol 96:235,236.
312. Almlid T (1981) Does enhanced antigenicity of semen increase the litter size in pigs? Z Tierzuchtg Zuchtgsbiol 98:1–10.
313. Blichfeldt T (1984) Effect of addition of antigen, adjuvant or mitogen to semen on embryonic survival in artificially inseminated gilts. Z Tierzuchtg Zuchtgsbiol 101:298–304.
314. Van der Lende T, Donker R, Hazeleger W (1986) Embryonic survival in the pig after insemination with antigen-enriched semen. Theriogenology 26:391–396.

315. Giles JR, Thompson LH, Arkins S, Camacho T, Eichen PA (1990) Effects of uterine infusion of non-viable semen, seminal plasma or egg albumin prior to breeding on the reproductive efficiency of gilts or sows. Can J Anim Sci 70:129–133.
316. Pang SF, Chow PH, Wong TM (1979) The role of the seminal vesicles, coagulating glands and prostate glands on the fertility and fecundity of mice. J Reprod Fertil 56:129–132.
317. Queen F, Dhabuwala CB, Pierrepoint CG (1981) The effect of removal of the various accessory sex glands on the fertility of male rats. J Reprod Fertil 62:423–436.
318. Davies DC, Hall G, Hibbit KG, Moore HDM (1975) The removal of the seminal vesicles from the boar and the effects on the semen characteristics. J Reprod Fertil 43:305–312.
319. Klonoff-Cohen HS, Savitz DA, Celafo RC, McCann MF (1989) An epidemiological study of contraception and preeclampsia. J Am Med Assoc 262:3143–3147.
320. Bellinge BS, Copeland CM, Thomas TD, Mazzucchelli RE, O'Neil G, Cohen MJ (1986) The influence of patient insemination on the implantation rate in an in vitro fertilization and embryo transfer program. Fertil Steril 46:2523–2526.
321. Marconi G, Auge L, Oses R, Qunitana R, Raffo F, Young E (1989) Does sexual intercourse improve pregnancy rates in gamete intrafallopian tube transfer? Fertil Steril 51:357–359.
322. Assheton R (1906) The morphology of the ungulate placenta. Phil Trans R Soc Lond (Biol) 198: 143–220.
323. Leiser R (1975) Kontaktaufnahme zwischen trophoblast und uterusepithel während der frühen implantation beim rind. Anat Histol Embryol 4:63–86.
324. King GJ (1993) Comparative placentation in ungulates. J Exp Zool 266:588–602.
325. Wooding FBP (1980) Electron microscope localisation of binucleate cells in the sheep placenta using phosphotungstic acid. Biol Reprod 22:357–365.
326. Wooding FBP (1983) Frequency and localization of binucleate cells in the placentomes of ruminnats. Placenta 4:527–540.
327. Atkinson BA, King GJ, Amoroso EC (1984) Development of the caruncular and intercaruncular regions in the bovine endometrium. Biol Reprod 30:763–774.
328. Wiley AA, Bartol FF, Barron DH (1987) Histogenesis of the ovine uterus. J Anim Sci 64: 1262–1269.
329. Van der Wielen AL, King GJ (1984) Intraepithelial lymphocytes in the bovine uterus during the oestrous cycle and early gestation. J Reprod Fertil 70:457–462.
330. Low BG, Hansen PJ, Drost M, Gogolin-Ewens KJ (1990) Expression of major histocompatiblity complex antigens on the bovine placenta. J Reprod Fertil 90:234–243.
331. Gogolin-Ewens KJ, Lee CS, Mercer WR, Brandon MR (1989) Site-directed differences in the immune response to the fetus. Immunology 66:312–317.
332. Staples LD, Heap RB, Wooding FBP, King GJ (1983) Migration of leukocytes into the uterus after acute removal of ovarian progesterone during early pregnancy in the sheep. Placenta 4: 339–350.
333. Lee CS, Meeusen E, Gogolin-Ewens K, Brandon MR (1992) Quantitative and qualitative changes in the intraepithelial lymphocyte population in the uterus of nonpregnant and pregnant sheep. Am J Reprod Immunol 28:90–96.
334. Meeusen E, Fox A, Brandon M, Lee CS (1993) Activation of uterine intraepithelial gamma-delta T cell receptor-positive lymphocytes during pregnancy. Eur J Immunol 23: 1112–1117.
335. Mackay CR, Maddox JF, Brandon MR (1987) A monoclonal antibody to the p220 component of sheep LCA identifies B-cells and a unique lymphocyte subset. Cell Immunol 110:46–55.
336. Kent JF (1952) The origin, fate and cytochemistry of the globule leucocyte of the sheep. Anat Rec 112:91–115.
337. Kellas LM (1961) An intra-epithelial granular cell in the uterine epithelium of some ruminant species during the pregnancy cycle. Acta Anat 44:109–130.
338. Wooding FBP, Flint APF (1994) Placentation, In: Marshalls Physiology of Reproduction, vol. 3 (Lamming CE, ed.), Chapman and Hall, London, pp. 230–460.
339. Lee CS, Wooding FBP, Morgan G (1995) Quantitative analysis of intraepithelial large granular lymphocyte distribution and maternofetal cellular interactions in the synepitheliochorial placenta of the deer. J Anat 187:445–460.
340. Mackay CR, Maddox JF, Brandon MR (1986) Three distinct subpopulations of sheep T lymphocytes. Eur J Immunol 16:19–25.
341. Hein WR, Mackay CR (1991) Prominence of gamma-delta T cells in the ruminant immune system. Immunol Today 12:30–34.

342. Guy-Grand D, Cerf-Bensussan N, Malissen B, Malassis-Seris ML, Briottet C, Vassalli P (1991) Two gut intraepithelial CD8+ lymphocyte populations with different T cell receptors: a role for the gut epithelium in T cell differentiation. J Exp Med 173:471–481.
343. Newton GR, Vallet JL, Hansen PF, Bazer FW (1989) Inhibition of lymphocyte proliferation by ovine trophoblast protein-1 and a high molecular weight glycoprotein produced by the peri-implantation sheep conceptus. Am J Reprod Immunol 19:99–107.
344. Skopets B, Li J, Thatcher WW, Roberts RM, Hansen PJ (1992) Inhibition of lymphocyte proliferation by bovine trophoblast protein-1 (type I trophoblast interferon) and bovine interferon-alpha$_{I}$1. Vet Immunol Immunopathol 34:81–96.
345. Tuo W, Ott TL, Bazer FW (1993) Natural killer cell activity of lymphocytes exposed to ovine, type I trophoblast interferon. Am J Reprod Immunol 29:26–34.
346. Hansen PJ (1995) Interactions between the immune system and the ruminant conceptus. J Reprod Fertil Suppl 49:69–82.
347. Imakawa K, Helmer SD, Nephew KP, Neka CS, Christenson RK (1993) A novel role for GM-CSF: enhancement of pregnancy specific interferon production, ovine trophoblast protein-1. Endocrinology 132:1869–1871.
348. Gottshall SL, Hansen PJ (1992) Regulation of leucocyte subpopulations in the sheep endometrium by progesterone. Immunology 76:636–641.
349. Low BG, Hansen PJ (1988) Actions of steroids and prostaglandins secreted by the placenta and uterus of the cow and ewe on lymphocyte proliferation in vitro. Am J Reprod Immunol Microbiol 18:71–75.
350. Monterroso VH, Hansen PJ (1993) Regulation of bovine and ovine lymphocyte proliferation by progesterone: modulation by steroid receptor antagonists and physiological status. Acta Endocrinol 129:532–535.
351. Olea-Serrano O, Devleeschower N, Leclerq G, Henson J-C (1985) Assay for estrogen and progesterone receptors of breast cancer cell lines in monolayer cultures. J Clin Oncol 21:965–973.
352. Staples LD, Binns RM, Heap RB (1983) Influence of certain steroids on lymphocyte transformation in sheep and goats studied in vitro. J Endocrinol 98:55–69.
353. Stephenson DC, Hansen PJ (1990) Induction by progesterone on immunosuppressive activity in uterine secretions of ovariectomized ewes. Endocrinology 126:3168–3178.
354. Skopets B, Hansen PJ (1993) Identification of the predominant proteins in uterine fluids of unilaterally pregnant ewes that inhibit lymphocyte proliferation. Biol Reprod 49:997–1007.
355. Segerson EC, Bazer FW (1989) High molecular weight basic and acidic immunosuppressive protein components in uterine secretions of pregnant cows. Biol Reprod 41:1014–1023.
356. Liu WJ, Hansen PJ (1995) Progesterone-induced secretion of dipeptidyl peptidase-IV (cluster differentiation antigen-26) by the uterine endometrium of the ewe and cow that costimulates lymphocyte proliferation. Endocrinology 136: 779–787.
357. Hegen M, Niedobitek G, Klein CE, Stein H, Fleischer B (1990) The T cell triggering molecule Tp103 is associated with dipeptidyl aminopeptidase IV activity. J Immunol 144:2908–2914.
358. Kameoka J, Tanaka T, Nojima Y, Schlossman SF, Morimoto C (1993) Direct association of adenosine deaminase with a T cell activation antigen, CD26. Science 261:466–469.
359. Fleischer B (1994) CD26: a surface protease involved in T-cell activation. Immunol Today 15: 180–184.
360. Classen L, Denker HW, Winterhager E (1987) Apical plama membrane-bound enzymes of rabbit uterine epithelium: pattern changes during the periimplantation phase. Histochemistry 87: 517–529.
361. Ohta N, Takahasi T, Mori T, Park MK, Kawashima S, Takahasi K, Kobayashi H (1992) Hormonal modulation of propylendopeptidase and dipeptidyl peptidase IV activities in the mouse uterus and ovary. Acta Endocrinol (Copenh) 127:262–266.
362. Betteridge KJ (1989) The structure and function of the equine capsule in relation to embryo manipulation and transfer. Equine Vet J (Suppl) 8:92–100.
363. Ginther OJ (1983) Fixation and orientation of the early equine conceptus. Theriogenology 19:613–623.
364. Enders AC, Liu IK (1991) Lodgement of the equine blastocyst in the uterus from fixation through endometrial cup formation. J Reprod Fertil (Suppl) 44:427–438.
365. van Niekerk CD, Allen WR (1975) Early embryonic development in the horse. J Reprod Fertil (Suppl) 23:495–498.
366. Steven D (1982) Placentation in the mare. J Reprod Fertil (Suppl) 31:41–55.
367. Allen WR, Moor RM (1972) The origin of equine endometrial cups. I. The production of PMSG by fetal trophoblast. J Reprod Fertil 29:313–316.

368. Allen WR, Hamilton DW, Moor RM (1973) The origin of equine endometrial cups. II. Invasion of the endometrium by trophoblast. Anat Rec 177:485–501.
369. Enders AC, Liu IKM (1991) Trophoblast-uterine interactions during equine chorionic girdle cell maturation, migration, and transformation. Am J Anat (192:366–381.
370. Allen WR (1979) Maternal recognition of pregnancy and immunological implications of trophoblast-endometrial interactions in equids, In: Maternal Recognition of Pregnancy. Ciba Foundation Symposium 64, Excerpta Medica, Amsterdam, pp. 323–352.
371. Antczak DF, Oriol JG, Donaldson WL, Polemen C, Stenzler L, Volsen SG, Allen WR (1987) Differentiation molecules of the equine trophoblast. J Reprod Fertil (Suppl) 35:371–378.
372. Licht P, Bona Gallo A, Aggerwal BB, Farmer SW, Castilno JB, Papkoff H (1979) Biological and binding activities of equine pituitary gonadotrophins and pregnant mare serum gonadotrophin. J Endocrinol 83:311–322.
373. Ginther OJ (1992) Reproductive Biology of the Mare: Basic and Applied Aspects, 2nd ed. Cross Plaines, WI.
374. Allen WR, Stewart F (1993) Equine chorionic gonadotropin, In: Equine Reproduction (McKinnon AO, Voss J, eds.), Lea and Febiger, Mavern, PA, pp. 81–96.
375. Hearn JP, Webley GE, Gidley-Baird AA (1991) Chorionic gonadotrophin and embryo-maternal recognition during the peri-implantation period in primates. J Reprod Fertil 92:497–509.
376. Bergfelt DR, Pierson RA, Ginther OJ (1989) Resurgence of the primary corpus luteum during pregnancy in the mare. Anim Reprod Sci 21:261–270.
377. Amoroso EC (1955) The endocrinology of pregnancy. Br Med Bull 17:717–125.
378. Grünig G, Triplett L, Canady LK, Allen WR, Antczak DF. (1995) The maternal leukocyte response to the endometrial cups in horses is correlated with the developmental stages of the invasive trophoblast cells. Placenta 16:539–559.
379. Antczak DF, Miller J, Remick L (1984) Lymphocyte alloantigens of the horse. II. Antibodies to ELA antigens produced during equine pregnancy. J Reprod Immunol 6:283–287.
380. Kydd J, Miller JM, Antczak DF, Allen WR (1982) Maternal anti-fetal cytotoxic antibody responses of equids during pregnancy. J Reprod Fertil (Suppl) 32:361–369.
381. Donaldson WL, Crump A, Zhang CH, Kornbluth J, Kamoun M, Davis W, Antczak DF (1988) At least two loci encode polymorphic class I MHC antigens in the horse. Anim Genet (19:379–390.
382. Allen WR, Kydd JH, Miller JM, Antczak DF (1984) Immunological studies on fetomaternal relationships in equine pregnancy, In: Immunological Aspects of Reproduction in Mammals (Crighton DB, ed.), Butterworths, London, pp. 183–193.
383. Sargent IL, Arenas J, Redman CWG (1987) Maternal cell-mediated sensitization to paternal HLA may occur, but it is not a regular event in normal human pregnancy. J Reprod Immunol 10:111–120.
384. Donaldson WL, Zhang CH, Oriol JG, Antczak DF (1990) Invasive equine trophoblast expresses conventional class I Major Histocompatibility Complex antigens. Development 110:63–71.
385. Crump A, Donaldson WL, Miller J, Kydd J, Allen WR, Antczak DR (1987) Expression of Major Histocompatibility Complex (MHC) antigens on equine trophoblast. J Reprod Fertil (Suppl) 35:379–388.
386. Kydd J, Butcher GW, Antczak DF, Allen WR (1991) Expression of major histocompatibility complex (MHC) class I molecules on early trophoblast. J Reprod Fertil (Suppl) 44:463–477.
387. Oriol JG, Donaldson WL, Dougherty DA, Antczak DF (1989) Molecules of the early equine trophoblast. J Reprod Fertil (Suppl) 44:455–462.
388. Antczak DF, Allen WR (1989) Maternal immunological recognition of pregnancy in equids. J Reprod Fertil (Suppl) 37:69–78.
389. Lea RG, Stewart F, Allen WR, Ohno I, Clark DA (1995) Accumulation of chromotrope 2R positive cells in equine endometrium during early pregnancy and expression of transforming growth factor-β2 (TGF-β2). J Reprod Fertil 103:339–347.
390. Lunn DP, McClure JT, Schobert S, Holmes A (1995) Abnormal patterns of equine leucocyte differentiation antigen expression in severe combined immunodeficiency foals suggests the phenotype of normal equine natural killer cells. Immunology 84:495–499.
391. Koets AP (1995) The equine endometrial cup reaction: A review. Vet Quart 17:21–29.
392. Allen WR (1982) Immunological aspects of the endometrial cup reaction and the effect of xenogeneic pregnancy in horses and donkeys. J Reprod Fertil (Suppl) 31:57–94.
393. Spincemaille J, Bouters R, Vandeplassche M, Bonte P (1975) Some aspects of endometrial cup formation and PMSG production. J Reprod Fertil 23:415–418.
394. Dhindsa DS, Dziuk PJ, Norton W (1967) Time of transuterine migration and distribution of embryos in the pig. Anat Rec 159:325–330.

395. Heuser CH, Streeter GL (1929) Early stages in the development of pig embryos, from the period of initial cleavage to the time of the appearance of the limb-buds. Contrib Embryol Carnegie Inst 20:1-29.
396. Samuel CA (1971) The development of pig trophoblast in ectopic sites. J Reprod Fertil 27:494-499.
397. Samuel CA, Perry JS (1972) The ultrastructure of pig trophoblast transplanted to an ectopic site in the uterine wall. J Anat 113:139-149.
398. King GJ (1988) Reduction in uterine intra-epithelial lymphocytes during early gestation in pigs. J Reprod Immunol 14:41-46.
399. Keys JL, King GJ (1990) Microscopic examination of porcine conceptus-maternal interface between d 10 and (19 of pregnancy. Am J Anat 188:221-238.
400. Swatman J, King GJ, Engelhardt H (1996) Leukocyte distribution in the pig uterus relative to sites of conceptus attachment during early pregnancy. Biol Reprod 54 (Suppl 1):abstract 475.
401. Vega-Lopez MA, Telemo E, Bailey M, Stevens K, Stokes CR (1993) Immune cell distribution in the small intestine of the pig: immunohistological evidence for an organized compartmentalization in the lamina propria. Vet Immunol Immunopathol 37:49-60.
402. Hammerberg C, Schurig G (1986) Characterisation of monoclonal antibodies directed against swine leukocytes. Vet Immunol Immunopathol 11:107-121.
403. Saalmller A, Hirt W, Reddehase MJ (1990) Porcine γ/δ T lymphocyte subsets differing in their propensity to home to lymphoid tissue. Eur J Immunol 20:2343-2346.
404. Croy BA, Wood W, King GJ (1987) Evaluation of intruterine immune suppression during pregnancy in a species with epitheliochorial placentation. J Immunol 139:1088-1095.
405. Hirt W, Saalmller A, Reddehase MJ (1990) Distinct γ/δ T cell receptors define two subsets of circulating porcine CD2-CD4-CD8- T lymphocytes. Eur J Immunol 20:265-269.
406. Mackay CR, Beya MF, Matzinger P (1989) Gamma-delta cells express a unique surface molecule during thymic development. Eur J Immunol (19:1477-1485.
407. Pescovitz MD, Lowman MA, Sachs DH (1988) Expression of T-cell associated antigens by porcine natural killer cells. Immunology 65:267-271.
408. Croy BA, Waterfield A, Wood W, King GJ (1988) Normal murine and porcine embryos recruit NK cells to the uterus. Cell Immunol 115:471-480.
409. Yu Z, Croy BA, Chapeau C, King GJ (1993) Elevated endometrial natural killer cell activity during early porcine pregnancy is conceptus-mediated. J Reprod Immunol 24:153-164.
410. King A, Birkby A, Loke YW (1989) Early human decidual cells exhibit NK activity against the K562 cell line but not first trimester trophoblast. Cell Immunol 118:337-344.
411. King A, Loke YW (1990) Human trophoblast and JEG choriocarcinoma cells are sensitive to lysis by IL-2-stimulated decidual NK cells. Cell Immunol 127:230-237.
412. Dato ME, Wierda WG, Kim YB (1992) A triggering structure recognized by G7 monoclonal antibody on porcine lymphocytes and granulocytes. Cell Immunol 140:468-477.
413. Wilson AD, Stokes CR, Bourne FJ (1986) Morphology and functional characteristics of isolated porcine intaepithelial lymphocytes. Immunology 59:109-113.
414. Cross JC, Roberts RM (1989) Porcine conceptuses secrete an interferon during the preattachment period of early pregnancy. Biol Reprod 40:1109-1118.
415. Mirando MA, Harney JP, Beers S, Pontzer CH, Torres BA, Johnson HM,Bazer FW (1990) Onset of secretion of proteins with antiviral activity by pig conceptuses. J Reprod Fertil 88:197-203.
416. La Bonnardiére C, Martinat-Botte F, Terqui M, Lefévre F, Zouari K, Martal J, Bazer FW (1991) Production of two species of interferon by Large White and Meishan pig conceptuses during the peri-attachment period. J Reprod Fertil 91:469-478.
417. Lefévre, F, Martinat-Botte F, Guillomot M, Zouari K, Charley B, La Bonnardiere C (1990) Interferon-gamma gene and protein are spontaneously expressed by the trophectoderm early in gestation. Eur J Immunol 20:2485-2490.
418. Lefévre F, Boulay V (1993) A novel and atypical type one interferon gene expressed by trophoblast during early pregnancy. J Biol Chem 268:19,760-19,768.
419. Dhindsa DS, Dziuk PJ (1968) Effects of pregnancy in the pig after killing embryos or fetuses in one uterine horn in early pregnancy. J Anim Sci 27:122-126.
420. Harney JP, Bazer FW (1989) Effect of porcine conceptus secretory proteins on interestrous interval and uterine secretion of prostaglandins. Biol Reprod 41:277-284.
421. Bazer FW, Ott TL, Spencer TE (1994) Pregnancy recognition in ruminants, pigs and horses: Signals from the trophoblast. Theriogenology 41:79-94.
422. D'Andrea S, Chousterman S, Flechon JE, La Bonnardiére C (1994) Paracrine activities of porcine trophoblastic interferons. J Reprod Fertil 102:185-194.

423. Zusman I, Engelhard D, Yaffe P, Ron A, Panet A, Ornoy A (1984) Effects of interferon and encephalomyocarditis virus on in vitro development of preimplantation mouse embryos with and without the zona pellucida. Teratology 29:405–409.
424. La Bonnardiére C (1993) No detection of interferon-γ activity during the early pregnancy in the mouse. Am J Reprod Immunol 30:26–31.
425. Johnston MI, Torrence PF (1984) The role of interferon-induced proteins, doublestranded RNA and 2′,5′-oligoadenylate in the interferon-mediated inhibition of viral translation, In: Interferon, vol. 3, Mechanisms of Production and Action (Friedman RM, ed.), Elsevier, B.V. Amsterdam, pp. 190–298.
426. Short, Jr EC, Geisert RD, Groothuis PG, Blair RM, Schmitt RAM, Fulton RW (1992) Porcine conceptus proteins: antiviral activity and effect on 2′,5′-oligoadenylate synthetase. Biol Reprod 46:464–469.
427. Vileck J, Gray TW, Rinderknecht E, Sevastopoulos CG (1985) Interferon gamma: A lymphokine for all seasons, In: Lymphokines, vol. 11 (Pick E, ed.), Academic, Harcourt Brace Jovanovich Publishers, Orlando, FL, pp. 1–32.
428. Reiter ZVI (1993) Interferon—a major regulator of natural killer cell-mediated cytotoxicity. J Interferon Res 13:247–257.
429. De Maeyer E, De Maeyer-Guignard J (1988) Interferons and Other Regulatory Cytokines. John Wiley, New York, pp. 91–113.

10 Secretion and Metabolism of Steroids in Subprimate Mammals During Pregnancy

Rodney D. Geisert, BS, MS, PHD
and *Alan J. Conley*, BVSC, MS, PHD

CONTENTS

INTRODUCTION

The establishment and maintenance of pregnancy in the majority of viviparous mammals evolved through utilization of steroids, namely progesterone, to regulate the maternal system during gestation *(1)*. Formation of the corpus luteum (CL) and progesterone release following ovulation of the Graafian follicle clearly have an established function in regulating myometrial contractility, uterine receptivity to the conceptus, and endometrial secretion for growth and development of the conceptus. Placental steroidogenesis and steroid metabolism also have evolved to varying degrees of necessity within the diverse mammalian species. Species vary not only in the sophistication of placental steroidogenic capabilities, but also the stage of gestation at which qualitative and quantitative changes in steroid metabolism are activated. For example, bovine and ovine species can maintain pregnancy following ovariectomy during the later stages of pregnancy in contrast to the pig and goat, which cannot, and in equine, the corpora lutea undergo a normal process of luteolysis during midgestation and become totally reliant on placental contributions of progesterone. The increased capacity to synthesize progesterone by the placenta of bovine, ovine, and equine species are adaptations by the fetal–placental unit to assert local progestational control during the last trimester of pregnancy. Placental steroidogenesis and metabolism play a vital role in fetal development and survival through steroid regulation of nutrient flow, be it by directing endometrial synthesis *(2–6)*, modulating blood flow to the utero-placental unit *(7,8)*, or providing one possible avenue for immunological regulation of the maternal immune system to prevent rejection of the fetal allograft *(9–12)*. The intent of the present chapter is to provide insight into our current knowledge concerning steroidogenesis and metabolism during pregnancy in various subprimate species.

SECRETION AND METABOLISM OF STEROIDS

Early Gestation

During the early stages of pregnancy, ovarian CL production of progesterone is essential for the establishment of a uterine environment permissive to conceptus implantation and placental attachment. In virtually all subprimate species, ovariectomy during the early stages of pregnancy invariably interferes with conceptus development and implantation. However, supplementation with progesterone alone is sufficient to permit the continuance of pregnancy to term in the majority of species. The mouse and rat are notable exceptions in that these species require a pulse of nidatory estrogen *(13)* in addition to progesterone therapy to replace the loss of ovarian estrogen synthesis, which is necessary to induce implantation *(14)*. Levasseur *(15)* proposed that the secretion of estrogen by either the ovary, conceptus, and/or endometrium during the period of implantation or, in the case of epitheliochorial placentation (placental attachment), suggests that metabolism of progestagens to estrogens serves an essential role in numerous eutherian mammals (Fig. 1). Although there are studies that provide exceptions or questions concerning the essential need for estrogen in implantation in some species *(16)*, there are also numerous species in which estrogen is a major player in this biological process.

Early peri-implantation mouse and rat blastocysts do not have the capacity to synthesize estrogen *(17,18)*, and are thus totally dependent on the proper timing of estrogen release from the ovaries (Fig. 1) to induce uterine receptivity for implantation and for the hemochorial type of placentation *(19,20)*. The lack of estrogen synthesis by unattached blastocysts in these species permits maternal control of implantation. Mouse and rat blastocysts can remain in a state of lactation-induced facultative dispause for many days following breeding of the dam shortly after parturition *(21)*, which can be mimicked through ovariectomy and progesterone administration *(20)*. Reactivation of blastocyst development occurs following weaning of the pups or treatment of the dam with estrogen. Rat and mouse blastocysts appear to have the capability to metabolize steroids, since 3β- and 17β-hydroxysteroid dehydrogenase are detected histochemically in peri-implantation blastocysts *(22)*. Although the ability of early mouse blastocysts to convert pregnenolone to progesterone has been questioned *(23)*, blastocysts have been demonstrated to convert pregnenolone to progesterone, which is rapidly metabolized to 5α-pregnan-3,20-dione and 3α-hydroxy-5α-pregnan-20-one *(24)*. The biological function of the rapid metabolism of progesterone by the developing mouse blastocyst has not been elucidated. However, the ability to regulate the concentration of progesterone in the microenvironment of the developing embryo may provide one mechanism to achieve local control over the maternal system. The maternal endometrium also has the capacity to metabolize steroids, since the rat uterus contains 5α-reductase, which produces the metabolite 3α-OH-5α-pregnan-20-one *(25)*. There are also indications of blastocyst–endometrial interactions for the conversion of estrone to estradiol and possible aromatization of testosterone *(15)*, which may serve as additional support to the ovary for the implantation process.

In contrast to the mouse and rat, rabbit and hamster blastocysts do not require a maternal source of estrogen for establishment of pregnancy. Rabbit and hamster blastocysts contain 3β- and 17β-hydroxysteroid dehydrogenases *(22)*, and can also synthesize estrogen from androgens *(26–28)*. Aromatase activity has been detected in rabbit blastocysts *(29,30)*, and there is a significant increase in aromatase activity and estrogen synthesis by rabbit blastocysts during the period of implantation (d 6–8). Blastocyst production of estrogen in the rabbit appears to be necessary for implantation, since treatment of blastocysts with

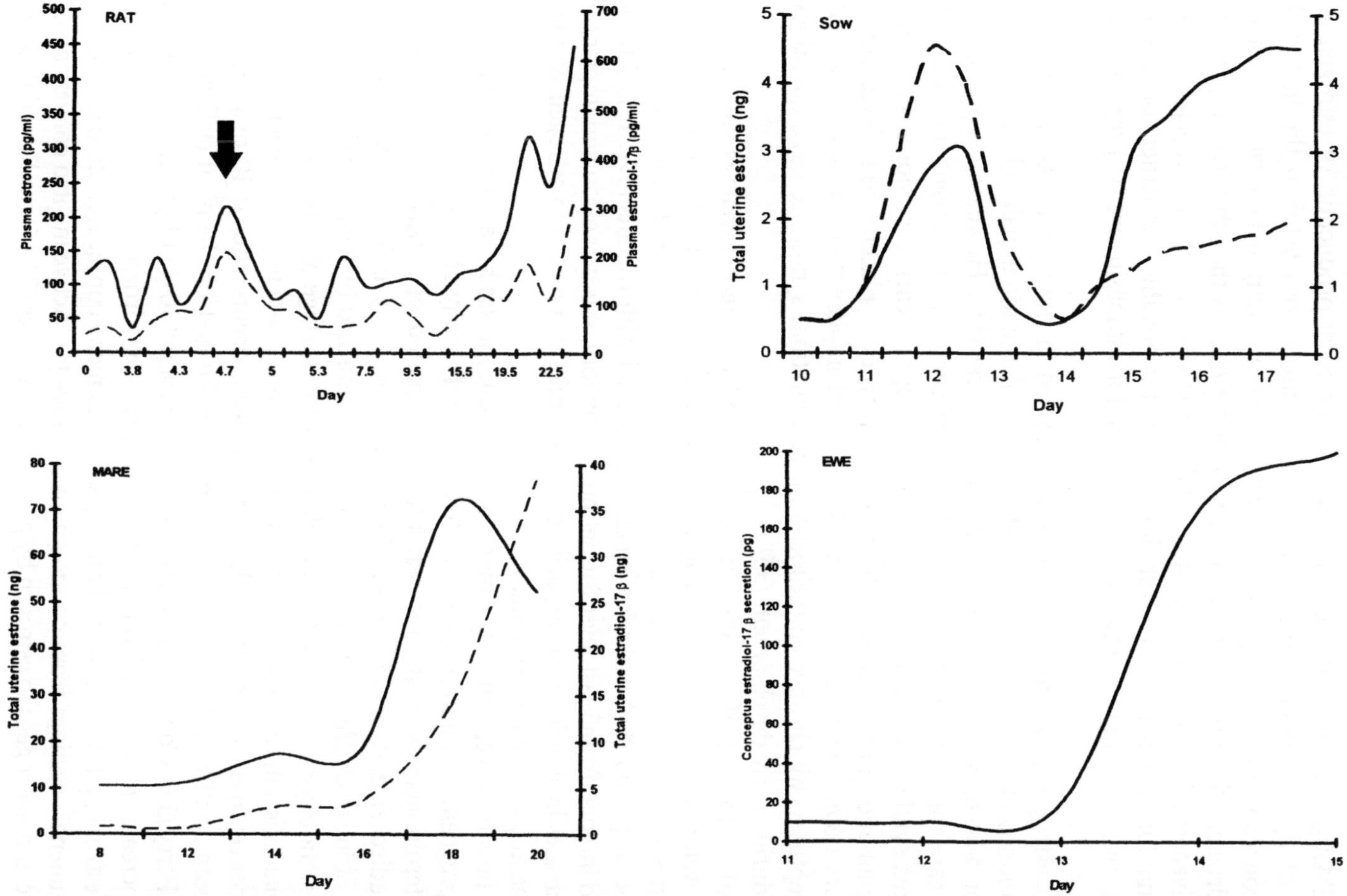

Fig. 1. Species comparison of estrogen involvement during early pregnancy. Ovarian estrogen production affects implantation in the rat as depicited by the nidatory increase in plasma estrone and estradiol-17b on d 4–5 (arrow). Conceptus secretion of estrogen occurs in the sow, mare, and ewe during critical stages of placental development and establishment of pregnancy. (Adapted from *41,43,72,86,214*)

an estrogen antagonist *(31)* hinders their ability to implant. However, administration of an aromatase inhibitor did not significantly affect conceptus development or implantation *(30)*. There is also evidence that the rabbit blastocysts can influence endometrial synthesis of estrogen from labeled progesterone and androstenedione in vitro *(32)*, which demonstrates the presence of cytochromes P450 17α-hydroxylase/C17,20-lyase ($P450_{17\alpha}$) and aromatase ($P450_{arom}$) in the endometrium. Low endometrial production of estrogen in the absence of the blastocyst also indicates possible interactions between the maternal uterus and conceptus in steroidogenesis. The rabbit endometrium metabolizes progesterone and androstenedione to a number of intermediates *(32)*. Although there is question of the effectiveness of estrogen or aromatase inhibitors in vivo, placental estrogen is essential for normal luteal function in the rabbit *(33)*, and it is possible that either conceptus, endometrial, and/or ovarian estrogens are necessary for establishment of pregnancy in this species.

Blastocyst estrogen production has been documented in the hamster *(28)*; however, estrogen is not necessary for implantation *(34)* nor is implantation impaired by the aromatase inhibitor 4-acetoxy-4-androstene-3,17-dione in the rat *(35)*. However, as previously mentioned, care must be taken regarding the effectiveness of the various inhibitors to block estrogen synthesis or action in utero. Thus, estrogen seems to be not essential for invasive implantation in all species with hemochorial types of placentation. Once more, estrogen is not necessarily restricted to invasive types of implantation, since porcine and equine conceptuses, which have epitheliochorial placentation, synthesize large quantities of estrogen during early development *(36)*.

In comparison to the peri-implantation period of rodents, steroidogenesis during early blastocyst development is basically similar among domestic farm species. However, conceptuses of these species remain unattached to the uterine surface epithelium for a much more protracted period (1–2 wk) of pregnancy compared with rodents *(37)*. It is during this extended interval from blastocyst formation to trophoblastic expansion and implantation that increases in steroidogenic capacity occur, especially in regard to estrogen synthesis by porcine and equine conceptuses.

With the possible exception of the mare, porcine conceptuses have a greater ability to metabolize pregnenolone and progesterone to estrogen than any other species reported at this time. Steroidogenesis during the peri-attachment period of conceptus development has been studied extensively in the pig. Estrogen synthesis by d 3–6 pig embryos was reported by Stone et al. *(38)*. However, this was not confirmed by a later study *(18)*. This period of gestation corresponds to the morula or blastocyst stage of embryo development prior to implantation in rodents. However, an enormous increase in steroidogenic capacity of porcine conceptuses, especially synthesis of estrogen, occurs after d 10 of gestation, which has been confirmed by numerous studies since the first biochemical evidence was reported by Perry *(39)*. Collection of uterine washings during d 10–18 of pregnancy revealed a marked increase in concentrations of pregnenolone, dehydroepiandrosterone, androstenedione, estrone, estradiol-17β, and estriol, as well as many conjugated steroids in comparison to lumenal washings from nonpregnant pigs *(40–43)*. Active in vitro conversion of progesterone and androgens to estrogen by porcine conceptuses *(27,44)* confirmed that the conceptus is the source of estrogen within the uterine lumen (Fig. 1). Likewise, no estrogen synthesis by endometrium was detected in those studies.

Synthesis of estrogen is stage-specific and is not detectable until the porcine conceptus has developed to approximately a 5-mm spherical diameter on d 11 of gestation with a

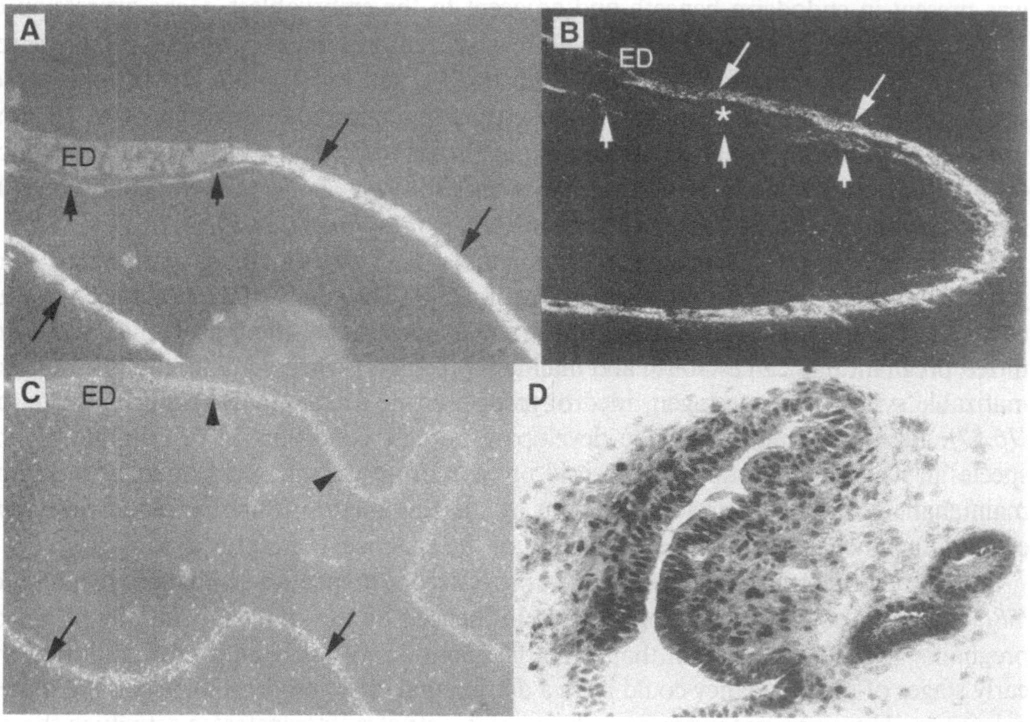

Fig. 2. Localization of cytochrome P450 17α-hydroxylase/17,20 lyase ($P450_{17\alpha}$) in the trophoblastic tissue of the porcine blastocyst by immunocytochemistry (**A** and **B**) and *in situ* hybridization (**C**), and immunocytochemical localization of nuclear estrogen receptor in the glandular and surface epithelium of the pig endometrium (**D**) on d 11 of pregnancy. Long arrows highlight $P450_{17\alpha}$ expression in the trophectoderm; short arrows indicate endoderm. Note the decrease in enzyme level adjacent to the embryonic disk (ED) of an elongated conceptus in plate B over the region of outgrowth of mesoderm (*), which corresponds to the relative lack of expression of $P450_{17\alpha}$ transcript (arrowheads) as shown by in situ hybridization in plate C.

notable surge in conceptus estrogen release occurring during the rapid transition from 10-mm ovoid to tubular and finally filamentous (150 mm in length) morphology on d 12 of gestation *(44–46)*. The detection of estrogen production at the 5-mm spherical stage corresponds to initiation of extra-embryonic mesodermal development between the trophectoderm and endoderm of the trophoblast *(45,47)*. Conceptus estrogen release rapidly declines on d 13 following trophoblast elongation until a second sustained increase is initiated on d 16 of gestation, where there is outgrowth of the allantoic sac from the hindgut *(41,42,46)*. The two periods of conceptus estrogen synthesis (Fig. 1) are essential for the maintenance of pregnancy in the pig *(48)*. Change in steroidogenesis by the porcine conceptus is correlated with the cellular content of $P450_{17\alpha}$ and $P450_{arom}$ *(49–52)*. Enzyme and gene localization is cell-specific, as $P450_{17\alpha}$ is restricted to trophoblast (Fig. 2A,B). As blastocyst development proceeds, particularly with formation of the mesoderm, $P450_{17\alpha}$ expression decreases in the trophoblast adjacent to the embryonic disk overlying the mesodermal cell layer (Fig. 2B). Expression of $P450_{17\alpha}$ protein (Fig. 2B) and mRNA (Fig. 2C) is maintained in the trophoblast furthest from the disk region. $P450_{arom}$ is present in both trophoblast and hypoblast with no staining for either enzyme detected in embryoblast or mesoderm. However, Conley et al. *(51)* indicated that the greatest expression of $P450_{arom}$

was present in endoderm beneath and adjacent to the embryoblast. Gene expression of $P450_{17\alpha}$ and $P450_{arom}$ as analyzed through reverse transcription-polymerase chain reaction (RT-PCR) parallels enzyme detection. Both $P450_{17\alpha}$ and $P450_{arom}$ are low in conceptuses smaller than 5–6 mm in diameter, but increase on conceptus development to 10 mm, followed by a greatly enhanced expression at the time of rapid trophoblastic elongation *(53,54)*. The marked decline in estrogen synthesis following conceptus elongation on d 12 is also consistent with decreased enzyme mRNA expression *(51,54,55)*.

Porcine conceptuses express genes for a number of enzymes involved with the steroidogenic pathway necessary for estrogen production *(56)*. The ability of the porcine conceptus to synthesize estrogen from various substrates is most likely the reason that ovariectomized pregnant pigs can establish and maintain pregnancy when administered the nonaromatizable synthetic progestagen, medroxyprogesterone acetate (MPA), during gestation *(16,57)*. Estrogen synthesis by the developing porcine conceptus is an example of one species in which, unquestionably, steroid production serves many major roles, including maintenance of the CL, protein secretion by the endometrium, uterine blood flow, placental attachment, and possibly elongation of the spherical conceptus itself *(48)*.

Porcine endometrial tissue does convert progesterone to inactive 5α-reduced metabolites *(58)*, but can also produce estrogen when influenced by the conceptus in later stages of pregnancy *(44)*. It would seem that the large quantities of estrogen produced during the early stages of pig pregnancy could have a detrimental effect on pregnancy and the maternal system. However, progesterone induces endometrial sulfotransferase activity in the pig *(59,60)* as well as other species with extended estrous cycles in comparison to the short estrous cycles of rodents *(61)*. High concentrations of sulfoconjugated estrone, estradiol, and estriol are detected in the uterine lumen *(41,43)* and plasma *(62)* of pigs during pregnancy. Induction of endometrial sulfotransferase activity during the period of conceptus estrogen synthesis allows the maternal system to regulate the activity of the steroid both within and outside the uterine environment and in target tissues that express sulfatase activity, such as the CL, hypothalamus, and mammary gland *(63)*.

The mare is another domestic species in which the conceptus has tremendous ability to synthesize estrogen during the preimplantation period. However, unlike the pig in which conceptus estrogen synthesis is essential for maintenance of the CL *(36)*, estrogen synthesis is not known to be involved directly with preventing luteolysis in the mare *(64)*. Estrogen maybe important for conceptus mobility within the uterine horns during the second week of pregnancy and subsequent fixation within the uterine horn, all of which are essential for the establishment of pregnancy *(65–67)*. Rapid trophoblast elongation in pigs permits contact with the vast surface area of the uterine horns. However, the mare conceptus remains spherical and migrates back and forth between the uterine horns until about d 18 of gestation to influence overall endometrial function until fixation within the uterus *(68)*. The mare's placental architecture is unique in that the spherical vesicle is covered by a thin acellular capsule during the period of uterine migration (d 10–16) and the yolk sac predominates from d 11 until being completely replaced by the allantoic sac on d 40 of gestation *(68)*.

Hydroxysteroid dehydrogenase enzyme activity has been detected in trophoblast tissue as early as d 8–13 in the mare *(69,70)*. However, there is a dramatic increase in estrone and estradiol-17β within the yolk sac fluid and uterine lumenal washings (Fig. 1) between d 12 and 14 of pregnancy *(71,72)*. Steroidogenic activity of the early equine conceptus has been established during this period of development, since progesterone and estrogen are synthesized by the developing conceptus *(71,73–76)*. Endometrial hydroxysteroid dehydrogenase is present within the uterine epithelium underlying the trophoblast during later (d 20) stages of gestation *(69)*, which may be involved with the increased conversion of estrone to estradiol detected in the uterine lumen following d 18 of pregnancy *(72)*. Interestingly, despite the large quantities of estrogen produced and released into the uterine lumen, an increase in either unconjugated or conjugated estrogen is not detected in maternal plasma until after d 30 of gestation *(77)*. Endometrial sulfotransferase and glucuronidase increase between d 18 and 36 of gestation in the mare *(75)*; however, an alteration in plasma concentrations of conjugated estrogen is not detected. It is possible that the yolk sac, along with the endometrium, can sequester the steroids, such as estrone sulfate, which is greatly elevated in the yolk sac. Thus, conjugation of estrogen appears to inhibit its ability to be transported across the yolk sac membrane *(75)*. Yolk sac control of estrogen release into the maternal compartments is consistent with the increase in plasma concentrations of conjugated and unconjugated estrogens during regression of the yolk sac and conversion from the choriovitelline placenta to chorioallantoic placenta in the mare. Early conceptus estrogen production in the mare does not regulate CL maintenance, but likely provides a means to establish local control over the uterine environment necessary for conceptus development and attachment.

Ovine and bovine conceptuses undergo trophoblast elongation into the ipsilateral and then the contralateral uterine horn several days prior to establishing an epitheliochorial placentation *(78,79)*, although over a much more protracted period of time compared to the pig. Although ovine and bovine conceptuses spend a similar period of time unattached within the uterine horn, they are devoid of significant aromatase activity in strong contrast to porcine and equine conceptuses. Estrogen synthesis by either the preattachment ovine or bovine conceptus is negligible *(27,80–82)*. Bovine conceptuses metabolize progesterone and androstenedione extensively to 5β-reduced steroids, and only androstenedione is converted to small quantities of estrone and estradiol-17β *(27,82)*. Very nominal concentrations of estrogen are present within the uterine washings collected during trophoblast expansion in either species *(83–86)*. Estrogen is luteolytic during the early weeks of pregnancy in both the ewe and cow *(87, see* Chapter 1). Therefore, adaptation of ruminant conceptuses to restrict aromatization at this sensitive time period would decrease possible endometrial prostaglandin release. Interestingly, the conceptus and the endometrium of the pregnant cow metabolize progesterone through a different pathway. The conceptus metabolizes progesterone to 5β-reduced and hydroxylated steroids, whereas endometrium produces 5α-reduced and hydroxylated steroids *(82)*. Eley et al. *(82)* suggest that conceptus 5β-reduced metabolites may inhibit uterine motility, stimulate erythropoeitic activity, and increase cellular transcription. These researchers also indicate that conceptus metabolism of progesterone to 5β-reduced steroids provides a mechanism to regulate estrogen production, and in addition to local progesterone metabolism by endometrium to 5α-reduced steroids with little steroid activity, allows the minute quantities of conceptus estrogens to stimulate endometrial function without inducing luteolysis. Nephew et al. *(86)* proposed that ovine conceptus estrogen synthesis during trophoblast elongation on d 14 (Fig. 1) stimulates intrauterine migration and placental attachment. The roles of 5α- and 5β-reduced steroids during gestation of ruminants have not been established. Following conceptus expansion throughout the uterine horns in both the cow and ewe, placental estrogen pro-

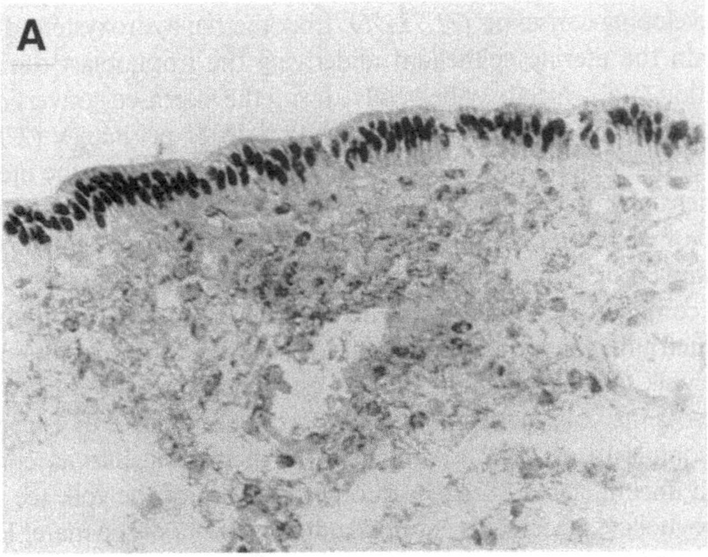

duction increases with development of the chorioallantois. Maternal peripheral plasma concentrations of conjugated and unconjugated estrogens are greatly elevated by 30 d of gestation *(88,89)*.

An alternative pathway of estrogen metabolism that has biological significance is production of catechol estrogens. The rapidly expanding porcine conceptus has a marked capacity to synthesize 2- and 4-hydroxyestradiol from d 10–14 of gestation, followed by a decline and a second increase on d 16 *(90)*. Chakraborty et al. *(90)* suggest that metabolism of estradiol into catechol estrogen's protects both the conceptus and uterus from oxidative damage. Catechol estrogens can also have a regulatory effect on uterine hyperemia and blood flow *(7)*, which are highly evident during trophoblast elongation and attachment in the pig, ewe, and cow *(83,91)*. Dey and Johnson *(20)* have also suggested roles for catechol estrogens in implantation of rodents.

Placental and Endometrial Steroid Receptors

Placental and endometrial steroid synthesis and metabolism regulate the multitude of biological functions essential for female fertility and survival of the developing conceptus through their respective nuclear receptors within the target tissues *(92,93)*. Progesterone and estrogen may have an autocrine effect on the placenta itself. Although estrogen receptor (ER) mRNA has been detected in mouse blastocysts through reverse transcriptase-PCR, clear evidence for placental ER or progesterone receptor (PR) is lacking during early conceptus development. Neither ER nor PR was detected in the trophoblast or placental tissue of either sheep, pig, or cat conceptuses by immunocytochemistry with specific antibodies *(94,* Geisert and Bazer, unpublished results) or in primates *(95)*. Reverse transcriptase-PCR has also failed to detect ER or PR mRNA in early porcine conceptuses *(96)*. Strong evidence that placental ER is not necessary for pregnancy in mice has been demonstrated through mutation of the ER gene *(97)*. Disruption of the ER gene does not affect development of homozygous mutant ER embryos; however, the adult females are infertile.

Although an essential need for the presence of placental PR and ER during pregnancy is questioned, endometrial PR and ER are unquestionably vital for regulation of fertility

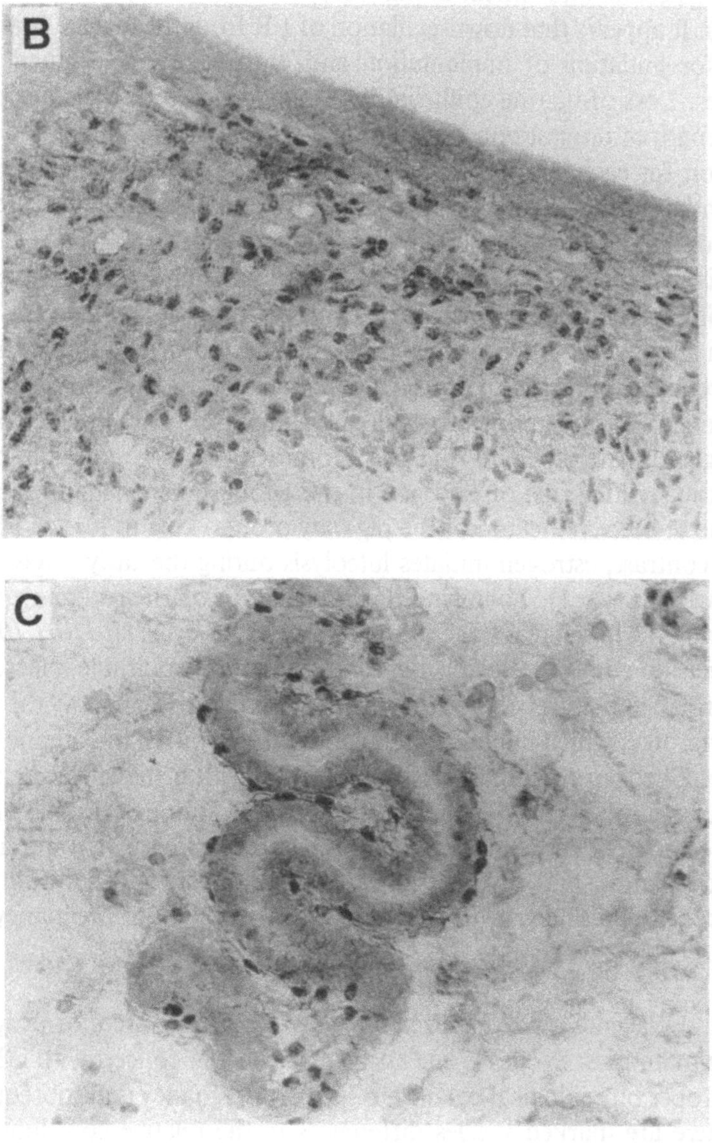

Fig. 3. Immunocytochemical localization of nuclear progesterone receptor in endometrial stroma, surface epithelium, and glandular epithelium on d 5 (**A**) and 12 (**B,C**) of the porcine estrous cycle. Note the loss of nuclear progesterone receptor from the surface (B) and glandular (C) epithelium on d 12. However, stromal staining remains detectable beneath the basement membrane of the epithelium.

and fetal survival in all mammalian species. Cell-specific changes in steroid receptors within stroma, endothelium, myometrium, surface epithelium, and glandular epithelium control conceptus development, implantation, placental attachment, and blood flow throughout gestation. Although there are similar alternations in uterine epithelial and stromal PR expression during pregnancy in the various species, there are temporal differences in timing for downregulation within the epithelium. Decline or loss of PR from the surface and glandular epithelium (Fig. 3) occurs in all species studied thus far and appears to be correlated with the time of implantation in the mouse *(98)*, rabbit *(99)*, and cat *(94)*, and placental attachment in pig *(100)*, ewe *(101–103)*, and cow (Geisert, unpublished results). It appears that downregulation of PR from the uterine epithelium may be a prerequisite for initiation of implantation and/or placental attachment in some mammalian species. Loss of uterine epithelial PR is independent of the conceptus, but dependent on the length of progesterone stimulation, which regulates the period of implantation or placentation for each species. Regulation of progesterone dominance over the uterus, which is essential for maintenance of pregnancy to term, is maintained through the continuation of stromal and myometrial PR expression.

Species display differential expression of endometrial ER during early pregnancy. Regulation of expression of epithelial ER plays an important role in the maintenance of pregnancy in species that have a more prolonged period of gestation (*see* Chapter 1). In the pig, conceptus production of estrogen maintains CL function and permits attachment of the trophoblast to the uterine lumenal epithelium *(36)*. The presence of ER within the surface and glandular epithelium (Fig. 2D) from d 10–18 of gestation in pigs *(104)* is consistent with the positive role of estrogen in the establishment of pregnancy. Increases in ER within the uterine epithelium of the pig may occur owing to loss of PR in this specific cell type. In contrast, estrogen initiates luteolysis during the early stages of pregnancy in ruminants (*see* Chapter 1). Following downregulation of PR, uterine epithelial ER also increases during the late-luteal stage of the ewe's estrous cycle *(101,103,105)* to permit follicular estrogens to stimulate the mechanism necessary for pulsatile release of endometrial prostaglandin $F_{2\alpha}$ and regression of the CL. During early pregnancy, the ovine conceptus secretes interferon τ, which inhibits upregulation of ER within the uterine epithelium *(101, 103,105,106)*. Estrogen receptor is also diminished within the surface epithelium during trophoblastic invasion in cats *(94)* and primates *(107)*. Although distinct differences in epithelial ER are apparent between species, ER is detectable in deep stroma surrounding uterine glands, capillaries, and myometrium of most species, which would allow placental estrogen to control uterine growth and blood flow throughout pregnancy.

Midgestation to Term

The CL and placenta are recognized as the two major sources of progesterone during pregnancy in mammals. Progesterone and estrogen act in concert with other hormones to maintain a proper physiological balance to support pregnancy and subsequent parturition. However, there are marked species differences in the relative contributions of CL and placenta to progesterone secretion at various stages of gestation. The CL is the sole source of progesterone throughout gestation in several species, but in other species, luteal function declines as pregnancy advances, and the placenta becomes the primary source of progesterone. The transition from luteal to placental progesterone production seems to depend on the establishment of the definitive, chorioallantoic placenta, and its subsequent rate of growth, which also varies among species. Placental mass is a major determinant of steroid secretory or metabolic capacity, although this association is strongest during periods of placental growth, which occurs earlier in gestation in some species. These few considerations provide a basis for understanding some of the divergent patterns in progesterone concentrations in the maternal circulation throughout gestation in mammals.

Historically, ovariectomy has been used to determine the need for luteal progesterone in the maintenance of pregnancy. The earliest time at which pregnancy survives in the absence of the CL is interpreted to indicate timing of the onset and adequacy of placental progesterone synthesis. Based on this approach, the ewe and the mare can maintain pregnancy without luteal progesterone during the latter half of gestation, but pig, goat, and dog were luteal-dependent throughout gestation. Several investigators used a systematic approach to establish the time of transition from luteal to placental progesterone synthesis. For instance, Casida and Warwick *(108)* ovariectomized (1 lutectomized) 11 ewes on various days from 30 to 125 postmating, and observed them for signs of abortion or normal lambing. Five ewes maintained term pregnancies, including two that were ovariectomized as early as d 55 and 64 of gestation, but the others aborted. The authors concluded that "the results establish the fact that in at least some cases the ewe can maintain pregnancy without the presence of corpora lutea after the 55th d of gestation." These results were confirmed later by Denamur and Martinet *(109)*. Similar studies established independence of pregnancy from luteal support as early as 70 d in pony mares *(110)* and by d 30 in guinea pigs *(111)*.

Opinions on the necessity for luteal support of pregnancy in cows are more divided. Hammond *(112)* first stated that the ovaries were essential for successful pregnancy in cattle, a view that has been widely held ever since. However, it was challenged by Raeside and Turner *(113)*, who noted that one heifer ovariectomized at 205 d of gestation delivered a live calf without any exogenous progesterone supplementation. McDonald et al. *(114)* used a similar approach and removed ovaries from cows at 60 d of gestation. Pregnancy was maintained with exogenous progesterone until discontinued at various stages of gestation. Progesterone withdrawal from two cows at 102 and 137 d of gestation caused abortion, but eight other heifers deprived of progesterone from as early as d 162 calved successfully with a mean gestation length of 267 $\pm$ 3 d. Other results were similar, but most indicated that parturition occurred in cows 1–2 wk prematurely in the absence of CL. Collectively, the success rate of pregnancy was better in ovariectiomized cattle than in ewes, yet cattle are still considered by many to be a CL-dependent species.

Observations of these investigators, particularly those studying the cow, do more than establish the necessity of luteal progesterone for the maintenance of pregnancy. They emphasize the importance of how progesterone is withdrawn, not just when, in relation to the survival of pregnancy. Specifically, rapid withdrawal of progesterone, e.g., ovariectomy, increases the likelihood of abortion, perhaps because stress increases the minimal requirements for progesterone for pregnancy maintenance. Glucocorticoid secretion by an active adrenal gland in response to surgical manipulation may directly inhibit placental progesterone synthesis and cannot be discounted as having a significant influence in this regard. However, if progesterone is withdrawn more slowly and with less stress, physiological needs may have a greater chance of being provided by the placenta and at earlier stages of pregnancy. This suggests that compensatory mechanisms exist that can respond to changes in steroid concentrations if given sufficient time.

The question of whether the placenta is the extragonadal source of progesterone in the absence of an active CL has been addressed in several ways. Some measured tissue concentrations of steroid, which were frequently low in the placenta *(115,116)*. More recently, arteriovenous differences in progesterone concentrations across various organs have been used to determine the relative contributions of the placenta and ovaries. Studying ewes with autotransplanted ovaries and adrenal glands, Harrison and Heap *(117)* estimated that placental progesterone synthesis exceeded the ovarian contribution by d 66 of pregnancy. Ricketts and Flint *(118)* confirmed these observations, and demonstrated that progesterone secretion by the gravid ovine uterus increased between d 60 and 70, and again between d 100 and term. Increases in progesterone secretion by cultured placental explants also occurred as gestation progressed. These studies were conducted with ovariectomized ewes in which pregnancy was maintained with a synthetic progestagen and, therefore, uncomplicated by luteal progesterone production. Together with other reports *(119)*, they firmly established the role of the placenta as an important steroid-secreting organ in the ewe.

Placental contributions to progesterone secretion during pregnancy have been studied in several species after removal of the CL. Illingworth and Deanesly *(120)* were among the first to use synthetic, nonmetabolizable progestagens to maintain pregnancy in animals after ovariectomy. Studies conducted in guinea pigs indicated that progesterone concentrations in systemic plasma were detectable from d 16–18 and increased thereafter, indicating the importance of nonluteal progesterone production in the maintenance of pregnancy. Sheldrick et al. *(121)* demonstrated a positive arteriovenous difference across the gravid uterus of goats that were ovariectomized and pregnancy maintained with synthetic progestagens. Craig *(122)* reported similar findings in the pig, which are consistent with reports of progesterone secretion by explants of porcine placenta collected at several stages of gestation *(123)*. Therefore, in at least two species known to require luteal progesterone throughout pregnancy, there is convincing evidence of placental progesterone secretion, but only after removal of the ovarian source.

Initial studies in the cow failed to demonstrate a positive venous minus arterial difference across the gravid bovine uterus or fetal placenta, leaving doubts regarding placental contributions to systemic levels of progesterone *(124,125)*. In fact, the consistency and magnitude of uptake of progesterone provided convincing evidence for significant uterine metabolism of steroids during pregnancy in the cow. Conley and Ford *(126)* attempted to minimize the influence of luteal progesterone production and endometrial progesterone metabolism in cows by measuring arteriovenous concentration differences in progesterone across single placentomes. Cows were treated with $PGF_{2\alpha}$ to eliminate luteal progesterone production at d 200 of gestation, which decreased systemic progesterone concentrations dramatically. However, caruncular venous progesterone concentrations were relatively unaffected, resulting in significant and positive venous–arterial concentration differences across the placentomes. Moreover, placental explants and in vitro perfused placentomes from $PGF_{2\alpha}$-treated cows synthesized more progesterone than those from control cows *(126)*. Tsumagari et al. *(127)* suggested that placental 3β-HSD activity was elevated during the last 3 mo of pregnancy, and others have demonstrated in vitro production of progesterone by bovine placental cells *(128–131)*. These results also suggest that pregnancy in cattle can be maintained by placental progesterone if luteolysis occurs after d 200 of gestation. Furthermore, these results suggest that placental progesterone production may increase in response to luteal demise. Results obtained from other species support this view. For instance, Bedwani and Marley *(132)* observed greater placental progesterone synthesis in ovariectomized than intact guinea pigs. Therefore, the placenta has an inherent ability for progesterone synthesis and secretion, which may increase after luteolysis, suggesting that communication exists between the ovary and the uterus to regulate progesterone production during pregnancy.

It is generally agreed that the rabbit, dog, cat, rat, and mouse require functional luteal tissue for pregnancy maintenance, but the placenta may contribute to progesterone production to a significant degree. Harterius *(133)* removed all but one fetus from pregnant, ovariectomized rats leaving all placental tissue in situ. He observed that pregnancy was maintained to term, suggesting that several placentae could maintain the viability of a single rat fetus. The steroid secretory capacity of the feline placenta remains controversial

(134); however, Courrier and Gros *(135)* noted a progestational effect of the placenta in ovariectomized cats. Other studies assert that placental tissues synthesize progesterone in vitro in many species *(136)*. Therefore, progesterone secretion by the placenta may represent a general characteristic, in which case, the constant need for luteal progesterone secretion may reflect the rate of progesterone metabolism in certain species.

The importance of progesterone metabolism during pregnancy is exemplified in the pregnant mare. Although the ovaries become dispensable quite early in equine pregnancy, doubt remains about whether or not placental progesterone synthesis accounts for the progestational state of the uterus. Short *(137)* reported that progesterone disappeared from the circulation of the mare as pregnancy progressed. The presence of progesterone in fetal cord blood at parturition and in placental tissues suggested that although progesterone was synthesized by the placenta, it was precluded from being secreted into the maternal compartment. Several later reports indicated a steady and substantial increase in concentrations of several progestagens in mares in the latter half of pregnancy *(138–141)*. These studies relied on radioimmunoassay for progesterone determination, and some doubt was expressed concerning the actual levels of progesterone owing to the possible presence of crossreacting metabolites. More recent studies have separated, identified, and quantified these progestagens using gas chromatography and mass spectrometry *(142)*. The results confirmed that maternal progesterone concentrations peak at d 150 and decline thereafter, presumably as a result of a reduction in luteal synthesis. Increases were observed in several progestagens, including 20α-hydroxy-5-pregnen-3-one, and 5α-pregnane-3β, 20β-diol, and 5α-dihydroprogesterone, coincident with the formation of the chorioallontoic placenta after d 50 of gestation. Presumably, these progestagens result from metabolism of fetal pregnenolone and placental progesterone by the endometrium or placenta itself *(142–144)*. The negative arterial–venous differences in pregnenolone concentrations in fetal cord blood are consistent with placental synthesis of progesterone, which can be reduced acutely by inhibitors of 3β-hydroxysteroid dehydrogenase *(145)*. The source of the high levels of circulating pregnenolone also encountered in the fetal lamb *(146)* is unknown. It is also possible that some or all of these progestagens have significant biological activity, but this remains to be determined. In any event, changes in sensitivity of the mare to uterotonic agents occurs around 320 d of gestation *(147)*. Importantly, progestagen levels decline around this time in anticipation of parturition *(142,144,148)*. Available results emphasize that steroid metabolism is an important determinant of the levels of hormone in fetal and maternal circulations, and ultimately, the endocrine response.

The extent and impact of progesterone metabolism has not been carefully studied in many species, with the notable exception of women *(149)*. The metabolic clearance rate of progesterone decreases markedly around d 20 of gestation in the guinea pig, coinciding with the initial rise in systemic progesterone concentrations *(150)* and placental progesterone synthesis *(120)*. Undoubtedly, the decrease in the metabolic clearance rate of progesterone is an important factor determining the adequacy of placental production for the maintenance of pregnancy after ovariectomy in this species. In contrast to pregnancy in the guinea pig, no substantial change occurs in the metabolic clearance rate of progesterone in ewes during gestation *(151)*. Studies by Sheldrick et al. *(152)* demonstrated that 5β-pregnane-3α, 20α-diol was a major product of the gravid uterus of the goat. In light of progesterone synthesis by the placenta *(121,153)*, the inability of the goat to maintain pregnancy after removal of the luteal source could be attributed, at least in part, to an increased rate of progesterone metabolism in does compared with ewes *(121)*. Thus, the rate of steroid metabolism also contributes to the adequacy of placental progesterone production for maintenance of pregnancy.

The preceding discussion emphasizes the importance of the contributions of the mammalian placenta to maintenance of pregnancy, which relies on a balance between progesterone synthesis and metabolism that exhibits marked differences among species. Unfortunately, the classical ablation approach cannot be used to study directly the significance of the placental contributions of steroids to pregnancy. Furthermore, the "luteal–placental shift" in progesterone production, often referred to in animals, was defined experimentally, and it is influenced by the method of luteal removal. Rarely, but for experimentation, is the burden of progesterone production borne by the placenta alone; therefore, the timing of the "luteal–placental shift" may reflect experimental design and may or may not address the endocrinology of pregnancy maintenance. In any case, the existence of placental and luteal sources of progesterone is entirely consistent with the idea that redundancy of function provides a safeguard against physiological/endocrinological failure and abortion.

Estrogen synthesis during fetal development is a relatively consistent feature of steroidogenesis in pregnancy, so much so that it has been suggested in the past that failure of estrogen synthesis might be lethal to the conceptus *(154)*. However, congenital deficiencies in the enzyme responsible for estrogen production in two human infants have been identified recently. The success of these pregnancies in the relative absence of conceptus-derived estrogen demonstrates that this is certainly not an absolute requirement in humans and, therefore, not in all mammalian species *(155)*. In contrast to progesterone synthesis, which appears to depend primarily on the CL or placenta, many different strategies seem to have evolved to accommodate estrogen production during pregnancy.

The mare provides a classic example of the complexity of estrogen synthesis during pregnancy. In fact, the identification of estrogen in the urine of pregnant women was soon followed by a similar observation in pregnant mares *(156)*. Hart and Cole *(157)* proposed that the equine placenta was the likely site of synthesis of estrogens. Meanwhile, Girard et al. *(158)* were the first to recognize that urine from pregnant mares contained novel steroids, the ring B unsaturated estrogens, the biochemical origin of which is still a mystery *(159)*. Later studies demonstrated that estrogen levels increase after 45 d with more marked increases occurring around d 90 of gestation in mares *(160)*. Fractionation of these steroids led to the suggestion that estrone sulfate was the predominant estrogen until peak levels were reached around d 200, and that equilin was present thereafter in equal or higher concentrations *(161,162)*. Total estrogens decrease from d 200 to term. Estradiol exhibits a similar pattern of change while remaining at levels approx 10-fold less than estrone for most of gestation *(160,162)*. These studies established that as with the progestagens, several unusual estrogens were synthesized and secreted during pregnancy in the mare.

The studies of Cole et el. *(163)* provided the first evidence of fetal gonadal involvement in estrogen synthesis during equine pregnancy, demonstrating that the levels of urinary estrogen were correlated with the growth of the fetal gonads. Several decades later, gonadectomy of fetal foals was shown to result in a rapid decline in circulating estrogen in mares, first suggested by Raeside et al. *(164)* and firmly established by Pashen and Allen *(165)*. The existence of an arteriovenous differences in fetal and maternal estrogen levels indicated a net output, which was consistent with placental synthesis of estrogen *(140)*. It is now generally accepted that equine fetal gonads secrete C-19 steroids, which are taken up and aromatized efficiently in the placenta of the pregnant mare *(166)*. The synthesis and secretion of steroids from one location, and their conversion to more or less active metabolites at another, sometimes peripheral site, is an important recurring feature of steroidogenesis *(167)*. The observations described above were particularly significant, because they established the concept that estrogen synthesis in the pregnant mare resulted from functional "cooperation" between the fetus and the placenta *(166,168)*, and stands as one of the best examples of this principle in animals. However, despite the considerable pharmacological importance of equine estrogens in relation to estrogen-replacement therapies in women, the physiological significance of the synthesis of these steroids in equine pregnancy remains unclear.

The need for estrogen synthesis during pregnancy in the rat is more obvious *(169)*. Estrogen is required for the maintenance of progesterone synthesis by CL during the last half of gestation in rats. The placenta plays a central role in the synthesis of estrogen during pregnancy in the rat, as in the mare, but with a slightly different twist. Specifically, rat trophoblastic giant cells of both the chorioallantois and the choriovitelline membranes *(170)* synthesize significant quantities of androgen from as early as d 12 of pregnancy *(171,172)*, but lack the ability to metabolize it to estrogen. Therefore, androgens secreted by the placenta into the maternal circulation are subsequently taken up and converted to estrogen by the ovaries *(173)*, principally in the CL *(169)*. This functional communication between the conceptus and the maternal ovary during pregnancy in the rat appears to regulate itself, such that estrogen exerts a negative effect on placental androgen synthesis. Moreover, as a feedback loop involving luteal and placental steroid production, it is reminiscent of the communication between bovine ovaries and placenta described for progesterone synthesis. The mechanistic basis of this phenomenon needs to be defined.

Estrogen synthesis is also observed during gestation in the pig, sheep, and cow, and these three species exhibit a similar temporal pattern of synthesis as determined by concentrations in fetal and, in most cases, maternal fluids. Estrogen synthesis in pregnancy occurs biphasically in all three of these species *(174)*. In particular, estrone sulfate concentrations increase in fetal fluids from as early as d 20 in the pig *(174)*, d 40 in the cow *(88,89,175)*, and d 35 in the ewe *(176)*. The first increase in estrogen secretion is only reflected in the maternal plasma of the sow, and is not apparent in the cow or ewe. However, it declines transiently in fetal fluids of all three species, preceding a secondary rise in estrogen, which is evident in maternal plasma around d 45, 70, and 50 in sows, cows, and ewes, respectively *(89,174,176)*. Consistent with these findings, porcine placenta secretes estrogen in vitro *(123)*, and aromatase activity and estrogen concentrations in bovine cotyledonary tissues also demonstrate a biphasic pattern during pregnancy *(177)*. The second sustained increase in maternal estrone sulfate in cows is accompanied by a similar increase in plasma androstenedione and testosterone concentrations, which continue to rise progressively from d 90 of gestation to term *(178)*. Robertson et al. *(174)* suggested that differences in rates of conjugation and deconjugation of estrogens by uterine or placental tissues favor the appearance of the early maternal rise in estrogen concentrations seen in the pig between d 25 and 30 of gestation. Knight *(123)* reported estrone release by porcine placental explants recovered at various days of gestation, the results of which were totally consistent with the data of Robertson et al. *(174)*. Similar in vitro studies on placental estrogen secretion have yet to be conducted using tissues collected throughout gestation in ruminant species. Moreover, the cellular site of steroidogenesis is in dispute. Dispersed cell cultures suggest that steroidogenesis in the ruminant placenta involves primarily binucleate cells *(179)*. However, immunolocalization of cytochrome P450 side-chain cleavage $P450_{scc}$ *(180)* and

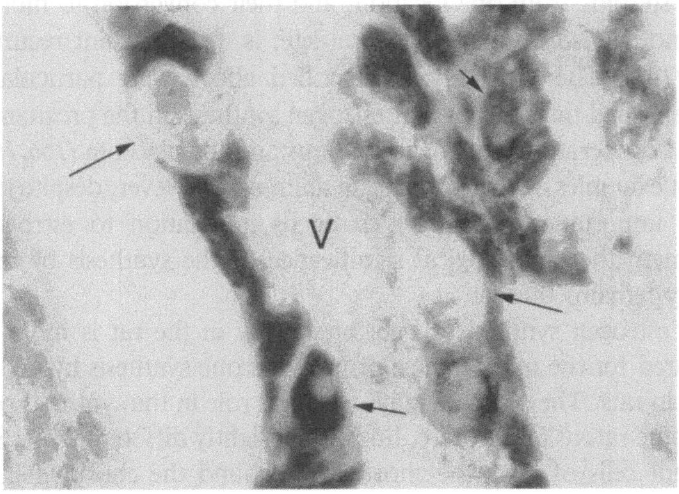

Fig. 4. Immunocytochemical localization of cytochrome P450 17α-hydroxylase/17,20 lyase ($P450_{17\alpha}$) in bovine trophoblast. Note fetal binucleate cells (long arrows) lack expression of $P450_{17\alpha}$ that is clearly present in uninucleate cells (short arrows) of a fetal villous (V).

$P450_{17\alpha}$ (Fig. 4) suggests that these enzymes are expressed by uninucleate, but not by binucleate cells of the bovine placenta. Systematic studies are required on different species throughout gestation to clarify these apparent discrepancies.

The tremendous progress in the identification and characterization of the many enzymes involved in steroid synthesis has made it possible to investigate the molecular regulation of steroidogenesis *(181)*. Cloning and in vitro expression have provided particularly important insights, one of the most notable relating to the synthesis of androgens from progestagens. Androgen synthesis is catalyzed by the cytochrome $P450_{17\alpha}$ *(182)*. Two reactions take place, the first involving hydroxylation of C-17, and the second cleavage of the C-17,20 bond (lyase). Fevold et al. *(183)* expressed rat, bovine and human $P450_{17\alpha}$ in nonsteroidogenic Cos-1 cells to examine enzymatic activity. Hydroxylase activity was equally efficient across species utilizing either pregnenolone or progesterone as substrate. However, lyase activity demonstrated distinct species preferences. The rat enzyme utilized both 17OH-pregnenolone and 17OH-progesterone for C-19 steroid synthesis (lyase activity). Although human and bovine $P450_{17\alpha}$ utilized 17OH-pregnenolone, neither enzyme was capable of efficient C-19 steroid synthesis from 17OH-progesterone *(184)*. Therefore, progesterone appears to be an efficient substrate for androstenedione synthesis in specific species (Fig. 5), namely rats, pigs, rabbits, horses, and guinea pigs, but not in human, bovine, ovine, or caprine *(184)*.

The physiological consequences of differential substrate utilization by $P450_{17\alpha}$ relative to the regulation of steroidogenesis may be profound *(184)*. With respect to pregnancy in particular, the characteristic specificity of the lyase activity potentially dictates the ability of the tissue to synthesize androgen and estrogen from progesterone. Moreover, this may be the most abundant substrate available in those species reliant on luteal progesterone secretion throughout pregnancy. Perhaps it is not a coincidence that several species capable of estrogen synthesis during blastocyst development (porcine, equine, and rabbit) are among those capable of utilizing progesterone as a substrate for androstenedione synthesis. In addition, the characteristics of rat $P450_{17\alpha}$ lyase activity also facilitate the use of

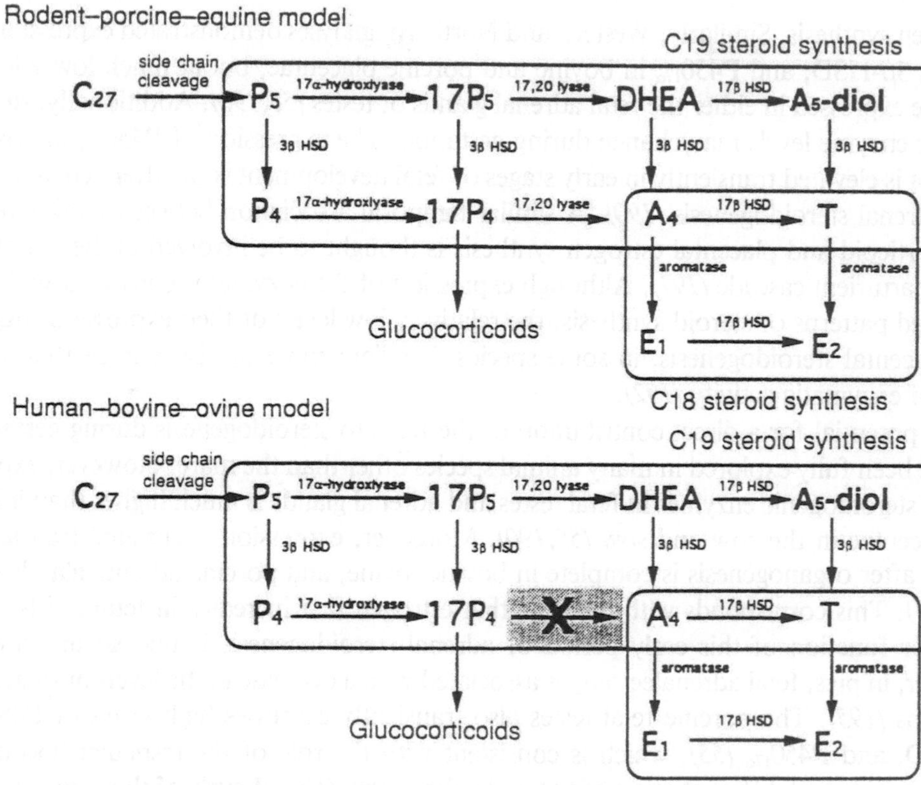

Fig. 5. Endocrine functions of the placenta steroidogenic pathways.

luteal progesterone for androstenedione synthesis in the rodent placenta after d 12 of gestation. Studies are required to determine whether or not luteal progesterone is utilized for C-19 and C-18 steroid synthesis during pregnancy in species other than the rat.

Regardless of substrate availability or utilization, the impact of estrogen synthesis is dependent on the local tissue expression of enzymes that further modify their form and bioactivity. The interconversion of estrone and estradiol is catalyzed by 17β-HSD enzymes, some of which have been cloned in recent years *(185)*. Oxidation or reduction is promoted by particular enzyme types within the family encoded by several related genes. As demonstrated for 3β-hydroxysteroid dehydrogenase (3β-HSD) isoforms *(186)*, expression of the 17β-HSD is expected to be tissue-specific within species, developmentally regulated, and exhibit complex regulation of gene expression. Estrogen availability is also influenced by the activities of conjugating and deconjugating enzymes *(187)*. Dwyer and Robertson *(188)* reported that the ratio of endometrial sulfotransferase to sulfatase increased with the stage of gestation in the ewe, but decreased in the sow. Consistent with this view, Knight *(123)* reported that sulfatase activity increased in the endometrium relative to placental activity in sows late in gestation. As noted, these species differences in estrogen conjugation may explain the appearance of conceptus estrogens in maternal plasma of the pig between d 25 and 30 of gestation *(174)*. The activities of these enzymes are undoubtedly important in determining the levels of active steroids at the cell and tissue level. Future studies will elucidate the significance of these enzymes in steroidogenesis during pregnancy.

Surprisingly few reports have documented levels of steroidogenic enzymes or their transcripts in the placenta. Durkee et al. *(189)* identified $P450_{scc}$ and $P450_{17\alpha}$ transcripts in rat placentae during the second half of gestation, consistent with studies demonstrating androgen synthesis. Similarly, Western and Northern analyses demonstrated expression of $P450_{scc}$, 3β-HSD, and $P450_{17\alpha}$ in bovine and porcine placentae, but at much lower levels than are expressed in either the fetal adrenal glands or testes *(55,190)*. Additionally, steroidogenic enzyme levels may change during gestation. The expression of $P450_{17\alpha}$ in bovine placenta is elevated transiently in early stages of fetal development soon after activation of fetal adrenal steroidogenesis *(190)*. A similar temporal association between fetal adrenal glucocorticoid and placental estrogen synthesis is thought to be involved in the initiation of the parturient cascade *(191)*. Although expression of the enzymes is consistent with the described patterns of steroid synthesis, the relatively low levels of their expression suggest that placental steroidogenesis, in some species, is reliant more on tissue mass than high levels of enzymatic activity *(192)*.

The potential for a direct contribution of the fetus to steroidogenesis during gestation has not been fully explored in many animal species other than the mare. However, expression of steroidogenic enzymes in fetal testes and adrenal glands is much higher than it is in the placentae in the cow and sow *(55,190)*. Moreover, expression is elevated transiently shortly after organogenesis is complete in bovine, ovine, and porcine adrenal glands *(55, 193,194)*. This corresponds with the time that estrogen first increases in fetal fluids. The effect or function of this early period of adrenal steroidogenesis is unclear at present; however, in pigs, fetal adrenalectomy is associated with a decrease in the levels of maternal estrogens *(195)*. The porcine fetal testes also transiently expresses high levels of $P450_{scc}$, 3β-HSD, and $P450_{17\alpha}$ *(55)*, which is consistent with the role of the testicular androgen secretion in sexual differentiation of the male phenotype *(196)*. Levels of these enzymes in porcine fetal testes increase again in late gestation when maternal concentrations of estrogens are rising *(55)*. In fact, synthesis and secretion of androgens by the fetus may provide substrates for placental aromatization to estrogen. Choong and Raeside *(197)* reported that estrogen concentrations in male placentas were higher than those in female placentae at d 100 of gestation in pigs, indicating that fetal testicular androgens provide substrate for placental aromatization to estrogen.

Whether or not fetal male androgen synthesis influences placental estrogen secretion, it may have other have important consequences in rodents. An effect of male proximity on sexual development of female rat fetuses was proposed to be owing to an androgen influence from adjacent male littermates *(198,199)*. This observation reinforces the claimed importance of placental aromatization in the clearance of fetal androgens, as evidenced by masculinization in female infants congenitally deficient in the aromatase enzyme. One of the major functions of $P450_{arom}$ expression in pregnancy in pigs may also be the elimination of androgens synthesized by male fetuses during sexual development and minimize effects of those androgens on female fetuses.

Trophoblast is a unique tissue, and it is becoming increasingly apparent that unique molecular mechanisms are involved in the regulation of placental function *(192)*. Studies to date suggest that steroidogenic enzyme expression in placental cells is not subject to acute stimulation by cAMP *(200)*, including in vitro cultures of bovine placenta *(131)*. Furthermore, the placenta may not express the recently identified StAR protein *(201)* involved in cholesterol transport to the inner mitochondrial membrane *(202)*. In addition, the placenta may not utilize the same trans-acting transcription factors, such as SF-1, that regulate steroidogenic enzyme expression in other organs *(200)*. For example, $P450_{17\alpha}$ expression reguires a unique transcriptional start site in pig trophoblast expression that is unrecognized in any steroidogenic tissue of other species *(203)*. Exon utilization controlling transcriptional expression of $P450_{arom}$ is conserved for the ovary, but is poorly conserved across exons utilized for $P450_{arom}$ expression in the placentae of cows, mares, and sows *(204)*. Collectively, these results indicate that placentae utilize a novel mechanism for regulation of transcription of steroidogenic enzymes *(192)*. In addition, they reinforce the importance of placental mass, rather than acute stimulation to induce higher levels of enzyme expression, in the control of placental steroid production.

The placenta deviates from the classical concept of a steroidogenic tissue that is based on studies on the gonads and adrenal glands. The isolation and characterization of unique placental isoforms of key steroidogenic enzymes are evidence of this fact *(184,185,205)*. Moreover, the expression of $P450_{scc}$ in rat decidua *(206)* and gut of mouse embryos *(207)*, $P450_{17\alpha}$ in the parietal cells of the stomach of the rat *(208)*, and $P450_{arom}$ in the porcine fetal adrenal gland *(209)* challenge our understanding of tissue-specific patterns of steroidogenic enzyme expression. The challenge of finding some unity in the species variability in placental steroidogenesis among the subprimate mammals may prove to be unrealistic. However, research will undoubtedly provide unprecedented insights into the developmental and evolutionary control of steroid biosynthesis.

Steroid Supplementation to Improve Establishment of Pregnancy

Attempts to increase embryonic survival in domestic farm animals through exogenous steroid therapy have been disappointing. Utilization of either progesterone or progesterone and estrogen supplementation to increase litter size in swine has not resulted in consistent, if any, improvements in the number of piglets born *(210)*. However, a combination of estrogen and progesterone therapy has increased placental weight *(210)*. Administration of estrogen can also have a detrimental effect on embryonic survival in the pig if given before conceptus production on d 11–12 of pregnancy *(210)*. In fact, consumption of the natural estrogenic componds, e.g., zearalenone found in moldy corn results in total embryonic loss if fed before d 11 of pregnancy.

Fluctuations in serum progesterone have also been implicated as possible limitations for early embryonic survival in the ewe and cow. Attempts to improve embryonic survival in ruminant species with steroid therapy also failed to have consistent results *(211–213)*. Studies in which progesterone had a positive effect on embryo survival in sheep have been associated with high levels of nutrition, which increases metablic clearance of progesterone *(211)*. Improvements in embryonic survival in both cattle and sheep through steroid supplementation are believed to be through effects on endometrium and its effects on early conceptus development and establishment of pregnancy.

Opportunities for decreasing embryonic mortality through steroid supplementation may be most successful in the mare. Progesterone administration has been used widely to reduce the incidence of early embryonic loss in mares *(68)*. However, evidence for actual improvement in pregnancy rates in mares with steroid therapy is clearly controversial. In cases of luteal insufficiency, detected through the monitoring of plasma progesterone, undersized embryos on d 11–15 of gestation or severe levels of endometrial cysts, progesterone supplementation may have beneficial effects on maintaining pregnancy in mares *(68)*. However, these physiological losses are a relatively minor cause of pregnancy failure in mares when compared to other pathological failures, such as that related to endometritis.

Progesterone therapy in all the domestic species is directed at improving deficiencies in luteal progesterone during early gestation. At this time, there has been no clear evidence that lack of placental steroidogenesis is responsible for pregnancy failure. The mare represents a species in which placental steroidogenesis would be essential to maintain pregnancy to term following regression of the CL during midgestation. Studies to evaluate the possibility that placental steroidogenic insufficiency contributes to late fetal loss have not been undertaken. However, it is entirely possible that a multitude of pathways and mechanisms developed throughout evolution of the mammalian fetal–placental unit have provided many safeguards to give the fetus the highest probability for successful delivery of an offspring.

REFERENCES

1. Guillette LJ (1989) The evolution of vertebrate viviparity: Morphological modifications and endocrine control, In: Complex Organismal Functions: Intergration and Evolution in Vertebrates (Wake DB, Roth G, eds.), John Wiley, New York, pp. 219–233.
2. Aitken RJ (1979) The hormonal control of implantation, In: Maternal Recognition of Pregnancy (Whelan J, ed.), Ciba Foundation Symposium 64, Excerptia Medica, Amsterdam, pp. 53–84.
3. Bazer FW (1975) Uterine protein secretion: Relationship to the development of the conceptus. J Anim Sci 41:1376–1382.
4. Beier HM (1985) Proteins and steroids in early pregnancy, In: Early Pregnancy Factors (Ellendroff F, Koch E, eds.), Perinatology Press, New York, pp. 1–12.
5. Roberts RM, Murray MK, Burke MG, Ketcham CM, Bazer FW (1987) Hormonal control and function of secretory proteins, In: Cell and Molecular Biology of the Uterus (Leavitt WW, ed.), Plenum, New York, pp. 137–150.
6. Roberts RM, Xie S, Trout WE (1992) Embryo-uterine interactions in pigs during the week 2 of pregnancy, In: Control of Pig Reproduction IV. The Journals of Reproduction and Fertility (Foxcroft GR, Hunter MG, Doberska C, eds.), Cambridge, pp. 171–186.
7. Ford SP (1989) Factors controlling uterine blood flow during estrus and early pregnancy, In: The Uterine Circulation (Rosenfeld CR, ed.), Perinatology, Ithaca, pp. 113–129.
8. Ford SP (1995) Control of Blood flow in the gravid uterine of domestic livestock species. J Anim Sci 73:1852–1860.
9. Staples LD, Binns RM, Heap RB (1983) Influence of certain steroids on lymphocyte transformation in sheep and goats studies in vitro. J Endocrinol 98:55–69.
10. Hansen PJ, Bazer FW, Segerson EC Jr. (1986) Skin graft survival in the uterine lumen of ewes treated with progesterone. Am J Reprod Immunol 12:48–54.
11. Van Vlasselaer P, Vandeputte M (1985) Local immune suppression by progesterone, In: Early Pregnancy Factors (Ellendroff F, Koch E, eds.), Perinatology, New York, pp. 89–92.
12. Szekeres-Bartho J, Chaouat G (1990) Lymphocyte-derived progesterone-induced blocking factor corrects resorption in a murine abortion system. Am J Reprod Immunol 23: 26–28.
13. Psychoyos A (1973) Hormonal control of egg ovoimplantation. Vitam Horm 31:201–256.
14. Yoshinaga K, Hawkins RA, Stocker JF (1969) Estrogen secretion by the rat ovary in vivo during the estrous cycle and pregnancy. Endocrinology 85:103–112.
15. Levasseur M-C (1984) The involvement of estradiol at the time of implantation in placental mammals. Anim Reprod Sci 7:467–488.
16. Heap RB, Flint APF, Gadsby JE (1981) Embryonic signals and maternal recognition, In: Cellular and Molecular Aspects of Implantation (Glasser SR, Bullock DW, eds.), Plenum, New York, pp. 311–326.
17. McCormack SA, Glasser SR (1981) Hormone production by rat blastocysts and midpregnancy trophoblasts in vitro, In: Cellular and Molecular Aspects of Implantation (Glasser SR, Bullock DW, eds.), Plenum, New York, pp. 461–463.
18. Niemann H, Freitag M, Elsaesser F (1989) The role of oestrogens in embryonic development. J Reprod Fertil Suppl. 38:73–83.
19. Singh MM, Booth WD (1979) Origin of oestrogen in preimplantation rabbit blastocysts. J Steroid Biochem 11:723–728.

20. Dey SK, Johnson DC (1986) Embryonic signals in pregnancy, In: Nidation: A Symposium Held in Honor of Professor M.C. Shelesnyak (Yoshinaga K, ed.), The New York Academy of Sciences, New York, pp. 49–62.
21. Surani MAH, Fishel SB (1981) Embryonic and uterine factors in delayed implantation in rodents. J Reprod Fertil (Suppl) 29:159–172.
22. Dickmann Z, Dey SK, Gupta JS (1976) A new concept: Control of early pregnancy steroid hormones originating in the preimplantation embryo. Vitam Horm 34:215–242.
23. Grube KE, Gwazdauskas FC, Lineweaver JA, Vinson WE (1978) Steroidogenic capabilities of the early mouse embryo. Steroids 32:345–354.
24. Wu JT, Liu ZH (1990) Conversion of pregnenolone to progesterone by mouse morulae and blastocysts. J Reprod Fertil 88:93–98.
25. Marrone BL, Karavolas HJ (1981) Progesterone metabolism by the hypothalamus, pituitary, and uterus of the rat during pregnancy. Endocrinology 109:41–45.
26. George FW, Wilson JD (1978) Estrogen formation in the early rabbit embryo. Science 199:200,201.
27. Gadsby JE, Heap RB, Burton RD (1980) Oestrogen production by blastocyst and early embryonic tissue of various species. J Reprod Fertil 60:409–417.
28. Sholl SA, Orsini MW, Hitchins DJ (1983) Estrogen synthesis and metabolism in the hamster blastocyst, uterus and liver near the time of implantation. J Steroid Biochem 19:1153–1161.
29. Hoversland RC, Dey SK, Johnson DC (1982) Aromatase activity in the rabbit blastocyst. J Reprod Fertil 66:259–263.
30. Wu JT, Lin GM (1982) Effect of aromatase inhibitor on oestrogen production in rabbit blastocysts. J Reprod Fertil 66:655–662.
31. Dey SK, Dickmann Z, Sen Gupta J (1976) Evidence that the maintenance of early pregnancy in the rabbit requires "blastocyst estrogen." Steroids 28:481–485.
32. Wise T, Heap RB (1983) Effects of the embryo on endometrial estrogen synthesis in the rabbit. Biol Reprod 28:1097–1106.
33. Gadsby JE, Keyes PL, Bill CH II (1983) Control of corpus luteum function in the pregnant rabbit: Role of estrogen and lack of a direct luteotropic role of the placenta. Endocrinology 113: 2255–2262.
34. Harper MJK, Dowd D, Elliot ASW (1969) Implantation and embryonic development in the ovariectomized-adrenalectomized hamster. Biol Reprod 1:253–257.
35. Brodie AMH, Wu J-T, Marsh DA, Brodie HJ (1978) Aromatase inhibitors III. Studies on the antifertility effect of 4-acetoxy-4-androstene-3,17-dione. Biol Reprod 18:365–370.
36. Geisert RD, Short EC, Morgan GL (1994) Establishment of pregnancy in domestic farm species, In: Embryonic Mortality in Domestic Species (Zavy MT, Geisert RD, eds.), CRC, Boca Raton, pp. 23–52.
37. Perry JS, Heap RB, Amoroso EC (1973) Steroid hormone production by pig blastocysts. Nature (Lond) 245:45–47.
38. Stone BA, Seamark RF, Kelly RW, Deam S (1986) Production of steroids and release of prostaglandins by spherical pig blastocysts in vitro. Aust J Biol Sci 39:283–293.
39. Perry JS (1981) The mammalian fetal membranes. J Reprod Fertil 62:321–335.
40. Zavy MT, Bazer FW, Thatcher WW, Wilcox CJ (1980) A study of prostaglandin F2α as the luteolysin in swine: Comparison of prostaglandin F, progestins, estrone and estradiol in uterine flushings from pregnant and non-pregnant gilts. Prostaglandins 20:837–851.
41. Geisert RD, Renegar RH, Thatcher WW, Roberts RM, Bazer FW (1982) Establishment of pregnancy in the pig. I. Interrelationships between preimplantation development of the pig blastocyst and uterine endometrial secretions. Biol Reprod 27:925–939.
42. Ford SP, Christenson RK, Ford JJ (1982) Uterine blood flow and uterine arterial, venous and luminal concentrations of oestrogens on Days 11, 13 and 15 after oestrus in pregnant and non-pregnant sows. J Reprod Fertil 64:185–190.
43. Stone BA, Seamark RF (1985) Steroid hormones in uterine washings and in plasma of gilts between days 9 and 15 after oestrus and between days 9 and 15 after coitus. J Reprod Fertil 75:209–221.
44. Fischer HE, Bazer FW, Fields MJ (1985) Steroid metabolism by endometrial and conceptus tissues during early pregnancy and pseudopregnancy in swine. J Reprod Fert 75:69–78.
45. Geisert RD, Brookbank JW, Roberts RM, Bazer FW (1982) Establishment of pregnancy in the pig: II. Cellular remodelling of the porcine blastocyst during elongation on day 12 of pregnancy. Biol Reprod 27:941–955.

46. Pusateri AE, Rothschild MF, Warner CM, Ford SP (1990) Changes in morphology, cell number, cell size and cellular estrogen content of individual littermate pig conceptuses on days 9 to 13 of gestation. J Anim Sci 68:3727–3735.
47. Stroband HWJ, Van der Lende T (1992) Embryonic and uterine development during early pregnancy. J Reprod Fertil (Suppl) 40:261–277.
48. Geisert RD, Zavy MT, Moffatt RM, Blair RM, Yellin T (1990) Embryonic steroids and the establishment of pregnancy. J Reprod Fertil (Suppl) 40:293–305.
49. King GJ, Ackerley CA (1985) Demonstrations of estrogen in developing pig trophectoderm and yolk sac endoderm between days 10 and 16. J Reprod Fertil 73:361–367.
50. Conley AJ, Christenson RK, Ford SP, Geisert RD, Mason JI (1992) Steroidogenic enzyme expression in porcine conceptuses during and after elongation. Endocrinology 131:896–902.
51. Conley AJ, Christenson RK, Ford SP, Christenson RK (1994) Immunocytochemical localization of cytochrome P450 17α-hydroxylase and aromatase in embryonic cell layers of elongating porcine blastocysts. Endocrinology 135:2248–2254.
52. Ko Y, Choi I, Green ML, Simmen FA, Simmen RCM (1994) Transient expression of the cytochrome P450 aromatase gene in elongating porcine blastocysts is correlated with uterine insulin-like growth factor levels during peri-implantation development. Mol Reprod Dev 37:1–11.
53. Yelich J, Pomp D, Geisert RD (1997) Detection of transcripts for retinoic acid receptors, retinal-binding protein, and transforming growth factors during rapid trophoblastic elongation in the porcine concepts. Biol Reprod 57:286–294.
54. Green ML, Simmen RCM, Simmen FA (1995) Developmental regulation of steroidogenic enzyme gene expression in the preiimplantation porcine conceptus: A paracrine role for insulin-like growth factor-I. Endocrinology 136:3961–3970.
55. Conley AJ, Rainey WE, Mason JI (1994) Ontogeny of steroidogenic enzyme expression in the porcine conceptus. J Mol Endocrinol 12:155–165.
56. Stromstedt M, Keeney DS, Waterman MR, Paria BC, Conley AJ, Dey SK (1996) Preimplantation mouse blastocysts fail to express CYP genes required for estrogen biosynthesis. Mol Reprod Dev 43:428–436.
57. Heap RB, Flint APF, Hartmann PE, Gadsby JE, Staples LD, Ackland N, Hamon M (1981) Oestrogen production in early pregnancy. J Endocrinol 89:77–94.
58. Henricks DM, Tindal DJ (1971) Metabolism of progesterone-4-[14^{C}] in porcine uterine endometrium. Endocrinology 89:920–924.
59. Pack BA, Brooks CL, Dukelow WR, Brooks SC (1979) The metabolism and nuclear migration of estrogen in porcine uterus throughout the implantation process. Biol Reprod 20:545–551.
60. Meyers SA, Lozon MM, Corombos JD, Saunders DE, Hunter K, Christensen C, Brooks SC (1983) Induction of porcine uterine estrogen sulfotransferase activity by progesterone. Biol Reprod 28:1119–1128.
61. Brooks SC, Pack BA, Rozhin J, Christensen C (1982) *In situ* control of estrogen activity by sulfurylation in uterus and other target tissues, In: Sulfate Metabolism and Sulfate Conjunction (Mulder GJ, Caldwell J, Van Kempen GMJ, Vonk RJ, eds.), Taylor & Francis, London, pp. 173–180.
62. Robertson HA, King GJ (1974) Plasma concentrations of progesterone, oestrone, oestradiol-17β and oestrone sulphate in the pig at implantation, during pregnancy and at parturition. J Reprod Fertil 40:133–141.
63. Heap RB, Perry JS, Burton RD, Gadsby JE, Wyatt C, Jenkin G (1977) Blastocyst steroidogenesis and embryo-maternal interactions in the establishment of pregnancy. In: Reproduction and Evolution (Calaby EH, Tyndale-Biscoe CH, eds.), Australian Academy of Science, Canberra, pp. 341–347.
64. Sharp DC III (1994) Embryonic mortality in the mare, In: Embryonic Mortality in Domestic Species (Zavy MT, Geisert RD, eds.), CRC, Boca Raton, pp. 141–152.
65. Ginther OJ (1993) Mobility of the equine conceptus. Theriogenology 19:603–611.
66. Leith GS, Ginther OJ (1985) Mobility of the conceptus and uterine contractions in the mare. Theriogenology 24, 701–711.
67. McDowell KJ, Sharp DC, Grubaugh W, Thatcher WW, Wilcox CJ (1988) Restricted conceptus mobility results in failure of pregnancy maintenance in mares. Biol Reprod 39:340–348.
68. Ginther OJ (1992) Embryology and placentation, In: Reproductive Biology of the Mare (Ginther OJ, ed.), Equiservices, Cross Plains, pp. 345–418.
69. Flood PF, Marrable AW (1975) A histochemical study of steroid metabolism in the equine fetus and placenta. J Reprod Fertil (Suppl) 2:569–573.

70. Paulo E, Tischner M (1985) Activity of Δ(5)3β-hydroxysteroid dehydrogenase and steroid hormones content in early preimplantation horse embryos. Folia Histochem Cytobiol 23:81–84.
71. Flood PF, Betteridge KJ, Irvine DS (1979) Oestrogens and androgens in blastocoelic fluid and cultures of cells from equine conceptus of 10–22 days gestation. J Reprod Fertil (Suppl) 27:414–420.
72. Zavy MT, Vernon MW, Sharp DC, Bazer FW (1984) Endocrine aspects of early pregnancy in pony mares: A comparison of uterine luminal and peripheral plasma levels of steroids during the estrous cycle and early pregnancy. Endocrinology 115:214–219.
73. Seamans KW, Fields MJ, Bazer FW, Vernon MW, Sharp DC (1979) In vitro aromatase activity of pregnant and nonpregnant equine endometrium and conceptus membranes [Abstract]. 71st Annual Meeting of Amer Soc Anim Sci, Tucson, AZ, p. 335.
74. Zavy MT, Mayer R, Vernon MW, Bazer FW, Sharp DC (1979) An investigation of the uterine luminal environment of nonpregnant and pregnant pony mares. J Reprod Fertil (Suppl) 27: 403–411.
75. Heap RB, Hamon M, Allen WR (1982) Studies on estrogen synthesis by the preimplantation equine conceptus. J Reprod Fertil (Suppl) 32:343–352.
76. Marsan C, Goff AK, Sirois J, Betteridge KJ (1987) Steroid secretion by different cell types of the horse conceptus. J Reprod Fertil (Suppl) 35:363–369.
77. Terqui M, Palmer E (1979) Oestrogen pattern during early pregnancy in the mare. J Reprod Fertil (Suppl) 27:441–446.
78. King GJ, Atkinson BA, Robertson HA (1992) Implantation and early placentation in domestic ungulates. J Reprod Fertil (Suppl) 31:17–30.
79. Betteridge KJ, Flechon J-E (1988) The anatomy and physiology of pre-attachment bovine embryos. Theriogenology 29:155–187.
80. Shemesh M, Milaquir G, Ayalon N, Hansel W (1979) Steroidogenesis and prostaglandin synthesis by cultured bovine blastocysts. J Reprod Fertil 56:181–185.
81. Chenault JR (1980) Steroid metabolism by the early bovine conceptus. 1. 5β-reducton of neutral C19 steroids. J Steroid Biochem 13:499–506.
82. Eley RM, Thatcher WW, Bazer FW, Fields MJ (1983) Steroid metabolism by the bovine uterine endometrium and conceptus. Biol Reprod 28:804–816.
83. Ford SP, Chenault JR, Christenson RK, Echternkamp SE, Ford SP (1981) Effects of preimplantation bovine and porcine conceptuses on blood flow and steroid content of the uterus, In: Cellular and Molecular Aspects of Implantation (Glasser SR, Bullock DW, eds.), Plenum, New York, pp. 436–438.
84. Reynolds LP, Magness RR, Ford SP (1984) Uterine blood flow during early pregnancy in ewes: Interaction between the conceptus and the ovary bearing the corpus luteum. J Anim Sci 58: 423–429.
85. Geisert RD, Zavy MT, Biggers BG, Garrett JE, Wettemann RP (1988) Characterization of the uterine environment during early conceptus expansion in the bovine. Anim Reprod Sci 16:11–25.
86. Nephew KP, McClure KE, Pope WF (1989) Embryonic migration relative to maternal recognition of pregnancy in sheep. J Anim Sci 67:999–1005.
87. Thatcher WW, Bazer FW, Sharp DC, Roberts RM (1986) Interrelationships between uterus and conceptus to maintain corpus luteum function in early pregnancy: sheep, cattle, pigs and horses. J Anim Sci 62:(Suppl) 2, 25–46.
88. Robertson HA, King GJ (1979) Conjugated and unconjugated oestrogens in fetal and maternal fluids of the cow throughout pregnancy. J Reprod Fertil 55:463–470.
89. Eley RM, Thatcher WW, Bazer FW (1979) Hormonal and physical changes associated with bovine conceptus development. J Reprod Fertil 55:181–190.
90. Chakraborty C, Dey SK, Davis DL (1989) Pattern and tissue distribution of catechol estrogen forming activity by pig conceptuses during the peri-implantation period. J Anim Sci 67:991–998.
91. Reynolds LP (1986) Utero-ovarian interactions during early pregnancy: Role of conceptus induced vasodilation. J Anim Sci 62 [Suppl] 2:47–61.
92. Katzenellenbogen BS (1980) Dynamics of steroid hormone receptor action. Ann Rev Physiol 42: 17–36.
93. Savouret JF, Misrahi M, Milgrom E (1990) Molecular action of progesterone. Int J Biochem 22: 579–594.
94. Li W, Boomsma RA, Verhage HG (1992) Immunocytochemical analysis of estrogen and progestin receptors in uteri of steroid-treated and pregnant cats. Biol Reprod 47:1073–1081.

95. Hild-Petito S, Verhage HG, Fazleabas AT (1992) Immunocytochemical localization of estrogen and progestin receptors in the baboon (*Papio anubis*) uterus during implantation and pregnancy. Endocrinology 130:2343–2353.
96. Yelich JV, Geisert RD, Pomp D (1997) Ontogeny of elongation and gene expression in the early developing porcine conceptus. Biol Reprod 57:1256–1265.
97. Lubahn DB, Moyer JS, Golding TS, Couse JF, Korach KS, Smithies O (1993) Alteration of reproductive function but not prenatal sexual development after insertional disruption of the mouse estrogen receptor gene. Proc Natl Acad Sci 90:11,162–11,166.
98. Ohta Y, Sato T, Iguchi T (1993) Immunocytochemical localization of progesterone receptor in the reproductive tract of adult female rats. Biol Reprod 48:205–213.
99. Gutierrez-Sagal R, Perez-Palacios G, Langley E, Pasapera AM, Castro I, Cerbon MA (1993) Endometrial expression of progesterone receptor and uteroglobin genes during early pregnancy in the rabbit. Mol Reprod Dev 34:244–249.
100. Geisert RD, Pratt TN, Bazer FW, Mayes JS, Watson GH (1994) Immunocytochemical localization and changes in endometrial progestin receptor protein during the porcine oestrous cycle and early pregnancy. Reprod Fertil Dev 6:749–760.
101. Zheng J, Johnson MJ, Redmer DA, Reynolds LP (1996) Estrogen and progesterone receptors, cell proliferation, and c-fos expression in ovine uterus during early pregnancy. Endocrinology 137: 340–348.
102. Ott TL, Zhou Y, Mirando MA, Stevens C, Harney JP, Ogle TF, Bazer FW (1993) Changes in progesterone and oestrogen receptor mRNA and protein during maternal recognition of pregnancy and luteolysis in ewes. J Mol Endocrinol 10:171–183.
103. Spencer TE, Bazer FW (1995) Temporal and spatial alterations in uterine estrogen receptor and progesterone receptor gene expression during the estrous cycle and early pregnancy in the ewe. Biol Reprod 53:1527–1543.
104. Geisert RD, Brenner RM, Moffatt RJ, Harney JP, Yellin T, Bazer FW (1993) Changes in oestrogen receptor protein, mRNA expression and localization in the endometrium of cyclic and pregnant gilts. Reprod Fertil Dev 5:247–260.
105. Cherny RA, Salamonsen LA, Findlay JK (1991) Immunocytochemical localization of oestrogen receptors in the endometrium of the ewe. Reprod Fertil Dev 3:321–331.
106. Spencer TE, Becker WC, George P, Mirando MA, Ogle TF, Bazer FW (1995) Ovine interferon-τ regulates expression of endometrial receptors for estrogen and oxytocin but not progesterone. Biol Reprod 53:732–745.
107. Brenner RM, West NB, McClellan MC (1990) Estrogen and progestin receptors in the reproductive tract of male and female primates. Biol Reprod 42:11–19.
108. Casida LE, Warwick EJ (1945) The necessity of the corpus luteum for the maintenance of pregnancy in the ewe. J Anim Sci 4:34–36.
109. Denamur R, Martinet J (1955) Effects de l'ovariectomie chez la brebis pendant la gestation. C R Acad Sci 149:2105–2107.
110. Holtan DW, Squires EL, Lapin DR, Ginther OJ (1979) Effect of ovariectomy on pregnant mares. J Reprod Fertil (Suppl) 27:457–463.
111. Csapo AI, Puri CP, Tarro S (1981) Relationship between timing of ovariectomy and maintenance of pregnancy in the guinea pig. Prostaglandins 22:131–140.
112. Hammond J (1927) The Physiology of Reproduction in the Cow. Cambridge, Cambridge University Press.
113. Raeside JI, Turner CW (1950) Progesterone in the maintenance of pregnancy in dairy heifers. J Anim Sci 9:681.
114. McDonald LE, Nichols RE, McNutt SH (1952) Studies on corpus luteum ablation and progesterone replacement therapy during prenancy in the cow. Am J Vet Res 13:446–451.
115. Short RV (1957) Progesterone and related steroids in the blood of domestic animals, In: Colloquia on Endocrinology: Hormones in Blood, vol 11 (Wolstenholme GEW, Miller ECP, eds.), Little, Brown and Company, Boston, pp. 362–398.
116. Melampy RM, Hearn WR, Rakes JM (1959) Progesterone content of bovine reproductive organs and blood during pregnancy. J Anim Sci 18:307–313.
117. Harrison FA, Heap RB (1978) Progesterone secretion during pregnancy in sheep with an autotransplanted adrenal and autotransplanted ovary. J Reprod Fertil 54:153–157.
118. Ricketts AP, Flint APF (1980) Onset of synthesis of progesterone by ovine placenta. J Endocrinol 86:337–347.

119. Flint APF (1983) Factors controlling placental endocrine function in domestic animals. Exp Endocrinol 5:75–95.
120. Illingworth DV, Deanesly R (1972) Maintenance of pregnancy by synthetic progestagens in guinea pigs ovariectomized before implantation; Progesterone-binding protein and placental progesterone secretion. J Endocrinol 54:435–444.
121. Sheldrick EL, Ricketts AP, Flint APF (1980) Placental production of progesterone in ovariectomized goats treated with a synthetic progestagen to maintain pregnancy. J Reprod Fertil 60: 339–348.
122. Craig VA (1982) Placental steroid metabolism in late pregnancy, In: Control of Pig Reproduction (Cole DJA, Foxcroft GR, eds.), Butterworth Scientific, London, pp. 405–418.
123. Knight JW (1994) Aspects of placental estrogen synthesis in the pig. Exp Clin Endocrinol 102: 175–184.
124. Comline RS, Hall LW, Lavelle RB, Nathanielsz PW, Silver M (1974) Parturition in the cow: Endocrine changes in animals with chronically implanted catheters in foetal and maternal circulation. J Endocrinol 63:451–472.
125. Ferrell CL, Ford SP, Prior RL, Christenson RK (1983) Blood flow, steroid secretion and nutrient uptake of the gravid bovine fetus. J Anim Sci 56:656–667.
126. Conley AJ, Ford SP (1987) Effect of prostaglandin F2α-induced luteolysis on in vivo and in vitro progesterone production by individual placentomes of cows. J Anim Sci 65:500–507.
127. Tsumagari S, Kamata J, Takagi K, Tanemura K, Yosai A, Takeishi M (1994) 3β-Hydroxysteroid dehydrogenase activity and gestagen concentrations in bovine cotyledons and caruncles during gestation and parturition. J Reprod Fertil 102:35–39.
128. Shemesh M, Hansel W, Strauss JF III (1984) Calcium dependent, cyclic nucleotide-independent steroidogenesis in bovine placenta. Proc Natl Acad Sci USA 80:6403–6407.
129. Reimers TJ, Ullman MB, Hansel W (1985) Progesterone production by bovine binucleate trophoblastic cells. Biol Reprod 33:1227–1236.
130. Shemesh M (1990) Production and regulation of progesterone in bovine corpus luteum and placenta in mid and late gestation: A personal review. Reprod Fertil Dev 2:129–135.
131. Shemesh M, Izhar M, Pasmanik M, Shore LS (1992) The regulation of steroidogenesis in the bovine placenta. J Physiol Pharmacol 43:153–163.
132. Bedwani JR, Marley PB (1971) Effects of ovariectomy and of various hormones on the synthesis of progesterone by guinea pig placenta in vitro. J Reprod Fertil 26:343–349.
133. Harterius HO (1936) Reduction of litter size and maintenance of pregnancy in the oophorectomized rat: Evidence concerning the endocrine role of the placenta. Am J Physiol 114:399–406.
134. Tsutsui T, Stabenfeldt GH (1993) Biology of ovarian cycles, pregnancy and pseudopregnancy in the domestic cat. J Reprod Fertil (Suppl) 47:29–35.
135. Courrier R, Gros G (1935) Contribution a l'endocrinologie de la grossesse chez la chatte. C R Acad Sci 120:5–7.
136. Matsumoto K, Yamane G, Endo H, Kotoh K, Okand K (1969) Conversion of pregnenolone to progesterone by rabbit placenta in vitro. Acta Endocrinol 61:577–584.
137. Short RV (1959) Progesterone in blood. IV. Progesterone in the blood of mares. J Endocrinol 19: 207–210.
138. Holtan DW, Nett TM, Estergreen VL (1975) Plasma progestagens in pregnant mares. J Reprod Fertil (Suppl) 23:419–424.
139. Ganjam JK, Kennym RM, Flickinger G (1975) Plasma progestins in cyclic, pregnant and postpartum mares. J Reprod Fertil (Suppl) 23:441–447.
140. Barnes RJ, Nathanielsz PW, Rossdale PD, Comline RS, Silver M (1975) Plasma progestagens and oestrogens in fetus and mother in late pregnancy. J Reprod Fertil [Suppl] 23:617–623.
141. Atkins DT, Harms PG, Sorenson Jr. AM, Fleeger JL (1976) Isolation, identification and quantitation of serum 5α-pregnane-3,20-dione and its relationship to progesterone in the pregnant mare. Steroids 28:867–880.
142. Holtan DW, Houghton E, Silver M, Fowden AL, Ousey J, Rossdale PD (1991) Plasma progestagens in the mare, fetus and newborn foal. J Reprod Fertil (Suppl) 44:517–528.
143. Moss GE, Estergreen VL, Becker SR, Grant BD (1979) The source of the 5α-pregnanes that occur during gestation in mares. J Reprod Fertil (Suppl) 27:511–519.
144. Hamon M, Clarke SW, Houghton E, Fowden AL, Silver M, Rossdale PD, Ousey JC, Heap RB (1991) Production of 5α-dihydroprogesterone during late pregnancy in the mare. J Reprod Fertil (Suppl) 44:529–535.

145. Fowden AL, Silver M (1987) Effects of inhibiting 3β-hydroxysteroid dehydrogenase on plasma progesterone and other steroids in the pregnant mare near term. J Reprod Fertil (Suppl) 35: 539–545.
146. Nathanielsz PW, Elsner C, Magyar D, Fridshal D, Freeman A, Buster JE (1982) Time trend analysis of plasma unconjugated and sulfoconjugated estrone and 3β Δ5-steroids in fetal in fetal and maternal sheep plasma in relation to spontaneous parturition at term. Endocrinology 110: 1402–1407.
147. Leadon DP, Rossdale PD, Jeffcoate LB, Allen WR (1982) A comparison of agents for inducing parturition in mares in the pre-viable and premature periods of gestation. J Reprod Fertil (Suppl) 32:597–602.
148. Seamans KW, Harms PG, Atkins DT, Fleeger JL (1979) Serum levels of progesterone, 5α-dihydroprogesterone and hydroxy-5α-pregnanones in the prepartum and postpartum equine. Steroids 33:55,56.
149. MacDonald PC, Dombroski RA, Casey ML (1991) Recurrent secretion of progesterone in large amounts: An endocrine/metabolic disorder unique to young women. Endocr Rev 12:372–401.
150. Challis JRG, Heap RB, Illingworth DV (1971) Concentrations of oestrogen and progesterone in the plasma of non-pregnant, pregnant and lactating guinea-pigs. J Endocrinol 51, 333–345.
151. Bedford CA, Harrison FA, Heap RB (1972) The metabolic clearance rate and production rate of progesterone and the conversion of progesterone to 20α-hydroxypregn-4-en-3-one in the sheep. J Endocrinol 55:105–118.
152. Sheldrick EL, Ricketts AP, Flint APF (1981) Placental production of 5β-pregnane-3α,20α-diol in goats. J Endocrinol 90:151–158.
153. Linzell JL, Heap RB (1968) A comparison of progesterone metabolism in the pregnant sheep and goat: Sources of production and an estimate of uptake by some target organs. J Endocrinol 41: 433–438.
154. Simpson ER, MacDonald PC (1981) Endocrine physiology of the placenta. Ann Rev Physiol 43: 163–188.
155. Simpson ER, Mahendroo MS, Means GD, Kilgore MW, Hinshelwood MM, Graham-Lorence S, Amarneh B, Ito Y, Fisher CR, Michael MD, Mendelson CR, Bulun SE (1994) Aromatase cytochrome P450, the enzyme responsible for estrogen biosynthesis. Endocr Rev 15:342–355.
156. Cole HH, Hart GH (1930) Sex hormones in the blood serum of mares. Am J Physiol 94:597–603.
157. Hart GH, Cole HH (1934) The source of oestrin in the pregnant mare. Am J Physiol 109:320–323.
158. Girard A, Sandulesco G, Friedenson A, Rutgers JJ (1932) Sur une nouvelle hormone sexuelle cristallisee retiree de l'urine de juments. C R Acad Sci 194:909.
159. Bhavnani BR (1988) The saga of the ring B unsaturated equine estrogens. Endocr Rev 9:396–416.
160. Nett TM, Holtan DW, Estergreen VL (1975) Oestrogens, LH, PMSG and prolactin in serum of pregnant mares. J Reprod Fertil (Suppl) 23:457–462.
161. Savard K (1961) The estrogens of the pregnant mare. Endocrinology 68:411–416.
162. Cox JE (1975) Oestrone and equilin in the plasma of the pregnant mare. J Reprod Fertil (Suppl) 23:463–446.
163. Cole HH, Hart GH, Lyons WR, Catchpole HR (1933) The development and hormonal content of fetal horse gonads. Anat Rec 56:275–293.
164. Raeside JI, Liptrap RM, Milne FJ (1973) Relationship of the fetal gonads to urinary estrogen excretion by the pregnant mare. Am J Vet Res 34:843–845.
165. Pashen RL, Allen WR (1979) The role of the fetal gonads and the placenta in steroid production, maintenance of pregnancy and parturition in the mare. J Reprod Fertil (Suppl) 27:499–509.
166. Pashen RL (1984) Maternal and foetal endocrinology during late pregnancy and parturition in the mare. Equine Veterinary Journal 16:233–238.
167. Labrie F (1991) Intracrinology. Mol Cell Endocrinol 78:C113–C118.
168. Mostl E (1994) The horse feto-placental unit. Exp Clin Endocrinol 102:166–168.
169. Gibori G, Khan I, Warshaw ML, McLeanm MP, Puryear TK, Nelson S, Durkee TJ, Azkar S, Steinschneider A, Rao MC (1988) Placental dervied regulators and the complex control of luteal cell function. Rec Prog Horm Res 44:377–429.
170. Johnson DC (1992) Cellular localization and factors controlling rat placental cytochrome P450 17α (CYP17): 17α-hydroxylase/C17,20-lyase activity. Biol Reprod 46:30–38.
171. Matt DW, MacDonald GJ (1984) In vitro progesterone and testosterone production by the rat placenta during pregnancy. Endocrinology 115:741–747.
172. Warshaw ML, Johnson DC, Kahn I, Eckstein B, Gibori G (1986) Placental secretion androgens in the rat. Endocrinology 119:2642–2648.

173. Jackson JA, Albrecht ED (1986) Estrogen regulates placental androstenedione production during rat pregnancy. Endocrinology 119:1052–1057.
174. Robertson HA, Dwyer RJ, King GJ (1985) Oestrogen in fetal and maternal fluids throughout pregnancy in the pig and comparisons with the ewe and cow. J Endocrinol 106:355–360.
175. Robertson HA, King GJ, Carnegie JA (1978) Appearance of oestrone sulphate in the allantoic fluid of the cow. J Endocrinol 79:243,244.
176. Carnegie JA, Robertson HA (1978) Conjugated and unconjugated estrogens in fetal and maternal fluids of the pregnant ewe: A possible role for estrone sulfate during early pregnancy. Biol Reprod 19:202–211.
177. Tsumagari S, Kamata J, Takagi K, Tanemura K, Yosai A, Takeishi M (1993) Aromatase activity and oestrogen concentrations in bovine cotylaedons and caruncles during gestation and parturition. J Reprod Fertil 98:631–636.
178. Gaiani R, Chiesa F, Mattioli M, Nannetti G, Galeati G (1984) Androstenedione and testosterone concentrations in plasma and milk of the cow throughout pregnancy. J Reprod Fertil 70:55–59.
179. Wooding FBP (1992) Current Topic: The synepitheliochorial placenta of ruminants: Binucleate cell fusions and hormone production. Placenta 13:101–113.
180. Ben-David E, Shemesh M (1990) Ultrastructural localization of cytochrome P450scc in the bovine placentome using protein A-gold technique. Biol Reprod 42:131–138.
181. Conley AJ, Mason JI (1990) Placental steroid hormones. Clin Endocrinol Metab 4:249–272.
182. Hall PF (1991) Cytochrome P-450 C_{21scc}: One enzyme with two actions: Hydroxylase and lyase. J Steroid Biochem Mol Biol 40:527–532.
183. Fevold HR, Lorence MC, McCarthy JL, Trant JM, Kagimoto M, Waterman MR, Mason JI (1989) Rat $P450_{17\alpha}$ from testis: Characterization of a full-length cDNA encoding a unique steroid hydroxylase capable of catalyzing both Δ4- and Δ5-steroid-17,20-lyase reactions. Mol Endocrinol 3:968–975.
184. Conley AJ, Bird IM (1997) The role of cytochrome P450 17alpha-hydroxylase and 3beta-hydroxysteroid dehydrogenase in the integration of gonadal and adrenal steroidogenesis via the delta-5 and delta-4 pathways. Biol Reprod 56:789–799.
185. Andersson S, Geissler WM, Patel S, Wu L (1995) The molecular biology of androgenic 17β-hydroxysteroid dehydrogenases. J Steroid Biochem Mol Biol 53:37–40.
186. Mason JI (1993) The 3β-hydroxysteroid dehydrogenase gene family of enzymes. TEM 4:199–203.
187. Hobkirk R (1985) Steroid sulfotransferases and steroid sulfate sulfatases: Characteristics and biological roles. Cell Biol 63:1127–1144.
188. Dwyer RJ, Robertson HA (1980) Oestrogen sulphatase and sulphotransferase activities in the endometrium of the sow and ewe during pregnancy. J Reprod Fertil 60:187–191.
189. Durkee TJ, McClean MP, Hales DB, Payne AH, Waterman MR, Khan I, Gibori G (1992) P45017α and P450scc gene expression and regulation in the rat placenta. Endocrinology 130:1309–1317.
190. Conley AJ, Head JR, Stirling D, Simpson ER, Mason JI (1992) Expression of steroidogenic enzymes in bovine placenta and fetal adrenals throughout gestation. Endocrinology 130:2641–2650.
191. Thorburn GD, Challis JRG, Currie WB (1977) Control of parturition in domestic animals. Biol Reprod 16:18–27.
192. Strauss JF III, Martinez F, Kiriakidou M (1996) Placental steroid hormone synthesis: Unique features and unanswered questions. Biol Reprod 54:303–311.
193. Lund J, Faucher DJ, Ford DP, Porter JC, Waterman, MR, Mason JI (1988) Developmental expression of bovine adrenalcortical steroid hydroxylases. J Biol Chem 263:16,195–16,201.
194. Tangalakis K, Coghlan JP, Crawford R, Hammond VE, Wintour EM (1990) Steroid hydroxylase gene expression in the ovine fetal adrenal gland following ACTH infusion. Acta Endocrinol 123: 371–377.
195. Randall GCB, Tsang BK (1986) Influence of the fetal pituitary-adrenal axis on fetal and maternal progesterone and unconjugated oestrogen concentrations in pigs. J Reprod Fertil (Suppl) 78: 65–72.
196. Saez JM (1994) Leydig cells: endocrine, paracrine, and autocrine regulation. Endocr Rev 15: 574–626.
197. Choong CH, Raeside JI (1974) Chemical determination of oestrogen distribution in the foetus and placenta of the domestic pig. Acta Endocrinol 77:171–185.
198. vom Saal FS (1981) Variation in phenotype due to random intrauterine positioning of male and female fetuses in rats. J Reprod Fertil 62:633–650.
199. vom Saal FS (1989) Sexual differentiation in litter bearing mammals: Influence of sex of adjacent fetuses. J Anim Sci 67:1824–1840.

200. Yamamoto T, Chapman BM, Clemens JW, Richards JS, Soares MJ (1995) Analysis of cytochrome P450 side-chain cleavage gene promoter activation during trophoblast cell differentiation. Mol Cell Endocrinol 113:183–194.
201. Clark BJ, Wells J, King SR, Stocco DM (1994) The purification, cloning and expression of a novel LH-induced mitochondrial protein in MA-10 mouse Leydig tumor cells: Characterization of the Steroidogenic Acute Regulatory protein (StAR). J Biol Chem 269:23,814–23,822.
202. Sugawa T, Holt JA, Driscoll D, Strauss III JF (1995) Human steroidogenic acute regulatory protein: Functional activity in Cos-1 cells, tissue-specific expression, and mapping of the structural gen to 8p11.2 and a pseudogene to chromosome 13. Proc Natl Acad Sci USA 92:4778–4782.
203. Chu X, Corbin CJ, Conley AJ (1994) A unique transcriptional start site for cytochrome P450 17α-hydroxylase (P450c17) in porcine trophoblast [Abstract]. Biol Reprod 50: (Suppl) 1, 50, 158.
204. Hinshelwood MM, Liu Z, Conley AJ, Simpson ER (1995) Demonstration of tissue-specific promoters in non-primate species that express aromatase cytochrome P450 ($P450_{arom}$) in placentae. Biol Reprod 53:1151–1159.
205. Corbin CJ, Khalil MW, Conley AJ (1995) Functional ovarian and placental isoforms of porcine aromatase. Mol Cell Endocrinol 113:29–37.
206. Schiff R, Arensburg J, Itin A, Keshet E, Orly J (1993) Expression and cellular localization of uterine side-chain cleavage cytochrome P450 messenger ribonucleic acid during early pregnancy in mice. Endocrinology 133:529–537.
207. Keeney DS, Ikeda Y, Waterman MR, Parker KL (1995) Cholesterol side-chain cleavage cytochrome P450 gene expression in the primitive gut of the mouse embryo does not require steroidogenic factor 1. Mol Endocrinol 9:1091–1098.
208. Le Goascogne C, Sananes N, Eychenne B, Gouezou M, Baulieu E-E, Robel P (1995) Androgen biosynthesis in the stomach: Expression of cytochrome P450 17α-hydroxylase/17,20-lyase messenger ribonucleic acid and protein, and metabolism of pregnenolone and progesterone by parietal cells of the rat gastric mucosa. Endocrinology 136:1744–1752.
209. Conley AJ, Corbin CJ, Hinshelwood MM, Liu Z, Simpson ER, Ford JJ, Harada N (1996) Functional aromatase expression in porcine adrenal gland and testis. Biol Reprod 54:497–505.
210. Pope WF (1994) Embryonic mortality in swine, In: Embryonic Mortality in Domestic Species (Zavy MT, Geisert RD, eds.), CRC, Boca Raton, pp. 53–78.
211. Nancarrow CD (1994) Embryonic mortality in the ewe and doe, In: Embryonic Mortality in Domestic Species (Zavy MT, Geisert RD, eds.), CRC, Boca Raton, pp. 79–98.
212. Ashworth CJ (1994) Nutritional factors related to embryonic mortality in domestic species, In: Embryonic Mortality in Domestic Species (Zavy MT, Geisert RD, eds.), CRC, Boca Raton, pp. 179–194.
213. Zavy MT (1994) Embryonic mortality in cattle, In: Embryonic Mortality in Domestic Species (Zavy MT, Geisert RD, eds.), CRC, Boca Raton, pp. 99–140.
214. Shaikh AA (1971) Estrone and estradiol levels in the ovarian venous blood from rats during the estrous cycle and pregnancy. Biol Reprod 5:297–307.

11 Secretion and Metabolism of Steroids in Primate Mammals During Pregnancy

Eugene D. Albrecht, PHD and Gerald J. Pepe, PHD

CONTENTS

INTRODUCTION

The principal steroid hormones produced by placenta and fetal adrenal gland during primate pregnancy are estrogen, progesterone, and the glucocorticosteroids. These hormones are critical to preparation of the uterus for implantation early in gestation, the maintenance of pregnancy thereafter, and the development of a healthy newborn at term (reviewed in *1,2*). For example, estrogen has a central integrative role in regulating key steps in the biosynthetic pathway for the formation of progesterone, a hormone essential to quiescence of the uterus and the maintenance of mammalian pregnancy. Progesterone, in turn, may have a role in immunosuppression to protect the developing conceptus from rejection by the maternal immune system. Estrogen and progesterone act in conjunction with prolactin, placental lactogen, and other hormones in development and preparation of the mammary gland for lactation. Estrogen also may stimulate utero-placental blood flow to provide nutrients and oxygen to the placenta and fetus for growth and development. Estrogen has been implicated in the cascade of events that initiate the process of labor. Finally, cortisol produced by the fetal adrenal gland has a critical role in the maturation of the lung and other organ systems in the developing fetus.

The present chapter will review the qualitative and quantitative nature of the biosynthetic and metabolic pathways involved in the production of estrogen and progesterone by the placenta and cortisol by the fetal adrenal gland during primate pregnancy. We will also review what is known about the developmental regulation of these steroid hormones in human and nonhuman primate pregnancy. Finally, the role of plasma steroid binding proteins on steroid hormone production rates and the influence that placental steroid hormone metabolism has on endocrine function in the fetus will be discussed.

STEROID HORMONE BIOSYNTHESIS

Cholesterol Uptake, Formation, and Intracellular Transport

During primate pregnancy, the ovary and placenta are major sites of estrogen and progesterone production, whereas the fetal adrenal produces cortisol and C_{19}-steroids as precursors for placental estrogen production. Cholesterol, the precursor for all steroid hormones, is derived either in the form of low-density lipoprotein (LDL) from the maternal circulation or *de novo* from acetate, depending on the organ and tissue involved. The uptake of LDL cholesterol within steroidogenic cells occurs via a receptor-mediated process, as originally shown in fibroblasts *(3)*, and free cholesterol is then liberated intracellularly via hydrolytic enzymes. The formation of cholesterol *de novo* from acetate depends on the rate-limiting enzyme 3-hydroxy-3-methylglutaryl coenzyme A (HMG CoA) reductase. The intracellular transport of free cholesterol then appears to involve its mobilization to the outer mitochondrial membrane and transfer from the outer to the inner mitochondrial membrane *(4)*. Although intracellular trafficking of cholesterol is not well understood, it may involve changes in cellular architecture, as well as specific regulatory factors, e.g., sterol carrier protein 2 (SCP 2) *(5–7)*. Because the aqueous space between the outer and inner mitochondrial membranes represents a major barrier for translocation of cholesterol, a hydrophobic compound, the production of steroids appears to be controlled by peptide factors that acutely regulate the translocation step. Several candidates have been proposed as acute steroid regulatory proteins in reproductive tissues, including steroidogenesis activator peptide (SAP) and steroidogenic acute regulatory (StAR) protein (*see 4, 8* for reviews). The StAR gene has been cloned *(9–11)* and is expressed in the ovary where it is increased by cAMP and stimulated pregnenolone synthesis *(4,11)*. However, StAR was not detected in the placenta *(11)*, and thus, it remains to be determined whether it or other regulatory cholesterol transport proteins have a role in steroidogenesis within the fetal–placental unit during primate pregnancy.

Steroidogenic Enzymes

Progesterone and Estrogen. Cholesterol is metabolized via a series of enzymes to form progesterone, the androgens, estrogens, and corticosteroids (Fig. 1). Most of these enzymes belong to the cytochrome P-450 family of oxidases, and many have been cloned and characterized in the human *(see 12,13)*. The conversion of cholesterol to pregnenolone is catalyzed by the mitochondrial P-450 cholesterol side-chain cleavage (P-450scc) enzyme system, which can only function in the mitochondrial environment *(14)*, and involves the 20α- and 22-hydroxylation of cholesterol, and scission of the cholesterol side chain between carbons 20 and 22. Within the mitochondria, electrons are transferred from NADPH, via adrenodoxin/ferredoxin reductase a flavoprotein, and adrenodoxin/ferredoxin an iron-sulfur protein, to P-450scc, which functions as a terminal oxidase and which is located on the matrix side of the inner mitochondrial membrane. The human P-450scc gene has been cloned, sequenced, and localized on human chromosome 5 *(15,16)*, and is transcribed into a single mRNA species and P-450scc protein product.

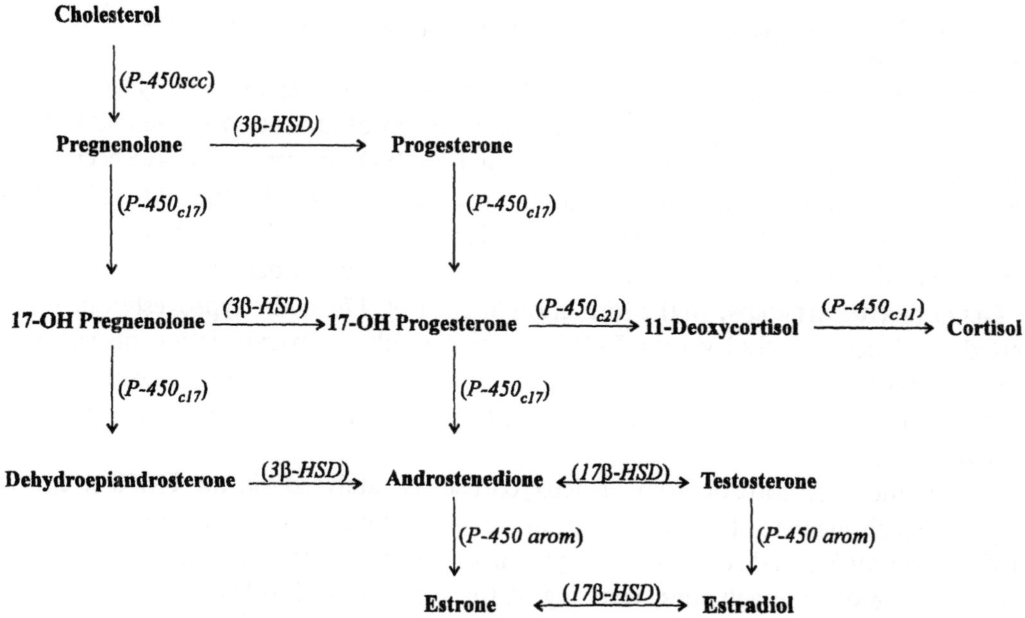

Fig. 1. Steroid biosynthetic pathway.

The Δ^5-3β-hydroxysteroid dehydrogenase/$\Delta^{5\text{-}4}$-isomerase (3β-HSD) enzyme converts the Δ^5-3β-hydroxysteroids, e.g., pregnenolone and dehydroepiandrosterone (DHA), to the Δ^4-3-ketosteroids, progesterone and androstenedione, respectively (Fig. 1). The 3β-HSD is located primarily in the microsomal cellular fraction, and catalyzes the dehydrogenation of carbon 3 and the isomerization of the double bond from steroid ring B to ring A. Two 3β-HSD genes and three related pseudogenes have been identified in humans *(17,18)*. In the human adrenal, only the type II 3β-HSD gene is expressed, whereas in the placenta, the type I is predominantly expressed. However, the types I and II can use either pregnenolone or DHA as substrates *(17)* and a single protein of 45,000-kDa mediates both dehydrogenase and isomerase activities *(19)*.

The conversion of the C_{21} steroids, pregnenolone and progesterone, to the C_{19} steroids, DHA and androstenedione (Fig. 1), is catalyzed by the P-450 17α-hydroxylase/17-20 lyase (P-450_{C17}), a single endoplasmic reticulum enzyme that results in 17α-hydroxylation to form the intermediates 17α-hydroxypregnenolone and 17α-hydroxyprogesterone, and scission of carbons 17 and 20. The P-450_{C17} enzyme also has a pivotal role in metabolizing progesterone to the glucocorticosteroids via 17α-hydroxylation only. A single P-450_{C17} gene has been cloned and sequenced in the human adrenal and testis, and lies on chromosome 10 *(20)*. A P-450 reductase flavoprotein receives electrons from NADPH and transfers them to the P-450_{C17}. The availability of electrons may determine whether the P-450_{C17} catalyzes 17α-hydroxylation only or C-17,20 scission as well *(21)*, and key amino acid residues of the enzyme may contribute to its catalytic activity and determine whether progesterone undergoes 17α- or 21-hydroxylation *(22)*.

The aromatization of the C_{19} steroids, androstenedione and testosterone, to the C_{18} steroids, estrone and estradiol, is catalyzed by a P-450 aromatase (P-450_{arom}). This enzyme catalyzes the double hydroxylation of the carbon 19 methyl group and hydroxylation of the carbon 2, resulting in the deletion of carbon 19 and aromatization of steroid ring A *(23,24)*. In this process, three electron pairs are transferred by P-450 reductase from three molecules of NADPH to P-450_{arom}. The human P-450_{arom} gene has been cloned and localized to chromosome 15 *(25,26)*.

A 17β-hydroxysteroid dehydrogenase (17β-HSD) enzyme mediates the hydroxylation/ oxidation of carbon 17, resulting in the interconversion of androstenedione and testosterone, and of estrone and estradiol (Fig. 1). Four 17β-HSD isoform types have been identified and cloned in various tissues, including the placenta *(27)*. All four 17β-HSDs utilize NAD(H) and/or NADP(H) as cofactors, and depending on which isoform is expressed in a particular tissue, result in reduction or oxidation as discussed below.

Glucocorticosteroids. In the formation of cortisol, 17α-hydroxyprogesterone is converted to 11-deoxycortisol via the P-450_{c21}, which results in hydroxylation of carbon 21 (Fig. 1). P-450 reductase transports electrons from NAPDH to P-450_{C21}. Although two P-450_{21} genes have been cloned, only one is active in humans *(28)*, and the second may be a pseudogene *(29)*.

The synthesis of cortisol from 11-deoxycortisol is catalyzed via the P-450_{C11} enzyme (Fig. 1), which mediates 11β-hydroxylation. A pair of tandomly duplicated genes located on chromosome 8 encode two forms of cytochrome P-450_{C11}, which also mediate 18-hydroxylase and 18-oxidase activities, resulting in the formation of aldosterone *(30–32)*. The P-450_{C11} is located on the inner mitochondrial membrane, and adrenodoxin and adrenodoxin reductase transfer electrons from NADPH to P-450_{C11}.

OVARIAN ESTROGEN AND PROGESTERONE PRODUCTION

The corpus luteum of pregnancy is the principal site of estrogen and progesterone biosynthesis in early stages of primate pregnancy. Consequently, ovariectomy results in a decline in estrogen and progesterone, and loss of pregnancy if performed in early gestation. For example, the ovary is required for steroidogenesis and pregnancy maintenance at least through d 40 (14% of gestation) in women *(33,34)*, d 20 (11% of gestation) in baboons *(35,36)*, and d 14-21 (11% of gestation) in rhesus monkeys *(37,38)*. At approximately the latter intervals in gestation in these primate species, the placenta assumes the role for the production of estrogen and progesterone.

Although luteinizing hormone (LH) is the initial luteotropic factor, the corpus luteum is rescued in early primate pregnancy by chorionic gonadotropin (CG), which then maintains the corpus luteum and stimulates the production of progesterone and estrogen *(39)*. LH/CG stimulate receptor-mediated LDL cholesterol uptake by the corpus luteum to promote steroidogenesis *(40)*. Interestingly, because the proliferative effects of CG on the corpus luteum are relatively short-lived, Christenson and Stouffer *(41)* have suggested that CG promotes further differentiation of existing cells in the corpus luteum of pregnancy, resulting in enhanced steroidogenesis.

PLACENTAL ESTROGEN BIOSYNTHESIS

Physiology of the Fetal-Placental Unit

Because the placenta in the human, baboon, and rhesus macaque does not express the P-450_{C17} enzyme necessary for C_{19} steroid formation *(42)*, it uniquely does not have the ability to form estrogen *de novo* during primate pregnancy. Consequently, the formation of placental estrogen in primates involves a functional fetal–placental unit, in which a major portion of the C_{19}-steroids, i.e., DHA and its sulfate DHAS, required for aromatization are derived from the fetal adrenal gland *(43,44)*. Thus, fetectomy causes a decrease in estrogen levels in the baboon *(45)* and rhesus monkey *(46,47)*. Moreover, fetal death during human *(48)* or rhesus monkey *(49,50)* pregnancy also results in a marked decline in estrogen. Because of the importance of the fetal adrenal to estrogen production in primates, suppression of the fetal pituitary–adrenocortical axis by the administration of the synthetic glucocorticosteroids betamethasone or dexamethasone also decreases placental estrogen production in humans *(51)*, baboons *(52,53)*, and rhesus monkeys *(54,55)*.

Approximately 40% of the estradiol and 90% of the estriol produced by the placenta during human pregnancy are derived from steroid precursors of fetal adrenal origin *(44)*, whereas the remainder originate from the maternal adrenals. Although a major proportion of the DHA and DHAS utilized for placental aromatization to estrogen in the baboon *(56)* is also derived from the fetus *(45,57)*, androstenedione is preferentially taken up from the maternal compartment for placental estrogen formation during baboon *(58)* and rhesus monkey *(59)* pregnancy. Consequently, the maternal adrenals also contribute, although to a lesser extent, C_{19} steroid precursors for placental estrogen production in nonhuman primates.

Patterns of Estrogen Production and Levels

During human placental development, stem-cell-like mononuclear cytotrophoblasts differentiate morphologically into multinucleated syncytiotrophoblasts *(60)*. As a consequence of this process *(60,61)*, and further functional differentiation *(62)*, syncytiotrophoblasts then produce extensive amounts of estrogen and progesterone, as well as the protein hormones. Although there are large amounts of estrone and estradiol synthesized during human pregnancy, because of extensive 16-hydroxylation in the fetal liver *(63)*, estriol is produced in great quantity during human *(64)*, as well as gorilla, orangutan, and chimpanzee *(65–67)* pregnancy. Because there is little or no 16-hydroxylase expressed in Old World monkeys, estriol is not produced, and thus estradiol is the major circulating estrogen and estrone the principal urinary estrogen metabolite in baboons *(68,69)*, rhesus monkeys *(70,71)*, vervet monkeys *(72)*, and langur monkeys *(73)*. Interestingly, in New World monkeys, e.g., marmosets, estradiol is the primary urinary metabolite of estrogen *(74,75)*, but in lion-tailed macques, estrone, estriol, 16α-hydroxyestrone, estradiol, and a flavonoid equol were identified in urine *(76)*. Consequently, with respect to the qualitative pattern of estrogen production, the Old World primates differ from the human in the ability to form extensive quantities of estriol.

Although in general there is a progressive increase in the circulating levels of the various estrogens with advancing primate pregnancy, there is considerable variability between primate species in the absolute levels. For example, in humans plasma unconjugated estrone, estradiol, and estriol concentrations reach maximum levels of 3–7, 6–30, and 6–20 ng/mL, respectively, near term *(77,78*, Fig. 2), whereas in the chimpanzee, the serum levels of these estrogens are lower *(67)*. In baboons, serum estradiol concentrations attain a maximum of 6–8 ng/mL at term *(68)*, whereas in rhesus monkeys, serum estradiol reaches a peak of < 1 ng/mL *(70)*.

An unequal distribution of estrogen secretion exists across the placenta during primate pregnancy. For example, Gurpide and coworkers *(79,80)* have shown that a larger proportion of estradiol than of estrone is released into the maternal compartment from the human placenta. Walsh and McCarthy *(81)* reported a similar phenomenon in the rhesus monkey,

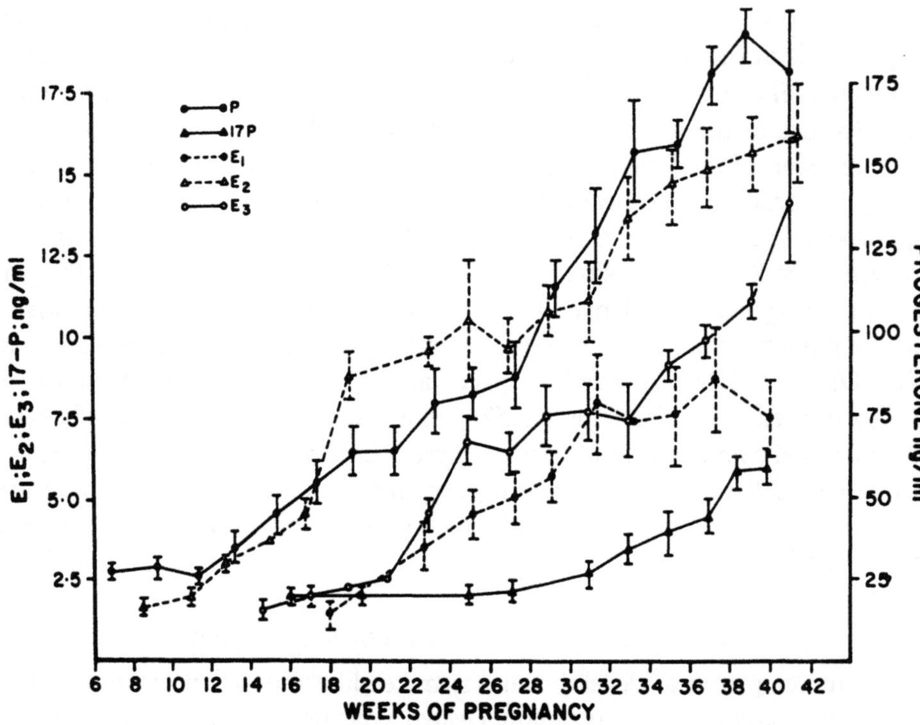

Fig. 2. Mean (± SE) plasma progesterone (P), 17-hydroxyprogesterone (17P), and unconjugated estrone (E_1), estradiol (E_2), and estriol (E_3) concentrations in human pregnancy. Reproduced with permission *(78)*.

and proposed that an estradiol carrier system may be involved in the preferential secretion of estradiol into the maternal circulation. However, the bidirectional secretion of estrogens could also reflect the fact that there are two different 17β-HSD enzymes catalyzing the oxidation-reduction of estradiol-estrone in the primate placenta *(82,83)* and that these enzymes are located in different subcellular compartments *(80)*. Thus, the placental 17β-HSD-1 enzyme, which preferentially catalyzes the reduction of estrone to estradiol, but does not utilize the carbon 19 androgens testosterone and androstenedione as substrates *(83)*, exists primarily in the cytosol. In contrast, placental 17β-HSD-2, which catalyzes the oxidation of estradiol to estrone *(83–85)* as well as that of testosterone to androstenedione and 20α-hydroxyprogesterone to progesterone *(84–87)*, has an extended hydrophobic amino-terminus *(88,89)*, and thus is primarily associated with the membranes of the endoplasmic reticulum *(84)*. Although it remains to be confirmed that 17β-HSD-1 and 2 reside in different components of the human and nonhuman primate placenta, the specific localization of 17β-HSD-2 to membrane fractions contiguous with the fetal capillaries would be consistent with the in vivo evidence demonstrating preferential secretion of estrone and androstenedione into the fetus. In addition, although studies in the baboon *(58)* and rhesus monkey *(59,81)* indicate that the differential secretion of estradiol-estrone between the maternal and fetal compartments is apparent at early, mid-, and late gestation, the ontogenesis and regulation of 17β-HSD-1 and 2 expression/localization in the human and nonhuman primate placenta remains to be elucidated. It is clear, however, that regardless of the underlying mechanisms, the bidirectional secretion of placental estrogens plays an important physiologic role in ensuring that the fetus is protected from the very high levels of bioactive estradiol produced by the placenta during primate pregnancy.

The principal means of excreting estrogen during primate pregnancy is via conjugation with glucuronic acid to form, for example, estriol-16-glucosiduronide, and sulfurylation to form estrogen sulfates. These conjugated estrogens are then excreted in urine in the latter water-soluble forms.

Regulation of Estrogen Production

Role of Utero–Placental Blow Flow. The formation of estrogen by the placenta is potentially regulated by placental mass *(90)*, the rate of utero–placental blood flow *(91,92)*, and/or availability of fetal adrenal C_{19} steroid precursors. Because there appears to be ample expression of the placental P-450_{arom} throughout primate gestation, this enzyme does not seem to be rate-limiting for the production of estrogen within the placenta.

It has been proposed *(91)* that placental clearance of steroid precursors through estrogen formation is directly related to utero–placental blood flow. This concept was initially put forth based on the finding that the placental utilization of DHAS for estradiol formation was greater than normal in pregnant women with twin gestations *(93)* and decreased in pregnancies complicated by pregnancy-induced hypertension *(94)*, a condition associated with a decrease in utero–placental perfusion. However, elegant studies conducted by Novy and coworkers *(95,96)* definitively showed in vivo that when utero–placental blood flow was reduced in baboons by graded reductions in maternal distal aortic blood flow, there was a corresponding decrease in the placental clearance of DHA through estradiol formation. Consequently, utero–placental perfusion has a significant role in regulating placental estrogen production in primates.

Fetal Adrenal C_{19}-Steroid Formation. Because the fetal adrenal provides a major portion of the precursors for estrogen synthesis within the placenta, growth and function of this gland greatly influence the production of placental estrogen during primate pregnancy. In support of this concept, an increase in fetal adrenal androgen production resulting from acute fetal hypoxemic stress in baboons causes a corresponding rise in maternal estrogen levels *(97)*. The fetal adrenal cortex of primates is comprised throughout gestation of a very unique fetal zone, which is the major source of the C_{19}-steroid substrates, e.g., DHA and DHAS *(98)*, and the mRNAs for the P-450scc and P-450_{c17} enzymes *(99)* involved in the formation of these estrogen precursors. There is a progressive increase in DHAS levels in the umbilical cord in the second half of human pregnancy *(100)*, apparently reflecting fetal adrenal growth. The definitive or neocortical zone, or an additional zone defined by Jaffe and coworkers *(99)* as the transitional zone, is the source of cortisol and develops relatively late in gestation. A number of studies have been conducted to elucidate the regulation of growth of and steroidogenesis within the primate fetal adrenal gland *(see 101,102*, for reviews).

Because the suppression of fetal pituitary ACTH secretion by the administration of synthetic glucocorticosteroids, e.g., betamethasone, during mid- to late gestation results in fetal adrenal atrophy in humans *(103)*, baboons *(52,53)*, and rhesus monkeys *(54,104)*, it is evident that fetal pituitary ACTH has a critical role in the maintenance and growth of the fetal adrenal gland in primates. Indeed, fetal anencephaly and, consequently, the absence of pituitary ACTH are associated with atrophy of the fetal adrenal gland and a striking decline in estrogen production in mid- to late gestation in humans *(105)* and rhesus monkeys *(49)*. Consequently, by stimulating fetal adrenal growth, and thus the overall capacity for C_{19} steroid formation, fetal ACTH has a major role indirectly in regulating placental estrogen biosynthesis.

ACTH also has an important role in regulating components of the steroid biosynthetic pathway within the primate fetal adrenal gland. A major source of cholesterol substrate for steroidogenesis within the human fetal adrenal is the receptor-mediated uptake of LDL. Thus, the addition of LDL to cultures of human fetal adrenal cells results in an increase in the formation of DHAS and cortisol *(106,107)*. ACTH has an important role in stimulating the receptor-mediated uptake of LDL by, and degradation of LDL within the human fetal adrenal to provide cholesterol substrate for steroidogenesis *(108,109)*. In addition, the *de novo* pathway for the formation of cholesterol may account for up to 30% of the daily secretion rate of DHAS and cortisol by the human fetal adrenal gland in culture *(110,111)*, and under these conditions, ACTH stimulates HMG CoA reductase, the rate-limiting enzyme for *de novo* steroidogenesis *(111)*. It appears, however, that the ACTH-stimulated LDL pathway is the preferred mechanism for fueling steroidogenesis in the primate fetal adrenal gland, because in the presence of ACTH and LDL, the HMG CoA reductase enzyme is not stimulated.

In addition to the provision of cholesterol substrate to the fetal adrenal cell, specific enzymes involved in C_{19}-steroid formation are regulated by ACTH. For example, the mRNAs for and activities of the P-450scc and P-450$_{C17}$ enzymes, and the hydroxysteroid-sulfotransferase (HST) enzyme that catalyzes the sulfurylation of DHA are stimulated in cultures of human fetal adrenal cells by ACTH *(112–114)*. Moreover, expression of the mRNAs for the ACTH receptor, P-450scc, and P-450$_{c17}$ in the fetal adrenal, along with serum estrogen levels, were suppressed in vivo in baboons by the administration of betamethasone and restored by ACTH *(53)*. Consequently, by stimulating fetal adrenal C_{19}-steroid formation, fetal ACTH has a pivotal role in regulating placental estrogen biosynthesis during primate pregnancy.

PLACENTAL PROGESTERONE BIOSYNTHESIS

Patterns of Progesterone Production and Levels

The production of placental progesterone progressively increases with advancing human gestation reaching a rate of over 200 mg/d at term *(115)* and a serum concentration of 150–175 ng/mL (*78;* Fig. 2) Chimpanzees also produce relatively large amounts of progesterone with serum levels approximating 50–120 ng/mL in late gestation *(67)*. In baboons, serum progesterone production rates also are significantly greater during pregnancy than in the menstrual cycle *(116,117)*, but serum progesterone levels plateau in the latter two-thirds of gestation to values that average 12 ng/mL *(45)*. In contrast, serum progesterone concentrations in rhesus monkeys approximate 3–4 ng/mL, values similar to those observed in the menstrual cycle *(118–120)*. Consequently, considering the quantities and pattern of progesterone production during primate pregnancy, the baboon appears to lie intermediate between humans, in whom there is a striking progressive increase in pregnancy and the rhesus macaque, in which there is no increase in pregnancy. Although there are differences in the quantities and profiles of progesterone and estrogen produced by the placenta between the various primates, it is important to note that substantially more progesterone and estrogen are produced during pregnancy than required to saturate the respective steroid receptors in target tissues and, consequently, to exert biologic effects.

The increase in the circulating concentrations of progesterone in primate pregnancy results from increased placental production and not decreased metabolism. For example, the metabolic clearance rate (MCR) of progesterone is not significantly different in nonpregnant and pregnant women *(115,121)* and baboons *(116)*. Splanchnic clearance of progesterone approximates 42% in pregnant women *(122)*. However, metabolism by extrahepatic tissues, e.g., brain, also contributes significantly to the clearance of progesterone *(123,124)*.

The levels of progesterone in the fetus are over twofold greater than in the mother during human *(125)*, baboon *(126)*, and rhesus monkey *(118)* pregnancy. Apparently, this in large part reflects a lower MCR of progesterone in the fetus than in the mother *(118)*. Although the transfer of progesterone across the placenta is bidirectional, at least in the rhesus monkey, the placenta is relatively impermeable to progesterone *(118)*.

In contrast to the striking decline in the peripheral levels of progesterone late in gestation in many laboratory species, e.g., the rat *(127)* and sheep *(128)*, there is no substantial change in the levels of progesterone or estrogen in the peripheral circulation in the immediate prepartum interval in humans *(78)*, baboons *(68)*, rhesus monkeys *(129)*, or several other primates *(130)*. Thus, although the precipitous decline in progesterone and rise in estrogen in many nonprimate species appear to be an integral part of the cascade of events leading to labor *(128)*, it is evident that the onset of labor in primates involves mechanisms other than a simple shift in the ratio of progesterone and estrogen.

The interconversion of progesterone and 20α-hydroxypregn-4-en-3-one is catalyzed via the 20α-hydroxysteroid dehydrogenase (20α-HSD) enzyme *(131,132)*. Although the equilibrium of the reaction typically favors progesterone *(133)*, there is a shift in the ratio of progesterone to 20α-hydroxypregn-4-en-3-one in umbilical cord serum in late baboon pregnancy, apparently reflecting enhanced secretion of the 20α-hydroxy metabolite into the fetal compartment *(126)* and extensive 20α-reduction of progesterone in the fetus *(134)*. It has been suggested *(135)* that increased metabolism of progesterone to its 20α-hydroxylated metabolite could cause a withdrawal of progesterone locally within the uterus, which might be important to the onset of labor.

The principal pathway for catabolism of progesterone in the human is via carbon 5 and carbon 20 reduction and hydroxylation to form pregnanediol, pregnanolone, and pregnanetriol. These metabolites are then conjugated to form sulfates and glucuronides, which are excreted primarily via urine.

Regulation of Progesterone Production

The LDL Pathway. The elegant studies of Simpson and coworkers *(136–138)* have shown that the utilization and metabolism of LDL for progesterone biosynthesis in human placental trophoblast cells in culture proceed according to the classical LDL pathway first described by Goldstein and Brown *(139)* in fibroblasts. Indeed, earlier studies conducted in vivo in pregnant women *(140,141)* and in vitro by perfusion of the human feto-placental unit *(142,143)* had shown that cholesterol was taken up from the maternal circulation by and utilized for progesterone formation within the placenta. Moreover, Winkel et al. *(138,144)* demonstrated that LDL uptake by human trophoblast cells in culture was mediated by saturable high-affinity binding, and LDL degradation occurred as a consequence of cellular uptake and internalization. A receptor-mediated pathway, involving coated pits and vesicles, endosomes, and lysosome-like bodies, has been shown ultrastructurally in human placental trophoblasts for the uptake of colloidal gold-conjugated LDL *(145)*. Henson and coworkers *(146)* have also demonstrated the existence of high-affinity receptor-mediated LDL uptake, i.e., binding and internalization, as well as LDL degradation by trophoblasts isolated from the baboon placenta. High density lipoprotein also increases progesterone secretion by human trophoblast cultures *(138,147)*, but is quantitatively much less effective than LDL. Although the *de novo* and de-esterification pathways represent additional sources of cholesterol in several tissues, these pathways do not appear to be major sources of cholesterol substrate for steroidogenesis within the primate placenta *(136,148)*. Consequently, the receptor-mediated LDL pathway is the principal source of cholesterol for the production of progesterone by the primate placenta.

Regulation by Estrogen

It has been well established during rat and rabbit pregnancy that estrogen is the major luteotropic stimulus resulting in maintenance of the corpus luteum and progesterone production (*see 149–151* for reviews). Estrogen stimulates the uptake of high-density lipoprotein cholesterol substrate *(152)* and P-450scc expression in the rat *(153)* and rabbit *(154)* corpus luteum, thereby promoting progesterone production. During mid- to late primate pregnancy, when the placenta is the principal source of progesterone, estrogen appears to have a similar regulatory role within trophoblasts (*see 1, 2* for reviews). In support of the latter concept, placental progesterone formation and serum progesterone concentrations were decreased in baboons by administration of the estrogen receptor antagonist ethamoxxytriphetal *(155–157)*, and this inhibitory effect was reversed by diethylstilbestrol *(158)*. Moreover, placental progesterone formation by human trophoblasts in culture was inhibited by an aromatase inhibitor and restored by estradiol *(159)*. A developmental increase in receptor-mediated LDL uptake *(160)* and LDL receptor *(161)*, and P-450scc *(62)* mRNA expression occurs in placental trophoblasts during the second half of baboon pregnancy when there is an increase in estrogen. The increases in LDL uptake and P-450scc are suppressed by antiestrogen, or fetectomy, which decreases the formation of estrogen, and reversed by estradiol *(157,162–164)*. In contrast, placental 3β-HSD and adrenodoxin mRNA expression, and 3β-HSD activity were not developmentally regulated or altered by antiestrogen treatment in baboons *(62,117)*. Therefore, inhibiting the action or levels of estrogen specifically blocked the developmental increase in placental LDL cholesterol uptake and expression of the P-450scc enzyme critical to the metabolism of cholesterol to pregnenolone within baboons (Fig. 3).

It appears, therefore, that an estrogen-dependent ontogenetic increase in key components of the progesterone biosynthetic pathway occurs within trophoblasts in the second half of primate pregnancy. Because these changes in endocrine function occurred specifically within syncytiotrophoblasts, it appears that although the morphological differentiation of cytotrophoblasts into syncytiotrophoblasts results in enhanced capacity for steroid and protein hormone biosynthesis *(60,61)*, there is further functional differentiation of syncytiotrophoblasts that results in enhanced upregulation of steroidogenesis.

Specific localization of the estrogen receptor has been shown by immunocytochemistry within the nuclei of human syncytiotrophoblasts in culture *(165)*, and the mRNA for the estrogen receptor *(166)* and specific estradiol binding *(167)* have been reported in the human placenta. Therefore, the primate placenta is an estrogen-responsive tissue.

In addition to the action of estrogen in trophoblasts, Carr and Simpson *(168,169)* have shown that estrogen and cortisol stimulated LDL cholesterol production by the human fetal liver, which is provided to the fetal adrenal gland as substrate for DHA/DHAS synthesis. These investigators have proposed, therefore, that the progressive increase in steroidogenesis within the fetal–placental unit results from a positive feedback system. However, estrogen also has a negative feedback action on ACTH-stimulated DHA/DHAS production by the baboon fetal adrenal, possibly to maintain the secretion of estrogen at a physio-

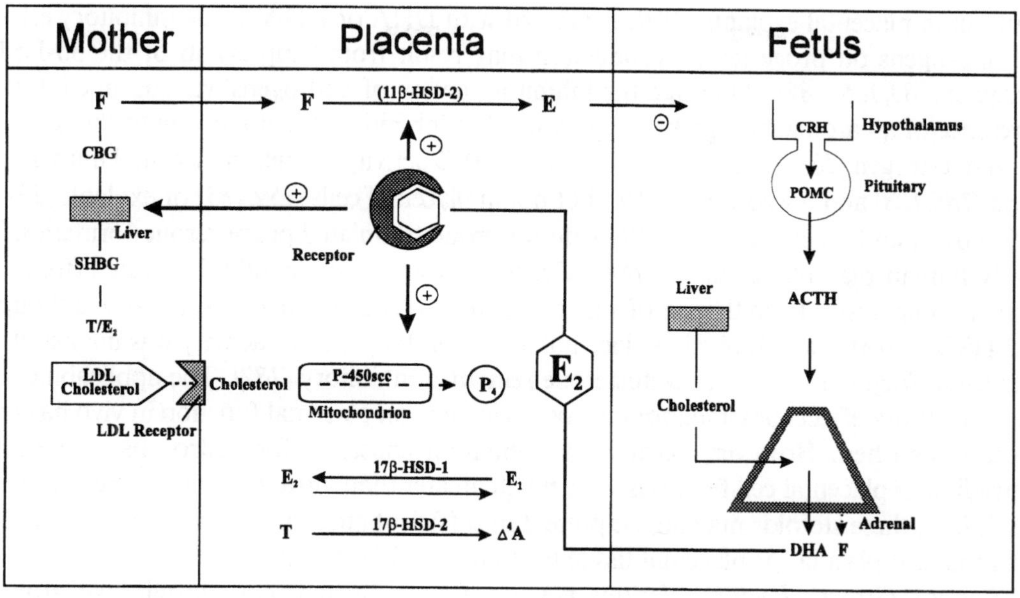

Fig. 3. Scheme for the production and metabolism of steroid hormones within the maternal, placental, and fetal compartments during primate pregnancy. Abbreviations: E_2, estradiol; E_1, estrone; P_5, pregnenolone; P_4, progesterone; F, cortisol; E cortisone; T, testosterone; Δ^4A, androstenedione; DHA, dehydroepiandrosterone.

logically normal level *(170–172)*. Consequently, a complex interaction of the placenta, fetal liver, and adrenal is operative during primate pregnancy, which is modulated by estrogen, and which apparently results in the normal balance of steroidogenesis.

ACTION OF cAMP. In cultures of human trophoblast cells, cAMP increases the secretion of progesterone and hCG *(173,174)* and the mRNAs for P-450scc *(175,176)*. Because the stimulatory effect of cAMP on progesterone formation was observed in cytotrophoblasts that were prevented from transforming into syncytiotrophoblasts, it was suggested that the cAMP-stimulated process was not dependent on syncytia formation. The cAMP-stimulated increase in P-450scc mRNA expression and progesterone secretion in human trophoblasts was suppressed by H-7 kinase inhibitor. Thus, the catalytic unit of protein kinases apparently is required *(175)*. Strauss and coworkers have postulated, therefore, that cAMP activates a protein kinase that phosphorylates a protein(s) integral to gene transcription of specific components of the progesterone pathway *(61,177)*.

Miller and coworkers *(178–180)* have extensively studied the transcriptional regulation of the P-450scc gene in the human placenta. Unique segments of the P-450scc promoter have been identified in the human placenta that are responsible for basal and cAMP-induced expression of the gene, and are very different from those in the adrenal or gonads *(178)*. A 55-kDa protein identified in the placenta, but not adrenal cells, appears to be a trans-acting factor required for placental P-450scc expression *(179)*. Therefore, the molecular mechanisms underlying the cAMP-mediated transcriptional activation of the P-450scc gene in trophoblast cells appear to be quite different from those in other steroid-secreting tissues.

OTHER FACTORS. *Androgens.* Inhibitory effects of androgens on progesterone secretion by the human placenta have been reported under in vitro conditions. For example, a significant decrease in progesterone formation occurs in term human placental cells *(181–183)*, but not in placental explants *(184)*, incubated with DHA or DHAS. The inhibitory effect of androgens on progesterone production may result from suppression of the 3β-HSD enzyme *(183,185–187)*. Although the inhibitory action of androgens was sustained in the presence of an aromatase blocker, suggesting that inhibition was not owing to the conversion to estrogen *(183)*, estradiol suppressed 3β-HSD activity in human placental mitochondria *(186,188)* and microsomes *(189)*, but not in placental cells *(159,183)* or explants *(184)*. Moreover, androstenedione and 19-nortestosterone stimulated progesterone formation in early human placental explants *(184)*. Consequently, the apparently disparate effects of steroids may result from the use of subcellular fractions and intact cells, because although 3β-HSD activity was inhibited in placental mitochondria, enzyme activity was unaltered in placental fragments, whereas testosterone remained inhibitory *(187)*. The applicability of the regulatory effects observed for androgens in vitro on placental function in vivo has not been established. However, because the inhibition constants for androgens, as well as estradiol, in placental cell fractions were much greater than intraplacental or plasma levels *(185,187)*, these steroids may not be present in sufficient amounts within human maternal or umbilical plasma, or placental tissue to decrease 3β-HSD activity.

Peptide Growth Factors. Various peptide growth factors, e.g., insulin-like growth factor-I (IGF-I) and IGF-II, are expressed *(190,191)* and have been reported to have stimulatory effects on P-450scc activity *(192)* within human trophoblasts. Epidermal growth factor (EGF) also has been observed to have stimulatory effects on progesterone formation in JEG-3 choriocarcinoma cells in culture *(193,194)*. The relative physiologic significance of peptide growth factors on placental progesterone production in primates and their potential interaction with the other factors that have been discussed above, however, remains to be determined.

ROLE OF PLASMA STEROID BINDING PROTEINS

Human and nonhuman primate plasma contains two glycoproteins, transcortin or corticosteroid binding globulin (CBG) and sex hormone binding globulin or testosterone-estradiol binding globulin (SHBG), that bind steroids with high affinity *(195–203)*. Of the physiologically important hormones circulating in plasma, CBG binds primarily cortisol and progesterone, whereas SHBG binds testosterone, dihydrotestosterone, and estradiol. Because steroid hormones are lipophilic and sparingly soluble in plasma, these proteins, as well as others, such as albumin, play an important role in transport of steroids throughout the body. It is well known, however, that the physiological actions of steroid hormones are elicited by that fraction circulating in plasma that is not bound (i.e., free) to high-affinity glycoproteins *(204)*. Thus in addition to facilitating transport, CBG and SHBG play important roles in regulating the level of unbound hormone available to the cell *(205, 206)*. Moreover, because binding to high-affinity proteins restricts the rate of hormone catabolism and thus elimination from the circulation, CBG and SHBG play a significant role in ensuring that hormone levels in the peripheral circulation are maintained relatively constant. Thus, these binding proteins also regulate the MCR and, consequently, the rate of hormone production *(207–210)*.

Recent studies have also demonstrated that in addition to binding steroid hormones, CBG and SHBG each bind to specific receptors on plasma membranes of various cells *(200,203,211)*, and it has been proposed that the steroid–glycoprotein complexes represent true physiologically active entities *(212)*. As pointed out by Strel'chyonok and Avvakumov

(212), evaluation of the biological functions regulated by CBG/SHBG–steroid complexes requires investigation of the structure and function of the membrane components involved and elucidation of the related multistep biochemical processes of transmembrane transport and signaling. Clearly, binding proteins play an important role in controlling cell function.

Corticosteroid Binding Globulin

The cDNA for human CBG has been isolated, and the sequence of the protein deduced from hepatic and pulmonary cDNAs *(213)*. In human and nonhuman primates, plasma CBG arises primarily from synthesis in and secretion by hepatocytes *(214–216)*, where both the protein and the mRNA have been detected *(203,217)*. Estrogen appears to play a significant role in regulating the plasma levels of CBG in women *(218)*, monkeys *(219)*, and baboons *(220,221)*, species in which administration of synthetic estrogens increases plasma CBG binding capacity, and results in a decrease in the MCR, but not the apparent secretion rate of adrenal cortisol *(220,222–224)*. Cortisol does not appear to increase CBG levels in the adult primate, since long term treatment with synthetic glucocorticoids did not alter CBG expression in baboons *(221)* or Japanese monkeys *(225)*. However, short-term treatment of rhesus macaques *(226)* and humans *(227,228)* with dexamethasone reduced CBG levels in nonpregnant adults by approx 30–40%.

In humans, presumably in response to the progressive increase in placental estradiol production, maternal plasma CBG levels increase markedly during the course of gestation with levels at term exceeding those in the nonpregnant state by approximately threefold *(229,230)*. CBG levels in pregnant rhesus monkeys *(231)*, squirrel monkeys *(232)*, and baboons *(220,233,234)* also exceed values in nonpregnant animals. However, in these nonhuman primates, CBG levels rise early in pregnancy, then plateau, and remain relatively elevated until very late in gestation at which time there appears to be a modest decline. This difference between the species does not reflect major changes in the nature of CBG, because the structural and functional characteristics of CBG are similar in human and several nonhuman primates *(235–238)*. Regardless of the pattern of secretion, because adrenal cortisol production is increased during primate pregnancy *(239)*, the gestational-induced increase in CBG in the baboon and human appears to ensure that the unbound levels of cortisol are only moderately elevated. In addition, because progesterone and cortisol bind to CBG with equal affinity *(230)*, the changes in CBG during primate pregnancy may also play a role in regulating the clearance and/or bioavailability of progesterone. Indeed, an experimental increase in serum cortisol levels in baboons decreases cortisol and increases progesterone MCR owing to the mutual interactions of these steroids with CBG *(233)*.

In contrast to the pattern of hepatic CBG synthesis/plasma concentrations in the mother, CBG levels in the primate fetus peak between early and midgestation, and then markedly decline thereafter *(219,220)*. In the baboon *(221)*, the decline in plasma CBG levels was owing to a decrease in fetal hepatic CBG expression and was associated with a change in the carbohydrate composition of circulating CBG. Thus, maturation of hepatic cells responsible for the adult pattern of CBG production and glycosylation occurs relatively late in gestation. It appears that the increase in hepatic CBG expression in the baboon fetus early in gestation is regulated by maternal cortisol *(221)*, which arrives in the fetus via transplacental passage *(240,241)*. Glucocorticoids also regulate fetal CBG expression and the pattern of glycosylation in the sheep *(217,242,243)*. The cortisol-induced increase in hepatic CBG synthesis early in gestation would presumably restrict cortisol availability to fetal tissues and thus may play a significant role in ensuring that maturation of organ systems regulated by cortisol does not occur prematurely (*see 2* for review). The decline in fetal CBG levels with advancing gestation may also play an important role in regulating the activity of the hypothalamic–pituitary–adrenocortical axis (HPAA) in the baboon *(2)* and sheep *(244)*. Thus, the decline in fetal CBG occurs concomitantly with a decrease in secretion of placental progesterone into the baboon fetus *(126)*, which would permit cortisol to bind to CBG. As a consequence, it would appear that the unbound levels of cortisol would be maintained despite a decline in CBG and, thus, permit maintenance of fetal pituitary ACTH secretion to drive maturation of the fetal adrenal gland. The factors regulating the decline in fetal CBG in late gestation remain to be elucidated.

Receptors for CBG have been isolated from plasma membranes of human liver, endometrium, and brush-border membranes of placental syncytiotrophoblasts *(212)*. In syncytiotrophoblast, binding of CBG did not restrict cortisol movement into the intravesicular space of isolated membrane vesicles. However, CBG complexed with cortisol also penetrated the syncytiotrophoblast membrane, and resulted in the activation of membrane adenylate cyclase and accumulation of cAMP within these cells. Interestingly, the presence of CBG decreased the oxidation of cortisol that was taken up by the microvesicles by more than 50%. It would appear therefore that CBG does not restrict cortisol uptake into the syncytiotrophoblast, but does protect the steroid from inactivation presumably by the 11β-hydroxysteroid dehydrogenase (11β-HSD) enzymes. It is apparent, therefore, that CBG is involved in the guided transport of cortisol to target cells and transmembrane transfer of cortisol and/or its hormonal signals. The potential relationship of these processes to placental growth and function remains to be elucidated.

Sex Hormone Binding Globulin

The cDNAs for human SHBG have been isolated from human liver cDNA libraries *(245–247)*, and the mRNA and protein detected in hepatic cells *(215,248)* and placenta *(249)*. SHBG is a dimeric 93-kDa glycoprotein with 68% homology to the androgen binding protein (ABP) produced by the Sertoli cells of the testis *(250)*. The molecular characteristics of SHBG are very similar in humans, baboons, and rhesus macaques *(251)*, and the protein is detected in the plasma of several mammalian species *(252)*. In contrast to the substantiated specific role of estrogen and perhaps glucocorticoids on hepatic CBG production, several other factors modulate hepatic SHBG. The latter include those that enhance (estrogen, thyroid hormone) or decrease (androgens, progestational agents, glucocorticoids, insulin, and IGF-I) SHBG levels and/or mRNA expression (*see 201* for review). Moreover, alterations in SHBG have been observed in many pathologic conditions, and measures of SHBG are often utilized clinically *(253–256)*.

In humans, plasma SHBG levels increase markedly during early to midgestation, and appear to plateau or increase only slightly thereafter *(257–259)*. Values of SHBG by midgestation are approximately three- to fourfold greater than those in the nonpregnant state *(257)*. In rhesus *(231)*, squirrel *(232)*, and cynomolgus *(260)* monkeys and baboons *(234)*, plasma SHBG levels also are greater in pregnancy and, like CBG, appear to increase early in gestation, plateau, and then decline by term to values that are equal to or lower than in the nonpregnant state *(232,261)*.

The increase in SHBG presumably plays a role in maintaining the peripheral levels of unbound and bound estradiol during early to late gestation. Although the unbound levels of estradiol appear to remain relatively low throughout most of human gestation *(262)*, they are two- to threefold higher near term than early midgestation in rhesus monkeys

(231). An increase in the unbound "free" levels of circulating estrogen late in gestation could be important to various physiologic parameters, e.g., mammary gland differentiation, uterine smooth muscle function, regulated by estrogen (*see 2* for review). The level of SHBG in the primate fetus in late gestation is much lower than in the maternal circulation *(261)*. Although estrone is preferentially secreted into the fetal circulation, estradiol concentrations continue to rise in the fetus throughout primate pregnancy *(1)*. Because fetal SHBG levels are relatively low late in gestation, it is possible that the fetus/fetal tissues are exposed to relatively high concentrations of unbound estradiol. The latter may play a role in eliciting the maturational events associated with fetal corticosteroid catabolism discussed below.

Similar to CBG, an equally important role of SHBG involves binding of the protein to membrane receptors *(201,263)*, which have been measured in human decidual endometrium and placental syncytiotrophoblast cells *(264,265)*. Moreover, the alternate N-terminal sequence of rat SHBG contains a nuclear targeting signal *(266)*, and it has been proposed that this sequence may act as a modulator of androgen receptor or estrogen receptor-mediated gene expression. Clearly, the role of SHBG binding to membrane receptors offers a potential new mechanism by which cell signaling is regulated by steroid hormones.

METABOLISM OF STEROID HORMONES

The metabolism of a steroid hormone either at its site of production (i.e., prior to secretion into the peripheral circulation) and/or in its target cell(s) ultimately determines the effective intracellular concentration of the hormone and, thus, its accessibility to its receptor and ability to affect target cell function. As discussed above, the ovary and placenta of human and nonhuman primates synthesize estradiol and progesterone, which are either secreted as such and/or first converted to their less potent metabolites estrone and 20α-OHP, respectively, by the enzymes 17β-HSD and 20α-HSD and then secreted. Peripheral target tissues also express the 17β-HSD and thus further regulate the effective concentration of bioactive estrogen and/or androgen reaching the nucleus. The maternal adrenal gland secretes cortisol throughout gestation, and this compound can be converted to its major metabolite cortisone by several maternal and fetal tissues, as well as the placenta, by the 11β-HSD enzymes. The latter is an important biological reaction, since cortisol, but not cortisone binds to the glucocorticoid receptor, i.e., cortisone is biologically inactive. It is apparent, therefore, that the expression of these various dehydrogenase enzymes in target tissues has the potential to modulate target tissue function critically.

Peripheral Metabolism of Androgens and Estrogens

Maternal Tissues. Based on in vitro and in vivo studies in humans *(267–271)* and rhesus monkeys *(272)*, in which differentially labeled steroid hormone pairs, such as testosterone–androstenedione or estradiol–estrone, were constantly infused, it has been demonstrated that the 17β-HSD enzymes are present in liver, kidney, and other organs in which blood flow is extensive. Although only a few studies have been performed during pregnancy, the conversion of androstenedione to testosterone in tissues of nonpregnant *(268)* and pregnant women *(92,273)* is similar. Therefore, it is possible that the level of 17β-HSD enzyme(s) in peripheral tissues is not altered during pregnancy, although this remains to be determined using more definitive experiments, including analyses of the mRNAs and peptide levels of 17β-HSD- 1 and 2.

The 17β-HSD-1 and 2 enzymes are also present in the uterus and breast of humans and rhesus monkeys *(274–280)*, and may act to modulate local concentrations of bioactive-bioinactive hormone in specific cell types of these tissues. For example, in breast the type I isoform of 17β-HSD, which catalyzes the formation of estradiol, is present primarily in breast adipose tissue, whereas the type II isoform acting to reduce estradiol to its less active metabolite estrone is present only in breast epithelial/glandular cells *(83)*. Consistent with enzyme studies, the 17β-HSD-2 appears to be the dominant isoform present in endometrium *(281)*, and its expression is regulated by progesterone in humans *(274,275,281)* and rhesus monkeys *(279,280)* during the luteal phase of the menstrual cycle. Unfortunately, there are no studies of the distribution or the regulation of 17β-HSD enzymes in estrogen target tissues of human and nonhuman primates during pregnancy.

Fetal Tissues. The metabolism of androgens by fetal tissues is particularly important to fetal development, because differentiation of the Wolffian structures and the primordia of the external genitalia/prostate *in utero* is regulated by testosterone, produced by the fetal testis, and dihydrotestosterone (DHT), respectively *(282)*. The conversion of testosterone to DHT is catalyzed by the enzyme 5α-reductase-type I in fetal skin of human and nonhuman primates and by the 5α-reductase-type II in the prostate *(283,284)*. The 5α-reductase enzymes are similar in human and cynomolgus monkeys *(285)*. In human and nonhuman primates, the female fetus is usually protected from testosterone and androstenedione of maternal origin *(286,287)*, presumably because these androgens are either catabolized by the placenta and/or fetal liver *(288)* and/or are converted to estrogens by placental aromatase *(59,289)*. Moreover, because the placenta expresses 17β-HSD-2, which actively oxidizes the C-17 hydroxyl of testosterone (or estradiol), any excess testosterone not aromatized by the placenta would be converted to the relatively weaker androgen androstenedione as has been demonstrated in the rhesus monkey *(287)*. Thus, although maternal testosterone, DHT, and androstenedione levels were elevated following maternal injection of testosterone to rhesus monkeys, only the levels of androstenedione were increased in the fetus. The absence of an increase in fetal testosterone levels in the presence of elevated levels of androstenedione suggests that the extensive amount of 17β-HSD enzyme activity measured in the primate fetal liver *(290)* is probably 17β-HSD-2. Consistent with this suggestion, in fetal baboons infused with radiolabeled androstenedione *(58)*, the percentage conversion of androstenedione to testosterone at mid- and late gestation was minimal.

Peripheral Metabolism of Cortisol and Cortisone

11β-Hydroxysteroid Dehydrogenase. There are at least two 11β-HSD enzymes (11β-HSD-1 and 2) that are the products of two different genes, catalyzing the oxidation-reduction of the glucocorticoids cortisol and cortisone in human and nonhuman primates *(2,291,292)*. It was originally shown that homogenates of human liver and kidney catalyzed both the oxidation and the reduction of cortisol-cortisone and utilized NADP(H) as cofactor preferentially *(293–296)*. This glucocorticoid oxido-reductase enzyme, termed 11β-HSD-1, was subsequently purified from rat liver and the gene cloned in the human *(297)* and baboon *(298)*. The cDNAs encoding 11β-HSD-1 have also been cloned from the human *(297)* and squirrel monkey *(299)*, and the predicted primary structure, which contains two consensus sites for *N*-glycosylation, is fairly well conserved. The enzyme exhibits a relatively low affinity (μ*M*) for substrate(s) *(300)* and utilizes NADP(H) as cofactor, and when expressed as a recombinant protein, catalyzes dehydrogenase and reductase reactions *(301)*.

The mRNA and peptide for 11β-HSD-1 have been detected in maternal liver, decidua, and placenta of the baboon *(302,303)*, human placenta *(304,305)*, and adult human liver, lung, decidua, ovary, and testis *(297,306,307)*. Interestingly, 11β-HSD-1 mRNA is not expressed in fetal tissues early in gestation, including in the liver or kidney of the baboon *(303)* or human *(304,306,308)*. However, 11β-HSD-1 peptide is expressed by late gestation in the baboon (Burch et al., in progress), and sheep *(309,310)* fetus. In the baboon placenta, the syncytiotrophoblast appears to be the predominant site of 11β-HSD-1 expression *(303)*.

The cDNAs for 11β-HSD-2 have been isolated from several mammalian species and the protein purified from the human placenta *(311–313)*. The cDNA for 11β-HSD-2 is only 20–25% homologous to that for 11β-HSD-1, but 37% identical to 17β-HSD-2 *(314)*. The deduced amino acid structure of 11β-HSD-2 is well conserved among the species and contains 396–404 amino acids with an apparent mol wt of 42,000 kDa. The enzyme has an affinity for substrate cortisol (< 100 n*M*) approaching that of the glucocorticoid and mineralocorticoid receptors *(313)*, utilizes NAD^+ as cofactor *(315)*, and is localized within the endoplasmic reticulum *(316)*. Unlike the relatively widespread tissue expression of 11β-HSD-1, 11β-HSD-2 expression is restricted to cells of the collecting duct of the adult and fetal kidney in humans *(304,317,318)*, and baboons *(303)* and to the syncytiotrophoblast of the human *(308,313,319,320)* and baboon *(303)* placenta. Because 11β-HSD-2 has such a high affinity for cortisol and only catalyzes the oxidation of cortisol to cortisone, its unique presence in the renal collecting duct and in the syncytiotrophoblast ensures that the concentrations of cortisol arriving at the renal mineralocorticoid receptor or into the fetus are relatively low. It has been proposed, therefore, that 11β-HSD-2-catalyzed conversion of cortisol to cortisone in these tissues plays an important physiologic role in renal *(321–323)* and fetal *(2)* function.

Regulation of Placental and Fetal 11β-HSD. In the baboon, the levels of the 11β-HSD-2 mRNA and protein in syncytiotrophoblast increase with advancing gestation *(303)*. Because NAD^+-dependent (i.e., 11β-HSD-2) enzyme activity is increased at midgestation in placentas of baboons treated with estradiol and decreased at term in animals in which estrogen was depleted *(324)*, it appears that estrogen regulates 11β-HSD-2 expression in baboon placental syncytiotrophoblast. Thus, the conversion of cortisol to cortisone by cultures of baboon syncytiotrophoblast was greater in cells obtained at term than at midgestation and increased in cells collected at midgestation following in vivo administration of estradiol *(325)*. The expression of 11β-HSD-2 also appears to be regulated by estrogen in fetal tissues. Thus, the conversion of cortisol to cortisone in the baboon fetus was enhanced twofold at midgestation when placental estrogen secretion into the fetus was increased *(326,327)* and decreased more than threefold in neonates delivered to mothers in which the action of estrogen was blocked by the estrogen receptor antagonist MER-25 *(328)*.

The syncytiotrophoblast levels of 11β-HSD-1 mRNA and peptide also increase with advancing stages of baboon gestation *(303)*. However, this increase may not reflect a direct effect of estrogen on the 11β-HSD-1 gene. Thus, the conversion of cortisone to cortisol (i.e., 11β-HSD-1 reductase) was similar in syncytiotrophoblast obtained from placentae of baboons at mid- and late gestation and at midgestation following maternal administration of estrogen *(325)*. Moreover, in baboon decidua, the conversion of cortisone to cortisol was not altered by estrogen *(325)*. The inability of estrogen to modulate placental/decidual catabolism of cortisone to cortisol is also manifest in the fetus. Thus, the conversion of cortisone to cortisol, which is negligible at midgestation, is not enhanced by estrogen treatment *(326)*. Although reduction of cortisone to cortisol by the fetus is increased late in gestation, this reaction was not altered in baboon neonates delivered to mothers treated with antiestrogen *(328)*. Thus, the factors regulating the ontogenesis of 11β-HSD-1 expression in placenta and fetal tissues remain to be elucidated.

Regulation of the Fetal HPAA by Estrogen-Induced Changes in Placental 11β-HSD. As discussed in Fetal Adrenal C_{19}-Steroid Formation, the fetal adrenal gland in primates does not initiate synthesis of cortisol until very late in gestation as a result of the lack of key enzymes, e.g., 3β-HSD, in the definitive zone. Although ACTH is considered essential to the growth and development of the fetal adrenal *(329)*, including induction of the ACTH receptor *(330)*, which is expressed by midgestation in the baboon *(331)*, our understanding of the factors regulating the activation of the pituitary–adrenocortical axis in the developing primate fetus is incomplete. Using in vivo approaches, we demonstrated that the pattern of cortisol-cortisone metabolism across the baboon placenta changed from preferential reduction (i.e., formation of cortisol) at midgestation to oxidation (i.e., formation of cortisone) near term *(240)*. Moreover, we demonstrated that this change was regulated by estrogen *(241)*, which stimulated the 11β-HSD-2 enzyme catalyzing cortisol oxidation within the syncytiotrophoblast *(324,325)*. Because the fetal pituitary of human and nonhuman primates is sensitive to feedback inhibition by synthetic glucocorticoids administered to the mother, we propose, as illustrated in Fig. 3, that this estrogen-induced change in placental metabolism of maternal glucocorticosteroids represents an active component in the sequence of events regulating fetal pituitary function. Although the interconversion of cortisol and cortisone within maternal tissues, such as the liver *(240,332)* and decidua *(325)*, does not change during baboon pregnancy, because of the preferential reduction of cortisone to cortisol by the placenta in early to midgestation, cortisol is the major steroid arriving within the fetal circulation at this time in pregnancy. We have proposed that this cortisol blocks fetal pituitary ACTH production and, thus, prevents the ACTH-dependent maturation of the fetal adrenal gland. With advancing gestation, the estrogen-induced increase in syncytiotrophoblast 11β-HSD-2/NAD^+-dependent conversion of cortisol to cortisone decreases transplacental secretion of cortisol into the fetus, which we propose activates fetal pituitary ACTH release and thus maturation of the fetal adrenal definitive zone (Fig. 3). Because estrogen simultaneously enhances 11β-HSD-2-catalyzed conversion of cortisol to cortisone in the fetus, this would also promote the release of ACTH by the fetal pituitary gland.

In support of this hypothesis, we have shown that proopiomelanocortin and ACTH expression in the fetal pituitary *(333)*, and the specific activities of the 3β-HSD and P-450c17 *(334)*, the cell signaling enzyme protein kinase A *(335)* ,and the ontogenesis of *de novo* cortisol production *(336)* in the baboon fetal adrenal at midgestation were increased to levels normally observed late in gestation by prematurely inducing placental NAD^+-dependent 11β-HSD-2 by the administration of estrogen. Clearly, the 11β-HSD enzymes controlling cortisol-cortisone metabolism within the placenta and fetus play an important physiologic role in ensuring the timely maturation of the fetus and its ability to exhibit adrenocortical self-sufficiency in the perinatal period.

SUMMARY

As summarized in Fig. 3, it is apparent that the production and metabolism of steroid hormones during primate pregnancy involve the collaborative actions of the mother, fetus, and placenta. In addition to the well-established functional interaction of the fetus and placenta with respect to estrogen production, estrogen stimulates the expression of the 11β-HSD enzymes controlling transplacental cortisol-cortisone metabolism, and thus activation and maturation of the fetal pituitary-adrenocortical axis. Consequently, the regulation of the fetal adrenal gland and its ability to synthesize glucocorticosteroids critical to fetal maturation is ultimately dependent on placental estrogen. Estrogen also regulates the uptake of LDL cholesterol and expression of the P-450scc enzyme catalyzing the synthesis of placental progesterone to promote the maintenance of pregnancy and stimulates hepatic cholesterol production to fuel adrenal steroidogenesis in the fetus. Selective distribution of the 17β-HSD enzymes in the placenta apparently ensures that estradiol is preferentially secreted into the maternal compartment, whereas highly active androgens, e.g., testosterone, are metabolized to androstenedione before entry into the fetus. Consequently, steroid-sensitive sexual differentiation of the fetus is not compromised. Estrogen also enhances maternal hepatic CBG and SHBG synthesis, resulting in an optimal balance of unbound:bound steroids to promote hormone bioactivity and bioavailability in target tissues. Clearly, the functional communication between the fetus and the placenta is extensive, and results in the timely regulation of steroidogenesis leading to the maintenance of pregnancy and maturation of a fully developed newborn.

ACKNOWLEDGMENTS

The excellent secretarial assistance of Wanda James with the computer preparation of the manuscript and illustrations is greatly appreciated. This work was supported in part by NIH Research Grant R01 HD-13294.

REFERENCES

1. Albrecht ED, Pepe GJ (1990) Placental steroid hormone biosynthesis in primate pregnancy. Endocr Rev 11:124–150.
2. Pepe GJ, Albrecht ED (1995) Actions of placental and fetal adrenal steroid hormones in primate pregnancy. Endocr Rev 16:608–648.
3. Brown MS, Kovanen PT, Goldstein JL (1979) Receptor-mediated uptake of lipoprotein-cholesterol and its utilization for steroid synthesis in the adrenal cortex. Recent Prog Horm Res 35: 215–257.
4. Stocco DM, Clark BJ (1996) Regulation of the acute production of steroids in steroidogenic cells. Endocr Rev 17:221–244.
5. Scallen TJ, Pastuszyn A, Noland BJ, Chanderbhan R, Kharroubi A, Vahoung GV (1985) Sterol carrier and lipid transfer proteins. Chem Phys Lipids 38:239–261.
6. Jefcoate CR, McNamara BC, Artemenko I, Yamazaki T (1992) Regulation of cholesterol movement to mitochondrial cytochrome P450scc in steroid hormone synthesis. J Steroid Biochem Mol Biol 43:751–767.
7. Reinhart MP (1990) Intracellular sterol trafficking. Experientia 46:569–611.
8. Miller WL (1995) Mitochondrial specificity of the early steps in steroidogenesis. J Steroid Biochem 55:607–616.
9. Clark BJ, Wells J, King SR, Stocco DM (1994) The purification cloning and expression of a novel luteinizing hormone-induced mitochondrial protein in MA-10 mouse. Leydig tumor cells. Characterization of the steroidogenic acute regulatory protein (StAR). J Biol Chem 269:28,314–28,322.
10. Sugawara T, Lin D, Holt JA, Martin KO, Javitt NB, Miller WL, Strauss JF III (1995) Structure of the human steroidogenic acute regulatory protein (StAR) gene: StAR stimulates mitochondrial cholesterol 27-hydroxylase activity. Biochemistry 34:12,506–12,512.
11. Sugawara T, Holt JA, Driscoll D, Strauss JF III, Lin D, Miller WL, Patterson D, Clancy KP, Hart IM, Clark BJ, Stocco DM et al. (1995) Human steroidogenic acute regulatory protein: functional activity in COS-1 cells, tissue specific expression, and mapping of the structural gene to 8p11.2 and a pseudogene to chromosome 13. Proc Natl Acad Sci USA 92:4778–4782.

12. Miller WL (1988) Molecular biology of steroid hormone synthesis. Endocr Rev 9:295–318.
13. Hanukoglu I (1992) Steroidogenic enzymes: structure, function, and role in regulation of steroid hormone biosynthesis. J Steroid Biochem Mol Biol 43:779–804.
14. Black SM, Harikrishna JA, Szklarz GD, Miller WL (1994) The mitochondrial environment is required for activity of the cholesterol side-chain cleavage enzyme, cytochrome P450scc. Proc Natl Acad Sci USA 91:7247–7251.
15. Chung BC, Matteson KJ, Voutilainen R, Mohandas TK, Miller WL (1986) Human cholesterol side-chain cleavage enzyme, P450scc: cDNA cloning, assignment of the gene to chromosome 15, and expression in the placenta. Proc Natl Acad Sci USA 83:8962–8966.
16. Morohashi K, Sogawa K, Omura T, Fujii-Kuriyama Y (1987) Gene structure of human cytochrome P-450(SCC), cholesterol desmolase. J Biochem 101:879–887.
17. Labrie F, Simard J, Luu-The V, Belanger A, Pelletier G (1992) Structure, function and tissue-specific gene expression of 3β-hydroxysteroid dehydrogenase/5-ene-4-ene isomerase enzymes in classical and peripheral intracrine steroidogenic tissues. J Steroid Biochem Mol Biol 43:805–826.
18. Simard J, Sanchez R, Durocher F, Rheaume E, Turgeon C, Labrie Y, Luu-The V, Mebarki F, Morel Y, Launoit Y, Labrie F (1995) Structure-function relationships and molecular genetics of the 3β-hydroxysteroid gene family. J Steroid Biochem Mol Biol 55:489–505.
19. Ishii-Ohba H, Inano H, Tamaoki B (1986) Purification and properties of testicular 3β-hydroxy-5-ene-steroid dehydrogenase and 5-ene-4-ene isomerase. J Steroid Biochem 25:555–560.
20. Picado-Leonard J, Miller WL (1987) Cloning and sequence of the human gene for P450c17 (steroid 17α-hydroxylase/17,20 lyase): similarity to the gene for P450c21. DNA 6:439–448.
21. Yanagibashi K, Hall PF (1986) Role of electron transport in the regulation of the lyase activity of C_{21} side-chain cleavage P-450 from porcine adrenal and testicular microsomes. J Biol Chem 261: 8429–8433.
22. Lin D, Zhang LH, Chiao E, Miller WL (1994) Modeling and mutagenesis of the active site of human $P450_{C17}$. Mol Endocrinol 8:392-402.
23. Fishman J, Goto J (1981) Mechanism of estrogen biosynthesis: participation of multiple enzyme sites in placental aromatase hydroxylations. J Biol Chem 256:4466–4471.
24. Fishman J, Rajo MS (1981) Mechanism of estrogen biosynthesis: stereochemistry of C-1 hydrogen elimination in the aromatization of 2β-hydroxy-19-oxoandrostenedione. J Biol Chem 256: 4472–4477.
25. Simpson ER, Evans CT, Corbin CJ, Powell FE, Ledesma DB, Mendelson CR (1987) Sequencing of cDNA inserts encoding aromatase cytochrome P-450 (P-450arom). Mol Cell Endocrinol 52:267–272.
26. Chen SA, Besman MJ, Sparkes RS, Zollman S, Klisak I, Mohandas T, Hall PF, Shively JE (1988) Human aromatase: cDNA cloning, Southern blot analysis and assignment of the gene to chromosome 15. DNA 7:27–38.
27. Luu-The V, Labrie C, Zhao HF, Couet J, Lachance Y, Simard J, LeBlanc G, Cote J, Berube G, Gagne R, Labrie F (1989) Characterization of cDNAs for human estradiol 17β-dehydrogenase and assignment of the gene to chromosome 17: evidence of two mRNA species with distinct 5′termini in human placenta. Mol Endocrinol 3:1301–1309.
28. Chung BC, Matteson KJ, Miller WL (1985) Cloning and characterization of the bovine gene for steroid 21-hydroxylase ($P450_{C21}$). DNA 4:211–219.
29. Bristow J, Gitelman SE, Tee MK, Staels B, Miller WL (1993) Abundant adrenal-specific transcription of the human P450C21A "pseudogene". J Biol Chem 268:12,919–12,924.
30. Nelson DR, Kamataki T, Waxman DJ, Guengerich FP, Estabrook RW, Feyereisen R, Gonzalez FJ, Coon MJ, Gunsalus IC, Gotoh O, Okuda K, Nebert DW (1993) The P450 superfamily: update on new sequences, gene mapping, accession numbers, early trivial names of enzymes, and nomenclature. DNA Cell Biol 12:1–51.
31. Kawamoto T, Mitsuuchi Y, Toda K, Miyahara K, Tokohama Y, Nakao K, Hosoda K, Yamamoto Y, Imura H, Shizuta Y (1990) Cloning of cDNA and genomic DNA for human cytochrome P-45011β. FEBS Lett 269:345–349.
32. Chua SC, Szabo P, Vitek A, Crzechik K-H, John M, White PC (1987) Cloning of cDNA encoding steroid 11β-hydroxylase $P450_{C11}$. Proc Natl Acad Sci USA 84:7193–7197.
33. Csapo AI, Pulkkinen MO, Ruttner B, Sauvage JP, Wiest WG (1972) The significance of the human corpus luteum in pregnancy maintenance. I. Preliminary studies. Am J Obstet Gynecol 112:1061–1067.
34. Berg AA, Thor L, Johansson EDB (1975) Luteectomy in early pregnancy. Ann Chir Gynaecol Fenn 64:249–251.

35. Castracane VD, Goldzieher JW (1986) Timing of the luteal-placental shift in the baboon (*Papio cynocephalus*). Endocrinology 118:506–512.
36. Hodges JK, Tarara R, Wangula C (1984) Circulating steroids and the relationship between ovarian and placental secretion during early and mid pregnancy in the baboon. Am J Primatol 7: 357–366.
37. Tullner WW, Hertz R (1966) Normal gestation and chorionic gonadotropin levels in the monkey after ovariectomy in early pregnancy. Endocrinology 78:1076–1078.
38. Bosu WTK, Johansson EDB (1975) Implantation and maintenance of pregnancy in mated rhesus monkeys following bilateral oophorectomy or luteectomy with and without progesterone replacement. Acta Endocrinol 79:598–609.
39. Stouffer RL, Ottobre JS, Vande Voort CA (1987) Regulation of the primate corpus luteum during early pregnancy, In: The Primate Ovary (Stouffer RL, ed.), Plenum, New York, pp. 207–220.
40. Carr BR, MacDonald PC, Simpson ER (1982) The role of lipoproteins in the regulation of progesterone secretion by the human corpus luteum. Fertil Steril 38:303–311.
41. Christenson LK, Stouffer RL (1996) Proliferation of microvascular endothelial cells in the primate corpus luteum during the menstrual cycle and simulated early pregnancy. Endocrinology 137:367–374.
42. Ainsworth L, Daenen M, Ryan KJ (1969) Steroid hormone transformations by endocrine organs from pregnant mammals. IV. Biosynthesis and metabolism of estrogens and progesterone by primate placental preparations in vitro. Endocrinology 84:1421–1429.
43. Diczfalusy E (1964) Endocrine function of the human fetal placental unit. Fed Proc 23:791–798.
44. Siiteri PK, MacDonald PC (1966) Placental estrogen biosynthesis during human pregnancy. J Clin Endocrinol Metab 26:751–761.
45. Albrecht ED, Haskins AL, Pepe GJ (1980) The influence of fetectomy at midgestation upon the serum concentrations of progesterone, estrone, and estradiol in baboons. Endocrinology 107: 766–770.
46. Tullner WW, Hodgen GD (1974) Effects of fetectomy on plasma estrogens and progesterone in monkeys (*Macaca mulatta*). Steroids 24:887–897.
47. Lanman JT, Thau R, Sundaram K, Brinson A, Bonk R (1975) Ovarian and placental origins of plasma progesterone following fetectomy in monkeys (*Macaca mulatta*). Endocrinology 96: 591–597.
48. Cassmer O (1959) Hormone production of the isolated human placenta. Acta Endocrinol Suppl 45:1–82.
49. Novy MJ, Walsh SW, Kittinger GW (1977) Experimental fetal anencephaly in the rhesus monkey: effect on gestational length and fetal and maternal plasma steroids. J Clin Endocrinol Metab 45: 1031–1038.
50. Bosu WT, Johansson ED, Gemzell C (1974) Influence of oophorectomy, luteectomy, foetal death and dexamethasone on the peripheral plasma levels of oestrogens and progesterone in the pregnant *Macaca mulatta*. Acta Endocrinol 75:601–616.
51. Challis J, Patrick J, Richardson B, Tevaarwerk G (1981) Loss of diurnal rhythm in plasma estrone, estradiol, and estriol in women treated with synthetic glucocorticoids at 34 and 35 weeks' gestation. Am J Obstet Gynecol 139:338–343.
52. Townsley JD (1976) Utilization of dehydroepiandrosterone and its sulphate for oestrogen production by pregnant baboons (*Papio papio*). Acta Endocrinol (Copenh) 81:830–838.
53. Aberdeen GW, Leavitt MG, Pepe GJ, Albrecht ED (1997) Effect of maternal betamethasone administration at midgestation on baboon fetal adrenal gland development and ACTH receptor messenger RNA expression. J Clin Endocrinol Metab (in revision).
54. Challis JRG, Davis IJ, Benirschke K, Hendrickx AG, Ryan KJ (1974) The effects of dexamethasone on plasma steroid levels and fetal adrenal histology in the pregnant rhesus monkey. Endocrinology 95:1300–1305.
55. Walsh SW, Resko JA, Grumbach MM, Novy MJ (1980) In utero evidence for a functional fetoplacental unit in rhesus monkeys. Biol Reprod 23:264–270.
56. Schut HAJ, Pepe GJ, Chez RA, Townsley JD (1978) Contribution of dehydroepiandrosterone and its sulfate to estradiol in baboon pregnancy. Am J Physiol 235:E78–E81.
57. Solomon S, Leung K (1972) Steroid hormones in nonhuman primates during pregnancy. Acta Endocrinol 166:178–190.
58. Waddell BJ, Albrecht ED, Pepe GJ (1992) Utilization of maternal and fetal androstenedione for placental estrogen production at mid and late baboon pregnancy. J Steroid Biochem Mol Biol 41: 171–178.

59. Walsh SW (1985) Regulation of progesterone and estrogen production during rhesus monkey pregnancy, In: Research in Perinatal Medicine (IV). Perinatal Endocrinology (Albrecht ED, Pepe GJ eds.), Perinatology, Ithaca, NY, pp. 219-242.
60. Kliman HJ, Nestler JE, Sermasi E, Sanger JM, Strauss JF III (1986) Purification, characterization, and *in vitro* differentiation of cytotrophoblasts from human term placentae. Endocrinology 118:1567-1582.
61. Strauss III JF, Kido S, Sayegh R, Sakuragi N, Gafvels ME (1992) The cAMP signalling system and human trophoblast function. Placenta 13:389-403.
62. Babischkin JS, Pepe GJ, Albrecht ED (1996) Developmental expression of placental trophoblast P-450 cholesterol side-chain cleavage, adrenodoxin and Δ^5-3β-hydroxysteroid dehydrogenase/isomerase messenger ribonucleic acids during baboon pregnancy. Placenta 17:595-602.
63. Milewich L, MacDonald PC, Carr BR (1986) Estrogen 16α-hydroxylase activity in human fetal tissues. J Clin Endocrinol Metab 63:404-406.
64. Adessi GL, Goutti-Coussieu C, Tran QN, Jayle MF (1976) Variations of the excretion curves of seven urinary estrogens during late pregnancy. Eur J Obstet Gynecol Reprod Biol 6:319-324.
65. Czekala NM, Benirschke K, McClure H, Lasley BL (1983) Urinary estrogen excretion during pregnancy in the gorilla (*Gorilla gorilla*), orangutan (*Pongo pygmaeus*) and the human (*Homo sapiens*). Biol Reprod 28:289-294.
66. Czekala NM, Hodges JK, Lasley BL (1981) Pregnancy monitoring in diverse primate species by estrogen and bioactive luteinizing hormone determinations in small volumes of urine. J Med Primatol 10:1-15.
67. Reyes FI, Winter JSD, Faiman C, Hobson WC (1975) Serial serum levels of gonadotropins, prolactin and sex steroids in the nonpregnant and pregnant chimpanzee. Endocrinology 96:1447-1455.
68. Albrecht ED, Townsley JD (1978) Serum estradiol in mid and late gestation and estradiol/progesterone ratio in baboons near parturition. Biol Reprod 18:247-250.
69. Merkatz IR, Beling CG (1969) Urinary excretion of oestrogens and pregnanediol in the pregnant baboon. J Reprod Fertil Suppl 6:129-133.
70. Hodgen GD, Dufau ML, Catt KJ, Tullner WW (1972) Estrogens, progesterone and chorionic gonadotropin in pregnant rhesus monkeys. Endocrinology 91:896-900.
71. Hopper BR, Tullner WW (1967) Urinary estrogen excretion patterns in pregnant rhesus monkeys. Steroids 9:517-527.
72. Setchell KDR, Bull R, Adlercreutz H (1980) Steroid excretion during the reproductive cycle and in pregnancy of the vervet monkey (*Cercopithecus aethiopus pygerythrus*). J Steroid Biochem 12: 375-384.
73. Shandilya LN, Ramaswami LS, Shandilya N (1976) Oestrogen metabolites in urine during the menstrual cycle, pregnancy and puerperium in the Indian hanuman langur (*Presbytis entellus entellus*). J Reprod Fertil 47:7-11.
74. Shackleton CHL (1974) Progesterone and oestrogen metabolism in the pregnant marmoset (*Callithrix jacchus*). J Steroid Biochem 5:597-600.
75. Eastman SAK, Makawiti DW, Collins WP, Hodges JK (1984) Pattern of excretion of urinary steroid metabolites during the ovarian cycle and pregnancy in the marmoset monkey. J Endocrinol 102:19-26.
76. Monfort SL, Thompson MA, Czekala NM, Kasman LH, Shackleton CHL, Lasley BL (1984) Identification of a non-steroidal estrogen, equol, in the urine of pregnant macaques: correlation with steroidal estrogen excretion. J Steroid Biochem 20:869-876.
77. Levitz M, Young BK (1977) Estrogens in pregnancy. Vitam Horm 35:109-148.
78. Tulchinksy D, Hobel CJ, Yeager E, Marshall JR (1972) Plasma estrone, estradiol, estriol, progesterone and 17-hydroxyprogesterone in human pregnancy. Am J Obstet Gynecol 112:1095-1100.
79. Gurpide E, Schwers J, Welch MT, Vande Wiele RL, Lieberman S (1966) Fetal and maternal metabolism of estradiol during pregnancy. J Clin Endocrinol Metab 26:1355-1365.
80. Gurpide E, Marks C, de Ziegler D, Berk PD, Brandes JM (1982) Asymmetric release of estrone and estradiol derived from labeled precursors in perfused human placentas. Am J Obstet Gynecol 144:551-555.
81. Walsh SW, McCarthy MS (1981) Selective placental secretion of estrogens into fetal and maternal circulations. Endocrinology 109:2152-2159.
82. Poutanen M, Isomaa V, Peltoketo H, Vihko R (1995) Role of 17β-hydroxysteroid dehydrogenase type 1 in endocrine and intracrine estradiol biosynthesis. J Steroid Biochem Mol Biol 55:525-532.
83. Blomquist CH (1995) Kinetic analysis of enzymic activities: Prediction of multiple forms of 17β-hydroxysteroid dehydrogenase. J Steroid Biochem Mol Biol 55:515-524.

84. Wu L, Einstein M, Geissler WM, Chan HK, Elliston KO, Andersson S (1993) Expression cloning and characterization of human 17β-hydroxysteroid dehydrogenase type 2, a microsomal enzyme possessing 20α-hydroxysteroid dehydrogenase activity. J Biol Chem 268:12,964–12,969.
85. Andersson S (1995) Molecular genetics of androgenic 17β-hydroxysteroid dehydrogenases. J Steroid Biochem Mol Biol 55:533–534.
86. Strickler RC, Tobias B (1980) Estradiol 17β-dehydrogenase and 20α-hydroxysteroid dehydrogenase from human placental cytosol: one enzyme with two activities? Steroids 36:243–253.
87. Blomquist CH, Lindemann NJ, Hakanson EE (1985) 17β-hydroxysteroid and 20α-hydroxysteroid dehydrogenase activities of human placental microsomes: kinetic evidence for two enzymes differing in substrate specificity. Arch Biochem Biophys 239:375–381.
88. Peltoketo H, Isomaa V, Maentausta O, Vihko R (1988) Complete amino acid sequence of human placental 17β-hydroxysteroid dehydrogenase deduced from cDNA. FEBS Lett 239:73–77.
89. Normand T, Husen B, Leenders F, Pelczar H, Baert J, Begue A, Flourens A, Adamski J, de Lanuoit Y (1995) Molecular characterization of mouse 17β-hydroxysteroid dehydrogenase IV. J Steroid Biochem Mol Biol 55:541–548.
90. Ogino M (1985) Productivity of estrogens by human placental organ culture at different stages of gestation. Endocrinol Jpn 32:607–613.
91. Everett RB, Porter JC, MacDonald PC, Gant NF (1980) Relationship of maternal placental blood flow to the placental clearance of maternal plasma dehydroisoandrosterone sulfate through placental estradiol formation. Am J Obstet Gynecol 136:435–439.
92. Edman CD, Toofanian A, MacDonald PC, Gant NF (1981) Placental clearance rate of maternal plasma androstenedione through placental estradiol formation: an indirect method of assessing uteroplacental blood flow. Am J Obstet Gynecol 141:1029–1037.
93. Worley RJ, Everett RB, Madden JD, MacDonald PC, Gant NF (1978) Fetal considerations. Metabolic clearance rate of maternal plasma dehydroisoandrosterone sulfate. Semin Perinatol 2:15–28.
94. Worley RJ, Everett RB, MacDonald PC, Gant NF (1975) Placental clearance of dehydroisoandrosterone sulfate and pregnancy outcome in three categories of hospitalized patients with pregnancy-induced hypertension. Gynecol Invest 6:28.
95. Fritz MA, Stanczyk FZ, Novy MJ (1985) Relationship of uteroplacental blood flow to the placental clearance of maternal dehydroepiandrosterone through estradiol formation in the pregnant baboon. J Clin Endocrinol Metab 61:1023–1030.
96. Fritz MA, Stanczyk FZ, Novy MJ (1986) Maternal estradiol response to alterations in uteroplacental blood flow. Am J Obstet Gynecol 155:1317–1325.
97. Shepherd RW, Stanczyk FZ, Bethea CL, Novy ML (1992) Fetal and maternal endocrine responses to reduced uteroplacental blood flow. J Clin Endocrinol Metab 75:301–307.
98. Seron-Ferre M, Lawrence CC, Siiteri PK, Jaffe RB (1978) Steroid production by definitive and fetal zones of the human fetal adrenal gland. J Clin Endocrinol Metab 47:603–609.
99. Mesiano S, Coulter CL, Jaffe RB (1993) Localization of cytochrome P450 cholesterol side-chain cleavage, cytochrome P450 17α-hydroxylase/17,20-lyase, and 3β-hydroxysteroid dehydrogenase isomerase steroidogenic enzymes in human and rhesus monkey fetal adrenal glands: reappraisal of functional zonation. J Clin Endocrinol Metab 77:1184–1189.
100. Parker CR Jr, Leveno K, Carr BR, Hauth J, MacDonald PC (1992) Umbilical cord plasma levels of dehydroepiandrosterone sulfate during human gestation. J Clin Endocrinol Metab 54:1216–1220.
101. Jaffe RB, Seron-Ferre M, Crickard K, Koritnik D, Mitchell BF, Huhtaniemi IT (1981) Regulation and function of the primate fetal adrenal gland and gonad. Recent Prog Horm Res 37:41–103.
102. Pepe GJ, Albrecht ED (1990) Regulation of the primate fetal adrenal cortex. Endocr Rev 11: 151–176.
103. Easterling WE Jr, Simmer HH, Dignam WJ, Frankland MV, Naftolin F (1966) Neutral C19-steroids and steroid sulphates in human pregnancy. II. Dehydroepiandrosterone sulfate, 16α-hydroxydehydroepiandrosterone and 16α-hydroxydehydroepiandrosterone sulfate in maternal and fetal blood of pregnancies with anencephalic and normal fetuses. Steroids 8:157–178.
104. Novy MJ, Walsh SW (1983) Dexamethasone and estradiol treatment in pregnant rhesus macaques: effects on gestational length, maternal plasma hormones, and fetal growth. Am J Obstet Gynecol 145:920–931.
105. Johannisson E (1979) Aspects of the ultrastructure and function of the human fetal adrenal cortex. Contrib Gynecol Obstet 5:109–130.
106. Simpson ER, Carr BR, Parker Jr CR, Milewich L, Porter JC, MacDonald PC (1979) The role of serum lipoproteins in steroidogenesis by the human fetal adrenal cortex. J Clin Endocrinol Metab 49:146–148.

107. Carr BR, Parker CR Jr, Milewich L, Porter JC, MacDonald PC, Simpson ER (1980) The role of low density, high density, and very low density lipoproteins in steroidogenesis by the human fetal adrenal gland. Endocrinology 106:1854–1860.
108. Carr BR, Porter JC, MacDonald PC, Simpson ER (1980) Metabolism of low density lipoprotein by human fetal adrenal tissue. Endocrinology 107:1034–1040.
109. Ohashi M, Carr BR, Simpson ER (1981) Effects of adrenocorticotropic hormone on low density lipoprotein receptors of human fetal adrenal tissue. Endocrinology 108:1237–1242.
110. Carr BR, Simpson ER (1981) *De novo* synthesis of cholesterol by the human fetal adrenal gland. Endocrinology 108:2154–2162.
111. Mason JI, Rainey WE (1987) Steroidogenesis in the human fetal adrenal: a role for cholesterol synthesized *de novo*. J Clin Endocrinol Metab 64:140–147.
112. Hornsby PJ, Aldern KA (1984) Steroidogenic enzyme activities in cultured human definitive zone adrenocortical cells: comparison with bovine adrenocortical cells and resultant differences in adrenal androgen synthesis. J Clin Endocrinol Metab 58:121–127.
113. Di Blasio AM, Voutilainen R, Jaffe RB, Miller WL (1987) Hormonal regulation of messenger ribonucoleic acids for P450scc (cholesterol side-chain cleavage enzyme) and P450c17 (17α-hydroxylase/17,20-lyase) in cultured human fetal adrenal cells. J Clin Endocrinol Metab 65:170–175.
114. Voutilainen R, Picado-Leonard J, DiBlasio AM, Miller WL (1988) Hormonal and developmental regulation of adrenodoxin messenger ribonucleic acid in steroidogenic tissues. J Clin Endocrinol Metab 66:383–388.
115. Lin TJ, Lin SC, Erlenmeyer F, Kline IT, Underwood R, Billiar RB, Little B (1972) Progesterone production rates during the third trimester of pregnancy in normal women, diabetic women, and women with abnormal glucose tolerance. J Clin Endocrinol Metab 34:287–297.
116. Albrecht ED, Townsley JD (1976) Metabolic clearance and production rates of progesterone in nonpregnant and pregnant baboons (*Papio papio*). Endocrinology 99:1291–1294.
117. Henson MC, Pepe GJ, Albrecht ED (1987) Transuterofetoplacental conversion of pregnenolone to progesterone in antiestrogen-treated baboons. Endocrinology 121:1265–1271.
118. Ducsay CA, Stanczyk FZ, Novy MJ (1985) Maternal and fetal production rates of progesterone in rhesus macaques: placental transfer and conversion to cortisol. Endocrinology 117:1253–1258.
119. Thau RB, Lanman JT, Brinson AO (1977) Metabolic clearance rates, production rates and concentrations of progesterone in pregnant rhesus monkeys. Biol Reprod 16:678–681.
120. Sholl SA, Wolf RC (1974) The metabolic clearance rate of progesterone in the pregnant rhesus monkey. Endocrinology 95:1287–1292.
121. Lin TJ, Billiar RB, Little B (1972) Metabolic clearance of progesterone in the menstrual cycle. J Clin Endocrinol Metab 35:879–886.
122. Little B, Billiar RB, Bougas J, Tait JF (1973) The splanchnic clearance rate of progesterone in patients with cardiac disease. J Clin Endocrinol Metab 36:1222–1229.
123. Billiar RB, Little B, Kline I, Reier P, Takaoka Y, White RJ (1975) The metabolic clearance rate, head and brain extractions, and brain distribution and metabolism of progesterone in the anesthetized, female monkey (*Macaca mulatta*). Brain Res 94:99–113.
124. Little B, Billiar RB, Rahman SS, Johnson WA, Takaoka Y, White RJ (1975) *In vivo* aspects of progesterone distribution and metabolism. Am J Obstet Gynecol 123:527–534.
125. Tulchinsky D, Okada DM (1975) Hormones in human pregnancy. IV. Plasma progesterone. Am J Obstet Gynecol 121:293–299.
126. Waddell BW, Pepe GJ, Albrecht ED (1996) Progesterone and 20α-hydroxypregn-4-en-3-one (20α-OHP) in the pregnant baboon: selective placental secretion of 20α-OHP into the fetal compartment. Biol Reprod 55:854–859.
127. Waddell BJ, Bruce NW (1989) Changes in the blood concentrations of progesterone and 20α-hydroxypreg-4-en-3-one during late pregnancy in the conscious rat: a specific role for metabolic clearance rate. Biol Reprod 40:1231–1236.
128. Challis JRG, Olson DM (1992) Parturition, In: The Physiology of Reproduction (Knobil E, Neill J, eds.), Raven, New York, p. 2177.
129. Walsh SW, Kittinger GW, Novy MJ (1979) Maternal peripheral concentrations of estradiol, estrone, cortisol and progesterone during late pregnancy in rhesus monkeys (*Macaca mulatta*) and after experimental fetal anencephaly and fetal death. Am J Obstet Gynecol 135:37–42.
130. Albrecht ED, Pepe GJ (1988) Endocrinology of Pregnancy, In: Nonhuman Primates in Perinatal Research (Brans YW, Kuehl, TJ, eds.), John Wiley, New York, pp. 13–78.
131. Little B, DiMartinis J, Nyholm B (1959) The conversion of progesterone to Δ^4-pregnene-20α-ol-3-one by human placenta *in vitro*. Acta Endocrinol (Copenh) 30:530–538.

132. Tseng L, Stolee A, Gurpide E (1972) *In vitro* measurements in human placenta and fetal membranes of rates of entry, metabolism and release of steroids. Endocrinology 90:405–414.
133. Rabe T, Kiesel L, Runnebaum B (1982) Partial characterization of the cytoplasmic 20α-hydroxysteroid dehydrogenase (EC 1.1.1.149) of the human placenta at term. J Steroid Biochem 16: 737–743.
134. Solomon S (1966) Formation and metabolism of neutral steroids in the human placenta and fetus. J Clin Endocrinol Metab 26:762–772.
135. Diaz-Zagoya JC, Wiest WG, Arias F (1979) 20α-Hydroxysteroid oxidoreductase activity and 20α-dihydroprogesterone concentration in human placenta before and after parturition. Am J Obstet Gynecol 133:673–676.
136. Simpson ER, Porter JC, Milewich L, Bilheimer DW, MacDonald PC (1978) Regulation by plasma lipoproteins of progesterone biosynthesis and 3-hydroxy-3-methyl glutaryl coenzyme A reductase activity in cultured human choriocarcinoma cells. J Clin Endocrinol Metab 47:1099–1105.
137. Simpson ER, Bilheimer DW, MacDonald PC, Porter JC (1979) Uptake and degradation of plasma lipoproteins by human choriocarcinoma cells in culture. Endocrinology 104:8–16.
138. Winkel CA, Gilmore J, MacDonald PC, Simpson ER (1980) Uptake and degradation of lipoproteins by human trophoblastic cells in primary culture. Endocrinology 107:1892–1898.
139. Goldstein JL, Brown MS (1974) Binding and degradation of low density lipoproteins by cultured human fibroblasts. Comparison of cells from a normal subject and from a patient with homozygous familial hypercholesterolemia. J Biol Chem 249:5153–5162.
140. Bloch K (1945) The biological conversion of cholesterol to pregnanediol. J Biol Chem 157:661–666.
141. Hellig H, Gattereau D, Lefebvre Y, Bolte E (1970) Steroid production from plasma cholesterol. I. Conversion of plasma cholesterol to placental progesterone in humans. J Clin Endocrinol Metab 30:624–631.
142. Telegdy G, Weeks JW, Lerner U, Stakemann G, Diczfalusy E (1970) Acetate and cholesterol metabolism in the human foeto-placental unit at midgestation. 1. synthesis of cholesterol. Acta Endocrinol (Copenh) 63:91–104.
143. Baird DT, Cockburn F, Galbraith A, Kelly R, Livingstone JR (1973) Formation of progesterone and pregnenolone from [4-^{14}C] cholesterol by the intact mid-term human foeto-placental unit perfused *in vitro*. J Endocrinol 56:187–202.
144. Winkel CA, Snyder JM, MacDonald PC, Simpson ER (1980) Regulation of cholesterol and progesterone synthesis in human placental cells in culture by serum lipoproteins. Endocrinology 106: 1054–1060.
145. Malassine A, Besse C, Roche A, Alsat E, Rebourcet R, Mondon F, Cedard L (1987) Ultrastructural visualization of the internalization of low density lipoprotein by human placental cells. Histochemistry 87:457–464.
146. Henson MC, Babischkin JS, Pepe GJ, Albrecht ED (1988) Effect of the antiestrogen ethamoxytriphetol (MER-25) on placental low density lipoprotein uptake and degradation in baboons. Endocrinology 122:2019–2026.
147. Rabe T, Kalbfleisch H, Haun A, Runnebaum B (1983) Influence of human lipoproteins on the progesterone synthesis of human term placenta in organ culture. Biol Res Pregnancy 4:75–83.
148. Simpson ER, Burkhart MF (1980) Acyl CoA: cholesterol acyl transferase activity in human placental microsomes: inhibition by progesterone. Arch Biochem Biophys 200:79–85.
149. Rothchild I (1981) The regulation of the mammalian corpus luteum. Recent Prog Horm Res 37: 183–298.
150. Holt JA (1989) Regulation of progesterone production in the rabbit corpus luteum. Biol Reprod 40:201–208.
151. Gibori G, Khan I, Warshaw ML, McLean MP, Puryear TK, Nelson S, Durkee TJ, Azhar S, Steinschneider A, Rao MC (1988) Placental-derived regulators and the complex control of luteal cell function. Recent Prog Horm Res 44:377–429.
152. Gibori G, Chen YD, Khan I, Azhar S, Reaven GM (1984) Regulation of luteal cell lipoprotein receptors, sterol contents, and steroidogenesis by estradiol in the pregnant rat. Endocrinology 114:609–617.
153. Goldring NB, Durica JM, Lifka J, Hedin L, Ratoosh SL, Miller WL, Orly J, Richards JS (1987) Cholesterol side-chain cleavage P450 messenger ribonucleic acid: evidence for hormonal regulation in rat ovarian follicles and constitutive expression in corpora lutea. Endocrinology 120:1942–1950.
154. Keyes PL, Kostyo JL, Hales DB, Chou SY, Constantino CX, Payne AH (1990) The biosynthesis of cholesterol side-chain cleavage cytochrome P-450 in the rabbit corpus luteum depends upon estrogen. Endocrinology 127:1186–1193.

155. Albrecht ED (1980) A role for estrogen in progesterone production during baboon pregnancy. Am J Obstet Gynecol 136:569–574.
156. Albrecht ED, Pepe GJ (1984) Effect of the antiestrogen ethamoxytriphetol (MER-25) and luteectomy on serum progesterone concentrations in pregnant baboons. Endocrinology 115:1717–1721.
157. Henson MC, Pepe GJ, Albrecht ED (1991) Regulation of placental low density lipoprotein uptake in baboons by estrogen: dose-dependent effects of the antiestrogen ethamoxytriphetol (MER-25). Biol Reprod 45:43–48.
158. Castracane VD, Goldzieher JW (1986) The relationship of estrogen to placental steroidogenesis in the baboon. J Clin Endocrinol Metab 62:1163–1166.
159. Wunsch DM, Anderson LD, Pepe GJ, Albrecht ED (1986) Regulation of progesterone formation by human placental cells in culture. Endocrinology 119:998–1003.
160. Henson MC, Pepe GJ, Albrecht ED (1992) Developmental increase in placental low density lipoprotein uptake during baboon pregnancy. Endocrinology 130:1698–1706.
161. Albrecht ED, Babischkin JB, Koos RD, Pepe GJ (1995) Developmental increase in low density lipoprotein receptor messenger ribonucleic acid levels in placental syncytiotrophoblasts during baboon pregnancy. Endocrinology 136:5540–5546.
162. Albrecht ED, Henson MC, Pepe GJ (1991) Regulation of placental low density lipoprotein uptake in baboons by estrogen. Endocrinology 128:450–458.
163. Babischkin JS, Pepe GJ, Albrecht ED (1997) Estrogen regulation of placental P-450 cholesterol side-chain cleavage enzyme messenger ribonucleic acid levels and activity during baboon pregnancy. Endocrinology 138:452–459.
164. Babischkin JS, Pepe GJ, Albrecht ED (1989) Regulation of progesterone biosynthesis by estrogen during baboon pregnancy: placental mitochondrial cholesterol side-chain cleavage activity in antiestrogen (ethamoxytriphetol, MER-25)-treated baboons. Endocrinology 124:1638–1645.
165. Billiar RB, Pepe GJ, Albrecht ED (1997) Immunocytochemical identification of the oestrogen receptor in the nuclei of cultured human placental syncytiotrophoblast. Placenta 18:365–370.
166. Chibbar R, Wong S, Miller FD, Mitchell BF (1995) Estrogen stimulates oxytocin gene expression in human chorio-decidua. J Clin Endocrinol Metab 80:567–572.
167. Kneussl ES, Ances IG, Albrecht ED (1982) A specific cytosolic estrogen receptor in human term placenta. Am J Obstet Gynecol 144:803–809.
168. Carr BR, Simpson ER (1982) Cholesterol synthesis in human fetal tissues. J Clin Endocrinol Metab 55:447–452.
169. Carr BR, Simpson ER (1984) Cholesterol synthesis by human fetal hepatocytes: effects of hormones. J Clin Endocrinol Metab 58:1111–1116.
170. Albrecht ED, Pepe GJ (1987) Effect of estrogen on dehydroepiandrosterone formation by baboon fetal adrenal cells *in vitro*. Am J Obstet Gynecol 156:1275–1278.
171. Pepe GJ, Waddell BJ, Albrecht ED (1989) Effect of estrogen on pituitary peptide-induced dehydroepiandrosterone secretion in the baboon fetus at midgestation. Endocrinology 125:1519–1524.
172. Albrecht ED, Henson MC, Walker ML, Pepe GJ (1990) Modulation of adrenocorticotropin-stimulated baboon fetal adrenal dehydroepiandrosterone formation in vitro by estrogen at mid-and late gestation. Endocrinology 126:3083–3088.
173. Caritis SN, Hirsch RP, Zeleznik AJ (1983) Adrenergic stimulation of placental progesterone production. J Clin Endocrinol Metab 56:969–972.
174. Feinman MA, Kliman HJ, Caltabiano S, Strauss III JF (1986) 8-Bromo-3′, 5′-adenosine monophosphate stimulates the endocrine activity of human cytotrophoblasts in culture. J Clin Endocrinol Metab 63:1211–1217.
175. Ringler GE, Kao LC, Miller WL, Strauss JF (1989) Effects of 8-bromo-cAMP on expression of endocrine functions by cultured human trophoblast cells. Regulation of specific mRNAs. Mol Cell Endocrinol 61:13–21.
176. Voutilainen R, Miller WL (1987) Coordinate tropic hormone regulation of mRNAs for insulin-like growth factor II and the cholesterol side-chain-cleavage enzyme, P-450scc, in human steroidogenic tissues. Proc Natl Acad Sci USA 84:1590–1594.
177. Nulsen JC, Woolkalis MK, Kopf GS, Strauss JF III (1988) Adenylate cyclase in human cytotrophoblasts: characterization and its role in modulating human chorionic gonadotropin secretion. J Clin Endocrinol Metab 66:258–265.
178. Moore CCD, Hum DW, Miller WL (1992) Identification of positive and negative placenta-specific basal elements and cyclic adenosine 3′, 5′-monophosphate response element in the human gene for P-450scc. Mol Endocrinol 6:2045–2058.

179. Hum DW, Aza-Blanc P, Miller WL (1995) Characterization of placental transcriptional activation of the human gene for P-450scc. DNA Cell Biol 14:451–463.
180. Bretano ST, Miller WL (1992) Regulation of human P450scc and adrenodoxin mRNAs in JEG-3 cytotrophoblast cells. Endocrinology 131:3010–3018.
181. Siiteri PK, Seron-Ferre M (1981) Some new thoughts on the fetoplacental unit and parturition in primates, In: Fetal Endocrinology (Novy MJ, Resko JA, eds.), Academic, New York, pp. 1–34.
182. Branchaud CL, Goodyer CG, Lipowski LS (1983) Progesterone and estrogen production by placental monolayer cultures: effect of dehydroepiandrosterone and luteinizing hormone-releasing hormone. J Clin Endocrinol Metab 56:761–766.
183. Grimshaw RN, Mitchell BF, Challis JR (1983) Steroid modulation of pregnenolone to progesterone conversion by human placental cells *in vitro*. Am J Obstet Gynecol 145:234–238.
184. Begum-Hasan J, Murphy BEP (1992) *In vitro* stimulation of placental progesterone production by 19-nortestosterone and C_{19} steroids in early human pregnancy. J Clin Endocrinol Metab 75: 838–845.
185. Townsley JD (1975) Inhibition of placental 3β-hydroxysteroid dehydrogenase by naturally occurring steroids. A potential mechanism regulating oestrogen synthesis from unconjugated precursors. Acta Endocrinol (Copenh) 69:740–748.
186. Rabe T, Kiesel L, Runnebaum B (1985) Regulation of human placental progesterone synthesis *in vitro* by naturally occurring steroids. J Steroid Biochem 22:657–664.
187. Raimondi SG, Olivier NS, Patrito LC, Flury A (1989) Regulation of the 3β-hydroxysteroid dehydrogenase activity in tissue fragments and microsomes from human term placenta: kinetic analysis and inhibition by steroids. J Steroid Biochem 32:413–420.
188. Das NP, Khan-Dawood FS, Dawood MY (1985) The effects of steroid hormones and gonadotropins on *in vitro* placental conversion of pregnenolone to progesterone. J Steroid Biochem 23: 517–522.
189. Depp R, Cox DW, Pion RJ, Conrad SH, Heinrichs WL (1973) Inhibition of the pregnenolone Δ^5-3β-hydroxysteroid dehydrogenase-$\Delta^{5\text{-}4}$ isomerase systems of human placenta and corpus luteum of pregnancy. Gynecol Invest 4:106–120.
190. Fant M, Munro H, Moses AC (1986) An autocrine/paracrine role for insulin-like growth factors in the regulation of human placental growth. J Clin Endocrinol Metab 63:499–505.
191. Han VK, Lund PK, Lee DC, D'Ercole AJ (1988) Expression of somatomedin/insulin-like growth factor messenger ribonucleic acids in the human fetus: identification, characterization, and tissue distribution. J Clin Endocrinol Metab 66:422–429.
192. Nestler JE, Williams T (1987) Modulation of aromatase and P450 cholesterol side-chain cleavage enzyme activities of human placental cytotrophoblasts by insulin and insulin-like growth factor I. Endocrinology 121:1845–1852.
193. Ritvos O (1988) Modulation of steroidogenesis in choriocarcinoma cells by cholera toxin, phorbol ester, epidermal growth factor and insulin-like growth factor I. Mol Cell Endocrinol 59:125–133.
194. Bahn RS, Speeg Jr KV, Ascoli M, Rabin D (1980) Epidermal growth factor stimulates production of progesterone in cultured human choriocarcinoma cells. Endocrinology 107:2121–2123.
195. Anderson DC (1974) Sex-hormone-binding globulin. Clin Endocrinol 3:69–96.
196. Brien TG (1981) Human corticosteroid binding globulin. Clin Endocrinol 14:193–212.
197. Englebienne P (1984) The serum steroid transport proteins: Biochemistry and clinical significance. Mol Aspects Med 7:313–396.
198. Heyns W (1977) The steroid binding β-globulin of human plasma. Adv Steroid Biochem Pharmacol 6:59–79.
199. Mercier-Bodard C, Renoir JM, Baulieu E (1981) Human sex steroid binding plasma protein. Horm Norm Abnorm Hum Tissue 2:25.
200. Rosner W (1990) The functions of corticosteroid-binding globulin and sex hormone-binding globulin: Recent advances. Endocr Rev 11:80–91.
201. Rosner W (1991) Plasma steroid-binding proteins. Endocrinol Metab Clin North Am 20:697–720.
202. Westphal U (1986) *Steroid Protein Interactions II*. Springer-Verlag, Berlin.
203. Hammond GL (1990) Molecular properties of corticosteroid binding globulin and the sex-steroid binding proteins. Endocr Rev 11:65–79.
204. Mendel CM (1989) The free hormone hypothesis: A physiologically based mathematical model. Endocr Rev 10:232–274.
205. Pardridge WM (1988) Selective delivery of sex steroid hormones to tissues in vivo by albumin and by sex hormone-binding globulin. Ann NY Acad Sci 538:173–192.

206. Ekins RP, Edwards PR (1988) Plasma protein-mediated transport of steroid and thyroid hormones. A Critique. Ann NY Acad Sci 538:193–203.
207. Bright GM (1995) Corticosteroid-binding globulin influences kinetic parameters of plasma cortisol transport and clearance. J Clin Endocrinol Metab 80:770–775.
208. Bright GM, Darmaun D (1995) Corticosteroid-binding globulin modulates cortisol concentration responses to a given production rate. J Clin Endocrinol Metab 80:764–769.
209. Petra PH, Stanczyk FZ, Namkung PC, Fritz FR, Novy MJ (1985) Direct influence of the sex steroid-binding protein (SBP) of plasma on the metabolic clearance rate of testosterone. J Steroid Biochem 22:739–746.
210. Namkung PC, Stanczyk FZ, Cook MJ, Novy MJ, Petra PH (1989) Half-life of plasma sex steroid-binding protein (SBP) in the primate. J Steroid Biochem 32:675–680.
211. Strel'chyonok OA, Avvakumov GV (1990) Specific steroid-binding glycoproteins of human blood plasma: novel data on their structure and function. J Steroid Biochem 35:519–534.
212. Strel'chyonok OA, Avvakumov GV (1991) Interaction of human CBG with cell membranes. J Steroid Biochem Mol Biol 40:795–803.
213. Hammond GL, Smith CL, Goping IS, Underhill DA, Harley MJ, Reventos J, Musto NA, Gunsalus GL, Bardin CW (1987) Primary structure of human corticosteroid binding globulin, deduced from hepatic and pulmonary cDNAs, exhibits homology with serine protease inhibitors. Proc Natl Acad Sci USA 84:5153–5157.
214. Weiser JN, Do YS, Feldman D (1979) Synthesis and secretion of corticosteroid-binding globulin by rat liver. J Clin Invest 63:461–467.
215. Khan MS, Knowles BB, Aden DP, Rosner W (1981) Secretion of testosterone-estradiol-binding globulin by a human hepatoma-derived cell line. J Clin Endocrinol Metab 53:448–449.
216. Khan MS, Aden DP, Rosner W (1984) Human corticosteroid binding globulin is secreted by hepatoma-derived cell line. J Steroid Biochem 20:677–678.
217. Challis JRG, Berdusco ETM, Jeffray TM, Yang K, Hammond GL (1995) Corticosteroid-binding globulin (CBG) in fetal development. J Steroid Biochem Mol Biol 53:523–527.
218. Musa BU, Doe RP, Seal US (1967) Serum protein alterations produced in women by synthetic estrogens. J Clin Endocrinol Metab 27:1463–1469.
219. Beamer NB, Hagemenas F, Kittinger GW (1972) Protein binding of cortisol in the rhesus monkey (*Macaca mulatta*). Endocrinology 90:325–327.
220. Oakey RE (1975) Serum cortisol binding capacity and cortisol concentration in the pregnant baboon and its fetus during gestation. Endocrinology 97:1024–1029.
221. Pepe GJ, Hodgert Jury H, Hammond GL, Albrecht ED (1996) Developmental regulation of corticosteroid-binding globulin biosynthesis in the baboon fetus. Endocrinology 137:3323–3328.
222. Billiar RB, Jassani M, Little B (1975) Estrogen and the metabolism of progesterone in vivo. Am J Obstet Gynecol 121:877–884.
223. Beitins IZ, Bayard F, Ances IG, Kowarski A, Migeon CJ (1973) The metabolic clearance rate, blood production, interconversion, and transplacental passage of cortisol and cortisone in pregnancy near term. Pediatr Res 7:509–519.
224. Pepe GJ, Johnson DK, Albrecht ED (1982) The effects of estrogen on cortisol metabolism in female baboons. Steroids 39:471–478.
225. Yamamoto S, Ohsawa N (1976) Effects of dexamethasone on the levels of plasma corticosteroid binding globulin in rats and monkeys. Biochem Biophys Res Commun 72:489–498.
226. Stanczyk FZ, Petra PH, Senner JW, Novy MJ (1985) Effect of dexamethasone treatment on sex steroid-binding protein, corticosteroid-binding globulin, and steroid hormones in cycling rhesus macaques. Am J Obstet Gynecol 151:464–470.
227. Schlechte JA, Hamilton D (1987) The effect of glucocorticoids on corticosteroid binding globulin. Clin Endocrinol 27:197–203.
228. Frairia R, Agrimonti F, Fortunati N, Fazzari A, Gennari P, Berta L (1988) Influence of naturally occurring and synthetic glucocorticoids on corticosteroid-binding globulin-steroid interaction in human peripheral plasma. Ann NY Acad Sci 538:287–303.
229. Doe RP, Fernandez R, Seal US (1964) Measurement of corticosteroid-binding globulin in man. J Clin Endocrinol Metab 24:1029–1039.
230. Westphal U (1971) Steroid-protein interactions, In: *Monographs on Endocrinology* (Gross F, Labhart A, Mann T, Samuels LT, Zander J eds.), Springer-Verlag, New York, pp. 209–236.
231. Stanczyk FZ, Hess DL, Namkung PC, Senner JW, Petra PH, Novy MJ (1986) Alterations in sex steroid-binding protein (SBP), corticosteroid-binding globulin (CBG), and steroid hormone concentrations during pregnancy in rhesus macaques. Biol Reprod 35:126–132.

232. Schiller HS, Holm RA, Sackett GP (1978) Alterations in steroid binding plasma proteins in *Macaca nemestrina* during pregnancy. Am J Physiol 234(5):E489–E493.
233. Pepe GJ, Albrecht ED, Townsley JD (1977) Serum cortisol levels affect the metabolic clearance rate of progesterone in female baboons. Steroids 30:561–568.
234. Stanczyk FZ, Namkung PC, Petra PH, Novy MJ (1986) Circulating sex steroid-binding protein (SBP) and corticosteroid-binding globulin (CBG) levels during pregnancy, infancy, and following estrogen treatment in the baboon, In: *Binding Proteins of Steroid Hormones* (Forest MG, Pugeat M, eds.), John Libbey, Paris, p. 634.
235. Robinson PA, Hawkey C, Hammond GL (1985) A phylogenetic study of the structural and functional characteristics of corticosteroid binding globulin in primates. J Endocrinol 104:251–257.
236. Klosterman LL, Murai JT, Siiteri PK (1986) Cortisol levels, binding, and properties of corticosteroid-binding globulin in the serum of primates. Endocrinology 118:424–434.
237. Pugeat M, Chrousos GP, Nisula BC, Loriaux DL, Brandon DD, Lipsett MB (1984) Plasma cortisol transport and primate evolution. Endocrinology 115:357–361.
238. Hammond GL, Smith CL, Lahteenmaki PLA, Grolla A, Warmels-Rodenhiser S, Hodgert H, Murai JT, Siiteri PK (1994) Squirrel monkey corticosteroid-binding globulin: Primary structure and comparison with the human protein. Endocrinology 134:891–898.
239. Pepe GJ, Albrecht ED (1985) Transplacental corticosteroid metabolism during baboon pregnancy, In: *Research in Perinatal Medicine (IV), Perinatal Endocrinology* (Albrecht ED, Pepe GJ, eds.), Perinatology, Ithaca, NY, pp. 201–217.
240. Pepe GJ, Albrecht ED (1984) Transuteroplacental metabolism of cortisol and cortisone during mid- and late gestation in the baboon. Endocrinology 115:1946–1951.
241. Pepe GJ, Waddell BJ, Stahl SJ, Albrecht ED (1988) The regulation of transplacental cortisol-cortisone metabolism by estrogen in pregnant baboons. Endocrinology 122:78–83.
242. Berdusco ETM, Hammond GL, Jacobs RA, Grolla A, Akagi K, Langlois D, Challis JRG (1993) Glucocorticoid-induced increase in plasma corticosteroid-binding globulin levels in fetal sheep is associated with increased biosynthesis and alterations in glycosylation. Endocrinology 132: 2001–2008.
243. Berdusco ETM, Milne WK, Challis JRG (1994) Low-dose cortisol infusion increases plasma corticosteroid-binding globulin (CBG) and the amount of hepatic CBG mRNA in fetal sheep on day 100 of gestation. J Endocrinol 140:425–430.
244. Berdusco ETM, Yang K, Hammond GL, Challis JRG (1995) Corticosteroid-binding globulin (CBG) production by hepatic and extra-hepatic sites in the ovine fetus; effects of CBG on glucocorticoid negative feedback on pituitary cells *in vitro*. J Endocrinol 146:121–130.
245. Hammond GL, Underhill DA, Smith CL, Goping IS, Harley MJ, Musto NA, Cheng CY, Bardin CW (1987) The cDNA-deduced primary structure of human sex hormone-binding globulin and location of its steroid-binding domain. FEBS Lett 215:100–104.
246. Que BG, Petra PH (1987) Characterization of a cDNA coding for sex steroid-binding protein of human plasma. FEBS Lett 219:405–409.
247. Gershagen S, Fernlund P, Lundwall A (1987) A cDNA coding for human sex hormone-binding globulin. Homology to vitamin K-dependent protein S. FEBS Lett 220:129–135.
248. Loukovaara M, Carson M, Adlercreutz H (1995) Regulation of production and secretion of sex hormone-binding globulin in HepG2 cell cultures by hormones and growth factors. J Clin Endocrinol Metab 80:160–164.
249. Larrea F, Diaz L, Carino C, Larriva-Sahd J, Carrillo L, Orozco H, Ulloa-Aguirre A (1993) Evidence that human placenta is a site of sex hormone-binding globulin gene expression. J Steroid Biochem Mol Biol 46:497–505.
250. Danzo BJ, Joseph DR (1994) Structure-function relationships of rat androgen-binding protein/human sex-hormone binding globulin: The effect of mutagenesis on steroid-binding parameters. Endocrinology 135:157–167.
251. Petra PH, Namkung PC, Senear DF, McCrae DA, Rousslang KW, Teller DC, Ross JBA (1986) Molecular characterization of the sex steroid binding protein (SBP) of plasma. Re-examination of rabbit SBP and comparison with the human, macaque and baboon proteins. J Steroid Biochem 25:191–200.
252. Corvol P, Bardin CW (1973) Species distribution of testosterone-binding globulin. Biol Reprod 8: 277–282.
253. Pasquali R, Casimirri F, De Iasio R, Mesini P, Boschi S, Chierici R, Flamia R, Biscotti M, Vicennati V (1995) Insulin regulates testosterone and sex hormone-binding globulin concentrations in adult normal weight and obese men. J Clin Endocrinol Metab 80:654–658.

254. Gafny M, Silbergeld A, Klinger B, Wasserman M, Laron Z (1994) Comparative effects of GH, IGF-I and insulin on serum sex hormone binding globulin. Clin Endocrinol 41:169–175.
255. Botwood N, Hamilton-Fairley D, Kiddy D, Robinson S, Franks S (1995) Sex hormone-binding globulin and female reproductive function. J Steroid Biochem Mol Biol 53:529–531.
256. Simmons D (1995) Interrelation between umbilical cord serum sex hormones, sex hormone-binding globulin, insulin-like growth factor I, and insulin in neonates from normal pregnancies and pregnancies complicated by diabetes. J Clin Endocrinol Metab 80:2217–2221.
257. O'Leary P, Boyne P, Flett P, Beilby J, James I (1991) Longitudinal assessment of changes in reproductive hormones during normal pregnancy. Clin Chem 37:667–672.
258. de Hertogh R, Thomas K, Vanderheyden I (1976) Quantitative determination of sex hormone-binding globulin capacity in the plasma of normal and diabetic pregnancies. J Clin Endocrinol Metab 42:773–777.
259. Uriel J, Dupiers M, Rimbaut C, Buffe D (1981) Maternal serum levels of sex steroid-binding protein during pregnancy. Br J Obstet Gynaecol 88:1229–1232.
260. Koritnik DR, Marschke KB (1986) Sex steroid hormone binding globulin levels and free 17β-estradiol and testosterone in Cynomolgus monkeys during different reproductive states. J Steroid Biochem 25:135–141.
261. Anderson DC, Lasley BL, Fisher RA, Shepherd JH, Newman L, Hendrickx AG (1976) Transplacental gradients of sex-hormone-binding globulin in human and simian pregnancy. Clin Endocrinol 5:657–669.
262. Motahashi T, Wu CH, Abdel-Rahman HA, Marymor N, Mikhail G (1979) Estrogen/androgen balance in health and disease. Am J Obstet Gynecol 135:89–95.
263. Porto CS, Lazari MFM, Abreu LC, Bardin CW, Gunsalus GL (1995) Receptors for androgen-binding proteins: Internalization and intracellular signalling. J Steroid Biochem Mol Biol 53: 561–565.
264. Strel'chyonok OA, Avvakumov GV, Survilo LI (1984) A recognition system for sex-hormone-binding protein-estradiol complex in human decidual endometrium plasma membranes. Biochim Biophys Acta 802:459–466.
265. Krupenko SA, Avvakumov GV, Strel'chyonok OA (1991) A transcortin-binding protein in the plasma membrane of human syncytiotrophoblast. Biochem Biophys Res Commun 177:834–839.
266. Joseph DR, Becchis M, Fenstermacher DA, Petrusz P (1996) The alternate N-terminal sequence of rat androgen-binding protein/sex hormone-binding globulin contains a nuclear targeting signal. Endocrinology 137:1138–1143.
267. Aoshima Y, Kochakian CD (1963) Activity, intracellular distribution and some properties of 17β-hydroxy-C19-steroid dehydrogenases in liver and kidney. Endocrinology 72:106–114.
268. Horton R, Tait JF (1966) Androstenedione production and interconversion rates measured in peripheral blood and studies on the possible site of its conversion to testosterone. J Clin Invest 45:301–313.
269. Baird DT, Horton R, Longcope C, Tait JF (1969) Steroid dynamics under steady-state conditions. Recent Prog Horm Res 25:611–664.
270. Rivarola MA, Singleton MA, Migeon CJ (1967) Splanchnic extraction and interconversion of testosterone and androstenedione in man. J Clin Invest 46:2095–2100.
271. Gurpide E (1975) Interpretation of isotopic data from blood-borne compounds, In: *Monographs on Endocrinology: Tracer Methods in Hormone Research* (Gross F, Labhort A, Lipsett MB, Mann T, Samuels LT, Zander J, eds.), Springer-Verlag, New York, pp. 105–147.
272. Heinrichs WL, Tabei T, Kuwabara Y, Resko JA, Petra PH, Shiller N, Namkung PC (1979) Differentiation and regulation of peripheral androgen metabolism in rats and rhesus monkeys. Am J Obstet Gynecol 135:974–983.
273. Belisle S, Lehoux JG, Brault J (1980) The metabolism of androstenedione in human pregnancy: The use of constant infusion of unlabeled steroid to assess its metabolic clearance rate, its production rate, and its conversion into androgens and estrogens. Am J Obstet Gynecol 136:1030–1035.
274. Tseng L, Gurpide E (1974) Estradiol and 20α-dihydroprogesterone dehydrogenase activities in human endometrium during the menstrual cycle. Endocrinology 94:419–423.
275. Tseng L, Gurpide E (1975) Induction of human endometrial estradiol dehydrogenase by progestins. Endocrinology 97:825–833.
276. Tseng L (1980) Hormonal regulation of steroid metabolic enzymes in human endometrium, In: *Advances in Sex Steroid Hormone Research* (Thomas JA, Singhal RL, eds.), Urban & Schwarzenbirg, Baltimore, pp. 329–361.

277. Tait GH, Newton CJ, Reed MJ, James VHT (1989) Multiple forms of 17β-hydroxysteroid oxidoreductase in human breast tissue. J Mol Endocrinol 2:71–80.
278. Mann VZ, Newton CJ, Tait GH (1991) 17β-hydroxysteroid dehydrogenase in human breast tissues: purification and characterization of soluble enzymes and the distribution of particulate and soluble forms in adipose, non-adipose and tumour tissues. J Mol Endocrinol 7:45–55.
279. Kreitman O, Kreitman-Gimbal B, Hodgen GD (1979) 17β-hydroxysteroid dehydrogenase in monkey endometrium: Characterization of enzyme activity and effects of estradiol alone or in combination with progesterone. Steroids 34:693–703.
280. Resko JA, Stadelman HL, Norman RL (1979) 17β-hydroxysteroid dehydrogenase activity in the pituitary gland and neural tissue of rhesus monkeys. J Steroid Biochem 11:1429–1434.
281. Casey ML, MacDonald PC, Andersson S (1994) 17β-hydroxysteroid dehydrogenase type 2: Chromosomal assignment and progestin regulation of gene expression in human endometrium. J Clin Invest 94:2135–2141.
282. Wilson JD (1978) Sexual differentiation. Ann Rev Physiol 40:279–306.
283. Thigpen AE, Silver RI, Guileyardo JM, Casey ML, McConnell JD, Russell DW (1993) Tissue distribution and ontogeny of steroid 5α-reductase isozyme expression. J Clin Invest 92:903–910.
284. Ellsworth K, Harris G (1995) Expression of the type 1 and 2 steroid 5α-reductases in human fetal tissues. Biochem Biophys Res Commun 215:774–780.
285. Levy MA, Brandt M, Sheedy KM, Holt DA, Heaslip JI, Trill JJ, Ryan PJ, Morris RA, Garrison LM, Bergsma DJ (1995) Cloning, expression and functional characterization of type 1 and type 2 steroid 5α-reductases from cynomolgus monkey: Comparisons with human and rat isoenzymes. J Steroid Biochem Mol Biol 52:307–319.
286. Resko JA, Ellinwood WE, Pasztor LM, Buhl AE (1980) Sex steroids in the umbilical circulation of fetal rhesus monkeys from the time of gonadal differentiation. J Clin Endocrinol Metab 50: 900–905.
287. Resko JA, Buhl AE, Phoenix CH (1987) Treatment of pregnant rhesus macaques with testosterone propionate: Observations on its fate in the fetus. Biol Reprod 37:1185–1191.
288. Resko JA, Abdelgadir SE, Connolly PB (1991) Androgen metabolism by hepatic and renal tissues of the fetal rhesus monkey. J Steroid Biochem Mol Biol 38:513–521.
289. Siiteri PK, MacDonald PC (1963) The utilization of circulating dehydroisoandrosterone sulfate for estrogen synthesis during human pregnancy. Steroids 2:713–730.
290. Resko JA, Stadelman HL (1982) 17β-hydroxysteroid dehydrogenase activity in tissues of fetal Rhesus Macaques. Proc Soc Exp Biol Med 171:233–237.
291. Monder C, White PC (1993) 11β-hydroxysteroid dehydrogenase. Vitam Horm 47:187–271.
292. Stewart PM (1994) 11β-hydroxysteroid dehydrogenase. Balliere's Clin Endocr Metab London, vol 8, pp. 357–378.
293. Bush IE, Mahesh VB (1959) Metabolism of 11-oxygenated steroids: Influences of the A/B ring junction on the reduction of 11-oxo groups. Biochem J 71:705–717.
294. Meigs RA, Engel LL (1961) The metabolism of adrenocortical steroids by human tissues. Endocrinology 69:152–162.
295. Monder C, Shackleton CHL (1984) Heterogeneity of 11β-hydroxysteroid dehydrogenase: fact or fancy? Steroids 44:383–417.
296. Monder C (1991) Heterogeneity of 11β-hydroxysteroid dehydrogenase in rat tissues. J Steroid Biochem Mol Biol 40:533–536.
297. Tannin GM, Agarwal AK, Monder C, New MI, White PC (1991) The human gene for 11β-hydroxysteroid dehydrogenase. Structure, tissue distribution, and chromosomal localization. J Biol Chem 266:16,653–16,658.
298. Davies WA, Luo H, Dong KW, Albrecht ED, Pepe GJ (1997) Cloning and expression of the 11β-hydroxysteroid dehydrogenase type 1 gene in the baboon. Mol Cell Endocrinol 127:201–209.
299. Moore CCD, Mellon SH, Murai JT, Siiteri PK, Miller WL (1993) Structure and function of the hepatic form of 11β-hydroxysteroid dehydrogenase in the squirrel monkey, an animal model of glucocorticoid resistance. Endocrinology 133:368–375.
300. Lakshmi V, Monder C (1988) Purification and characterization of the corticosteroid 11β-dehydrogenase component of the rat liver 11β-hydroxysteroid dehydrogenase complex. Endocrinology 123:2390–2398.
301. Agarwal AK, Tusiep-Luna MT, Monder C, White PC (1990) Expression of 11β-hydroxysteroid dehydrogenase using recombinant vaccinia virus. Mol Endocrinol 4:1827–1832.

302. Pepe GJ, Waddell BJ, Burch MG, Albrecht ED (1996) Interconversion of cortisol and cortisone in the baboon placenta at midgestation: Expression of 11β-hydroxysteroid dehydrogenase type 1 messenger RNA. J Steroid Biochem Mol Biol 58:403–410.
303. Pepe GJ, Babischkin JS, Burch MG, Leavitt MG, Albrecht ED (1996) Developmental increase in expression of the messenger ribonucleic acid and protein levels of 11β-hydroxysteroid dehydrogenase types 1 and 2 in the baboon placenta. Endocrinology 137:5678–5684.
304. Stewart PM, Whorwood CB, Mason JI (1995) Type 2 11β-hydroxysteroid dehydrogenase in foetal and adult life. J Steroid Biochem Mol Biol 55:465–471.
305. Sun K, Yang K, Challis JRG (1997) Differential expression of 11β-hydroxysteroid dehydrogenase types 1 and 2 in human placenta and fetal membranes. J Clin Endocrinol Metab 82:300–305.
306. Stewart PM, Murry BA, Mason JI (1994) Human kidney 11β-hydroxysteroid dehydrogenase is a high affinity nicotinamide adenine dinucleotide-dependent enzyme and differs from the cloned type I isoform. J Clin Endocrinol Metab 79:480–484.
307. Stewart PM, Krozowski Z, Gupta A, Milford DV, Howie A, Sheppard MC, Whorwood CB (1996) Hypertension in the syndrome of apparent mineralocorticoid excess due to mutation of the 11β-hydroxysteroid dehydrogenase type 2 gene. Lancet 347:88–91.
308. Stewart PM, Murry BA, Mason JI (1994) Type 2 11β-hydroxysteroid dehydrogenase in human fetal tissues. J Clin Endocrinol Metab 78:1529–1532.
309. Yang K, Smith CL, Dales D, Hammond GL, Challis JRG (1992) Cloning of an ovine 11β-hydroxysteroid dehydrogenase complementary deoxyribonucleic acid: Tissue and temporal distribution of its messenger ribonucleic acid during fetal and neonatal development. Endocrinology 131:2120–2126.
310. Yang K (1995) Co-expression of two distinct isoforms of 11β-hydroxysteroid dehydrogenase in the ovine placenta. J Steroid Biochem Mol Biol 52:337–343.
311. Albiston AL, Obeyesekere V, Smith R, Krozowski Z (1994) Cloning and tissue distribution of the human 11β-hydroxysteroid dehydrogenase type 2 enzyme. Mol Cell Endocrinol 105:R11–R17.
312. Brown RW, Chapman KE, Kotelevtsev Y, Yau JLW, Lindsay RS, Brett L, Leckie C, Murad P, Lyons V, Mullins JJ, Edwards CRW, Seckl JR (1996) Cloning and production of antisera to human placental 11β-hydroxysteroid dehydrogenase type 2. Biochem J 313:1007–1017.
313. Brown RW, Chapman KE, Murad P, Edwards CRW, Seckl JR (1996) Purification of 11β-hydroxysteroid dehydrogenase type 2 from human placenta utilizing a novel affinity labeling technique. Biochem J 313:997–1005.
314. Agarwal AK, Rogerson FM, Mune T, White PC (1995) Analysis of the human gene encoding the kidney isozyme of 11β-hydroxysteroid dehydrogenase. J Steroid Biochem Mol Biol 55:473–479.
315. Brown RW, Chapman KE, Edwards CRW, Seckl JR (1993) Human placental 11β-hydroxysteroid dehydrogenase: Evidence for and partial purification of a distinct NAD-dependent isoform. Endocrinology 132:2614–2621.
316. Naray-Fejes-Toth A, Fejes-Toth G (1996) Subcellular localization of the type 2 11β-hydroxysteroid dehydrogenase. A green fluorescent protein study. J Biol Chem 271:15,436–15,442.
317. Whorwood CB, Mason J, Ricketts M, Howie A, Stewart PM (1995) Detection of human 11β-hydroxysteroid dehydrogenase isoforms using RT-PCR and localization of the type 2 isoform to renal collecting ducts. Mol Cell Endocrinol 110:R7–R11.
318. Roland BL, Funder JW (1996) Localization of 11β-hydroxysteroid dehydrogenase type 2 in rat tissues: *In situ* studies. Endocrinology 137:1123–1128.
319. Krozowski Z, Albiston AL, Obeyesekere V, Andrews RK, Smith RE (1995) The human 11β-hydroxysteroid dehydrogenase type II enzyme: Comparisons with other species and localization to the distal nephron. J Steroid Biochem Mol Biol 55:457–464.
320. Krozowski Z, Maguire JA, Stein-Oakley AN, Dowling J, Smith RE, Andrews RK (1995) Immunohistochemical localization of the 11β-hydroxysteroid dehydrogenase type II enzyme in human kidney and placenta. J Clin Endocrinol Metab 80:2203–2209.
321. Ulick S, Levine LS, Gunczler P, Zanconato G, Ramirez LC, Rauh W, Rosler A, Bradlow HL, New MI (1979) A syndrome of apparent mineralocorticoid excess associated with defects in the peripheral metabolism of cortisol. J Clin Endocrinol Metab 49:757–764.
322. Funder JW, Pearce PT, Smith R, Smith I (1988) Mineralocorticoid action: target tissue specificity is enzyme not receptor mediated. Science 242:583–585.
323. Seckl JR, Brown RW (1994) 11β-hydroxysteroid dehydrogenase: on several roads to hypertension. J Hypertens 12:105–112.
324. Baggia S, Albrecht ED, Pepe GJ (1990) Regulation of 11β-hydroxysteroid dehydrogenase activity in the baboon placenta by estrogen. Endocrinology 126:2742–2748.

325. Baggia S, Albrecht ED, Babischkin JS, Pepe GJ (1990) Interconversion of cortisol and cortisone in baboon trophoblast and decidua cells in culture. Endocrinology 127:1735–1741.
326. Waddell BJ, Albrecht ED, Pepe GJ (1988) Effect of estrogen on the metabolism of cortisol and cortisone in the baboon fetus at midgestation. Biol Reprod 38:1006–1011.
327. Waddell BJ, Albrecht ED, Pepe GJ (1988) Metabolism of cortisol and cortisone in the baboon fetus at midgestation. Endocrinology 122:84–88.
328. Albrecht ED, Johnson DK, Pepe GJ (1981) Effect of maternal administration of the antiestrogen ethamoxytriphetol throughout the last third of baboon gestation upon neonatal corticoid production. Steroids 37:45–50.
329. Jaffe RB, Mulchahey JJ, DiBlasio AM, Martin MC, Blumenfeld Z, Dumesic DA (1988) Peptide regulation of pituitary and target tissue function and growth in the primate fetus. Recent Prog Horm Res 44:431–549.
330. Mesiano S, Fujimoto VY, Nelson LR, Lee JY, Voytek CC, Jaffe RB (1996) Localization and regulation of corticotropin receptor expression in the midgestation human fetal adrenal cortex: Implications of *in utero* homeostasis. J Clin Endocrinol Metab 81:340–345.
331. Albrecht ED, Aberdeen GW, Babischkin JS, Tilly JL, Pepe GJ (1996) Biphasic developmental expression of adrenocorticotropin receptor messenger ribonucleic acid levels in the baboon fetal adrenal gland. Endocrinology 137:1292–1298.
332. Pepe GJ, Ehrenkranz RA, Townsley JD (1976) The metabolic clearance rates and interconversion of cortisol and cortisone in pregnant and nonpregnant baboons. Endocrinology 99:597–601.
333. Pepe GJ, Davies WA, Albrecht ED (1994) Activation of the baboon fetal pituitary-adrenocortical axis at midgestation by estrogen: Enhancement of fetal pituitary proopiomelanocortin mRNA expression. Endocrinology 135:2581–2587.
334. Pepe GJ, Albrecht ED (1991) Activation of the baboon fetal pituitary-adrenocortical axis at midgestation by estrogen: Adrenal Δ^5-3β-hydroxysteroid dehydrogenase and 17α-hydroxylase-17,20-lyase activity. Endocrinology 128:2395–2401.
335. Davies WA, Berghorn KA, Albrecht ED, Pepe GJ (1993) Developmental regulation of protein kinase-A and -C activities in the baboon fetal adrenal. Endocrinology 132:2491–2497.
336. Pepe GJ, Waddell BJ, Albrecht ED (1990) Activation of the baboon fetal hypothalamic-pituitary-adrenocortical axis at midgestation by estrogen-induced changes in placental corticosteroid metabolism. Endocrinology 127:3117–3123.

12 Endocrine Maturation of the Fetus

Stuart B. Hooper, PHD, and Ian R. Young, PHD

CONTENTS

INTRODUCTION

Throughout gestation the fetus grows and develops in a warm and protected environment. It receives oxygen and nutrients from the mother, across the placenta, via the umbilical circulation and the fluid surrounding the fetus (amniotic fluid) acts as a hydrostatic brace, which protects the fetus from outside physical influences. However, at the time of birth the fetus must have grown and developed, and its physiological systems must be sufficiently mature to survive in the extrauterine environment for a given level of parental care. Clinically, one of the greatest problems facing modern human obstetrics is the premature birth of infants that are too immature to survive in the extrauterine environment without intensive and expensive postnatal treatments.

In terms of fetal development, the term "maturation" is relatively vague, and as a process, it is often difficult to distinguish it from growth and functional development. However, in broad terms, it is usually described as changes that facilitate survival following the transition from intra- to extrauterine existence. It is important to note that some of these changes are not conducive to continued intrauterine existence (e.g., switching of hemoglobin subtypes), which necessitates that they occur late in gestation near the time of birth. Based on this interpretation of maturation, we consider that, teleologically, it makes sense that many of the maturational events that must occur in the fetus are linked to the events that precipitate normal labor.

It is now evident that many maturational changes occur in the fetus that facilitate its survival postnatally, and that these changes are linked to the same endocrinological processes that lead to the onset of labor. However, within the limits of this chapter, it is not possible to describe all of the maturational changes that occur in the fetus before birth, since this in itself would constitute a whole book. Instead, we have decided to focus on what we consider are two of the most important maturational processes that must occur within the fetus for survival of the newborn. The original studies of Liggins et al. *(1–4)* demonstrated that a functional fetal hypothalamic–pituitary–adrenal (HPA) axis is essential for the normal initiation of labor, and it is now evident that this axis must also mature before it is capable of initiating the process of parturition and inducing maturation of other physiological systems. One such system is the maturation of the lung. It is commonly recognized that the immediate success of the transition from a fetus to an air-breathing newborn is more dependent on the lungs than on any other organ. Consequently, in this chapter, we have focused on the maturation and development of the HPA axis and on the factors that determine adequate respiratory function in the newborn.

MATURATION OF THE FETAL HPA AXIS

Glucocorticoids produced by the fetal adrenal cortex are essential for the induction of parturition in many species and play a vital role in the maturation of organ systems, which are needed for postnatal survival. In the sheep, fetal plasma cortisol concentrations increase over the last weeks of gestation and interruption of the fetal HPA axis by lesion of the paraventricular nuclei *(5)*, hypophysectomy *(3,4)*, hypothalamo–pituitary disconnection *(6,7)*, or adrenalectomy *(8)* prevents parturition. The importance of fetal glucocorticoid status for perinatal survival was recently underlined when it was shown that although capable of leading apparently normal lives postnatally, mice lacking corticotrophin-releasing hormone (CRH) cannot survive birth unless supplementary glucocorticoid is supplied *(9)*. The birth of an appropriately developed and viable neonate thus depends on the timely maturation of the fetal HPA axis, although the degree to which the fetal HPA axis determines the onset of labor differs between species *(10)*.

In addition to ensuring neonatal viability and synchronizing fetal maturation with birth, the fetal HPA axis is capable of responding to intrauterine stressors, including hypoxemia, hypoglycemia, infection, and hypotension. Since these and other stressors may assail the fetus during gestation and at birth, it is important to understand the nature of the fetal response to stress and the way it changes with maturation of the HPA axis.

In recent years, considerable emphasis has been placed on the regulation of basal cortisol secretion. This is the key determinant of fetal maturation and, in some species, of parturition itself. A particular focus has been the paradoxical ability of the fetal HPA axis to overcome the negative feedback effects of cortisol and generate an exponential increase in plasma cortisol concentrations over the last week or two of gestation. Because the peripartum period requires major physiological adaptations and often involves actual harm to the fetus, attention has also been directed to stress-induced cortisol secretion. The themes of basal and stress-induced activity within the fetal HPA axis will recur throughout this contribution. Since the development of the fetal HPA axis and parturition have recently been the subject of authoritative reviews *(10–12)*, we shall emphasize subsequent findings and current issues. Most experimental data have been derived from the fetal sheep, and most of what follows necessarily relies on that model. Parallels and contrasts between the ovine and human models will be discussed.

The HPA Axis in Early to Midgestation

STRUCTURE AND TISSUE CONSTITUENTS. The pituitary of the fetal sheep is present, and the hypophyseal portal system is patent by 45 d of gestational age (DGA) *(13–15)*. CRH, a known hypothalamic releasing factor for ACTH, is present in the PVN of the fetal hypothalamus by 49 DGA *(16)*, and CRH receptors are present in the fetal pituitary by d 65 *(17)*. Arginine vasopressin (AVP) is also believed to function as a releasing factor for ACTH and is present in hypothalamic extracts by 70 DGA *(18)*. The pituitary corticotrophs contain cleavage products of pro-opiomelanocortin (POMC), the ACTH precursor molecule, by 38 DGA *(19,20)*, and the mRNA encoding POMC was detectable by 60 DGA, the earliest age studied by Matthews et al. *(21)*.

The fetal adrenal glands are present by 28 DGA *(22)* and contain the steroidogenic enzymes needed for cortisol secretion by d 40 *(23)*. The essential components of a functional HPA axis appear to be present soon after the tissues are differentiated and well in advance of any likely occasion for their use by the fetus.

Adrenal Responsiveness. Adrenal cortisol production in vitro is very high early in gestation *(23,24)*, and the responsiveness of adrenal cells to ACTH between 40 and 50 DGA exceeds that at any other age. Consistent with this pattern, mRNAs encoding key steroidogenic enzymes in adrenal tissue were detectable by 42 DGA by *in situ* hybridization *(22)*. Adrenal cells from fetuses aged between 90 and 120 DGA are relatively refractory to stimulation by ACTH with responsiveness returning after 120 d. The loss of adrenal responsiveness is reflected in a reduction of ACTH receptor numbers *(25)*, impaired coupling of ACTH receptors to the adenylate cyclase system *(26)*, and lowered activity of key steroidogenic enzymes *(27)*. The pools of mRNA encoding these enzymes are also reduced *(22)*. The factor(s) controlling the loss and return of adrenal responsiveness to ACTH are considered to be key elements for our understanding of the prepartum cortisol surge.

Physiological Regulation of the HPA Axis in Midgestation. As early as 65 DGA, the basal activity of the fetal HPA axis is subject to negative feedback by glucocorticoid. Maternally administered dexamethasone suppressed ACTH and cortisol concentrations in fetal plasma *(28)*. The adrenal tissue content of mRNAs coding for 17α-hydroxylase and cholesterol side-chain cleavage enzyme were also dramatically reduced in dexamethasone-treated fetuses compared to saline-treated controls *(28)*.

The technical difficulty of cannulating sheep fetuses before 70 DGA has limited physiological studies before that time, but by 74–84 d, the fetus can mount both ACTH and cortisol responses to exogenous CRH and AVP *(29)*. The removal of blood equivalent to 6.6% of the body wt of acutely anesthetized fetuses at this age was associated with an increase in plasma ACTH concentration. Thus, the midgestation fetus can respond to severe physiological stress, although it is unclear in this case to what extent the increase in plasma ACTH concentration reflects a reduction in the initial volume of distribution of ACTH caused by the hypovolaemia. Basal ACTH concentrations are low in fetuses of this age, and basal cortisol concentrations decreased further over the range of 74–84 DGA. This suggests that adrenal responsiveness to ACTH was decreasing over this period.

It has been proposed that the relative refractoriness of the fetal adrenal during the 90–120 d period is owing to hyposecretion of ACTH with consequent reductions in the level of expression of the steroid synthetic enzymes *(29–31)*. This suggestion is supported by studies in which 24-h infusion of ACTH at moderately supraphysiological doses induced mRNAs encoding side-chain cleavage enzyme and 17α-hydroxylase in the fetal adrenal during this quiescent, midgestation period *(32)*. Although this proposal is well supported, there is reason to believe that it may not be the sole explanation for the midgestation refractory period.

Durand and coworkers have shown that cAMP secretion, an important index of maturation of fetal adrenocortical cells, increases spontaneously during the initial 6 d of culture, even in the absence of ACTH. The pattern of steroid metabolism in such cells was also consistent with a spontaneous maturation in vitro, which led to the postulation that an in vivo inhibitor of adrenal maturation may exist *(33)*. This proposal may be related to the suggestion that POMC and perhaps other high-mol-wt precursors of ACTH might be endogenous inhibitors of ACTH action in fetal sheep *(34–36)*. The emergence of the fetal

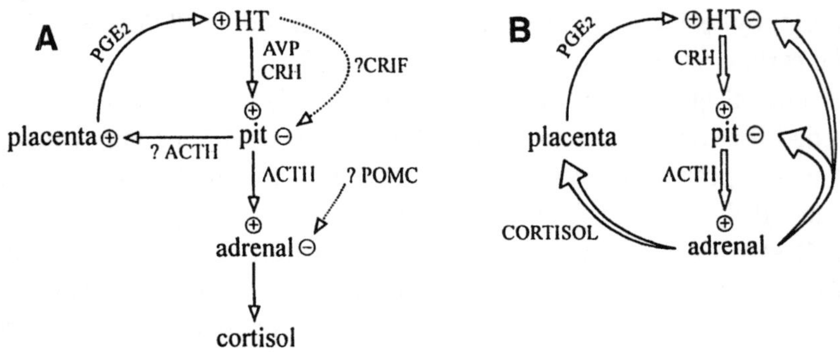

Fig. 1. Developmental changes in the control of fetal HPA function. **(A)** D 100, **(B)** d 140. Over the periods depicted in these schematic diagrams, several important changes occur in the control of HPA function. The level of central drive to the fetal pituitary increases with a consequent increase in plasma cortisol concentrations. At d 100, cortisol output is insufficient to activate negative feedback, but by d 140, negative feedback is clearly demonstrable. The increased central drive at d 140 may reflect increased secretion of hypothalamic-releasing factors and withdrawal of the putative CRIF. The resultant increased drive to the fetal adrenal is associated with rising basal cortisol concentrations. This change induces placental enzymes (especially 17-hydroxylase/C-17,20 lyase and aromatase). Estrogen production increases at the expense of progesterone, favoring the induction of type 2 cyclooxygenase. Plasma PGE_2 concentrations increase accordingly, maintaining a tonic stimulus to the fetal hypothalamus and closing the positive feedback loop.

adenal gland from its unresponsive state around d 120 may depend on the balance between increasing endogenous drive from the hypothalamo–pituitary unit on one hand and the negative influence of the postulated inhibitor on the other. This hypothesis will be further addressed in a subsequent section (*see* Fig. 1).

Pituitary-Placental Interactions in Midgestation. The onset of refractoriness in the fetal HPA axis occurs simultaneously with a significant increase in the placental secretion of progesterone, estrogens, and prostaglandin (PG) E_2 between 90 and 120 DGA. Although fetal hypophysectomy after this period did not produce consistent effects on these parameters, different results were obtained when hypophysectomy was done in midgestation *(37)*. Ewes bearing hypophysectomized fetuses failed to exhibit the usual increases in oestrone sulfate and PGE_2, and the accompanying increase in progesterone was also significantly impaired. Clearly, the fetal pituitary exerts control over the developmentally regulated induction of the enzymes responsible for placental steroidogenesis and PGE_2 output (Fig. 1).

It is unclear whether a causal link exists between the simultaneous increase in placental hormone production and the onset of adrenal refractoriness in the fetus. However, evidence gained from older fetuses suggests that crosstalk between the fetal pituitary and placenta does occur, and that it affects hormones believed to be involved in the maturation of the fetal HPA axis.

The Significance of the Fetal Role in Placental Hormone Synthesis

Control of Placental PGE_2 Production. As noted in the preceding section, fetal hypophysectomy abolished the normal midgestation increase in PGE_2 concentrations in maternal plasma *(37)*. Although fetal hormone concentrations were not determined in that study, it was subsequently shown that the late gestation increase in fetal PGE_2 concentrations was similarly abolished after fetal hypophysectomy at 125 DGA or fetal hypothalamo–pituitary disconnection (HPD) at 125 or 135 DGA *(38,39)*. The main source of PGE_2 in pregnant ewes and their fetuses is the placenta *(40–43)*, and these findings therefore confirm the fetal pituitary as the main determinant of placental PGE_2 production.

To date, no formal investigation has addressed the identity of the fetal pituitary factor(s) controlling placental PGE_2 production. One likely candidate for this role is fetal ACTH, as indicated by a study *(38)* involving two groups of hypophysectomized fetuses; one group received chronic, low-dose ACTH replacement and the other a saline infusion. Although not statistically significant, the PGE_2 concentrations in the ACTH-infused fetuses tended to be greater than in control fetuses. This suggested that fetal ACTH may be a trophic factor for PGE_2 which is supported by the finding that fetuses adrenalectomized at 115 DGA had increased basal PGE_2 concentrations (9.9 ± 3.3 n*M* at d 120–130, whereas intact controls had 3.7 ± 0.5 n*M*, $P < 0.001$; Young and Hollingworth, unpublished observations). These adrenalectomized fetuses had increased plasma ACTH concentrations (1551 ± 454 vs 114 ± 18 pg/mL), and the finding of increased PGE_2 in the plasma of these fetuses is consistent with the hypothesis that ACTH drives placental PGE_2 synthesis. Contrary to this suggestion, a 2-d cortisol infusion did not reduce PGE_2 concentrations of adrenalectomized fetuses although it did reduce ACTH to control values (Young and Hollingworth, unpublished data). Furthermore, hypothalamo–pituitary disconnected fetuses had reduced PGE_2 concentrations, but their plasma ACTH concentrations were normal *(39)*.

Because PGE_2 is a very potent activator of the fetal HPA axis and because it is present at significant concentrations in the fetal circulation *(42,44,45)*, the finding that the fetal pituitary controls the concentration of PGE_2 in the fetal circulation may be critical to our understanding of the maturation of the fetal HPA axis. It will, therefore, be important to clarify which pituitary hormone(s) control its secretion.

Negative Feedback Control of Cortisol Secretion

Sites of Cortisol Negative Feedback. Placement of dexamethasone implants adjacent to the paraventricular nucleus (PVN) of fetal sheep did not affect basal ACTH secretion, but abolished the ACTH response to hypotension, hypoxemia, and CRH *(46)*. This treatment also reduced the expression of mRNAs for CRH in the PVN *(47)*. Similarly, it has also been shown that cortisol infusion attenuated the increase in CRH mRNA seen in hypoxemic fetuses *(48)*. This is in accord with the finding of glucocorticoid receptors in the PVN *(49)*, and together, these findings suggest that glucocorticoid negative feedback is integrated within the PVN and that secretagogs or neurohormones (CRH and AVP) originating in the PVN are responsible for stimulus-induced ACTH secretion. CRH and AVP immunostaining in the median eminence were reduced in dexamethasone-treated animals, suggesting that the dexamethasone implants tonically reduced the hypothalamic drive to the fetal pituitary. It is unclear, however, why the pituitary response to exogenous CRH was attenuated when basal ACTH concentrations and POMC mRNA content were unaffected. Loss of responsiveness to exogenous CRH suggests a direct effect of glucocorticoid on the pituitary, perhaps by diffusion from the implant.

There is ample evidence from in vitro studies for glucocorticoid feedback at the pituitary level. The fetal pituitary has glucocorticoid receptors *(50,51)*, and cortisol treatment of cultured pituitary cells reduces POMC mRNA and ACTH secretion *(52)*. It has also been shown that cells treated with dexamethasone had reduced responsiveness to secre-

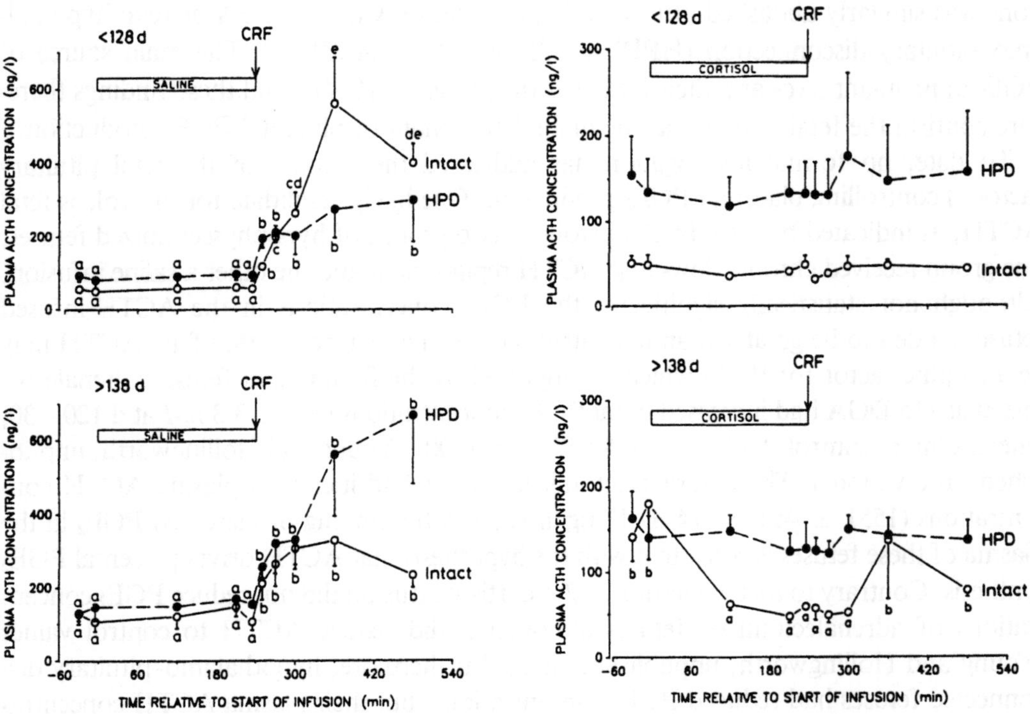

Fig. 2. Sites of cortisol negative feedback on basal and CRF-stimulated ACTH secretion. The left-hand panels illustrate the developmental changes in ACTH response to CRF under control conditions (saline infusion). Points within a panel sharing a lower-case letter are not significantly different from each other. In the upper panel, immature intact fetuses mount a large and prolonged ACTH response. Older fetuses (lower panel) show a truncated response attributable to negative feedback by the endogenous cortisol secreted in response to the initial phases of the ACTH response. This feedback does not occur in the HPD fetuses, which display an enhanced ACTH response at the older age, indicating that the hypothalamus is the site of the feedback observed in the older, intact fetuses.

The right-hand panels show the sites of feedback of exogenous cortisol (4-h infusion) on basal ACTH secretion and the ACTH responses to CRF. At the late gestational age (lower panel), cortisol infusion causes a reduction in basal ACTH concentrations in intact fetuses only, indicating that the hypothalamus is the major site of cortisol feedback on basal ACTH secretion. At both gestational ages, the HPD fetuses fail to respond to CRF after cortisol infusion, implicating the pituitary as a major site of feedback on CRF-induced ACTH secretion. At the early gestational age, basal ACTH concentration in HPD fetuses exceeds that in intact fetuses, suggesting the existence of a hypothalamic inhibitor of ACTH secretion (CRIF). Reproduced with permission *(55)*.

tagogs, although there was no reduction in basal secretion *(53)*. To overcome some of the disadvantages of dispersed and cultured cells, fresh pituitary slices have been studied in a perifusion system *(54)*. It was found that after 120 DGA, a 30-min exposure to 100 n*M* of cortisol significantly reduced ACTH secretion.

In chronically catheterized fetal sheep, disconnection of the fetal pituitary from hypothalamic inputs completely abolishes the inhibitory effect of a 4-h cortisol infusion on basal plasma ACTH concentrations. This shows that glucocorticoid negative feedback at the hypothalamus is sufficient to account for the observed negative feedback effects of high cortisol concentrations on basal ACTH secretion *(55)* (Figs. 2 and 3). In addition to its effects on basal ACTH output, glucocorticoid pretreatment also attenuates stimulus-

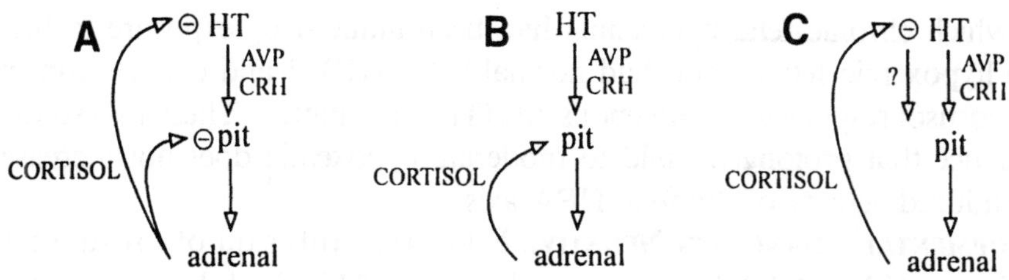

Fig. 3. Major sites of cortisol feedback following acute increases in plasma cortisol under different conditions of the HPA axis in late gestation. (**A**) Basal, (**B**) CRH-stimulated, (**C**) stress-induced. The main site of feedback on basal secretion is the hypothalamus (A), whereas the pituitary is also sensitive to negative feedback as indicated by the impaired response to CRH after acute increases in plasma cortisol (A and B). Glucocorticoid feedback on ACTH release in response to physiological stressors is effected through the hypothalamus (C).

induced ACTH secretion in fetal sheep. The ACTH response to CRH was abolished or attenuated by cortisol priming in both hypothalamo–pituitary disconnected fetuses and intact controls, implicating the pituitary as an important site of glucocorticoid feedback on CRH-induced ACTH secretion (Figs. 2 and 3). The usual marked ACTH responses to hypoxemia and hypoglycemia were also abolished in HPD fetuses, confirming the essential role of the hypothalamus in stress-induced ACTH secretion.

Differential Effects of Glucocorticoid Feedback on Basal and Stimulus-Induced ACTH Secretion. It has been observed repeatedly that periods of elevated plasma cortisol exceeding a few hours are not associated with suppressed basal ACTH concentrations, but stress-stimulated ACTH responses are blunted or abolished *(11)*. Recent reports confirm these broad conclusions *(46,56)*, although basal ACTH is suppressible by large (6×) increases in plasma cortisol late in gestation *(48)*. Interestingly, these infusions did not reduce either CRH mRNA in fetal PVN or glucocorticoid receptor mRNA in the fetal pituitary *(51)*, although the *in situ* hybridization methods used to quantify these parameters may not be sufficiently sensitive to detect small changes. The hypoxia-induced increase in CRH mRNA content of the fetal PVN was significantly attenuated by a sixfold increase in cortisol at 135 d, reinforcing the earlier conclusion that cortisol feedback on stress-induced ACTH secretion is effected through the hypothalamus, at least in part *(46)* (Fig. 3).

Elevated cortisol concentrations, resulting from an injection of CRH, have been shown to abolish the ACTH response to a second CRH challenge given 6 h after the first injection, suggesting that pituitary responsiveness to CRH was reduced *(57)*. This bears out the finding that glucocorticoid feedback acts via a short feedback loop to inhibit CRH-induced ACTH secretion *(55)*. In an accompanying study, these workers found that similar pretreatment with CRH did not affect the ACTH response to hypotension 6 h later *(57,58)*. The combined results of the two studies suggest that stress induces a stronger stimulus to ACTH secretion than can be accounted for by CRH alone. This conclusion is consistent with findings in adult sheep *(59)*.

Although most studies of the effects of physiological stressors on fetal HPA function have utilized relatively short periods of exposure to the stressor, an interesting recent study investigated the effect of chronic, naturally occurring hypoxemia on the fetus *(60)*. Basal ACTH and cortisol concentrations of the hypoxemic fetuses did not differ from those of control fetuses, and the responses of ACTH and cortisol to exogenous CRH were also similar to those of normoxemic controls. The conclusions resembled those of another study in which chronic fetal hypoxemia had been induced by exposure to high altitude *(61)*. The hypoxemic fetuses also had normal basal ACTH and cortisol concentrations, and their cortisol responses to exogenous ACTH were blunted. These two studies provide good evidence that prolonged, mild to moderate hypoxemia does not increase basal or stimulus-induced activity of the fetal HPA axis.

Developmental Changes in Negative Feedback. Infusion of low-dose cortisol at 121–135 d or at 132–142 d did not suppress basal ACTH in fetal sheep. The effect of cortisol on hypotension-induced ACTH release differed markedly at the two GA ranges. At the earlier GA, the feedback threshold was very low, but at the later GA, the ACTH response was unaffected by very high cortisol concentrations *(62,63)*. These results indicate that the fetal HPA axis escapes from cortisol negative feedback around 140 DGA. However, not all subsequent studies have yielded results consistent with that interpretation. A 4-h cortisol infusion, between 138 and 142 DGA, has been shown to suppress basal ACTH (Fig 2), although ACTH was unaffected by the same cortisol infusion regime before 128 DGA *(55)*. At the earlier age, cortisol pretreatment had abolished the CRH-induced ACTH response, but the same treatment after 138 DGA did not prevent an increase in plasma ACTH. The effects of raising fetal cortisol concentrations by CRH treatment on subsequent ACTH responses to a further CRH challenge or to hypotension have also been studied at two gestational ages *(57,58)*. At 103–113 DGA, the initial CRH treatment induced little increase in plasma cortisol, but a sustained increase in ACTH. However, at 133–139 DGA, the cortisol response was greater and sustained, whereas the peak ACTH response appeared reduced in amplitude and duration compared to that at the earlier age. At the later GA, the ACTH response to a second CRH challenge was abolished.

Taken together, these results indicate that although not as sensitive to glucocorticoid feedback, the fetal HPA axis retains its negative feedback response to cortisol well after the age at which endogenous cortisol concentrations have started their prepartum increase, i.e., after 135 DGA. Thus, the loss of HPA sensitivity to cortisol is not absolute and cannot fully explain the paradoxical, simultaneous increases in ACTH and cortisol in late gestation. The activity of the HPA axis is enhanced in late gestation, and several hypotheses have been advanced to explain the relative increase in glucocorticoid feedback threshold.

Mechanisms of Altered Glucocorticoid Feedback in Late Gestation. The fetus requires increased plasma cortisol in the immediate prepartum period to promote maturation of organ systems needed for extrauterine survival. To achieve this and to initiate the parturient process, the drive to the fetal adrenal must be maintained in the presence of increasing cortisol concentrations. Thus, it has been proposed that the sites of glucocorticoid feedback are in some way protected from the increased plasma cortisol concentrations, blunting the feedback response.

One mechanism by which glucocorticoid negative feedback may be moderated is to limit the bioavailability of glucocorticoid to its receptors in cells of the CNS, which transduce the plasma glucocorticoid concentrations. Increasing circulating concentrations of corticosteroid binding globulin (CBG) would be expected to moderate the effects of high cortisol concentrations in this way. It has long been established that the plasma corticosteroid binding capacity of fetal sheep increases toward term *(64,65)*. More recent studies have shown that hepatic CBG mRNA and plasma corticosteroid binding capacity are positively regulated by synthetic glucocorticoid late in gestation and by cortisol at physiological concentrations at 100 DGA. This contrasts with the situation in the adult, where increased plasma glucocorticoid inhibits CBG synthesis *(66,67)*.

CBG added to the medium of cultured fetal pituitary cells significantly reduced the ability of cortisol to inhibit CRH-stimulated ACTH secretion, strengthening the proposal that bioavailability of cortisol is a factor in modulating the cortisol feedback threshold in late gestation *(68)*. It should be noted that in these in vitro experiments, the pituitary cells were exposed directly to CBG, and direct effects of CBG on those cells cannot be excluded. This situation may apply to pituitary cells in vivo, because of the sinusoidal nature of this tissue, but not to other cells located behind the blood–brain barrier, which are also involved in transducing plasma cortisol concentrations and modulating negative feedback. Glucocorticoid feedback on basal ACTH secretion occurs predominantly above the level of the pituitary (Fig. 2); *(55)*, and it is there that an effect of any agent thought to attenuate feedback should be sought. Nonetheless, increased plasma CBG reduces plasma free cortisol and, hence, the cortisol concentration affecting cells within the CNS.

A reduction in the availability of cortisol to target cells in the HPA axis may result in a similar reduction in its availability to other target cells where its presence is required. To overcome this objection to CBG as a principal modulator of glucocorticoid feedback, one must assume differences in the delivery of cortisol to its target cells inside and outside the HPA axis. It has been proposed that CBG is produced locally within the pituitary. If this mechanism can be demonstrated in the pituitary and in other glucocorticoid-sensitive cells of the HPA axis, it could explain the apparent selectivity of CBG for these tissues.

An alternative mechanism whereby cortisol feedback may be blunted is metabolism of the cortisol molecule in the cytoplasm of target cells, preventing its binding to the nuclear receptor. 11-β hydroxysteroid dehydrogenase (11-β HSD) metabolizes cortisol to its relatively inactive metabolite cortisone and could potentially fulfill this function. The enzyme is expressed in fetal hypothalamus and pituitary, and its expression and activity in pituitary, including the pars intermedia, increase with gestational age *(69,70)*. The expression of 11-β HSD mRNA in fetal pituitary was not affected by a 12-h cortisol infusion, and the mechanism underlying the developmental increase in this parameter is unknown.

Glucocorticoid receptor numbers and expression in fetal pituitary increase toward term *(49,51)*, and receptor number in hypothalamus do not alter at this time. This rules out downregulation of these receptors as an explanation for impaired glucocorticoid feedback.

Results published to date are consistent with a blunting of cortisol feedback or an increase in the set point of its threshold through increases in plasma CBG and hypothalamic and pituitary 11-β HSD. However, they are observational and do not permit an appreciation of the magnitude and importance of these proposed effects. An assessment of the importance of 11-β HSD and CBG in fetal life is possible if these factors can be specifically removed. An inhibitor of 11-β HSD is available, but experimental reduction or elimination of CBG is not likely in the foreseeable future.

The apparent, partial escape from negative feedback during the last day of gestation may reflect increased drive to the fetal HPA axis. This could alter the balance of stimulatory and inhibitory influences, and result in an alteration in the set point of the cortisol feedback threshold. It is essential, therefore, to consider the sources that may contribute positively to increased drive within the HPA axis in late gestation.

Positive Feedback in the HPA-Placental Unit

Although the fetal HPA axis clearly exhibits negative feedback regulation on ACTH secretion, the continuing increase in ACTH and cortisol over the last week of gestation indicates that positive drives within the system override the effects of negative feedback at this time. The onset of labor, which results from this process, is a unique, explosive event in the life of the individual. Physiological processes that have involved a buildup of positive drives and end suddenly in a singular event (e.g., ovulation or parturition) may involve positive feedback control systems. Apart from these general characteristics of the fetal HPA axis in late gestation, positive feedback is likely to be involved at specific loci in the control systems.

Glucocorticoid Positive Feedback at the Hypothalamo-Pituitary Unit. Only negative effects of cortisol on ACTH secretion have been demonstrated in vivo. However, there is evidence that cortisol may induce maturation of pituitary corticotrophs. The corticotrophs fall into two histologically distinct types: fetal and adult *(20)*. The proportion of adult-type cells within the fetal pituitary can be accelerated by intrafetal cortisol infusion at d 115 GA and inhibited by fetal adrenalectomy *(71)*. The ability of exogenous cortisol to accelerate the disappearance of fetal type cells was maintained in HPD fetuses, although a corresponding increase in the percentage of adult-type cells could not be demonstrated. On balance, it appears that cortisol does act directly on the fetal pituitary to mature the corticotroph population, although a complementary hypothalamic effect cannot be excluded.

Glucocorticoid Positive Feedback at the Adrenal Cortex. Intrafetal infusions of the 11-β hydroxylase inhibitor metyrapone negates the growth-promoting action of $ACTH_{1-24}$ on the fetal adrenal gland *(2)*. This suggested that unlike humans (e.g., in congenital adrenal hyperplasia), the adrenal gland of the fetal sheep requires cortisol synthesis for its own growth. It was shown subsequently that pretreatment of fetuses with dexamethasone enhanced their adrenal responsiveness to an ACTH challenge. Analogous results have been achieved in vitro *(72,73)*. Considered together, these disparate findings suggest that cortisol produced within the fetal adrenal acts directly on the adrenal cortical cells to enhance their secretory capacity and responsiveness.

ACTH Positive Feedback at the Hypothalamo-Pituitary Unit. It has been suggested that ACTH stimulates its own secretion from the fetal pituitary. This hypothesis arose from studies that examined the effect of $ACTH_{1-24}$ infusion (10 mg/h) into hypophysectomized and intact fetal sheep. In the hypophysectomized sheep, the infusion yielded plasma-immunoactive ACTH concentrations with a mean value of 512 pg/mL, whereas infusion into intact fetuses resulted in a mean value of 1817 pg/mL *(74,75)*. These differences did not appear to be owing to methodological reasons, since the plasma half-life of ACTH immunoactivity was the same in both groups of fetuses. In keeping with the suggestion that endogenous ACTH secretion was stimulated in intact fetuses, chromatography of plasma from hypophysectomized fetuses revealed only $ACTH_{1-24}$, but intact fetuses had large quantities of higher-mol-wt ACTH-immunoactive species. Further, the ACTH concentrations fluctuated widely in intact, but not in hypophysectomized fetuses, again suggesting endogenous secretion. These results have traditionally been interpreted as reflecting ACTH-induced ACTH secretion, with the action of ACTH being directly at the hypothalamo-pituitary unit. Given this observation and our findings of pituitary-dependent PGE_2 secretion, it is possible that ACTH acts at the placenta via a long positive feedback loop to induce its own secretion. It is, therefore, important that the site and mechanism of ACTH action in inducing its own release be determined.

Positive Feedback of Placental PGE_2 and Pituitary ACTH. Recent endeavors in our laboratory have focused on the role of placental PGE_2 in the onset of parturition. In particular, we have investigated the hypothesis that PGE_2 plays a role in activating and supporting the HPA axis.

In late gestation, fetal PGE_2 concentrations increase in parallel with those of ACTH and cortisol *(39)*. This increase is dependent on an intact hypothalamo-pituitary unit, because hypophysectomy or HPD results in low fetal PGE_2 levels, which do not increase as expected in late gestation *(37,39)*. Further, the expression of cyclooxygenase, the prostaglandin synthetic enzyme, is decreased in placental tissue after fetal hypophysectomy *(76)*.

Following fetal adrenalectomy, PGE_2 concentrations are elevated and increase in parallel with ACTH, suggesting that ACTH may be the pituitary factor responsible for placental PGE_2 synthesis (our unpublished observations). In addition to fetal PGE_2 concentrations being dependent on an intact hypothalamus and pituitary, we have demonstrated that PGE_2 is a potent stimulator of ACTH secretion (Fig. 1). Acute PGE_2 infusion dramatically increases fetal ACTH and cortisol concentrations at all gestational ages studied, from 120 d until term *(45)*. The increase in ACTH was far greater than that obtained with maximal doses of CRH. Similar changes in fetal ACTH and cortisol levels were detected in fetuses receiving chronic infusions of PGE_2, and physiologically normal labor was initiated in these animals after 16 d of infusion *(77)*. This was 10 d earlier than for saline-infused control fetuses. We have recently shown that PGE_2 does not release ACTH in HPD fetuses. Thus PGE_2 at physiologically relevant concentrations exerts its action on the fetal HPA axis predominantly through the hypothalamus. This is consistent with results obtained recently in rats *(78–80)* and confirms the conclusions of a previous study in fetal sheep *(81)*.

We propose that pituitary ACTH stimulates placental PGE_2 secretion. In turn, we postulate that PGE_2 acts via a long positive feedback loop on the hypothalamus to stimulate further ACTH secretion and, hence, further placental PGE_2 secretion. The long latency between starting our chronic PGE_2 infusion and labor suggests that PGE_2 functions as an amplifier of other positive drives within the fetal HPA axis and does not directly activate the parturient mechanism.

ACTH and Modulators of Its Adrenal Actions

ACTH is believed to play a crucial part in the reawakening of the fetal adrenal from its midgestation "off" period and the subsequent increase in activity of the HPA axis. During midgestation the fetal adrenal can be activated prematurely by ACTH infusion, setting in motion the characteristic sequence of events leading to labor. This observation, together with the low plasma concentrations of ACTH at this time, suggest that an increase in ACTH secretion is all that is required for activation of the parturient process. Although such an increase undoubtedly occurs in late gestation, other factors appear to modulate the response of the system. In particular, high-mol-wt ACTH precursors have been proposed as endogenous ACTH antagonists *(34,35,82,83)*.

ACTH AND THE TIMING OF ADRENAL ACTIVATION. Plasma cortisol concentrations in fetal sheep begin to increase around d 125, although they are not significantly increased until about 10 d later. The temporal profile of plasma ACTH concentrations varies according to the specificity of the assays used. Some RIAs use antisera that although raised against $ACTH_{1\text{-}24}$, crossreact significantly with high-mol-wt ACTH-containing species. These assays typically measure basal concentrations in late gestation fetal plasma in the range 70–150 pg/mL *(12)*. Other assays, predominantly commercially available kits and two-site immunoradiometric assays *(12,39,84,85)*, measure lower concentrations around 20–30 pg/mL. It appears that the latter assays are more specific for low-mol-wt $ACTH_{1\text{-}39}$.

The less specific assays usually do not detect significant increases in ACTH immunoreactivity before the last few days of gestation, but use of the more specific assays suggests that plasma ACTH begins to increase around 2–3 wk before labor *(5,12,39,84,86)*. Because the initial stages of these increases are gradual, it has not been conclusively established that the increase in ACTH secretion precedes adrenal activation.

The fetal pituitary exhibits a peculiarly increased responsiveness at 120 DGA, a few days before the earliest suggested increase in cortisol concentrations. This hyperresponsiveness manifests itself by unusually large increases in ACTH concentrations when secretagogs are given, together with an increase in the proportion of ACTH in low-mol-wt forms *(45,84,87,88)*. The timing of this event coincides with the emergence of enhanced drive to the fetal pituitary in adrenalectomized fetuses. Prior to d 120, such fetuses do not exhibit increased ACTH secretion, indicating that cortisol negative feedback does not normally contribute to regulation of ACTH before this time. Their cortisol concentrations do not differ from those of intact fetuses at 120 d. Thus it seems that some factor unrelated to cortisol increases the drive to the fetal hypothalamus at this time. The fetal adrenal is relatively unresponsive at d 120, but a subtle increase in the secretion rate or bioactivity of ACTH may suffice to restore adrenal function. The subsequent decrease in pituitary responsiveness would then be explicable by cortisol negative feedback.

It has been proposed that the emergence of central drive to ACTH secretion is a maturation-related event, possibly depending on increased fetal demand for nutrients and mediated by PGE_2 *(44,89,90)*. The increased activity of the fetal hypothalamo–pituitary axis at 120 d may also reflect a reduction in the secretion of a proposed corticotrophin release inhibiting factor (CRIF). The existence of such a factor has been proposed, partly on the basis that ACTH secretion in adult sheep increases when the neural connections between the hypothalamus and the pituitary are severed by HPD surgery *(91)*. We have repeatedly demonstrated the same phenomenon in the fetus *(7,92)*. The possibility must be considered that ACTH secretion may be controlled by hypothalamic inhibitory factors as well as by the accepted releasing factors (Fig. 1).

High-Mol Wt ACTH Precursors as Modulators of ACTH Action. Since the early proposals of Jones and Roebuck *(34,35)*, considerable evidence has accumulated to suggest that high-mol-wt precursors of ACTH act as physiological antagonists of ACTH action on the adrenal cortex. The proportion of low-mol-wt ACTH immunoreactivity in fetal plasma and in medium from perifused pituitaries increases toward term *(84,85,93)*. The concentration of high-mol-wt ACTH precursors in fetal plasma is surprisingly high, variously reported as 7–30 times that of $ACTH_{1\text{-}39}$ at term. The high-mol-wt forms appear to have little or no effect on fetal adrenal cells *(82)*, but they may act as competitive inhibitors of ACTH action. The presence of POMC or pro-ACTH at physiologically relevant concentrations significantly attenuated the cortisol responses of cultured fetal adrenal cells to ACTH. Interestingly, the high-mol-wt precursors had no such inhibitory effect on ACTH-stimulated cortisol secretion by adult adrenal cells. The inhibitory effect of high-mol-wt forms on ACTH-induced cortisol secretion has been confirmed by acute infusion experiments in the calf in vivo *(36)*.

A series of recent publications shows that the ratio of bioactive (as assessed by cortisol output from rat adrenal cells) to immunoactive ACTH in fetal plasma increases toward term and also increases with severity of acutely applied stress. The ACTH assay used in these studies recognizes high-mol-wt ACTH precursors, and the results are congruent with other studies in which the ratio of low-mol-wt to high-mol-wt ACTH-containing species exhibits similar patterns *(34,84,85,87)*. Carr et al. *(84)* found that the ratio of $ACTH_{1\text{-}39}$ to its precursors increased acutely in response to CRH. Together, these results strongly suggest that much of the immunoassayable ACTH in basal fetal plasma samples is attributable to high-mol-wt forms that are not bioactive.

The low-mol-wt and high-mol-wt forms of ACTH may be differentially secreted by the anterior and intermediate lobes of the fetal pituitary. It has been suggested that the majority of β-endorphin (β-EP) immunoactivity in fetal plasma under basal conditions was of intermediate lobe origin, but that the anterior pituitary is responsible for the increased β-EP concentrations observed when the fetus is stressed *(94,95)*. By analogy, and because the intermediate lobe of the fetal pituitary expresses POMC very strongly, it is tempting to speculate that a significant proportion of the basally secreted high-mol-wt ACTH immunoreactive species in fetal plasma also originates from the intermediate lobe. The stimulus-induced increase in ACTH immunoreactivity presumably originates from the anterior lobe. These hypotheses have not been formally addressed, but call for prompt attention.

There is now a considerable body of evidence that the ratio of high-mol-wt to low-mol-wt ACTH-containing species in fetal plasma is an important regulator of adrenal steroidogenesis. POMC processing is different in the anterior and intermediate lobes of the fetal pituitary. Two enzymes known as prohormone convertases- (PC) 1 and 2 are involved *(96–98)*. PC1 occurs predominantly in the anterior lobe and its action releases ACTH, but PC2 further processes ACTH to smaller forms (α-MSH and CLIP). PC2 is believed to be preferentially expressed in the intermediate lobe. Thus, the majority of low-mol-wt ACTH in fetal plasma probably originates from the anterior lobe, whereas the site of high-mol-wt precursor secretion is not clear. The patterns of POMC processing and the factors controlling secretion of its cleavage products from the anterior and intermediate lobes require urgent clarification. It is possible that the differential expressions of PC1 and PC2 are more important for the activation of the fetal adrenal than is POMC expression.

Adrenal Responsiveness to ACTH and the Timing of Parturition

It has long been considered that the emergence of adrenal responsiveness to ACTH is a prime determinant of the timing of parturition *(11,12)*. The responsiveness of the ovine fetal adrenal to ACTH increases after d 125, and this change coincides with an increase in both the numbers of ACTH receptors and their coupling to the intracellular adenylate cyclase *(11,12,99)*. This change can be induced prematurely by intrafetal ACTH infusion, and it appears spontaneously when fetal adrenal cells are cultured in vitro, suggesting the existence of an in vivo inhibitor of ACTH action and adrenal maturation *(33,100)*. Whether this putative inhibitor is a high-mol-wt precursor of ACTH remains to be established.

Summary of Developmental Changes in the Fetal HPA Axis

The preceding discussion suggests the following outline on development of the fetal HPA axis:

Before d 90, ACTH and cortisol concentrations are low, but adrenal responsiveness to ACTH is very high.

Between 90–120 d, drive to the fetal corticotrophs remains low, the fetal adrenal is unresponsive, and cortisol negative feedback is not operative.

Around d 120, hypothalamic drive increases, the fetal pituitary becomes very responsive to hypothalamic secretagogs, but the adrenal has not been exposed to sufficient ACTH to permit adrenal responsiveness to develop.

Between d 125 and 135, adrenal responsiveness increases, basal plasma cortisol concentrations increase, and negative feedback damps the pituitary response to hypothalamic stimuli.

In the period from d 135 to term, ACTH receptor numbers increase, as does their linkage to the steroidogenic machinery within the adrenal cortical cell. As a result, the expression and activities of the key steroidogenic enzymes, cholesterol side-chain cleavage enzyme, and 17α hydroxylase also increase. Cortisol concentrations increase in turn, and their negative feedback effects on ACTH secretion are reduced or overridden by increased hypothalamic drive.

During the last day of fetal life, ACTH secretion continues to increase, and cortisol output is maximal. Placental secretion of PGE_2 increases dramatically, amplifying the hypothalamic drive to the corticotrophs.

Comparison of the Human with the Ovine Model

Postmaturity in human fetuses has long been associated with anencephaly, especially in cases where the fetal pituitary is absent *(101,102)*. Hypopituitarism owing to hypothalamic deficiency is not consistently associated with prolonged gestation, but the relationship appears stronger in cases of pituitary aplasia *(103)*. Nonetheless, the human fetal pituitary does not exert such absolute control over the onset of labor as does that of the fetal sheep. Pituitary aplasia in the human does not prolong gestation indefinitely, and spontaneous labor can occur, although somewhat late. The fetal pituitary appears to contribute to the parturient event, perhaps imposing some precision on its timing, but other intrauterine factors ensure that labor is initiated.

The role of fetal cortisol in the initiation of labor in humans is also less clear than it is in the sheep. Congenital deficiencies of key enzymes in the cortisol synthetic pathway do not necessarily prevent or even delay labor in humans. Although parturition can occur, neonatal survival is compromised in conditions that severely reduce the glucocorticoid status of the neonate. These conditions include adrenal and pituitary agenesis *(104–106)*. In other conditions, including some of the congenital adrenal enzyme defects, cortisol may not be secreted. Instead certain members of its less bioactive precursors are secreted, which may suffice for pulmonary maturation. Neonatal survival thus depends on a degree of maturation of the fetal HPA axis. Consistent with this requirement, fetal glucocorticoid concentrations increase over the final weeks of normal human gestation *(107)*.

Although a clear association between development of the fetal HPA axis and the timing of human birth has proven elusive, there is strong evidence that hormones of the HPA axis are expressed by the placenta and fetal membranes. CRH is expressed in human placenta, amnion, and decidua *(108)* and its concentrations in maternal plasma increase markedly during gestation, peaking at labor *(109,110)*. High maternal plasma CRH concentrations in late gestation are associated with early delivery *(109)*. CRH secreted by the placenta may thus be a significant factor in the onset of human labor, a view that is reinforced by experimental studies suggesting mechanisms of CRH action.

Administration of CRH to cultured placental, decidual, or amnion cells causes an increase in their secretion of $PGF_{2\alpha}$ and PGE_2, suggesting an effect of CRH on cyclooxygenase content and activity in these tissues. Interestingly, the ability of CRH to stimulate PG production by placenta was inhibited by anti-ACTH antiserum, suggesting that ACTH mediates the CRH effect, at least in that tissue *(111,112)*. The placenta also expresses POMC *(113–115)*, which increases the likelihood of a link between CRH, ACTH, and prostaglandin production. In addition to its ability to enhance prostaglandin production, CRH also potentiates the positive inotropic effect of $PGF_{2\alpha}$ on human myometrium, further strengthening its link with the onset of labor *(116,117)*.

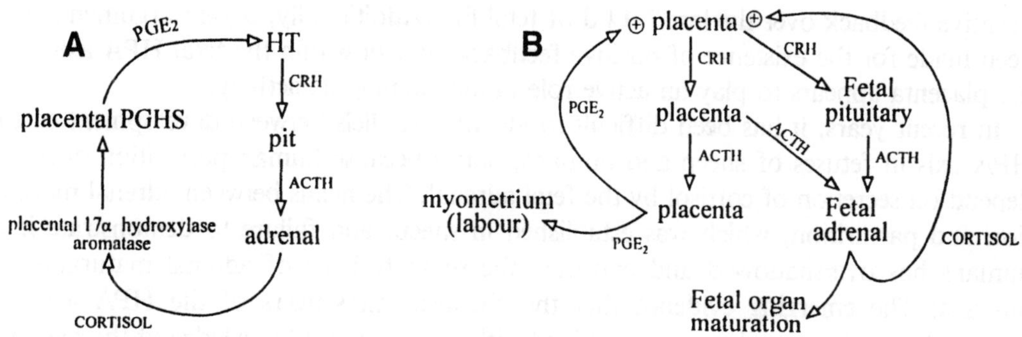

Fig. 4. Proposed differential control of the ovine and human fetal HPA axes at term. (**A**) Ovine, (**B**) human. In the ovine fetus (A), the fetal HPA axis functions as it does in the adult, with tonic drive amplified by placental PGE_2 secretion. Earlier in gestation, this PGE_2 secretion depends on fetal pituitary function, but at term, it is markedly enhanced by changes in placental steroidogenic enzyme expression resulting from the increased cortisol concentrations, which occur at this time. The main source of CRH in the human feto-placental unit may be the placenta. CRH acts on the fetal pituitary and, perhaps, the placenta to release ACTH. This, in turn, acts on the fetal adrenal to increase cortisol secretion and on the placenta to increase prostaglandin secretion. PGE_2 and cortisol both act on the placenta to potentiate the effects of CRH, closing the proposed positive feedback loop.

Although a strong case is emerging for placental CRH as a determinant of labor in the human, its role in endocrine maturation and its actions on the HPA axis of the fetus are less clear. Cortisol stimulates CRH production by amnion and placental cells *(111,118)*, and CRH secreted by the placenta is biologically active, presumably stimulating ACTH secretion from the fetal pituitary. A positive feedback control system may thus be postulated, involving the fetal pituitary, adrenal, and placenta, and resulting in activation of the fetal HPA axis. The theoretical possibility that this system also activates the parturient mechanism is less likely, because the fetal HPA axis normally plays a limited part in this process (Fig. 4).

The probable multiple roles of CRH in human parturition and fetal development would most likely have gone undiscovered had it not been shown that activation of the fetal HPA axis is a prerequisite for these processes in sheep. There are fascinating parallels between the hormones used to induce fetal maturation and parturition in these two species, irrespective of their sites of synthesis. The fetal sheep develops with a fully functional, self-contained HPA axis, whereas the human appears to rely on stimulation from a transient organ, the placenta, whose influence ceases at birth. The evolutionary significance and selective advantages of the two strategies may be related to the differences in fetal maturity at birth. The fetal lamb is precocial and relatively self-reliant at birth, except for its nutritional needs. The lamb, therefore, has more need for a functional stress axis than does a human infant who is born with a very immature forebrain and whose homeostasis depends heavily on maternal protection.

Summary

The ovine fetal HPA axis possesses the regulatory systems demonstrated by adults and undoubtedly functions autonomously long before the end of gestation. It also exhibits several features unique to fetal life. These include the enigmatic period of adrenal quiescence, which terminates around d 120, and its escape from the consequences of cortisol negative feedback over the last 7–14 d of fetal life. Additionally, cogent arguments have been made for the existence of positive feedback control within the fetal HPA axis, and the placenta appears to play an active role in maintaining its activity.

In recent years, it has been difficult to identify parallels between development of the HPA axis in fetuses of sheep and humans, partly because human parturition does not depend on secretion of cortisol by the fetal adrenal. The nexus between adrenal maturation and parturition, which was established in sheep, and failure to demonstrate it in humans has overshadowed and confused the separate issue of adrenal maturation in humans. The emerging evidence that the chemical messengers of the HPA axis are secreted by the human placenta, combined with our improved knowledge of their actions in fetal sheep, raise the intriguing possibility that nature has recruited different structures, but retained the same compounds to achieve maturation of the HPA axis in both species.

ENDOCRINE REGULATION OF FETAL LUNG MATURATION

At birth, survival of the newborn is critically dependent on the ability of its lung to function as an organ of gas exchange. Before birth, the fetal lungs are liquid-filled; gas exchange occurs at the placenta and the fetus receives oxygenated blood via the umbilical circulation. Consequently, the successful transition from an intrauterine to an extrauterine existence is largely dependent on the ability of the fetal lungs to assume a role that they have not previously performed. To exchange gases after birth effectively, the lungs must be:

1. Of an appropriate size;
2. At an appropriate level of structural and biochemical maturity; and
3. Cleared of liquid.

For example, a mature lung at birth contains millions of thin-walled alveoli, which create a sufficiently large surface area for gas exchange, dense capillary networks closely surround each alveolus, the connective tissue framework that supports the airways and blood vessels is sufficiently elastic, and the alveolar epithelial cells are able to synthesize and release surfactant into the lung lumen. Many of these features, which greatly facilitate the ability of the lung to exchange gases after birth, occur late in gestation and are closely linked to the endocrinological changes associated with the initiation of parturition. For instance, the preparturient increase in circulating corticosteroids is considered to play an important role in increasing potential airspace volume, the structural changes that lead to an increase in lung compliance, surfactant synthesis, and the reabsorption of liquid from the airways.

The precise mechanisms that control the progressive growth, structural maturation, and cellular differentiation of the lung throughout its development are largely unknown. However, they undoubtedly include a mixture of endocrine and physical factors, mesodermal/epithelial cell interactions, cell–cell and cell-substrate interactions, and cell-specific expression of transcription factors, which either activate or repress genes. Although it is well known that endocrine factors play an important role in fetal lung development, the pervasiveness of their influence becomes apparent when their roles are discussed in terms of the primary factors that determine the growth, structure, and cellular identity of the fetal lung. Thus, it is important to discuss the role of endocrine factors in the growth, structural development, differentiation of epithelial cell types, and in the preparation for air breathing after birth.

Stages of Fetal Lung Development

The development of the lung can be subjectively divided into four or five stages depending on the species; embryonic, pseudoglandular, canalicular, and saccular/alveolar stages *(119–122)*. The stage of lung development at birth varies in different species from relatively immature in rats and mice to quite mature in sheep. Presumably in sheep, there is an evolutionary advantage to having a mature lung at birth, so that the level of gas exchange sufficiently matches the respiratory demands required for survival. Thus, it is important to recognize that the level of lung development at birth differs markedly among species. At the normal time of birth in humans (40 wk), the lung is at the beginning of the alveolar stage of development, which continues postnatally for many years *(119–121)*. Thus, babies born prematurely (at 24–28 wk of gestation) have lungs that, at least in the peripheral margins, are in the canalicular stage of development and, therefore, have poorly developed terminal air sacs.

Embryonically, the lung originates as an outgrowth of the primitive foregut, which progressively elongates and branches to form the extensive respiratory tree; these epithelial tubes grow into the surrounding mesodermal tissue which is poorly vascularized *(see 119–122)*. The subsequent stages of lung development are characterized by: 1) Growth and subsequent ramification of the major conducting airways (glandular stage); 2) Expansion of the peripheral airway units caused by growth and subdivision of the epithelial tubes, as well as thinning and vascularization of the mesenchymal tissue adjacent to the developing airways (canalicular stage); and 3) The formation of secondary crests which compartmentalizes the terminal "airway" units, and, as gestation proceeds, these crests, become increasingly higher and both the epithelium and interstitium progressively thin (saccular/alveolar stage) *(see 119–122)*.

Fetal Lung Growth

Throughout gestation, the future airways of the fetal lungs are filled with liquid (lung liquid) and the presence of this liquid is critical for normal fetal lung growth and development *(see 123,124)*. It was once assumed that lung liquid was inhaled amniotic fluid, and that the fetal lungs develop in a collapsed state and inflate at birth when the first breath of air is taken. However, the findings that liquid accummulates in the lung lumen following tracheal ligation *(125,126)* and that lung liquid has a totally different ionic composition to amniotic fluid *(127)* clearly indicate that lung liquid is not inhaled amniotic fluid. It is now well recognized that lung liquid is a secretory product of the pulmonary epithelium *(128, 129)*, which leaves the lungs via the trachea and is either swallowed or enters the amniotic sac *(130)*. Furthermore, rather than being collapsed during fetal life, the fetal lungs are expanded by the liquid that occupies the future airways *(see 123,124)*. Indeed, during late gestation, the fetal lungs are expanded to a volume that is approximately double (~50 mL/kg vs ~25 mL/kg) the analogous volume (functional residual capacity [FRC]) in the air-filled lung of the newborn (*see 123*; Fig. 5). In the fetus, this high degree of lung expansion is critical for its growth and functional development, and is dependent on both the secretion of lung liquid and the restriction of its loss from the future airways *(see below)*.

Control of Fetal Lung Liquid Secretion. The secretion of fetal lung liquid is considered to result from the net movement of Cl^- across the pulmonary epithelium into the lung lumen *(129)*. This model is based on that proposed for Cl^- secretion in the shark rectal gland *(131)* and predicts that Na^+/K^+ ATPase, which is located on the basolateral surface

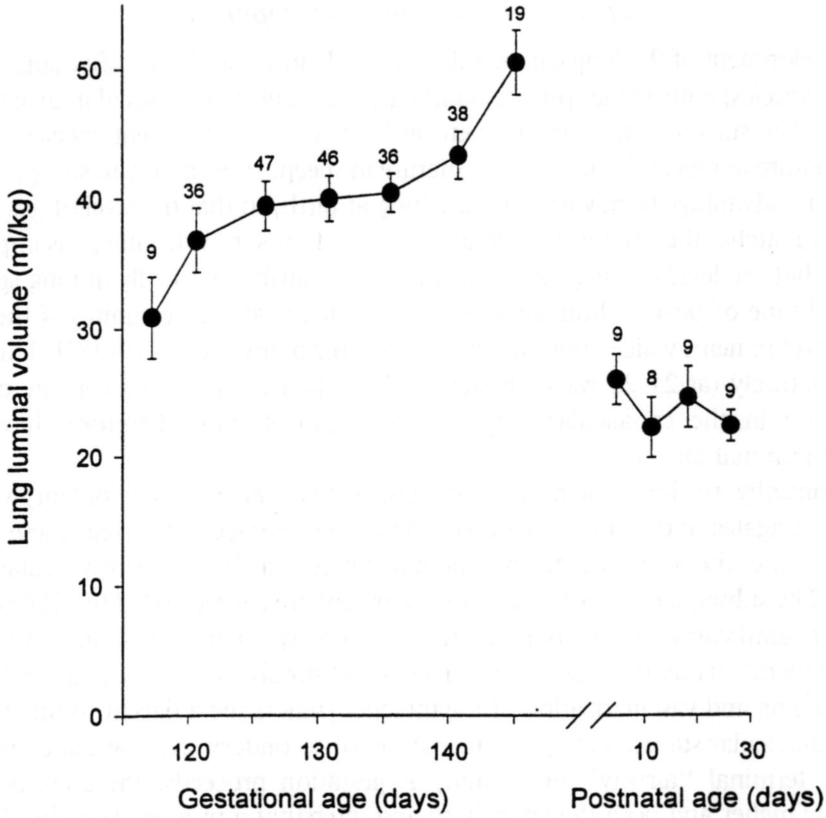

Fig. 5. Changes in lung liquid volume over the last third of gestation in fetal sheep. The volume (mL/kg) of fetal lung liquid, measured by the dye-dilution technique, during the last half of gestation in fetal sheep. For comparison, postnatal measurements of lung volume (functional residual capacity) were made in newborn lambs using an He dilution technique *(see 123,124)*.

of pulmonary epithelial cells, provides the electrochemical gradient for Na^+ to enter the cell coupled to Cl^-. Cl^- is considered to exit the cell and enter the lung lumen down its electrochemical gradient. The resultant net movement of Cl^- into the lung lumen most probably provides the osmotic gradient for the movement of water in the same direction *(129)* (Fig. 6).

The rate of secretion of fetal lung liquid is strongly influenced by endocrine factors. Both epinephrine *(132–134)* and arginine vasopressin *(135,136)* are potent inhibitors of fetal lung liquid secretion, and their inhibitory effects increase markedly over the last 2 wk before birth. The increased inhibitory effect of these hormones is thought to be primarily responsible for the inhibition of secretion and the reabsorption of lung liquid at birth *(129,136)*, and is considered to be mediated by increased circulating fetal corticosteroids before birth *(136,137)*. This response is believed to be an important maturational event prior to birth, which facilitates the transition of the lung to a gas exchange organ at birth, as described in more detail later. Intravenous infusions of epidermal growth factor (EGF) have also been shown to inhibit fetal lung liquid secretion *(138)*, although it is unclear whether the effect of EGF is mediated by an associated increase in epinephrine release. In addition, both cortisol and aldosterone, at least in vitro, have been shown to inhibit lung liquid secretion late in gestation in fetal guinea pigs *(139)*, although an inhibitory effect of cortisol is not supported by in vivo data in fetal sheep *(140,141)*.

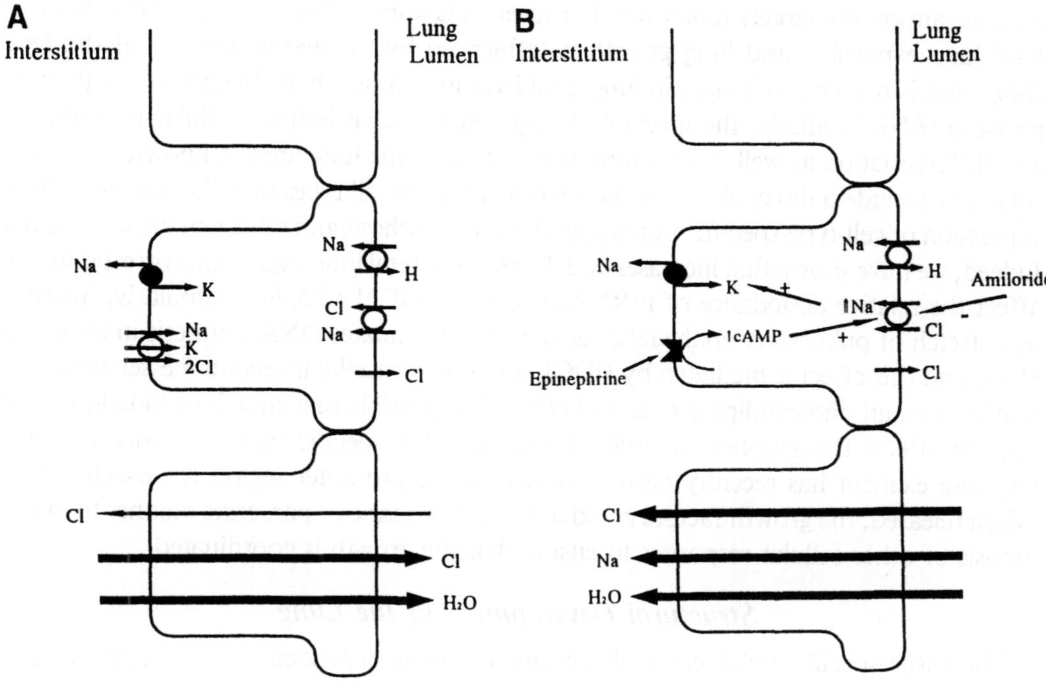

Fig. 6. Proposed model for fetal lung liquid secretion and reabsorption. Diagrammatic representation of the current model of lung liquid secretion and reabsorption in the fetus. **(A)** Lung liquid secretion: Pulmonary epithelial cells are connected by tight junctions at the luminal surface, thereby separating the lung lumen from the interstial space. Na/K ATPase, located on the basolateral surface of the epithelial cells, generates the gradient for Na to enter the cell linked with Cl and K. Cl then is thought to move out of the cell, down its electrochemical gradient, through specific channels located on the apical surface. The net movement of Cl into the lung lumen provides the osmotic gradient for the movement of water in the same direction. **(B)** Lung liquid reabsorption: Late in gestation, stimulation of pulmonary epithelial cells by epinephrine or AVP increases intracellular cAMP concentrations, which activates amiloride-inhibitable Na channels in the apical membrane. The resulting increase in intracellular Na ions increases the activity of Na/K ATPase, which promotes a net increase in Na and Cl flux away from the lung lumen, thereby reversing the osmotic gradient across the epithelium.

Fetal Lung Liquid and Lung Growth. The growth and structural development of the fetal lung is dependent on the degree to which it is expanded by liquid. Deflation of the fetal lung, caused by draining the lung of liquid, retards structural development of the lung and causes an abrupt cessation of fetal lung growth *(142–144)*. On the other hand, increasing the level of fetal lung expansion, by obstructing the efflux of lung liquid via the trachea, enhances its structural development and is a potent stimulus for its growth *(142, 143,145)*. Thus, any condition that influences the volume of liquid retained within the fetal lungs will affect their growth and structural development; some of these conditions include congenital diaphragmatic hernia, oligohydramnios, pleural effusions, and certain skeletal and neuromuscular disorders.

Increases in fetal lung expansion, caused by obstructing the fetal trachea, induces a rapid acceleration in lung growth, which begins within 2 d *(146)* and is completed within 7 d, at which time there is a 70% increase in cell number *(145,147)*. The integrative mechanisms that lead to alterations in fetal lung growth in response to alterations in fetal lung expansion are largely unknown. However, it is known that the relationship between fetal lung expansion and lung growth is influenced by the gestational age of the fetus *(146)*, and is related to changes in lung liquid volume rather than changes in intraluminal pressure *(147)*. Similarly, the mechanisms by which stretch induces cellular proliferation and differentiation as well as structural maturation of the lung are not known. However, they may include a direct effect on the genome in some cell types directly causing mitosis, expression of cell-type-specific proteins, and/or the synthesis and release of growth factors. Indeed, we have shown that increases and decreases in fetal lung expansion correspondingly affect the relative abundance of mRNAs encoding IGF-II *(145,148)*. Similarly, intermittent stretch of pulmonary epithelial cells in culture stimulates DNA synthesis in these cells *(149)*, and this effect is mediated by PDGF and the intracellular second messengers, tyrosine kinase and phospholipase C and D *(150)*. It is possible that stretch of individual cells directly affects transcription of mRNA encoding for specific proteins, since a stretch response element has recently been identified in the promoter region for α-actin *(151)*. When released, the growth factors could act in an autocrine or paracrine manner to induce mitosis or other cellular responses to ensure that the growth is coordinated.

Structural Development of the Lung

The tissue-specific architecture of the lung is largely dependent on the presence of an extracellular matrix (ECM) and on cell-to-cell and cell-substrate adhesion properties. The components of the ECM are synthesized by a variety of cell types within the lung and provide the structural support to which the lung cells attach *(152,153)*. Consequently, the ECM plays an integral role in lung physiology from early stages in its growth and development, through to its function as a gas-exchange organ in the adult. Indeed, different components of the ECM are considered to be critically involved with cell migration, branching morphogenesis, cellular proliferation, and cytodifferentation as well as being a prinicpal determinant of the elasticity (compliance) of the lung *(153–155)*. The ECM of the lungs is comprised of collagen (principally types I, III, V, and VI), elastin, glycoproteins (e.g., fibronectin and laminin) and proteoglycans *(152,153)*. At the level of the peripheral airway units, these components form the epithelial and endothelial basement membranes, and the structural fibers that course through the interstitium located at the interalveolar septa; these connect with axial fibers running in parallel to major conducting airways and blood vessels, and are further braced by connective tissue elements projecting in from the pleura *(152,153)*. Thus, major alterations in the architecture of the lung, as occurs during lung development, must include remodeling of the ECM.

There is now good evidence demonstrating that corticosteroids are intimately involved in the structural maturation of the fetal lung. The increase in fetal plasma cortisol concentrations prior to parturition is thought to play an important role in maturing the lung by altering its structure. This leads to an increase in potential airspace volume, a reduction in gas-diffusing distances, and an increase in tissue compliance. For example, over the last third of gestation in fetal sheep, the volume of the future airspace increases from 25–30 to 250–300 mL *(123)*, which is associated with an increase in alveolar surface area and reduced interalveolar tissue distances *(122)*. This gestational age-related increase in lung liquid volume and secretion rate is enhanced by the infusion of cortisol, which prematurely increases circulating fetal plasma cortisol concentrations *(140)*. On the other hand, removal of the principal source of circulating cortisol in the fetus, by adrenalectomy, greatly diminishes the gestational age-related increase in fetal lung liquid volume and secretion rate *(141)*. However, because the treatments used in these studies also altered the circulating concentrations of the thyroid hormone, triiodothyronine (T3), it is possible that this hormone is also involved in these changes in lung liquid volume (potential airspace volume).

Fetal hypophysectomy, which also decreases circulating fetal plasma cortisol concentrations and prolongs gestation in fetal sheep, markedly alters fetal lung architecture, such that the lungs appear structurally immature. Following fetal hypophysectomy, at the time of expected birth, the interalveolar walls of the fetal lung were thicker, compared with controls, and the volume density of septal tissue was greater, i.e., the potential airspace volume was reduced *(156)*. These characteristics were very similar to the structural characteristics observed in immature lungs from much younger fetuses *(156)*. Infusions of either cortisol or ACTH, which would be expected to stimulate endogenous cortisol release, into hypophysectomized fetuses over 3–4 d, reduced interalveolar wall thicknesses and the volume density of septal tissue to control levels *(156)*. This indicates that over the last third of gestation in fetal sheep, structural development of the lung is dependent on the progressive increase in circulating endogenous fetal cortisol concentrations. Thyroidectomy, on the other hand, had no detectable effect on lung structure in this study, although this procedure retarded structural development of the lung in another *(157)*. It is interesting that sustained deflation of the lung during the last third of gestation in fetal sheep causes identical changes in lung structure as that reported for corticosteroid withdrawal *(142)*.

Corticosteroid infusions into fetal monkeys *(158)* and sheep *(159)* and single im injections of betamethasone into fetal sheep *(160)* cause an increase fetal lung compliance (of saline-filled lungs), principally as a result of structural changes *(158,159)*. The increase in lung compliance occurs within 48 h and is associated with an increase in ventilatory efficiency in prematurely delivered newborn lambs *(160,161)*. The combination of betamethasone and thyroxine (T_4) treatment enhanced the effect of betamethasone alone *(161)*. Consequently, the increase in lung liquid volume over the last third of gestation *(123,141)* is probably owing to alterations in lung structure, leading to an increase in potential airspace volume and lung compliance, resulting from the endogeneous increase in circulating corticosteroids in combination with elevated T_3 concentrations *(140,141)*. Indeed, because the intraluminal pressure measured during periods of apnea *(162)* remains relatively constant during late gestation, owing to continued lung liquid secretion, an increase in lung tissue compliance must be associated with an increase in lung liquid volume to sustain the intraluminal pressure. However, lung liquid volume is unlikely to increase late in gestation as a result of compliance changes if the trans-thoracic pressure gradient is increased by external factors; for example, during oligohydramnios, the trans-thoracic pressure gradient is increased because of increased ventral flexion of the fetal abdomen leading to a decrease in lung volume *(163)*.

The mechanisms by which cortisosteroids affect fetal lung structure and tissue compliance are not known, but most probably include remodeling of the ECM. Over the last third of gestation in fetal sheep, the content of collagen, and particularly elastin, increases markedly in lung parenchyma, with most of the increase occurring over the last 25–30 d *(164)*. Similarly, it has been shown that fetal lung elastin mRNA levels increase markedly over the last third of gestation in fetal sheep, and in particular, tropoelastin (elastin precursor) production peaks just before the time of birth *(165)*. This period of gestation coincides with the exponential increase in cortisol concentrations circulating in fetal plasma and a large increase in lung liquid volume *(123,141)*. Thus, because the components of the lung ECM are rapidly turned over, at least in culture *(166,167)*, it is likely that endocrine factors like cortisol induce remodeling of the ECM by altering expression of its specific components *(168)*. Altering the rate of ECM turnover via altering the expression of metalloproteinases or their specific inhibitors may also contribute to the remodeling *(169)*. On the other hand, although dexamethosone treatment in fetal rats on d 17 of gestation had no effect on elastin content (as measured by desmosine content) at the time of birth, a reduction was observed by d 10 after birth, which persisted until d 30 *(170)*. The reasons for the discrepancy between this finding and the findings of a large increase in elastin production in association with the exponenial rise in endogenous cortisol concentrations are unclear. Whatever the reasons, it is likely that endogenous glucocorticoids play an important role in regulating the ECM of the lung, and therefore, influence its structure and thus its ability to function as a gas-exchange organ after birth. It is possible that the glucocorticoids act directly on specific cell types within the lung to effect these changes, or their effects are mediated via other endocrine factors, including epidermal growth factor *(171)*, transforming growth factor *(172)*, and fibroblast-pneumonocyte factor *(173)*. It is possible that these growth factors act in a paracrine fashion to modulate the action of both glucocorticoids and physical influences, like alterations in lung expansion, which would explain the similarity in the effect of these stimuli on lung architecture and cellular differentiation.

Epithelial Cell Differentiation

The mechanisms that regulate lung epithelial cell differentiation are largely unknown. However, these mechanisms are of considerable interest, because appropriate epithelial cell differentiation is critical for respiratory function both in the neonate and adult. Indeed, type I epithelial cells make up >90% of the surface area of the lung and, therefore, are intimately involved in gas exchange. Type II cells, on the other hand, produce surfactant, which is critical for lowering surface tension forces at the air–liquid interface *(see 174)*.

Differentiation of the epithelial cells lining the peripheral airway units begins during the canalicular stage of lung development in sheep *(122)*. Initially, most epithelial cells within the terminal airways are undifferentiated *(122)* with near-equal numbers of type I and type II epithelial cells *(122,156)*. As gestation and structural development of the lung proceed, the undifferentiated cells progressively differentiate and the density of type II cells decrease such that at term, there are approximately twice as many type I as type II cells *(156)*. Although it is widely considered that both types of differentiated epithelial cells arise as daughter cells from proliferating type II stem cells *(175)*, recent studies, which have examined the expression of cell-specific markers from very early in gestation, indicate that this concept is not entirely accurate *(176)*. Indeed, Alcorn et al. *(122)* first observed the presence of type I epithelial cells at an earlier period in gestation than type II epithelial cells in fetal sheep lungs. Whatever the mechanisms that control lung epithelial cell differentiation, they are influenced by both corticosteroids *(156)* and the degree of fetal lung expansion *(142)*. Fetal hypophysectomy, which prevents the normal gestational age-related increase in fetal plasma cortisol concentrations and the onset of labor, prevents the gestational age-related decrease in type II cell density at the expected time of birth *(156)*. However, the infusion of ACTH and cortisol into hypophysectomized fetuses reduced the density of type II cells to control levels at the expected time of birth *(156)*. Similar results occur following alterations in fetal lung expansion, indicating that there may be a common link between changes in lung expansion and the action of corticosteroids. Deflation of the fetal lung, by draining the lung of liquid, increases the density of type II epithelial cells, whereas increasing the degree of lung expansion reduces the density of type II epithelial cells *(142)*.

Preparation for Air-Breathing After Birth

The Clearance of Lung Liquid at Birth. At birth, when the umbilical cord is severed, the lungs must be cleared of liquid so that air can enter the lungs and respiratory gases diffuse across the alveolar epithelium. Thus, the pulmonary epithelium must transform from a secretory epithelium in the fetus to one that predominantly absorbs liquid in the newborn. One of the primary mechanisms by which lung liquid is cleared from the airways is the result of reabsorption in response to the very high circulating concentrations of epinephrine and arginine vasopressin at the time of labor *(133,177)*.

Epinephrine and AVP are considered to inhibit fetal lung liquid secretion in vivo, via activation of amiloride-inhibitable Na^+ channels in the apical (luminal) surface of pulmonary epithelial cells *(129,178,179)*. This is thought to increase the net movement of Na^+ into the cell, resulting in an increase in the activity of Na^+/K^+ ATPase, which actively transports Na^+ out of the cell across the basolateral surface. The net result is increased Na^+ and Na^+-coupled Cl^- flux *(129)* from lung lumen to plasma, which opposes the osmotic gradient across the epithelium (Fig. 6). The inhibitory effects of both AVP and epinephrine on the secretion rate of fetal lung liquid clearly increase with increasing gestational age *(132–134,136)*, although at any gestational age (GA), the relative potency of epinephrine appears to be greater than that of AVP *(133,136)*. The inhibitory effect of these hormones on fetal lung liquid secretion increases exponentially toward term *(133,136)*, indicating that this is another maturational process late in gestation that facilitates the transition of the lung to a gas-exchange organ after birth. Indeed, the inhibitory effects of AVP on fetal lung liquid secretion closely parallel the preparturient increase in fetal plasma cortisol concentrations, indicating that cortisol may be involved in this process *(136)*.

Studies have now revealed that the fetal hormonal environment necessary for maturing the fetal lungs, both in respect of their surfactant production *(see below)* and increased tissue compliance, is also important for maturing the lung liquid reabsorptive response to epinephrine and AVP. Removal of the fetal thyroid gland abolished the increased reabsorptive effects of the pulmonary epithelium to epinephrine, and the infusion of triiodothyronine (T_3) restored this response *(180)*. In addition, relatively short-term (3-d) infusions of both cortisol and T_3 can prematurely increase the inhibitory effect of epinephrine on fetal lung liquid secretion, although neither hormone had an independent effect *(137)*. However, more recent studies have shown that longer-term (10-d) infusions of cortisol into the fetus, which mimicked the normal preparturient increase of this hormone in fetal plasma, greatly enhanced the inhibitory effect of epinephrine on fetal lung liquid secretion *(140)*. In addition, fetal adrenalectomy, which removes the principal source of circulating cortisol in the fetus late in gestation, greatly reduced the inhibitory effect of epinephrine on fetal lung liquid secretion *(141)*. However, neither of these studies *(140,141)* could separate the individual effects of cortisol and T_3, since circulating T_3 concentrations were increased by cortisol infusions and reduced by adrenalectomy. Nevertheless, it was *(140,141)* concluded that the preparturient increase in fetal plasma cortisol concentrations, and the associated endocrine changes, increased the sensitivity of the lung liquid secretory mechanism to adrenaline and presumably AVP *(181)*. It was further speculated that this was a maturational process that facilitated the clearance of lung liquid at the time of birth in preparation for the onset of air breathing.

Surfactant Biosynthesis and Release. Surfactant is a complex mixture of both lipids and protein (~87% phospholipids and ~10% protein), which is synthesised by type II epithelial cells and is released into the lung lumen by exocytosis *(see 174,182)*. The presence of surfactant within alveoli is essential for normal respiratory function after birth, principally owing to its inherent ability to form a monolayer at the air–liquid interface. This monolayer acts to greatly reduce surface tension forces at the air–liquid interface, and thereby prevents alveoli from collapsing at end expiration and importantly prevents smaller alveoli from emptying into larger ones *(174)*.

Undoubtedly, a large component of the respiratory distress that occurs in infants born prematurely (Neonatal Respiratory Distress Syndrome [RDS]) results from lungs that are too immature to produce sufficient amounts of surfactant. The original observation that glucocorticoid administration in sheep not only induced premature parturition, but also enhanced fetal lung maturation *(1)* prompted much research into the hormonal regulation (particularly by glucocorticoids) of surfactant synthesis. The regulation of surfactant biosynthesis includes regulating expression of the surfactant protein (SPA, SPB, and SPC) genes as well as the synthesis and activity of enzymes involved in phospholipid biosynthesis *(183)*. The expression of the surfactant proteins in fetal lung tissue increases with advancing gestation *(184,185)*, and the concentrations of SPA and SPB in amniotic fluid increase over the last third of gestation in humans *(186)*. Furthermore, the expression of the surfactant proteins can be induced by glucocorticoids *(183,187)*, presumably via glucocortocoid response elements that have been identified in the 5′-flanking regions of the genes encoding for SPA and SPB *(see 183)*. Although SPA is also expressed in a gestational age-dependent manner, its pattern of expression is different from that of SPB and SPC, at least in humans *(184,185)* and rats *(176)*. This indicates that expression of the different surfactant proteins can be differentially controlled; indeed, SPA expression is believed to be principally controlled by cAMP-mediated factors, including PGE_2 *(183)*, which also increases exponentially before birth *(42,188)*. Many of the enzymes critical for phospholipid biosynthesis also increase in the lung before birth, and their expression is increased by glucocorticoid administration *(see 182)*. Similarly, the presence of the fetal thyroid gland appears to be necessary for normal maturation of the fetal lung surfactant system *(157)*. This finding, and the fact that thyroid hormones potentiate the effect of corticosteroids *(189)*, has resulted in clinical trials using combined corticosteroids and thyroid hormones to reduce the incidence of repiratory distress in premature infants *(see 190)*.

It has also been demonstrated that indices of fetal lung maturity (e.g., pressure–volume curves and tissue and lavage fluid content of saturated phosphatidylcholine) are more closely related to fetal plasma cortisol concentrations than gestational age *(191)*. Consequently, it is highly likely that the endogenous increase in fetal plasma cortisol concentrations is an important factor in attaining functional lung maturity in late gestation. This contention is supported by numerous clinical trials demonstrating that maternal glucocorticoid treatment can successfully reduce the incidence of RDS in infants born prematurely *(192,193)*.

Summary

In summary, effective gas exchange in the newborn is largely dependent on whether appropriate growth, structural maturation, and cellular differentiation of the lung have occurred during fetal life. In particular, the future airways must have branched to an appropriate number, the lung must have grown to an appropriate size, and structural modification must have occurred within the terminal airways to increase surface area, reduce gas-diffusing distances, and increase tissue compliance. Furthermore, appropriate differentiation and maturation of the epithelial cells must have occurred within the terminal airways to ensure that appropriate levels of surfactant are synthesized and released, and that the surface area is sufficiently large. Considerable evidence has accumulated to indicate that the preparturient increase in circulating corticosteroids within the fetus is intimately involved in many of the processes that are essential for the establishment of effective gas exchange after birth. However, it is important to note that many other hormones are likely to be involved in, or to influence, fetal lung maturation, including thyroid hormones, epidermal growth factor, catecholamines, estrogens, prolactin, and insulin.

REFERENCES

1. Liggins GC (1969) Premature delivery of foetal lambs infused with glucocorticoids. J Endocrinol 45:515–523.
2. Liggins GC (1968) Premature parturition after infusion of corticotropin or cortisol in foetal lambs. J Endocrinol 42:323–325.
3. Liggins GC, Kennedy PC (1968) Effects of electrocoagulation of the foetal lamb hypophysis on growth and development J Endocrinol 40:371–381.
4. Liggins GC, Kennedy PC, Holm LW (1967) Failure of initiation of parturition after electrocoagulation of the pituitary of the fetal lamb. Am J Obstet Gynecol 98:1080–1086.
5. McDonald TJ, Nathanielsz PW (1991) Bilateral destruction of the fetal paraventricular nuclei prolongs gestation in sheep. Am J Obstet Gynecol 165:764–770.
6. Antolovich GC, Clarke IJ, McMillen IC, Perry RA, Robinson PM, Silver M, Young R (1990) Hypothalamo-pituitary disconnection in the fetal sheep. Neuroendocrinology 51:1–9.
7. Antolovich GC, McMillen IC, Robinson PM, Silver M, Young IR, Perry RA (1991) The effect of hypothalamo-pituitary disconnection on the functional and morphologic development of the pituitary-adrenal axis in the fetal sheep in the last third of gestation. Neuroendocrinology 54: 254–261.
8. Drost M, Holm LW (1968) Prolonged pregnancy in ewes after foetal adrenalectomy. J Endocrinol 40:293–296.
9. Mugila L, Jacobson L, Dikkes P, Majzoub JA (1995) Corticotropin-releasing hormone deficiency reveals major fetal but not adult glucocorticoid need. Nature 373:427–432.
10. Liggins GC, Thorburn GD (1994) Initiation of parturition, In: Marshall's Physiology of Reproduction (Iamming GE, ed.), Chapman & Hall, London, pp. 863–1002.
11. Challis JRG, Brooks AN (1989) Maturation and activation of hypothalamic-pituitary-adrenal function in fetal sheep. Endocr Rev 10:182–203.
12. Thorburn GD, Liggins GC (1994) Role of the fetal pituitary-adrenal axis and placenta in the initiation of parturition, In: Marshall's Physiology of Reproduction (Iamming GE, ed.), Chapman & Hall, London, pp. 1003–1036.
13. Levidiotis M, Oldfield B, Wintour ME (1987) Corticotrophin-releasing factor and arginine vasopressin fibre projections to the median eminence of fetal sheep. Neuroendocrinology 46:453–456.
14. Matwijiw I, Thliveris JA, Faiman C (1988) Ontogenesis of the hypothalamo-pituitary portal vasculature in the ovine fetus [Abstract]. Clin Invest Med 10:B71,R418.
15. Levidiotis ML, Wintour EM, McKinley MJ, Oldfield BJ (1988) Hypothalamic–hypophyseal vascular connections in the fetal sheep. Neuroendocrinology 49:47–50.
16. Watabe T, Levidiotis ML, Oldfield B, Wintour EM (1991) Ontogeny of corticotrophin-releasing factor (CRF) in the ovine fetal hypothalamus—use of multiple CRF antibodies. J Endocrinol 129: 3–35.
17. Lu F, Yang K, Challis JRG (1991) Characteristics and developmental changes of corticotrophin-releasing hormone-binding sites in the fetal sheep anterior pituitary gland. J Endocrinol 130: 223–229.
18. Currie IS, Brooks AN (1992) Corticotrophin-releasing factors in the hypothalamus of the developing fetal sheep. J Dev Physiol 17:241–246.
19. Mulvogue HM, McMillen IC, Robinson PM, Perry RA (1986) Immunocytochemical localization of protMSH,tMSH, ACTH and bendorphin/blipotrophin in the fetal sheep pituitary: an ontogenetic study. J Dev Physiol 8:355–368.

20. Perry RA, Mulvogue HM, McMillen IC, Robinson PM (1985) Immunohistochemical localization of ACTH in the adult and fetal pituitary. J Dev Physiol 7:397–404.
21. Matthews SG, Han X, Lu F, Challis JRG (1994) Developmental changes in the distribution of pro-opiomelanocortin and prolactin mRNA in the pituitary of the ovine fetus and lamb. J Mol Endocrinol 13:175–185.
22. Tangalakis K, Coghlan JP, Connell J, Crawford R, Darling P, Hammond VE, Haralambidis J, Penschow J, Wintour EM (1989) Tissue distribution and levels of gene expression of three steroid hydroxylases in ovine fetal adrenal glands. Acta Endocrinol (Copenh) 120:225–232.
23. Wintour EM, Brown EH, Denton DA, Hardy KJ, McDougall JG, Oddie CJ, Whipp GT (1975) The ontogeny and regulation of corticosteroid secretion by the ovine foetal adrenal. Acta Endocrinol 79:301–316.
24. Glickman JA, Challis JRG (1980) The changing response pattern of sheep fetal adrenal cells throughout the course of gestation. Endocrinology 106:1371–1376.
25. Durand P (1979) ACTH receptor levels in lamb adrenals at late gestation and early neonatal states. Biol Reprod 20:837–845.
26. Durand P, Cathiard AM, Morera AM, Dazord A, Saez JM (1981) Maturation of adrenocorticotropin-sensitive adenylate cyclase of ovine fetal adrenal during late pregnancy. Endocrinology 108:2114–2119.
27. Manchester EL, Challis JRG (1982) The effects of adrenocorticotropin, guanylylimidodiphosphate, dibutyryl adenosine 3′,5′-monophosphate and exogenous substrates on corticosteroid output by ovine fetal adrenal cells at different times in pregnancy. Endocrinology 111:889–895.
28. Tangalakis K, Crawford R, McFarlane AC, Wintour EM (1994) Regulation of steroid hydroxylase gene expression in the ovine fetal adrenal gland at 0.4 gestation. Mol Cell Endocrinol 103: 21–27.
29. McFarlane AC, Potocnik S, Towstoless M, Moritz K, Wintour EM (1995) Pituitary-adrenal function in the immature ovine foetus. J Endocrinol 145:455–460.
30. Wintour EM, Crawford R, McFarlane A, Moritz K, Tangalakis K (1995) Regulation and function of the fetal adrenal gland in sheep. Endocr Res 21:81–89.
31. McFarlane AC, Cooper EJ, Fernley RT, Watabe T, Wintour EM (1995) Comparative response of the immature and mature ovine fetus to corticotrophin-releasing hormone (CRH). Reprod Fertil Dev 7:75–82.
32. Tangalakis K, Coghlan JP, Crawford R, Hammond VE, Wintour EM (1990) Steroid hydroxylase gene expression in the ovine fetal adrenal gland following ACTH infusion. Acta Endocrinol 123: 371–377.
33. Durand P, Cathiard AM, Saez JM (1982) In vitro maturation of ovine fetal adrenal cells adenylate cyclase: corticotropin-dependent and independent development of the response to corticotropin. Biochem Biophys Res Commun 106:8–15.
34. Roebuck MM, Jones CT, Holland D, Silman R (1980) In vitro effects of high molecular weight forms of ACTH on the fetal sheep adrenal. Nature 284:616–618.
35. Jones CT, Roebuck MM (1980) ACTH peptides and the development of the fetal adrenal. J Steroid Biochem 12:77–82.
36. Jones CT, Edwards AV, Tindell D (1992) Inhibitory effects of proopiomelanocortin on cortical and medullary activity in the calf adrenal. J Dev Physiol 17:69–73.
37. Deayton JM, Young IR, Thorburn GD (1993) Early hypophysectomy of sheep fetuses—effects on growth, placental steroidogenesis and prostaglandin production. J Reprod Fertil 97:513–520.
38. Jacobs RA, Young IR, Hollingworth SA, Thorburn GD (1994) Chronic administration of low doses of adrenocorticotrophin to hypophysectomized fetal sheep leads to normal term labour. Endocrinology 134:1389–1394.
39. Deayton JM, Young IR, Hollingworth SA, White A, Crosby SR, Thorburn GD (1994) Effect of late hypothalamo-pituitary disconnection on the development of the HPA axis in the ovine fetus and the initiation of parturition. J Neuroendocrinol 6:25–31.
40. Kelleman A, Binienda Z, Ding XY, Rittenhouse L, Mitchell M, Nathanielsz PW (1992) Prostaglandin production in the umbilical and uterine circulations in pregnant sheep at 129-136 days gestation. J Dev Physiol 17:63–67.
41. Mitchell MD (1991) The regulation of placental eicosanoid biosynthesis. Placenta 12:557–572.
42. Fowden AL, Harding R, Ralph MM, Thorburn GD (1987) The nutritional regulation of prostaglandin E concentrations in the fetus and pregnant ewe during late gestation. J Physiol 394:1–12.
43. Rice GE, Payne MJ, Wong MH, Thorburn GD (1992) Immunoreactive prostaglandin G/H synthase content increases in ovine cotyledons during late gestation. Placenta 13:429–437.

44. Thorburn GD, Hollingworth SA, Hooper SB (1991) The trigger for parturition in sheep: fetal hypothalamus or placenta? J Dev Physiol 15:71–79.
45. Hollingworth SA, Deayton JM, Young IR, Thorburn GD (1995) Prostaglandin E2 administered to fetal sheep increases the plasma concentrations of adrenocorticotropin (ACTH) and the proportion of ACTH in low molecular weight forms. Endocrinology 136:1233–1240.
46. McDonald TJ, Hoffmann GE, Myers DA, Nathanielsz PW (1990) Hypothalamic glucocorticoid implants prevent fetal ovine adrenocorticotropin secretion in response to stress. Endocrinology 127:2862–2868.
47. Myers DA, McDonald TJ, Dunn TG, Moss GE, Nathanielsz PW (1992) Effect of implantation of dexamethasone adjacent to the paraventricular nucleus on messenger ribonucleic acid for corticotropin-releasing hormone and proopiomelanocortin during late gestation in fetal sheep. Endocrinology 130:2167–2172.
48. Matthews SG, Challis JRG (1995) Regulation of CRH and AVP mRNA in the developing ovine hypothalamus: effects of stress and glucocorticoids. Am J Physiol 268:E1096–E1107.
49. Yang K, Jones SA, Challis JRG (1990) Changes in glucocorticoid receptor number in the hypothalamus and pituitary of the sheep fetus with gestational age and after adrenocorticotropin treatment. Endocrinology 126:11–17.
50. Yang K, Hammond GL, Challis JRG (1992) Characterization of an ovine glucocorticoid receptor cDNA and developmental changes in its mRNA levels in the fetal sheep hypothalamus, pituitary gland and adrenal. J Mol Endocrinol 8:173–180.
51. Matthews SG, Yang K, Challis JRG (1995) Changes in glucocorticoid receptor mRNA in the developing ovine pituitary and the effects of exogenous cortisol. J Endocrinol 144:483–490.
52. Lu F, Yang K, Challis JRG (1994) Regulation of ovine fetal pituitary function by corticotrophin-releasing hormone, arginine vasopressin and cortisol in vitro. J Endocrinol 143:199–208.
53. Schwartz J, Ash P, Ford V, Raff H, Crosby S, White A (1994) Secretion of adrenocorticotrophin (ACTH) and ACTH precursors in ovine anterior pituitary cells: actions of corticotrophin-releasing hormone, arginine vasopressin and glucocorticoids. J Endocrinol 140:189–195.
54. McMillen IC, Merei JJ (1993) Effect of gestational age, CRF and cortisol on ACTH secretion from slices of fetal sheep pituitaries in an in vitro perifusion system. Neuroendocrinology 58: 564–569.
55. Ozolins IZ, Young IR, McMillen IC (1990) Effect of cortisol infusion on basal and corticotropin-releasing factor (CRF)-stimulated plasma ACTH concentrations in the sheep fetus after surgical isolation of the pituitary. Endocrinology 1274:1833–1840.
56. Zehnder TJ, Valego NK, Rose JC (1994) The effects of chronically elevated plasma cortisol on the bioactive and immunoreactive corticotropin secretory responses to hemorrhage in the fetal sheep at 0.70 gestation. Am J Obstet Gynecol 171:1251–1256.
57. Kerr DR, Castro MI, Rawashdeh NM, Rose JC (1992) ACTH and cortisol responses to sequential CRF injections in fetal sheep. Am J Physiol 262:E319–E324.
58. Kerr DR, Castro MI, Valego NK, Rawashdeh NM, Rose JC (1992) ACTH and cortisol responses to hypotension in fetal sheep after a prior CRF injection. Am J Physiol 262:E325–E329.
59. Canny BJ, Clarke IJ, Funder JW (1990) Adrenocorticotropin responses to endogenous and exogenous secretagogues in the sheep: specificity of glucocorticoid action. Neuroendocrinology 51: 181–189.
60. Kerr DR, Castro MI, Valego NK, Rawashdeh NM, Rose JC (1992) Corticotropin and cortisol responses to corticotropin-releasing factor in the chronically hypoxemic ovine fetus. Am J Obstet Gynecol 167:1686–1690.
61. Harvey LM, Gilbert RD, Longo LD, Ducsay CA (1993) Changes in ovine fetal adrenocortical responsiveness after long-term hypoxemia. Am J Physiol 264:E741–E747.
62. Wood CE (1986) Sensitivity of cortisol-induced inhibition of ACTH and renin in fetal sheep. Am J Physiol 250:R795–R802.
63. Wood CE (1988) Insensitivity of near term fetal sheep to cortisol: Possible relation to the control of parturition. Endocrinology 122:1565–1572.
64. Ballard PL, Kitterman JA, Bland RD, Clyman RI, Gluckman PD, Platzker ACG, Kaplan SL, Grumbach MM (1982) Ontogeny and regulation of corticosteroid binding globulin capacity in plasma of fetal and newborn lambs. Endocrinology 110:359–366.
65. Fairclough RJ, Liggins GC (1975) Protein binding of plasma cortisol in the foetal lamb near term. J Endocrinol 67:333–341.
66. Berdusco ETM, Hammond GL, Jacobs RA, Grolla A, Akagi K, Langlois D, Challis JRG (1993) Glucocorticoid-induced increase in plasma corticosteroid binding globulin levels in fetal sheep is

associated with increased biosynthesis and alterations in glycosylation. Endocrinology 132: 2001–2008.
67. Berdusco ETM, Milne WK, Challis JRG (1994) Low-dose cortisol infusion increases plasma corticosteroid binding globulin (CBG) and the amount of hepatic CBG mRNA in fetal sheep on day 100 of gestation. J Endocrinol 140:425–430.
68. Berdusco ETM, Yang K, Hammond GL, Challis JRG (1995) Corticosteroid binding globulin (CBG) production by hepatic and extra-hepatic sites in the ovine fetus: effects of CBG on glucocorticoid negative feedback on pituitary cells in vitro. J Endocrinol 146:121–130.
69. Yang K, Smith CL, Dales D, Hammond GL, Challis JRG (1992) Cloning of an ovine 11B-hydroxysteroid dehydrogenase complementary deoxyribonucleic acid: tissue and temporal distribution of its messenger ribonucleic acid during fetal and neonatal development. Endocrinology 131: 2120–2126.
70. Yang K, Matthews SG, Challis JRG (1995) Developmental and glucocorticoid regulation of pituitary 11B-hydroxysteroid dehydrogenase 1 gene expression in the ovine fetus and lamb. J Mol Endocrinol 14:109–116.
71. Antolovich GC, Perry RA, Trahair JF, Silver M, Robinson PM (1989) The development of corticotrophs in the fetal sheep pars distalis: the effect of adrenalectomy or cortisol infusion. Endocrinology 124:1333–1339.
72. Challis JRG, Huhtanen D, Sprague C, Mitchell BF, Lye SJ (1985) Modulation by cortisol of adrenocorticotropin-induced activation of adrenal function in fetal sheep. Endocrinology 116:2267–2272.
73. Darbeida H, Durand P (1990) Mechanism of glucocorticoid enhancement of the responsiveness of ovine adrenocortical cells to adrenocorticotropin. Biochem Biophys Res Commun 166:1183–1191.
74. Jones CT, Kendall JZ, Ritchie JWK, Robinson JS, Thorburn GD (1978) Adrenocorticotrophin and corticosteroid changes during dexamethasone infusion to intact and synacthen infusion to hypophysectomized foetuses. Acta Endocrinol 87:203–211.
75. Jones CT, Johnson P, Kendall JZ, Ritchie JWK, Thorburn GD (1978) Induction of premature parturition in sheep: adrenocorticotrophin and corticosteroid changes during infusion of Synacthen into the foetus. Acta Endocrinol 87:192–202.
76. Rice GE, Wong MH, Hollingworth SA, Thorburn GD (1990) Prostaglandin G/H synthase activity in ovine cotyledons: a gestational profile. Eicosanoids 3:231–236.
77. Young IR, Deayton JM, Hollingworth SA, Thorburn GD (1996) Continuous intrafetal infusion of prostaglandin E2 prematurely activates the hypothalamo-pituitary-adrenal axis and induces parturition in the sheep. Endocrinology 137:2424–2431.
78. Watanabe T, Morimoto A, Sakata Y, Murakami N (1990) ACTH response induced by interleukin-1 is mediated by CRF secretion stimulated by hypothalamic PGE. Experientia 46:481–484.
79. Watanobe H, Takebe K (1994) Effects of intravenous administration of interleukin-1-beta on the release of prostaglandin E2, corticotrophin releasing factor and arginine vasopressin in several hypothalamic areas of freely moving rats: estimation by push–pull perfusion. Neuroendocrinology 60:8–15.
80. Swain MG, Maric M, Carter L (1995) Defective interleukin-1-induced ACTH release in cholestatic rats: impaired hypothalamic PGE2 release. Am J Physiol 268:G404–G409.
81. Brooks AN (1993) Prostaglandin E2 stimulates adrenocorticotrophin and cortisol secretion via a hypothalamic site of action in fetal sheep. J Dev Physiol 18:173–177.
82. Schwartz J, Kleftogiannis F, Jacobs RA, Thorburn GD, Crosby SR, White A (1995) Biological activity of adrenocorticotropic hormone precursors on ovine adrenal cells. Am J Physiol 268: E623–E629.
83. Saphier PW, Glynn BP, Woods RJ, Shepherd DAL, Jeacock MK, Lowry PJ (1993) The contribution of elevated levels of N-terminal pro-opiomelanocortin peptides in fetal sheep plasma to adrenal gland development and the pre-parturient cortisol surge, In: 12th Joint Meeting of British Endocrine Societies, March 29–April 1, 1993; Liverpool, England, p. 12.
84. Carr GA, Jacobs RA, Young IR, Schwartz J, White A, Crosby S, Thorburn GD (1995) Development of adrenocorticotropin-(1-39) and precursor peptide secretory responses in the fetal sheep during the last third of gestation. Endocrinology 136:5020–5027.
85. Saphier PW, Glynn BP, Woods RJ, Shepherd DAL, Jeacock MK, Lowry PJ (1993) Elevated levels of N-terminal pro-opiomelanocortin peptides in fetal sheep plasma may contribute to fetal adrenal gland development and the preparturient cortisol surge. Endocrinology 133:1459–1461.
86. Hennessy DP, Coghlan JP, Hardy KJ, Wintour EM (1982) Development of the pituitary–adrenal axis in chronically cannulated ovine fetuses. J Develop Physiol 4:339–352.

87. Ozolins IZ, Antolovich GC, Browne CA, Perry RA, Robinson PM, Silver M, McMillen IC (1991) Effect of adrenalectomy or long term cortisol or adrenocorticotropin (ACTH)- releasing factor infusion on the concentration and molecular weight distribution of ACTH in fetal sheep plasma. Endocrinology 129:1942–1950.
88. Norman LJ, Challis JRG (1987) Synergism between systemic corticotropin-releasing factor and arginine vasopressin on adrenocorticotropin release in vivo varies as a function of gestational age. Endocrinology 120:1052–1058.
89. Thorburn GD (1992) The placenta, PGE2 and parturition. Early Hum Dev 29:63–73.
90. Young IR, Thorburn GD (1994) Prostaglandin E2, fetal maturation and ovine parturition. Aust NZ J Obstet Gynecol 34:342–346.
91. Engler D, Pham T, Liu JP, Fullerton MJ, Clarke IJ, Funder JW (1990) Studies of the regulation of the hypothalamic-pituitary-adrenal axis in sheep with hypothalamic-pituitary disconnection. II. Evidence for in vivo ultradian hypersecretion of proopiomelanocortin peptides by isolated anterior and intermediate pituitary. Endocrinology 127:1956–1966.
92. Antolovich GC, McMillen IC, Robinson PM, Silver M, Young IR, Perry RA (1992) Effect of cortisol infusion on the pituitary-adrenal axis of the hypothalamo-pituitary-disconnected fetal sheep. Neuroendocrinology 56:312–319.
93. McMillen IC, Merei JJ, White A, Crosby S, Schwartz J (1995) Increasing gestational age and cortisol alter the ratio of ACTH precursors:ACTH secreted from the anterior pituitary of the fetal sheep. J Endocrinol 144:569–576.
94. Stark RI, Wardlaw SL, Daniel SS (1986) Characterization of plasma B-endorphin immunoactivity in the fetal lamb: effects of gestational age and hypoxia. Endocrinology 119:755–761.
95. Wardlaw SL, Stark RI, Daniel S, Frantz AG (1981) Effects of hypoxia on β-endorphin and β-lipotropin release in fetal, newborn and maternal sheep. Endocrinology 108:1710–1715.
96. Seidah NG, Fournier H, Boileau G, Benjannet S, Rondeau N, Chretien M (1959) The cDNA structure of the porcine pro-hormone convertase PC2 and the comparative processing by PC1 and PC2 of the N-terminal glycopeptide segment of porcine POMC. FEBS Lett 310:235–239.
97. Benjannet S, Rondeau N, D R, Chretien M, Seidah NG (1991) PC1 and PC2 are proprotein convertases capable of cleaving proopiomelanocortin at distinct pairs of basic residues. Proc Natl Acad Sci USA 88:3564–3568.
98. Seidah NG, Marcinkiewicz M, Benjannet S, Gasper L, Beaubien G, Mattei MG, Lazure C, Mbikay M, Chretien M (1991) Cloning and primary sequence of a mouse candidate prohormone convertase PC1 homologous to PC2, furin, and kex2: distinct chromosomal localization and messenger RNA distribution in brain and pituitary compared to PC2. Mol Endocrinol 5:111–122.
99. Durand P, Cathiard AM, Saez JM (1985) Involvement of the regulatory protein (Ns) in the maturation of ACTH-sensitive adenylate cyclase of ovine fetal adrenal during late gestation. Mol Cell Endocrinol 39:145–150.
100. Cathiard AM, Crozat A, Durand P, Saez JM (1985) in vitro spontaneous and adrenocorticotropin-dependent maturation of the steroidogenic pathway of ovine fetal adrenal cells. Endocrinology 116:585–590.
101. Malpas P (1933) Postmaturity and malformations of the foetus. J Obstet Gynecol 40:1046–1053.
102. Anderson ABM, Laurence KM, Turnbull AC (1969) The relationship in anencephaly between the size of the adrenal cortex and the length of gestation. J Obstet Gynecol 76:196–199.
103. de Zegher F, Kaplan SL, Grumbach MM, Van den Berghe G, Francois I, Vanhole C, Devlieger H (1995) The foetal pituitary, postmaturity and breech presentation [comment]. Acta Paediatr 84: 1100–1102.
104. Sadeghi-Nejad A, Senior B (1974) A familial syndrome of isolated aplasia of the anterior pituitary. J Pediatr 84:79–84.
105. Pakravan P, Kenny FM, Depp R, Allen RG (1974) Familial congenital absence of adrenal glands; evaluation of glucocorticoid, mineralocorticoid and estrogen metabolism in the perinatal period. J Pediatr 84:74–78.
106. Heinrichs C, de Zegher F, Vansnick F, Vokaer A, Christophe C, Frankenne F (1994) Fetal hypopituitarism: perinatal endocrine and morphological studies in two cases. Acta Paediatr 83: 448–451.
107. Fencl M, Stillman RJ, Cohen J, Tulchinsky D (1980) Direct evidence of sudden rise in fetal corticoids late in human gestation. Nature 287:225–226.
108. Jones SA, Brooks AN, Challis JRG (1989) Steroids modulate corticotropin-releasing hormone production in human fetal membranes and placenta. J Clin Endocrinol Metab 68:825–830.

109. Chan EC, Smith R, Lewin T, Brinsmead MW, Zhang HP, Cubis J, Thornton K, Hurt D (1993) Plasma corticotropin-releasing hormone, beta-endorphin and cortisol inter-relationships during human pregnancy. Acta Endocrinol 128:339–344.
110. Goland RS, Wardlaw SL, Blum M, Tropper PJ, Stark RI (1988) Biologically active corticotropin-releasing hormone in maternal and fetal plasma during pregnancy. Am J Obstet Gynecol 159: 8848–8890.
111. Jones SA, Challis JRG (1990) Steroid, corticotrophin-releasing hormone, ACTH and prostaglandin interactions in the amnion and placenta of early pregnancy in man. J Endocrinol 125: 153–159.
112. Jones SA, Challis JRG (1990) Effects of corticotropin-releasing hormone and adrenocorticotropin on prostaglandin output by human placenta and fetal membranes. Gynecol Obstet Invest 29:165–168.
113. Chen CLC, Chang CC, Krieger DT, Bardin CW (1986) Expression and regulation of proopiomelanocortin-like gene in the ovary and placenta: comparison with the testis. Endocrinology 18: 2382–2389.
114. Chan EC, Smith R (1992) b-endorphin immunoreactivity during human pregnancy. J Clin Endocrinol Metab 75:1453–1458.
115. Davies JJ, Falconer J, Zhang HP, Chan EC, McLean M, Smith R (1991) Perifused ovine placental tissue secretes b-endorphin immunoreactivity. Reprod Fertil Dev 3:397–404.
116. Potestio FA, Zakar T, Olson DM (1988) Glucocorticoids stimulate prostaglandin synthesis in human amnion cells by a receptor-mediated mechanism. J Clin Endocrinol Metab 67:1205–1210.
117. Benedetto C, Petraglia F, Marozio L, Chiarolini L, Florio P, Genazzani AR, Massobrio M (1994) Corticotropin-releasing hormone increases prostaglandin F2a activity on human myometrium in vitro. Am J Obstet Gynecol 171:126–131.
118. Robinson BG, Emanuel RL, Frim DM, Majzoub JA (1988) Glucocorticoid stimulated expression of corticotropin-releasing hormone gene in human placenta. Proc Natl Acad Sci USA 85:5244–5248.
119. Langston C, Thurlbeck WM (1982) Lung growth and development in late gestation and early postnatal life. Perspectives in Pediatric Pathology 7:203–235.
120. Burri PH (1984) Fetal and Postnatal Development of the Lung. Annu Rev Physiol 46:617–628.
121. Hodson WA (1992) Normal and abnormal structural development of the lung, In: Fetal and Neonatal Physiology (Polin RA, Fox WW, eds.), W.B. Saunders, Philadelphia, pp. 771–782.
122. Alcorn DG, Adamson TM, Maloney JE, Robinson PM (1981) A morphologic and morphometric analysis of fetal lung development in the sheep. Anat Rec 201:655–667.
123. Hooper SB, Harding R (1995) Fetal lung liquid: a major determinant of the growth and functional development of the fetal lung. Clin Exp Pharmacol Physiol 22:235–247.
124. Harding R, Hooper SB (1996) Regulation of lung expansion and lung growth before birth. J Appl Physiol 81:209–224.
125. Jost A, Policard A (1948) Contribution expérimentale a l'étude du développement prénatal du poumon chez le lapin. Archives D'Anatomie Microscopique 37:323–332.
126. Carmel JA, Friedman F, Adams FH (1965) Fetal tracheal ligation and lung development. Am J Dis Child 109:452–2456.
127. Adamson TM, Boyd RDH, Platt HS, Strang LB (1969) Composition of alveolar liquid in the foetal lamb. J Physiol 204:159–168.
128. Olver RE, Strang LB (1974) Ion fluxes across the pulmonary epithelium and the secretion of lung liquid in the foetal lamb. J Physiol 241:327–357.
129. Olver RE, Ramsden CA, Strang LB, Walters DV (1986) The role of amiloride-blockable sodium transport in adrenaline-induced lung liquid reabsorption in the fetal lamb. J Physiol 376:321–340.
130. Harding R, Sigger JN, Wickham PJD, Bocking AD (1984) The regulation of flow of pulmonary fluid in fetal sheep. Respir Physiol 57:47–59.
131. Silva P, Stoff J, Field M, Fine L, Forrest JN, Epstein FH (1977) Mechanism of active chloride secretion by shark rectal gland: role of Na-K-ATPase in chloride transport. Am J Physiol 233: F298–F306.
132. Walters DV, Olver RE (1978) The role of catecholamines in lung liquid absorption at birth. Pediatr Res 12:239–242.
133. Brown MJ, Olver RE, Ramsden CA, Strang LB, Walters DV (1983) Effects of adrenaline and of spontaneous labour on the secretion and absorption of lung liquid in the fetal lamb. J Physiol 344: 137–3152.
134. Hooper SB, Harding R (1989) Effects of β-adrenergic blockade on lung liquid secretion during fetal asphyxia. Am J Physiol 257:R705–R710.

135. Perks AM, Cassin S (1982) The effects of arginine vasopressin and other factors on the production of lung fluid in fetal goats. Chest 81S:63S–65S.
136. Wallace MJ, Hooper SB, Harding R (1990) Regulation of lung liquid secretion by arginine vasopressin in fetal sheep. Am J Physiol 258:R104–R111.
137. Barker PM, Walters DV, Markiewicz M, Strang LB (1991) Development of the lung liquid reabsorptive mechanism in fetal sheep: synergism of triiodothyronine and hydrocortisone. J Physiol 433:435–449.
138. Kennedy KA, Wilton P, Mellander M, Rojas J, Sundell H (1986) Effect of epidermal growth factor on lung liquid secretion in fetal sheep. J Dev Physiol 8:421–433.
139. Kindler PM, Chuang DC, Perks AM (1993) Fluid production by in vitro lungs from near-term fetal guinea pigs: effects of cortisol and aldosterone. Acta Endocrinol 129:169–177.
140. Wallace MJ, Hooper SB, Harding R (1995) Effects of elevated fetal cortisol concentrations on the volume, secretion and reabsorption of lung liquid. Am J Physiol 269:R881–R887.
141. Wallace MJ, Hooper SB, Harding R (1996) Role of the adrenal glands in the maturation of lung liquid secretory mechanisms in fetal sheep. Am J Physiol 270:R1–R8.
142. Alcorn D, Adamson TM, Lambert TF, Maloney JE, Ritchie BC, Robinson PM (1977) Morphological effects of chronic tracheal ligation and drainage in the fetal lamb lung. J Anat 123:649–660.
143. Moessinger AC, Harding R, Adamson TM, Singh M, Kiu GT (1990) Role of lung fluid volume in growth and maturation of the fetal sheep lung. J Clin Invest 86:1270–1277.
144. Nardo L, Hooper SB, Harding R (1994) Fetal lung hypoplasia can be reversed by short-term obstruction of the fetal trachea in fetal sheep. Pediatr Res 38:690–696.
145. Hooper SB, Han VKM, Harding R (1993) Changes in lung expansion alter pulmonary DNA synthesis and IGF-II gene expression in fetal sheep. Am J Physiol 265:L403–L409.
146. Keramidaris E, Hooper SB, Harding R (1996) Effect of gestational are on the increase in fetal lung growth following tracheal obstruction. Exp Lung Res 22:283–298.
147. Nardo L, Hooper SB, Harding R (1997) Stimulation of lung growth by tracheal obstruction in fetal sheep: relation to luminal pressure and lung liquid volume. Pediatr Res, in press.
148. Harding R, Hooper SB, Han VKM (1993) Abolition of fetal breathing movements by spinal cord transection leads to reductions in fetal lung liquid volume, lung growth and IGF-II gene expression. Pediatr Res 34:148–153.
149. Liu M, Skinner SJM, Xu J, Han RNN, Tanswell AK, Post M (1992) Stimulation of fetal rat lung cell proliferation in vitro by mechanical stretch. Am J Physiol 263:L376–L383.
150. Liu M, Xu J, Liu J, Kraw ME, Tanswell AK, Post M (1996) Mechanical strain-enhanced fetal lung cell proliferation is mediated by phospholipases C and D and protein kinase C. Am J Physiol 268:L729–L738.
151. Carson JA, Yan Z, Booth FW, Coleman ME, Schwartz RJ, Stump CS (1995) Regulation of skeletal α-actin promoter in young chickens during hypertrophy caused by stretch overload. Am J Physiol 268:C918–C924.
152. Clark JG, Kuhn C, III, McDonald JA, Mecham RP (1983) Lung connective tissue. Int Rev Connect Tissue Res 10:249–331.
153. Schellenberg JC (1986) The development of connective tissue and its role in pulmonary mechanics, In: Respiratory Control and Lung Development in the Fetus and Newborn (Johnston BM, Gluckman PD, eds.), Perinatology, Ithaca, pp. 3–62.
154. Spooner BS, Faubion JM (1980) Collagen involvement in branching morphogenesis of embryonic lung and salivary gland. Dev Biol 77:84–102.
155. Nardell EA, Brody JS (1982) Determinants of mechanical properties of rat lung during postnatal development. J Appl Physiol 53:140–148.
156. Crone RK, Davies P, Liggins GC, Reid L (1983) The effects of hypophysectomy, thyroidectomy, and postoperative infusion of cortisol or adrenocorticotrophin on the structure of the ovine fetal lung. J Dev Physiol 5:281–288.
157. Erenberg A, Rhodes ML, Weinstein MM, Kennedy RL (1979) The effect of fetal thyroidectomy on ovine fetal lung maturation. Pediatr Res 13:230–235.
158. Mitzner W, Johnson JWC, Scott R, London WT, Palmer AE (1979) Effect of betamethasone on pressure-volume relationship of fetal rhesus monkey lung. J Appl Physiol 47:377–382.
159. Liggins GC, Schellenberg JC, Finberg K, Kitterman JA, Lee CH (1985) The effects of ACTH-124 or cortisol on pulmonary maturation in the adrenalectomized ovine fetus. J Dev Physiol 7:105–111.
160. Jobe AH, Polk D, Ikegami M, Newnham J, Sly P, Kohen R, Kelly R (1993) Lung responses to ultrasound-guided fetal treatments with corticosteroids in preterm lambs. J Appl Physiol 75: 2099–2105.

161. Polk DH, Ikegami M, Jobe AH, Newnham J, Sly P, Kohen R, Kelly R (1996) Postnatal lung function in preterm lambs: effects of a single exposure to betamethasone and thyroid hormones. Am J Obstet Gynecol 172:872–881.
162. Vilos GA, Liggins GC (1982) Intrathoracic pressures in fetal sheep. J Dev Physiol 4:247–256.
163. Harding R, Hooper SB, Dickson KA (1990) A mechanism leading to reduced lung expansion and lung hypoplasia in fetal sheep during oligohydramnios. Am J Obstet Gynecol 163:1904–1913.
164. Schellenberg J-C, Liggins GC (1987) Elastin and collagen in the fetal sheep lung. I. Ontogenesis. Pediatr Res 22:335–338.
165. Shibahara S, Davidson JM, Smith K, Crystal RG (1981) Modulation of tropoelastin production and elastin messenger ribonucleic acid activity in developing sheep lung. Biochemistry 20:6577–6584.
166. Rannels DE, Dunsmore SE, Grove RN (1992) Extracellular matrix synthesis and turnover by type II pulmonary epithelial cells. Am J Physiol 262:L582–L589.
167. Dunsmore SE, Rannels DE (1996) Turnover of extracellular matrix by type II pulmonary epithelial cells. Am J Physiol 268:L336–L346.
168. Dunsmore SE, Rannels SR, Grove RN, Rannels DE (1995) Adrenal hormone regulation of extracellular matrix synthesis by type II cells. Am J Physiol 268:L885–L893.
169. Minoo P, Penn R, deLemos DM, Coalson JL, DeLemos RA (1993) Tissue inhibitor of metalloproteinase-1 mRNA is specifically induced in lung tissue after birth. Pediatr Res 34:729–734.
170. Schellenberg JC, Liggins GC, Stewart AW (1987) Growth, elastin concentration, and collagen concentration of perinatal rat lung: effects of dexamethasone. Pediatr Res 21:603–607.
171. Goetzman BW, Read LC, Plopper CG, Tarantal AF, Nascimento CG, Merritt TA, Whitsett JA, Styne D (1994) Prenatal exposure to epidermal growth factor attenuates respiratory distress syndrome in rhesus infants. Pediatr Res 35:30–36.
172. DiMari SJ, Howe AM, Haralson MA (1991) Effects of transforming growth factor- on collagen synthesis by fetal rat lung epithelial cells. Am J Respir Cell Mol Biol 4:455–462.
173. Smith BT, Post M (1989) Fibroblast-pneumonocyte factor. Am J Physiol 257:L174–L178.
174. Possmayer F (1982) The perinatal lung, In: The Biochemical Development of the Fetus and Neonate (Jones CT, ed.), Elsevier Biomedical, Amsterdam, pp. 337–391.
175. Adamson IYR, Bowden DH (1975) Derivation of type I epithelium from type 2 cells in the developing rat lung. Lab Invest 32:736–745.
176. Brody JS, Williams MC (1992) Pulmonary alveolar epithelial cell differentiation. Annu Rev Physiol 54:351–371.
177. Stark RI, Daniel SS, Husain KM, James LS, Vande Wiele RL (1979) Arginine vasopressin during gestation and parturition in sheep fetus. Biol Neonate 35:235–241.
178. Hooper SB, Wallace MJ, Harding R (1993) Amiloride blocks the inhibition of fetal lung liquid secretion caused by AVP but not by asphyxia. J Appl Physiol 74:111–115.
179. Cassin S, Perks AM (1993) Amiloride inhibits arginine vasopressin-induced decrease in fetal lung liquid secretion. J Appl Physiol 75:1925–1929.
180. Barker PM, Brown MJ, Ramsden CA, Strang LB, Walters DV (1988) The effect of thyroidectomy in the fetal sheep on lung liquid reabsorption induced by adrenaline or cyclic AMP. J Physiol 407:373–383.
181. Cassin S, DeMarco V, Perks AM, Kuck H, Ellis TM (1994) Regulation of lung liquid secretion in immature fetal sheep: hormonal interaction. J Appl Physiol 77:1445–1450.
182. Rooney SA, Young SL, Mendelson CR (1994) Molecular and celluar processing of lung surfactant. FASEB J 8:957–967.
183. Mendelson CR, Boggaram V (1991) Hormonal control of the surfactant system in fetal lung. Annu Rev Physiol 53:415–440.
184. Ballard PL (1989) Hormonal control of lung maturation. Perinatal Endocrinology 3:723–753.
185. Ballard PL (1989) Hormonal regulation of pulmonary surfactant. Endocr Rev 10:165–181.
186. Pryhuber GS, Hull WM, Fink I, McMahan MJ, Whitsett JA (1991) Ontogeny of surfactant proteins A and B in human amniotic fluid as indices of fetal lung maturity. Pediatr Res 30:597–605.
187. Beers MF, Shuman H, Liley HG, Floros J, Gonzales LW, Yue N, Ballard PL (1997) Surfactant protein B in human fetal lung: Developmental and glucocorticoid regulation. Pediatr Res 38:668–675.
188. Fowden AL, Harding R, Ralph MM, Thorburn GD (1989) Nutritional control of respiratory and other muscular activities in relation to plasma prostaglandin E in the fetal sheep. J Dev Physiol 11:253–262.

189. Warburton D, Parton L, Buckley S, Cosico L, Enns G, Saluna T (1988) Combined effects of corticosteroid, thyroid hormones, and -agonist on surfactant, pulmonary mechanics, and -receptor binding in fetal lamb lung. Pediatr Res 24:166–170.
190. Liggins GC (1994) Fetal lung maturation. Aust NZ J Obstet Gynecol 34:247–250.
191. Kitterman JA, Liggins GC, Campos GA, Clements JA, Forster CS, Lee CH, Creasy RK (1981) Prepartum maturation of the lung in fetal sheep: relation to cortisol. J Appl Physiol 51:384–390.
192. Liggins GC, Howie RN (1972) A controlled trial of antepartum glucocorticoid treatment for prevention of the respiratory distress syndrome in premature infants. Pediatrics 50:515–525.
193. Doyle LW, Kitchen WH, Ford GW, Rickards AL, Kelly EA (1989) Antenatal steroid therapy and 5-year outcome of extremely low birth weight infants. Obstet Gynecol 73:743–746.

13 Development and Function of the Fetal Endocrine System

Tom E. Porter, PhD

CONTENTS

Pregnancy is associated with numerous changes in maternal endocrine function and development of the fetal endocrine system. Although some intercommunication exists between the maternal and fetal endocrine systems, the placenta serves as an effective barrier to many potential maternal–fetal hormonal interactions. This chapter will focus on the ontogeny of fetal hormone production, regulation of fetal hormone synthesis, and fetal requirements for hormone secretion. Each of the major endocrine systems will be examined. Although the discussion will concentrate on evidence obtained during human fetal development, supplemental information from studies of fetal development in sheep and rodents, the two most widely used experimental models for fetal endocrine function, will be examined.

PITUITARY GLAND

The pituitary gland is located immediately beneath the hypothalamus of the brain, and it has been referred to as the master gland because of its integral role in regulating other endocrine organs during postpartum life. The pituitary gland of rodents and other mammals is composed of cellular anterior and intermediate lobes and a posterior lobe, which is a neural extension of the hypothalamus. In humans, the intermediate lobe appears only briefly during development and then regresses. Interestingly, the intermediate lobe reappears during pregnancy in women, although its significance is not known. The anterior pituitary or adenohypophysis secretes six major hormones, adrenocorticotropin (ACTH), follicle-stimulating hormone (FSH), luteinizing hormone (LH), thyroid-stimulating hormone (TSH), growth hormone (GH), and prolactin (PRL). Each hormone is produced by a separate cell type, with the exception of FSH and LH, which are produced by the same cells. Secretion of each hormone in adult animals is regulated by stimulatory or inhibitory secretagogs produced by the hypothalamus, and positive or negative feedback loops involving hormones of pituitary target glands. During embryonic development, the adenohypophysis arises from a folding of ectoderm toward the neural plate. Classically, oral ectoderm was thought to form the adenohypophysis, whereas neural ectoderm formed the posterior pituitary, or neurohypophysis. However, more recent evidence from chick embryogenesis indicates that the anterior pituitary also arises from the neural ridge *(1–3)*. This folded ectoderm, Rathke's pouch, makes contact with a down growth from the diencephalon called the infundibulum. Formation of Rathke's pouch occurs by 5 wk of gestation in humans *(4)*. The anterior wall of Rathke's pouch proliferates to form the anterior pituitary gland. In most species studied, ACTH-producing corticotrophs differentiate shortly after formation of Rathke's pouch. Differentiation of gonadotrophs, thyrotrophs, somatotrophs, and lactotrophs follows that of corticotrophs, and in most species, occurs in that order. Gonadotroph differentiation begins shortly after formation of Rathke's pouch, with the appearance of cells containing the shared α-subunit of the glycoprotein hormones. Indeed, contact of oral and neural ectoderm may be the inductive signal for gonadotroph differentiation, since the α-subunit gene is expressed in nearly all cells immediately after formation of Rathke's pouch in rodents *(5)*. It is not surprising that thyrotrophs are thought to differentiate from gonadotrophs or a common precursor cell type during development, because the secretory product of thyrotrophs, TSH, shares the same α-subunit as LH and FSH. Somatotroph differentiation follows thyrotroph differentiation, and occurs by wk 10 of fetal development in humans *(6,7)* and d 18 (out of 21) in rats *(8)*. Lactotrophs are the final cell type to differentiate in the anterior pituitary, and this occurs by wk 16 in humans *(9)* and around birth in rats *(10,11)*.

Evidence for cellular lineage relationships among the anterior pituitary cell types comes from transgenic mice in which the developmental homeobox gene Lhx3 was mutated. Lhx3 activates the promoter for the α-subunit of the glycoprotein hormones, LH, FSH, and TSH, and this transcription factor also interacts with another transactivating protein, Pit-1, to regulate GH and PRL gene expression. In these animals, only corticotrophs differentiated *(12)*. In addition, the anterior pituitaries of these animals were grossly underdeveloped. These findings indicate that each of the anterior pituitary cell types may differentiate from an Lhx3-expressing stem cell. The low numbers of corticotrophs that differentiate in the Lhx3-mutated mouse are the most likely candidates as the anterior pituitary stem cells. A direct lineage relationship has been established between somatotrophs and lactotrophs. Elimination of somatotrophs in transgenic mice during fetal development resulted in lactotroph ablation as well *(13)*, indicating that lactotrophs arise from cells that formerly produced GH. In contrast to this direct lineage of lactotrophs from somatotrophs, the precursor cell types for each of the other anterior pituitary cell types have not been identified conclusively. It is unlikely that hypothalamic stimulation is necessary for induction of cellular differentiation within the anterior pituitary, since all five cell types are present in anencephalic human fetuses *(7)*, which lack a brain, including the hypothalamus. However, homeostatic control of pituitary hormone secretion later during fetal development likely involves hypothalamic input.

ACTH is the first functional hormone secreted by the anterior pituitary during fetal development. ACTH is the principal stimulator of adrenal glucocorticoid synthesis, and as a result is involved in regulation of metabolism and mediation of stress responses in adults. Synthesis of ACTH begins by 9 wk of gestation in humans *(14)*, 110 d in sheep *(15)*, and 14 d in rats *(16)*, gestation lasting approx 275 d in humans, 147 d in sheep, and 21 d in rats. Levels of ACTH in the fetal circulation increase during late gestation in sheep *(15)* and humans *(17)*. Secretion of ACTH in the fetus is stimulated by hypothalamic corticotropin-releasing hormone (CRH) and inhibited by adrenal glucocorticoids, as it is in adults *(18–20)*. Elevation of plasma ACTH concentrations during late gestation may be involved in increasing fetal adrenal cortisol secretion associated with parturition. However, the pulsatile frequency and amplitude of ACTH levels do not correlate with those for cortisol in fetal sheep *(21)*, suggesting that increased ACTH secretion is not the driving force behind elevated glucocorticoid production at term. Rather, evidence exists indicating that elevated cortisol levels associated with parturition may result from increased sensitivity of the fetal adrenal gland to ACTH stimulation *(22)*. Fetal secretion of ACTH is likely necessary for normal adrenal development, since adrenal involution occurs by 20 wk of gestation in the anencephalic fetus, where ACTH production is low *(23,24)*.

Secretion of the gonadotropins, LH and FSH, begins shortly after that of ACTH *(25)*. The gonadotropins are heterodimeric glycoprotein hormones consisting of unique β-subunits and a common α-subunit. The α-subunit is also shared by TSH and human chorionic gonadotropin (hCG). The gonadotropins regulate gonadal steroidogenesis, follicular maturation, ovulation, and spermatogenesis in adults. Circulating levels of fetal LH and FSH increase to high concentrations during midgestation in humans *(25)* and sheep *(26)*. A sexual dimorphism in gonadotropin levels exists during the second trimester in humans, with concentrations of LH and FSH being greater in female fetuses than in male fetuses *(25,27,28)*. A similar sexual dimorphism in gonadotropin levels has been noted in fetal sheep during midgestation, except that levels of FSH are higher in females, whereas concentrations of LH are greater in males *(26)*. Greater production of inhibin by fetal testes than fetal ovaries likely contributes to this sexual dimorphism in FSH secretion in humans *(29,30)*. Similarly, higher testosterone production in males at midterm may suppress LH levels below those in females. Hypothalamic gonadotropin-releasing hormone (GnRH) has been documented to stimulate gonadotropin secretion in fetal sheep *(31,32)*. Similar involvement of GnRH in stimulating fetal LH and FSH secretion has been suggested in humans, since gonadotropin levels are low in anencephalic fetuses *(33)*. During the third trimester in humans and late gestation in sheep, gonadotropin levels decrease to virtually nondetectable levels in response to maturation of the negative-feedback loop involving gonadal steroids *(25,27,34)*. Despite this characteristic pattern of gonadotropin levels during mammalian gestation, fetal sexual differentiation does not depend on pituitary production of gonadotropins. The first 14 wk of gestation in humans are critical for sexual differentiation, and during this time, hCG is the predominant gonadotropin present in the circulation. In contrast to this lack of involvement of pituitary gonadotropins in gonadal differentiation, evidence from anencephalic fetuses suggests that growth of the ovaries and testes is affected by fetal pituitary gonadotropin secretion during midgestation *(35,36)*.

TSH increases thyroid hormone production in adults, and as a result, this pituitary hormone is involved in modulating metabolic rate during periods of growth and in response to temperature stress. Secretion of TSH begins by wk 10 of gestation in humans *(37)*, and circulating levels of TSH increase between wk 26 and 36 of gestation *(38,39)*, when they reach adult levels. No obvious differences exist between sexes in this ontogenic profile. Concentrations of TSH and thyroxine are positively correlated during this period, indicating that TSH likely functions in fetal humans to regulate thyroid hormone secretion. Evidence from rats and sheep confirms a role for pituitary TSH in fetal thyroid function *(40–42)*, and indicates that pituitary thyrotrophs respond to negative feedback from thyroid hormones and feed-forward stimulation by hypothalamic thyrotropin-releasing hormone (TRH), although TSH secretion appears to be regulated primarily by thyroid hormone negative feedback rather than TRH stimulation *(41)*.

GH, or somatotropin, stimulates long bone growth and muscle weight gain in postpartum mammals. GH also plays a role in metabolic regulation, producing diabetogenic, lipolytic, and antilipogenic effects. Many of these GH effects are mediated by production of insulin-like growth factor-I (IGF-I) by the liver or other GH target tissues, such as the epiphyseal growth plates. Pituitary production of GH occurs by wk 10 of fetal development in humans *(6,7)*. Levels of GH in the fetal circulation increase through wk 19–25 of gestation, but decrease prior to delivery *(43,44)*. Circulating concentrations of GH also decline on the day of parturition in rats *(45)* and during the final week of gestation in sheep *(46)*. Studies with fetal sheep indicate that GH is secreted in a pulsatile manner, as it is in adults, with one pulse occurring about every 2 h *(32)*. Peak levels of GH were higher in male fetal sheep than in females *(46)*. As in adults, GH release from fetal somatotrophs is stimulated by hypothalamic GH-releasing hormone (GHRH), and inhibited by hepatic IGF-I and hypothalamic somatostatin *(47–50)*. Although responsiveness to GHRH stimulation occurs early in development, responsiveness to inhibition of GH release by somatostatin and IGF-I is delayed until late gestation. This may account in part for the general increase in circulating concentrations of GH during gestation and the decline in GH levels prior to parturition.

A definitive role for GH in fetal growth has not been established. In fact, newborns with idiopathic GH deficiencies are only marginally smaller, by about one standard deviation, than normal infants. Growth deficiencies are not readily apparent until after birth. In contrast, fetal GH production may play an important role in metabolic regulation and tissue differentiation within the fetus. For example, serum GH concentrations in sheep are higher in fetuses of undernourished mothers than in those fed ad libitum *(51)*. In addition, fetal hypophysectomy in sheep caused accumulation of substantial subcutaneous fat, whereas GH administration abolished this increase *(52)*. Growth and differentiation of small intestinal explants from fetal rats transplanted under the renal capsule of hypophysectomized adult hosts were dependent on GH administration *(53)*, suggesting a role for GH in development of the gastrointestinal system. However, potentially the most exciting role for fetal GH is in the differentiation of pancreatic islet β-cells and the relative response of these cells to changes in glucose concentration. Support for such a role comes primarily from cell-culture studies. GH was shown to increase the insulin response of human fetal pancreatic islet cells to glucose in vitro *(54,55)*. In addition, GH stimulated pancreatic β-cell mitosis in cultures of rat pancreatic islet cells *(56)*. Based on these findings, further examination of the actions of fetal GH on β-cell differentiation and function is warranted.

Numerous functions have been ascribed to PRL, most notably the regulation of lactation and corpora luteal function in adult females. Evidence also exists that PRL may function in osmoregulation and as an immunomodulator. Prolactin secretion begins by wk 16 of gestation in humans, and serum PRL concentrations increase after 21 wk of gestation until term *(57–60)*. Similar increases in plasma PRL have been noted in fetal sheep before parturition *(61)* and in fetal rhesus monkeys during late gestation *(62)*. No differences in this profile are evident between the sexes *(63)*. This increase apparently does not involve hypothalamic input, since it is also observed in anencephalic human fetuses.

Rather, it may result from a late gestational increase in placental estrogen production, a known stimulator of PRL synthesis. Plasma PRL concentrations exhibit a 24-h rhythm in fetal sheep *(64)*. However, surgical disconnection of the hypothalamus and pituitary abolished this rhythm, indicating hypothalamic involvement in the rhythmic secretion of fetal PRL *(65)*. Treatment of human mothers with bromocryptine (a dopaminergic agonist) suppressed fetal PRL *(66)*, and treatment of sheep fetuses with TRH increased PRL levels *(67)*, suggesting that fetal PRL secretion is suppressed by dopamine and stimulated by TRH, as it is in adults.

Although no definitive role for PRL in fetal development has been established, the increase in PRL levels during late gestation in humans, sheep, and monkeys suggests a role in late development. Addition of PRL to human amniotic membranes in culture decreased the permeability of the membranes to water *(68)*, and cord serum PRL levels correlated with amniotic fluid osmolality *(69)*, indicating that PRL may function to regulate fetal water and electrolyte balance. However, the most promising role for fetal PRL production relates to maturation of the fetal lungs. Specifically, synthesis of surfactant glycerophospholipids and proteins is stimulated by PRL *(70)*, and the risk for respiratory distress syndrome is higher for newborns whose PRL levels were low during late gestation *(71)*. In hypophysectomized fetal sheep, administration of PRL, along with glucocorticoids and thyroxine, is necessary to induce lung maturation *(72)*.

The posterior pituitary or neurohypophysis releases two principal hormones, arginine vasopressin (AVP) and oxytocin (OT). AVP is also referred to as antidiuretic hormone, and is the primary regulator in adults of renal tubule water reabsorption, thereby controlling blood volume and osmolality. This same system functions during fetal development. A thorough review of the endocrine regulation of renal function during fetal development is beyond the scope of this chapter, but this topic has been reviewed elsewhere *(73)*. The posterior pituitary arises from a down growth of the infundibulum of the hypothalamus by 37 d postconception *(74,75)*. Regulation and effects of AVP during fetal development have been reviewed *(76)*. AVP is detectable in the neurohypophysis by 10 wk of gestation in humans *(77)*. However, final maturation of AVP production occurs after birth, since the number of AVP-expressing neurons at term is substantially less than in adults *(78)*. AVP secretion is regulated by osmolar and blood volume changes from midgestation on in sheep *(76,79)*, and administration of AVP to fetal sheep induces changes in blood pressure, heart rate, and cardiac output. AVP has also been shown to increase fetal glomerular filtration rate, increase urine osmolality, and decrease urine output in fetal sheep *(80)*. Responsiveness to AVP increases with gestational age *(80)*. By wk 11 of gestation in humans, OT is present in the neurohypophysis. The ratio of OT to AVP increases in sheep and human fetuses during gestation *(77)*. Although OT has been suggested as a modulator of adrenal function and parturition, a definitive role for OT in fetal physiology of primates is not known. The role of OT in initiating parturition is discussed in Chapter 18.

RENIN–ANGIOTENSIN SYSTEM

In addition to AVP release from the neurohypophysis, the other principal modulator of renal function in adults is the renin–angiotensin system. Angiotensinogen is produced primarily in the liver and is the initial substrate for this system. Angiotensinogen is cleaved in the kidney by the enzyme renin to form angiotensin I, and angiotensin I is converted to the active hormone angiotensin II by angiotensin-converting enzyme. Renin is produced primarily in the juxtaglomerular cells of the kidney, whereas angiotensin-converting enzyme is located in the vascular endothelium throughout the body, including the kidneys and lungs. In adults, angiotensin II increases blood pressure within 15 s. This system seems to differentiate early on during embryogenesis, and its role in regulating renal function and blood pressure increases during gestation. Fetal development and function of the renin–angiotensin system have been reviewed recently *(81)*. During development of the rat, angiotensinogen is produced as early as d 11 of gestation *(82)*, and angiotensinogen production increases substantially during the last third of gestation *(83–85)*. Renin expression is initially restricted to the renal artery on d 17 of rat development *(86)*, but later during fetal and postnatal development, renin production occurs in the juxtaglomerular cells *(87,88)*. In humans, renin production in the kidney begins by the 8th wk of gestation *(89)*. Concentrations of renin in fetal kidneys are higher than in adults and increase during gestation *(90)*. Similarly, angiotensin II levels in the fetal circulation are higher than in adults. Studies of the actions of the renin–angiotensin system during fetal development have been conducted in sheep. The effects of angiotensin II on vasoconstriction and renal function are minimal during early gestation, but increase with fetal maturation. A thorough discussion of endocrine control of fetal renal function is available *(73)*.

THYROID GLAND

The thyroid gland is located in the neck on either side of the upper trachea, just below the larynx. The principal products of the thyroid gland, thyroxine (T_4), and its most active metabolite, triiodothyronine (T_3), regulate basal metabolic rate. Thus, the thyroid gland, and conversion of T_4 to T_3 by type I monodeiodinase in the liver play integral roles in regulating growth rate and mediating metabolic stress responses in postpartum animals. Development and function of the fetal thyroid gland have been reviewed in detail *(91)*. The thyroid gland develops from the endoderm of the buccal cavity, and is well developed by wk 7 of gestation in humans *(37)*. Thyroid function and synthesis of thyroid hormones occurs by wk 10 of gestation. Pituitary TSH is not necessary for thyroid development during the first half of gestation *(37,91)*. However, thyroid hormone production is stimulated by TSH during fetal development, as it is in adults. As discussed earlier, pituitary TSH secretion is responsive to TRH stimulation during the third trimester in humans. During fetal development of sheep, the thyroid gland becomes progressively responsive to TSH stimulation *(92)*. Increased sensitivity of the fetal thyroid to TSH is also likely to occur in humans, since circulating levels of T_4 increase in the absence of elevations in TSH concentrations during late gestation *(39)*. Fetal serum concentrations of T_4 are low before 16 wk of gestation and increase from there to a high plateau at 34–36 wk of gestation *(91)*. Serum concentrations of T_3 are low before 30 wk of gestation, when they begin to increase until term *(93)*. Similarly, in fetal sheep, T_3 levels increase during the last week of gestation *(94)*. In contrast, levels of T_3 do not increase appreciably until after birth in the rat *(95)*. The placenta actively transports iodide to the fetus, providing an abundant source for fetal thyroid hormone production *(91)*. Concentrations of TSH, T_4, and T_3 increase dramatically and transiently at birth in most mammals. Hepatic type I monodeiodinase activity increases twofold during the last third of gestation in sheep *(96,97)*, undoubtedly contributing to the rise in serum T_3 levels toward term. Type II monodeiodinase is expressed in the brain and pituitary gland, and converts T_4 to T_3 within these target tissues for local effects during fetal development. Concentrations of type II tissue monodeiodinase are high during midgestation in sheep, prior to an increase in circulating T_3 levels *(97)*, thus supplying these tissues with T_3 early on. Unlike larger peptide hormones, thyroid hormones should readily pass between the maternal and fetal circulations. However, fetal thyroid hormone levels are regulated independently of maternal concentrations. The placenta and fetal membranes of rats and sheep contain large amounts of type III monodeiodinase, which converts T_4 to reverse T_3 (rT_3), a relatively inactive metabolite. The presence of a monodeiodinase enzyme in the placenta and fetal membranes may contribute to the separation of maternal and fetal thyroid function *(91)*. However, transfer of small amounts of maternal T_4 and T_3 to the fetal circulation was observed in human fetuses with thyroid agenesis. In contrast to humans, substantial transfer of thyroid hormones from maternal to fetal circulation occurs in the rat *(95,98)*.

Although thyroid hormone receptors have been identified in human fetal brain, heart, and lung, the role of thyroid hormones in human fetal development is not clear. Human infants born athyroid show few, if any, signs of hypothyroidism *(91)*. However, modest deficiencies in bone epiphyseal plate maturation were noted in about half of athyroid human infants at birth *(93,99)*. Classical features of hypothyroidism or cretinism develop later during neonatal life. Thus, either human fetal development does not depend greatly on thyroid hormones, or the modest amounts of maternal thyroid hormones passing the placenta are sufficient for normal development. In contrast to human fetal growth, development of the fetal sheep is greatly affected by fetal hypothyroidism. Decreased growth and bone maturation are evident in thyroidectomized fetal sheep by 90–100 d of gestation *(91)*. Fetal thyroid hormone production at term seems to function in lung maturation, and administration of TRH, which passes freely across the placenta, is being explored as a treatment for premature infants at risk for respiratory distress syndrome *(100)*. In the fetal sheep, thyroidectomy at 95–99 d of gestation results in decreased surfactant production *(101)*.

PARATHYROID GLAND AND CALCIUM HOMEOSTASIS

The parathyroid glands lie adjacent to the thyroid gland. The principal product of the parathyroid glands, parathyroid hormone (PTH), controls the balance of calcium (Ca^{2+}) in the blood, that in the bone, and that secreted by the kidneys in adult animals. Disruption of Ca^{2+} homeostasis by parathyroidectomy results in tetany and, ultimately, death. Thus, a similar balance of Ca^{2+} homeostasis must exist during fetal development. Maintenance of Ca^{2+} in the fetal circulation is also essential for fetal bone mineralization. The mammalian placenta actively transports Ca^{2+} from the maternal circulation into the fetal circulation, forming a Ca^{2+} gradient across the placenta, with Ca^{2+} concentrations being greater in the fetal circulation than in the maternal circulation. Similarly, magnesium (Mg^{2+}) and phosphate (PO_4^{2-}) are transferred across the placenta to the fetal circulation. Active transport of Ca^{2+} across the placenta is thought to be regulated by a product of the fetal parathyroid glands in primates and other mammals. Maintenance of higher concentrations of Ca^{2+} and Mg^{2+} in the fetal circulation by a product of the fetal parathyroid glands has been well documented in sheep, and a thorough review of this topic is available *(102)*. Fetal Ca^{2+} concentrations increase above those in the maternal circulation by 5 wk of gestation in sheep, shortly after development of the parathyroid glands. Reabsorption of fetal bone Ca^{2+} apparently does not contribute to this increase in plasma Ca^{2+}. Production of PTH begins around wk 10 of gestation in humans *(103)*, but levels of PTH in the circulation are low throughout fetal development *(104)*. Thyroparathyroidectomy in fetal sheep, in combination with T_4 replacement, results in reduced bone mineralization

(102) and decreased Ca^{2+} and Mg2 concentrations by 50 and 20%, respectively. Interestingly, treatment with PTH does not reverse the effect of parathyroidectomy. Rather, the active hormone secreted by the fetal parathyroid gland of sheep appears to be a PTH-related protein (PTHrP). PTHrP shares N-terminal homology with PTH, and PTHrP or a similar compound is produced by the fetal parathyroid gland. A PTHrP has been localized in the parathyroid gland of fetal lambs from 116 d of gestation and lambs up to 6 mo of age, but not in parathyroid glands of adult sheep. These results suggest that parathyroid regulation of calcium homeostasis may involve a shift in the active hormone secreted during development from PTHrP in fetal growth to PTH in later postnatal life. Levels of PTH and PTHrP in the fetal circulation increase in response to decreased plasma Ca^{2+} concentrations *(105–107)*. Synthesis of PTHrP has also been identified in the placenta *(108,109)*, indicating that sites of PTHrP production other than the parathyroid gland may be involved in fetal Ca^{2+} homeostasis.

Mineral homeostasis during fetal development also involves metabolites of vitamin D, as it does in adults. Vitamin D metabolites increase the capacity of target tissues to transport Ca^{2+}. These primary targets in adults include the gut epithelium and the renal tubule system. The active metabolite of vitamin D, 1,25-dihydroxyvitamin D_3, is produced in the fetal kidney and liver *(110)*, and nephrectomy in fetal sheep decreases circulating Ca^{2+} levels *(111)*. Fetal concentrations of 1,25-dihydroxyvitamin D_3 are regulated independently of those in the maternal circulation *(112)*. Furthermore, receptors for 1,25-dihydroxyvitamin D_3 and the mediator of its actions, calbindin D28, are also found in the fetal kidney *(113)*, indicating that this system likely functions during fetal development as it does in adults. Expression of calbindin D28 in the fetal kidney is apparently unaffected by maternal vitamin D levels *(114)*, suggesting fetal autonomy of calcium transport regulation. In addition, receptors for 1,25-dihydroxyvitamin D_3 are located in the placenta *(115)*, indicating that this hormone likely contributes to regulating placental Ca^{2+} transport. However, additional research is needed regarding the regulation of placental transport of vitamin D, fetal metabolism of vitamin D to 1,25-dihydroxyvitamin D_3, and production of calbindin D28 in fetal tissues.

ADRENAL GLAND

The adrenal glands, located superior to the kidneys, are divided into a medulla and cortex. The adrenal medulla is effectively an extension of the sympathetic nervous system, and releases the catecholamines epinephrine, norepinephrine, and dopamine. The adrenal cortex secretes glucocorticoid and mineralocorticoid steroid hormones. In adult mammals, the cortex is divided into three zones, the outer zona glomerulosa, middle zona fasciculata, and inner zona reticularis. Although production of the mineralocorticoid aldosterone is restricted to the zona glomerulosa, glucocorticoid synthesis occurs in all three zones. In adults, the adrenal glands are essential in mediating stress responses, and in regulating carbohydrate metabolism and sodium balance. As in adults, cortical and medullary tissue exists in the fetal adrenal gland, although adrenal zonation is not complete until after birth. Instead, the majority of the large cortex is referred to as fetal adrenal cortex, which undergoes rapid degeneration after birth. The principal product of the fetal adrenal cortex is the sex steroid dehydroisoandrosterone (DHA).

Development and function of fetal medullary tissue have been described in detail *(116)*. In addition to the adrenal medulla, extraadrenal, medullary-like chromaffin tissue exists during fetal development, and this chromaffin tissue is located primarily at the origin of the inferior mesenteric artery. This tissue first appears by 8 wk of gestation in humans, and catecholamine-containing cells are evident by 9–11 wk. This extraadrenal chromaffin tissue persists to term and degenerates after birth. The catecholamine content of this extra-adrenal tissue exceeds that of the adrenal glands throughout gestation and is maximal around birth. In contrast to this extraadrenal chromaffin tissue, the adrenal medulla remains immature during most of fetal development. Formation of the adrenal medulla begins around 7 wk of gestation in humans, with the number of medullary chromaffin cells increasing through the next 4–5 wk. Formation of the adrenal medulla and catecholamine synthesis is dependent on fetal pituitary ACTH and adrenal glucocorticoid secretion. Secretion of catecholamines during fetal development is stimulated by hypoxia, and increased norepinephrine and epinephrine secretion redirects blood flow toward the heart and brain. Levels of glucose in the fetal circulation are dependent on those in the maternal circulation. However, fetal chromaffin tissue responds to hypoglycemia, and infusion of epinephrine in fetal sheep increases blood glucose levels. Thus, some degree of autonomy exists in the regulation of fetal blood glucose levels by chromaffin tissue, primarily the extraadrenal chromaffin tissue. Fetal chromaffin tissue may also function in lung maturation. Catecholamines have been shown in rabbits to increase lung surfactant secretion in vitro, and infusion of epinephrine into fetal sheep increased lung surfactant secretion. Thus, the fetal adrenal medulla and extraadrenal chromaffin tissue serve at least two functions during fetal development.

Substantial effort has been invested toward the study of adrenal cortical development in primates and sheep, and excellent reviews of the development and role of fetal adrenal glucocorticoid production are available *(117–119)*. Fetal cortisol production is involved in fetal lung maturation and liver glycogen synthesis. Production of cortisol by the fetal adrenal is also involved in stimulating parturition in sheep. The fetal adrenal gland increases in size dramatically during the last third of gestation in humans and nonhuman primates *(118)* and in sheep *(119)*. Similarly, production of glucocorticoids by the fetal adrenal is low through most of fetal development and increases toward term. Growth of the adrenal gland during late gestation is dependent on pituitary ACTH secretion. An intriguing change in anterior pituitary processing of the preprohormone pro-opiomelanocortin (POMC) from production primarily of melanocyte-stimulating hormone (MSH) and corticotropin-like intermediate lobe peptide (CLIP) to mainly ACTH occurs prior to parturition. This switch in the major product of POMC processing to ACTH has been proposed to stimulate adrenal cortical maturation around wk 25 of human gestation. As mentioned earlier, the fetal adrenal gland develops normally in anencephalic human fetuses through 14–17 wk of gestation, with involution occurring by wk 20. Thus, factors other than pituitary secretions are likely important in early fetal adrenal development.

Adrenal glucocorticoid synthesis is regulated during fetal development as it is in adults. Low-density lipoprotein (LDL) produced in the liver provides most of the cholesterol substrate for fetal adrenal steroidogenesis *(118)*, but *de novo* synthesis of cholesterol also occurs in the fetal adrenal. Fetal adrenal steroidogenesis is stimulated primarily by ACTH during late fetal development. However, during most of fetal development, adrenal steroidogenesis appears to be regulated by factors in addition to ACTH. These may include MSH and CLIP as discussed previously. In addition, other non-POMC hormones have been implicated, including hCG, GH, and PRL. The capacity of the fetal adrenal to produce cortisol is low through most of fetal development. Instead, the principal steroid produced by the fetal adrenal is DHA, which serves as a substrate for placental estrogen production. Substantial adrenal glucocorticoid production is not necessary during most of fetal development, since sufficient cortisol crosses the placenta in humans and nonhuman primates to maintain homeostasis. The contribution of maternal cortisol to fetal cortisol concentrations changes during development, with nearly all cortisol in the fetal circulation arising from placental transport at midgestation and less than half being of maternal origin near term. Changes in placental metabolism of glucocorticoids also occur during gestation. During midgestation, placental metabolism favors the conversion of inactive cortisone to cortisol, whereas conversion of cortisol to cortisone prevails near term. This transition in glucocorticoid metabolism is likely induced by increasing estrogen concentrations during later gestation.

A role for increased fetal cortisol production in stimulating parturition in sheep is well documented *(119,120)*. The adrenal glands develop by d 28 of gestation in sheep, and the weight of the adrenal glands increases during the last 15–20 d of pregnancy. As in primates, circulating levels of cortisol increase dramatically during the last 25 d of gestation. The majority of the cortisol in the circulation prior to this age arises from maternal transfer across the placenta. Fetal adrenalectomy does not affect circulating cortisol levels until d 135 of gestation in sheep. The increase in cortisol levels near term reflects increased concentrations of ACTH and an increased responsiveness of the adrenal gland to ACTH stimulation during this period of development. The number of adrenal ACTH receptors increases fivefold between 123 d of gestation and birth, with the majority of this increase occurring during the final 5 d of fetal development. Apparently, pituitary responsiveness to CRH increases prior to heightened responsiveness of the adrenal gland to ACTH stimulation, on d 125–130 and d 135–140, respectively *(119)*. In contrast, negative feedback of glucocorticoids on fetal ACTH release is diminished during the final 5 d of pregnancy. In short, late gestation in sheep is associated with a sequential maturation of the fetal hypothalamo-pituitary–adrenal axis that ultimately leads to stimulation of parturition.

ENDOCRINE PANCREAS AND GLUCOSE HOMEOSTASIS

The pancreas is located between the major duodenal loop of the small intestine. The majority of the pancreas, or exocrine pancreas, secretes digestive enzymes and buffers into the lumen of the small intestine to aid in digestion. Interspersed within the tissue of the exocrine pancreas lie the islets of Langerhans, which constitute the endocrine pancreas. In adults, the endocrine pancreas constitutes about 1–2% of the entire pancreas. Four cell types make up the pancreatic islets, the α-cells, which produce glucagon, the β-cells, which secrete insulin, the D-cells, which release somatostatin, and the F-cells, which make pancreatic polypeptide. Insulin and glucagon regulate blood glucose concentrations, whereas somatostatin and pancreatic polypeptide modulate insulin and glucagon release and gastric secretions, respectively. Insulin acts to decrease blood glucose levels by increasing hepatic and muscle glucose uptake, but glucagon increases blood glucose levels by stimulating hepatic glycogenolysis and gluconeogenesis. In addition, elevated blood glucose levels stimulate insulin secretion and inhibit glucagon release. Elevated amino acid concentrations stimulate the release of insulin and glucagon, whereas somatostatin inhibits secretion of both hormones.

The pancreas develops during wk 4 of gestation in humans and by d 10 of gestation in rodents (reviewed in *121)*. Endocrine cells can be detected soon after the tissue first develops. Both endocrine and exocrine pancreas develop from endodermal epithelium, a process induced by associated mesenchyme. Initially, the endocrine cells occur individually and are associated with the developing pancreatic ducts of the exocrine pancreas. These cells migrate and proliferate during later gestation to form islets characteristic of the endocrine pancreas in adults. The initial endocrine cells appear to express both insulin and glucagon. Cells producing somatostatin or pancreatic polypeptide differentiate later. Glucagon-containing α-cells predominate during early gestation, with insulin-containing β-cells becoming more prominent later in gestation. Similarly, pancreatic insulin content increases during gestation *(122)*. Changes also occur in responsiveness of pancreatic β-cells to glucose, with glucose having minimal effects on insulin secretion during fetal development *(123,124)*, although the concentration of glucose necessary to elicit a response is similar to that in adults *(125)*. In contrast, chronically high levels of glucose can affect fetal insulin secretion, as during gestational diabetes where fetal insulin secretion is increased *(123)*. Insulin found in the fetal circulation is of fetal origin, since insulin does not cross the placenta. In contrast to its relative insensitivity to changes in blood glucose concentrations, insulin secretion is stimulated effectively during fetal development by the amino acids arginine and leucine and by glucagon. Of these, glucagon is the most consistent secretagog for insulin during fetal development. In addition, fetal β-cells are relatively insensitive to inhibitory effects of somatostatin *(126)*. Pancreatic glucagon synthesis begins between wk 6 and 8 of human gestation, and concentrations of glucagon in the pancreas increase during gestation to levels higher than those found in adults. Glucagon is found in the fetal circulation from wk 15, and levels increase during gestation. As with insulin, glucagon does not cross the placenta, indicating that these levels reflect fetal glucagon secretion.

Glucose is transported across the placenta from maternal to fetal circulation. Levels of glucose in the fetus are lower than those in the maternal circulation, but changes in fetal glucose concentrations are in parallel with alterations in maternal blood glucose levels. Owing to this constant supply of glucose to the fetus, gluconeogenesis in the fetus is minimal. In contrast, glycogen synthesis in the liver increases toward term, and hepatic glycogen synthesis during late fetal development is stimulated by insulin *(123)*. In short, it is doubtful whether the low levels of insulin in the fetal circulation during early to mid-gestation play an important role in fetal glucose homeostasis. However, the contribution of insulin to this process increases during late gestation, especially during the perinatal period. The involvement of glucagon in fetal glucose homeostasis is also unclear. Infusion of glucagon into fetal sheep resulted in only modest increases in blood glucose concentrations *(123)*. However, the response may be diminished owing to counteracting effects of glucagon-stimulated insulin secretion. In contrast, a role for glucagon in maintaining blood glucose levels immediately after birth is well documented in humans, sheep, and rats *(123)*. This perinatal period is also associated with the onset of gluconeogenesis.

GONADS AND SEXUAL DIFFERENTIATION

Significant advances in the genetic and molecular basis for mammalian sexual differentiation have occurred recently. A thorough review of this process is beyond the scope of this chapter, but detailed reviews of the molecular events involved are available *(127–129)*. The process of mammalian sexual differentiation begins with expression of the Sry gene on the short arm of the Y chromosome. The SRY gene product is a DNA binding protein that is expressed in the undifferentiated primordial cells of male gonads just before morphological differentiation. Differentiation of the testes is associated with production of anti-

Müllerian hormone (AMH), also referred to as Müllerian-inhibiting substance. AMH is produced by the Sertoli cells and induces regression of the Müllerian duct. Testicular production of AMH begins by d 12 of fetal development in the mouse and continues after differentiation of the testes. However, the function of AMH during late gestation is not known. Interestingly, ovarian AMH production occurs after birth, and levels increase toward adult age in humans. However, the function of AMH in adult females is unclear. Differentiation of the testes during fetal development is also associated with production of androgens by the Leydig cells, which stimulate masculinization of the external genitalia and differentiation of the Wolffian duct. Differentiation of the gonadal primordial cells to the ovary, or the absence of gonads, leads to female-type differentiation. Thus, ovarian hormone secretion is not needed for female development during fetal life. By wk 5 of gestation in humans, the undifferentiated gonad contains primordial germ cells and mesenchyme of the gonadal ridge. The first morphologically distinct structure of the male gonad, the presence of Sertoli cells, occurs by 6–7 wk of gestation in humans. Differentiation of Leydig cells from mesenchyme occurs by wk 8. Testosterone secretion by the Leydig cells also begins during the 8th wk of gestation in humans and by d 15 in rats. Testosterone secretion is maximal during wk 12–14 in humans and d 18–20 in rats, decreasing to low levels during late gestation and the neonatal period. Levels of testosterone production by the fetal testes are regulated by hCG, and concentrations of hCG in the fetal circulation are maximal at 10 wk of gestation. Testicular hCG receptors are highest in concentration between wk 15 and 20 of fetal development. As mentioned earlier in this chapter, testicular hormone production likely suppresses pituitary gonadotropin secretion, since fetal LH and FSH concentrations are lower in male fetuses than in females during the second trimester. During late gestation, levels of testosterone, inhibin, LH, and FSH are similar between the sexes. Pituitary gonadotropins are likely not important during early and midgestation, when hCG levels dominate. However, a role for pituitary gonadotropin secretion during late gestation is evident, since gonadal development is diminished during the third trimester in anencephalic human fetuses. In the undifferentiated ovary, primordial follicles do not appear until wk 13 of gestation, preantral follicles form by wk 24, and antral follicles are present near term. In contrast to fetal testes, fetal ovaries do not produce significant amounts of steroid hormones during early or midgestation. Low steroid production by the ovaries is likely owing to the absence of hCG and FSH receptors in fetal ovaries in early and midgestation.

EPILOGUE

This chapter reviewed endocrine function during fetal development. A thorough review of such a broad subject was not intended. Thus, many details of each endocrine system were omitted. Rather, a general overview of the ontogeny and function of the fetal endocrine system was provided. The ontogeny and function of the fetal endocrine system is summarized in Table 1. Although much of our understanding of fetal endocrinology is derived from experimental models, this tabular summary concentrates on human fetal development for the sake of simplicity. Close inspection of the ontogeny of the fetal endocrine system reveals that production of the majority of hormones initiates during a relatively narrow window of fetal development, between 6 and 11 wk of gestation in humans. This close association of differentiation of different endocrine elements suggests that hormones from one endocrine gland may affect the ontogeny of other endocrine systems, just

Table 1
Ontogeny and Function of Fetal Hormone Production

Hormone	*Ontogenic profile in humans*	*Proposed function*
AMH	Production occurs by wk 5 in males	Male gonadal differentiation
Insulin	Secretion begins by 6–8 wk, but is low until birth	Glucose homeostasis
Glucagon	Secretion begins by 6–8 wk and increases during gestation	Glucose homeostasis and insulin secretion
Testosterone	Secretion occurs by 8 wk, increases through wk 12–14, and is low thereafter	Development of male genetalia
Angiotensin	Production begins by 8 wk and increases during gestation	Vasoconstriction and renal function
ACTH	Production begins by 9 wk and increases during late gestation	Adrenal development
Cortisol	Low levels produced by wk 9	Surfactant production
	Secretion increases toward term	Initiation of parturition
Epinephrine	Synthesis begins by 9 wk.	Glucose homeostasis
LH/FSH	Synthesis begins during wk 9 and is greatest during midgestation	Gonadal growth
TSH	Secretion begins by wk 10 and increases by late gestation	Thyroid function
T_4/T_3	Secretion begins by 10 wk and increases during late gestation	Lung maturation and fetal growth and metabolism
GH	Production initiates during wk 10, increases during gestation, but declines prior to birth	Fetal metabolism
PTH/ PTHrP	Production begins by wk 10, but PTHrP predominates during fetal development	Bone mineralization and Ca^{2+} homeostasis
AVP	Production begins by wk 10 and fluctuates with changes in blood volume	Blood volume and osmolality
OT	Synthesis begins by wk 11 and increases just prior to delivery	Parturition?
PRL	Secretion occurs by wk 16 and increases during late gestation	Lung maturation

as intercommunication among endocrine glands exists in adults. Further research is needed to clarify whether communication between endocrine glands leads to functional development of a complete endocrine system within a relatively short period of fetal development.

REFERENCES

1. Takor-Takor T, Pearse AGE (1975) Neuroectodermal origin of avian hypothalamo-hypophyseal complex: the role of the ventral neural ridge. J Embryol Exp Morphol 34:311–326.
2. Couly G, LeDouarin NM (1985) Mapping of the early neural primordium in quail-chick chimeras. I. Developmental relationships between placodes, facial ectoderm, and prosencephalon. Dev Biol 110:422–439.
3. Couly G, Le Douarin NM (1988) Mapping of the early neural primordium in quail-chick chimeras. II. The prosencephalic neural plate and neural folds: implications for the genesis of cephalic human congenital abnormalities. Dev Biol 120:198–214.

4. Ikeda H, Suzuki J, Sasano N, Niizuma H (1988) The development and morphogenesis of the human pituitary gland. Anat Embryol 178:327–336.
5. Simmons DM, Voss JW, Ingraham HA, Holloway JM, Broide RS, Rosenfeld MG, Swanson LW (1990) Pituitary cell phenotypes involve cell-specific Pit-1 mRNA translation and synergistic interactions with other classes of transcription factors. Genes Dev 4:695–711.
6. Asa SL, Kovacs K, Laszlo FA, Domokos I, Ezrin C (1986) Human fetal adenohypophysis: histologic and immunocytochemical analysis. Neuroendocrinology 43:308–316.
7. Begeot M, Dubois MP, Dubois PM (1977) Growth hormone and ACTH in the pituitary of normal and anencephalic fetuses: immunocytochemical evidence for hypothalamic influences during development. Neuroendocrinology 24:208–220.
8. Frawley LS, Hoeffler JP, Boockfor FR (1985) Functional maturation of somatotropes in fetal rat pituitaries: analysis by reverse hemolytic plaque assay. Endocrinology 116:2355–2360.
9. Baker BL, Yu YY (1977) An immunocytochemical study of human pituitary mammotropes from fetal life to old age. Am J Anat 148:217–239.
10. Hoeffler JP, Boockfor FR, Frawley LS (1985) Ontogeny of prolactin cells in neonatal rats: initial prolactin secretors also release growth hormone. Endocrinology 117:187–195.
11. Watanabe YG, Daikoku S (1979) An immunohistochemical study on the cytogenesis of adenohypophysial cells in fetal rats. Dev Biol 68:557–567.
12. Sheng HZ, Zhadanov AB, Mosinger B Jr, Fujii T, Bertuzzi S, Grinberg A, Lee EJ, Huang SP, Mahon KA, Westphal H (1996) Specification of pituitary cell lineages by the LIM homeobox gene Lhx3. Science 272:1004–1007.
13. Borrelli E, Heyman RA, Arias C, Sawchenko PE, Evans RM (1989) Transgenic mice with inducible dwarfism. Nature 339:538–541.
14. Kastin AJ, Gennser G, Arimura A, Miller MC III, Schally AV (1968) Melanocyte-stimulating and corticotrophic activities in human foetal pituitary glands. Acta Endocrinol 58:6–10.
15. Carr GA, Jacobs RA, Young IR, Schwartz J, White A (1995) Development of adrenocorticotropin-(1-39) and precursor peptide secretory responses in the fetal sheep during the last third of gestation. Endocrinology 136:5020–5027.
16. Voss JW, Rosenfeld MG (1992) Anterior pituitary development: short tales from dwarf mice. Cell 70:527–530.
17. Economides DL, Nicolaides KH, Linton EA, Perry LA, Chard T (1988) Plasma cortisol and adrenocorticotropin in appropriate and small for gestational age fetuses. Fetal Ther 3:158–164.
18. Robinson PM, Silver M, McMillen IC (1991) Effect of adrenalectomy or long term cortisol or adrenocorticotropin (ACTH)-releasing factor infusion on the concentration and molecular weight distribution of ACTH in fetal sheep plasma. Endocrinology 129(4):1942–1950.
19. Rose JC, Turner CS, Ray D, Rawashdeh N (1988) Evidence that cortisol inhibits basal adrenocorticotropin secretion in the sheep fetus by 0.70 gestation. Endocrinology 123:1307–1313.
20. Wood CE, Rudolph AM (1983) Negative feedback regulation of adrenocorticotropin secretion by cortisol in ovine fetuses. Endocrinology 112:1930–1936.
21. Apostolakis EM, Longo LD, Veldhuis JD, Yellon SM (1992) Dissociation of pulsatile cortisol and adrenocorticotropin secreton in fetal sheep during late gestation. Endocrinolgy 130(5): 2571–2578.
22. Rose JC, Meis PJ, Urban RR, Greiss FC Jr (1982) *In vivo* evidence for increased adrenal sensitivity to adrenocorticotropin-(1-24) in the lamb fetus late in gestation. Endocrinology 111:80–85.
23. Angevine DM (1938) Pathological anatomy of hypophysis and adrenals in anencephaly. Arch Pathol 26:507–518.
24. Young MC, Laurence KM, Hughes IA (1989) Relationship between fetal adrenal morphology and anterior pituitary function. Hormone Res 32:130–135.
25. Kaplan SL, Grumbach MM (1976) The ontogenesis of human foetal hormones. II. Luteinizing hormone (LH) and follicle stimulating hormone (FSH). Acta Endocrinol 81:808–829.
26. Mesiano S, Hart CS, Heyer BW, Kaplan SL, Grumbach MM (1991) Hormone ontogeny in the ovine fetus. XXVI. A sex difference in the effect of castration on the hypothalamic-pituitary gonadotropin unit in the ovine fetus. Endocrinology 129:3073–3079.
27. Beck-Peccoz P, Padmanabhan V, Baggiani AM, Cortelazzi D, Buscaglia M, Medri G, Marconi AM, Pardi G, Beitins IZ (1991) Maturation of hypothalamic-pituitary-gonadal function in normal fetuses: circulating levels of gonadotropins, their common α-subunit and free testosterone, and discrepancy between immunological and biological activities of circulating follicle-stimulating hormone. J Clin Endocrinol Metab 73:525–532.

28. Clements JA, Reyes FI, Winter JS, Faiman C (1976) Studies of human sexual development. III. Fetal pituitary and serum and amniotic fluid concentrations of LH, CG, and FSH. J Clin Endocrinol Metab 42:919
29. Rabinovici J, Goldsmith PC, Robert VJ, Vaughan J, Vale W, Jaffe RB (1991) Localization and secretion of inhibin/activin subunits in the human and subhuman primate fetal gonads. J Clin Endocrinol Metab 73:1141–1149.
30. Rabinovici J, Jaffe RB (1990) Development and regulation of growth and differentiation in human and subhuman primate fetal gonads. Endocr Rev 11:532–557.
31. Clark SJ, Hauffa BP, Rodens KP, Styne DL, Kaplan SL, Grumbach MM (1989) Hormone ontogeny of the ovine fetus. XIX. The effect of a potent luteinizing hormone-releasing factor agonist on gonadatropin and testosterone release in the fetus and neonate. Pediatr Res 25:347–352.
32. Albers N, Bettebdorf M, Herrmann H, Kaplan SL, Grumbach MM (1993) Hormone ontogeny in the ovine fetus, XXVII. Pulsatile and copulsatile secretion of luteinizing hormone, follicle-stimulating hormone, growth hormone, and prolactin in late gestation: a new method for the analysis of copulsatility. Endocrinology 132:701–709.
33. Kaplan SL, Grumbach MM, Aubert ML (1976) The ontogenesis of pituitary hormones and hypothalamic factors in the human fetus: Maturation of central nervous system regulation of anterior pituitary function. Recent Prog Horm Res 32:161–243.
34. Massa G, de Zegher F, Vanderschueren-Lodeweyckx M (1992) Serum levels of immunoreactive inhibin, FSH and LH in human infants at preterm and term birth. Biol Neonate 61:150–155.
35. Baker TG, Scrimgeour JB (1980 Development of the gonad in normal and anencephalic human fetuses. J Reprod Fertil 60:193–199.
36. Zondek LH, Zondek T (1983) Ovarian hilar cells and testicular Leydig cells in anencephaly. Biol Neonate 43:211–219.
37. Fisher DA, Dussault J (1974) Development of the mammalian thyroid gland, In: Handbook of Physiology: Endocrinology III. The Thyroid (Greer MA, Solomon DH, eds.), American Physiological Society, Washington DC, pp 21–38.
38. Thorpe-Beeston JG, Nicolaides KH, Felton CV, Butler J, McGregor AM (1991) Maturation of the secretion of thyroid hormone and thyroid-stimulating hormone in the fetus. N Engl J Med 324:532–536.
39. Klein AH, Oddie TH, Parslow M (1982) Developmental changes in pituitary-thyroid function in the human fetus and newborn. Early Hum Dev 6:321–330.
40. Kawaoi A, Tsuneda M (1986) Effects of thyroidectomy and administration of propylthiouracil (PTU) or thyrotropin (TSH) to pregnant rats on the functional development of the fetal thyroid gland: an immunohistochemical study. Endocrinol Jpn 33:835–841.
41. Tonooka N, Greer MA (1978) Evidence that control of fetal thyrotropin secretion is independent of both the fetal and maternal hypothalamus. Endocrinology 102:852–858.
42. Rodriguez-Garcia M, Jolin T, Santos A, Perez-Castillo A (1995) Effect of perinatal hypothyroidism on the developmental regulation of rat pituitary growth hormone and thyrotropin genes. Endocrinology 136:4339–4350.
43. Bona G, Aquili C, Ravanini P, Gallina MR, Cigolotti AC, Zaffaroni M, Paniccia P, Mussa F (1994) Growth hormone, insulin-like growth factor-I and somatostatin in human fetus, newborn, mother plasma and amniotic fluid. Panminerva Med 36:5–12.
44. Salardi S, Orsini LF, Cacciari E, Righetti F, Donati S, Mandini M, Cicognani A, Bovicelli L (1991) Growth hormone, insulin-like growth factor-I, insulin and C-peptide during human fetal life: in-utero study. Clin Endocrinol 34:187–190.
45. Kishi K, Hirashiba M, Hasegawa Y (1991) Gestational profiles of rat placental lactogen-II (rPL-II) and growth hormone (GH) in maternal and fetal serum, amniotic fluid, and placental tissue. Endocrinol Jpn 38:589–595.
46. Bassett NS, Gluckman PD (1986) Pulsatile growth hormone secretion in the ovine fetus and neonatal lamb. J Endocrinol 109:307–312.
47. de Zegher F, Daaboul J, Grumbach MM, Kaplan SL (1989) Hormone ontogeny in the ovine fetus and neonate. XXII. The effect of somatostatin on the growth hormone (GH) response to GH-releasing factor. Endocrinology 124:1114–1117.
48. Gluckman PD, Grumbach MM, Kaplan SL (1981) The neuroendocrine regulation and function of growth hormone and prolactin in the mammalian fetus. Endocr Rev 2:363–395.
49. Gluckman PD, Uthne K, Styne DM, Kaplan SL, Rudolph AM, Grumbach MM (1979) Hormone ontogeny in the ovine fetus. IV. Serum somatomedin activity in the fetal and neonatal lamb and

pregnant ewe: correlation with maternal and fetal growth hormone, prolactin, and chorionic somatomammotropin. Pediatr Res 13:194–196.
50. Goodyer CG, Branchaud CL, Lefebvre Y (1993) Effects of growth hormone, GH-releasing factor and somatostatin on GH secretion from early to midgestation human fetal pituitaries. J Clin Endocrinol Met 76:1259–1264.
51. Bauer MK, Breier BH, Harding JE, Veldhuis JD, Gluckman PD (1995) The fetal somatotropic axis during long term maternal undernutrition in sheep: evidence for nutritional regulation in utero. Endocrinology 136:1250–1257.
52. Stevens D, Alexander G (1986) Lipid deposition after hypophysectomy and growth hormone treatment in the sheep fetus. J Dev Physiol 8:139–145.
53. Cooke PS, Yonemura CU, Russell SM, Nicoll CS (1986) Growth and differentiation of fetal rat intestine transplants: dependence on insulin and growth hormone. Biol Neonate 49:211–218.
54. Otonkoski T, Knip M, Wong I, Simell O (1988) Effects of growth hormone and insulin-like growth factor I on endocrine function of human fetal islet-like cell clusters during long-term tissue culture. Diabetes 37:1678–1683.
55. Sandler S, Anderson A, Korsgren O, Tollemar J, Peterson B, Groth CG, Hellerstrom C (1987) Tissue culture of human fetal pancreas: growth hormone stimulates the formation and insulin production of islet-like cell clusters. J Clin Endocrinol Met 65:1154–1158.
56. Scharfmann R, Basmaciogullari A, Czernichow P (1990) Effect of growth hormone and glucose on rat islet cells replication using 5-bromo-2-deoxyuridine incorporation. Diabetes Res 15:137–141.
57. Fukaya T, Furuhashi N, Shinkawa O, Kono H, Takahashi T, Suzuki M (1984) The human fetal prolactin and estradiol levels, and their correlationship. Tohoku J Exp Med 143:87–92.
58. Suganuma N, Seo H, Yamamoto N, Kikkawa F, Oguri H, Narita O, Tomoda Y, Matsui N (1989) The ontogeny of growth hormone in the human fetal pituitary. Am J Obst Gynecol 160:729–733.
59. Root AW (1976) Growth hormone and prolactin in fetus. Prog Clin Biol Res 10:107–126.
60. Aubert MJ, Grumbach MM, Kaplan SL (1975) The ontogenesis of human fetal hormones. III. Prolactin. J Clin Invest 56:155–164.
61. McMillen IC, Jenkin G, Robinson JS, Thorburn GD (1983) Concentrations of prolactin in the plasma of fetal sheep and in amniotic fluid in late gestation and during dexamethasone-induced parturition. J Endocrinol 99:107–114.
62. SeronFerre M, Monroe SE, Hess D, Parer JT, Jaffe RB (1979) Prolactin concentrations in the monkey fetus during the last third of gestation. Endocrinology 104:1243–1246.
63. Yuen BH, Mincey EK (1987) Human chorionic gonadotropin, prolactin, estriol, and dehydroepiandrosterone sulfate concentrations in cord blood of premature and term newborn infants: relationship to the sex of the neonate. Am J Obst Gynecol 156:396–400.
64. Vergara M, Parraguez VH, Riquelme R, Figueroa JP, Llanos AJ, Seron-Ferre M (1989) Ontogeny of the circadian variation of plasma prolactin in sheep. J Dev Physiol 11:89–95.
65. Houghton DC, Young IR, McMillen IC (1995) Evidence for hypothalamic control of the diurnal rhythms in prolactin and melatonin in the fetal sheep during late gestation. Endocrinology 136: 218–223.
66. Roti E, Robuschi G, Alboni A, d'Amato L, Montermini M, Gardini E, Salvi M, Borciani E, Dall'Aglio E, Bisi S (1986) Human foetal prolactin but not thyrotropin secretion is decreased by bromocriptine. Acta Endocrinol 112:35–41.
67. Thomsett MJ, Marti-Henneberg C, Gluckman PD, Kaplan SL, Rudolph AM, Grumbach MM (1980) Hormone ontogeny in the ovine fetus. VIII. The effect of thyrotropin-releasing factor on prolactin and growth hormone release in the fetus and neonate. Endocrinology 106:1074–1078.
68. Leontic EA, Tyson JE (1977) Prolactin and fetal osmoregulation: water transport across isolated human amnion. Am J Physiol 232:R124–R127.
69. Pullano JG, Cohen-Addad N, Apuzzio JJ, Ganesh VL, Josimovich JB (1989) Water and salt conservation in the human fetus and newborn. I. Evidence for a role of fetal prolactin. J Clin Endocrinol Metab 69:1180–1186.
70. Mendelson CR, Boggaram V (1991) Hormonal control of the surfactant system in the fetal lung. Ann Rev Physiol 53:415–440.
71. Parker CR, MacDonald PC, Guzick DS, Porter JC, Rosenfeld CR, Hauth JC (1989) Prolactin levels in umbilical cord blood of human infants: relation to gestational age, maternal complications, and neonatal lung function. Am J Obst Gynecol 161:795–802.
72. Schellenberg J-C, Liggins GC, Manzai M, Kitterman JA, Lee CC (1988) Synergistic hormone effects on lung maturation in fetal sheep. J Appl Physiol 65:94–100.

73. Robillard JE, Nakamura KT (1988) Hormonal regulation of renal function during development. Biol Neonate 53:201–211.
74. Wittkowski WH, Schulze-Bonhage AH, Bockers TM (1992) The pars tuberalis of the hypophysis: A modulator of the pars distalis? Acta Endocrinol 126:285–290.
75. Yokoh Y (1968) The early development of the nervous system in man. Acta Anat (Basel) 71: 492–518.
76. Ervin MG, Kullama LK, Ross MG, Leake RD, Fisher DA (1993) Vasopressin receptors and effects during fetal development. Regul Pep 45:203–208.
77. Skowsky WR, Fisher DA (1977) Fetal neurohypophyseal arginine vasotocin in man and sheep. Pediatr Res 11:627–630.
78. Swaab DF, Hofman MA, Honnebier MB (1990) Development of vasopressin neurons in the human suprachiasmatic nucleus in relation to birth. Brain Res Dev Brain Res 52:289–293.
79. Weitzman RE, Fisher DA, Robillard J, Erenberg A, Kennedy R, Smith F (1978) Arginine vasopressin response to an osmotic stimulus in the fetal sheep. Pediatr Res 12:35–38.
80. Bell RJ, Congiu M, Hardy KJ, Wintour EM (1984) Gestation dependent aspects of the response of the ovine fetus to the osmotic stress induced by maternal water deprivation. Q J Exp Physiol 69:187–195.
81. Gomez RA, Norwood VF (1995) Developmental consequences of the renin-angiotensin system. Am J Kidney Dis 26:409–425.
82. Lee HU, Campbell DJ, Habener JF (1987) Developmental expression of the angiotensinogen gene in rat embryos. Endocrinology 121:1335–1342.
83. Gomez RA, Cassis L, Lynch KR, Chevalier RL, Wilfong N, Carey RM, Peach MJ (1988) Fetal expression of the angiotensinogen gene. Endocrinology 123:2298–2302.
84. Kalinyak JE, Hoffman AR, Perlman AJ (1991) Ontogeny of angiotensinogen mRNA and angiotensin II receptors in rat brain and liver. J Endocrinol Invest 14:647–653.
85. Everett AD, Chevalier RL, Gomez RA (1991) Hepatic angiotensinogen gene regulation in the fetal and pregnant rat. Pediatr Res 30:252–255.
86. Richoux AS, Amsaguine S, Grignor G, Bouhnik J, Menrad J, Corvol P (1987) Earliest renin-containing cell differentation during ontogenesis in the rat. Histochemistry 88:41–46.
87. Pupilli C, Gomez RA, Tuttle JB, Peach MJ, Carey RM (1991) Spatial association of renin-containing cells and nerve fibers in developing rat kidney. Pediatr Nephrol 5:690–695.
88. Gomez RA, Chevalier RL, Sturgill BC, Johns DW, Peach MJ, Carey RM (1993) Maturation of the intrarenal renin distribution in Wister-Kyoto rats. J Hypertens 4:S31–S33.
89. Celio MR, Groscurth P, Inagami T (1985) Ontogeny of renin immunoreactive cells in the human kidney. Anat Embryol 173:149–155.
90. Taylor GM, Peart WS, Porter KA (1986) Concentration and molecular forms of active and inactive renin in human fetal kidney, amniotic fluid and adrenal gland: Evidence for renin-angiotensin system hyperactivity in 2nd trimester of pregnancy. J Hypertens 4:121–129.
91. Fisher DA, Polk DH (1989) Development of the thyroid. Baillieres Clin Endocrinol Metab 3: 627–652.
92. Klein AH, Fisher DA (1980) Thyrotropin releasing hormone stimulated pituitary and thyroid gland responsiveness and 3, 5, 3′-triiodothyronine supression in fetal and neonatal lambs. Endocrinology 106:697–701.
93. Fisher DA, Klein AH (1981) Thyroid development and disorders of thyroid function in the newborn. N Engl J Med 304:702–712.
94. Klein AH, Oddie TH, Fisher DA (1978) Effect of parturition on serum iodothyronine concentrations in fetal sheep. Endocrinology 103:1453–1457.
95. Morreale de Escobar G, Obregon MJ, Ruiz de Ona C, Escobar del Rey F (1988) Transfer of thyroxine from the mother to the rat fetus near term: effects on brain 3,5,3′-triiodothyronine deficiency. Endocrinology 122:1521–1531.
96. Polk DH, Wu SY, Fisher DA (1986) Serum thyroid hormone and tissue 5′-monodeiodinase activity in acutely thyroidectomized newborn lambs. Am J Phys 14:E151–E155.
97. Polk DH, Wu SY, Wright C (1988) Ontogeny of thyroid hormone effect on tissue 5′-monodeiodinase activity in fetal sheep. Am J Phys 17:E337–E341.
98. Obregon MJ, Mallol J, Pator R (1984) L-Thyroxine and 3,5,3′-triiodothyronine in rat embryos before onset of fetal thyroid function. Endocrinology 114:305–307.
99. Letarte J, Guyda H, Dussault JH (1980) Clinical, biochemical and radiological features of neonatal hypothyroid infants, In: Neonatal Screening (Dussault JH, Burrow GN, eds.), Raven, New York, pp 225–236.

100. O'Brien WF (1991) Use of TRH in the fetus to advance lung maturity. Adv Exp Med Biol 299: 243–250.
101. Erenberg A, Rhodes ML, Weinstein MM, Kennedy RL (1979) The effect of fetal thyroidectomy on ovine fetal lung maturation. Pediatr Res 13:230–235.
102. MacIsaac RJ, Heath JA, Rodda CP, Moseley JM, Care AD, Martin TJ, Caple IW (1991) Role of the fetal parathyroid hormone-related protein in the regulation of placental transport of calcium, magnesium and inorganic phosphate. Reprod Fertil Dev 3:447–457.
103. LeroyerAlizon E, David L, Anast CS, Dubois PM (1981) Immunocytochemical evidence for parathyroid hormone in human fetal parathyroid glands. J Clin Endocrinol Metab 52:513–516.
104. Seki K, Furuya K, Makimura N, Mitsui C, Hirata J, Nagata I (1994) Cord blood levels of calcium-regulating hormones and osteocalcin in premature infants. J Perinatal Med 22:189–194.
105. Abbas SK, Ratcliffe WA, Moniz C, Dixit M, Caple IW, Silver M, Fowden A, Care AD (1994) The role of parathyroid hormone-related protein in calcium homeostasis in the fetal pig. Exp Physiol 79:527–536.
106. Wadsworth JC, Kronfeld DS, Ramberg Jr CF (1982) Parathyrin and calcium homeostasis in the fetus. Biol Neonate 41:101–109.
107. Pitkin RM, Reynolds WA, Williams GA, Kawahara W, Bauman AF, Hargis GK (1980) Maternal and fetal parathyroid hormone responsiveness in pregnant primates. J Clin Endocrinol Metab 51:1044–1047.
108. Rodda CP, Kubota M, Heath JA, Ebeling PR, Moseley JM, Care AD, Caple IW, Martin TJ (1988) Evidence for a novel parathyroid hormone-related protein in fetal lamb parathyroid glands and sheep placenta: comparisons with a similar protein implicated in humoral hypercalcemia of malignancy. J Endocrinol 117:261–271.
109. Abbas SK, Pickard DW, Illingworth D, Storer J, Purdie DW, Moniz C, Dixit M, Caple IW, Ebeling PR, Rodda CP, Martin TJ, Care AD (1990) Measurement of parathyroid hormone-related protein in extracts of fetal parathyroid glands and placental membranes. J Endocrinol 124:319–325.
110. Takeuchi A, Okano T, Sekimoto H, Kobayashi T (1994) The enzymatic formation of 1 alpha, 25-dihydroxyvitamin D3 from 25-dihydroxyvitamin D3 in the liver of fetal rats. Comp Biochem Phys 109:1–7.
111. Ross R, Care AD, Robinson JS, Pickard DW, Weatherley AJ (1980) Perinatal 1,25-dihydroxycholecalciferol in the sheep and its role in the maintenance of the transplacental calcium gradient. J Endocrinol 87:17P,18P.
112. Ross R, Halbert K, Tsang RC (1989) Determination of the production and metabolic clearance rates of 1,25-dihydroxyvitamin D3 in the pregnant sheep and its chronically catheterized fetus by primed infusion technique. Pediatr Res 26:633–638.
113. Johnson JA, Grande JP, Roche PC, Sweeney WE, Avner ED, Kumar R (1995) 1-alpha, 25-dihydroxyvitamin D3 receptor ontogenesis in fetal renal development. Am J Physiol 269:F419–F428.
114. Shameley DR, Buffenstein R, Veale G, Pettifor JM (1993) Maternal vitamin D status has no effect on the ontogeny of calcium-binding proteins in the duodenum, kidney and cerebellum of fetal mice. J Endocrinol 139:473–478.
115. Ross R, Florer J, Halbert K, McIntyre L (1989) Characterization of 1,25-dihydroxyvitamin D3 receptors and in vivo targeting of [3H]-1,25-dihydroxyvitamin D3 in the sheep placenta. Placenta 10:553–567.
116. Phillipe M (1983) Fetal catecholamines. Am J Obstet Gynecol 146:840–855.
117. Liggins GC (1994) The role of cortisol in preparing the fetus for birth. Reprod Fertil Dev 6: 141–150.
118. Pepe GJ, Albrecht ED (1990) Regulation of the primate fetal adrenal cortex. Endocr Rev 11: 151–171.
119. Challis JRG, Brooks AN (1989) Maturation and activation of hypothalamic-pituitary-adrenal function in fetal sheep Endocr Rev 10:182–204.
120. Liggins GC, Fairclough RJ, Grimes SA, Kendall JZ, Knox BS (1973) The mechanism of initiation of parturition in the ewe. Recent Prog Horm Res 29:111–159.
121. Slack JMW (1995) Developmental biology of the pancreas. Development 121:1569–1580.
122. Schaeffer LD, Wilder ML, Williams RH (1973) Secretion and content of insulin and glucagon in human fetal pancreas slices in vitro. Proc Soc Exp Biol Med 143:314–319.
123. Sperling MA (1994) Carbohydrate metabolism: insulin and glucagon, In: Maternal-Fetal Endocrinology, 2nd ed. (Tulchinsky D, Little AB, eds.), WB Saunders, Philadelphia, pp. 379–400.
124. Hellerstrom C, Swenne I (1991) Functional maturation and proliferation of fetal pancreatic beta cells. Diabetes 2:89–93.

125. Simpson AM, Tuch BE (1995) Control of insulin biosynthesis in the human fetal beta cell. Pancreas 11:48–54.
126. Otonkoski T, Anderson S, Simell O (1993) Somatostatin regulation of beta-cell function in the normal human fetuses and in neonates with persistent hyperinsulinemic hypogylcemia. J Clin Endocrinol Met 76:184–188.
127. Haqq CM, King CY, Ukiyama E, Falsafi S, Haqq TN, Donahoe PK, Weiss MA (1994) Molecular basis of mammalian sexual determination: activation of mullerian inhibiting substance gene expression by SRY. Science 226:1494–1499.
128. Voutilainen R (1992) Differentiation of the Fetal Gonad. Horm Res 38(suppl 2):66–71.
129. Huhtaniemi I (1994) Fetal testis—a very special endocrine organ. Eur J Endocrinol 130:25–31.

14 Endocrine Control of Parturition

Robert E. Garfield, PHD, *George Saade,* MD, *and Kristof Chwalisz,* MD, PHD

CONTENTS

INTRODUCTION

Parturition is the process that starts with uterine contractions and cervical dilation, and ends with delivery of the fetus and placenta. It is a procedure that involves progression of uterine contractility from inactive to vigorously active, and requires softening and opening of the previously rigid and closed cervix. These crucial steps are thought to be regulated by the coordinated changes in various systems, including interactions among humoral, neurogenic, and immunologic control mechanisms. The means by which the myometrium and cervix achieve conversion to their final stages is the key to understanding parturition. In the past, many studies have demonstrated that changes in hormones, cytokines, prostaglandins (PGs), and so forth, play important roles in the initation of labor. More recently, nitric oxide has emerged as a possible element of control.

The myometrium contracts in response to the underlying electrical activity that is present in bursts of action potentials. The force, duration, and frequency of contractions are directly related to the characteristics of these electrical bursts, which increase tremendously during labor (Fig. 1). The cervix, on the other hand, softens as pregnancy reaches term, mainly because of a decrease in collagen concentration (Fig. 2). In this brief chapter, we will outline some of the important mechanisms that are thought to regulate the myometrial and cervical functions during pregnancy and parturition. For more detailed discussion of the proposed mechanisms, the reader is referred to the reviews at the end of the chapter in the Reference Section.

HUMORAL CONTROL OF LABOR

Role of Steroid Hormones

It is widely accepted that endocrine systems control the onset of labor. This theory holds that hormones interact with the uterus to maintain quiescence, and that at term, an

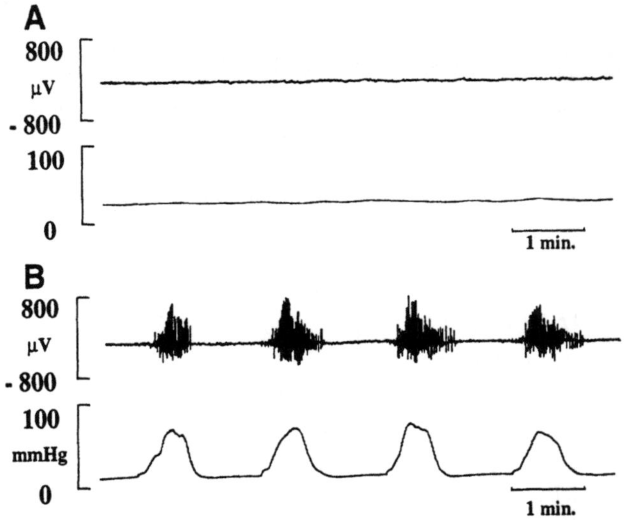

Fig. 1. Electromyographic (EMG) activity as recorded by electrodes placed on the rat uterine wall during labor (top tracings in **A** and **B**) and intrauterine pressure measured with an intrauterine pressure transducer (bottom tracings in A and B); (A) shows lack of activity recorded prior to term (d 15 of pregnancy). Note that the periodic increases in pressure correspond to bursts of EMG activity (B) recorded from an animal in spontaneous labor at term.

alteration in hormone levels enhances uterine contractility and initiates labor *(1)*. In some animals, such as rats, rabbits, sheep, and various other species, a pronounced decline in progesterone levels (progesterone withdrawal) occurs prior to labor. However, this is not the case in primates or guinea pigs *(2,3)*. Although serum progesterone levels decrease in some species, estrogen levels increase prior to labor in all species studied. This has led to speculation that either rising levels of estrogen or estrogen precursors, or a change in the estrogen:progesterone ratio initiates labor *(1,2,4–6)*. Progesterone and estrogen as signals for parturition will be discussed later in this chapter.

Progesterone. Progesterone plays a pivotal role in establishing and maintaining pregnancy. During early pregnancy, progesterone is essential for the entire implantation process. Later in gestation, progesterone maintains the pregnancy by acting predominantly on the cervix and myometrium. In addition, there is some evidence that progesterone has an immunosuppressive effect and may regulate the cytokine network in the uterus. Finally, progesterone may play an important role in the maternal cardiovascular adaptation during pregnancy.

According to Csapo, progesterone is the major hormone responsible for the quiescent state of the uterine musculature *(1)*. He believed that progesterone withdrawal changes the uterus from an inert state to a highly active organ by both increasing uterine responsiveness (owing to the lowering of the threshold for excitation by oxytocic agents) and inducing the release of "intrinsic uterine stimulants." However, Csapo's "progesterone block theory" was based primarily on the results of experiments performed in rabbits and rats. In these two species, the corpus luteum is the major source of peripheral progesterone, and parturition is preceded by luteolysis and a sudden progesterone withdrawal with a concomitant increase in estradiol *(4)*. In humans, nonhuman primates, and guinea pigs, there is no progesterone decrease prior to the onset of labor. In contrast, in humans, there is a sustained increase in peripheral progesterone concentrations up to the time of birth. In addition, progesterone supplementation fails to prolong pregnancy in either primates or

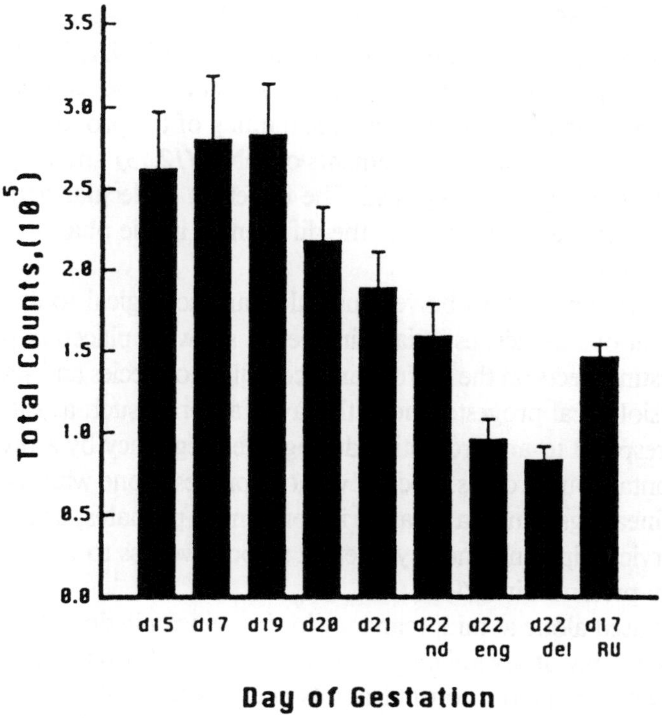

Fig. 2. Light-induced fluorescence from rat cervical tissue measured at various stages of pregnancy. The fluorescence is thought to represent changes in collagen content of the cervix (d22nd = d 22 nondelivery; d22eng = d 22 pups engaged in cervical canal; d22del = d 22 following delivery of one to three pups; d17RU = measurements made at d 17 following RU 486 treatment). Total fluorescent counts are represented by means ± SEM. From ref. *(116)*.

guinea pigs. These observations suggest that progesterone withdrawal does not play a significant role in the initiation of parturition in primates and guinea pigs. However, alterations in progesterone activity, binding to its receptor and response elements, or interaction of progesterone with other proteins (e.g., transacting factors), rather than changes in peripheral progesterone concentrations, may be more important in controlling parturition in these species. The fact that antiprogestins induce labor in all species investigated to date, including nonhuman primates and humans, supports the assumption of a commanding role for progesterone in this process. Studies of induction of parturition in guinea pigs and primates, as well as clinical studies with RU 486 and other progesterone antagonists show that these compounds clearly increase myometrial responsiveness and induce cervical ripening during midpregnancy as discussed in the next section of this chapter. Furthermore, some antiprogestins (e.g., onapristone) are highly effective in inducing preterm parturition in guinea pigs, Tupajas, and monkeys (species with no progesterone withdrawal at term).

Progesterone Antagonists. Until the synthesis of the first progesterone antagonist (antiprogestin) RU 486 more than a decade ago *(7)*, the exact mechanism of progesterone action, particularly in the pregnant uterus, was poorly understood. RU 486 (mifepristone) and ZK 98 299 (onapristone) are the antiprogestins most thoroughly investigated to date *(8,9)*. Both compounds bind with high affinity to progesterone and glucocorticoid receptors, and show antiprogestagenic and antiglucocorticoid effects in vivo. The antiglucocorticoid activity of onapristone is, however, significantly less than that of RU 486 *(8,10)*. The molecular mechanisms of action of onapristone and RU 486 seem to be different. Since RU 486 facilitates binding of the progesterone receptor to DNA, it may act as a mixed agonist/antagonist *(11)*. On the other hand, onapristone (and certain other 13α-configurated progesterone antagonists), impairs the binding of the progesterone receptor (PR) complexes to progesterone-responsive elements of DNA *(12,13)* and may be regarded as a "pure" progesterone receptor antagonist. The different molecular actions of these two compounds may in part explain some of the differences in the pharmacodynamic effects in the pregnant uterus.

Antiprogestins have proven to be very useful pharmacological tools to define progesterone action in various tissues, especially in species showing placental progesterone synthesis. Antiprogestin effects on the uterus vary according to species and stage of pregnancy. Species with physiological progesterone withdrawal at term (such as rats, rabbits, sheep, pigs, and cows) respond to antiprogestins during late pregnancy by a preterm parturition similar to the spontaneous process. Species without progesterone withdrawal prior to parturition (e.g., guinea pigs, Tupaja belangeri, nonhuman primates, and humans) react by an increase in cervical ripening and myometrial responsiveness to contractilie agents, but not necessarily by preterm birth *(9)*.

Antiprogestins used alone at midpregnancy in the guinea pig do not consistently lead to delivery. There is a delay of several days *(10)* in those animals that deliver. The increase in peripheral plasma prostaglandin concentrations in rats within 1–3 d of antiprogestin treatment has not been detected in guinea pigs *(3,10)*. This indicates that progesterone antagonists in guinea pigs do not effectively induce the release of endogenous uterotonins, such as PGs and oxytocin. In monkeys, RU 486 does not successfully induce labor when given alone during late pregnancy *(14-16)*. However, it is highly effective in combination with oxytocin *(14)*. In contrast, studies done in early gestation in guinea pigs and monkeys indicate that the antiprogestins alone effectively result in termination of pregnancy. In guinea pigs, the progestins R5020 and gestodene totally inhibit the labor-inducing activity of onapristone, which clearly indicates that this action is mediated by the PR *(9,17)*.

A number of in vitro *(18)* and in vivo studies have clearly shown that antiprogestins given during advanced pregnancy increase myometrial responsiveness to uterotonic agents, including prostaglandins *(10)* and oxytocin in all species investigated to date *(9)*. This effect is particularly pronounced in species showing no spontaneous progesterone withdrawal prior to parturition, such as guinea pigs and nonhuman primates. About a 30-fold increase in uterine responsiveness to oxytocin was found in guinea pigs at midpregnancy (d 42–43 post coitus) after onapristone priming *(19)*. Normally, at this stage of pregnancy, the uterus is insensitive to oxytocin and even very high doses do not effectively induce abortion without antiprogestin priming. An increase in myometrial responsiveness to oxytocin and PGs after antiprogestin priming has also been demonstrated in monkeys and in a number of clinical studies using RU 486 *(9)*.

Studies with the antiprogesterones clearly show that these agents prime the myometrium for labor. Treatment with these agents produce all the changes in the muscle cells that prepare them for effective contractions and labor. These include changes in cell-to-cell contacts, receptors, ion channels, and so on, to be described later.

Another possibility of functional progesterone withdrawal during parturition might be the downregulation of myometrial PR. In the nonpregnant human uterus, the cellular distribution of estrogen receptors (ERs) and PRs in the human endometrium, as assessed by immunohistology, shows a cyclic pattern during the menstrual cycle. Both glandular and stromal cell expression of ERs increase during the proliferative phase and then gradually decline to undetectable levels during the midluteal phase. A similar pattern of change occurs for PR expression in the endometrial epithelium, but PRs are maintained in the stroma throughout the luteal phase, although at slightly lower levels *(20)*. These changes reflect an increase in serum progesterone concentrations, since it is well established that progesterone downregulates the expression of both ERs and PRs at the genomic level. However, the downregulation of PRs in the uterus prior to parturition has never been convincingly demonstrated in primates.

The PR consists of two isoforms: an A-receptor (hPR-A), which contains 933 amino acids, and a B-receptor (hPR-B), which lacks the N-terminal 164 amino acids *(21)*. The B-receptor functions as a hormone-dependent positive regulator of specific progesterone-induced genes, whereas the A-receptors can inhibit the activity of B-receptors *(22,23)*, and other members of the steroid receptor family, including ERs. The ratio of B- to A-receptors in the progesterone target tissue may, therefore, determine its response to progestational and antiprogestational agents. The expression of PR isoforms changes during the human menstrual cycle *(24)*. However, very little is known about their role in the pregnant uterus.

Progesterone and Antiprogestins Effects in the Cervix. The maturation process known as cervical ripening is an integral part of the preparatory changes preceding the onset of labor. The cervix, which consists mainly of connective tissue, changes considerably in preparation for labor. This change involves softening, shortening, and dilatation. Cervical ripening is an active biochemical process that involves a complex cascade of degradative enzymes and an alteration in the synthesis of extracellular matrix proteins and glycoproteins *(25)*. There is evidence that progesterone may prevent cervical ripening.

Animal and clinical studies with antiprogestins indicate that progesterone plays a significant role in the control of cervical ripening during pregnancy. The ripening effect of antiprogestins in guinea pigs has been well established *(9)*. Morphological and biochemical studies in guinea pigs *(19,26,27)* have demonstrated that there is an increase in collagenolysis within the cervix at term and following antiprogestin treatment. The available experimental and clinical data indicate that the action of antiprogestins on the cervix is independent of endogenous PG production, since the prostaglandin synthase inhibitors do not block this effect *(19,28,29)*.

Liggins *(30)* proposed that cervical ripening is similar to an inflammatory reaction. This process involves an infiltration of white blood cells into the cervix of women at term, accompanied by both dissolution of the connective tissue matrix around polymorphonuclear leukocytes and an increase in activated and degranulated eosinophiles *(31,32)*. A similar reaction occurs in the pregnant guinea pig cervix after onapristone *(26)*, independent of PGs. The action of antiprogestins on the cervix seems to be mediated through enzymatic activity of inflammatory cells and chemotactic agents, such as cytokines (e.g., IL-8, IL-1β) *(17,19)*. Cytokines are clearly involved in cervical ripening during normal parturition. Cervical explants from pregnant rabbits *(33)* and pregnant women *(34)* are capable of producing vast amounts of IL-1 and IL-8, respectively. Recent morphological and biomechanical studies demonstrate the efficacy of topically administered IL-8 and IL-1β in inducing cervical ripening in pregnant guinea pigs *(35)*. Progesterone inhibits and RU 486 stimulates IL-8 release in human choriodecidual cells in vitro *(36)*. Thus, progesterone may act as an immunosuppressor in the cervix, whereas antiprogestins may activate the cytokine cascade and neutrophil migration. Neutrophils and macrophages are well-known sources of collagenases and other enzymes capable of digesting extracellular matrix proteins. These cells are also a rich source of nitric oxide as discussed later.

Estrogens. There is evidence to suggest that estrogens are required in the preparation of the myometrium for parturition *(1,2,5)*. Estrogen levels in the maternal blood are elevated during pregnancy and increase further at term. Rising estrogen levels have been suggested to control various processes in the myometrium, including stimulating growth of the uterus, numbers of stimulatory receptors, prostaglandin synthesis, and myometrial excitability through changes in resting membrane potential and propagation of electrical signals *(5,6)*.

However, treatment of many species (i.e., guinea pigs and primates, including humans) with estrogen during pregnancy fails to induce labor. These studies indicate that estrogens alone do not initiate labor, but may assist in preparing the uterus for efficient contraction during labor.

Estrogens can directly stimulate a number of genes in the uterus. However, the transcriptional activity of ERs is generally suppressed in the presence of progesterone. This can be achieved either by downregulation of ERs, or by the direct interaction between PRs and ERs, or other transcription factors. Therefore, estrogens are unlikely to exhibit their stimulatory activity when progesterone levels are high. Parturition studies in primates and guinea pigs using estrogen, progesterone antagonists, and progesterone synthase inhibitors *(37)* strongly indicate that progesterone inhibition is a much more powerful signal for the conversion of a quiescent uterus to labor than the estrogen treatment.

Knockout studies of the ER show that female mice are infertile indicating the important role of estrogen in conception, whereas heterozygous mice have normal fertility and pregnancy *(38,39)*. On the other hand, overexpression of the ER gene in transgenic mice causes dystocia and disrupts labor *(38)*. Furthermore, estrogens completely inhibit preterm birth in rats and guinea pigs treated with antiprogesterones *(40–43)*. How these effects are achieved is not known. The above results indicate the need for additional studies on the effects of estrogens during parturition.

Androgens. Physiologically, testosterone is not a uniquely male hormone. It is well documented that testosterone levels increase prior to parturition in some species *(44)*. The biosynthetic pathway of the steroids includes the conversion of testosterone to estrogens by the aromatase enzyme present in the ovary and placental trophoblast. Testosterone is also converted into a more potent androgen, dihydrotestosterone, by two isoforms of 5α-reductase. Recent studies in mice with an induced null mutation in the 5α-reductase type I gene indicate that two-thirds of the pregnant females fail to go into spontaneous labor at term *(44)*. This parturition defect can be reversed by the administration of a 5α-reduced androgen, 5α-androstan-3α, 17β (3α Andiol). These studies suggest that 5α-reduced androgens play essential, but as yet undetermined roles in parturition in mice. It remains to be determined what role these androgens have in other species. It is possible that the 5α-reductase androgens function as endogenous antiprogesterone compounds at the level of the progesterone receptor *(44)*. It is unlikely that the role of androgens in parturition is mediated through the androgen receptors, since female mice deficient in the androgen receptor have normal gestations *(45)*. The concept that labor may be initiated by changes in androgens needs to be investigated further, especially as it relates to their interaction with other mechanisms.

Effect on Dyhydroepiandrosterone Sulfate (DHEAS) on Cervical Ripening

In the 1960s and 1970s, injections of DHEAS were used clinically to assess placental function in complicated pregnancies. Using it for this purpose, some investigators also found that it induced cervical ripening *(46,47)*. In contrast to other agents used to ripen the cervix, DHEAS requires multiple injections and a lag period of several days for any effect. This drawback limits its clinical usefulness, but may be important in supporting a physiological role for DHEAS, since cervical ripening in normal human pregnancy seems to occur over a period of several days. In normal pregnancies, it has been demonstrated that the cervical changes preceding the onset of labor are associated with a significant elevation in maternal plasma levels of DHEAS, but not estradiol, estriol, or progesterone *(48)*. A separate study found that umbilical artery DHEAS levels are higher in laboring patients compared to women who were not in labor, indicating that the increase in DHEAS may be triggered by the fetus *(49)*. This increase in the sulfated steroids, but not in their precursors raises the possibility that it may be owing to changes in the sulfatase enzyme activity. In the primate sampled longitudinally during pregnancy, increases in fetal plasma DHEAS, estrone, and estradiol precede the onset of labor and the rise in amniotic prostaglandin F2α metabolites *(50)*. All of these results point to an essential role for the fetal adrenal in determining the timing of delivery in normal pregnancy.

Peptide, Protein, and Fatty Acid Hormones

Oxytocin and relaxin are peptide hormones that stimulate and inhibit uterine contractility, respectively. Oxytocin is synthesized by the pituitary, and the oxytocin gene is also expressed in the uterine wall during pregnancy *(51,52)*. Oxytocin is thought to be required for the initiation of labor through action on myometrial oxytocin receptors, which are upregulated at term *(4)*. Relaxin, on the other hand, is believed to inhibit uterine contractions and to aid in cervical dilation through modulation of connective tissue *(53)*. Whether oxytocin and relaxin play essential roles during labor is not known. It is noteworthy that patients with oxytocin deficiency secondary to a pituitary disorder still proceed into spontaneous onset of labor. Very recently, it was shown that in mice lacking the oxytocin gene (knockout), the duration of pregnancy was normal, which suggests that oxytocin is not essential for the onset of labor in mice *(54)*. Whether the expulsion process (duration of parturition) is disturbed in this situation remains to be established.

PGs are produced by all tissues. PGs increase in the uterus and amniotic fluid during labor. PGs have long been known to stimulate uterine contractility, and their importance in parturition has been well documented *(55–57)*. In addition, cyclooxygenase (COX) inhibitors have been used clinicaly to inhibit labor *(58)*. Other studies suggest that PGs may only be involved in the late stages of labor to reinforce uterine contractions *(59)*. Recently MacDonald and colleagues suggested that PGs are not important in the initiation of labor *(60)*. Based on differences in amniotic fluid PG levels between the forebag and the fundal compartment, they hypothesized that the increase in amniotic fluid PGs reported by other investigators was the consequence of cervical dilatation rather than the initiating event.

PGs, which have been thought for a long time to be the key mediators of cervical ripening, do not modulate antiprogestin effects in the cervix, as demonstrated in guinea pigs *(19)*, rats, and humans *(61)*. Apparently, there are other local mediators that are more important than PGs, at least during antiprogestin-induced cervical ripening. It should also be noted that NO increases PG production in some tissues *(62,63)*. It seems unlikely that PGs are the main physiological mediators of cervical ripening, since they also produce uterine contractions. On the other hand, NO relaxes the uterus while softening the cervix as discussed later.

COX enzymes convert arachidonic acid to PGH,, which is then further metabolized to various PGs, prostacyclins, and tromboxanes. Two isoforms of COX have been identified *(64,65)*. COX-1 is constitutively expressed, and COX-2 is induced in cells exposed to proinflammatory agents, such as cytokines and endotoxins. The exact role of COX-1 and COX-2 in the uterus and their function during pregnancy have not been established. However, several studies indicate that COX enzymes are gestatively regulated *(64–71)*. The control of PG synthesis by constitutive (COX 1) and cytokine-induced (COX 2) enzymes is very similar to the regulation of NO, which is either constitutive or inducible.

In pregnant sheep, all fetal tissues (amnion, allantochorion, and cotyledons) contain COX-1 with minimal regulation of this isoform during late pregnancy. In contrast, COX-2, which is expressed only in cotyledons, increases gradually during advanced pregnancy (from days 120–139 of gestation), with most marked expression at term, indicating that the increase in PGs that occurs in sheep at term is predominantly owing to the upregulation of COX-2 in fetal cotyledons *(67)*. Similarly, an increase in COX-2 mRNA expression was found in the amnion epithelium in women during labor *(68,69)*, and COX-2 mRNA levels in human amnion correlated with enzyme activity *(69)*. In summary, COX-2 seems to be responsible for the increase in amniotic fluid PG concentrations detected prior to and during the onset of spontaneous labor in both sheep and women. Recently, we determined that the specific COX-2 inhibitor flosulide (ZK 38 997; CGP 28238) *(70)* inhibited onapristone-induced preterm labor in guinea pigs, but had no effect on spontaneous parturition *(71)*. Clearly, further studies are needed to define the role of COX-2 in the initiation of normal parturition and in preterm labor. Nevertheless, the development of specific COX-2 inhibitors opens new perspectives for the treatment and prevention of preterm labor and preterm birth.

Cytokines are protein hormones that have been linked with the immune system. The effector phases of both natural and specific immunity are mediated in part by cytokines. Cytokines are a diverse group of substances that include the interferons (IFNs), tumor necrosis factor (TNF), interleukins (Ils), transforming growth-factor (TGF), colony-stimulating factors (CSFs), and many others. It is interesting to note that cytokines and progesterone are involved in many steps in female reproduction, and may interact at several levels during gestation.

Lipopolysaccharides (LPS), also called endotoxin, are derived from bacterial cell walls, and stimulate the production of cytokines from mononuclear phagocytes, B-cells, and mast cells. LPS and cytokines are also known to stimulate NO by activation of the inducible form of NO synthase (NOS) *(see* Nitric Oxide *below)*.

Nitric Oxide

NO controls contractility of many smooth muscles *(72–79)*. It is synthesized from the amino acid L-arginine, a step that requires one of three NOS isoforms. NO acts on many pathways in smooth muscle cells to produce relaxation *(80,81)*. Our studies, done in vitro and in vivo using rats and guinea pigs, and in vitro, using human myometrial strips, indicate that an L-arginine–NO pathway exists in the uterus, and that this system inhibits uterine contractility *(82–83)*. Authentic NO, NO donors (nitroglycerin or sodium nitroprusside), and L-arginine cause rapid and reversible suppression of uterine contractions. The relaxation effect of L-arginine can be reversed by NOS inhibitors, such as L-nitroarginine methyl ester (L-NAME). Methylene blue, an inhibitor of cGMP, counteracts the suppressive effects of NO on uterine contractility (Fig. 3). Measurements of NO as total

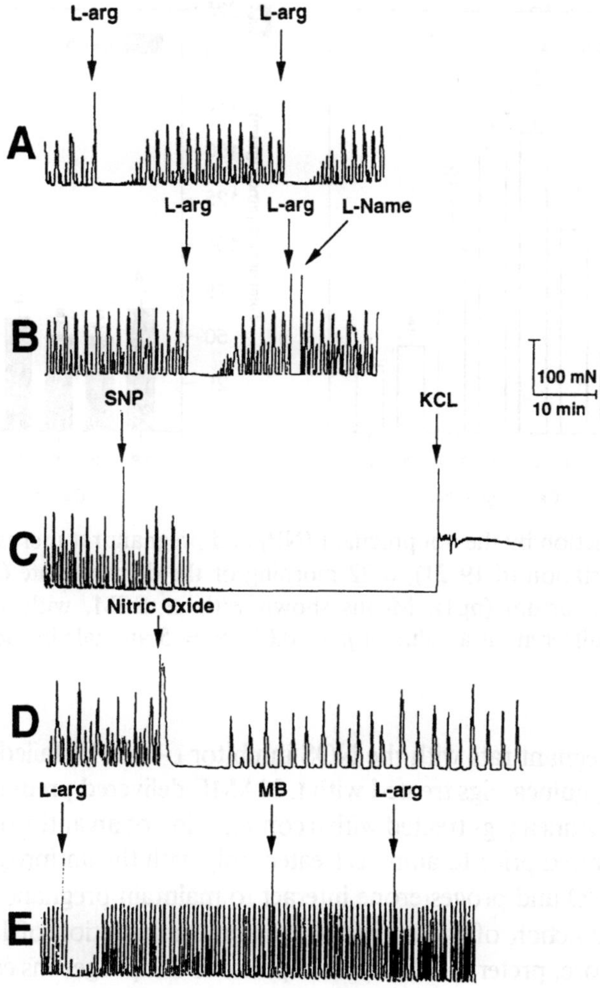

Fig. 3. The effect of L-arginine, L-NAME, methylene blue. and sodium nitroprusside on spontaneously contracting uterine strips from rat uterus obtained on d 18 of pregnancy. Application of L-arginine to a muscle bath resulted in immediate relaxation (10–15 min in duration) **(A)**. The effect of L-arginine was antagonized by L-NAME when added during an L-arginine-induced relaxation **(B)**. Inhibition of L-arginine effects with methylene (MB) **(E)**, and the effects of SNP **(C)** and NO **(D)** are shown. These are typical recordings, and each upstroke from baseline represents a contraction.

nitrites in uterine tissues confirm that the rat and human uterus produce NO during pregnancy. NO production is decreased in the uterus and increased in the cervix during labor (Fig. 4). The sensitivity of the myometrium to inhibition by NO is increased during pregnancy prior to the onset of labor. However, experiments using myometrial strips from rats and humans taken during labor show that the suppressive effects of NO are attenuated. These results indicate that the NO system is present in the uterus and that it may be important in maintaining uterine quiescence. A downregulation of this system at term may initiate abor. The sensitivity of the uterus to NO donors is much lower when compared to vascular tissue (Fig. 5). This indicates that large amounts of NO (from iNOS?) are required to inhibit uterine contractility. This also suggests that NO donors used to inhibit conractility could have vascular effects.

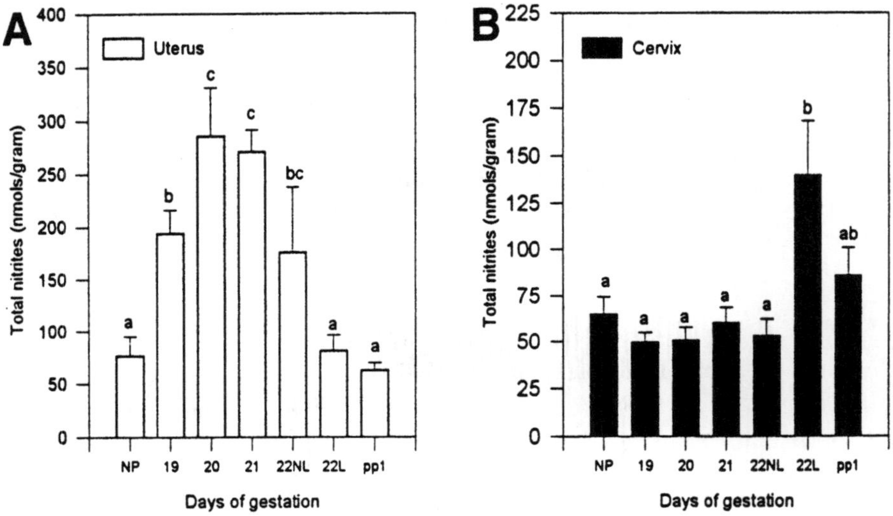

Fig. 4. Nitrite production by the nonpregnant (NP) and pregnant rat uterus (panel **A**) and cervix (panel **B**) during gestation (d 19–21), d 22 morning of the delivery date (22NL), term delivery (22L), and 1 d postpartum (pp1). Means shown with ± SEM, with at least one common superscript are not different at a value of $p < 0.05$. $N = 5$ animals in each group.

Treatment of pregnant rats with the NOS inhibitor L-NAME failed to alter the time of delivery. However, guinea pigs treated with L-NAME delivered prematurely *(85)*. In addition, both rats and guinea pigs treated with a combination of an antiprogestin (onapristone) and L-NAME delivered prior to animals treated only with the antiprogestin *(84,85)*. These studies show that NO and progesterone interact to maintain pregnancy. The inhibition of NO potentiates the action of the antiprogestins on the initiation of labor in guinea pigs and rats. Furthermore, preterm delivery in response to antiprogestins can be inhibited with combinations of NO donors and progestins, but not with NO donors alone in rats (Garfield et al., unpublished observations).

NO is known to be produced by several isoforms of NOS (mNOS or iNOS, an inducible form found in macrophages; bNOS, found in brain; and eNOS, located primarily in endothelial cells). Using immunoblot techniques and RT-PCR, our results showed that iNOS is the dominant isoform present in the uterus *(86)*. The mRNA and protein for iNOS increase throughout pregnancy until term, at which time they decline in the uterus and rise in the cervix (Fig. 6). iNOS levels also decline when preterm labor is initiated with antiprogestins *(86)*. These studies provide strong evidence that NO released through the action of iNOS plays important regulatory roles in the uterus during pregnancy. The changes in iNOS in the uterus during pregnancy are in agreement with results from other studies in rats *(87)* and rabbits *(88)*. Another mechanisms by which NO production may be regulated during pregnancy is through changes in concentrations of its precursor L-arginine. Weiner et al. *(89)* have shown that myometrial arginase activity in guinea pigs increases throughout gestation, peaking close to term.

The inducible NOS, iNOS, always produces large amounts of NO when it is present in cells. It is induced (upregulated) by some cytokines (IL-1, IFNγ, TNF-γ) and inhibited by others (IL-4, IL-10, TGF-β) *(73)*. The expression of iNOS is also increased by endotoxins, such as LPS. The iNOS was first described in immune cells (macrophages), but was later

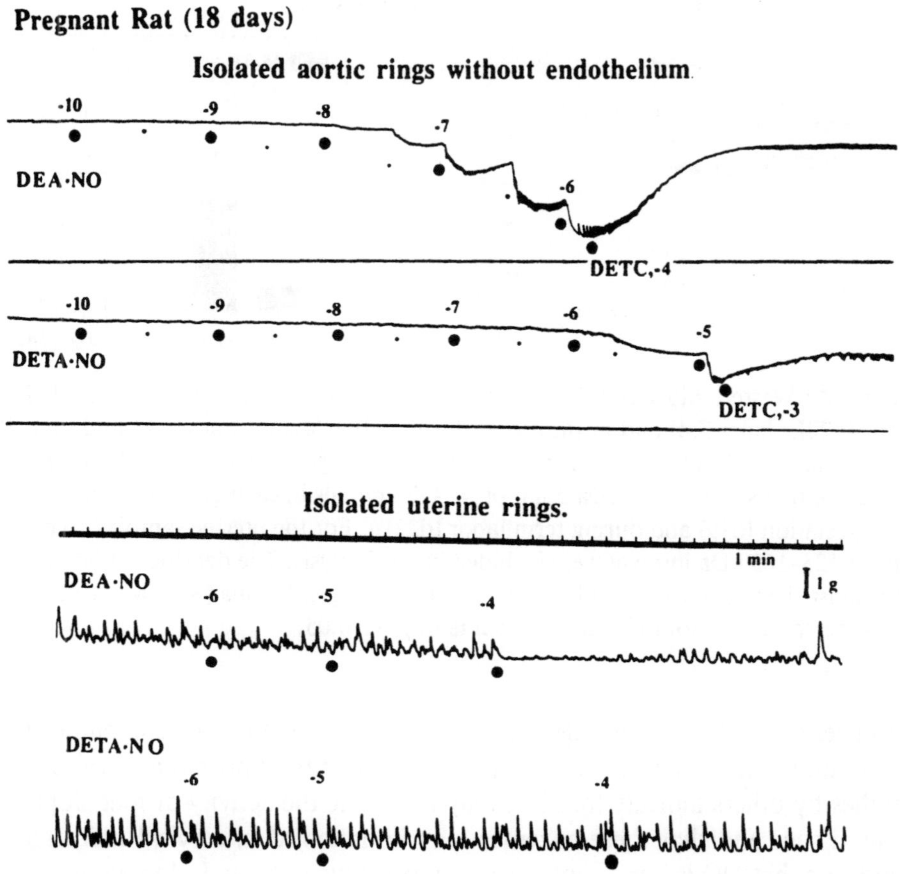

Fig. 5. Contractile responses of rat aorta (top tracings) and uterine strips (bottom tracings) to NO donors (2-[*N,N*-diethylamino]-diazenolate-2-oxide, DEA-NO; [z]-1-[2-{2-aminoethyl}-*N*-{2-ammonioethyl} amino] diazen-1, 2-diolate, DETA-NO). Aortic rings were precontracted with phenylephrine. Uterine activity represents spontaneous contractility. Diethyldithiocarbamic acid (DETC, an NO scavenging agent) was added following the highest dose of DEA-NO. Note the rapid increase in tension after DETC.

identified in epithelial cells, hepatocytes, myocytes, chondrocytes, and bone-forming cells (osteoblasts and osteoclasts). NO released in large quantities through the action of iNOS can destroy parasites and bacteria. This pathway has been suggested to be most crucial in the defense against invading pathogenic organisms. This system also plays a significant role in tissue rejection. Some cytokines (IL-1 and TNF-α), thought to be involved in preterm labor resulting from reproductive tract infections *(89,90)*, may act through NO.

The distribution of iNOS in the uterus in not known. However, recent studies suggest that iNOS may also be present in trophoblast cells *(36)*. These findings indicate that iNOS may be important in suppression of the immune response invoked by the fetal semiallograph and that placental NO may be important in the inhibition of uterine contractility. It has long been recognized that the placenta produces substances that maintain uterine quiescence, but this has often been attributed to the synthesis of steroids (progesterone).

We also examined the function of NO on the cervix during pregnancy. Unlike the uterus, the cervical content of NO and iNOS increases at the end of pregnancy, parallelling the

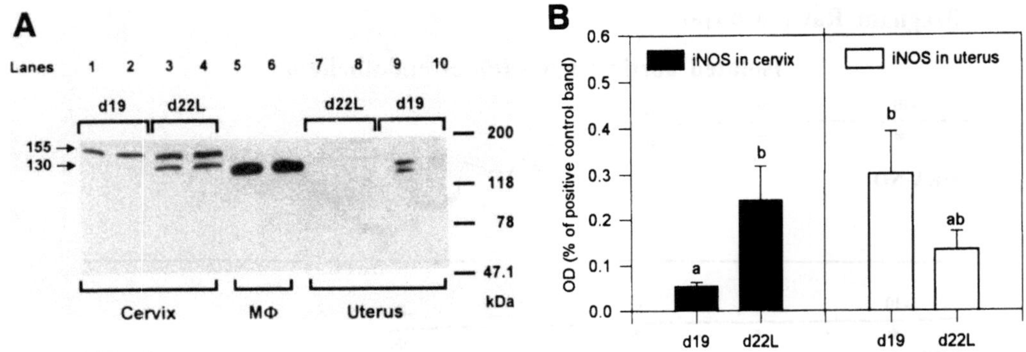

Fig. 6. Panel **A**: Western blots of iNOS in rat cervix on d 19 of gestation (d19: lanes 1, 2), during term labor (d22L: lanes 3,4) and in rat uterus during labor (d22L: lanes 7, 8) and on d 19 (d19: lanes 9,10). Lanes 5, 6: mouse macrophage lysate (MΦ) (positive control). Panel **B**: Densitometric measurements of the 130-kDa band (n = 4–7 animals in each group) in cervix and uterus on d 19 of gestation (d19) and during term labor (d22L). For the uterine samples on d 19, all the bands in the 125–165 kDa interval were included in the analysis. The densities of bands were normalized against the positive control band within the same gel. Means (± SEM) with at least one common superscript are not different at a value of $p < 0.05$.

increase in cervical extensibility (Figs. 4B,6B) *(86)*. Treatment of rats and guinea pigs with either NOS inhibitors or NO donors, respectively, inhibits or promotes cervical softening *(91)*. Studies by others indicate that NO may modulate the activity of metalloproteinases in various tissues and that these enzymes may be involved in cervical maturation. Our results indicate that NO is important in cervical ripening at the end of pregnancy, and that NO is differentially regulated in the uterus and cervix during pregnancy. Since NO synthesis by iNOS is stimulated by cytokines, which are known to control cervical softening, it is possible that NO may be the final common pathway in the induction of metalloproteinases and the breakdown of collagen.

NO may, therefore, be involved in cervical ripening as a local mediator of the inflammatory cascade during term labor and preterm birth. To evaluate this hypothesis, we applied the NO donor sodium nitroprusside (SNP) locally on the pregnant guinea pig cervix, and detected a significant increase in cervical extensibility. Evaluation by electron microscopy revealed a pronounced cervical ripening accompanied by dissolution of collagen fibers, stromal edema, arterial dilatation, and tissue infiltration by macrophages, lymphocytes, and granulocytes *(71)*. It is quite clear from these studies that NO exerts a powerful physiological function during cervical ripening acting probably at the end of the inflammatory cascade. NO may act in concert with PGE2 by inducing local vasodilatation, increasing vascular permeability and leading to leukocyte infiltration, all of which occur during cervical ripening. In addition, NO may directly regulate the activity of metalloproteinases which breakdown connective tissue within the cervix, similar to its action in other tissues *(92–95)*.

Exactly what controls NO synthesis in the cervix is not known. Although PGs can stimulate NO production *(96,97)* and NO can increase PG production *(60,61)*, there is evidence (as noted earlier) that PGs are not required for cervical ripening. On the other hand, cytokines do seem to be necessary for cervical ripening. It is possible that cytokines modulate stages between the rigid and soft cervix by acting on iNOS either to inhibit or stimulate NO synthesis.

TFG-β appears to control the formation of extracellular matrix proteins in a variety of tissues. TGF-β has been termed "the master switch" of fibrosis *(98)*. TGF-β increases renal type IV collagen and fibronectin *(98)*, and it also stimulates mesangial matrix proteoglycans *(100)*. TGF-β also reduces proteinase activity and enhances tissue inhibitors of metalloproteins (TIMP) *(101)*. Fibrosis and scarring are also associated with increased levels of TGF-β *(100,102)*.

TGF-β and various peptides inhibit NO synthesis *(103)*. The promoter region of the NOS gene contains IFNγ response elements, and is also under control by NF-kβ and AP-1 (sites for steroid regulation) transcription factors *(104)*. NO is now known to regulate gene expression *(105)*, and the gene transcription may be mediated by guanylate cyclase or changes in activation of NF-kβ. In vascular tissues, NO inhibits macrophage-CSF transcription by interfering with NF-kβ activation *(106,107)*.

NO has been shown recently to modulate extracellular matrix biosynthesis and degradation. Treatment of aging NMRI mice with L-arginine decreases the content of kidney collagen *(108)*. Similarly, L-arginine reduced heart collagen accumulation and decreased the incidence of cardiomyopathy in diabetic db/db mice *(94)*. NO-generating compounds inhibit collagen and protein synthesis by cultured vascular smooth muscle cells *(95)*. In addition, induction of iNOS activity or treatment with NO donor agents increased activity of the ECM proteolytic enzymes, collagenase, and stromelysin in cultured chondrocytes *(109)*.

There is evidence that PGs and NO reciprocally regulate one another in some tissues *(62,96)*. In some systems, PGs seem to stimulate NO synthesis and NO seems to increase PG synthesis. In other tissues, however, PGs inhibit NO synthesis *(110)*. Since PGs and NO are thought to stimulate and inhibit, respectively, uterine contractility, such a reciprocal relationship in the uterus would result in contractile disorder. A rise in PGs at term would be expected to increase NO production. However, NO synthesis and iNOS levels are decreased at term *(86)*. Moreover, NO levels are elevated prior to term when PG levels are lower. Similarly, treatment with NO donors, NO inhibitors, PGs, and PG inhibitors would be expected to result in uterine contractile chaos if such an association existed. Also, evidence that cytokines stimulate both COX-2 and NOS enzymes simultaneously is incompatible with the theory that PGs and NO are simultaneously important in controlling uterine contractility.

If PGs inhibit NO release, this might explain the inverse relationship between PG and NO levels at term. However, this would not be compatible with the changes in endogenous or exogenous effects of PGs and NO in the cervix. Our studies indicate that LPS stimulates NO production in the nonpregnant uterus, but fails to produce significant increases in NO in late pregnancy. However, LPS significantly increased cervical NO synthesis in both nonpregnant and late pregnant females *(86)*. These studies demonstrate that iNOS and its activity are increased in the uterus during pregnancy, perhaps to their full potential. In the cervix, NOS activity may not increase to its maximum until near term. This could mean that treatments to elevate cytokines would not increase uterine NO release, but cervical NO could be elevated.

We conclude that NO plays a significant role in the functional control of the female reproductive tract by inhibiting uterine contractility to aid in maintaining pregnancy. At term, NO levels decline in the uterus, but rise in the cervix. This combination of events allows labor to proceed and assists the uterus to contract and the cervix to dilate, resulting in a coordinated progress of labor. The exact mechanism of the differential NO production in the uterus and cervix is not known, but may be related to the influx of monocytes into the cervix at the end of gestation and downregulation of iNOS activity in the uterus.

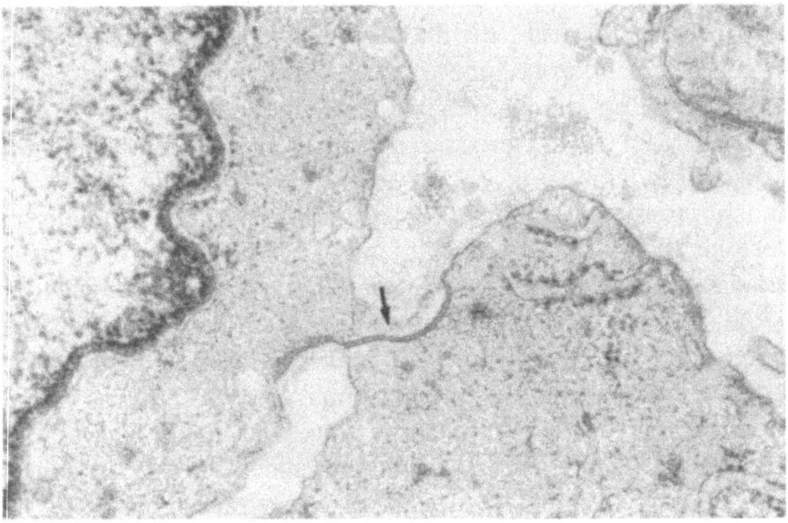

Fig. 7. Electron photomicrograph of a gap junction (arrow) between two uterine muscle cells from pregnant rabbit at term fixed during spontaneous parturition (×71,000).

FUNDAMENTAL MECHANISMS REGULATING UTERINE CONTRACTILITY

The myometrium is composed of billions of smooth muscle cells. The basic process that controls a uterine contraction is the underlying electrical activity in the form of action potentials. Action potentials usually occur together in a group, called a burst. The number of bursts in a given time determines the frequency of uterine contractions, whereas the duration of the burst determines the duration of the contraction. The force generated by the whole uterus, or the amplitude of a contraction, is dependent on the propagation of action potentials from cell to cell and the amount of muscle mass involved *(5,6)*.

Many studies indicate that myometrial cells are coupled electrically via gap junctions (Figs. 7 and 8) composed of connexin proteins. The grouping of connexins provides channels of low electrical resistance between cells, and thereby furnishes pathways for the efficient conduction of action potentials. Throughout most of pregnancy, in all species studied, the cell-to-cell channels or contacts are low, indicating poor coupling and low electrical conductance. This condition favors quiescence of the muscle and the maintenance of pregnancy. However, at term the cell junctions increase and form an electrical syncytium required for effective contractions (Figs. 9 and 10). The presence of the contacts seems to be controlled by changing estrogen and progesterone levels affecting the uterus.

Functional studies of electrical coupling between myometrial cells are few. Recently, we examined the currents between pairs of freshly isolated rat myometrial cells using double whole-cell patch-clamp techniques *(111)*. These studies showed that during term as well as preterm labor, junctional conductance is significantly elevated in cells of the longitudinal and circular muscle layers (32 to 26 nS) compared to the antepartum or postpartum periods (4–7 nS) (Fig. 11). The conductance values measured during labor correspond to those reported for connexin 43 (Cx43), the protein component of the gap junctions in several tissues. These findings demonstrate that heightened electrical coupling between myometrial cells of the uterine wall emerges at the end of pregnancy in preparation for the massive, coordinated contractions of labor.

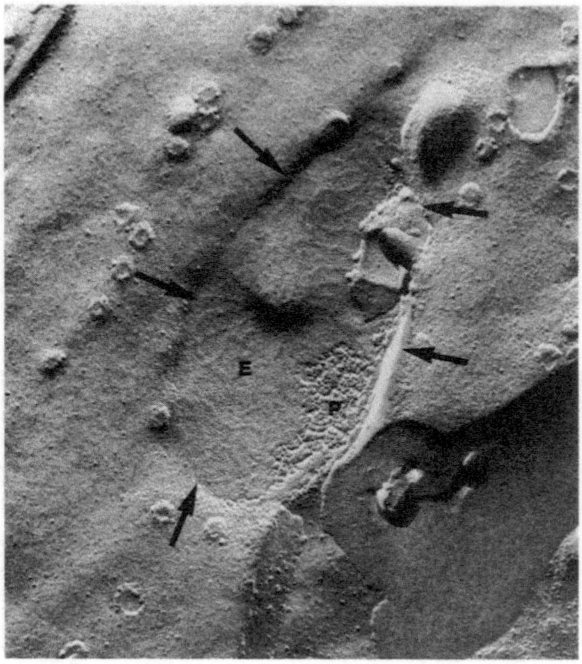

Fig. 8. Uterine gap junction. Electron micrograph of a freeze-fracture replicate showing an oval-shaped gap junction between muscle cells of the rat uterus. The fracture plane passed between cell membranes within the region of the gap junction (between arrows) to reveal the protoplasmic (P) and exoplasmic face (E). Note the pits in the E-face of junction and the aggregation of particles (connexins) in the P-face (× 105,000).

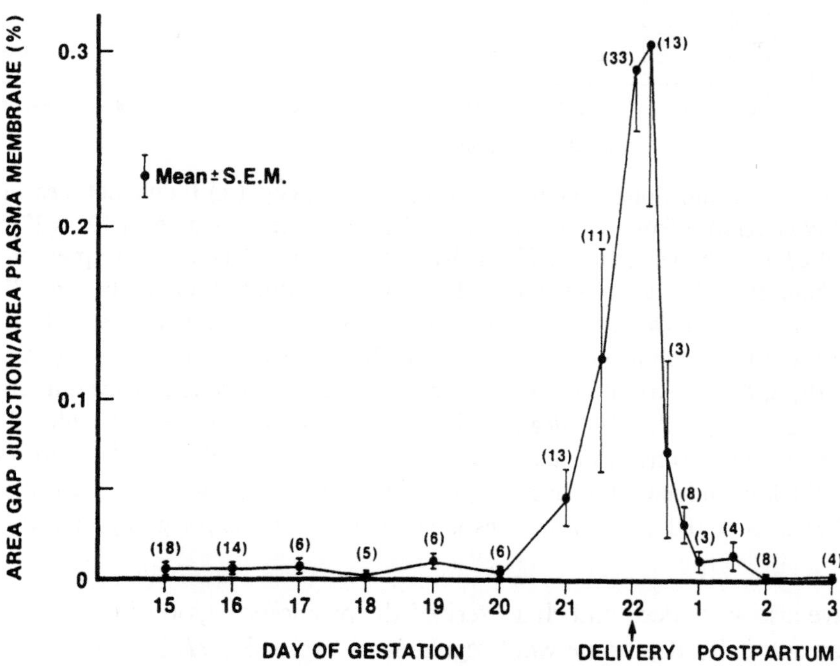

Fig. 9. Changes in gap junctions in the rat myometrium during gestation and postpartum. Shown is area of gap junction as a percentage of plasma membrane area vs day of pregnancy and postpartum.

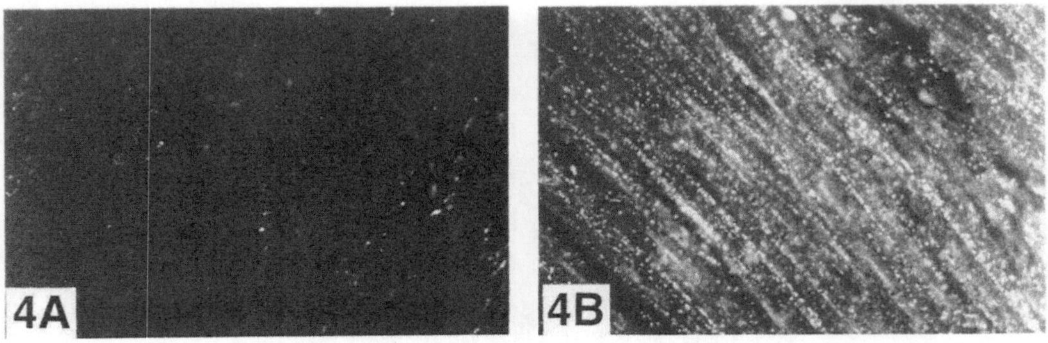

Fig. 10. Effect of onapristone on gap junctions in late pregnant guinea pigs. Immunocytochemical staining with antibodies to connexin 43 was used. Light micrograph (1000x) of myometrial tissue from a control animal on d 45 of pregnancy (**A**) and from an animal at the same stage of gestation after 2 d of treatment with 10.0 mg onapristone subcutaneously (**B**). Note the lack of staining in (**A**) and the abundance of bright fluorescent spots, which represent gap junctions in (**B**).

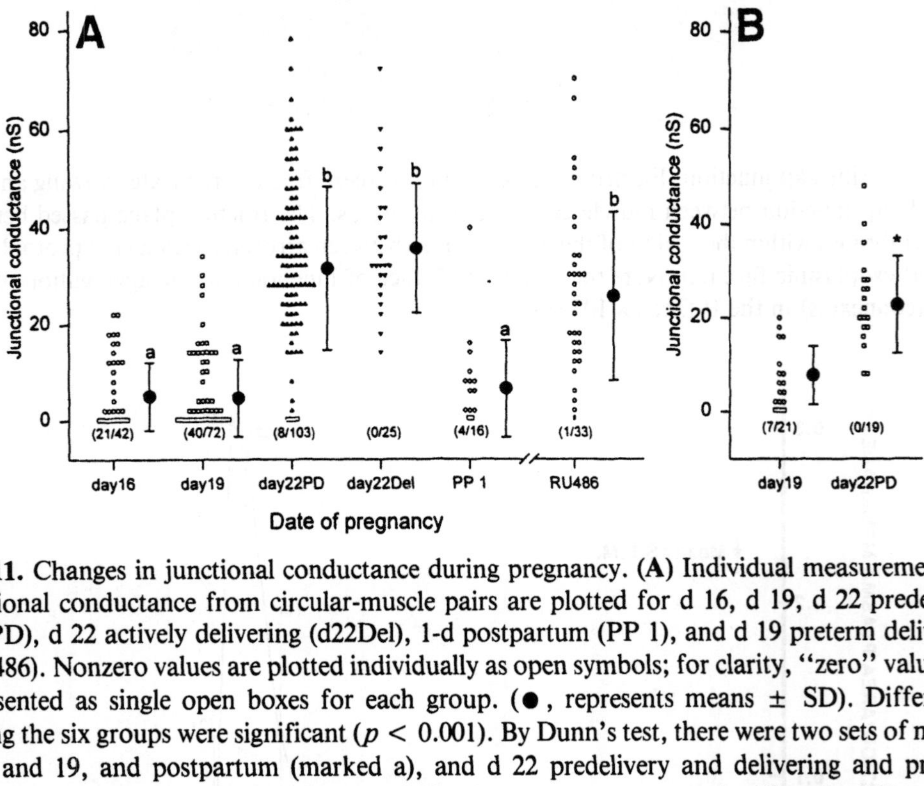

Fig. 11. Changes in junctional conductance during pregnancy. (**A**) Individual measurements of junctional conductance from circular-muscle pairs are plotted for d 16, d 19, d 22 predelivery (d22PD), d 22 actively delivering (d22Del), 1-d postpartum (PP 1), and d 19 preterm delivering (RU 486). Nonzero values are plotted individually as open symbols; for clarity, "zero" values are represented as single open boxes for each group. (●, represents means ± SD). Differences among the six groups were significant ($p < 0.001$). By Dunn's test, there were two sets of means, d 16 and 19, and postpartum (marked a), and d 22 predelivery and delivering and preterm delivering (RU 486) (marked b). Means within the same set were not significantly different; all other pairwise comparisons of means are different at the $p < 0.05$ level of significance. (**B**) In cells from the longitudinal layer, average junctional conductance was higher for the d 22 cells than d 19 cells ($p < 0.05$, two-tailed t-test). The number of rats per group ranged from 3–31.

We have also sequenced and characterized the promoter region of the Cx43 protein in the human uterus to determine what regulates its expression *(112)*. The evidence so far indicates that transcription of the Cx43 gene is induced through activation of protein kinase C in human myometrial cells, and that the induction involves upregulation and stimulation of c-jun and c-fos through binding to an AP-1 site located in the proximal

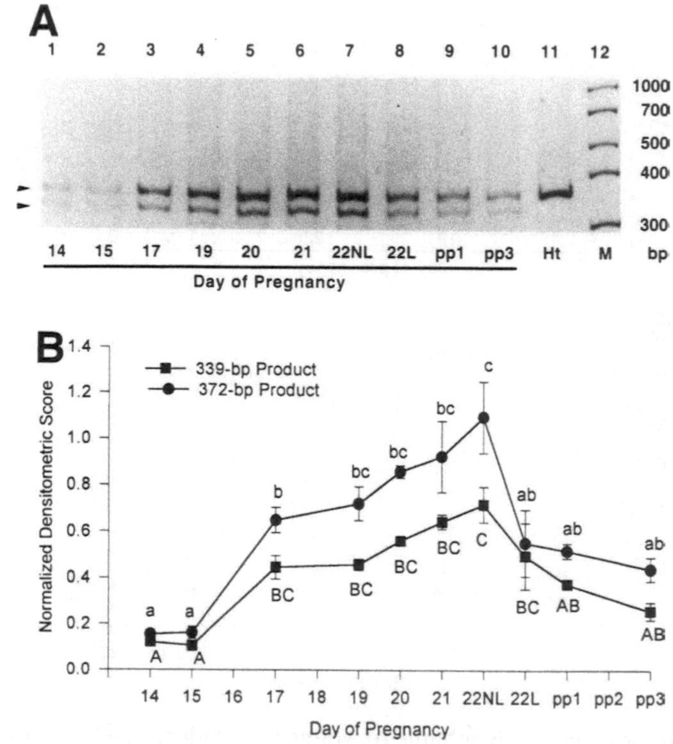

Fig. 12. RT-PCR products of Ca^{2+} channel α_1-subunit mRNA from rat myometrium at different times of pregnancy. **A**: lanes 1–10, products from myometrial RNAs at different days of pregnancy (NL, nonlabor: L, labor; pp, postpartum); lane 11: product from rat cardiac RNA; lane 12, molecular size markers (BioMarker Low; Bio Ventures, Murfreesboro, TN). The two arrowheads point to the 372- and 339-bp product bands. **B**: gestational changes of Ca^{2+} channel α_1-subunit mRNA levels in rat myometrium as measured by RT-PCR. Photographs of PCR product bands were scanned, and densities of bands were normalized. For points (n = 3–5 animals) lacking an SE bar, error was smaller than or equal to size of symbol. Values with different lower-or upper-case letters indicate significant differences compared with other time- points for 372 or 339 bp, respectively.

region of the gene. The function of the AP-1 site suggests that steroid hormones may regulate Cx43 expression by production of c-fos or c-jun. These studies may lead to a better understanding of how steroid hormones regulate this crucial step in the initiation of labor in humans.

As action potentials propagate over the surface of a myometrial cell, the depolarization causes voltage-dependent Ca^{2+} channels (VDCC) to open. When this occurs, Ca^{2+} enters the muscle cell down its chemical gradient to activate the myofilaments and provoke a contraction. We have recently demonstrated by RT-PCR that the expression of VDCC subunits in the rat myometrium increases during term and preterm labor *(113)* (Figs. 12 and 13). The increased expression, which appears to be controlled by progesterone withdrawal, may facilitate uterine contractility during labor by increasing portals for Ca^{2+} entry.

MODEL FOR CONTROL OF PARTURITION

The above studies indicate that the myometrium undergoes a series of changes at term that place it at a higher level of excitability and responsiveness (Fig. 14). This preparatory

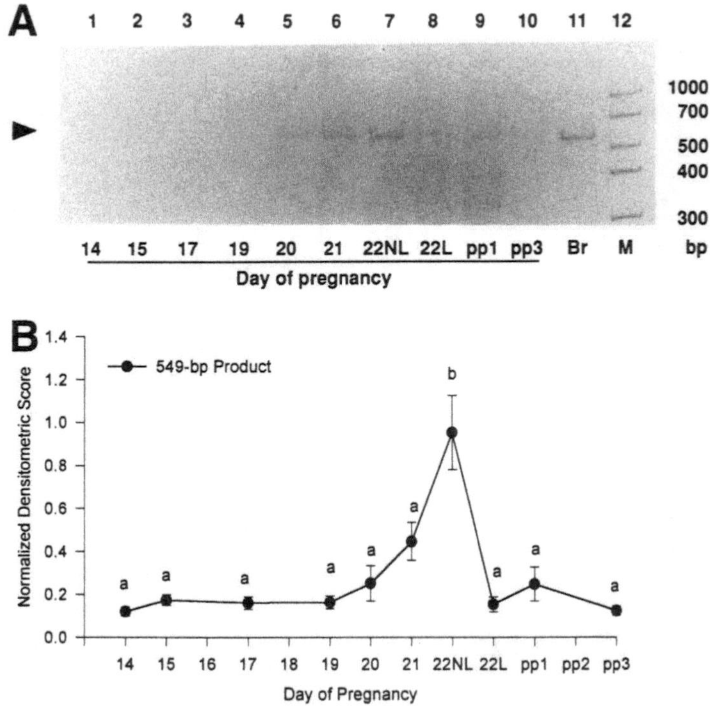

Fig. 13. RT-PCR products of B-subunit of voltage-dependent Ca^{2+} channels from rat myometrium at different times of pregnancy. **A**: photograph of a gel stained with ethidium bromide. A single 549-bp product (arrowhead) is visible in all lanes at different days of gestation (d 14–22; NL, nonlabor; L, labor) and postpartum (pp; d 1 and 3). **B**: Quantitative data based on densiometric scanning of bands at various times of gestation and postpartum. Values (n = 3–5 animals) with different lower-case letters indicate significant ($p < 0.05$) differences at different times of pregnancy.

process (conversion or conditioning step) involves changes in transduction mechanisms and the synthesis of several new proteins, including connexins, ion channels, and receptors for agonists or antagonists *(6)*. The preparatory step appears to be irreversible and in most animals is controlled by the estrogen/progesterone ratio.

Cervical ripening and weakening of the fetal membranes are also part of the preparatory process preceding labor. Both the cervix and fetal membranes contain high amounts of connective tissue composed mainly of collagen. The biochemical processes that control remodeling of the cervix by the end of gestation are unknown, but the steps are thought to be similar to an inflammatory reaction involving recruitment of monocytes, release of degradative enzymes, and breakdown of connective tissue (*see above* and *9*).

Studies in different pregnant animal models show that antiprogestins exhibit predominantly conditioning (preparatory) effects by inducing cervical ripening and myometrial responsiveness. The major mechanism of antiprogestin action on the late pregnant uterus may be to induce gap junction protein synthesis, an essential step responsible for phasic and coordinated responses to uterotonins. In addition, antiprogestins also downregulate the L-arginine–NO–cGMP system, which is partly responsible for uterine relaxation and may stimulate myometrial calcium channel biosynthesis and thereby increase the excitability of myometrial cells. A second important component of the conditioning effect of antiprogestins is cervical ripening, which may be mediated by cytokines (IL-8, IL-1, and so on).

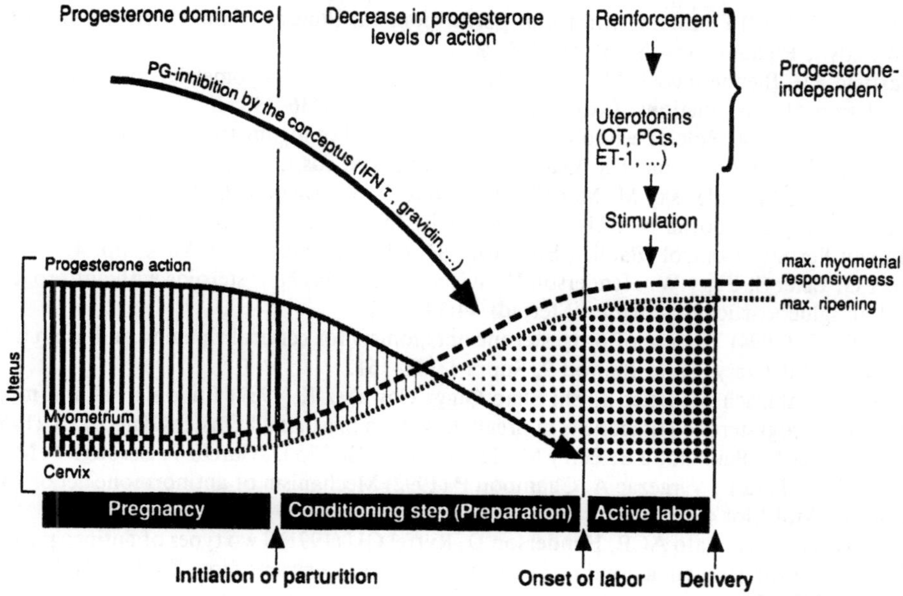

Fig. 14. Model of parturition showing stages along the horizontal axis and changes in the myometrium and cervix in relationship to progesterone action.

The downregulation of the cytokines during pregnancy may be the result of the immunosuppressive action of progesterone.

For many years, labor was considered as the transition from an inactive to an active myometrium by the addition of a uterotonin or withdrawal of tonic inhibition. These models neither defined precisely the uterine stages of labor nor the action of progesterone. We suggest that the uterus (myometrium and cervix) undergoes a conditioning (preparatory) step, which prepares it for labor and delivery (Fig. 14) *(114)*. This step may be induced by antiprogestin treatment even in species without progesterone withdrawal, but which may require another mechanism responsible for the reduction in progesterone action on the uterus. This mechanism might involve either changes in progesterone receptor numbers and function, or there may be a physiologically functional antiprogestin present.

The mechanism(s) controlling the release of uterotonins (e.g., prostaglandins, oxytocin, endothelin), which eventually lead to forceful contractions of the uterus (active labor), may not be dependent on progesterone. These uterotonins may be inhibited by fetal and/or placental factors during pregnancy (example IFNτ during early pregnancy in sheep; *115*). A release of this inhibition may exist at term. This concept would explain why onapristone alone, which may be considered a "pure" progesterone receptor antagonist, is effective in inducing preterm labor in guinea pigs and nonhuman primates.

REFERENCES

1. Csapo AI (1981) Force of labor, In: Principles and Practice of Obstetrics and Perinatology, vol. 2 (Iffy L, Kaminetzky HA, eds.), John Wiley, New York, pp. 761–799.
2. Thorburn GD, Challis JRG (1979) Endocrine control of parturition. Physiol Rev 59:863–918.
3. Elger W, Chwalisz K, Fahnrich M, Hasan SH, Laurent D, Beier S, Ottow E, Neef G, Garfield RE (1990) Studies on labor conditioning and labor inducing effects of antiprogesterones in animal models, In: Uterine Contractility: Mechanisms of Control (Garfield RE, ed.), Serono, Norwell, MA, pp. 153–176.

4. Soloff MS (1989) Endocrine control of parturition, In: Biology of the Uterus (Wynn RM, Jollie WP, eds.), Plenum, New York, pp. 559–607.
5. Garfield RE, Blennerhassett MG, Miller SM (1988) Control of myometrial contractility: Role and regulation of gap junctions. Oxford Rev Reprod Biol 10:436–490.
6. Garfield RE (1994) Role of cell-to-cell coupling in control of myometrial contractility and labor, In: Control of Uterine Contractility (Garfield RE, Tabb TN, eds.), CRC, Boca Raton, FL, pp. 40–81.
7. Phillibert D, Moguilewsky M, Mary M, Lecagque D, Tournemine C. Secchi J, Deraedt R (1985) Pharmacological profile of RU 486 in animals, In: The Antiprogestrone Steroid RU 486 and Human Fertility Control (Baulieu EE, Segal SJ, eds.), Plenum, New York, pp. 49–68.
8. Neef G, Beier S, Elger W, Henderson D, Wiechert R (1984) New steroids with antiprogestational and antiglucocorticoid activities. Steroids 44:349–372.
9. Chwalisz K (1994) The use of progesterone antagonists for cervical ripening and as an adjunct to labour and delivery. Hum Reprod 9, Suppl 1:131–161.
10. Elger W, Fahnrich M, Beier S, Shi Shao Qing, Chwalisz K (1987) Endometrial and myometrial effects of progesterone antagonists in pregnant guinea pigs. Am J Obstet Gynecol 157:1065–1074.
11. Gronemeyer H, Benhamou B, Berry M, Bocquel MT, Gofflo D, Garcia T, Lerouge T, Metzger D, Meyer ME, Tora L, Vergezac A, Chambon P (1992) Mechanism of antihormone action. J Steroid Biochem Mol Biol 41:217–221.
12. Klein-Hitpass LA, Cato ACB, Henderson D, Ryffel GU (1991) Two types of antiprogestins identified by their differentail action in transcriptionally active extracts from T47D cells. Nucleic Acids Res 19:1227–1234.
13. Horwitz KB (1992) The molecular biology of RU486. Is there a role for antiprogestins in the treatment of breast cancer? Endocr Rev 13(2):146–163.
14. Wolf JP, Sinosich MJ, Anderson T, Ulmann A, Baulieu EE, Hodgen GF (1989) Progesterone antagonist (RU 486) for cervical dilatation, labor induction, and delivery in monkeys: Effectiveness in combination with oxytocin. Am J Obstet Gynecol 160:45–47.
15. Wolf JP, Simon J, Itskovitz J, Sinosich MJ, Ulmann A, Baulieu EE, Hodgen GD (1993) Progesterone antagonist RU 486 accomodates, but does not induce labour and delivery in primates. Hum Reprod 8:759–763.
16. Haluska GJ, Stanczyk FZ, Cook MJ, Novy MJ (1987) Temporal changes in uterine activity and prostaglandin response to RU486 in rhesus macaques in late gestation. Am J Obstet Gynecol 157: 1487–1495.
17. Chwalisz K (1993) Role of progesterone in the control of labor, In: Basic Mechanisms Controlling Term and Preterm Labor (Chwalisz K, Garfield RE, eds.), Ernst Schering Research Foundation Workshop 7, Springer Verlag, Berlin, pp. 97–163.
18. Garfield RE, Beier S (1989) Increased myometrial responsiveness to oxytocin during term and preterm labor. Am J Obstet Gynecol 161:454–461.
19. Chwalisz K, Hegele-Hartung, Schulz R, Qing S-S, Louton PT, Elger W (1991) Progesterone control of cervical ripening—experimental studies with the progesterone antagonists onapristone, lilopristone and mifepristone, In: The Extracellular Matrix of the Uterus, Cervix and Fetal Membranes: Synthesis, Degradation and Hormonal Regulation (Leppert P, Woessner F, eds.), Perinatology, Ithaca, NY, pp. 119–131.
20. Lessey BA, Killman AP, Metzger DA, Haney AF, Greene GL, McCarty KS Jr (1988) Immunohistochemical analysis of human uterine estrogen and progesterone receptors throughout the menstrual cycle. Journal of Clinical Endocrinol Metab 67(2):334–340.
21. Horwitz KB, Alexander PS (1993) In situ photolinked nuclear progesterone receptors of human breast cancer cells; subunit molecular weights after transformation and translocation. Endocrinology 113:2195–2201.
22. Sartorius CA, Tung L, Takimoto GS, Hoertwitz KB (1993) Antagonist-occupied human progesterone receptors bound to DNA are functionally switched to transcriptional agonists by cAMP. J Biol Chem 5:9262–9269.
23. Vegato E, Shabhaz MM, Wen DX, Goldman ME, O'Malley BW, McDonnell DP (1993) Human progesterone receptor A form is a cell and promoter-specific repressor of human progesterone receptor B function. Mol Endocrinol 7:1244–1255.
24. Feil PD, Clarke CL, Satyaswaroop PG (1988) Progestin-mediated changes in progesterone receptor forms in the normal human endometrium. Endocrinology 123:2506–2513.
25. Leppert PC (1992) Cervical softening, effacement and dilatation: A complex biochemical cascade. J Maternal Fetal Med 1:213–223.

26. Hegele-Hartung C, Chwalisz K, Beier HM, Elger W (1989) Ripening of the uterine cervix of the guinea pig after treatment with the progesterone antagonist onapristone (ZK 98299): an electron microscopic study. Hum Reprod 4:369–377.
27. Rajabi M, Solomon S, Poole R (1991) Biochemical evidence of collagenase-mediated collagenolysis as a mechanism of cervical dilatation at parturition in the guinea pig. Biol Reprod 45:764–772.
28. Cabrol D, Carbonne B, Bienkiewicz A, Dallot E, Alj AE, Cedard L (1991) Induction of labour and cervical maturation using mifepristone (RU 486) in the late pregnant rat. Influence of a cyclooxygenase inhibitor (diclofenac). Prostaglandins 42:71–79.
29. Radestadt A, Bygdeman M (1992) Cervical softening with mifepristone (RU 486) after pretreatment with naproxen. A double-blind randomized study. Contraception 45:221–227.
30. Liggins GC (1981) Cervical ripening as an inflamatory reaction, In: The Cervix in Pregnancy and Labour (Ellwood DA, Anderson ABM, eds.), Churchil Livingstone, Edinburgh, pp. 1–9.
31. Jungueira LCU, Zugaib M, Montes GS, Toledo OMS, Kristzan RM, Shigihara KM (1980) Morphologic and histochemical evidence for the occurrence of collagenolysis and for the role of neutrophylic polymorphnuclear leukocytes during cervical dilatation. Am J Obstet Gynecol 138: 273–281.
32. Osmers R, Rath W, Adelmann-Grill BC, Fittkow C, Kuloczik M, Szeverenyi M, Tschesche H, Kuhn W (1992) Origin of cervial collagenase during parturition. Am J Obstet Gynecol 166:1455–1460.
33. Hiro D, Hioro D, Ojima Y, Mori Y (1988) Spontaneous production of interleukin 1-like factors from pregnant rabbit uterine cervix. Am J Obstet Gynecol 159:261–265.
34. Barclay CG, Brennand JE, Kelly RW, Calder AA (1993) Interleukin-8 production by the human cervix. Am J Obstet Gynecol 169:625–632.
35. Chwalisz K, Benson M, Scholz P, Daum J, Beier HM, Hegele-Hartung C (1994b) Cervical ripening with the cytokines interleukin 8 (IL-8), interleukin 1β (IL-1β) and tumor necrosis factor alpha (TNF-α) in guinea pigs. Hum Reprod 9:2173–2181.
36. Kelly RW, Leask R, Calder AA (1992) Choriodecidual production of interleukin-8 and the mechanism of parturtion. Lancet 339:776–777.
37. Novy MJ, Haluska GJ (1993) New perspectives on estrogen, progesterone, and oxytocin action in primate parturition, In: Basic Mechanisms Controlling Term and Preterm Birth (Chwalisz K, Garfield RE, eds.), Springer-Verlag, New York, pp. 163–195.
38. Korach KS (1994) Insights from the study of animals lacking functional estrogen receptor. Science 266(5190):1524–1527.
39. Korach KS, Couse JF, Curtis SW, Washburn TF, Lindzey J, Kimbro KS, Eddy EM, Migliaccio S, Snedeker SM, Lubahn DB, Schomberg DW, Smith EP (1996) Estrogen receptor gene disruption: molecular characterization and experimental and clinical phenotypes. Recent Prog in Horm Res 51:159–186.
40. Garfield RE (1998) Effects of antiprogesterone compounds on uterine contractility, In: Hormone Antagonists for Fertility Regulation (Puri CP, Van Look PFA, eds.), Indian Society for the Study of Reproduction and Fertility, Bombay, India, pp. 63–85.
41. Garfield RE, Gasc JM, Baulieu EE (1987) Effects of the antiprogesterone RU 486 on preterm birth in the rat. Am J Obstet Gynecol 157:1281–1285.
42. Yallampalli C, Byam-Smith M, Garfield RE (1994) Nitric oxide controls uterine relaxation during pregnancy but not during labor: role of nitric oxide in the maintenance of pregnancy and initiation of labor, In: Biology of Nitric Oxide: Physiological and Clinical Aspects, vol. 3. Portland Press, London, pp. 192–198.
43. Chwalisz K, Stockemann K, Fuhrmann U, Fritzemeier KH, Einspanier A, Garfield RE (1995) Mechanism of action of antiprogestins in the pregnant uterus. Ann NY Acad Sci 761:202–224.
44. Mahendroo MS, Cala KM, Russell DW (1996) 5a-Reduced androgens play a key role in murine parturition. Mol Endocrinol 10:380–392.
45. Lyon MF, Gleniser PH (1980) Reduced reproductive performance in androgen-resistant. Tfm/Tfm female mice. Proc R Soc Lond (B) 208:1–12.
46. Mochizuki M, Honda T, Deguchi M, Morikawa H, Tojo S (1978) A study on the effect of dehydroepiandrosterone sulfate on so-called cervical ripening. Acta Obstet Gynecol Scand 57:397–401.
47. Sasaki K, Nakano R, Kadoya Y, Iwao M, Shima K, Sowa M (1982) Cervical ripening with dehydroepiandrosterone sulphate. Br J Obstet Gynaecol 89:195–198.
48. Zuidema LJ, Khan-Dawood F, Dawood MY, Work BA (1986) Hormones and cervical ripening: dyhydroepiandrosterone sulfate, estradiol, estriol, and progesterone. Am J Obstet Gynecol 155: 1252–1254.

49. Chang RJ, Buster JE, Blakely JL, Okada DM, Hobel CJ, Abraham GE, Marshall JR (1976) Simultaneous comparison of Δ5-3b-hydroxysteroid levels in the fetoplacental circulation of normal pregnancy in labor and not in labor. J Clin Endocrinol Metab 42:744–751.
50. Walsh SW, Stanczyk F, Novy MJ (1984) Daily hormonal changes in the maternal, fetal and amniotic fluid compartments before parturition in a primate species. J Clin Endocrinol Metab 58: 629–639.
51. Lefebvre DL, Giaid A, Bennett H, et al (1992) Oxytocin gene expression in the rat uterus. Science 256:1553–1555.
52. Mitchell BF, Chibbar R (1995) Synthesis and metabolism of oxytocin in late gestation in human decidua. Adv Exp Med Biol 395:365–380.
53. Sherwood OD, Downing SJ, Guico-Lam ML, Hwang J-J (1990) Relaxin promotes diverse physiological processes in the pregnant rat, In: Uterine Contractility (Garfield RE, ed.), Serono Symposia, Norwell, MA, pp. 237-252.
54. Nishimori K, Young LJ, Guo Q, Wang Z, Insel TR, Matzuk MM (1996) Oxytocin is required for nursing but is not essential for parturition or reproductive behavior. Proc Natl Acad Sci USA 93(21):11,699–11,704.
55. Bleasdale JE, DiRenzo GC (1989) Fetal influence on huma parturition, In: Fetal Medicine Reviews (Rodeck C, ed.), Blackwell, London, pp. 242–288.
56. Mitchell MD (1988) Sources of eicosanoids within the uterus during pregnancy, In: The Onset of Labor: Cellular and Integrative Mechanisms (McNellis D, Challis J, MacDonald P, Nathanielsz P, Robert J, eds.), Perinatology, Ithaca, NY, pp. 165–181.
57. Challis JRG, Olson DM (1988) Parturition, In: The Physiology of Reproduction (Knobil E, Neill J, eds.), Raven, New York, pp. 2177–2216.
58. Higby K, Xenakis EMG, Pauerstein CJK (1993) Do tocolytic agents stop preterm labor? A critical and comprehensive review of efficacy and safety. Am J Obstet Gynecol 168:1247–1259.
58a. Bennett PR, Henderson DJ, Moore GE (1992) Changes in expression of the cyclooxygenase gene in human fetal membranes and placenta with labor. Am J Obstet Gynecol 167:212–216.
59. Cox SM, King MR, Casey ML, MacDonald PC (1993) Interleukin-1β, -1α, and -6 and Prostaglandins in Vaginal/Cervical Fluids of Pregnant Women before and during Labor. J Clin Endocrinol Metab 77:805–815.
60. Bygdeman M, Swahn M-L, Gemzell-Danielsson K, Svalander P (1993) Mode of Action of RU 486. Ann Med 25:61–64.
61. Salvemini D, Misko T, Masferrer JL, Seibert K, Currie MG, Needleman P (1993) Nitric oxide activates cyclooxygenase enzymes. Proc Natl Acad Sci USA 90:7240–7244.
62. Salvemini D, Seibert K, Masferrer JL, Misko T, Currie MG and Needleman P (1994) Endogenous nitric oxide enhances prostaglandin production in a model of renal inflammation. J Clin Invest 93:1940–1947.
63. Xie W, Chipman JG, Robertson DL, Erickson RL (1991) Expression of a mitogen-responsive gene encoding prostaglandin synthase is regulating by mRNA splicing. Proc Natl Acad Sci USA 88:2692–2696.
64. Sirois J, Richards JS (1992) Purification and characterization of a novel, distinct isoform of prostaglandin endoperoxide synthase induced by human chorionic godadotropin in granulosa cells of rat preovulatory follicles. J Biol Chem 267:6382–6388.
65. Vane JR (1971) Inhibition of prostaglandin synthesis as a mechanism of action for aspirin-like drugs. Nature 231:232–237.
66. Wimsatt J, Nathanielsz PW, Sirois J (1993) Induction of prostaglandin endoperoxide synthase isoform-2 in ovin cotyledonary tissues during late gestation. Endocrinology 133:1068–1073.
67. Slater DM, Berger LC, Newton R, Moore GE, Bennett PR (1995) Expression of cycooxygenase types 1 and 2 in human fetal membranes at term. Am J Obstet Gynecol 172:77–82.
68. Hirst JJ, Teixeira FJ, Zakar T, Olson DM (1995) Prostaglandin endoperoxide-H synthase and-messenger ribonucleic acid levels in human amnion with spontaneous labor onset. J Clin Endocrinol Metab 80:517–523.
69. Klein T, Nüsing RM, Pfeilschifter J, Ullrich V (1994) Selective inhibition of cyclooxygenase 2. Biochem Pharmacol 48:1605–1610.
70. Shi Shao Qing, Diel P, Fritzemeier KH, Garfield RE, Chwalisz K (1996) The specific cyclooxygenase-2 (COX-2) inhibitor flosulide inhibits antiprogestin-induced preterm birth. J Soc Gyncol Invest 3 (Suppl): 540.
71. Furchgott RF, Vanhoutte PM (1989) Endothelium-derived relaxing and contracting factors. FASEB J 3:2007–2018.

72. Ignarro LJ, Kadowitz PJ (1985) The pharmacological and physiological role of cyclic GMP in vascular smooth muscle relaxation. Ann Rev Pharm Toxicol 25:171–191.
73. Moncada S, Palmer RMG, Higgs EA (1991) Nitric oxide: physiology, pathophysiology and pharmacology. Pharmacol Rev 43:109–142.
74. Sanders KM, Ward SM (1992) NO as a mediator of nonadrenergic noncholinergic neurotransmission. Am J Physiol 262:G379–G392.
75. Li CG, Rand MJ (1991) Evidence that part of the NANC relaxant response of guinea-pig trachea to electrical field stimulation is mediated by NO. Br J Pharm 102:91–94.
76. Kannan MS, Johnson DE (1991) Functional innervation of pig tracheal smooth muscle: neural and non-neural mechanisms of relaxation. J Pharm Exp Therap 260:1180–1184.
77. Kannan MS, Johnson DE (1992) Nitric oxide mediates the neural nonadrenergic, noncholinergic relaxation of pig tracheal smooth muscle. Am J Physiol 262:L511–L514.
78. Pickard RS, Powell PH, Zar MA (1991) The effect of inhibitors of NO biosynthesis and cyclic GMP formation on nerve-evoked relaxation of human covernosal smooth muscle. Br J Pharm 104:755–759.
79. Moncada S. Higgs EA (1993) The L-arginine-nitric oxide pathway. N Engl J Med 329:2002–2012.
80. Ignarro LG (1989) Biological actions and properties of endothelium-derived nitric oxide formed and released from artery and vein. Cir Res 65:1–21.
81. Izumi H, Yallampalli C, Garfield RE (1993) Gestational changes in L-arginine-induced relaxation of pregnant rat and human myometrial smooth muscle. Am J Obstet Gynecol 169:1327–1337.
82. Vane IR (1994) The Croonian Lecture (1993) The endothelium: maestro of the blood circulation. Phil Trans R Soc London, pp. 225–246.
83. Yallampalli C, Buhimschi I, Chwalisz K, Garfield RE, Dong Y-L (1996) Preterm birth in rats produced by synergistic action of a nitric oxide inhibitor (NG-nitro-L-arginine methyl ester) and an antiprogestin (onapristone). Am J Obstet Gynecol 175:207–212.
84. Chwalisz K, Shi S-S, Garfield RE (1997) Inhibition of nitric oxide (NO) production increases the labor-inducing activity of antiprogestins in guinea pigs. 17th Annual Meeting of Society of Perinatal Obstetricians, Abstract #368, Anaheim, CA, January 20–25, 1997.
85. Buhimschi I, Ali M, Jain V, Chwalisz K, Garfield RE (1996) Differential regulation of nitric oxide in the uterus and cervix during pregnancy and labor. Hum Reprod 11(8):1755–1766.
86. Natuzzi ES, Ursell PC, Harrison M, Buscher C, Riemer RK (1993) Nitric oxide synthase activity in the pregnant uterus decreases at parturition. Biochem Biophys Res Commun 194:108–114.
87. Sladek SM, Regenstrin AC, Lykins D, Roberts JM (1993) Nitric oxide synthase activity in pregnant rabbit uterus decreases on the last day of pregnancy. Am J Obstet Gynecol 169:1285–1291.
88. Weiner CP, Knowles RG, Stegink LD, Dawson J, Moncada S (1996) Myometrial arginase activity increases with advancing pregnancy in the guinea pig. Am J Obstet Gynecol 174:779–782.
89. Romero R, Mazor M (1988) Infection and preterm labor. Clin Obstet Gynecol 31:553–584.
90. Shi S-Q, Beier HM, Garfield RE, Chwalisz K (1996) Local application of an nitric oxide (NO) donor induces cervical ripeing. J Soc Gynecol Invest 3, 2(Suppl): 462.
91. Tasikiran D, Stefanovic-Racic M, Georgescu H, Evans C (1994) Nitric oxide mediates suppression of cartilage proteoglycan synthesis by interleukin-1. Biochem Biophys Res Commun 200: 142–148.
92. Evans CH, Stefanovic-Racic M, Lancaster J (1995) Nitric oxide and its role in orthopaedic disease. Clin Orthop Related Res 312: 275–294.
93. Khaidar A, Marx M, Lubec B, Lubec G (1994) L-arginine reduced heart collagen accumulation in the diabetic db/db mouse. Circulation 90:479–483.
94. Koplakov V, Gordon D, Kulik T (1995) Nitric oxide-generating compound inhibit total protein and collagen synthesis in cultured vascular smooth muscle cells. Circ Res 76:305–309.
95. Milano S, Arcoleo F, Dieli M, D'Agostino R, D'Agostino P, De Nucci G, Cillari E (1995) Prostaglandin E2 regulates inducible nitric oxide synthase in the murine macrophage cell line J774. Prostaglandins 49(2):105–115.
96. Di Rosa M, Ialenti A, Ianaro A, Sautebin L (1995) Interaction between nitric oxide and cyclooxygenase pathways. Prostaglandins, Leukotriens and Essential Fatty Acids 54,4:229–238.
97. Bienkowski RS and Gotkin MG (1995) Control of collagen deposition in mammalian lung. Proc Soc Exp Biol Med 209(2):118–140.
98. Border WA and Ruoslahti E (1990) Transforming growth factor-beta 1 induces extracellular matrix formation in glomerulonephritis. Cell Differ Dev 32(3):425–431.
99. Border WA, Okuda S, Languino LR, Ruoslahti E (1990) Transforming growth factor-beta regulates production of proteoglycans by mesangial cells. Kidney Int 37(2):689–695.

100. Slavin J, Unemori E, Hunt, TK Amento E (1994) Transforming growth factor beta (TGF-beta) and dexamethasone have direct opposing effects on collagen metabolism in low passage human dermal fibroblasts in vitro. Growth Factors 11(3):205–213.
101. Border WA, Noble NA (1995) Targeting TGF-beta for treatment of disease. Nature Med 1(10): 1000–1001.
102. Pfeilschifter J, Vosbeck K (1991) Transforming growth factor beta 2 inhibits interleukin 1 beta- and tumour necrosis factor alpha-induction of nitric oxide synthase in rat renal mesangial cells. Biochem Biophys Res Commun 175(2):372–329.
103. Nathan C, Xie QW (1994) Nitric oxide synthases: roles, tolls and controls. Cell 78(6) 915–918.
104. Peunova N, Enikolopov G (1995) Nitric oxide triggers a switch to growth arrest during differentiation of neuronal cells. Nature 375(6526):68–73.
105. Peng HB, Libby P, Liao JK (1995) Induction and stabilization of I kappa B alpha by nitric oxide mediates inhibition of NF-kappa B. J Biol Chem 270(23):14,214–14,219.
106. Peng HB, Rajavashisth TB, Libby P, Liao JK (1995) Nitric oxide inhibits macrophage-colony stimulating factor gene transcription in vascular endothelial cells. J Biol Chem 270(28):17,050–17,055.
107. Lubec B, Golej J., Marx M, Weninger M, Hoeger H (1995) L-arginine reduces kidney lipid peroxidation, glycoxidation and collagen accumulation in the aging NMRI mouse. Renal Phys Biochem 18(2):97–102.
108. Murrell GA, Jang D, Wiliams RJ (1995) Nitric oxide activates metalloprotease enzymes in articular cartilage. Biochem Biophys Res Commun 206(1):15–21.
109. Sautebin L, Ialentia A, Ianaro A and Di Rosa M (1995) Endogenous nitric oxide increases prostaglandin biosynthesis in carrageenin rat paw oedema. Eur J Pharmacol 286:219–222.
110. Miyoshi H, MB Boyle, MacKay L, Garfield RE (1996) Voltage-clamp studies of gap junctions between uterine muscle cells during term and preterm labor. Biophys J 71:1324–1334.
111. Geimonen E, Echetebu C, Jiang W, Ali M, Fishmann GI, Garfield RE, Anderson J (1996) Activation of protein kinase C in human uterine smooth muscle induces connexin43 gene transcription through an AP-1 site in the promoter sequence. J Biol Chem 271:23,667–23,674.
112. Tezuka N, Ali M, Chwalisz K, Garfield RE (1995) Changes in transcripts encoding calcium channel subunits of rat myometrium during pregnancy. Am J Physiol 269 (Cell Physiol 38):C1008–C1017.
113. Garfield RE, Yallampalli C (1993) Control of myometrial contractility and labor, In: Basic Mechanisms Controlling Term and Preterm Birth (Chwalisz K, Garfield RE, eds.), Springer-Verlag, NY, pp. 1–28.
114. Bazer FW, Simmen RCM, Simmen FA (1991) Comparative aspects of concepts signals for maternal recognition of pregnancy. Proc NY Acad Sci 622:202–211.
115. Glassman W, Byam-Smith M, Garfield RE (1995) Changes in rat cervical collagen during gestation and following antiprogesterone treatment as measured in vivo with light induced autofluorescence. Am J Obstet Gynecol 173:1550–1556.

15 Multiple Physiological Effects of Relaxin During Pregnancy

O. David Sherwood, PHD

CONTENTS

INTRODUCTION

Overview

In 1926, Hisaw *(1)* discovered relaxin by observing that the injection of serum obtained from pregnant guinea pigs or rabbits into virgin guinea pigs shortly after estrus induced a relaxation of the pubic ligament. Relaxin is produced in the reproductive tract of several laboratory, domestic, and primate species during pregnancy. The source of the relaxin that is secreted into the peripheral blood varies among species; for example, it is the corpora lutea in rats and pigs, the placentae in rabbits, and the uterus in guinea pigs *(2)*. Since the mid-1970s when highly purified relaxin preparations began to be described *(2)*, great progress has been made toward an understanding of the chemistry and physiology of relaxin. It is now recognized that there is extraordinary diversity among species in not only the source of relaxin, but also in its structure, regulation of synthesis and secretion, and physiological effects during pregnancy. This diversity mandates that rigorous study of relaxin be done on a species-by-species basis.

The physiology of relaxin has been studied most extensively in rats and pigs, because the corpora lutea in both species contain enough relaxin during late pregnancy to enable its isolation in quantities sufficient for physiological studies. Additionally, the source of relaxin can be removed in these two species in order to determine the physiological roles of relaxin during pregnancy.

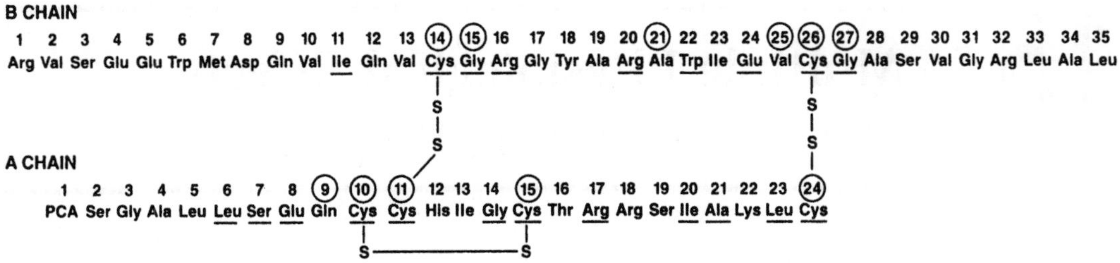

Fig. 1. Covalent structure of rat relaxin *(3)*. Numbers of residues that are identical in rat relaxin and rat insulin are circled. Residues that are identical in rat relaxin and porcine relaxin *(4,5)* are underlined.

Structures of Rat and Porcine Relaxin

Relaxin has structural features that resemble those of insulin (Fig. 1). The lengths of the A- and B-chains and also the locations of the disulfide bonds closely correspond in the two hormones. These similar structural features coupled with the discovery of at least one common intron site in relaxin and insulin genes *(6)* are the basis for the generally held view that relaxin and insulin evolved from a common ancestral gene. There is, however, only about 25% identity in the amino acid sequences of rat relaxin and rat insulin, and extensive experimentation has failed to demonstrate that relaxin and insulin share common biological effects *(2)*.

There is striking variation in the primary structure of relaxin among species *(2)*. Rat relaxin and porcine relaxin, for example, share only about 40% amino acid sequence homology, and the homology is largely confined to the half cystine and glycine residues (Fig. 1). Because of this extraordinary structural variation among species, relaxin from the species of interest should be used when feasible to determine the physiological effects of the hormone.

Secretion of Rat and Porcine Relaxin

The corpora lutea in pregnant rats and pigs both store and secrete relaxin following its production during pregnancy. A portion of the relaxin accumulates in membrane-bound storage granules within luteal cells until 2–3 d before birth when the luteal cells degranulate and ovarian relaxin levels decline precipitously (*2*; Fig. 2A,C).

The profile of relaxin secretion in the rat differs from that in the pig until 2–3 d before delivery when surges occur in both species. In the rat, relaxin is secreted in relatively high levels throughout the last half of the 23-d gestation period. Blood levels of relaxin increase rapidly beginning on d 10 and exceed 40 ng/mL from d 14 to d 20 (*7*; Fig. 2B). In the pig, low levels of relaxin (~150 pg/mL) are detectable in the peripheral blood by d 6 of the 114-d gestation period, and blood levels increase gradually to only about 10 ng/mL by d 110 of pregnancy (*11,12*; Fig. 2D).

Regulation of luteal function in the rat and pig differs remarkably throughout nearly all of pregnancy. In the rat, relaxin synthesis and secretion are promoted by an unknown placental factor(s) that acts in concert with estrogen *(2,13,14)*. The conceptuses are not required for the synthesis or secretion of relaxin in pigs. Luteal function was maintained beyond 100 d following either hysterectomy or the administration of estrogen during the luteal phase of the estrous cycle, and relaxin levels in both the corpora lutea and the peripheral blood of the pseudopregnant gilts were similar to those in pregnant pigs *(10,12)*.

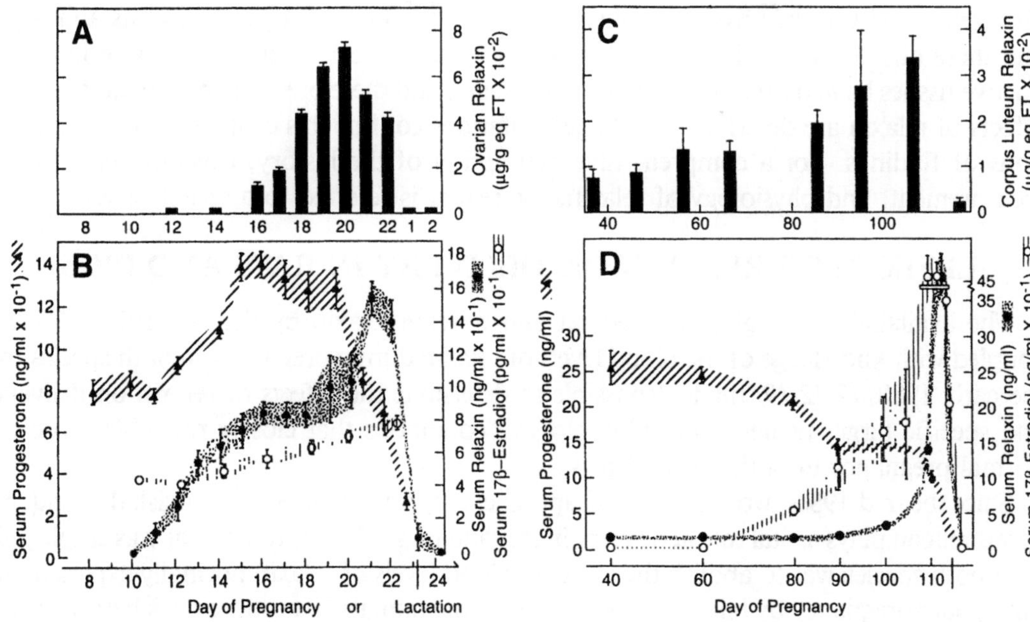

Fig. 2. **(A)** Mean (+ SE) relaxin immunoactivity levels in extracts of ovaries obtained from rats during pregnancy. FT, fresh tissue. (Redrawn from *[7]* with permission.) **(B)** Mean (±) relaxin, progesterone, and estrogen levels in the peripheral sera of rats during pregnancy. (Redrawn from *[7–9]* with permission.) **(C)** Mean (+ SE) relaxin bioactivity levels in extracts of corpora lutea obtained from pigs during pregnancy. (Redrawn from *[10]* with permission.) **(D)** Mean (±) relaxin, progesterone, and estradiol levels in peripheral sera of pigs during pregnancy. (Redrawn from *[11]* with permission.)

The degranulation of luteal cells and surge in serum relaxin levels that occur during the 2–3 d before birth in rats and pigs (Fig. 2B,D) coincide temporally with the marked decline in serum progesterone levels that occurs at functional luteolysis and is required for delivery to occur in both species. The factors that trigger luteolysis differ, at least in part, between the two species. In rats, the timing of the luteolytic process with its concomitant antepartum surge in relaxin secretion is tied to the photoperiod *(2)*. In pigs, the timing of luteolysis is not tightly regulated by the photoperiod *(15)*.

Serum levels of estrogen increase during the second half of pregnancy in rats (Fig. 2B) and after d 80 of pregnancy in pigs (Fig. 2D). In rats, it is the developing ovarian follicles that are the primary source of the circulating estrogen, whereas, in pigs, it is the placentae. Estrogen is either required for or enhances the expression of relaxin's biological activity on several of relaxin's target tissues in both the rat and the pig.

Scope of the Chapter

This chapter places major emphasis on recent advances in our understanding of the diverse physiological effects of relaxin during pregnancy in primiparous Sprague-Dawley-derived rats and primiparous crossbred pigs. The chapter emphasizes studies that employed highly purified relaxin and were conducted in vivo with pregnant animals under experimental conditions that closely resemble those that occur in untreated intact pregnant animals. The chapter first summarizes recent studies that establish a long-suspected role of relaxin, namely, that of enabling normal delivery. The best-understood effects of relaxin are those on the reproductive tract and mammary apparatus, and they are described next.

Differences exist in the physiological effects of relaxin during pregnancy in rats and pigs, and these differences are indicated. Numerous biological effects of relaxin on nonreproductive tissues have been discovered in recent years, and these presently poorly understood effects of relaxin are described last. Page limitations confine this chapter to brief descriptions of findings. For a comprehensive description of the history, isolation, chemistry, measurement, and physiology of relaxin, the reader is referred to a recent review *(2)*.

EFFECTS OF RELAXIN ON DELIVERY IN RATS AND PIGS

The availability of highly purified rat and porcine relaxin by the late 1970s *(16–18)* coupled with knowledge of the blood levels of relaxin during pregnancy in both species by the early 1980s *(7,12,19)* made it possible to determine the effects of relaxin on delivery and specific target tissues under physiological conditions that closely resemble those of normal pregnancy in both rats and pigs.

Since the mid-1980s two experimental approaches have been used to establish that endogenous relaxin plays a vital role at delivery in rats and pigs. The approach that was employed with both species was to abolish the elevated blood levels of relaxin normally experienced during late pregnancy by bilaterally ovariectomizing animals 10 or more days before term. Throughout the remainder of pregnancy, animals were given hormone replacement therapy with progesterone plus estrogen (rats) or progesterone only (pigs) in doses that provide blood levels closely resembling those that occur during late pregnancy in intact rats and pigs. When progesterone was withdrawn from these relaxin-deficient animals in order to mimic luteolysis and initiate parturition, the duration of delivery was markedly prolonged and the incidence of live births was extremely low. When hormone replacement therapy included physiological levels of highly purified porcine relaxin, however, the duration of delivery and the incidence of live births were restored to values similar to those of controls *(20–22*, Fig. 3).

Additionally, a highly specific and noninvasive experimental approach was used to examine the influence of relaxin on delivery in rats. A monoclonal antibody (MAb) developed to rat relaxin, designated MCA1 *(23)*, was administered once daily throughout the second half of gestation to neutralize the biological actions of endogenous relaxin. Controls received either phosphate-buffered saline (PBS, vehicle control) or an MAb for fluorescein (MCAF; MAb control). Findings were similar to those obtained with the ovariectomized pregnant rat *(20,21)*. Following passive immunization of rat relaxin, the onset of delivery was delayed, the duration of delivery was markedly prolonged, and the incidence of live pups at birth was low as compared to the PBS and MCAF controls *(24)*.

EFFECTS OF RELAXIN ON THE REPRODUCTIVE TRACT

Effects of Relaxin on the Uterus

Uterine Contractility. In 1950, Krantz et al. *(25)* discovered that iv administration of crude porcine relaxin to estrogen-primed guinea pigs inhibited spontaneous uterine contractility. Numerous investigators subsequently confirmed this effect of relaxin on uterine contractility both in vitro and in vivo with experiments that employed nonpregnant animals *(2)*. Following relaxin's isolation, its role on uterine contractility during rat pregnancy was investigated.

Rat. The frequency of uterine contractions diminishes throughout the second half of pregnancy, and there is strong evidence that relaxin plays a major role in restraining

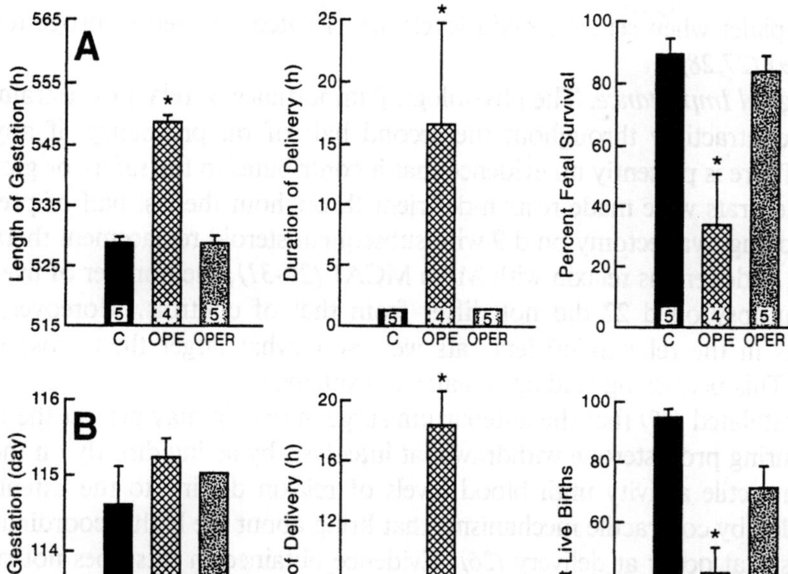

Fig. 3. **(A)** The influence of relaxin on birth in rats. Pregnant rats were bilaterally ovariectomized (O) on d 9 and given progesterone (P) implants (four SILASTIC implants each containing 60 mg P) and an estrogen (E) implant (one SILASTIC implant containing 2 μg 17β-estradiol, which was replaced with a SILASTIC implant containing 12 μg 17β-estradiol on d 18). Highly purified porcine relaxin (R; *16*) was administered to group OPER from d 9 through delivery at a dose of 1 μg/h via miniature osmotic pump. P implants were withdrawn on the evening of d 21 to mimic the decline in serum progesterone levels that normally occurs at luteolysis. Means (+ SE) are for the number of animals shown at the base of each bar. Asterisk indicates a significant difference from intact controls (C) and group OPER ($P < 0.05$) (From *[20]* with permission.) **(B)** The influence of relaxin on birth in pigs. Pregnant pigs were bilaterally ovariectomized (O) on d 105 and given 100 mg progesterone (P) intramuscularly in 4 mL of corn oil at 12-h intervals from d 105–112 and, in addition, one of the following injection regimens: highly purified porcine relaxin (R; group OPR) or R vehicle (group OP). Group OPR received 1 mg of porcine relaxin *(16)* intramuscularly in 1 mL of 0.9% saline at 6-h intervals from d 105 until birth. The control group (C) was sham-ovariectomized on d 105 and received the P and R vehicles thereafter. Means (+ SE) are for 5 animals/group. Asterisk indicates a significant difference from intact controls (group C) and group OPR ($P < 0.05$). (From *[22]* with permission.)

uterine contractility during this approx 10-d period *(26)*. When rats were ovariectomized on d 9 and given replacement therapy with progesterone and estrogen, the frequency of uterine contractions was approximately twice that of intact controls. When replacement therapy included the ovarian steroids plus highly purified porcine relaxin, however, the frequency of uterine contractions did not differ from that of controls.

Pig. The influence of relaxin on uterine contractility in the pregnant pig has received little experimental attention. Relaxin may restrain uterine activity during the antepartum period when serum relaxin levels surge. The electrical activity and contractile activity of the myometrium remain low as late as the period between 24 and 10 h before the expulsion of the first piglet when serum relaxin levels are elevated and serum progesterone levels have declined *(27,28)*.

Physiological Importance. The physiological importance of relaxin's restraining effects on uterine contractility throughout the second half of rat pregnancy, if any, remains unknown. There is presently no evidence that it contributes to the safety or growth of the fetuses. When rats were made relaxin-deficient throughout the last half of pregnancy by either employing ovariectomy on d 9 with subsequent steroid replacement therapy *(20)* or neutralizing endogenous relaxin with MAb MCA1 *(29–31)*, the number of live fetuses (*in utero*) at autopsy on d 22 did not differ from that of controls. Moreover, the mean fetal weights in the relaxin-deficient rats were somewhat larger than those in controls *(20,29–31)*. This perplexing finding remains unexplained.

It was postulated *(32)* that the antepartum surge in relaxin may protect the fetuses and placentae during progesterone withdrawal at luteolysis by acting directly on the uterus to restrain contractile activity until blood levels of relaxin decline to the extent that they are overridden by contractile mechanisms that bring about the highly coordinated uterine contractions that occur at delivery *(26)*. Evidence obtained in rats does not support the hypothesis that endogenous circulating relaxin influences the timing of birth through direct restraining effects on uterine contractile activity. Neutralization of relaxin during the antepartum period did not influence the time of onset of labor *(24,33)*.

Mechanism of Action. Phosphorylation of myosin 20-kDa light chains by the enzyme myosin light-chain kinase (MLCK) is required for smooth muscle contraction. Activation of MLCK is a sequential process requiring the elevation of intracellular calcium (Ca^{2+}) levels. Calcium first binds to the calcium regulatory protein calmodulin to form a Ca^{2+}• calmodulin complex. This complex then binds to the inactive subunit of MLCK to form the active holoenzyme complex Ca^{2+}•calmodulin•MLCK required for phosphorylation of the 20-kDa light chain of myosin *(34,35)*.

Relaxin acts directly on the uterine myometrium *(2)*. There is considerable evidence that relaxin initiates its effects on rat myometrial contractility, at least in part by activating adenylyl cyclase and thereby generating cAMP *(36,37)*. One intracellular mechanism whereby relaxin-induced cAMP elevation appears to mediate its effects is through activation of protein kinase A *(38)* and subsequent phosphorylation of the catalytic subunit of MLCK *(39)*. Phosphorylation of MLCK reduces its affinity for its modulator Ca^{2+}• calmodulin and thereby inhibits formation of the active Ca^{2+}•calmodulin•MLCK complex *(39)*. Activation of protein kinase A may also inhibit uterine contractility by bringing about a reduction in intracellular Ca^{2+} levels and thereby inhibiting formation of the active Ca^{2+}•calmodulin•MLCK complex. The protein kinase A inhibitor H-8 reduces the ability of relaxin to inhibit oxytocin-induced increases in Ca^{2+} and inositol triphosphate *(40)*. Furthermore, recent evidence indicates that relaxin stimulates myometrial calcium-activated potassium channel activity via protein kinase A *(41)*, and these channels may control Ca^{2+} concentrations by regulating myometrial cell resting membrane potential *(42)*.

It has also been postulated that relaxin's actions on uterine contractility may be mediated in part at the level of the plasma membrane by opening ATP-sensitive K^+ channels *(43)*. For more comprehensive descriptions of the action of relaxin on uterine contractions, the reader is referred to recent reviews *(2,34,35)*.

Uterine Metabolic Effects. In 1957, Steinetz et al. *(44)* first demonstrated that relaxin has rapid general metabolic effects on the uterus (uterotropic effects). Uterine water content, wet weight, dry weight, glycogen content, and nitrogen content increased to maximal

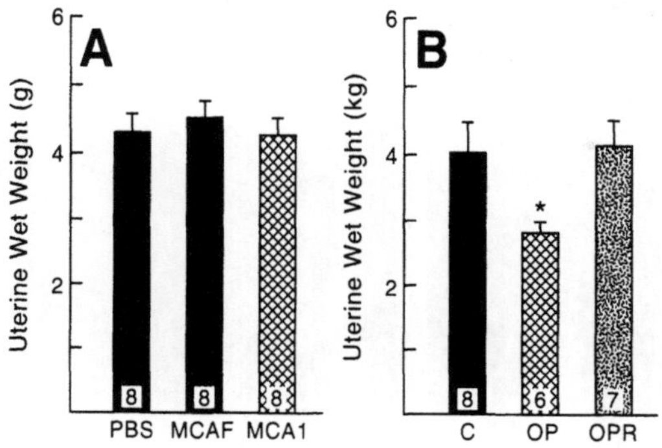

Fig. 4. (**A**) The influence of neutralization of endogenous relaxin throughout the second half of pregnancy on uterine wet weight in rats. Five milligrams of highly purified MAb for rat relaxin (MCA1), 5 mg of highly purified MAb for fluorescein (MCAF, MAb control), and 0.5 mL phosphate-buffered saline (PBS, vehicle control) were injected via tail vein once daily from d 12–22 of pregnancy. Uteri were removed at 1200 h on d 22. Means (+ SE) are for the number of animals shown at the base of each bar. (Zhao and Sherwood, unpublished.) (**B**) The influence of relaxin on uterine wet weight in pregnant pigs. Pregnant pigs were bilaterally ovariectomized (O) on d 40 and given 50 mg progesterone (P) intramuscularly in 2 mL of corn oil at 12-h intervals from d 38–110, and in addition, one of the following injection regimens: highly purified porcine relaxin (R, group OPR) or R vehicle (group OP). Group OPR received relaxin *(16)* intramuscularly in 2 mL physiological saline at 6-h intervals in doses that increased as pregnancy progressed (0.1 mg for d 40–80, 0.25 mg for d 81–100, and 0.5 mg for d 101–110). The control group (C) was sham-ovariectomized on d 40, and received progesterone and relaxin vehicles thereafter. Means (+ SE) are for the number of animals shown at the base of each bar. Asterisk indicates a significant difference from intact controls (group C) and group OPR ($P < 0.05$). (From *[49]* with permission.)

levels within 6–12 h following the administration of impure porcine relaxin to ovariectomized estrogen-primed rats. The uterotropic effects of relaxin were confirmed in the late 1980s and early 1990s with highly purified porcine relaxin in nonpregnant rats *(45)* and pigs *(46–48)*. These findings prompted studies aimed at determining if endogenous relaxin has uterotropic effects in pregnant rats and pigs.

Rat. The high levels of relaxin in the peripheral blood do not appear to have uterotropic effects during the second half of rat pregnancy. When rats were made relaxin-deficient throughout the second half of pregnancy by neutralizing endogenous relaxin with MAb MCA1, the wet weights of the uteri did not differ from those of relaxin-replete controls on d 22 of pregnancy (*29* and Fig. 4A).

It is possible that endogenous relaxin from a source other than the corpora lutea has uterotropic effects during rat pregnancy. Fields et al. *(50)* demonstrated relaxin immunostaining in antimesometrial epithelial cells at implantation sites during the second half of pregnancy, and this putative relaxin may act locally via paracrine mechanisms. Consistent with this possibility, uterine growth in the gravid horn of unilaterally pregnant rats far exceeded that in the nongravid horns during the second half of pregnancy *(51)*.

Pig. Unlike the rat, endogenous circulating relaxin does promote growth of the pig uterus. When gilts were bilaterally ovariectomized on d 40 and given hormone replacement therapy with either progesterone or progesterone plus porcine relaxin in doses that provided plasma hormone levels resembling those in intact conrols, the wet weights of the

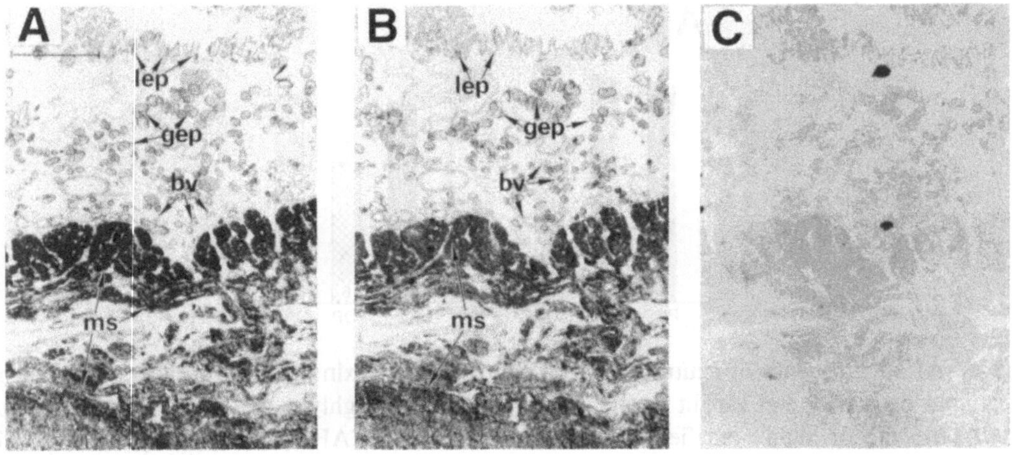

Fig. 5. The localization of relaxin binding sites in the uterus of a d 110 pregnant pig. Relaxin binding was observed in uteri incubated with biotinylated relaxin (**A**). Tissue sections incubated with biotinylated relaxin showed binding in the presence of a 2000-fold excess of porcine insulin (**B**), but not in the presence of a 2000-fold excess of porcine relaxin (**C**). ms, myometrial smooth muscle; bv, blood vessels; lep, luminal epithelial cells; gep, glandular epithelial cells. Bar in A = 997 μm and all panels are the same magnification. (From *[49]* with permission.)

uteri of relaxin-deficient pigs were significantly lower than those of both intact controls and relaxin-treated ovariectomized gilts on d 110 of pregnancy (Fig. 4B).

Physiological Importance. The physiological importance of relaxin's uterotropic effects in the pregnant pig remains unknown. Through these effects, relaxin may assist with the accommodation of the growing fetuses and placentas. If that is the case, these effects do not appear to be vital. Litter size, fetal viability, fetal wet weight, and placental wet weight in pigs made relaxin deficient by ovariectomy on d 40 of pregnancy did not differ from those in intact controls on d 110 *(49)*.

Mechanism of Action. Relaxin appears to act directly on the uterus to bring about its uterotropic effects in pigs. A biotinylated relaxin probe that retains biological activity *(52,53)* was used to demonstrate specific and saturable binding of relaxin in the uterus of the pregnant pig (Fig. 5). Within the endometrium, relaxin binding sites were localized on both luminal and glandular epithelial cells as well as on cells associated with blood vessels. Within the myometrium, relaxin binding sites were localized on smooth muscle cells. Molecular events that occur following relaxin binding are not well understood. There is evidence that relaxin promotes both hypertrophy and hyperplasia of the uterus in non-pregnant pigs *(46,47)*. Following the administration of porcine relaxin every 6 h for 54 h, the wet weight, dry weight, water content, protein content, and DNA content of uteri from relaxin-treated animals exceeded those of uteri from untreated controls.

It is well established that estrogen alone has marked uterotropic actions in both rats (54) and pigs *(47,48)*. The interactive effects of estrogen and relaxin on growth of the uterus are not well understood. Whereas investigators reported that estrogen pretreatment is not essential for relaxin to exert uterotropic effects in nonpregnant rats *(55,56)* and pigs *(46,47)*, others reported that estrogen priming is essential for these effects in pigs *(48)*. There is limited evidence that progesterone, when given in conjunction with estrogen, may augment relaxin's uterotropic effects in pigs *(47,48)*, but not in rats *(57)*.

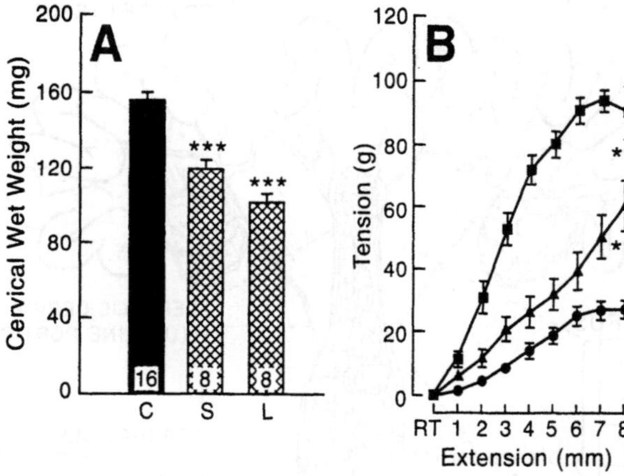

Fig. 6. The influence of neutralization of endogenous relaxin on the wet weight and extensibility of the rat cervix. The rats were administered MCA1 daily as described in the legend to Fig. 4A. **(A)** Mean (+ SE) wet weight of cervices obtained from control rats (C) and rats treated with MCA1 either during the 3-d antepartum period (short treatment, S) or throughout the second half of pregnancy (long treatment, L). Cervices were removed at 1200 h on d 22. Means are for the number of animals shown at the base of each bar. **(B)** Mean (± SE) tension at extension of the cervices from the three groups for eight successive 1-mm extensions at 30-min intervals. RT, resting tension. Asterisks indicate a significant difference from controls ($P < 0.001$). (Redrawn from *[29,33]* with permission.)

Effects of Relaxin on the Cervix

In the late 1950s and early 1960s, it was shown that partially purified porcine relaxin promotes growth and softening of the cervix in rats *(54,58)* and pigs *(59)*. Moreover, studies in the 1980s demonstrated that the progressive growth and softening of the cervix that occur from d 12 until term in rats *(33)* and from d 80 until term in pigs *(11)* coincide with elevated blood levels of relaxin and estrogen in both species (Fig. 2). Studies in the late 1980s and early 1990s established that endogenous relaxin plays a major role in bringing about these cervical modifications during pregnancy in both the rat and the pig.

RAT. Both rats that were ovariectomized on d 9 and given hormone replacement therapy throughout the second half of pregnancy *(20,60,61)* and intact rats that were made relaxin deficient by neutralizing endogenous relaxin with MAb MCA1 either throughout the second half of pregnancy *(29)* or during the antepartum period *(33)* were used to establish that relaxin plays a major role in promoting the growth and softening of the cervix that occurs throughout the last half of pregnancy. The effects of neutralization of endogenous relaxin throughout the second half of pregnancy and during the antepartum period on cervical wet weight and extensibility (degree of softening) are shown in Fig. 6. Both cervical wet weight and extensibility were markedly lower in relaxin-deficient MCA1-treated rats than in controls.

PIG. The cervix in the pregnant pig, which is about 15 cm long and characterized by rounded prominences on its internal surface, consists of a uterine portion (cephalic cervix) and a vaginal portion (caudal cervix; Fig. 7). The time-course of changes in the physical properties of the cervix was demonstrated *(11)* by employing 1-cm segments of cervical tissue collected as shown in Fig. 7. After d 80 of pregnancy, marked increases in the wet weight, lumen diameter, and extensibility occur in the uterine portion of the cervix, whereas moderate increases occur in the vaginal portion of the cervix (Fig. 8). By d 110

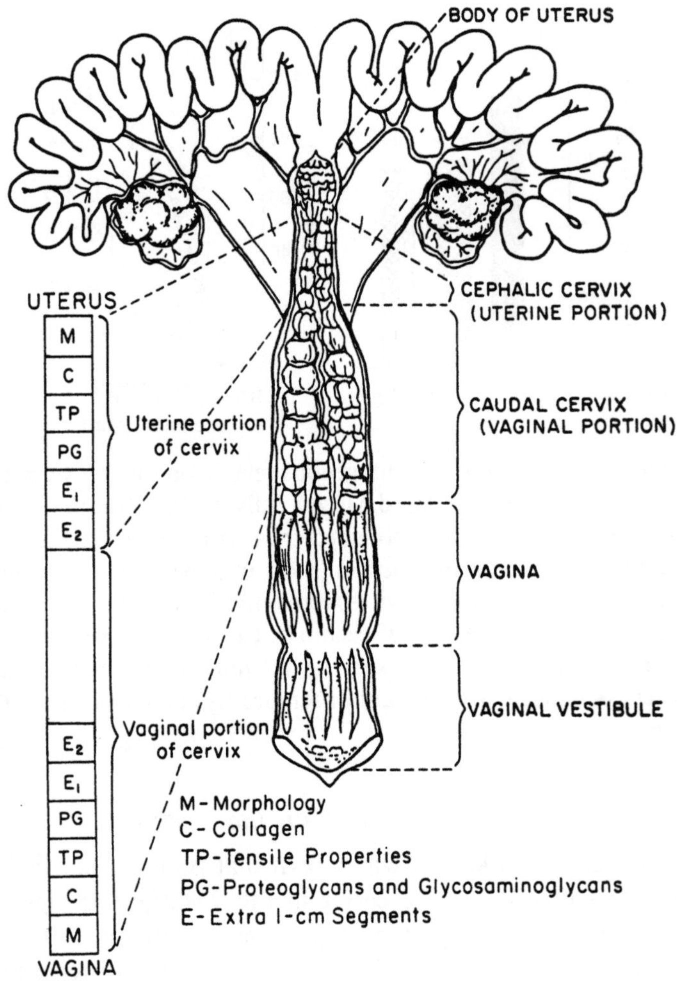

Fig. 7. Diagram of the female pig reproductive tract. To examine the physical properties, biochemical composition, and histological characteristics of the cervix, adjacent 1-cm segments of both the uterine and vaginal portions of the cervix were collected. (From *[11]* with permission.)

these physical properties of the uterine portion of the cervix are similar to those of the vaginal portion. In view of its relatively firm consistency and small lumen throughout most of pregnancy, it was concluded that the uterine portion of the cervix plays a more important role than the vaginal cervix in protecting the uterus and its contents during pregnancy *(11)*.

Experiments with pigs that were ovariectomized on d 100 and given subsequent hormone replacement therapy with either progesterone or progesterone plus relaxin established that relaxin plays a major role in promoting the changes in the physical properties of both the uterine and the vaginal portions of the cervix that occur during the last third of pregnancy in pigs *(62)*. Mean values for cervical wet weight, lumen diameter, and extensibility were significantly lower in relaxin-deficient gilts than in intact control gilts. Hormone replacement therapy that included relaxin restored these physical properties of the cervix to values that did not differ from those in intact controls (Fig. 8). The extent to which relaxin promoted modifications of the physical properties was far greater in the uterine portion than the vaginal portion of the cervix (Fig. 8).

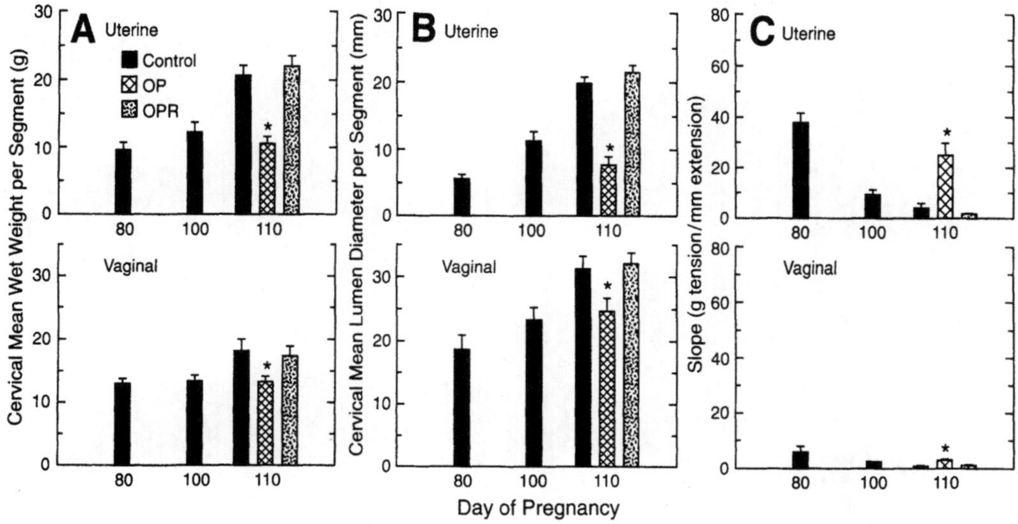

Fig. 8. The influence of relaxin on the **(A)** wet weight, **(B)** lumen diameter, and **(C)** extensibility (slope [g of tension/mm extension]) of 1-cm segments from the uterine and vaginal portions of the cervix. Pregnant pigs were bilaterally ovariectomized (O) on d 100 and given 50 mg progesterone (P) intramuscularly in 2 mL corn oil at 12-h intervals from d 98–110 and, in addition, one of the following injection regimens: highly purified porcine relaxin (R, group OPR) or R vehicle (group OP). Group OPR received 1 mg of porcine relaxin *(16)* intramuscularly in 2 mL of 0.9% saline at 6-h intervals from 1200 h on d 100 until 0600 h on d 110. The control group was sham-ovariectomized on d 100 and received P and R vehicles thereafter. Means (+ SE) are for 5 or 6 animals/group. Asterisk indicates a significant difference from intact controls and group OPR ($P < 0.05$). (Redrawn from *[62]* with permission.)

Physiological Significance. It is likely that relaxin facilitates rapid and safe delivery in rats *(20,21,24,33)* and pigs *(22)* mainly through its dramatic effects on growth and softening of cervix. The observation that passive immunization of rats against endogenous relaxin throughout the second half of pregnancy not only inhibits growth and softening of the cervix, but also disrupts birth more profoundly than does deprivation of relaxin during the antepartum period is consistent with this view *(33)*.

Mechanism of Action. Efforts to understand mechanisms at the cellular and molecular levels whereby relaxin modifies the cervix in rats and pigs have determined relaxin's effects on the histological characteristics and biochemical composition of the cervix, identified the cervical cells that contain relaxin binding sites, and examined the roles that estrogen and progesterone play in relaxin's effects on the cervix. The findings with the two species are generally similar, and they are described together.

Relaxin plays a major role in bringing about the remodeling that occurs within the cervix during pregnancy in rats *(63)* and pigs *(64)*. Light microscopic analysis of cervices removed on d 22 from rats in which endogenous relaxin was neutralized with MAb MCA1 throughout the second half of pregnancy identified several histological characteristics that differed markedly from those of cervices removed from control rats (63). The collagen fiber bundles in MCA1-treated rats failed to disperse or to become as disorganized as did those in controls (compare Fig. 9B to 9A). Elastin fibers were more prevalent, longer, and exhibited more interdigitation in relaxin-deficient MCA1-treated rats than in controls (compare Fig. 9D to 9C). The cross-sectional areas of arteries in the MCA1-treated rats were smaller than in controls. The area of luminal involutions was smaller in MCA1-treated

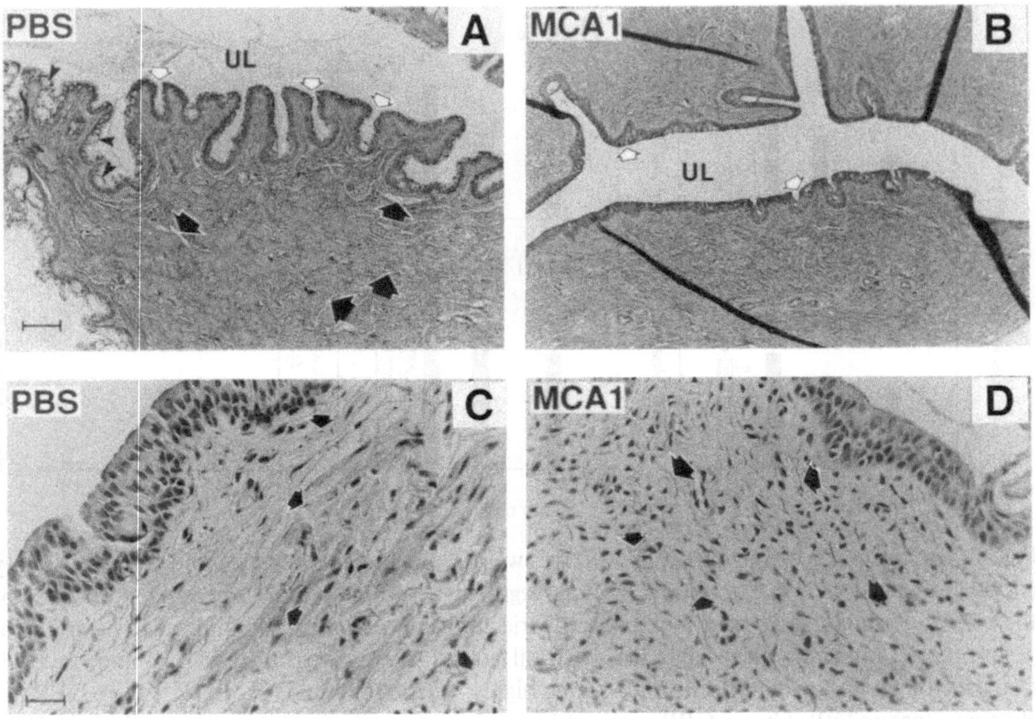

Fig. 9. The influence of neutralization of endogenous relaxin with MAb MCA1 for rat relaxin throughout the second half of pregnancy on the histological characteristics of the rat cervix on d 22 of pregnancy. Animals were injected with MCA1 and phosphate-buffered saline (PBS) as described in the legend to Fig. 4A. **(A)** PBS control. Disruption of the connective tissue matrix is indicated by many spaces between the collagen fiber bundles (large closed arrows). Note the large luminal epithelial cell involutions (open arrows) and large vacuolated epithelial cells that appear to be secreting a mucus-like material (small closed arrow heads). UL, cervical lumen. **(B)** MCA1-treated. The connective tissue matrix is more compact, the luminal epithelial cell involutions are smaller, and the epithelial cells are less vacuolated than seen in A. Bar in A = 400 μm. A and B are the same magnification. **(C)** PBS control. Note many small pieces of elastin fibers (closed arrows) and scant amount of long elastin fibers. Interdigitation of elastin fibers is not apparent. **(D)** MCA1-treated. Long strands of elastin fibers (large closed arrows) and interdigitation of elastin fibers (small closed arrows) are more numerous than in C. Bar in C = 40 μm. C and D are the same magnification. (From *[63]* with permission.)

rats than in controls. Finally, there were fewer vacuolated epithelial cells that appeared to be secreting a polysaccharide-rich material (presumably mucin) in MCA1-treated rats than in controls (compare Fig. 9B to 9A). In the pig, relaxin also brings about dispersion and disorganization of the collagen fiber bundles *(64)*.

Relaxin also plays a major role in promoting changes in the biochemical composition of the cervix that occur during late pregnancy in rats *(20,33,61)* and pigs *(65)*. Relaxin promotes increased cervical wet weight, percent hydration, dry weight, glycosaminoglycans (dermatan sulfate, heparan sulfate, hyaluronic acid) content, and DNA content. Relaxin has little, if any, effect on cervical collagen content. Therefore, the ratio of glycosaminoglycans to collagen increases in relaxin-replete rats *(61)* and pigs *(65)* during late pregnancy.

How the relaxin-dependent changes in the histological characteristics and biochemical composition contribute to the alteration in the tensile properties of the cervix remains to be established. The dispersion and reduction in organization of collagen fiber bundles may allow the fibers to be readily pulled past one another as the fetus enters the cervix during labor. It is presently not known if the elastin fibers that are prevalent in the rat cervix assist in maintaining a rigid connective tissue matrix. If that is the case, the relaxin-dependent reduction in length and interdigitation of elastin fibers may also contribute to increased cervical extensibility.

The relaxin-induced increase in glycosaminoglycans may play an important role in the alteration in the organization of collagen fibers. It was postulated that the highly hydrated hyaluronic acid may accumulate in the interstices among collagen fibrils and thereby disperse them or prevent their aggregation *(66)*. The predominant cervical proteoglycan is dermatan sulfate proteoglycan, which consists of a core protein with a mol wt of approx 50,000 and a single glycosaminoglycan chain of about the same mol wt *(65,67)*. Dermatan sulfate binds to specific sites (so-called d bands) at regular intervals along collagen fibrils in tendon and skin *(68)*. It was postulated that the increased ratio of dermatan sulfate proteoglycan to collagen in the cervix during late pregnancy may increase the coating of collagen fibrils with the dermatan sulfate proteoglycan molecules *(61,69)*. According to this hypothesis, the high charge density of the sulfated glycosaminoglycans chain causes mutual repulsion of the dermatan sulfate proteoglycan molecules, and thereby fosters increased separation and random orientation of collagen fibrils.

Relaxin-induced enlargement of the cervical arteries may contribute to the increased water content of the cervix that occurs during late pregnancy and/or migration into the cervix of nonresident cells that may contribute to remodeling of the cervix. In humans, there is evidence that cervical softening may be brought about, at least in part, by collagenolysis that is triggered by collagenase released from polymorphonuclear leukocytes that migrate into the cervix at term *(70,71)*. There is currently no evidence that nonresident cells contribute to cervical softening in rats and pigs. The enlarged luminal involutions that occur in the rat may provide sufficient luminal surface area to enable expansion of the cervix to a circumference required for rapid and safe delivery of the fetuses.

A fundamental step toward an understanding of the mechanism(s) whereby relaxin initiates growth and softening of the cervix is to identify the target cells for relaxin in the cervix. In the mid-1990s, biotinylated porcine relaxin was employed with an immunohistochemical procedure at the light microscope level to identify cells that contain relaxin receptors in the rat *(52)* and pig *(53)* cervix. In both species, specific and saturable binding was associated with the epithelial cells that line the cervical lumen as well as with circular smooth muscle cells, longitudinal smooth muscle cells, and cells associated with blood vessels (Fig. 10). Whereas specific binding of the biotinylated relaxin also appeared to be associated with fibroblasts and perhaps other cell types within the cervical stroma, examination of the binding of biotinylated relaxin at the electron microscope level is required to be certain that is the case. The molecular events triggered by relaxin binding are unknown. The observation that relaxin receptors are associated with several cell types can be interpreted to suggest that relaxin's dramatic effects on growth and softening of the cervix are attributable to multiple paracrine interactions between cells and the extracellular matrix.

A comprehensive understanding of hormonal control of cervical growth and softening requires knowledge of the effects of estrogen and progesterone as well as those of relaxin. It is known that estrogen independently promotes growth of the cervix in rats *(54,58)* and pigs *(72)*, but has little, if any effect on the extensibility of the cervix in the two species *(54, 58,72,73)*. Progesterone alone does not promote growth of the cervix in rats *(54,58)* or pigs *(72)*, and has little effect on cervical softening in the two species *(54,58,72)*. The combined

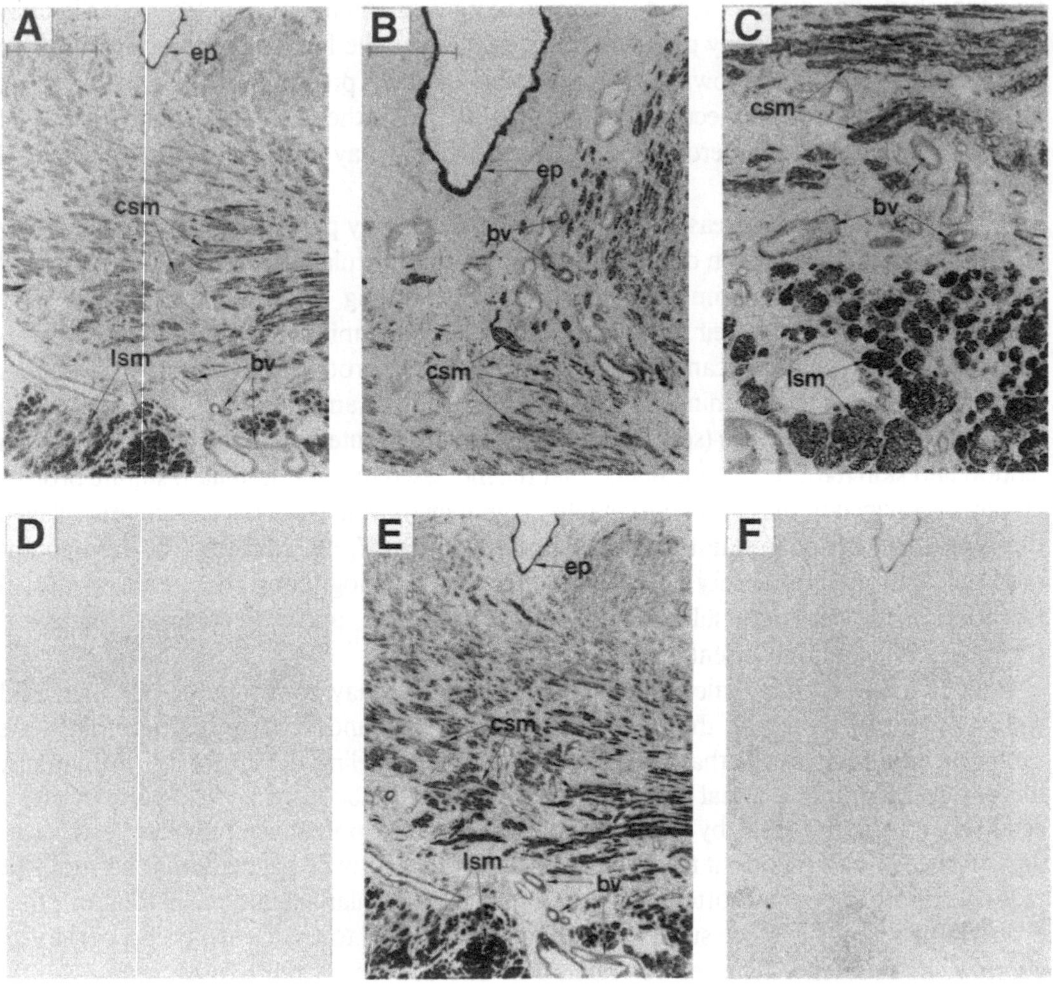

Fig. 10. Localization of relaxin binding sites in the cervix of a d 110 intact pregnant pig. Relaxin binding was localized in cervices incubated with biotinylated relaxin (**A–C; B** and **C** are a higher magnification of luminal and peripheral areas of A, respectively), but not in cervices incubated with unmodified porcine relaxin (**D**). Tissue sections incubated with biotinylated relaxin showed binding in the presence of a 2000-fold excess of porcine insulin (**E**), but not in the presence of a 2000-fold excess of porcine relaxin (**F**). lsm, longitudinal smooth muscle; csm, circular smooth muscle; bv, blood vessels; ep, epithelial cells. Bar in A = 1970 μm and panels A and D–F are the same magnification. Bar in B = 493 μm and panels B and C are the same magnification. (From *[53]* with permission.)

effects of relaxin, estrogen, and progesterone on the cervix have received little experimental attention. Relaxin's effects on the cervix are estrogen-dependent in the rat *(54,58)*, but not in pigs *(72,73)*. Whether estrogen augments relaxin's effects on growth and softening of the cervix in the pig *(72,73)* as it does in the rat *(54)* remains unresolved. Whereas there are data supporting the view that progesterone augments relaxin's effects on cervical softening in the rat *(60)* and pig *(72)*, not all findings support this view *(54,58,73)*.

Effects of Relaxin on the Vagina

In 1987, Vasilenko and Mead *(74)* reported that 6 h following a single sc injection of porcine relaxin into ovariectomized and estrogen-pretreated nonpregnant rats, the vaginal

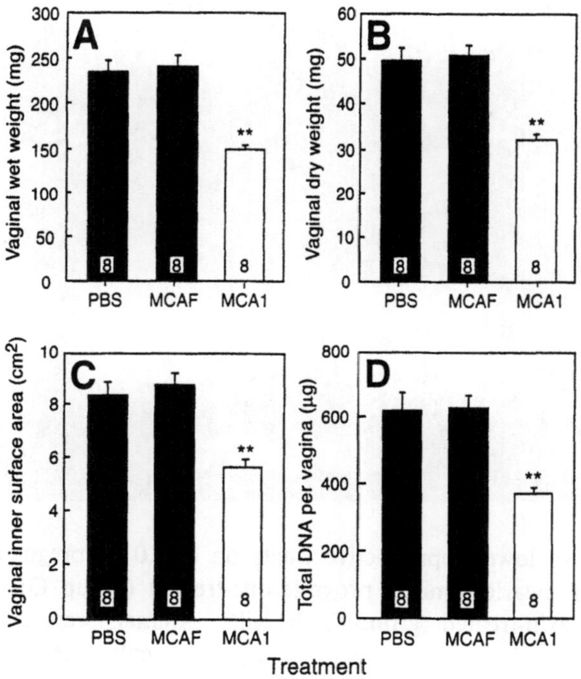

Fig. 11. The influence of neutralization of endogenous rat relaxin with MAb MCA1 throughout the second half of pregnancy on the (**A**) wet weight, (**B**) dry weight, (**C**) inner surface area, and (**D**) DNA content of vaginas removed on d 22 of pregnancy. The rats were administered MCA1, MCAF, and PBS daily as described in the legend to Fig. 4A. Means (+ SE) are for 8 rats/group. Asterisks indicate a significant difference from controls ($P < 0.01$). (Redrawn from *[75]* with permission.)

wet weight, dry weight, percent hydration, total protein, and total glycogen were increased. In the mid-1990s, studies were conducted to determine if endogenous relaxin promotes growth of the vagina in pregnant rats and pigs.

Rat. Both rats that were ovariectomized on d 9 and given hormone replacement therapy throughout the second half of pregnancy *(20)*, and intact rats that were administered MAb MCA1 for rat relaxin throughout the second half of pregnancy *(75)* were used to establish that endogenous relaxin plays a major role in promoting growth of the vagina during pregnancy (Fig. 11). The vaginal wet weight, dry weight, inner surface area, and DNA content in relaxin-deficient MCA1-treated rats were significantly lower than those of vehicle- and MAb-treated controls.

Pig. Relaxin also promotes growth of the vagina in pregnant pigs. When pigs were ovariectomized on d 40 of pregnancy and given hormone replacement throughout the remainder of pregnancy as described in the legend to Fig. 4B, the wet weights of vaginas removed on d 110 of pregnancy from ovariectomized pigs given progesterone only were approx 70% of both intact controls and ovariectomized pigs treated with progesterone plus relaxin *(49)*. The influence of relaxin deprivation throughout the last 70 d of gestation on the size of the lower reproductive tract in the pig is shown in Fig. 12.

Physiological Significance. The physiological significance of relaxin's effects on the vagina in rats and pigs cannot be readily differentiated experimentally from relaxin's effects on the cervix. Nevertheless, it seems reasonable to postulate that relaxin-induced growth of the vagina contributes to rapid and safe delivery of the fetuses *(20–22,24)*.

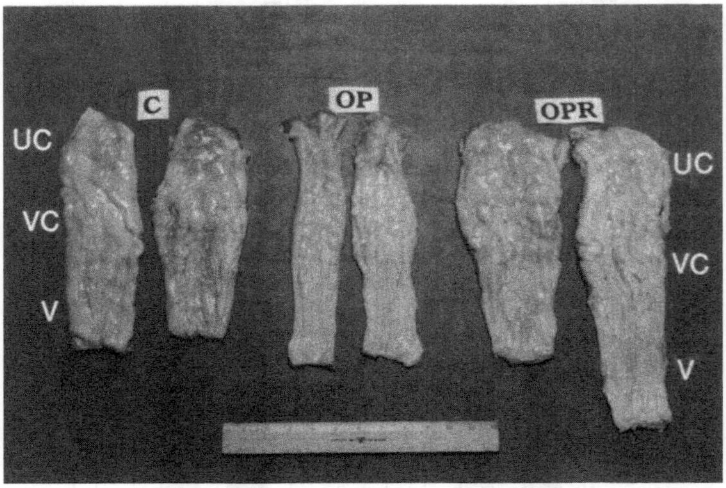

Fig. 12. Representative lower reproductive tracts on d 110 of pregnancy from sham-ovariectomized (group C), ovariectomized progesterone-treated (group OP), and ovariectomized progesterone plus relaxin-treated (group OPR) gilts. Animals were sham-ovariectomized or ovariectomized on d 40 of gestation and given hormone replacement therapy as described in the legend to Fig. 4B. uc, uterine cervix; vc, vaginal cervix; v, vagina. (From *[49]* with permission.)

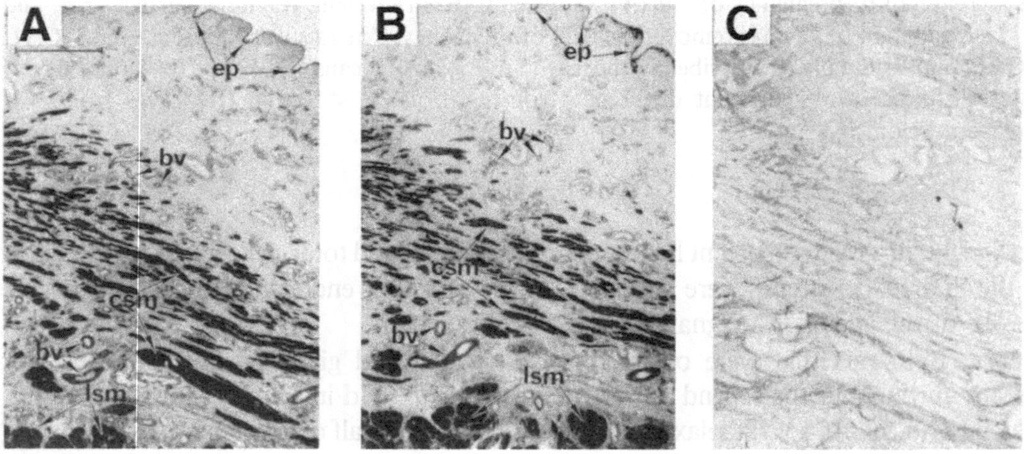

Fig. 13. Localization of relaxin binding sites in the vagina of a d 110 pregnant pig. Relaxin binding was observed in vaginas incubated with biotinylated relaxin (**A**). Tissue sections incubated with biotinylated relaxin showed binding in the presence of a 2000-fold excess of porcine insulin (**B**), but not in the presence of a 2000-fold excess of porcine relaxin (**C**). lsm, longitudinal smooth muscle; csm, circular smooth muscle; bv, blood vessels; ep, epithelial cells; Bar in A = 1987 μm. All panels are the same magnification. (From *[49]* with permission.)

Mechanism of Action. Little is known concerning the mechanism of action of relaxin on the vagina. It seems likely that relaxin initiates its effects by acting directly on the vagina. Specific and saturable relaxin binding sites were found associated with luminal epithelial cells, circular and longitudinal smooth muscle cells, and cells associated with blood vessels within the rat vagina as well as the pig vagina (Fig. 13). The extent to which relaxin interacts with estrogen and/or progesterone, if any, to bring about its effects on the vagina in rats and pigs has not been examined.

EFFECTS OF RELAXIN ON MAMMARY APPARATUS

Sporadic reports that porcine relaxin administration promotes lobulo-alveolar growth in rats *(2)* began with a publication by Hamolsky and Sparrow in 1945 *(76)*. These infrequent and inconsistant studies triggered efforts in the early 1990s aimed at determining if endogenous relaxin plays a role in promoting the development of the mammary glands in pregnant rats and pigs.

Effects of Relaxin on Mammary Glands

RAT. Relaxin has little, if any, effect on the growth of the mammary glands in pregnant rats. When endogenous relaxin was neutralized with MAb MCA1 throughout the second half of pregnancy, the wet weights of mammary glands removed on d 22 did not differ from those of controls *(77)*. Nevertheless, the histological characteristics of mammary glands in the relaxin-deficient MCA1-treated rats differed from those in controls; that is, the collagen fiber bundles were more compact and elastin fibers exhibited greater density, length, and interdigitation. Additionally, the number of alveoli within connective tissue surrounding lactiferous ducts in mammary glands was smaller in MCA1-treated rats than in controls *(77)*.

PIG. As with cervical growth and softening, mammary lobulo-alveolar development begins at about d 80 of pregnancy in primiparous gilts *(78)*. Hurley et al. *(79)* discovered that relaxin plays a major role in promoting mammary gland parenchyma development in the pregnant pig. When gilts were ovariectomized on d 100 and given progesterone only, development of mammary parenchyma was markedly lower than in intact controls *(79)*. In contrast, when replacement therapy included relaxin, the mammary parenchyma appeared as well developed as that in intact controls (Fig. 14).

PHYSIOLOGICAL SIGNIFICANCE. The physiological significance of relaxin's effects on the mammary glands in rats and pigs remains to be established. Whereas it might be presumed that the marked relaxin-dependent growth of the mammary parenchyma that occurs during late pregnancy in pigs is necessary for normal lactational performance, a recent study *(80)* indicates that may not be the case. Gilts were ovariectomized on d 100 and given hormone replacement therapy with progesterone to maintain pregnancy until d 113, when they were delivered by cesarean section and given colostrum-replete foster litters (born of untreated mothers) to nurse from d 1 to d 28 of lactation. In spite of the fact that prepartum mammary development was negligible in the relaxin-deficient gilts as compared to sham ovariectomized controls, stimulation of the nipples by the nursing piglets overcame the relaxin-dependent deficiency. There was no effect of treatment on average piglet weight, time piglets spent on udder, piglet mortality, and mammary cross-sectional area on d 28 of lactation. Nevertheless, this study *(80)* does not rule out the possibility that relaxin-dependent prepartum growth of the mammary glands is essential for normal lactational performance in gilts. Since the piglets had access to colostrum from their own dams, who delivered naturally before being fostered onto experimental sows, the study did not allow for an assessment of treatment effects on colostrum availability.

Mechanism of Action. There is good evidence that relaxin initiates its effects by acting directly on the mammary glands in both rats and pigs. Specific and saturable relaxin binding sites were localized in epithelial cells in both lactiferous ducts and lobulo-alveolar structures as well as in cells associated with blood vessels *(52,53)*. There is evidence that the relaxin binding sites are functional relaxin receptors. When a dose of relaxin too low to elevate relaxin levels in the peripheral blood was infused into one mammary gland, only

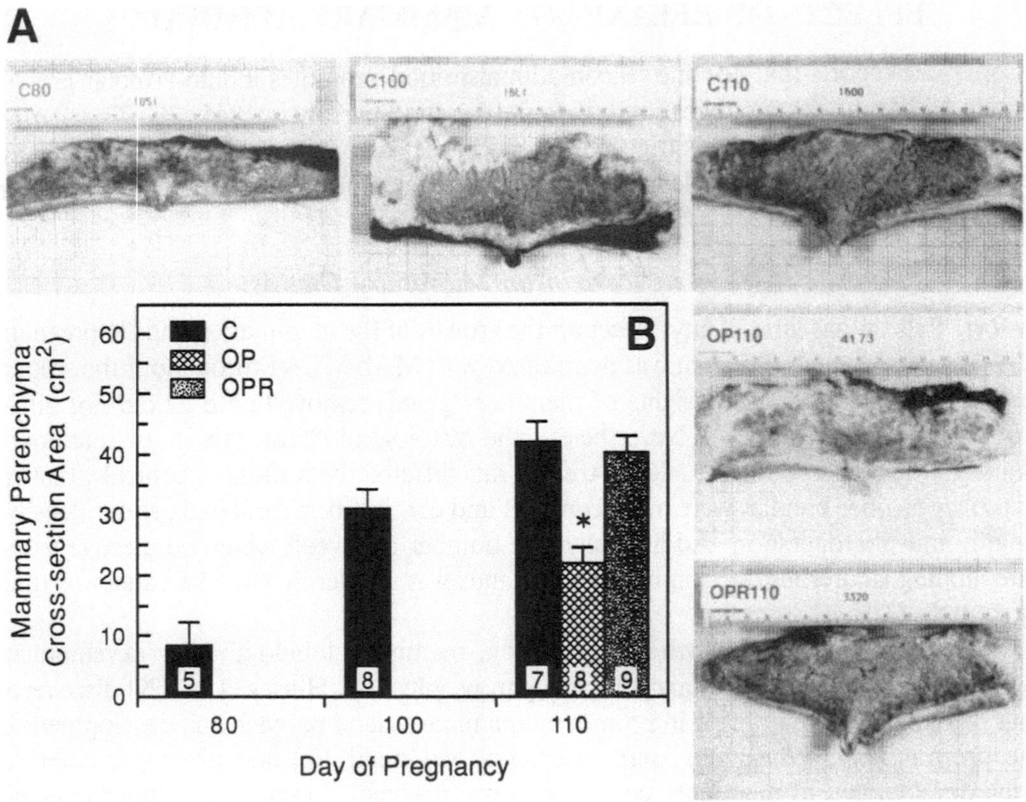

Fig. 14. (A) Photographs of transverse cross-sections of mammary glands from gilts during late gestation. Representative mammary glands are from intact control gilts on d 80 (C80), 100 (C100), and d 110 (C110); ovariectomized progesterone-treated gilts on d 110 (OP110), and ovariectomized progesterone plus relaxin-treated gilts on d 110 (OPR110). Sham surgery or bilateral ovariectomy was performed on d 100 of gestation. Ovariectomized gilts were treated with either progesterone (50 mg intramuscularly in 2 mL corn oil at 12-h intervals) or with progesterone plus highly purified porcine relaxin (*16*; 1 mg intramuscularly in 2 mL physiological saline at 6-h intervals) from d 100–110 of pregnancy. (**B**) Mean (+ SE) cross-section areas of mammary parenchymal tissue from the five groups of gilts in (**A**). The number of animals is given at the base of each bar. Asterisk indicates significant difference from groups C110 and OPR110 ($P < 0.05$). (Redrawn from *[79]* with permission.)

local mammary lobule-alveolar development occurred *(53a)*. Recently, the influence of relaxin, estrogen, and progesterone on mammary parenchyma development was examined, individually and in combination, in ovariectomized sexually mature, nonpregnant gilts *(81)*. Relaxin alone had little effect on mammary development, and estrogen alone stimulated mammary development only modestly. Combined treatment with relaxin and estrogen, however, stimulated mammary development markedly. Progesterone alone had no effect on lobulo-alveolar development. As in the pig cervix, combined treatment with relaxin and progesterone reduced the organization of the collagen fibers within the stroma *(81)*.

Effects of Relaxin on Mammary Nipples

Rat. Hwang et al. *(77)* discovered that relaxin plays a major role in promoting the development of the mammary nipples in rats. Development of the mammary nipples

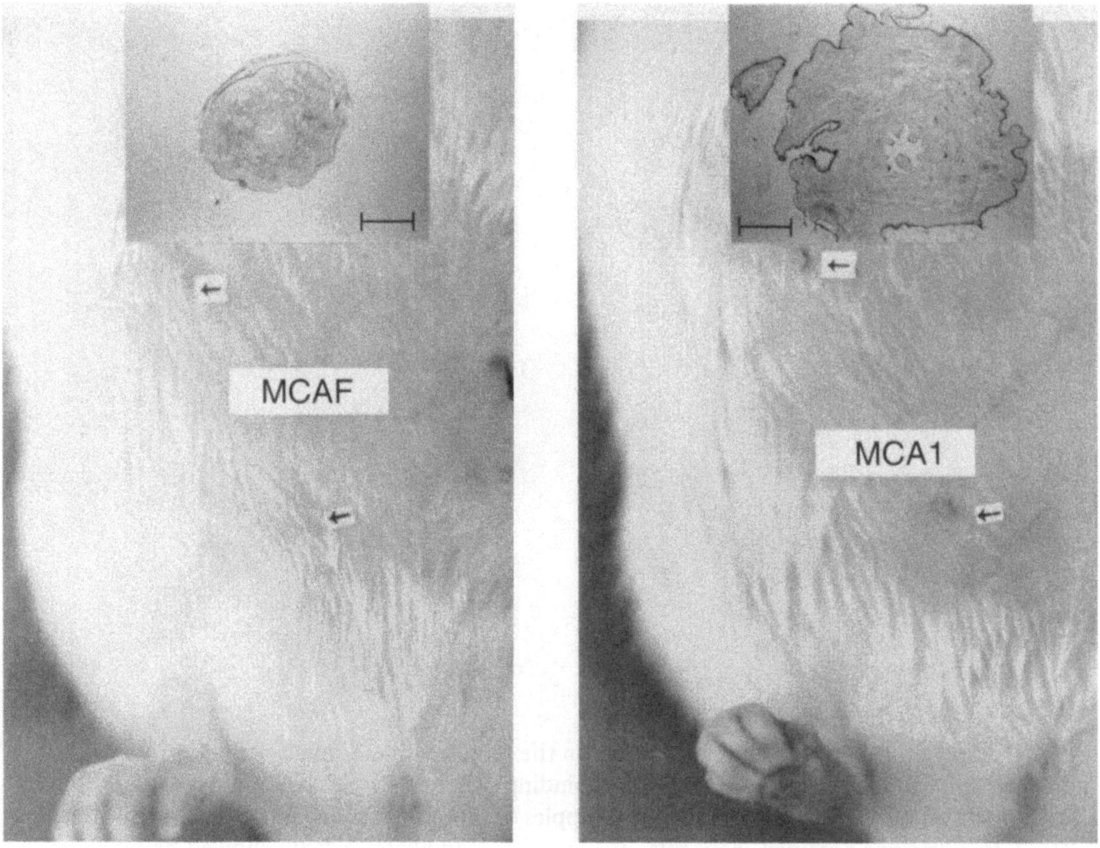

Fig. 15. Representative photographs of nipples (arrows) of d 22 pregnant rats following the administration of 5 mg of MAb for rat relaxin (MCA1) or 5 mg of MAb for fluorescein (MCAF antibody control) from d 12–22. Animals were treated as described in the legend to Fig. 4A. Insets show cross-sections of the midpoint of nipples. Bar = 300 μm. (From *[82]* with permission.)

nearly fails to occur in rats when relaxin is neutralized with MAb MCA1 throughout the second half of pregnancy (*77,82*; Fig. 15).

Pig. There is evidence *(53a)* that relaxin contributes to the development of the nipples of primiparous pigs. Nipple development is less dependent on relaxin in pregnant pigs *(53a, 79,80)*, however, than it is in pregnant rats *(77,82)*.

Physiological Significance. In rats, relaxin-dependent growth of the mammary nipples is vital. The nipples are so small at term in relaxin-deficient dams that pups cannot attach to them. As a consequence, the pups fail to obtain milk, stimulate prolactin release, and stimulate postpartum mammary gland development *(77,82)*.

Unlike rats, the nipples of relaxin-deficient gilts are moderately well developed near term *(79,80)*. Therefore, the comparatively modest relaxin-dependent portion of the growth of the nipples that occurs during pregnancy in primiparous pigs is not required for normal lactational performance. Piglets were readily able to grasp the nipples, obtain adequate milk, and stimulate postpartum mammary gland development when fostered to ovariectomized gilts that were relaxin-deficient during late pregnancy *(80)*.

Mechanism of Action. The initial effort to understand the mechanism(s) whereby relaxin brings about its striking effect on nipple development in pregnant rats examined

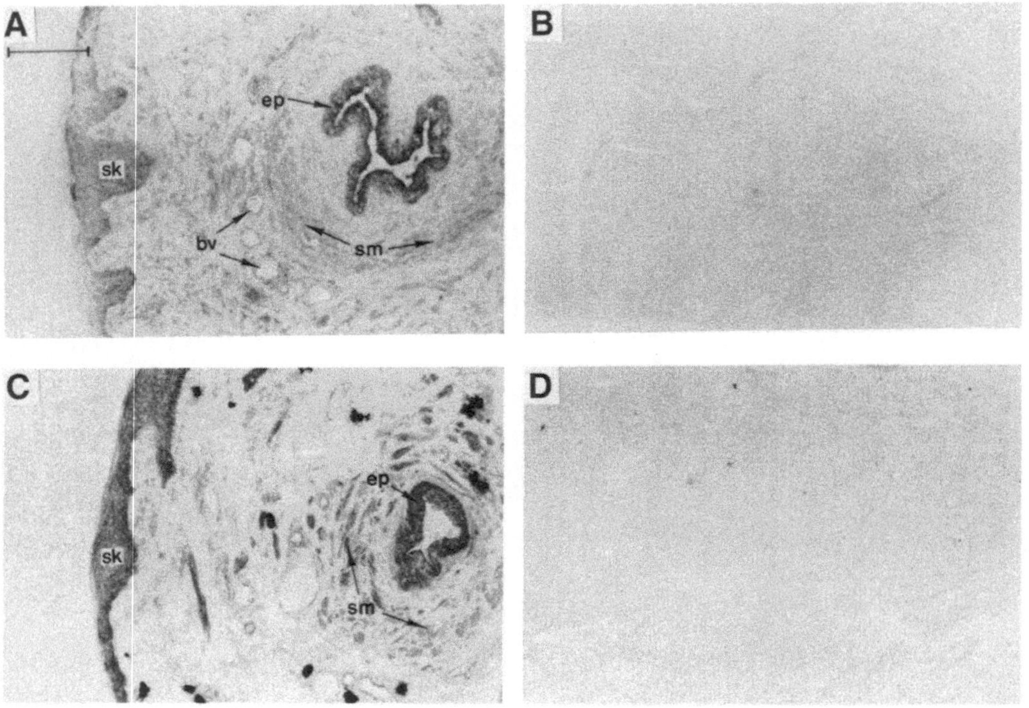

Fig. 16. Localization of relaxin binding sites in the nipples of d 18 intact pregnant rats 1 h after the injection of biotinylated relaxin. Relaxin binding was localized in the nipples of rats administered biotinylated relaxin (**A**), but not in the nipples of rats administered unlabeled porcine relaxin (**B**). Tissue sections obtained from rats injected with biotinylated relaxin showed binding in the presence of a 500-fold excess of porcine insulin (**C**), but not in the presence of a 500-fold excess of porcine relaxin (**D**). sm, smooth muscle; ep, epithelial cells; bv, blood vessels; sk, skin. Bar in A = 444 μm. All panels are the same magnification. (From *[52]* with permission.)

the influence of neutralization of endogenous relaxin with MAb MCA1 on the histology of the nipple *(82)*. Relaxin promotes modifications that are similar to its effects on the histological characteristics of the mammary glands and cervix; namely, collagen fibers become dispersed, elastin fibers become short, and the cross-sectional area of blood vessels increases. There is strong evidence that relaxin promotes nipple development through direct actions on the nipples in rats *(52,83)* and pigs *(49)*. Specific and saturable binding of biotinylated relaxin was localized in the lactiferous duct epithelial cells, smooth muscle cells, cells associated with blood vessels, and skin of nipples obtained from intact rats and pigs during late pregnancy (Fig. 16). Additionally, subcutaneous administration of a low dose of porcine relaxin at the base of the left abdominal nipple of ovariectomized nonpregnant rats for 5 d promoted significant growth of that nipple relative to its right counterpart (Fig. 17).

Little is known concerning the roles that estrogen and progesterone play in nipple development during pregnancy in rats and pigs. One study of the combined effects of relaxin and estrogen was conducted in nonpregnant rats *(83)*. Whereas estrogen is required for relaxin's effects on growth of the rat cervix, relaxin-induced growth of the rat mammary nipples occurs in the absence of estrogen priming (Fig. 17).

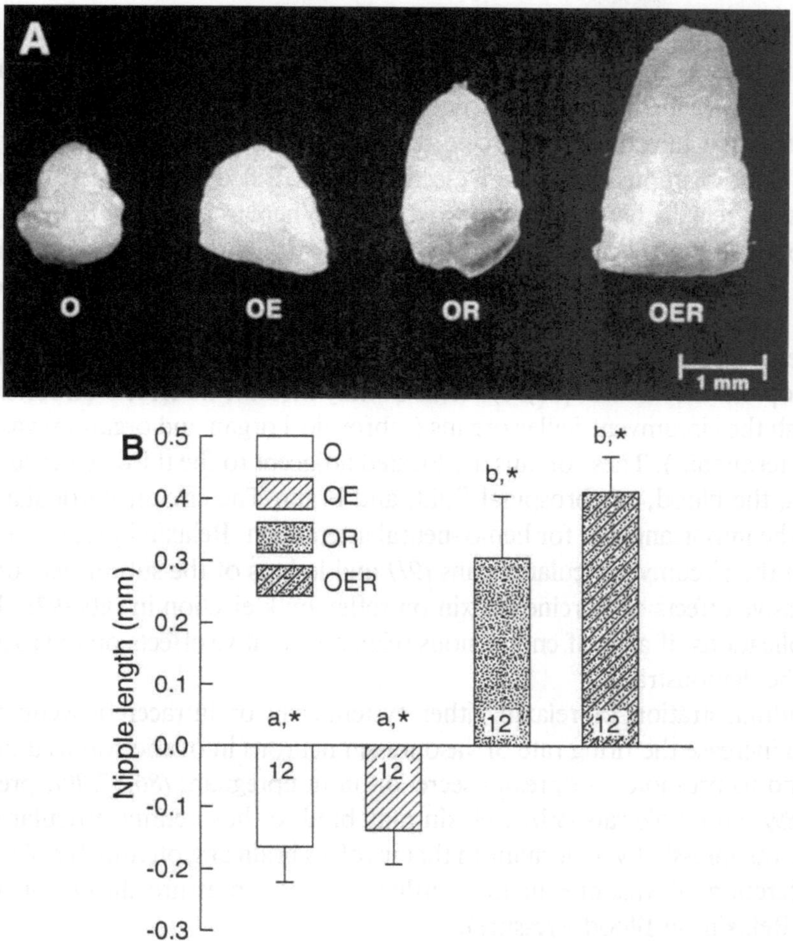

Fig. 17. Influence of local administration of relaxin on mammary nipple development in rats. Ninety-day-old nonpregnant rats were ovariectomized (d 0) and received either one daily 0.1 mL sc injection of the estrogen vehicle corn oil (groups O and OR) or 0.05 μg 17 β-estradiol (groups OE and OER) from d 6–16 postsurgery. Rats were injected with either the relaxin vehicle 0.05 mL 5% beeswax in corn oil (groups O and OE) or 12.5 μg porcine relaxin (*16*; groups OR and OER) at the base of the left abdominal nipple from d 11–16 postsurgery. **(A)** Photomicrographs of representative left abdominal nipples removed on d 16 postsurgery from rats in groups O, OE, OR, and OER. **(B)** Mean (± SE) differences in the lengths of the left (treated) vs the right (untreated) abdominal nipples within the same animal. Twelve rats were used in each group. Groups significantly different from one another are indicated with different superscript letters ($P < 0.05$). Differences in lengths that were significantly different from zero are indicated with an asterisk ($P < 0.05$). Because of tissue damage, local injections of relaxin vehicle, with or without estrogen treatment (groups O and OE), resulted in significantly smaller left (relaxin vehicle-treated) than right (untreated) controls. (Redrawn from *[83]* with permission.)

ADDITIONAL EFFECTS OF CIRCULATING RELAXIN

Beginning in the mid-1980s, effects of highly purified relaxin on the brain, cardiovascular system, skin, and intestine were reported. Since most of these effects were identified in the rat employing experimental conditions that do not enable conclusions concerning their existence or physiological importance during pregnancy, they are mentioned briefly here.

Central Effects of Relaxin

Effect of Relaxin on Oxytocin and Vasopressin Secretion. In 1984, Summerlee and coworkers *(84)* provided the first evidence that relaxin may have effects on the brain when they reported that injections of porcine relaxin into either the cerebral ventricles or the peripheral blood disrupted reflex milk ejection in rats. Since then, numerous putative central effects of relaxin have been reported *(85)*. Whereas it was initially reported that relaxin suppressed reflex milk ejection by acting centrally to suppress oxytocin secretion *(85)*, more recent studies provide evidence that relaxin increases the firing rate of oxytocin neurons in lactating rats *(86)* and increases the secretion of oxytocin in rats *(86–89)*. There is limited evidence that relaxin may suppress reflex milk ejection by activating a central inhibitory opioid mechanism *(88,90)*. Relaxin may mediate its effects on reflex milk ejection through the circumventricular organs (subfornical organ and organum vasculosum of the lamina terminalis). These organs are located adjacent to the third ventricle at the interface among the blood, cerebrospinal fluid, and brain. The circumventricular organs are thought to be important sites for hemo–neural interaction. Relaxin binding sites have been localized in the circumventricular organs *(91)* and lesions of the subfornical organ negate the suppressive effects of porcine relaxin on reflex milk ejection in rats *(92)*. The physiological implications, if any, of endogenous relaxin's putative effects on oxytocin secretion remain to be demonstrated.

Acute administration of relaxin either systemically or intracerebroventricularly was reported to increase the firing rate of vasopressin neurons in ovariectomized nonpregnant rats *(86)* and to promote vasopressin secretion in nonpregnant *(86,87,89)*, pregnant *(89)*, lactating *(89)*, and male rats *(93)*. Relaxin may bind to the circumventricular organs *(91)* and release vasopressin by a mechanism that involves brain angiotensin-II *(87,94)*. Relaxin-induced secretion of vasopressin may influence blood pressure during pregnancy (*see* Effects of Relaxin on Blood Pressure).

Effect of Relaxin on Drinking. During the second half of rat pregnancy, the increase in daily water consumption is temporally closely correlated with elevated serum relaxin levels *(7,31)*. Two experimental approaches provided evidence that this increase in water consumption is mediated in part by relaxin. Intracerebroventricular administration of porcine relaxin prompted a dramatic dipsogenic effect in female and male rats *(95,96)*. Furthermore, rats in which endogenous relaxin was neutralized with MAb MCA1 throughout the second half of pregnancy consumed less water than did relaxin-replete controls *(31)*. The dipsogenic effect of relaxin along with its capacity to promote vasopressin secretion has been postulated to account for the increase in blood volume, decrease in plasma osmolality, and increase in circulating concentrations of plasma vasopressin that occur during rat pregnancy *(95,97)*. The central dipsogenic effect of relaxin appears to be mediated by the central angiotensin system *(95)*.

Effect of Relaxin on Prolactin, Growth Hormone, and Lutenizing Hormone Secretion. Human and porcine relaxin were reported to stimulate the secretion of prolactin in anterior pituitary cell cultures obtained from the rat *(98)* and the pig *(99)*, respectively. Intravenous infusion of human relaxin in rhesus monkeys during the midluteal phase of the menstrual cycle reportedly stimulated both prolactin and growth hormone secretion *(100)*, and intracerebroventricular administration of porcine relaxin in hysterectomized pigs stimulated prolactin secretion *(101)*. Whereas acute iv administration of porcine relaxin reduced the frequency of LH pulses in ovariectomized rats, it stimulated LH secretion when the animals were pretreated with estrogen and progesterone *(102)*. In contrast, relaxin failed to influence LH secretion in midluteal phase monkeys *(100)* or from rat *(98)* and pig *(99)* pituitary cells in culture. The physiological implication, if any, of endogenous relaxin's putative effects on prolactin, growth hormone, and luteinizing hormone secretion remains to be demonstrated.

Effects of Relaxin on the Cardiovascular System

Effects of Relaxin on Blood Pressure. Injection of porcine relaxin either intravenously *(87,89,93,94,103)* or intracerebroventricularly *(93,94)* increased systemic arterial blood pressure in anesthetized *(87,89,94,103)* and unanesthetized *(93)* rats. Elevated serum vasopressin levels may be responsible because administration of a vasopressin (V1) receptor antagonist before relaxin treatment markedly attenuated relaxin-induced elevation of blood pressure *(93,94,103)*.

Presently, reports concerning the influence of relaxin on blood pressure during pregnancy are not consistent. The fall in systolic blood pressure near term in relaxin-deficient ovariectomized normotensive Wistar-Kyoto rats was greater than in sham-operated controls *(104)*, and this finding can be interpreted to indicate that endogenous relaxin has a pressor effect during late pregnancy. The injection of synthetic human relaxin into intact normotensive pregnant Sprague-Dawley rats, however, did not influence arterial pressure *(105)*.

Effects of Relaxin on Heart Contractility. Human relaxin bound with specificity to the atrium in female and male rat hearts *(106)* and brought about dose-dependent and marked increases in both the rate of contraction of the right atrium and the force of electrically stimulated contractions of the left atrium in vitro *(107,108)*. Increased heart rate followed acute iv administration of both porcine relaxin *(103)* and human relaxin *(93)* to nonpregnant rats. Also, sc infusion of human relaxin for 1 or 2 wk increased heart rate in nonpregnant female rats *(108)*. One report indicated that iv injection of human relaxin to intact rats on d 19 of pregnancy did not influence heart rate *(105)*. Administration of relaxin intracerebroventricularly provided limited evidence that relaxin may also act centrally to influence heart rate *(93)*. It was reported that relaxin increases heart rate by modulating calcium current in rabbit cardiac pacemaker cells via a cAMP-dependent mechanism *(109)*.

Effects of Relaxin on Blood Vessel Dilation. Relaxin has marked dilatory effects on the microvessels of the rat mesocecum *(110)*, mouse mammary gland *(111)*, rat cervix *(63)*, and rat mammary nipples *(82)*. Relaxin was reported to increase coronary blood flow in isolated rat and guinea pig hearts through stimulation of nitric oxide production *(112)*. Relaxin may dilate blood vessels by directly inhibiting the contraction of smooth muscle cells that surround blood vessels *(33)*.

Effects of Relaxin on Blood Platelets. Porcine relaxin was reported to depress aggregation of isolated human and rabbit platelets in vitro through a mechanism that involved stimulation of nitric oxide *(113)*. Furthermore, the administration of porcine relaxin to rats reduced the number of circulating platelets and their release from spleen megakaryocytes *(114)*.

Effect of Relaxin on the Integumentary System

Both local intradermal injection *(115)* and subcutaneous systemic infusion *(116)* of porcine relaxin increased skin expansion in pigs. Also, sc systemic infusion of human relaxin decreased collagen accumulation in two rodent models of fibrosis *(117)*, and human relaxin downregulated collagen synthesis in human normal dermal fibroblasts *(118)* and scleroderma fibroblasts *(119)* in vitro. Specific and saturable relaxin binding sites were demonstrated in the skin of rats *(52)* and pigs *(53)*.

Effects of Relaxin on Intestine Contractility

In 1991 Del-Angel-Meza et al. reported that rat relaxin reduces both the amplitude and frequency of rat small intestine spontaneous contractility both in vitro and in vivo *(120)*. Consistent with this discovery, porcine relaxin inhibited the amplitude of pig small intestine spontaneous contractility in vitro, and specific and saturable relaxin binding sites were found associated with longitudinal and circular smooth muscle cells as well as muscularis mucosa of pig small intestine (Min and Sherwood, unpublished).

PARACRINE EFFECTS OF UTERINE RELAXIN

The pig endometrium produces relaxin during early pregnancy. It was postulated that this relaxin, which is localized in greatest quantities in luminal epithelial cells on about d 16, may play a local role in stimulating uterine growth and function at implantation *(121)*. There may also be local roles for uterine relaxin during late pregnancy. Relaxin immunostaining is present in uterine endometrial epithelial cells during the second half of pregnancy in rats *(122)*. In pregnant humans, low amounts of relaxin are produced in the maternal decidual cells and placenta *(123)*. It was postulated *(124)* that through its effects on the extracellular matrix, decidual and/or placental relaxin assists with the rupture of fetal membranes at term. Several observations are consistent with that possibility. The addition of human relaxin to human chorioamnionic membranes reduced their tensile strength and elastic modulis in vitro *(125)*. Also, the secretion of plasminogen activator and collagenase into the medium increased when porcine relaxin was added to cultures of human amnion and chorion cells *(124)*. Finally, expression of the relaxin gene as well as genes for several matrix metalloproteinase enzymes that degrade the extracellular matrix components collagen, proteoglycans, fibronectin, and laminin were elevated in human chorion-decidua near term *(126)*.

CONCLUSIONS

Studies conducted since the early 1980s have established that endogenous relaxin has vital physiological roles during pregnancy in rats and pigs. In both species, relaxin promotes growth and softening of the cervix, and thereby facilitates rapid and safe delivery. Relaxin also promotes growth of the mammary nipples in both species, and relaxin-dependent nipple growth is required for normal lactational performance in rats. Studies in the mid-1990s demonstarted that endogenous relaxin has additional effects on the reproductive tract during pregnancy in pigs and rats. In pigs, relaxin promotes growth of the uterus and vagina, and in rats relaxin promotes growth of the vagina. There are also striking differences in the physiological effects of endogenous relaxin between rats and pigs. Endogenous relaxin promotes marked growth of the uterus and mammary glands in pigs, but not in rats. Whereas it seems likely that endogenous relaxin has vital physiological effects during pregnancy in additional mammalian species, the extraordinary variation in relaxin's effects on the reproductive system among species *(2)* makes extrapolation of findings in rats and pigs to other species inadvisable. The physiological role(s) of relaxin during pregnancy must be determined experimentally for each species of interest.

It is now well established that relaxin administration induces diverse physiological effects on organs and tissues other than those of the reproductive tract and mammary apparatus. To date, however, it remains to be demonstrated that endogenous relaxin's putative effects on sites, such as the brain, heart, blood vessels, skin, and intestine, are of physiological importance.

Other fundamental questions concerning the physiological role(s) of relaxin during pregnancy remain to be answered. Is the restraint of spontaneous myometrial contractility by endogenous relaxin of physiological importance during pregnancy? What is the physiological role of the apparent small quantities of relaxin produced in the uterine endometrium during pregnancy in rats and pigs? Both the similarity of relaxin's effects on histological characteristics of the cervix and mammary nipples in pregnant rats and pigs and the similarity of the cell types that bind relaxin in reproductive tissues in these two species indicate that relaxin may bring about its effects in different target tissues by similar molecular mechanisms. What are those molecular mechanisms? In conclusion, studies during the past 15 years pushed ajar the door to an understanding of the physiological roles of relaxin to reveal that the hormone is vital and has diverse effects. Nevertheless, we remain at the threshold in our endeavors to understand this fascinating hormone.

ACKNOWLEDGMENTS

I thank the College of Medicine Word Processing Center for typing this manuscript and the School of Life Sciences Artist Service for help in preparing the graphics. L. Burger, G. Min, and S. Zhao are also thanked for reading the manuscript and providing helpful advice for its improvement.

REFERENCES

1. Hisaw, FL (1926) Experimental relaxation of the pubic ligament of the guinea pig. Proc Soc Exp Biol Med 23:661–663.
2. Sherwood, OD (1994) Relaxin, In: The Physiology of Reproduction, second ed. (Knobil E, Neill JD, eds.), Raven, New York, pp. 861–1009.
3. John MJ, Borjesson BW, Walsh JR, Niall HD (1981) Limited sequence homology between porcine and rat relaxins: implications for physiological studies. Endocrinology 108:726–729.
4. Schwabe C, McDonald JK, Steinetz BG (1976) Primary structure of the A chain of porcine relaxin. Biochem Biophys Res Commun 70:397–405.
5. Schwabe C, McDonald JK, Steinetz BG (1977) Primary structure of the B chain of porcine relaxin. Biochem Biophys Res Commun 75:503–510.
6. Hudson P, Haley J, John M, Cronk M, Crawford R, Haralambidis J, Tregear G, Shine J, Niall H (1983) Structure of a genomic clone encoding biologically active human relaxin. Nature 301: 628–631.
7. Sherwood OD, Crnekovic VE, Gordon WL, Rutherford JE (1980) Radioimmunoassay of relaxin throughout pregnancy and during parturition in the rat. Endocrinology 107:691–698.
8. Pepe GJ, Rothchild I (1974) A comparative study of serum progesterone levels in pregnancy and in various types of pseudopregnancy in the rat. Endocrinology 95:275–279.
9. Taya K, Greenwald GS (1981) *In vivo* and *in vitro* ovarian steroidogenesis in the pregnant rat. Biol Reprod 25:683–691.
10. Anderson LL, Ford JJ, Melampy RM, Cox DF (1973) Relaxin in porcine corpora lutea during pregnancy and after hysterectomy. Am J Physiol 225:1215–1219.
11. Eldridge-White R, Easter RA, Heaton DM, O'Day MB, Petersen GC, Shanks RD, Tarbell MK, Sherwood OD (1989) Hormonal control of the cervix in pregnant gilts. I. Changes in the physical properties of the cervix correlate temporally with elevated serum levels of estrogen and relaxin. Endocrinology 125:2996–3003.

12. Anderson LL, Adair V, Stromer MH, McDonald WG (1983) Relaxin production and release after hysterectomy in the pig. Endocrinology 113:677–686.
13. Golos TG, Sherwood OD (1982) Control of corpus luteum function during the second half of pregnancy in the rat: a direct relationship between conceptus number and both serum and ovarian relaxin levels. Endocrinology 111:872–878.
14. Lao Guico MS, Sherwood OD (1985) Effect of oestradiol-17β on ovarian and serum concentrations of relaxin during the second half of pregnancy in the rat. J Reprod Fertil 74:65–70.
15. First NL, Bosc MJ (1979) Proposed mechanisms controlling parturition and the induction of parturition in swine. J Anim Sci 48:1407–1421.
16. Sherwood OD, O'Byrne EM (1974) Purification and characterization of porcine relaxin. Arch Biochem Biophys 160:185–196.
17. Sherwood OD (1979) Purification and characterization of rat relaxin. Endocrinology 104:886–892.
18. Walsh JR, Niall HD (1980) Use of an octadecylsilica purification method minimizes proteolysis during isolation of porcine and rat relaxins. Endocrinology 107:1258–1260.
19. Sherwood OD, Chang CC, BeVier GW, Dziuk PJ (1975) Radioimmunoassay of plasma relaxin levels throughout pregnancy and at parturition in the pig. Endocrinology 97:834–837.
20. Burger LL, Sherwood OD (1995) Evidence that cellular proliferation contributes to relaxin-induced growth of both the vagina and the cervix in the pregnant rat. Endocrinology 136:4820–4826.
21. Downing SJ, Sherwood OD (1985) The physiological role of relaxin in the pregnant rat. I. The influence of relaxin on parturition. Endocrinology 116:1200–1205.
22. Nara BS, Welk FA, Rutherford JE, Sherwood OD, First NL (1982) Effect of relaxin on parturition and frequency of live births in pigs. J Reprod Fertil 66:359–365.
23. Lao Guico-Lamm M, Voss EW Jr, Sherwood OD (1988) Monoclonal antibodies specific for rat relaxin. I. Production and characterization of monoclonal antibodies that neutralize rat relaxins bioactivity *in vivo*. Endocrinology 123:2472–2478.
24. Lao Guico-Lamm M, Sherwood OD (1988) Monoclonal antibodies specific for rat relaxin. II. Passive immunization with monoclonal antibodies throughout the second half of pregnancy disrupts birth in intact rats. Endocrinology 123:2479–2485.
25. Krantz JC, Bryant HH, Carr CJ (1950) The action of aqueous corpus luteum extract upon uterine activity. Surg Gynecol Obstet 90:372–375.
26. Downing SJ, Sherwood OD (1985) The physiological role of relaxin in the pregnant rat. II. The influence of relaxin on uterine contractile activity. Endocrinology 116:1206–1214.
27. Taverne MAM, Naaktgeboren C, Elsaesser F, Forsling ML, van der Weyden GC, Ellendorff F, Smidt D (1979) Myometrial electrical activity and plasma concentrations of progesterone, estrogens, and oxytocin during late pregnancy and parturition in the miniature pig. Biol Reprod 21: 1125–1134.
28. Watts AD, Flint APF, Foxcroft GR, Porter DG (1988) Plasma steroid, relaxin and dihydro-keto-prostaglandin F-2α changes in the minipig in relation to myometrial electrical and mechanical activity in the pre-partum period. J Reprod Fertil 83:553–564.
29. Hwang JJ, Sherwood OD (1988) Monoclonal antibodies specific for rat relaxin. III. Passive immunization with monoclonal antibodies throughout the second half of pregnancy reduces cervical growth and extensibility in intact rats. Endocrinology 123:2486–2490.
30. Kuenzi MJ, Sherwood OD (1992) Monoclonal antibodies specific for rat relaxin. VII. Passive immunization with monoclonal antibodies throughout the second half of pregnancy prevents development of normal mammary nipple morphology and function in rats. Endocrinology 131: 1841–1847.
31. Zhao S, Malmgren CH, Shanks RD, Sherwood OD (1995) Monoclonal antibodies specific for rat relaxin. VIII. Passive immunization with monoclonal antibodies throughout the second half of pregnancy reduces water consumption in rats. Endocrinology 136:1892–1897.
32. Porter DG (1979) The myometrium and the relaxin enigma. Anim Reprod Sci 2:77–96.
33. Hwang J-J, Shanks RD, Sherwood OD (1989) Monoclonal antibodies specific for rat relaxin. IV. Passive immunization with monoclonal antibodies during the antepartum period reduces cervical growth and extensibility, disrupts birth, and reduces pup survival in intact rats. Endocrinology 125:260–266.
34. Downing SJ, Hollingsworth M (1993) Action of relaxin on uterine contractions—a review. J Reprod Fertil 99:275–282.
35. Sanborn BM, Anwer K, Monga M, Wen Y, Singh SP, Meera P, Oberti C, Toro L, Stefani E (1995) Mechanisms controlling the acute effects of relaxin on the myometrium, In: Progress in

Relaxin Research (MacLennan AH, Tregear GW, Bryant-Greenwood GD, eds.), Global Publications Services, River Edge, NJ, pp. 289–297.

36. Sanborn BM, Kuo HS, Weisbrodt NW, Sherwood OD (1980) The interaction of relaxin with the rat uterus. I. Effect on cyclic nucleotide levels and spontaneous contractile activity. Endocrinology 106:1210–1215.
37. Hsu CJ, McCormack SM, Sanborn BM (1985) The effect of relaxin on cyclic adenosine 3′,5′-monophosphate concentrations in rat myometrial cells in culture. Endocrinology 116:2029–2035.
38. Kemp BE, Niall HD (1981) Effect of relaxin on the activation of cAMP-dependent protein kinase in rat uterus, In: Relaxin (Bryant-Greenwood GD, Niall HD, Greenwood FC, eds.), Elsevier/North Holland, New York, pp. 273–275.
39. Nishikori K, Weisbrodt NW, Sherwood OD, Sanborn BM (1983) Effects of relaxin on rat uterine myosin light chain kinase activity and myosin light chain phosphorylation. J Biol Chem 258: 2468–2474.
40. Anwer K, Hovington JA, Sanborn BM (1990) Involvement of protein kinase A in the regulation of intracellular free calcium and phosphoinositide turnover in rat myometrium. Biol Reprod 43: 851–859.
41. Meera P, Anwer K, Monga M, Oberti C, Stefani E, Toro L, Sanborn BM (1995) Relaxin stimulates myometrial calcium-activated potassium channel activity via protein kinase A. Am J Physiol 269:C312–C317.
42. Anwer K, Oberti C, Perez GJ, Perez-Reyes N, McDougall JK, Monga M, Sanborn BM, Stefani E, Toro L (1993) Calcium activated K^+ channels as modulators of human myometrial contractile activity. Am J Physiol 265: C976–C985.
43. Downing SJ, Hollingsworth M (1991) Antagonism of relaxin by glibenclamide in the uterus of the rat *in vivo*. Br J Pharmacol 104:71–76.
44. Steinetz BG, Beach VL, Blye RP, Kroc RL (1957) Changes in the composition of the rat uterus following a single injection of relaxin. Endocrinology 61:287–292.
45. Vasilenko P, Mead JP, Weidmann JE (1986) Uterine growth promoting effects of relaxin: a morphometric and histological analysis. Biol Reprod 35:987–995.
46. Hall JA, Cantley TC, Day BN, Anthony RV (1990) Uterotropic actions of relaxin in prepubertal gilts. Biol Reprod 42:769–774.
47. Hall JA, Cantley TC, Galvin JM, Day BN, Anthony RV (1992) Influence of ovarian steroids on relaxin-induced uterine growth in ovariectomized gilts. Endocrinology 130:3159–3166.
48. Zaleski HM, Winn RJ, Jennings RL, Dziuk PJ, Sherwood OD (1995) Effects of relaxin administration in early gestation or prior to mating on uterine length and fetal survival in gilts. Biol Reprod 52:1389–1394.
49. Min G, Hartzog MG, Jennings RL, Winn RJ, Sherwood OD (1997) Evidence that the endogenous relaxin promotes growth of the vagina and uterus during pregnancy in gilts. Endocrinology 138:560–565.
50. Fields PA, Lee AB, Haab LM, Hwang J-J, Sherwood OD (1992) Evidence for a dual source of relaxin in the pregnant rat: immunolocalization in the corpora lutea and endometrium. Endocrinology 130:2985–2990.
51. Vasilenko P, Adams WC, Frieden EH (1981) Uterine size and glycogen content in cycling and pregnant rats: influence of relaxin. Biol Reprod 25:162–169.
52. Kuenzi MJ, Sherwood OD (1995) Immunohistochemical localization of specific relaxin-binding cells in the cervix, mammary glands, and nipples of pregnant rats. Endocrinology 136: 1367–1373.
53. Min G, Sherwood OD. Identification of specific relaxin-binding cells in the cervix, mammary glands, nipples, small intestine, and skin of pregnant pigs. Biol Reprod 55:1243–1252.

53a. Min G (1997) Identication of relaxin-target tissues and target cells in the pig. University of Illinois at Urbana-Champaign. Ph.D. Dissertation, pp. 77–104.

54. Kroc RL, Steinetz BG, Beach VL (1959) The effects of estrogens, progestagens, and relaxin in pregnant and nonpregnant laboratory rodents. Ann NY Acad Sci 75: 942–980.
55. Frieden EH, Adams WC (1985) Stimulation of rat uterine collagen synthesis by relaxin. Proc Soc Exp Biol Med 180:39–43.
56. Vasilenko P, Frieden EH, Adams WC (1980) Effect of purified relaxin on uterine glycogen and protein in the rat. Proc Soc Exp Biol Med 163:245–248.
57. Adams WC, Hanousek CA, Frieden EH (1989) Progesterone inhibits the uterotrophic effect of relaxin in immature rats. Proc Soc Exp Biol Med 191:159–162.

58. Cullen BM, Harkness RD (1960) The effect of hormones on the physical properties and collagen content of the rat's uterine cervix. J Physiol 152:419–436.
59. Zarrow MX, Neher GM, Sikes D, Brennan DM, Bullard JF (1956) Dilatation of the uterine cervix of the sow following treatment with relaxin. Am J Obstet Gynecol 72:260–264.
60. Downing SJ, Sherwood OD (1985) The physiological role of relaxin in the pregnant rat. III. The influence of relaxin on cervical extensibility. Endocrinology 116:1215–1220.
61. Downing SJ, Sherwood OD (1986) The physiological role of relaxin in the pregnant rat. IV. The influence of relaxin on cervical collagen and glycosaminoglycans. Endocrinology 118:471–479.
62. O'Day MB, Winn RJ, Easter RA, Dziuk PJ, Sherwood OD (1989) Hormonal control of the cervix in pregnant gilts. II. Relaxin promotes changes in the physical properties of the cervix in ovariectomized hormone-treated pregnant gilts. Endocrinology 125:3004–3010.
63. Lee AB, Hwang J-J, Haab LM, Fields PA, Sherwood OD (1992) Monoclonal antibodies specific for rat relaxin. VI. Passive immunization with monoclonal antibodies throughout the second half of pregnancy disrupts histological changes associated with cervical softening at parturition in rats. Endocrinology 130:2386–2391.
64. Winn RJ, O'Day-Bowman MB, Sherwood OD (1993) Hormonal control of the cervix in pregnant gilts. IV. Relaxin promotes changes in the histological characteristics of the cervix that are associated with cervical softening during late pregnancy in gilts. Endocrinology 133:121–128.
65. O'Day-Bowman MB, Winn RJ, Dziuk PJ, Lindley ER, Sherwood OD (1991) Hormonal control of the cervix in pregnant gilts. III. Relaxins influence on cervical biochemical properties in ovariectomized hormone-treated pregnant gilts. Endocrinology 129:1967–1976.
66. Golichowski AM, King SR, Mascaro K (1980) Pregnancy-related changes in rat cervical glycosaminoglycans. Biochem J 192: 1–8.
67. Kokenyesi R, Woessner JF Jr (1989) Purification and characterization of a small dermatan sulphate proteoglycan implicated in the dilatation of the rat uterine cervix. Biochem J 260:413–419.
68. Scott JE (1988) Proteoglycan-fibrillar collagen interactions. Biochem J 252:313–324.
69. Kokenyesi R, Woessner JF Jr (1990) Relationship between dilatation of the rat uterine cervix and a small dermatan sulphate proteoglycan. Biol Reprod 42:87–97.
70. Junqueira LCU, Zugaib M, Montes GS, Toledo OMS, Krisztán RM, Shigihara KM (1980) Morphologic and histochemical evidence for the occurrence of collagenolysis and for the role of neutrophilic polymorphonuclear leukocytes during cervical dilation. Am J Obstet Gynecol 138: 273–281.
71. Osmers R, Rath W, Adelmann-Grill BC, Fittkow C, Kuloczik M, Szevernyi M, Tschesche H, Kuhn W (1992) Origin of cervical collagenase during parturition. Am J Obstet Gynecol 166:1455–1460.
72. Winn RJ, Baker MD, Sherwood OD (1994) Individual and combined effects of relaxin, estrogen, and progesterone in ovariectomized gilts. I. Effects on the growth, softening, and histological properties of the cervix. Endocrinology 135:1241–1249.
73. Hall JA, Anthony RV (1993) Influence of ovarian steroids on relaxin-induced distensibility and compositional changes in the porcine cervix. Biol Reprod 48:1348–1353.
74. Vasilenko P, Mead JP (1987) Growth-promoting effects of relaxin and related compositional changes in the uterus, cervix and vagina of the rat. Endocrinology 120:1370–1376.
75. Zhao S, Kuenzi MJ, Sherwood OD (1996) Monoclonal antibodies specific for rat relaxin. IX. Evidence that endogenous relaxin promotes growth of the vagina during the second half of pregnancy in rats. Endocrinology 137:425–430.
76. Hamolsky M, Sparrow RC (1945) Influence of relaxin on mammary development in sexually immature female rats. Proc Soc Exp Biol Med 60:8–9.
77. Hwang J-J, Lee AB, Fields PA, Haab LM, Mojonnier LE, Sherwood OD (1991) Monoclonal antibodies specific for rat relaxin. V. Passive immunization with monoclonal antibodies throughout the second half of pregnancy disrupts development of the mammary apparatus and, hence, lactational performance in rats. Endocrinology 129:3034–3042.
78. Kensinger RS, Collier RJ, Bazer FW, Ducsay CA, Becker HN (1982) Nucleic acid, metabolic and histological changes in gilt mammary tissue during pregnancy and lactogenesis. J Anim Sci 54: 1297–1308.
79. Hurley WL, Doane RM, O'Day-Bowman MB, Winn RJ, Mojonnier LE, Sherwood OD (1991) Effect of relaxin on mammary development in ovariectomized pregnant gilts. Endocrinology 128: 1285–1290.
80. Zaleski HM, Winn RJ, Jennings RL, Sherwood OD (1996) Effects of relaxin on lactational performance in ovariectomized gilts. Biol Reprod 55:671–675.

81. Winn RJ, Baker MD, Merle CA, Sherwood OD (1994) Individual and combined effects of relaxin, estrogen, and progesterone in ovariectomized gilts. II. Effects on mammary development. Endocrinology 135:1250–1255.
82. Kuenzi MJ, Sherwood OD (1992) Monoclonal antibodies specific for rat relaxin. VII. Passive immunization with monoclonal antibodies throughout the second half of pregnancy prevents development of normal mammary nipple morphology and function in rats. Endocrinology 131: 1841–1847.
83. Kuenzi MJ, Connolly BA, Sherwood OD (1995) Relaxin acts directly on rat mammary nipples to stimulate their growth. Endocrinology 136:2943–2947.
84. Summerlee AJS, O'Byrne KT, Paisley AC, Breeze MF, Porter DG (1984) Relaxin affects the central control of oxytocin release. Nature 309:372–374.
85. Geddes BJ, Summerlee AJS (1995) The emerging concept of relaxin as a centrally acting peptide hormone with hemodynamic actions. J Neuroendocrinol 7:411–417.
86. Way SA, Leng G (1992) Relaxin increases the firing rate of supraoptic neurones and increases oxytocin secretion in the rat. J Endocrinol 132:149–158.
87. Geddes BJ, Parry LJ, Summerlee AJS (1994) Brain angiotension-II partially mediates the effects of relaxin on vasopressin and oxytocin release in anesthetized rats. Endocrinology 134:1188–1192.
88. Way SA, Douglas AJ, Dye S, Bicknell RJ, Leng G, Russell JA (1993) Endogenous opiod regulation of oxytocin release during parturition is reduced in ovariectomized rats. J Endocrinol 138:13–22.
89. Parry LJ, Poterski, RS, Summerlee AJS (1994) Effects of relaxin on blood pressure and the release of vasopressin and oxytocin in anesthetized rats during pregnancy and lactation. Biol Reprod 50:622–628.
90. Jones SA, Summerlee AJS (1987) Effects of chronic infusion of porcine relaxin on oxytocin release in lactating rats. J. Endocrinol 114:241–246.
91. Osheroff PL, Phillips HS (1991) Autoradiographic localization of relaxin binding sites in rat brain. Proc Natl Acad Sci USA 88:6413–6417.
92. Summerlee AJS, O'Byrne KT, Jones SA, Eltringham L (1987) The subfornical organ and relaxin-induced inhibition of reflex milk ejection in lactating rats. J Endocrinol 115:347–353.
93. Yang RH, Bunting S, Wyss JM, Berecek KH, Zhang L, Jin H (1995) Pressor and bradycardic effects of centrally administered relaxin in conscious rats. Am J Hypertens 8:375–381.
94. Parry LJ, Summerlee AJS (1991) Central angiotensin partially mediates the pressor action of relaxin in anesthetized rats. Endocrinology 129:47–52.
95. Summerlee AJS, Robertson GF (1995) Central administration of porcine relaxin stimulates drinking behavior in rats: an effect mediated by central angiotensin II. Endocrine 3: 377–381.
96. Thornton SN, Fitzsimons JT (1995) The effects of centrally administered porcine relaxin on drinking behaviour in male and female rats. J Neuroendocrinol 7:165–169.
97. Weisinger RS, Burns P, Eddie LW, Wintour EM (1993) Relaxin alters the plasma osmolality-arginine vasopressin relationship in the rat. J Endocrinol 137:505–510.
98. Sortino MA, Cronin MJ, Wise PM (1989) Relaxin stimulates prolactin secretion from anterior pituitary cells. Endocrinology 124:2013–2015.
99. Musah AI, Barsness BD, Schrank GD (1995) Antirelaxin and relaxin on prolactin and gonadotropin secretion *in vitro* from porcine pituitary cells. Anim Reprod Sci 40:239–247.
100. Bethea CL, Cronin MJ, Haluska GJ, Novy MJ (1989) The effect of relaxin infusion on prolactin and growth hormone secretion in monkeys. J Clin Endocrinol Metab 69:956–962.
101. Li Y, Huang C, Klindt J, Anderson LL (1993) Stimulation of prolactin secretion in the pig: central effects of relaxin and the antiprogesterone RU 486. Endocrinology 133:1205–1212.
102. Summerlee AJS, Mumford AD, Smith MS (1991) Porcine relaxin affects the release of luteinizing hormone in rats. J Neuroendocrinol 3:133–138.
103. Parry LJ, Poterski RS, Summerlee AJS, Jones SA (1990) Mechanism of the haemotensive action of porcine relaxin in anaesthetized rats. J Neuroendocrinol 2:53–58.
104. Ahokas RA, Sibai BM, Anderson GD (1989) Lack of evidence of a vasodepressor role for relaxin in spontaneously hypertensive and normotensive pregnant rats. Am J Obstet Gynecol 161:618–622.
105. Ward DG, Cronin MJ, Baertschi AJ (1991) Lack of cardiovascular and vasopressin responses to human relaxin in conscious late pregnant rats. Am J Physiol 261:H206–H211.
106. Osheroff PL, Cronin MJ, Lofgren JA (1992) Relaxin binding in the rat heart atrium. Proc Natl Acad Sci USA 89:2384–2388.
107. Kakouris H, Eddie LW, Summers RJ (1992) Cardiac effects of relaxin in rats. Lancet 339: 1076–1078.

108. Ward DG, Thomas GR, Cronin MJ (1992) Relaxin increases rat heart rate by a direct action on the cardiac atrium. Biochem Biophys Res Commun 186:999–1005.
109. Han X, Habuchi Y, Giles WR (1994) Relaxin increases heart rate by modulating calcium current in cardiac pacemaker cells. Circ Res 74:537–541.
110. Bigazzi M, Del Mese A, Petrucci F, Casali R, Novelli GP (1986) The local administration of relaxin induces changes in the microcirculation of the rat mesocaecum. Acta Endocrinol 112:296–299.
111. Bani G, Bani Sacchi T, Bigazzi M, Bianchi S (1988) Effects of relaxin on the microvasculature of mouse mammary gland. Histol Histopathol 3:337–343.
112. Bani Sacchi T, Bigazzi M, Bani D, Mannaioni PF, Masini E (1995) Relaxin-induced increased coronary flow through stimulation of nitric oxide production. Br J Pharmacol 116:1589–1594.
113. Bani D, Bigazzi M, Masini E, Bani G, Bani Sacchi T (1995) Relaxin depresses platelet aggregation: in vitro studies on isolated human and rabbit platelets. Lab Invest 73:709–716.
114. Bani D, Maurizi M, Bigazzi M (1995) Relaxin reduces the number of circulating platelets and depresses platelet release from megakaryocytes: studies in rats. Platelets 6:330–335.
115. Osetinsky GV, Marion MS, McCaffrey TV (1988) Modification of collagen in tissue expansion. Surg Forum 39:559–561.
116. Kibblewhite D, Larrabee WF Jr, Sutton D (1992) The effect of relaxin on tissue expansion. Arch Otolaryngol Head Neck Surg 118:153–156.
117. Unemori EN, Beck LS, Lee WP, Xu Y, Siegel M, Keller G, Liggitt HD, Bauer EA, Amento EP (1993) Human relaxin decreases collagen accumulation in vivo in two rodent models of fibrosis. J Invest Dermatol 101:280–285.
118. Unemori EN, Amento EP (1990) Relaxin modulates synthesis and secretion of procollagenase and collagen by human dermal fibroblasts. J Biol Chem 265:10,681–10,685.
119. Unemori EN, Bauer EA, Amento EP (1992) Relaxin alone and in conjunction with interferon-γ decreases collagen synthesis by cultured human scleroderma fibroblasts. J Invest Dermatol 99: 337–342.
120. Del-Angel-Meza AR, Beas-Zárte C, Alfaro FL, Morales-Villagran A (1991) A simple biological assay for relaxin measurement. Comp Biochem Physiol 99:35–39.
121. Knox RV, Zhang Z, Day BN, Anthony RV (1994) Identification of relaxin gene expression and protein localization in the uterine endometrium during early pregnancy in the pig. Endocrinology 135:2517–2525.
122. Fields PA, Lee AB, Haab LM, Hwang J-J, Sherwood OD (1992) Evidence for a dual source of relaxin in the pregnant rat: immunolocalization in the corpora lutea and endometrium. Endocrinology 130:2985–2990.
123. Hansell DJ, Bryant-Greenwood GD, Greenwood FC (1991) Expression of the human relaxin H1 gene in the decidua, trophoblast and prostate. J Clin Endocrinol Metab 72:899–904.
124. Bryant-Greenwood GD, Greenwood FC (1988) Postulated roles for luteal or decidual relaxins at parturition in the pregnant sow and woman, In: The Physiology and Biochemistry of Human Fetal Membranes (Mitchell BF, ed.), Perinatology, Ithaca, NY, pp. 141–156.
125. Petersen LK, Helmig R, Oxlund H, Vogel I, Uldbjerg N (1994) Relaxin (hRLX-2)-induced weakening of human fetal membranes *in vitro*. Eur J Obstet Gynecol 57:123–128.
126. Bryant-Greenwood GD, Yamamoto SY (1995) Control of peripartal collagenolysis in the human chorion-decidua. Am J Obstet Gynecol 172:63–70.

16 Placental Lactogen and Growth Hormone

Regulation and Action

Russell V. Anthony, PHD, *Sean W. Limesand,* MS, *Michael D. Fanning,* PHD, *and Rongti Liang,* PHD

Contents

INTRODUCTION

The importance of the anterior pituitary-derived hormones, growth hormone (GH), and prolactin (PRL) in regulating postnatal growth and lactogenesis is well documented in a variety of species. However, the necessity of GH and PRL in stimulating fetal growth and mammogenesis during pregnancy is more controversial. For example, the lack of effect of anencephaly or congenital absence of the pituitary gland on human fetal growth rate led to the conclusion *(1)* that fetal development occurs independent of fetal pituitary-derived GH. Yet infants with idiopathic GH defeciency *(2)* or GH receptor dysfunction *(3)* exhibit clinical in utero growth retardation, suggesting that in fact GH may have actions within fetal tissues. Furthermore, the importance of these hormones during pregnancy may vary between species. In cattle and sheep, the inhibition of PRL secretion during pregnancy does not impede mammary development *(4)*, whereas in hypophysectomized rats lobulo-alveolar growth is stimulated with exogenous PRL *(5)*. The difficulty in defining the requisite roles for GH and PRL during pregnancy at least in part results from the fact that during pregnancy placental-derived members of the GH/PRL gene family are produced, which have common functions providing sufficient redundancy to enhance the likelihood of an optimal pregnancy outcome.

The placenta of most eutharian mammals are known to synthesize and secrete members of the GH/PRL gene family. Included in this diverse gene family are the placental lactogens (PL), placental growth hormone-variant (GH-V) and the prolactin-related proteins *(6,7)*. Whereas PL's have been identified and characterized in primates, rodents and domestic ruminants, GH-V appears to exist only in primates and the various prolactin-related proteins have been identified only in rodents and ruminants *(6, 7)*. Differences also exist between species in the number and primary structure of the PL's produced. As described in this volume *(8)* all rodent species examined to date produce at least two PL's along with various prolactin-related proteins, whereas, as will be discussed in this chapter, primates and ruminants secrete a single PL. As structural diversity is a hallmark of the placental members of this gene family, functional diversity also likely exists between the various members of this family. However, primate and ruminant PL's may have similar roles in fetal growth regulation and mammogenesis although they are structurally distinct. Accordingly, the aim of this chapter is to review the synthesis and secretion, mechanism of action and the biological activities of primate and ruminant PLs.

SYNTHESIS AND SECRETION

As alluded to in the introduction, primate and ruminant PLs are structurally divergent, yet their biological functions during pregnancy may be quite similar. Primate PL's are structurally more similar to GH than they are to PRL, whereas the PLs produced by cattle and sheep placenta are structurally more similar to PRL. In addition to PL, primate placenta synthesize and secrete GH-V, a homolog for which has yet to be clearly identified in non-primate species.

Biochemical Characteristics

Primates. Human PL (hPL) was the first PL purified *(9, 10)* and is still the most extensively studied, although PLs have been identified, partially characterized or purified in the chimpanzee and orangutan *(11)*, baboon *(12)*, and rhesus monkey *(13, 14)*. The primary structure of mature hPL consists of 191 amino acids, with two disulfide loops *(15, 16)* formed between Cys^{53} and Cys^{165}, and between Cys^{182} and Cys^{189}. Human PL and pituitary-derived growth hormone share 167 out of 191 amino acids in identical locations within their respective primary sequences *(15, 16)*, but when conservative amino acid substitutions are taken into consideration, the overall sequence homology between hPL and GH is approximately 96% *(15)*. The other placenta-derived member of this family, human GH-V (hGH-V, *17*), diverges in amino acid sequence from pituitary-derived GH (GH-N) at only 13 locations, one of which, a switch from Leu to Asn at position 140 provides a site for N-linked glycosylation in GH-V *(18)*. Additionally, differential splicing of the hGH-V mRNA can result in the retention of intron 4, and this mRNA (hGH-V2) is predicted to encode a 26,000 M_r membrane-anchored polypeptide *(19)*. The high degree of similarity in the primary amino acid sequences of hGH-N, hGH-V and hPL, especially the location of the disulfide bonds, suggests that hGH-V and hPL share the four-helical bundle topography described for hGH-N *(20)*. This bundle stucture is somewhat unusual in that the first two α-helices run up whereas the last two α-helices run down, rather than the more typical up-down-up-down configuration. It is not clear what overall conformation is taken by the product of the hGH-V2 mRNA.

Ruminants. Placental lactogens have been purified from placenta of cattle *(21)*, goats *(22)*, and sheep *(23)*, and the primary amino acid sequences of bovine PL (bPL; *24, 25*) and ovine PL (oPL; *26, 27*) have been determined. Bovine PL contains 200 amino acids in its primary sequence *(24)*, but is secreted as multiple isoforms (32–34,000 M_r; *21*) containing both N- and O-linked oligosaccharide chains *(28)*. Whereas bPL is a glycosylated secretory protein, oPL is a nonglycosylated polypeptide *(29)* comprised of 198 amino acids

(27) with an apparent M_r of 22,000 *(29)*. Similar to oPL, caprine PL has an apparent M_r of 22,500 *(22)* and there is no evidence that it is glycosylated. In contrast to hPL, both bPL and oPL are more similar in their respective amino acid sequences *(30)* with PRL (48–50%) than they are to GH (≈24%). This similarity includes the approximate location of 6 Cys residues in ruminant PLs and PRLs, which provides for the formation of 3 disulfide bridges rather than the two found in GH and hPL. Although bPL and oPL are more similar to each other (≈66%) than they are to other members of their respective gene family, the divergence in the primary amino acid sequences of these two polypeptides is considerably greater than the interspecific divergence (≈99% sequence identity) of either ruminant PRL or GH. Analysis of sequence similarity between bPL and oPL *(31)* indicated that the rate of synonymous substitution is much less than the nonsynonymous substitution rate (ratio of 1:1.75), suggesting that the more rapid rate of evolution exhibited between these two ruminant PLs as compared to ruminant PRL or GH may have resulted from adaptive pressure.

As stated earlier, production of a GH-V by ruminant placentae has not been described. However, recent data *(32)* suggests that GH is produced by the sheep placenta early in pregnancy. These investigators *(32)* provided immunoblot and immunohistochemical evidence that GH is produced by the syncytium and trophectoderm from d 35–50 of gestation. Interestingly, an ≈22,000 M_r polypeptide was detected during this time frame and an ≈28,000 M_r polypeptide was detected throughout pregnancy by immunoblot analysis, the latter of which was not detected when a highly purified antibody raised against recombinant pituitary-derived ovine GH was used. Furthermore, ovine GH mRNA was only detectable by Northern blot analysis through d 50 of gestation, and the three cDNAs generated from placental mRNA were identical or very similar to cDNAs derived from pituitary mRNA, leaving the origin of the 28,000 M_r GH-like polypeptide in question. Other than the primary amino acid sequences derived from the cDNAs of the ≈22,000 M_r form of placental GH, no structural features of either immunoreactive polypeptide are known.

Gene Organization and Transcriptional Regulation

Of the placental members of this gene family, the organization and transcriptional regulation of the human PL genes have been the most extensively studied. The lack of information on ruminant PL gene transcription is in part due to the relative time frame in which these began to be examined at the molecular level, but is also a function of the lack of ruminant-derived chorionic cell lines in which to examine tissue-specific transcriptional control. Regardless, a thorough understanding of the transcriptional regulation which provides placenta-specific expression of these genes is an important prerequisite if clinical modulation of placental gene expression is a desirable endpoint. Owing to the transient nature of the placenta, in many regards it is an ideal target for gene therapy, and placental gene expression could potentially be regulated to correct placental deficiencies that result in intra-uterine growth retardation or other suboptimal pregnancy outcomes.

PRIMATES. Human chromosome 17 *(33)* contains a 66 kb gene cluster that includes the genes encoding hGH-N, hGH-V and the three hPL genes *(34,35)*. It is believed that duplication of a common ancestoral gene *(36)* approx 350 million yr ago (Fig. 1) led to the formation of the GH/PL and PRL precursor genes, which then segregated onto two separate chromosomes *(34,37)*. Duplication of the GH/PL ancestoral gene, giving rise to the "pre-GH" and "pre-PL" genes (Fig. 1), likely occurred after the separation of the main order of mammals *(38)*, and the hPL genes arose after the divergence of rodents and primates some 80 million yr ago *(39)*. Two additional duplication events within the last 10–15 million yr *(34,*

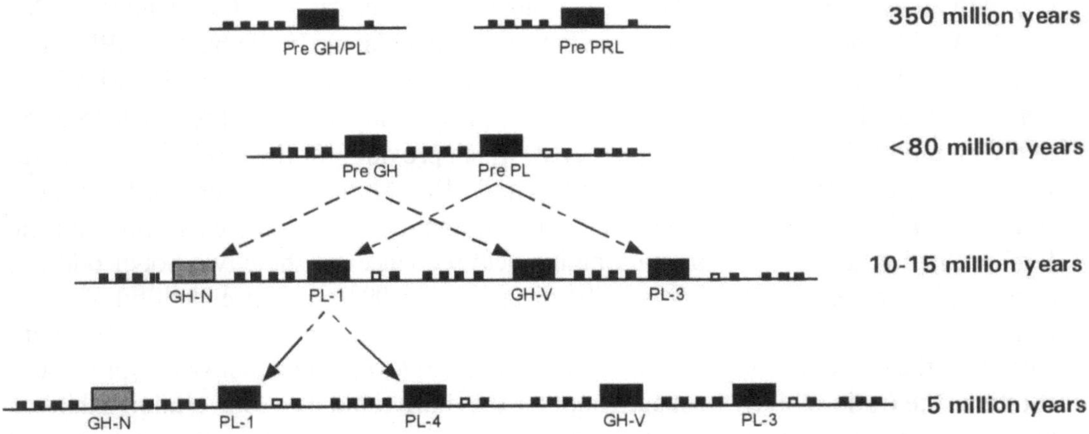

Fig. 1. Schematic of the proposed evolution of the human GH/PL locus located on chromosome 17. A primordial gene gave rise to the GH/PRL and PRL precursor genes, and the GH/PL gene locus evolved from a series of duplication events (as depicted) of the ancestral GH/PL gene. Repetitive *Alu* sequences (small boxes) predisposed the locus to unequal recombination or duplication events. (Adapted from ref. *40*).

35) resulted in the formation of the five gene cluster as we know it today (Fig. 1). The first generated the hGH-N and hGH-V genes from the "pre-GH" gene, and the hPL-1/hPL-4 and hPL-3 genes from the "pre-PL" gene. The final recombination likely occurred within the last five million years and resulted in the hPL-1 and hPL-4 genes (Fig. 1).

Approximately 21% of this five gene locus is comprised of 48 copies of the 300 base pair (bp) *Alu* sequence *(35)*, which likely predisposed this locus to chromosomal misalignment, resulting in the unequal recombination or duplication events. *Alu* sequences flank the 5′ and 3′-ends of the large sequences that were duplicated, and partial *Alu* sequences flank the 3′-end of the PL genes, representing differences between the resultant GH and PL genes *(40)*. This difference might explain the absence of the PL gene 3′-enhancer region (see below) in the hGH genes and the absence of placental expression of hGH-N.

If this scenario of gene duplication is correst, hPL-1 and hPL-4 should be more similar to each other than either are to hPL-3. Indeed this is not the case, since hPL-4 shares greater overall sequence identity with hPL-3 *(40)*, but downstream from the fourth intron, the hPL-1 gene becomes more similar to the hPL-4 gene. It has been suggested *(40)* that the hPL-4 gene was derived from duplication of the hPL-1/hPL-4 precursor gene, and that a gene conversion event may have occurred in the fourth intron of hPL-4, resulting in it's upstream region being more similar in sequence to the hPL-3 gene. Regardless of how the three hPL genes were derived, only hPL-3 and hPL-4 have been shown to be transcriptionally active *(41,42)*. The polypeptide encoded by the hPL-3 and hPL-4 genes only differ at position -24 of the signal peptide *(41)*, where an alanine in hPL-3 is replaced with a proline in hPL-4, such that mature hPL generated by either gene possesses the same amino acid sequence. In contrast, the hPL-1 gene has been considered a psuedogene resulting from a G to A transversion at the second intron splice donor site *(35,40)*, rendering it nonfunctional in the production of hPL. Indeed, no mRNA transcripts from the hPL-1 gene were detected *(40,41)*, and reversion of this mutation did not restore hPL expression in transfected COS-7 cells *(42)*, suggesting that the splice mutation in the hPL-1 gene may not be the only reason for it's inactivity. However, transcripts from the hPL-1

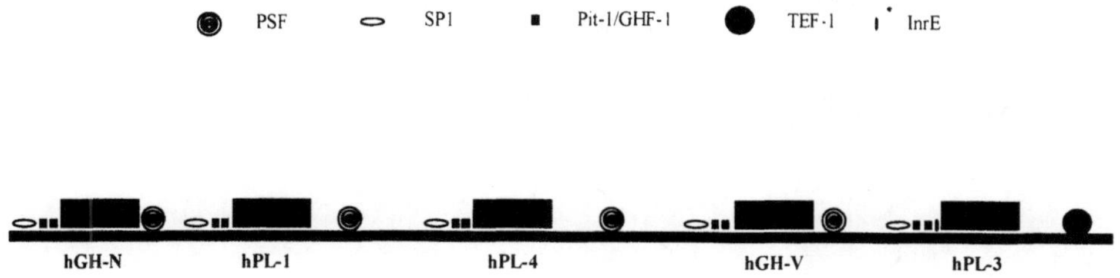

Fig. 2. Diagram of the GH/PL locus, showing the relative location of common transcriptonal response elements (SP1 and Pit-1/GHF-1) as well as those involved in the transcriptional regulation (PSF, TEF-1 and InrE) of the placentally-expressed genes.

gene have been identified in a placental cDNA library *(35)*, one which used an alternative splice site and others which resulted from incomplete processing of heterogenous nuclear RNAs. As yet, it is not clear if a polypeptide can be synthesized in vivo from hPL-1 gene-derived transcripts.

This five gene locus provides an interesting paradigm of transcriptional regulation, in that all of the genes except hGH-N are transcribed solely by the placenta. Yet, the proximal 500 bp of 5′-flanking sequences from the hGH-N, hPL-3 and hPL-4 genes share ≈94% sequence identity *(43)*. Within the upstream promoter region of the hGH-N gene (Fig. 2) resides two cis-acting elements for the pituitary-specific transcription factor GHF-1 (or Pit-1; *44–46*), and GHF-1 has been reported to bind the hPL-3 promoter *(47)* although GHF-1 is not thought to be expressed in trophoblast cells. Additionally, within this proximal 5′-flanking region, reside response elements for the ubiquitous transcription factor Sp1 (Fig. 2). Sp1 binds to the hGH-N *(47)*, hPL-3 *(48)* and hPL-4 *(49)* promoter sequences and appears to be required for initiation of hPL-3 gene transcription *(50)*. The Sp1 response element (GGGAGG) is a variant of the normal Sp1 response element (GGGCGG;51), and resides within a region (-142 to -129 bp) required for basal promoter activity of the hPL-3 gene *(48)*. Additional trans-acting factors have been observed to bind the proximal 5′-flanking region of the hGH gene, including the upstream stimulating factor/adenovirus major-late transcription factor (USF/MLTF), nuclear factor-1 (NF-1) and activator protein-2 (AP-2; *52–54*), and DNAse footprint analyses indicate similar protection patterns for the hPL-3 and hGH-N promoters *(47)*. Human GH-N and PL gene expression is also modulated by cAMP, thyroid hormone and glucocorticoids and their respective cis-acting elements have been mapped within 200 bp of proximal 5′-flanking sequence and the first intron by DNAse footprinting *(55–58)*. Interestingly, when the 500 bp upstream regions of hGH-N and hPL-4 are used in reporter constructs in rat pituitary GC cells, the hGH-N promoter activity is inhibited by thyroid hormone *(59)* and hPL-4 promoter activity is stimulated *(60)*. Although the sequence of the hGH-N and hPL promoter regions are nearly identical, there exists slight differences within their respective thyroid hormone response elements, which have been postulated *(61)* as the reason behind the differential responses to thyroid hormone.

Additional regulation of hPL gene expression resides further upstream of the proximal 500 bp 5′-flanking region. A region between -500 and -1200 bp, relative to the transcriptional start site, confers responsiveness to 1,25-dihyroxyvitamin D_3 *(62)*. This region contains a consensus Vitamin D response element, comprised of a direct repeat motif separated by three bp. Interleukin-6 (IL-6) has also been identified as a positive regulator of hPL gene expression *(63)*. The hPL gene 5′-flanking region contains three NF-IL6 binding sites in the region between -1134 and -1097 bp, and these sites were shown to be

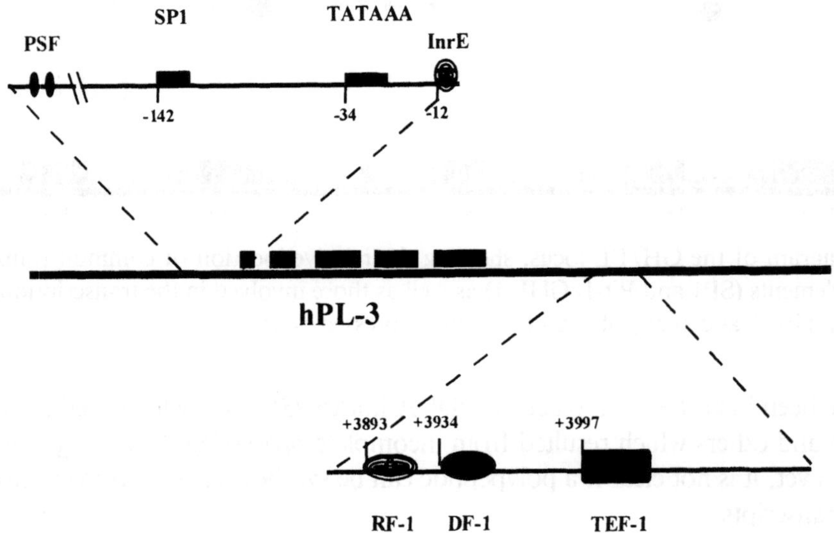

Fig. 3. Schematic of the hPL-3 gene, including the location of elements involved in the cell-specific expression of hPL-3. These include both positive (InrE, DF-1 and TEF-1) and negative (PSF and RF-1) regulatory elements, located either upstream or downstream of the structural gene.

active binding domains via transient transfection and gel-mobility shift assays *(63)*, suggesting that the three NF-IL6 response elements are at least in part responsible for IL-6's effect on hPL expression.

The aforementioned cis-acting elements involved in the transactivation of the hGH-N and hPL genes reside within the 5′-flanking sequences and do not appear to explain the regulation required for trophoblast-specific expression of hPL. Indeed, the tissue specific positive-transcriptional regulation of hPL expression appears to reside within a domain located ≈2.2 Kb downstream of the structural gene (Fig. 3). A 1022 bp segment of the hPL-3 3′-flanking sequence has been shown to direct trophoblast-specific expression *(64)*, and the enhancer activity appears to reside within a 138 bp fragment (nucleotides 103–241) of the larger domain *(65)*. DNAase footprint analysis *(65)* of this region identified a 22 bp element that is bound by nuclear proteins of trophoblast and nontrophoblast-lineage (HeLa) cells, which encodes a transcriptional enhancer factor-1 (TEF-1; Fig. 3) binding motif *(66)*. Similar enhancer sequences are observed in the 3′-flanking domains of the hPL-1 and hPL-4 genes, but their functional significance if any appears to be minor relative to the enhancer activity observed with the hPL-3 gene downstream segment *(64,67)*. Since TEF-1 protein is found in nontrophoblast derived cells *(66)*, and the enhancer activity exhibited by the TEF-1 element is less than that observed with larger portions of this domain *(68)*, the cell-specificity of this response element has been questioned. However, differences in gel-shift assay affinities and patterns of DNAase-1 hypersensitivity between HeLa and trophoblast cell nuclear extracts led Walker et al. *(65)* to suggest that a placental-specific TEF-1-like protein may exist. Alternatively, it is likely that more than one cis-acting element within this 3′-flanking region is involved in providing trophoblast-specific transactivation.

Further examination of the hPL-3 enhancer region supports the latter hypthesis, and it appears that more than one cis-acting element is involved. Four protein binding sites (designated DF-1 to DF-4) have been identified within the hPL-3 enhancer *(67)*, but only two of these (DF-3 and DF-4) seemed to be required for trophoblast-specific transactivation. DF-4 includes the TEF-1 (or TEF-1-like) protein binding site described earlier (Fig. 3), and

DF-3 includes the positive-regulatory element (DF-1) described by Lytras and Cattini *(68)*. These two cis-elements act in synergy to provide transactivation of a heterologous promoter in trophoblast-derived cells *(67)*, whereas an additional cis-element (RF-1; *68*) located just 5′ to DF-3 appears to act as a repressor. The RF-1 and DF-3 elements (Fig. 3) appear to act together in the formation of a protein-DNA complex, or they compete for the same nuclear proteins in a cell-specific manner *(68)*. It is thought that DF-3 acts to derepress RF-1, allowing full activity of the hPL-3 enhancer (TEF-1/DF-4). However, when cells are cotransfected with TEF-1 expression vectors and promoter constructs containing the TEF-1 binding site, promoter activity is repressed rather than being enhanced *(69)*. These investigators *(69)* identified an unrelated protein (CSEF-1) which competed with TEF-1 for it's binding domain, and suggested that TEF-1 and CSEF-1 may possess mutually exclusive actions on hPL promoter activity. It is possible that CSEF-1 is the TEF-1-like activity suggested earlier *(65)* and may be actually responsible for the positive-transcriptional regulation of this downstream element.

Of interest is the fact that transrepression of the hPL promoter by TEF-1 *(69)*, appears to be mediated by TEF-1 interactions with the TATA Binding Protein (TBP) likely disrupting formation of the preinitiation complex *(70)*. On the other hand, the TATA box (Fig. 3) and an initiator element (InrE; *71*), located between the TATA box and the transcriptional start site (-15 to + 1), are required for full basal-promoter activity and enhancer-mediated transactivation in trophoblast cells. An $\approx$70,000 M_r protein binds specifically to the InrE, and appears to be preferentially expressed in cells of trophoblast-lineage (BeWo and JEG-3; *71*). In addition to its role in the formation of a functional transcription initiation complex, InrE also appears to play a role in determining the fidelity of the transcriptional start site.

The previous discussion has focused on factors that drive trophoblast-specific expression of hPL. However, due to the sequence and functional similarity of the proximal 5′-flanking region of the hPL and hGH genes, it must be asked why the placental members of this locus are not expressed in the pituitary. Recent evidence *(72)* indicates that a 263 bp domain located $\approx$2 Kb 5′ of the hPL and hGH-V genes serves as a functional repressor of the hPL-4 proximal promoter in pituitary cells. Within this domain reside two elements (Fig. 3), designated PSF-A and PSF-B, which interact with the nuclear protein PSF-1 in rat pituitary (GC) cells, but not in human choriocarcinoma (JEG-3) cells. Combined, all of these studies suggest that hPL expression is regulated by a complex of positive and negative cis-acting elements, located both upstream and downstream of the structural genes, which act to ensure it's expression solely in the placenta. Additional regulatory factors could also be involved, since all of these elements have been defined by in vitro methods, and confirmation of the necessity and relative importance of each element may not be readily addressed by a transgenic model.

Ruminants. The genes encoding bPL *(73)* and oPL *(74)* have been structurally characterized, both of which are comprised of five exons spanning 10–12 Kb of DNA. As might be expected, due to the sequence similarity between the ruminant PL's and PRL's *(30)*, the bPL gene is linked to the bPRL gene on chromosome 23 *(75)*, but similar data for oPL has yet to be reported. Although bPL is likely encoded by a single copy gene *(73)*, as is oPL *(76)*, evidence exists for differential splicing and allelic variants with the bPL gene *(73,77)*. The proximal 5′-flanking sequences of bPL and oPL share significant sequence identity ($\approx$86%), and have several putative cis-acting elements in common *(74)* as determined by computer analyses. As alluded to earlier, little has been reported regarding the transcriptional regulation of the bPL and oPL genes. Recently, our laboratory *(76)* began examining the ability of the oPL 5′-flanking sequence to direct trophoblast cell-specific

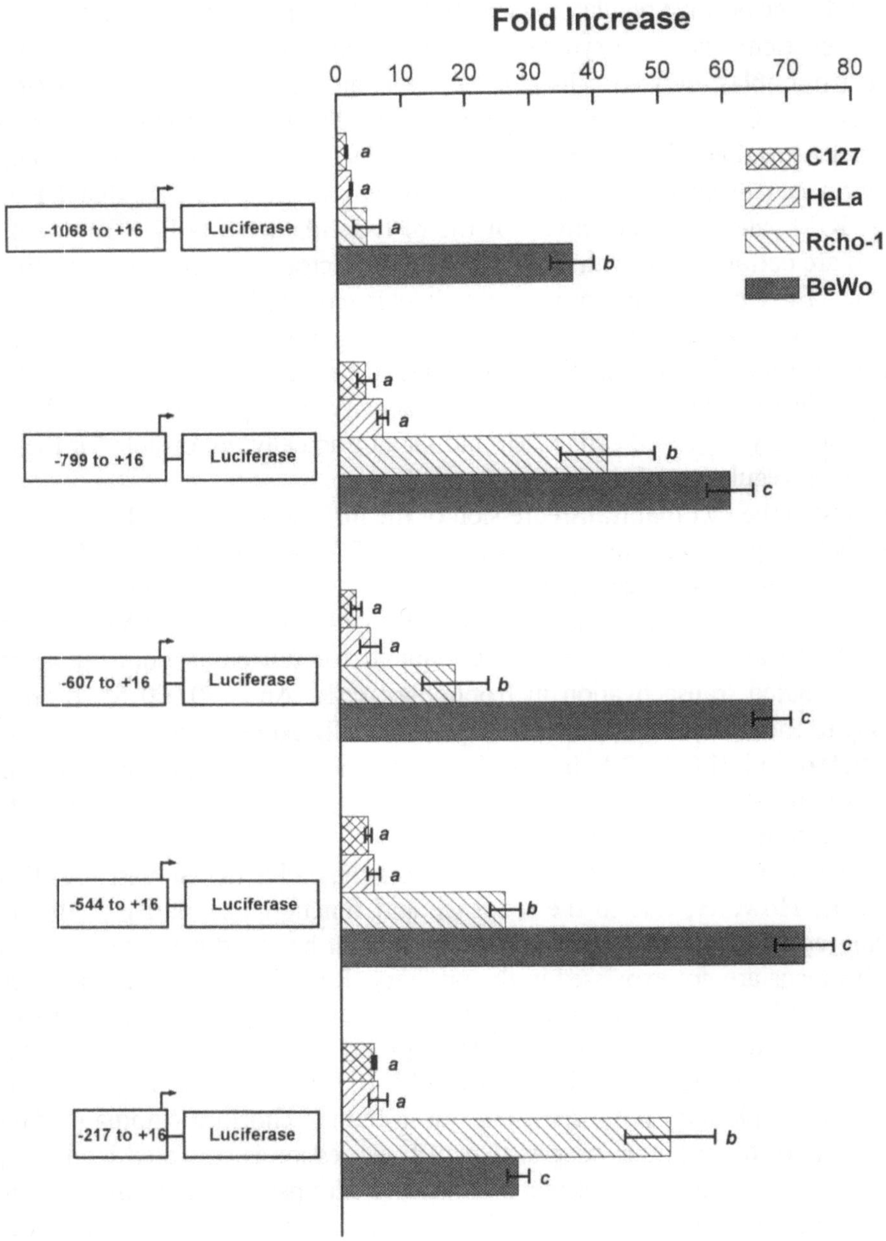

Fig. 4. Transactivation of firefly luciferase in trophoblast-derived (Rcho-1 and BeWo) and non-trophoblast-derived (C127 and HeLa) cells, as influenced by various domains of the oPL 5′-flanking sequence. All constructs were cotransfected with a control plasmid (pβgal) for normalization on transfection efficiency, and the data are expressed as "fold-increase" over the promoterless vector. Values with different superscripts for a given construct are statistically different ($P \leq .05$). These data indicate that trophoblast cell-specific transcription of the oPL gene may be mediated by *cis*-acting elements within -1068 bp of the transcriptional start site (position + 1). (Derived from ref. *76*).

transactivation, using human (BeWo) and rat (Rcho-1) choriocarcinoma cells. As depicted in Fig. 4 *(76)*, elements within the proximal ≈ 1 Kb of 5′-flanking seqence of the oPL gene appear to provide trophoblast cell-specific transactivation of the reporter gene. In general, the degree of transactivation for the various deletion mutants (Fig. 4) suggests that cis-acting elements residing between -799 and + 16 bp relative to the oPL gene transcriptional start site are acting in a trophoblast specific fashion. However, the pattern of expression generated by these constructs indicates that they respond somewhat differently between the two choriocarcinoma cell lines. This raises the question as to whether the transcriptional regulation of oPL is more similar in nature to humans or rodents.

To begin to address this question, DNAse footprint analysis of the ≈ 1 Kb 5′-flanking sequence was conducted with sheep chorionic binucleate cell nuclear extracts *(78)*, which revealed a variety of protected sequences. The various protected sites include 10 GATA factor recognition sites and a proximal AP-2 site, and both types of cis-elements exhibited specificity of binding with the sheep nuclear proteins in gel-mobility shift assays. As indicated earlier, the hPL gene 5′-flanking sequence includes an AP-2 site *(52–54)*, as does the human chorionic gonadotropin α and β-subunit genes which are also produced by syncytiotrophoblast cells *(79)*. The expression of AP-2 is increased when primary cultures of human cytotrophoblasts differentiate into syncytiotrophoblasts, suggesting that this trans-acting factor may play a common role in trophoblast cell differentiation and subsequent gene expression. Furthermore, GATA factors have been implicated in the transcriptional regulation of mouse placental lactogen-I *(80)* and the human chorionic gonadotropin α-subunit *(81)* genes. These data suggest that at least some commonality exists in the transcriptional regulation of placental hormones amongst these three divergent species. However, it is too early to know how critical a role the GATA and AP-2 cis-acting elements play in placenta-specific expression of the ruminant PL genes.

Cell-Specific and Temporal Expression

From the previous discussions regarding the transcriptional regulation of human and ruminant PL's, we have alluded to the fact that these placental hormones are produced by a subpopulation of placental cells, namely syncytiotrophoblast cells in humans and chorionic binucleate cells in ruminants. Furthermore, the placenta-derived members of this gene family in rodents are primarily derived from an analogous subpopulation of cells, that being the trophoblast giant cells *(6)*. The development and differentiation of these particular cell types appears to drive the expression of these hormones, and as discussed below, likely determines the concentration profiles observed.

Placental lactogen. Human PL is detectable in the placenta by d 18 of pregnancy *(82)*, can be detected in maternal circulation by the 3rd week, increases exponentially during the first trimester, and then more gradually until term reaching values of 5–10 μg/mL *(83,84)*. *In situ* hybridization and immunocytochemistry studies clearly identify the syncytiotrophoblasts as the major site of hPL production *(85)*, but before wk 6 of gestation the cytotrophoblasts of the developing placenta appear to be the site of production *(86)*, suggesting a developmental switch in hPL expression. By the end of pregnancy, hPL mRNA accounts for approx 5% of placental mRNA *(35)*, yielding upwards of 1.0 g of hPL each day *(87,88)*. The content of hPL mRNA within individual syncytiotrophoblast cells does not appear to change during the course of pregnancy *(85)*, but the amount of syncytiotrophoblast tissue increases *(89)* as gestation progresses, which could explain the fivefold increase in hPL mRNA concentration from the first to the last trimester *(90)*. One may infer from these data that hPL is constitutively expressed following syncytiotrophoblast formation, and it's synthesis may not be subject to a great deal of regulation. A variety of growth factors, secretogogs and metabolic regulators have been implicated in the regulation of hPL's secretion rate, but no clear regulatory control has been established *(91)*. Although hPL's synthesis rate and concentration in maternal blood is quite high, it's concentration in fetal blood ranges from 4–500 ng/mL between wk 12 and 20 of gestation *(92)*, and is only 20–30 ng/mL at term *(93)*. Since there appears to be no direct transfer of hPL from the maternal to the fetal circulation *(88)*, separate routes of secretion must exist for hPL entering the two vascular compartments. However, the mechanism by which hPL is routed into either the maternal or fetal vasculature has not been elucidated.

Placental lactogen can be localized within the trophectoderm as early as d 16 in sheep *(94)* and by d 18 in cattle *(95)*, but can not be detected in maternal sera until later in pregnancy. Both bovine *(96)* and ovine *(97)* PL are produced by chorionic binucleate cells, which are likely functional analogs of human syncytiotrophoblast cells. Chorionic binucleate cells are believed *(98)* to migrate out of the chorionic epithelium, fusing with uterine epithelium to form either trinucleated cells or a syncytium, and providing an avenue by which ruminant PL's are delivered to maternal vasculature. Although the route of secretion of PL into maternal circulation is likely quite similar for cattle and sheep, the concentration of PL achieved in maternal circulation is different. Bovine PL can be detected in maternal serum by the 4th month of gestation *(99)*, but concentrations remain low (≤ 3 ng/mL) throughout gestation *(100)*. On the other hand, oPL is detectable in maternal serum by d 50 *(101,102)*, and it's concentration increases throughout gestation reaching levels ≥ 1 μg/mL near term *(97)*. Maternal sera oPL concentrations are reflected by the amount of oPL mRNA in cotyledonary tissue during mid- and late gestation *(97)*, and the gestational increase appears to be a function of increasing numbers of chorionic binucleate cells rather than greater oPL expression by individual binucleate cells. Similar data are not available for bPL, but it appears that both hPL *(85)* and oPL *(97)* are essentially consituitively expressed by their cell of origin following differentiation of that respective placental cell type. Fetal sera concentrations of both bPL *(99)* and oPL *(97)* reach peak values by mid-gestation, and stay constant or decline slightly during the remainder of gestation. As in the human, the transfer of oPL from the maternal to the fetal circulation is negligible *(103)*, indicating a distinct secretion pathway towards the fetal portion of the placental vasculature. Although fetal sera concentrations of oPL do not increase after mid-gestation *(97)*, this does not mean that the secretion of oPL into fetal vasculature plateaus. Indeed, the rate of entry of oPL into fetal circulation increases with increasing gestational age *(104)*, suggesting a correlation between the entry rate and oPL mRNA concentrations.

Placental growth hormone. As stated earlier in the section entitled Primates, the human placenta expresses hGH-V and hGH-V2 which are derived from a different gene than the one encoding pituitary-derived GH. Similar to hPL, hGH-V is synthesized by placental syncytiotrophoblast cells *(105,106)*, but unlike hPL, hGH-V does not appear to be secreted into fetal vasculature *(107)*. This raises an interesting question as to how the two placental hormones, derived from the same gene locus and cell of origin, can have directionally distinct secretion routes. This could result from different subpopulations of syncytiotrophoblasts, some producing hPL and others hGH-V, but as yet no evidence is available to support this hypothesis. Regardless, hGH-V becomes detectable in maternal serum between 21 and 26 weeks of gestation and becomes the predominant form of hGH in maternal circulation during the second half of pregnancy *(107,108)*. During the latter half of pregnancy, hGH-V concentrations in maternal sera increase reaching ≈ 20 ng/mL by wk 36, whereas hGH-N concentrations become quite low.

Owing to the recent discovery of GH expression in sheep placenta *(32)*, nothing is known about it's specific cell of origin or it's secretion profile. The fact that GH is expressed by nonprimate placentae, suggests that placental expression of GH may play a role in the establishment or maintenance of pregnancy that is not met by PL. The secretion pattern of hGH-V and hPL are similar, except that hGH-V does not get into fetal circulation. In sheep, placental GH expression appears to occur only during the first trimester, whereas oPL is expressed throughout gestation. Collectively, these data could lead to the conclusion that placentally-derived GH may serve different functions in humans and sheep, and these functions may or may not overlap with those of their respective PL. More effort is needed to more clearly define the synthesis, secretion, regulation, and biological actions of hGH-V and placental-oGH.

MECHANISM OF ACTION

Characterization of the specific mechanism of action for placental members of this gene family has been hampered by the lack of information pertaining to the receptors through which their actions are mediated. Placental lactogens were often initially purified using heterologous GH or PRL radioreceptor assays, and hPL, bPL and oPL are capable of binding their respective species GH receptor (GHR; *109–111*). This, coupled with the fact that a structurally unique PL receptor (PLR) has yet to be purified and characterized, has led to the widely held hypothesis that non-rodent PL's exert their actions through the GHR. Even if this hypothesis is wrong, and a specific PLR exists, it is likely that it will be quite similar to the GHR or prolactin receptor (PRLR).

Primates

Owing to the high degree of structural similarity amongst hGH, hGH-V and hPL, one could surmise that all three ligands may be acting through a single membrane-bound receptor (e.g. human GHR). Indeed, both hGH and hPL are capable of binding the human GHR *(109)*, although hPL binds with 2,300-fold weaker affinity than does hGH. The GHR is a member of the cytokine receptor superfamily, which is comprised of single-transmembrane domain receptors that lack intrinsic tyrosine kinase domains. The human GHR is comprised of three domains: a 246-amino acid extracellular domain; a short transmembrane domain; and a 350-amino acid intracellular domain required for signal transduction *(112,113)*. When hGH interacts with it's receptor, one molecule of hormone is bound by two molecules of receptor (1:2 stoichiometry; *113*), and this ligand-induced dimerization of the receptor is necessary for activation of the GHR-associated signal transduction cascade *(114,115)*. As illustrated in Fig. 5, Janus kinase 2 (JAK2) is a GHR-associated, GH-activated tyrosine kinase that serves as the initial step in cellular activation in GH responsive cells *(116)*. Upon ligand-induced dimerization of the GHR, JAK2 and/or JAK1 is activated, thereby phosphorylating itself and the GHR (Fig. 5). Furthermore, this initial activation step stimulates *(117)* the tyrosine phosphorylation of latent cytoplasmic transcripition factors known as "signal transducers and activators of transcription" (Stat) proteins-1 (Stat-1), -3 (Stat-3) and -5 (Stat 5). Stat-protein phosphorylation results in their translocation to the nucleus, where Stat proteins serve as trans-acting factors *(118)* to stimulate GH-target gene expression (Fig. 5). Furthermore, GHR activation (Fig. 5) leads to the phosphorylation of insulin receptor substrate (IRS) -1 and -2 *(119)*, as well as Src-homology domain proteins that are involved in the Ras-MAP kinase pathway. Activation of IRS-1 and -2 is not only important for insulin signaling, but also provides a binding site for the regulatory subunit of phosphatidylinositol 3-kinase (PI-3 kinase; Fig. 5) which may be involved in mediating some of GH's effects on metabolism.

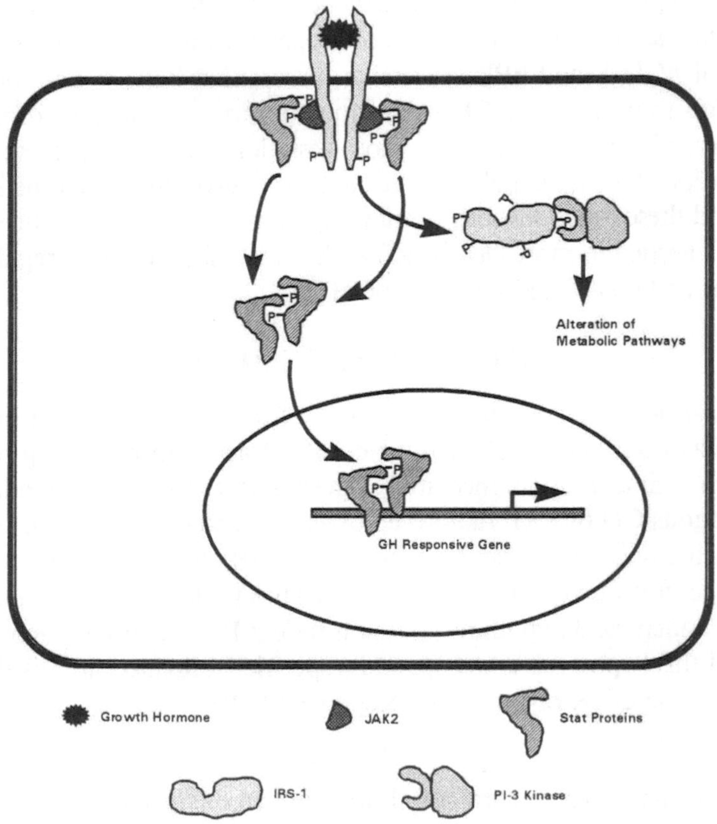

Fig. 5. Schematic of the signal transduction cascade mediated by growth hormone. Growth hormone induces receptor dimerization, which leads to the activation of the JAK/Stat pathway, as well as activation of insulin receptor substrate-1 (IRS-1) and phosphatidylinositol 3-kinase (PI-3 kinase). Stat proteins serve as trans-acting factors in responsive-gene transcriptional regulation, whereas PI-3 kinase may be involved in altering metabolic pathways of the responsive cell.

Considerable insight into the mechanism of action of the GHR has been obtained during the last several years, but the question remains as to whether or not the placental members of this hormone family (i.e., hGH-V and hPL) act solely through the GHR. When GHR mRNAs were described that lacked the exon 3 sequence *(120)*, it was suggested that the receptor encoded by this mRNA may be a specific receptor for either hGH-V or hPL. Besides being expressed in the placenta, this form of GHR mRNA is also expressed in a variety of fetal tissues *(121)*. Since hGH-V does not appear to be present in fetal circulation *(107)*, it is unlikely that this splice-variant encodes a specific hGH-V receptor. Furthermore, since deletion of exon 3 only results in a 22-amino acid deletion from the NH_2-terminus of the GHR, which does not alter the binding affinity of the receptor for hGH *(122)*, it is unlikely that this mRNA encodes a specific hPL receptor.

Specific binding of hGH has been demonstrated *(123)* with human fetal liver microsomes, and specific binding of hPL has been demonstrated with the microsomal fraction of human fetal liver and fetal skeletal muscle *(123)*. The hGH binding sites in fetal liver exhibited sixfold greater affinity for hGH than for hPL, and the hPL binding sites showed a ninefold greater affinity for hPL than for hGH. These differences in relative affinity, coupled with the fact that no specific binding was identified for hGH in fetal skeletal muscle, suggests that the respective binding sites or receptors are different. This conclusion is supported by the fact that the GHR can be immunolocalized in fetal liver, pancreas, kidney, skin, and cerebral cortex, but not in fetal skeletal or cardiac muscle, adrenal, intestine, lung, or epiphyseal growth plate tissue *(124)*. However, the mRNA encoding the human GHR has been identified *(121)* in muscle, adrenal, intestine, and lung tissue. These data could be interpreted to suggest that the mRNA detected in tissues like muscle, by reverse transcriptase-polymerase chain reaction (RT-PCR), encodes a variant form of the GHR capable of greater affinity for hPL. Eight different variants of the GHR mRNA were identified in an adult liver cDNA library *(125)*, all of which varied in the 5′-untranslated sequence of the mRNA, which is encoded entirely by exon 1 *(126)* of the human GHR gene. Further RT-PCR analysis of GHR mRNA expression in fetal and adult tissues *(127)* indicates that the "V1" form of exon 1 is only expressed in postnatal liver, whereas the "V3" form could be identified in a variety of fetal and postnatal tissues. The functional significance of the differential transcription and/or processing of the GHR gene, leading to the use of the "V1" form of exon 1 is not known. It is possible that use of various exon 1 sequences could provide a mechanism for post-transcriptional regulation of GHR translation. Regulation of the translational efficiency could explain why some fetal tissues contain GHR mRNA, but do not synthesize sufficient quantities of the receptor to allow detection by more conventional methods *(123,124)*.

As yet, it is not clear if there is a distinct receptor for hPL in fetal tissues. Receptor binding studies *(123)* indicate that there may be a specific-hPL receptor, but it has not been purified or characterized. Recent evidence *(128)* suggests that hPL is capable of stimulating the phosphorylation of uncharacterized intracellular proteins, as well as the JAK-Stat pathway proteins. However, it can not be ascertained if these phosphoproteins are only responsive to hPL, since comparable experiments were not conducted with hGH or human PRL. If these phosphorylation events are only responsive to hPL, this adds further evidence for a specific hPL receptor. Regardless of the outcome, concerted effort needs to be placed on unequivocally identifying the receptor through which hPL exerts it's actions, such that our understanding of hPL's mechanism of action can move forward.

Ruminants

Considerably more evidence is available to support the existence of a structurally distinct PL receptor in ruminants. There is essentially no specific binding of ovine GH (oGH) or ovine PRL (oPRL) in fetal liver until near term *(128,129)*, yet there is significant and saturable binding of oPL to fetal liver microsomes during the latter two-thirds of gestation *(129,130)*. The oPL binding site in fetal liver *(129,130)* exhibits high-affinity ($K_d \approx 0.12$–0.5 n*M*), and increases in number per cell *(130)* as gestation progresses. Cross linking studies *(131,132)* indicated that the oPL binding site had an apparent M_r of 39–44,000, which is considerably smaller than the M_r of the GHR, but is similar in size to the proteolytically cleaved extracellular domain of the GHR *(112)*. Partial purification of the oPL binding site in fetal and maternal liver has been reported *(133)*, but unfortunately no amino acid sequence data are available on this receptor.

If late gestation (125–135 d post coitus) fetal liver is used, cross-linking and immunoprecipitation experiments suggest *(134)* that oPL and oGH are able to bind identical or very similar receptors. However, even at this later stage of gestation, the amount of specific binding of oGH (1.2 ± 0.4%) was considerably less than the amount of oPL binding (7.6 ± 2.4%). These investigators *(134)* suggested that the difference in the amount of

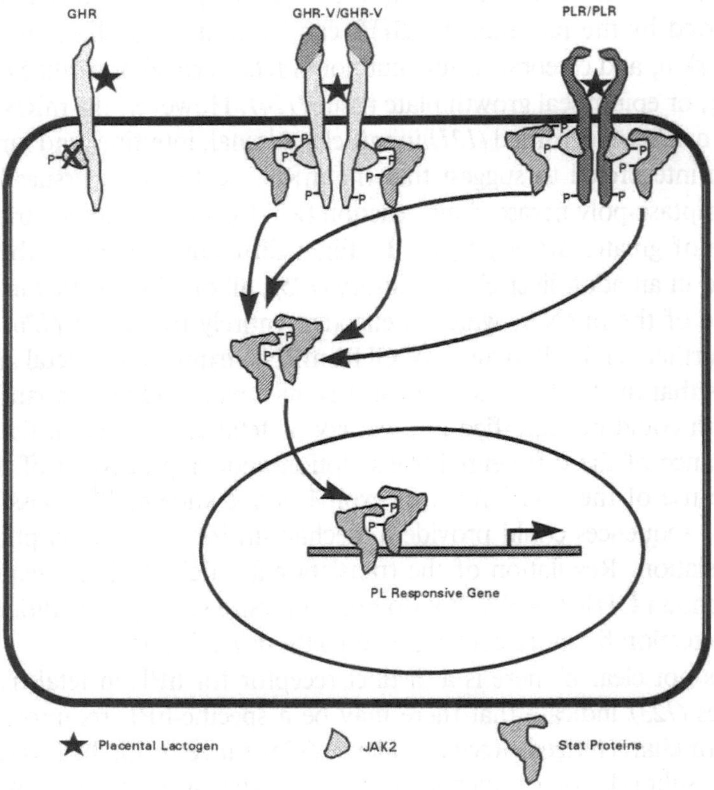

Fig. 6. Possible scenarios through which PLs may mediate their actions. Placental lactogens could act through a variant of the GHR (GHR-V) or through a structurally-distinct PL receptor (PLR). If PL acts by binding a single monomer of the GHR, as indicated in cattle (110), it is unlikely that the signal transduction cascade would be activated.

specific binding could be a function of oPL binding the ovine GHR with a 1:1 stoichiometry rather than the 1:2 stoichiometry normally exhibited with the GHR. This interpretation is not consistent with data obtained with Chinese hamster ovary (CHO) cells expressing the ovine GHR *(111)*. With these cells, oGH exhibited greater affinity (K_d = 0.30 n*M*) for the receptor than did oPL (K_d = 0.76 n*M*), yet both ligands bound the same number of receptors per cell. If oPL interacted with the ovine GHR in a 1:1 stoichiometry, and oGH with a 1:2 stoichiometry, one would expect oPL to bind more receptor molecules per cell given nearly equivalent affinities for the receptor.

Although specific binding of oGH can not be demonstrated with fetal liver microsomes until late gestation, GHR mRNA has been detected in fetal liver and skeletal muscle tissues *(135,136)* as early as 60 d post coitus *(137)*. The mRNA expressed throughout most of gestation is ≈300 nucleotides larger than the mRNA expressed in adult liver *(137)*, and does not possess the same exon 1 sequence. This raises the possibility that the "variant" exon 1 *(137)* provides an alternative translational start site for the oGHR in fetal liver. Such a scenario could provide an NH_2-terminal extension to the oGHR (Fig. 6), thereby changing the receptor's conformation in a fashion that generated a specific-binding site for oPL but interfered with oGH's binding. This is an attractive hypothesis from the standpoint that a single gene could be developmentally switched from providing PL responsiveness during fetal life to GH responsiveness during postnatal life. An alternative exon 1 (exon 1B) has been isolated from sheep skeletal muscle *(138)*, which possesses a translation initiation codon with features of a preferred site *(139)*. However, there is an inframe translation stop codon, such that an autonomous open-reading frame resides within exon 1B. Furthermore, the GC-rich nature of exon 1B coupled with the short autonomous open-reading frame may inhibit translational efficiency *(140)* of the GHR, whose normal translation initiation site is located in exon 2-derived sequence. We have recently determined (L.C. Richter and R.V. Anthony, unpublished results) that exon 1B is expressed throughout gestation in ovine fetal liver, and confirmed our earlier results *(137)* that exon 1A is not expressed until approx 120 d of gestation. If our interpretation of the structural properties of exon 1B is correct, in that it may inhibit the translational effeciency of the oGHR mRNA, this could explain why GHR mRNA is detected in fetal liver at a time when specific oGH binding can not be demonstrated *(130,137)*.

Clearly there is a developmental or gestational age induced switch in the transcription and/or splicing of the oGHR mRNA. Interestingly, the appearance of exon 1A occurs late in gestation, and may be driven by the maturation of other fetal systems. In sheep, fetal cortisol concentrations increase during the last 10–15 d of gestation *(141)*, and it was recently demonstrated *(142)* that cortisol infusion before 130 d of gestation stimulated the expression of oGHR mRNA. However, it is not clear from these studies *(142)* whether the gestational age and cortisol induced increases in GHR mRNA expression are related to the appearance of exon 1A. This response may result from cortisol induced maturation of hepatic function, since similar responses are seen with the prolactin receptor mRNA *(143)*. However, we have preliminary data (L.C. Richter and R.V. Anthony, unpublished results) indicating that cortisol treatment of fetal hepatocyte cultures (100 d of gestation) will induce expression of exon 1A-containing oGHR mRNA. Regardless of whether this is a direct action of cortisol, the "switching on" of exon 1A late in gestation is an important developmental phenomenon that requires further investigation.

Specific binding sites for bPL *(144,145)* have been identified in uterine endometrium, which possess little affinity for bovine GH or PRL. However, mRNA encoding the bovine GHR and PRLR have been detected in endometrium, corpus luteum, and maternal and fetal liver *(146)*. Bovine PL is capable of binding both the GHR *(110)* and the PRLR *(146)*, such that without purification and characterization of the bPL-specific binding sites identified *(144,145)*, it is difficult to discern if there is a structurally distinct bPL receptor. When bPL binds the GHR, it does so in a 1:1 stoichiometry rather than the 1:2 stoichiometry observed with GH *(110)*. Furthermore, competition with monoclonal antibodies indicate *(110)* that bPL may be interacting at a different site on the receptor than is GH. As illustrated in Fig. 6, bPL binding to a single monomer of the bovine GHR may not be sufficient to activate the GHR signal transduction cascade. Ligand-induced dimerization of the receptor is believed to be necessary for activation of signal transduction *(114,115)*, which suggests that bPL binding to the bovine GHR in a 1:1 stoichiometry is insufficient to activate the JAK/Stat pathway (Fig. 6). However, recent real-time kinetic measurements *(147)* utilizing surface plasmon resonance indicates that the ligand-induced receptor dimerization may be quite transitory in nature, especially if ligand and receptor are derived from the same species. These data could be interpreted to suggest that the 1:1 stoichiometry observed for the bPL:bovine GHR interaction *(110)* may be misleading, in that a transient 1:2 interaction may have been missed by the techniques employed. If that is in fact the case, it could be possible for bPL to exert it's actions through the bovine GHR. However, recent experiments *(148)* using a Baf cell line expressing the bovine GHR indicate that bPL is unable to induce tyrosine phosphorylation of JAK2 and Stat 5, but bovine

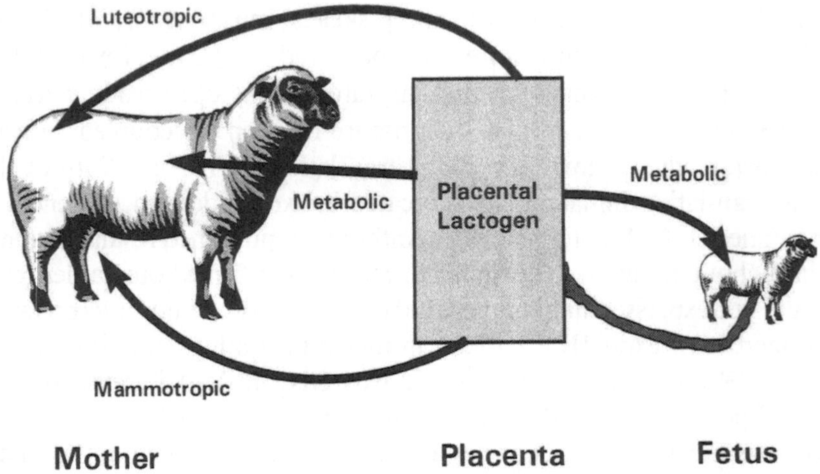

Fig. 7. Maternal and fetal sites where PLs have inferred actions. Human and ruminant PLs have been implicated in modulating maternal mammogenesis, metabolism and steroidogenesis, while also having direct actions on the fetal liver to stimulate fetal metabolism and growth factor production. However, many of these actions have been inferred from *in vitro* experiments, often using heterologous (interspecific) tissues.

GH stimulated the phosphorylation of both. These data fit with the model (Fig. 6) that bPL binds the bovine GHR in a 1:1 stoichiometry and is unable to induce signal transduction through this interaction.

In summary, there is evidence in humans, cattle and sheep for a structurally distinct PL receptor (Fig. 6). This receptor is likely related to the GHR or PRLR, and should induce the JAK/Stat signal transduction cascade as does GH and PRL. However, this has yet to be definitively demonstrated in any of the three species. Furthermore, there is considerable evidence that suggests that human and ruminant PL's can bind and possibly act through their respective species GHR. It is also possible that GHR mRNA exist with exon 1 sequences that encode an NH_2-terminal extension, such that the conformation of the receptor is altered in a fashion to generate a PL-specific receptor (Fig. 6). All of these possibilities (Fig. 6) need to be investigated further, but we must keep in mind that we may be dealing with an inherently redundant system which may continue to interfere with our ability to define "specific" mechanisms of action. Redundancy is becoming commonplace as the "true" biology of various systems are defined, and it is entirely possible that PL, placenta-derived GH and pituitary-derived GH may all serve within a redundant system aimed at maintaining the homeorrhetic environment necessary for optimal outcome of pregnancy. Therefore, confusion over each ligands specific mechanism of action may not be that surprising.

BIOLOGICAL ACTIVITIES

The exact biological function(s) of the placental members of this gene family has yet to be clearly defined in any species. As depicted in Fig. 7, diverse roles for PL have been inferred for the maternal and fetal systems, whereas hGH-V is assumed to have the same biological actions of pituitary-derived GH. A good portion of the evidence used to infer the biological actions of PL has been derived from in vitro systems, often using heterologous sources of ligand and tissue. This has made it difficult to clearly interpret the impact of the results, such that some of the inferred roles of PL may not pertain to all species. Furthermore, the relative diversity in the primary structure of PL in humans, cattle and sheep may indicate that the "true" biological function(s) of PL differs between these species.

Maternal System

The biological actions of PL within the mother may include stimulating gonadal steroidogenesis, modulating maternal metabolic pathways and augmenting mammogenesis (Fig. 7). As discussed earlier, at least in humans and sheep, the amount of PL in the maternal circulation is quite high (100's ng/mL), especially when compared to the K_d of the PL binding sites described in maternal and fetal tissues. This relationship, between circulating concentrations of PL and the K_d of it's binding site, is such that administration of additional PL into what may already be a saturated system is unlikely to yield readily interpretable results. Consequently, in the absence of PL-deficient models, it will be difficult to define the specific role and necessity of PL within the maternal system.

Steroidogenesis. Although there is good evidence for direct luteotropic actions by one or more of the mouse PLs *(149)* and for bPL *(150)*, evidence for direct luteal support by human and sheep PLs is lacking. For example, hPL treatment is unable to extend the luteal phase of the menstrual cycle in women when human chorionic gonadotropin can *(151)*, and there is an absence of hPL binding sites in the corpus luteum (CL) at the end of pregnancy *(152)*. Furthermore, in nonpregnant women, hPL did not stimulate progesterone secretion, but did stimulate insulin-like growth factor (IGF)-II secretion from granulosa cells *(153)*. These latter data indicate that hPL could have actions on the ovary, but not in stimulating luteal progesterone production. In sheep, ovarian infusion of oPL does not increase progesterone secretion *(154)*, does not inhibit the luteolytic actions of prostaglandin $F_2\alpha$ *(154)*, and short-term immunoneutralization of the oPL in maternal circulation does not alter the blood concentrations of progesterone *(155)*. The lack of luteal support provided by hPL and oPL may not be all that surprising since there is not a full-gestational requirement for CL-derived progesterone in these species.

In cattle, the CL is required for the maintenance of pregnancy throughout most of the 280 d gestation. Injections of bPL will increase luteal size and plasma concentrations of progesterone *(150)*, as well as reduce the size of the largest follicle. However, some but not all of these effects were also obtained with bGH injections, and the bovine GHR has been demonstrated in luteal tissue *(156)*. Although the presence of bovine GHR has been demonstrated in luteal tissue by immunohistochemistry *(156)*, little to no specific-binding of bGH to luteal microsomes could be demonstrated *(150)*, whereas specific-binding of bPL was demonstrable. It is possible the bPL is exerting it's actions on the CL through the PRLR, since PRLR mRNA is present in bovine luteal tissue and bPL will compete with equal affinity with bovine PRL for the PRLR expressed in COS cells *(146)*. However, the fact that GH can elicit many of the same effects as bPL infers that the two ligands may be acting through the same receptor. Furthermore, GH is luteotropic in sheep *(157)*, a species in which PL does not appear to have a luteotropic function (*see* above). Together, these data indicate that GH is a luteotropic agent, and that the actions of bPL may in fact be mediated through the GHR which it is capable of binding *(110)*.

Metabolism. Placental lactogen has been considered a partitioning agent that serves to regulate nutrient supply for fetal growth. During the third trimester, basal and glucose-stimulated insulin secretion increases, some tissues become resistant to insulin, glucose tolerance is impaired and lipid mobilization is increased, all changes proposed *(158)* to be mediated by PL. These metabolic changes are aimed at providing a ready source of glucose for the fetus, and although a variety of in vitro and in vivo experiments have been performed to assess PLs ability to mediate these changes, it is still difficult to sort out which of these maternal adaptations are mediated specifically by PL and which are mediated by GH or GH-V.

In humans, the ability of hPL to augment glucose-stimulated insulin secretion has varied amongst experiments *(159–161)*, and the variation may result from the GH status of the individuals studied (e.g. normal vs hypopituitary). However, in vitro treatment of human pancreatic islets with hPL resulted in increased insulin secretion *(162)*, suggesting that in fact hPL has direct insulinotropic actions. Human PL has also been implicated in reducing carbohydrate tolerance, as defined by an abnormal elevation in blood glucose concentrations following bolus glucose delivery. Carbohydrate tolerance is reduced in diabetic patients *(160,161)* followng hPL treatment, but the results in non-diabetics has been variable *(158,160,161,163)*. A reduction in carbohydrate tolerance could result from a lack of insulin secretion, or from resistance to insulin's actions. If hPL is in fact insulinotropic *(162)*, any reduction in carbohydrate tolerance is likely to result from hPL-induced insulin resistance. Unfortunately, insulin resistance has not been demonstrated in humans, although in rats, hPL reduces the sensitivity of the liver *(164)* to insulin while enhancing insulin sensitivity in adipose tissue *(165)*.

In sheep, infusion of partially purified oPL for 8 h in fasting pregnant and nonpregnant ewes resulted in reduced plasma concentrations of glucose and an increase in plasma insulin concentrations *(166)*. However, infusion of a placental extract, enriched for oPL *(167)*, for 36 h resulted in increased plasma glucose concentrations and decreased plasma insulin. Short-term (12 h) immunoneutralization of maternal oPL did not affect whole body glucose utilization, but significantly increased plasma insulin concentrations *(155)*. The first report agrees with the putative insulin-stimulatory actions of hPL (*see* above), but the latter two reports do not. All three reports differed in their experimental approaches, purity of oPL, pregnancy status and gestational age, making it difficult to draw any solid conclusions. Insulin secretion in response to a 2 h hyperglycemic clamp *(168)* reduces in magnitude as gestation increases. The gestational-age related change in glucose-stimulated insulin secretion *(168)* correlates with increasing oPL concentrations in maternal blood, and if this is a response to oPL, the results agree with the latter two reports *(155,167)*. However, another factor which needs to be considered when interpreting such experiments is the nutritional status of the experimental animals. In ewes, fasting will increase oPL concentration in both maternal and fetal circulation *(169)*, and reduce the concentration of oPL binding sites in maternal and fetal liver *(170)*. This latter effect of fasting can be reversed by glucose infusion *(170)*, indicating that not only is oPL's secretion regulated by nutrition but also it's function.

Studies examining the effects of PL on lipid metabolism in humans and sheep have generally suggested that it is lipolytic. Increased lipolysis and reesterification of fatty acids is observed during late pregnancy *(171)*, allowing free fatty acids to be used as a maternal energy source during fasting, or for the building of energy stores during periods of adequate nutrition. Relative to lipolysis, hPL increases basal lipolysis in vitro *(172)*, and in vivo treatment results in increased concentrations of nonesterified fatty acids (NEFA), ketones and glycerol in circulation *(173,174)*. However, these in vivo lipolytic effects of hPL have not been observed in all studies *(163,175)*. The esterification of NEFA into triglycerides is enhanced by insulin-stimulated glucose uptake by adipocytes, which is increased by hPL treatment of human and rat adipose tissue *(176,177)*, an action which could enhance maternal energy stores. Contrasting results have been obtained with oPL, in that one study indicated reduced plasma NEFA concentrations *(167)* and the other demonstrated increased plasma NEFA concentrations *(168)* following oPL infusion. Short-term immunoneutralization of maternal oPL resulted in a trend for reduced plasma NEFA concentrations *(155)*, which agrees with one of the previous studies *(168)* and the data obtained in humans *(173,174)*. However, oPL did not stimulate lipolysis in omental adipose tissue obtained from pregnant ewes *(178)*. As with the studies on carbohydrate metabolism, differences in the physiological status of the experimental animals, source of tissue and purity of the PL preparation, make drawing firm conclusions difficult. As mentioned earlier, the relationship between the endogenous concentration of hPL or oPL and the K_d of their respective binding sites, needs to be considered when evaluating the results of in vivo experiments. In other words, additional ligand is unlikely to stimulate responses if the receptors are already saturated by endogenous ligand. Furthermore, it may not be safe to assume that nonpregnant subjects will respond, or are capable of responding, to PL administration in the same fashion as pregnant individuals would be.

Cattle differ from either humans or sheep from the standpoint that maternal concentrations of bPL do not reach the high levels that hPL and oPL do during late pregnancy. For this reason, the pregnant cow may be a good model to examine the influence of PL on maternal intermediary metabolism, assuming that bPL is similar in it's actions. When bPL was administered to pregnant or nonpregnant, nonlactating cows, no effect was seen on the concentrations of plasma glucose, insulin, NEFA or tri-iodothyronine, whereas bGH increased all of these parameters *(179)*. In contrast, both bPL and bGH increased plasma concentrations of insulin-like growth factor (IGF) -I and IGF-II *(179)*. The increase in plasma IGF-I concentrations was also observed when nonpregnant heifers were injected with bPL *(150)*. The impact on IGF secretion in cattle may infer that at least part of PL's actions may be mediated by indirectly acting through the IGFs. However, in pregnant ewes (d 101–107 of pregnancy) hepatic IGF-I mRNA expression was not altered by oPL administration *(180)*, nor were IGF-I plasma concentrations increased *(181)* in response to 5 d of oPL administration during early lactation (d 17 of lactation). These last reports do not fit with the hypothesis of oPL altering maternal metabolism by inducing IGF expression, but the physiological status of these ewes (i.e., endogenous oPL concentrations and pregnancy status) may have impacted the results. Further studies are needed before firm conclusions can be drawn, and a PL deficient pregnancy may be needed to assess the full impact of PL on maternal metabolism.

Mammogenesis. As the name implies, PLs may have actions either on the development (mammogenesis) or the function (lactogenesis) of the mammary gland. In cattle and sheep, induction of mammogenesis is inhibited in nongravid females by administration of bromocryptine *(4)*, but the absence of prolactin secretion during pregnancy does not impede mammogenesis *(4)* suggesting the presence of a conceptus-derived mammotropic agent. Bovine PL stimulates DNA synthesis in mammary tissue explanted into athymic nude mice *(182)*, and similar results were obtained with hPL when human breast tissue derived from the periphery of benign tumors was transplanted in athymic nude mice *(183)* or subjected to tissue culture for 2 d *(184)*. Furthermore, in heifers induced to lactate, bPL injections increased total mammary DNA content and blood sera concentratons of α-lactalbumin *(185)*. Interestingly, bPL was more potent than PRL in stimulating DNA accretion and less potent than PRL in stimulating α-lactalbumin, which may suggest that PL may play a greater role in mammogenesis than lactogenesis. Recent results *(186)* indicate that bPL is capable of increasing milk yield 22% in heifers induced to lactate, but this increase was not statistically significant, and may again infer a greater role in mammogenesis.

Although little is known about hPL's ability to stimulate mammogenesis and lactogenesis, the data described above support the hypothesis that bPL is mammotropic in nature. However, the evidence for a mammotropic role is not as strong in sheep. Ovine PL is not as efficient as PRL in stimulating β-casein mRNA transcription in ewe mammary gland explants *(187)*, and it does not compete for PRL binding sites in mammary tissue *(188)*. Furthermore, treating ewes during early lactation with oPL *(181)* failed to increase milk yield and mammary gland weight, but both parameters were increased by treatment with bGH. Unfortunately, these experiments were really designed to address the lactogenic properties of oPL, rather than any possible mammogenic properties. Clearly, in all three species, more research is needed before any mammotropic role can be definitively assigned to PL.

Fetal System

The function of GH and PL within the fetus has generated considerable interest for a number of years. Much of the interest in PLs function within the fetus was generated by the concept that fetal pituitary-derived GH was unnecessary for normal fetal growth rate *(1)*. This concept was augmented by the lack of specific-GH binding sites in fetal sheep liver *(128–131)*, and the presence of specific binding sites for PL. The presence of GHR *(123,124)* or GHR mRNA *(121,135–137)* in fetal tissues, and the occurrence of clinical in utero growth retardation in infants with idiopathic GH deficiency *(2)* or GHR dysfunction *(3)*, suggests that GH may play a larger role in regulating fetal growth than earlier data indicated. Unfortunately, the specific actions of GH within the fetus are only now being examined, and little is known about the specific roles of hPL and bPL within the fetus.

Ovine PL stimulates amino acid uptake *(189)*, IGF-II secretion *(190)*, glycogen synthesis *(191)* and ornithine decarboxylase activity *(192)* in fetal rat tissues, but analogous treatment with GH is without effect. However, interpretation of these results must be moderated by the realization that oPL is not acting through oPL-specific receptors in these tissues. At least one of these actions has been recapitulated using fetal sheep tissues. Ovine fetal hepatocytes respond to oPL in a dose-dependent fashion by increasing the incorporation of glucose into glycogen, resulting in greater total cellular glycogen content *(193)*. Glycogenesis was also stimulated by oGH and oPRL, but oGH possessed only 12% of oPL's potency and oPRL possessed only 4% of oPL's potency. Coinciding with these data, is the ability of hPL, but not hGH, to stimulate the secretion of IGF-I, IGF-II and IGF-binding proteins (IGFBP) by human fetal fibroblasts *(194)*. From these studies, it has been suggested *(195)* that many of PLs somatogenic activities are mediated by IGFs.

Recent in vivo experiments designed to test this hypothesis have resulted in contrasting results. Short-term (24 h) infusion of recombinant oPL (roPL) into late-gestation fetal sheep did not alter plasma concentrations of IGF-I, IGF-II, insulin, NEFA and glucose *(196)*, although IGFBP-3 was reduced by 30%. However, long-term infusion (14 d) of oPL beginning on d 122 of gestation, resulted in elevated fetal plasma IGF-I with no effect on plasma IGFBP-2 *(197)*. Additionally, this infusion scheme resulted in greater liver glycogen accumulation *(197)*, which agrees with the earlier in vitro results *(193)*. The differing results from these studies may be a function of duration of treatment. What this may infer is that PL acts to modulate the fetal environment over the long-term, rather than responding to acute fluctuations in nutrient supply. Recent data *(198)* provide evidence for PLs ability to modulate systems or alter set-points. When postnatal lambs (3 d of age) were treated with oPL for 21 d, daily energy intake and live-weight gain were increased through 9 mo of age *(198)*. Similar effects were not seen with bGH treatment, and oPL clearly reset some form of appetite control. These data fit well with the hypothesis that PL serves in a long-term modulatory role of fetal growth, which is consistent with the concept of providing the proper homeorrhetic environment necessary for optimal fetal growth rates.

SUMMARY AND FUTURE DIRECTIONS

Human and ruminant GH and PL provide an interesting paradigm of structure, mechanism of action and biological function during pregnancy. Human PL is structurally very similar to GH, whereas ruminant PLs are more similar to PRL. However, both human and ruminant PLs may act through the GHR to elicit their effects, and may have similar roles during pregnancy. We have learned a great deal about their structures and secretion patterns, and are beginning to understand the transcriptional regulation of human and sheep PL. These latter efforts are needed if we hope to genetically manipulate the expression of these hormones. Such genetic manipulation could be used to provide a "deficient" system for analysis of biological function during pregnancy, or could provide the basis for future interventions to treat intrauterine growth retardation. The specific mechanism of action of PL is not known, and concerted effort is needed to structurally characterize the PL-specific binding sites that have been identified. Expression cloning is one approach that could be used to define the functional binding site for PL. Effort is also needed in determining the functional relevance of the "variant exon 1" containing GHR mRNA. Are they translated into functional GHR, or do these sequences provide for post-transcriptional down-regulation of the GHR? The answer to this question will provide insight into the role of GH within the fetus. Furthermore, determining what is responsible for the developmental "turn on" of the adult-liver specific GHR mRNA should provide insight into the regulation of fetal maturation, as well as possibly providing the base knowledge for designing better methods for the care of premature infants. Finally, well designed experiments which take into consideration the pregnancy and nutritional status of the subjects are needed to define function of these hormones. To define the function of PL within the mother, a PL deficient model is needed. As yet, gene ablation experiments are only feasible in mice, but recent progress suggests that this technology may soon be feasible in other animal models. In summary, although approximately three decades of research has been devoted to understanding the role of GH and PL during pregnancy, in many ways we are still infants in our understanding of their relative significance.

REFERENCES

1. Browne CA, Thorburn GD (1989) Endocrine control of fetal growth. Biol Neonate 55:331–346.
2. Gluckman PD, Gunn AJ, Wray A, Cutfield WS, Chatelain PG, Guilbaud O, Ambler GR, Wilton P, Albertson-Wikland K (1992) Congenital idiopathic growth hormone deficiency associated with prenatal and early postnatal growth failure. J Pediatr 121:920–923.
3. Rosenfeld RG, Rosenbloom AL, Guevara-Aguirre J (1994) Growth hormone (GH) insensitivity due to primary GH receptor deficiency. Endocr Rev 15:369–390.
4. Schams D, Russe I, Schallenberger E, Prokopp S, Chan JSD (1984) The role of steroid hormones, prolactin and placental lactogen on mammary gland development in ewes and heifers. J Endocrinol 102:121–130.
5. Talwalker PK, Meites J (1961) Mammary lobulo-alveolar growth induced by anterior pituitary hormones in adreno-ovariectomized-hypophysectomized rats. Proc Soc Exp Biol Med 107: 880–883.

6. Soares MJ, Faria TN, Roby KF, Deb S (1991) Pregnancy and the prolactin family of hormones: coordination of anterior pituitary, uterine, and placental expression. Endocr Rev 12:402–423.
7. Roberts RM, Anthony RV (1994) Molecular biology of trophectoderm and placental hormones. In: Findlay JK (ed) Molecular Biology of the Female Reproductive System. Academic Press, San Diego, 395–440.
8. Soares MJ, Dai G, Orwig GE (1997) The rodent placental prolactin gene family and pregnancy, In: Endocrinology of Pregnancy (Bazer FW, ed.), Humana, Totowa, NJ.
9. Ito Y, Higashi K (1961) Studies on the prolactin-like substance in human placenta II. Endocrinol Jpn 8:279–287.
10. Josimovich JB, MacLaren JA (1962) Presence in the human placenta and term serum of a highly lactogenic substance immunologically related to pituitary growth hormone. Endocrinology 71: 209–220.
11. Forsyth IA (1986) Variation among species in the endocrine control of mammary growth and function: the roles of prolactin, growth hormone, and placental lactogen. J Dairy Sci 69:886–903.
12. Josimovich JB, Levitt MJ, Stevens VC (1973) comparison of baboon and human placental lactogen. Ann NY Acad Sci. 148:488–500.
13. Shome B, Friesen HG (1971) Purification and characterization of monkey placental lactogen. Endocrinology 89:631–641.
14. Vinik AI, Kaplan SL, Grumbach MM (1973) Purification, characterization and comparison of immunological properties of monkey chorionic somatomammotropin with human and monkey growth hormone, human chorionic somatommotropin and ovine prolactin. Endocrinology 92: 1051–1064.
15. Bewley TA, Dixon JS, Li CH (1972) Sequence comparison of human pituitary growth hormone, human chorionic somatomammotropin, and ovine pituitary growth and lactogenic hormones. Int J Pept Protein Res 4:281–287.
16. Li CH, Dixon JS, Chung D (1973) Amino acid sequence of human chorionic somatomammotropin. Arch Biochem Biophys 155:95–110.
17. Cooke NE, Ray J, Watson MA, Estes PA, Kuo BA, Liebhaber SA (1988) Human growth hormone gene and the highly homologous growth hormone variant gene display different splicing patterns. J Clin Invest 82:270–275.
18. Ray J, Jones BK, Liebhaber SA, Cooke NE (1989) Glycosylated human growth hormone variant. Endocrinology 125:566–568.
19. Cooke NE, Ray J, Emery JG, Liebhaber SA (1988) Two distinct species of human growth hormone-variant mRNA in the human placenta predict the expression of novel growth hormone proteins. J Biol Chem 263:9001–9006.
20. DeVos AM, Ultsch M, Kossiakoff AA (1992) Human growth hormone and extracellular domain of its receptor: crystal structure of the complex. Science 255:306–312.
21. Murthy GS, Schellenberg C, Friesen HG (1982) Purification and characterization of bovine placental lactogen. Endocrinology 111:2117–2124.
22. Currie WB, Card CE, Michel FJ, Ignotz G (1990) Purification, partial characterization, and development of a specific radioimmunoassay for goat placental lactogen. J Reprod Fertil 90: 25–36.
23. Martal J, Djiane J (1975) Purification of lactogenic hormone in sheep placenta. Biochem Biophys Res Commun 65:770–778.
24. Schuler LA, Shimomura K, Kessler MA, Zieler CG, Bremel RD (1988) Bovine placental lactogen: molecular cloning and protein structure. Biochemistry 27:8443–8448.
25. Yamakawa M, Tanaka M, Koyama M, Kagesato Y, Watahiki M, Yamamoto M, et al. (1990) Expression of new members of the prolactin growth hormone gene family in bovine placenta. J Biol Chem 265:8915–8920.
26. Colosi P, Thordarson G, Hellmiss R, Singh K, Forsyth LA, Gluckman P, et al. (1989) Cloning and expression of ovine placental lactogen. Mol Endocrinol 3:1462–1469.
27. Warren WC, Liang R, Krivi GG, Siegel NR, Anthony RV (1990) Purification and structural characterization of ovine placental lactogen. J Endocrinol 126:141–149.
28. Byatt JC, Welply JK, Leimgruber RM, Collier RJ (1990) Characterization of glycosylated bovine placental lactogen and the effect of enzymatic deglycosylation on receptor binding and biological activity. Endocrinology 127:1041–1049.
29. Warren WC, Keisler DH, Anthony RV (1990) Synthesis and secretion of ovine placental lactogen and its biochemical properties. Dom Anim Endocrinol 7:331–342.
30. Anthony RV, Liang R, Kayl EP, Pratt SL (1995) The growth hormone/prolactin gene family in ruminant placentae. J Reprod Fertil Suppl. 49:83–95.

31. Wallis M (1993) Remarkably high rate of molecular evolution of ruminant placental lactogens. J Mol Evolution 37:86–88.
32. Lacroix MC, Devinoy E, Servely JL, Puissant C, Kann G (1996) Expression of the growth hormone gene in ovine placenta: detection and cellular localization of the protein. Endocrinology 137:4886–4892.
33. Owerbach D, Rutter W, Martial J, Baxter J (1980) Genes for growth hormone, chorionic somatomammotropin, and growth hormone-like gene are on chromosome 17 in humans. Science 209:289–292.
34. Barsch GS, Seeburg PH, Gelinas RE (1983) The human growth hormone gene family: structure and evolution of the chromosomal locus. Nucleic Acids Res 11:3939–3958.
35. Chen EY, Liao YC, Smith DH, Barrera-Saldana HA, Gelinas RE, Seeburg PH (1989) The human growth hormone locus nucleotide sequence, biology, evolution. Genomics 4:479–497.
36. Niall HD, Hogan ML, Sauer R, Rosenblum IY, Greenwood FC (1971) Sequences of pituitary and placental lactogenic and growth hormones: evolution from a primordial peptide by gene reduplication. Proc Natl Acad Sci USA 68:866–869.
37. Miller WL, Eberhardt NL (1983) Structure and evolution of the growth hormone gene family. Endocr Rev 4:97–130.
38. Wallis M (1981) The molecular evolution of pituitary growth hormone, prolactin, and placental lactogen: A protein family showing variable rates of evolution. J Mol Evol 17:10–15.
39. Moore DD, Conkling MA, Goodman HM (1982) Human growth hormone: a multigene family. Cell 29:285–296.
40. Hirt H, Kimelman J, Birnbaum MJ, Chen EY, Seeburg PH, Eberhardt NL, et al. (1987) The human growth hormone gene locus, structure, evolution, allelic variations. DNA 6:59–70.
41. Barrera-Saldana HA, Seeburg PH, Saunders GF (1983) Two structurally different genes produce the same secreted human placental lactogen hormone. J Biol Chem 258:3787–3793.
42. Resendez-Perez D, Ramirez-Solis R, Varela-Echavarria A, Martinez-Rodrigues HG, Barrera-Saldana HA (1990) Coding potential of transfected human placental lactogen genes. Nucleic Acids Res 18:4665–4670.
43. Selby MJ, Barta A, Baxter JD, Bell GI, Eberhardt NL (1984) Analysis of a major human chorioic somatomammotropin gene. J Biol Chem 259:13,131–13,138.
44. Bodner M, Castrillo J-L, Theill LE, Deerinck T, Ellisman M, Karin M (1988) The pituitary-specific transcription factor GHF-1 is a homeobox-containing protein. Cell 55:505–518.
45. Ingraham HA, Chen R, Mangalam HJ, Elsholtz HP, Flynn SE, Lin CR, Simmons DM, Swanson L, Rosenfeld MG (1988) A tissue-specific transcription factor containing a homeodomain specifies a pituitary phenotype. Cell 55:519–529.
46. Karin M, Castrillo J-L, Theill LE (1990) Growth hormone gene regulation: a paradigm for cell-type-specific gene activation. Trends Genet. 6:92–96.
47. Lemaigre FP, Peers B, Lafontaine DA, Mathy-Hartert M, Rousseau GG, Belayew A, et al. (1989) Pituitary-specific factor binding to the human prolactin, growth hormone, placental lactogen genes. DNA 8:149–159.
48. Fitzpatrick SL, Walker WH, Saunders GF (1990) DNA sequences involved in the transcriptional activation of a human placental lactogen gene. Mol Endocrinol 4:1815–1826.
49. Tansey WP, Catanzaro DF (1991) Spl and thyroid hormone receptor differentially activate expression of human growth hormone and chorionic somatomammotropin genes. J Biol Chem 266:9805–9813.
50. Letovsky J, Dynan WS (1989) Measurements of the binding of transcription factor Spl to a single GC box recognition sequence. Nucleic Acids Res 17:2639–2653.
51. Kadonaga JT, Jones KA, Tjian R (1986) Promoter-specific activation of RNA polymerase II transcription by Spl. Trends Biochem 11:20–25.
52. Peritz LN, Fodor EJB, Silversides DW, Cattini PA, Baxter JD, Eberhardt NL (1988) The human growth hormone gene contains both positive and negative control elements. J Biol Chem 263: 5005–5007.
53. Lemaigre FP, Courtois SJ, Lafontaine DA, Rousseau GG (1989) Evidence that the upstream stimulatory factor, the Spl transcription factor bind in vitro to the promoters of the human-growth-hormone gene. Eur J Biochem 181:555–561.
54. Courtois SJ, Lafontaine DA, Lemaigre FP, Durviaux SM, Rousseau GG (1990) Nuclear factor-1 and activator protein-2 bind in a mutually exclusive way to overlapping promoter sequences and trans-activate the human growth hormone gene. Nucleic Acids Res 18:57–64.
55. Slater EP, Rabenau O, Karin M, Baxter JD, Beato M (1985) Glucocorticoid receptor binding and activation of a heterologous promoter by dexamethasone by the first intron of the human growth hormone gene. Mol Cell Biol 5:2984–2992.

56. Barlow JW, Voz MLJ, Eliard PH, Mathy-Hartet M, DeNayer P, Economidis IV, et al. (1986) Thyroid hormone receptors bind to defined regions of the growth hormone and placental lactogen genes. Proc Natl Acad Sci USA 83:9021–9025.
57. Dana S, Karin M (1989) Induction of human growth hormone promoter activity by the adenosine 3′,5′-monophosphate pathway involves a novel responsive element. Mol Endocrinol 3:815–821.
58. Nickel BE, Cattini PA (1991) Tissue specific expression and thyroid hormone regulation of the endogenous placental growth hormone variant and chorionic somatomammotropin genes in a human choriocarcinoma cell line. Endocrinology 128:2353–2359.
59. Cattini PA, Anderson TR, Baxter JD, Mellon P, Eberhardt NL (1986) The human growth hormone gene is negatively regulated by triiodothyronine when transfected into rat pituitary tumor cells. J Biol Chem 261:13,367–13,372.
60. Cattini PA, Eberhardt NL (1987) Regulated expression of chimaeric genes containing the 5′-flanking regions of human growth hormone-related genes in transiently transfected rat anterior pituitary tumor cells. Nucleic Acids Res 15:1297–1309.
61. Voz ML, Peers B, Belayew A, Martial JA (1991) Characterization of an unusual thyroid response unit in the promoter of the human placental lactogen gene. J Biol Chem 266:13,397–13,408.
62. Stephanou A, Ross R, Handwerger S (1994) Regulation of human placental lactogen expression by 1,25-dihydroxyvitamin D3. Endocrinology 135:2651–2656.
63. Stephanou A, Handwerger S (1995) The nuclear factor NF-IL6 activates human placental lactogen gene expression. Biochem Biophys Res Commun 206:215–222.
64. Rogers BL, Sobnosky MG, Saunders GF (1986) Transcriptional enhancer within the human placental lactogen and growth hormone multigene cluster. Nucleic Acids Res 14:7647–7659.
65. Walker WH, Fitzpatrick SL, Saunders GF (1990) Human placental lactogen transcriptional enhancer. J Biol. Chem 265:12,940–12,948.
66. Davidson I, Xiao JH, Rosales R, Staub A, Chambon P (1988) The HeLa cell protein TEF-1 binds specifically and cooperatively to two SV40 motifs of unrelated sequence. Cell 54:931–942.
67. Jacquemin P, Oury C, Peers B, Morin A, Belayew A, Martial JA (1994) Characterization of a single strong tissue-specific enhancer downstream from the three human genes encoding placental lactogen. Mol Cell Biol 14:93–103.
68. Lytras A, Cattini PA (1994) Human chorionic somatomammotropin gene enhancer activity is dependent on the blockade of a repressor mechanism. Mol Endocrinol 8:478–489.
69. Jiang S-W, Eberhardt NL (1995) Involvement of a protein distinct from transcription enhancer factor-1 (TEF-1) in mediating human chorionic somatomammotropin gene enhancer function through the GT-IIC enhanson in choriocarcinoma and COS cells. J Biol Chem 270:13,906–13,915.
70. Jiang S-W, Eberhardt NL (1996) TEF-1 transrepression in BeWo cells is mediated through interactions with the TATA-binding protein, TBP. J Biol Chem 271:9510–9518.
71. Jiang S-W, Shepard AR, Eberhardt NL (1995) An initiator element is required for maximal chorionic somatomammotropin gene promoter and enhancer function. J Biol Chem 270:3683–3692.
72. Nachtigal MW, Nickel BE, Cattini PA (1993) Pituitary-specific repression of placental lactogen members of the human growth hormone gene family. J Biol Chem 268:8473–8479.
73. Kessler MA, Schuler LA (1991) Structure of the bovine placental lactogen gene and alternative splicing of transcripts. DNA Cell Biol 10:93–104.
74. Liang R, Anthony RV (1993) Characterization of the gene encoding ovine placental lactogen. Biol Reprod 48(Suppl 1):177. (Abstract)
75. Dietz AB, Georges M, Threadgill DW, Womack JE, Schuler LA (1992) Somatic cell mapping, polymorphism, and linkage analysis of bovine prolactin-related proteins and placental lactogen. Genomics 14:137–143.
76. Liang R (1995) Molecular cloning and characterization of the ovine placental lactogen gene. Ph.D. Dissertation, University of Missouri, Columbia.
77. Yamakawa M, Tanaka M, Koyama M, Kagesto Y, Watahiki M, Yamamoto M, et al. (1990) Expression of new members of the prolactin growth hormone gene family in bovine placenta. J Biol Chem 265:8915–8920.
78. Limesand SL, Liang R, Anthony RV (1997) Identification of cis-acting elements involved in modulating transcription of the ovine placental lactogen gene. The Endocrine Society 79th Annual Meeting and Abstracts, Abstract #P2-440, p. 394.
79. Johnoson W, Albanese C, Handwerger S, Williams T, Pestell RG, Jameson JL (1997) Regulation of the human chorionic gonadotropin α- and β-subunit promoters by AP-2. J Biol Chem 272: 15,405–15,412.

80. Ng Y-K, George KM, Engel JD, Linzer DIH (1994) GATA factor activity is required for the trophoblast-specific transcriptional regulation of the mouse placental lactogen I gene. Development 120:3257–3266.
81. Steger DJ, Hecht JH, Mellon PL (1994) GATA-binding proteins regulate the human gonadotropin α-subunit gene in the placenta and pituitary gland. Mol Cell Biol 14:5592–5602.
82. Beck JS (1970) Time of appearance of human placental lactogen in the embryo. N Engl J Med 283:189–190.
83. Biswas S, Hindocha P, Dehurst CJ (1972) Human chorionic somatomammotropin in serum and urine in various stages of pregnancy: its correlation with enzymes and oestrogens. J Endocrinol 54:251–261.
84. Braunstein GD, Rasor JL, Engvall E, Wade ME (1980) Interrelationships of human chorionic gonadotropin, human placental lactogen, and pregnancy-specific β_1-glycoprotein throughout normal human gestation. Am J Obstet Gynecol 138:1205–1213.
85. Hoshina M, Boothby M, Boime I (1982) Cytological localization of chorionic gonadotropin α and placental lactogen mRNAs during development of the human placenta. J Cell Biol 93:190–198.
86. Maruo T, Ladines-Llave CA, Matsuo H, Manalo AS, Mochizuki M (1992) A novel change in cytological localization of human chorionic gonadotropin and human placental lactogen in first-trimester placenta in the course of gestation. Am J Obstet Gynecol 167:217–222.
87. Beck P, Daughaday WH (1967) Human placental lactogen: studies of its acute metabolic effects and disposition in normal man. J Clin Invest 46:103–110.
88. Kaplan SL, Gurpide E, Sciarra JJ, Grumbach MM (1968) Metabolic clearance rate and production rate of chorionic growth hormone-prolactin in late pregnancy. J Clin Endocrinol Metab 28:1450–1460.
89. Pierce GB, Midgley AR (1963) The origin and function of human syncytiotrophoblast giant cells. Am J Pathol 43:153–173.
90. Boime I, Boothby M, Hoshina M, Daniels-McQueen S, Darnell R (1982) Expression and structure of human placental hormone genes as a function of placental development. Biol Reprod 26:73–91.
91. Handwerger S (1991) Clinical counterpoint: The physiology of placental lactogen in human pregnancy. Endocr Rev 12:329–336.
92. Hill DJ, Freemark M, Strain AJ, Handwerger S, Milner RDG (1988) Placental lactogen and growth hormone receptors in human fetal tissues: relationship to fetal plasma human placental lactogen concentrations and fetal growth. J Clin Endocrinol Metab 66:1283–1290.
93. Crosignani PG, Nencioni T, Brambati B (1972) Concentration of chorionic gonadotrophin and chorionic somatomammotropin in maternal serum, amniotic fluid and cord blood serum at term. J Obstet Gynaecol Br Commonw 79:122–126.
94. Carnegie JA, Chan JSD, McCully ME, Robertson HA, Friesen HG (1982) The cellular localization of chorionic somatomammotrophin in ovine chorion. J Reprod Fertil 66:9–16.
95. Kessler MA, Duello TM, Schuler LA (1991) Expression of prolactin-related hormones in the early bovine conceptus, and potential for paracrine effect on the endometrium. Endocrinology 129: 1885–1895.
96. Milosavljevic M, Duello TM, Schuler LA (1989) In situ localization of two prolactin-related messenger ribonucleic acids to binucleate cells of bovine placentomes. Endocrinology 125:883–889.
97. Kappes SM, Warren WC, Pratt SL, Liang R, Anthony RV (1992) Quantification and cellular localization of ovine placental lactogen messenger ribonucleic acid expression during mid- and late gestation. Endocrinology 131:2829–2838.
98. Wooding FBP (1992) Current topic: the synepitheliochorioal placenta of ruminants: binucleate cell fusions and hormone production. Placenta 13:101–113.
99. Beckers JF, deCoster R, Wouters-Ballman P, Fromont-Lienard C, van der Zwalman P, Ectors F (1982) Dosage radioimmunologique de l'hormone placentaire somatotrope et mammotrope bone. Ann Med Vet 126:9–21.
100. Wallace CR (1993) Concentrations of bovine placental lactogen in dairy and beef cows across gestation. Dom Anim Endocrinol 10:67–70.
101. Handwerger S, Chrenshaw C, Maurer WF, Barrett J, Hurley TW, Golander A, Fellows RE (1977) Studies on ovine placental lactogen secretion by homologous radioimmunoassay. J Endocr 72:27–34.
102. Martal J, Djiane J (1977) The production of chorionic somatomammotrophin in sheep. J Reprod Fertil 49:285–289.
103. Reddy S, Watkins WB (1983) Plasma clearance and distribution of ^{125}I-ovine placental lactogen in sheep. Aust J Exp Biol Med Sci 61:301–310.

104. Schoknecht PA, Currie WB, Bell AW (1992) Kinetics of placental lactogen in mid- and late gestation ovine fetuses. J Endocrinol 133:95–100.
105. Jara CS, Salud AT, Bryant-Greenwood GD, Pirens G, Hennen G, Frankenne F (1989) Immunocytochemical localization of the human growth hormone variant in the human placenta. J Clin Endocrinol Metab 69:1069–1072.
106. Liebhaber SA, Urbanek M, Ray J, Tuan RS, Cooke NE (1989) Characterization and histologic localization of human growth hormone-variant gene expression in the placenta. J Clin Invest 83:1985–1991.
107. Frankenne F, Closset J, Gomez F, Scippo ML, Smal J, Hennen G (1988) The physiology of growth hormones (Ghs) in pregnant women and partial characterization of the placental GH variant. J Clin Endocrinol Metab 66:1171–1180.
108. Hennen G, Frankenne F, Closset J, Gomez F, Pirens G, El Khayat N (1985) A human placental GH: increasing levels during second half of pregnancy with pituitary GH suppression as revealed by monoclonal antibody radioimmunoassays. Int J Fertil 30:27–33.
109. Lowman HB, Cunningham BC, Wells JA (1991) Mutational analysis and protein engineering of receptor-binding determinants in human placental lactogen. J Biol Chem 266:10,982–10,988.
110. Staten MR, Byatt JC, Krivi GG (1993) Ligand-specific dimerization of the extracellular domain of the bovine growth hormone receptor. J Biol Chem 268:18,467–18,473.
111. Fiddes RJ, Brandon MR, Adams TE (1992) Functional expression of an ovine growth hormone receptor in transfected Chinese hamster ovary cells. Mol Cell Endocrinol 86:883–889.
112. Leung DW, Spencer SA, Cachianes G, Hammonds RG, Collins C, Henzel WJ, Barnard R, Waters MJ, Woods WI (1987) Growth hormone receptor and serum binding protein: Purification, cloning and expression. Nature 330:537–543.
113. Cunningham BC, Ultsch M, de Vos AM, Mulkerrin MG, Clausser KR, Wells JA (1991) Dimerization of the extracellular domain of the human growth hormone receptor by a single hormone molecule. Science 254:821–825.
114. Ishizaka-Ikeda E, Fukunaga R, Wood WI, Goeddel DV, Nagata S (1993) Signal transduction mediated by growth hormone receptor and its chimeric molecules with the granulocyte colony-stimulating factor receptor. Proc Natl Acad Sci USA 90:123–127.
115. Ilondo MM, Damholt AB, Cunningham BA, Wells JA, De Meyts P, Shymko RM (1994) Receptor dimerization determines the effects of growth hormone in primary rat adipocytes and cultured human IM-9 lymphocytes. Endocrinology 134:2397–2403.
116. Argetsinger LS, Campbell GS, Yang X, Wittuhun BA, Silvennoinen O, Ihle JN, et al. (1993) Identification of JAK2 as a growth hormone receptor-associated tyrosine kinase. Cell 74: 237–244.
117. Smit LS, Meyer DJ, Billestrup N, Norstedt G, Schwartz J, Carter-Su C (1996) The role of growth hormone (GH) receptor and JAK1 and JAK2 kinases in the activation of Stats 1, 3, and 5 by GH. Mol Endocrinol 10:519–533.
118. Gronowski AM, Rotwein P (1994) Rapid changes in nuclear protein tyrosine phosphorylation after growth hormone treatment in vivo. J Biol Chem 269:7874–7878.
119. Carter-Su C, King AP, Argetsinger LS, Smit LS, Vanderkuur J, Campbell GS (1996) Signalling pathway of GH. Endocrine J 43 (Suppl.):S65–S70.
120. Urbanek M, MacLeod JN, Cooke NE, Liebhaber SA (1992) Expression of a human growth hormone (hGH) receptor isoform is predicted by tissue-specific alternative splicing of exon 3 of the hGH receptor gene transcript. Mol Endocrinol 6:279–287.
121. Zogopoulos G, Figueiredo R, Jenab A, Ali Z, Lefebvre Y, Goodyer CG (1996) Expression of exon3-retaining and -deleted human growth hormone receptor messenger ribonucleic acid isoforms during development. J Clin Endocrinol Metab 81:775–782.
122. Urbanek M, Russell JE, Cooke NE, Liebhaber SA (1993) Functional characterization of the alternatively spliced, placental human growth hormone receptor. J Biol Chem 268:19,025–19,032.
123. Hill DJ, Freemark M, Strain AJ, Handwerger S, Milner RDG (1988) Placental lactogen and growth hormone receptors in fetal tissues: relationship to fetal plasma human placental lactogen concentrations and fetal growth. J Clin Endocrinol Metab 66:1283–1290.
124. Hill DJ, Riley SC, Bassett NS, Waters MJ (1992) Localization of the growth hormone receptor, identified by immunocytochemistry, in second trimester human fetal tissues and placenta throughout gestation. J Clin Endocrinol Metab 75:646–650.
125. Pekhletsky RI, Chernov BK, Rubtsov PM (1992) Variants of the 5′ untranslated sequence of human growth hormone receptor mRNA. Mol Cell Endocrinol 90:103–109.
126. Godowski PJ, Leung DW, Meacham LR, Galgani JP, Hellmiss R, Keret R, et al. (1989) Characterization of human growth hormone receptor gene and demonstration of a partial gene deletion in two patients with Laron-type dwarfism. Proc Natl Acad Sci USA 86:8063–8087.

127. Zogopoulos G, Albrecht S, Pietsch T, Alpert L, von Schweinitz D, Lefebvre Y, Goodyer CG (1996) Fetal- and tumor-specific regulation of growth hormone receptor messenger RNA expression in human liver. Cancer Res 56:2949–2953.
128. Gluckman PD, Butler JH, Elliot TB (1983) The ontogeny of somatotropic binding sites in ovine hepatic membranes. Endocrinology 112:1607–1612.
129. Freemark M, Comer M, Handwerger S (1986) Placental lactogen and growth hormone receptors in sheep liver: striking differences in ontogeny and function. Am J Physiol 251:E328–E333.
130. Pratt SL, Kappes SM, Anthony RV (1995) Ontogeny of a specific high-affinity binding site for ovine placental lactogen in fetal and postnatal liver. Dom Anim Endocrinol 12:337–347.
131. Freemark M, Comer M, Korner G, Handwerger S (1987) A unique placental lactogen receptor: Implications for fetal growth. Endocrinology 120:1865–1872.
132. Freemark M, Comer M, Korner G (1988) Differential solubilization of placental lactogen and growth hormone-binding sites: Further evidence for a unique PL receptor in fetal and maternal liver. Endocrinology 122:2771–2779.
133. Freemark M, Comer M (1989) Purification of a distinct placental lactogen receptor, a new member of the growth hormone/prolactin receptor family. J Clin Invest 83:883–889.
134. Breier BH, Funk B, Surus A, Ambler GR, Wells CA, Waters MJ, et al. (1994) Characterization of ovine growth hormone (oGH) and ovine placental lactogen (oPL) binding to fetal and adult hepatic tissue in sheep: evidence that oGH and oPL interact with a common receptor. Endocrinology 135:919–928.
135. Adams TE, Baker L, Fiddes RJ, Brandon MR (1990) The sheep growth hormone receptor: molecular cloning and ontogeny of mRNA expression in the liver. Mol Cell Endocrinol 73:135–145.
136. Klempt M, Bingham B, Breier BH, Baumbach WR, Gluckman PD (1993) Tissue distribution and ontogeny of growth hormone receptor messenger ribonucleic acid and ligand binding to hepatic tissue in the midgestation sheep fetus. Endocrinology 132:1071–1077.
137. Pratt SL, Anthony RV (1995) The growth hormone receptor messenger ribonucleic acid present in ovine fetal liver is a variant form. Endocrinology 136:2150–2155.
138. Adams TE (1995) Differential expression of growth hormone receptor messenger RNA from a second promoter. Mol Cell Endocrinol 108:23–33.
139. Kozak M (1991) An analysis of vertebrate mRNA sequences: intimations of translational control. J Cell Biol 115:887–903.
140. Geballe AP, Morris DR (1994) Initiation codons within 5′-leaders of mRNAs as regulators of translation. Trends Biochem Sci 19:159–164.
141. Challis JRG, Brooks AN (1989) Maturation and activation of hypothalamic-pituitary-adrenal function in fetal sheep. Endocrine Rev 10:182–210.
142. Li J, Owens JA, Owens PC, Saunders JC, Fowden AL, Gilmour RS (1996) The ontogeny of hepatic growth hormone receptor and insulin-like growth factor I gene expression in the sheep fetus during late gestation: developmental regulation by cortisol. Endocrinology 137:1650–1657.
143. Phillips ID, Anthony RV, Butler TG, Ross JT, McMillen IC (1997) Hepatic prolactin receptor gene expression increases in the sheep fetus before birth and after cortisol infustion. Endocrinology 138:1351–1354.
144. Galosy SS, Gertler A, Elberg, Laird DM (1991) Distinct placental lactogen and prolactin (lactogen) receptors in bovine endometrium. Mol Cell Endocrinol 78:229–236.
145. Kessler MA, Duello TM, Schuler LA (1991) Expression of prolactin-related hormones in the early bovine conceptus, and potential for paracrine effects on the endometrium. Endocrinology 129: 1885–1895.
146. Scott P, Kessler MA, Schuler LA (1992) Molecular cloning of the bovine prolactin receptor and distribution of prolactin and growth hormone receptor transcripts in fetal and utero-placental tissues. Mol Cell Endocrinol 89:47–58.
147. Gertler A, Grosclaude J, Strasburger CJ, Nir S, Djiane J (1996) Real-time kinetic measurements of the interactions between lactogenic hormones and prolactin-receptor extracellular domains from several species support the model of hormone-induced transient receptor dimerization. J Biol Chem 271:24,482–24,491.
148. Warren WC, Huynh M, Paik K, Pegg G, Byatt JC, Staten NR (1997) Evaluation of bovine placental lactogen (bPL) and somatotropin (bST) utilizing a bST receptor expressing lymphoid cell line. The Endocrine Society 79th Annual Meeting and Abstracts, Abstract #P2-212, p. 337.
149. Galosy SS, Talamantes F (1995) Luteotropic actions of placental lactogens at midpregnancy in the mouse. Endocrinology 136:3993–4003.
150. Lucy MC, Byatt JC, Curran TL, Curran DF, Collier RJ (1994) Placental lactogen and somatotropin: hormone binding to the corpus luteum and effects on growth and function of the ovary in heifers. Biol Reprod 50:1136–1144.

151. Stock RJ, Josimovich JB, Kosor B, Klopper A, Wilson GR (1971) The effect of chorionic gonadotropin and chorionic somatomammotropin on steroidogenesis in the corpus luteum. J Obstet Gyn Br Comm 78:549–553.
152. Goldsmith LT, Hochman JA, Weiss G (1978) Effect of human placental lactogen upon the corpus luteum of late pregnancy. Gyn Obstet Invest 9:210–218.
153. Ramasharma K, Li CH (1987) Human pituitary and placental hormones control human insulin-like growth factor II secretion in human granulosa cells. Proc Natl Acad Sci USA 84:2643–2647.
154. Schramm W, Friesen HG, Robertson HA, McCracken JA (1984) Effects of exogenous ovine placental lactogen on luteolysis induced by prostaglandin $F_{2\alpha}$ in sheep. J Reprod Fertil 70: 557–565.
155. Waters MJ, Oddy VH, McCloghry CE, Gluckman PD, Duplock R, Owens PC, et al. (1985) An examination of the proposed roles of placental lactogen in the ewe by means of antibody neutralization. J Endocrinol 106:377–386.
156. Lucy MC, Collier RJ, Kitchell MI, Dibner JJ, Hauser SD, Krivi GG (1993) Immunohistochemical and nucleic acid analysis of somatotropin receptor populations in the bovine ovary. Biol Reprod 48:1219–1227.
157. Juengel JL, Nett TM, Anthony RV, Niswender GD (1997) Effects of luteotrophic and luteolytic hormones on expression of mRNA encoding insulin-like growth factor I and growth hormone receptor in the ovine corpus luteum. J Reprod Fertil 110:291–298.
158. Grumbach MM, Kaplan SL, Sciarra JJ, Burr IM (1968) Chorionic growth hormone-prolactin (CGP): secretion, disposition, biological activity in man, and postulated function as the "growth hormone" of the second half of pregnancy. Ann NY Acad Sci 148:501–531.
159. Josimovich JB, Mintz DH (1968) Biological and immunochemical studies on human placental lactogen. Ann NY Acad Sci 148:488–500.
160. Samaan N, Yen SCC, Gonzalez D, Pearson OH (1968) Metabolic effects of placental lactogen (HPL) in man. J Clin Endocrinol Metab 28:485–591.
161. Kalkhoff RK, Richardson BL, Beck P (1969) Relative effects of pregnancy, human placental lactogen and predisolone on carbohydrate tolerance in normal and subclinical diabetic subjects. Diabetes 18:153–175.
162. Brelje TC, Schapp DW, Lacy PE, Ogren L, Talamantes F, Robertson M, et al. (1993) Effect of homologous placental lactogens, prolactins, and growth hormones on islet B-cell division and insulin secretion in rat, mouse, and human islets: implication for placental lactogen regulation of islet function during pregnancy. Endocrinology 132:879–887.
163. Beck P, Daughaday WH (1967) Human placental lactogen: studies of its acute metabolic effects and disposition in normal man. J Clin Invest 46:103–110.
164. Sladek CD (1975) The effects of human chorionic somatomammotropin and estradiol on gluconeogenesis and hepatic glycogen formation in the rat. Horm Metab Res 7:50–54.
165. Leake NH, Burt RL (1969) Effect of HPL and pregnancy on glucose uptake in rat adipose tissue. Am J Obstet Gynecol 103:39–43.
166. Handwerger S, Fellows RE, Crenshaw MC, Hurley T, Barrett J, Maurer WF (1976) Ovine placental lactogen: acute effects on intermediary metabolism in pregnant and non-pregnant sheep. J Endocrinol 69:133–137.
167. Thordarson G, McDowell GH, Smith SV, Iley S, Forsyth IA (1987) Effects of continuous intravenous infusion of an ovine placental extract enriched in placental lactogen on plasma hormones, metabolites and metabolic biokinetics in non-pregnant sheep. J Endocrinol 113:277–283.
168. Regnault TRH (1997) Orchestrated partitioning of maternal nutrients during ovine pregnancy. Ph.D. Dissertation, University of Western Sydney-Hawkesbury.
169. Brinsmead MW, Bancroft BJ, Thorburn GD, Waters MJ (1981) Fetal and maternal ovine placental lactogen during hyperglycaemia, hypoglycaemia and fasting. J Endocrinol 90:337–343.
170. Freemark M, Keen A, Fowlkes J, Mularoni T, Comer M, Grandis A, et al. (1992) The placental lactogen receptor in maternal and fetal sheep liver: regulation by glucose and role in the pathogenesis of fasting during pregnancy. Endocrinology 130:1063–1070.
171. Kalkhoff RK, Kissebah AH, Kim H-J (1978) Carbohydrate and lipid metabolism during normal pregnancy: relationship to gestational hormone action. Semin Perinatol 2:291–307.
172. Williams C, Coltart TM (1978) Adipose tissue metabolism in pregnancy: the lipolytic effect of human placental lactogen. Br J Obstet Gynaecol 85:43–46.

173. Grumbach MM, Kaplan SL, Abrams CL, Bell JJ, Conte FA (1966) Plasma free fatty acid response to the administration of chorionic "growth hormone-prolactin." J Clin Endocrinol Metab 26:478–482.
174. Berle P (1973) Comparative studies on the metabolic effects of some parameters of carbohydrate and lipid metabolism after intravenous administration of human placental lactogen, human prolactin and growth hormone. Acta Endocrinol 173(Suppl.):104.
175. Berle P, Finsterwalder E, Apostolakis M (1974) Comparative studies on the effect of human growth hormone, human prolactin and human placental lactogen on lipid metabolism. Horm Metab Res 6:347–350.
176. Leake NH, Burt RL (1969) Effect of HPL and pregnancy on glucose uptake in rat adipose tissue. Am J Obstet Gynecol 103:39–43.
177. Recio F, Knight BL, Osorio C, Myant NB (1979) The effect of human placental lactogen upon the metabolism of rat and human adipose tissue. Rev Esp Fisiol 35:143–152.
178. Iliou JP, Demarne Y (1987) Evolution of the sensitivity of isolated adipocytes of ewes to the lipolytic effects of different stimuli during pregnancy and lactation. Int J Biochem 19:253–258.
179. Byatt JC, Eppard PJ, Veenhuizen JJ, Sorbet RH, Buonomo FC, Curran DF, et al. (1992) Serum half-life and in vivo actions of recombinant bovine placental lactogen in the dairy cow. J Endocrinol 132:185–193.
180. Currie MJ, Bassett NS, Breier BH, Klempt M, Min SH, Mackenzie DD, et al. PD (1996) Differential effects of maternal ovine placental lactogen and growth hormone (GH) administration on GH receptor, insulin-like growth factor (IGF)-1 and IGF binding protein-3 gene expression in the pregnant and fetal sheep. Growth Reg 6:123–129.
181. Min SH, Mackenzie DD, McCutcheon SN, Breier BH, Gluckman PD (1997) Comparative effects of recombinant ovine placental lactogen and bovine growth hormone on galactopoiesis in ewes. J Dairy Sci 80:640645.
182. Vega JR, Shefield LG, Bremel RD (1989) Bovine placental lactogen stimulates DNA synthesis of bovine mammary tissue maintained in athymic nude mice. Proc Soc Exp Biol Med 192:135–129.
183. McManus MJ, Welsch CW (1984) The effect of estrogen, progesterone, thyroxine, and human placental lactogen on DNA synthesis of human breast ductal epithelium maintained in athymic nude mice. Cancer 54:1920–1927.
184. Welsch CW, Dombroske SE, McManus MJ (1978) Effects of insulin, human placental lactogen and human growth hormone on DNA synthesis in organ cultures of benign human breast tumours.
185. Byatt JC, Eppard PJ, Veenhuizen JJ, Curran TL, Curran DF, McGrath MF, et al. (1994) Stimulation of mammogenesis and lactogenesis by recombinant bovine placental lactogen in steroid-primed dairy heifers. J Endocrinol 140:33–43.
186. Byatt JC, Sorbet RH, Eppard PJ, Curran TL, Curran DF, Collier RJ (1997) The effect of recombinant bovine placental lactogen on induced lactation in dairy heifers.
187. Severly J-L, Emane NM, Houdebine L-M, Djiane J, Delouis C, Kelly PA (1983) Comparative measurements of the lactogenic activity of ovine placental lactogen in rabbit and ewe mammary gland. Gen Comp Endocrinol 51:255–262.
188. Emane MN, Delouis C, Kelly PA, Djiane J (1986) Evolution of prolactin and placental lactogen receptors in ewes during pregnancy and lactation. Endocrinology 118:695–700.
189. Freemark M, Handwerger S (1983) Ovine placental lactogen, but not growth hormone, stimulates amino acid transport in fetal rat diaphragm. Endocrinology 120:402–404.
190. Adams SO, Nissley SP, Handwerger S, Rechler MM (1983) Developmental patterns of insulin-like growth factor-1 and -II synthesis and regulation in rat fibroblasts. Nature 302:150–152.
191. Freemark M, Handwerger S (1984) Ovine placental lactogen stimulates glycogen synthesis in fetal rat hepatocytes. Am J Physiol 246:E21–E24.
192. Hurley TW, Thadani P, Kuhn CM, Schanberg SM, Handwerger S (1980) Differential effects of placental lactogen, growth hormone and prolactin on rat liver ornithine decarboxylase activity in the perinatal period. Life Sci 27:2269–2275.
193. Freemark M, Handwerger S (1986) The glycogenic effects of placental lactogen and growth hormone in ovine fetal liver are mediated through binding to specific fetal ovine placental lactogen receptors. Endocrinology 118:613–618.
194. Hill DJ, Camacho-Hubner C, Rashid P, Strain AJ, Clemmons DR (1989) Insulin-like growth factor (IGF)-binding protein release by human fetal fibroblasts: dependency on cell density and IGF peptides. J Endocrinol 122:87–98.

195. Handwerger S (1991) Clinical counterpoint: the physiology of placental lactogen in human pregnancy. Endocrine Rev 12:329–336.
196. Oliver MH, Harding JE, Breier BH, Evans PC, Gallaher BW, Gluckman PD (1995) The effects of ovine placental lactogen infusion on metabolites, insulin-like growth factors and binding proteins in the fetal sheep. J Endocrinol 144:333–338.
197. Schoknecht PA, McGuire MA, Cohick WS, Currie WB, Bell AW (1996) Effect of chronic infusion of placental lactogen on ovine fetal growth in late gestation. Dom Anim Endocrinol 13:519–528.
198. Min SH, Mackenzie DD, Breier BH, McCutcheon SN, Gluckman PD (1996) Growth-promoting effects of ovine placental lactogen (oPL) in young lambs: comparison with bovine growth hormone provides evidence for a distinct effect of oPL on food intake. Growth Reg 6:144–151.

17 Stromal-Epithelial Cell Communication in the Female Reproductive Tract

Paul S. Cooke, PHD, David L. Buchanan, MS, Takeshi Kurita, PHD, Dennis B. Lubahn, PHD, and Gerald R. Cunha, PHD

CONTENTS

INTRODUCTION

The female reproductive organs undergo well-characterized structural and functional changes during the estrous or menstrual cycles and the establishment and maintenance of pregnancy. These reproductive tract changes are primarily under the control of hormones such as estrogens, specifically estradiol 17-β (E2), and progesterone (P). Owing to the critical role of E2 and P in the normal functioning of the female reproductive tract, as well as the role of these hormones in the etiology and progression of various diseases of the reproductive organs, it is important to understand the cellular and molecular mechanisms by which these hormones act.

It is well known that interactions between epithelium and connective tissue stroma or between epithelium and mesenchyme, the undifferentiated embryonic/fetal precursor of stroma, are critical for the development of a large number of organs *(1–3)*. Recent evidence indicates that these stromal-epithelial interactions may be involved in mediating hormonal responses in the female reproductive tract. This chapter will review the evidence suggesting that stromal-epithelial interactions are critical mediators of E2 and P actions in the epithelium of the uterus, vagina, and mammary glands, and will provide evidence indicating that stromal-epithelial interactions could also be important in androgenic responses in these organs. Since stromal-epithelial interactions are reciprocal, we will also review data on the role of epithelium in regulating stromal differentiation. In addition, evidence suggesting that growth factors are the critical mediators of stromal-epithelial interactions will be reviewed, along with evidence implicating different growth factors in various aspects of this stromal-epithelial communication.

HORMONAL CONTROL OF REPRODUCTIVE TRACT FUNCTION

The estrous or menstrual cycle is characterized by cyclic changes in E2 and P. The effects of E2 predominate during the preovulatory period, as granulosa and thecal cells in the developing follicles produce increasing quantities of E2. Following ovulation, serum concentrations of E2 decrease sharply, but the newly formed corpora lutea secrete increasing amounts of P, which serves to prepare the endometrial lining for implantation in the event that conception has occurred.

These hormonal changes during the estrous cycle and pregnancy result in dramatic alterations in cell proliferation, morphology and secretory activity in target female reproductive organs such as the uterus, vagina, oviduct, and mammary glands. These changes have been most thoroughly documented using rodent model systems, while information in other species is much less extensive. The discussion presented here will concentrate on rodent systems because the vast majority of work on stromal-epithelial interactions has been done in rodents.

Stromal (connective tissue) and epithelial changes during the estrous cycle and early pregnancy in the intact female have been described *(4)*, but these studies are difficult to interpret not only because of the concomitant presence of E2 and P, but also because of the constantly changing levels of both of these hormones during the estrous cycle and establishment of pregnancy. To obviate this problem, extensive use has been made of the ovariectomized mouse or rat model, where the effects of E2 and/or P can be elucidated in a more defined endocrine environment. Studies using ovariectomized mice and rats have indicated that E2 is a potent inducer of epithelial proliferation *(5)*, and that P antagonizes this effect *(6)*. These results correlate well with the observed peak in luminal epithelial proliferation in rodents when E2 levels are maximal at about the time of ovulation *(4)*, and the subsequent decline in uterine luminal epithelial proliferation during the period when E2 falls and P increases.

In the rodent uterus, E2 also regulates epithelial integrity since luminal epithelium undergoes atrophic changes following estrogen withdrawal. These changes include decreases in cell height, microvilli and overall metabolic and synthetic activity, accompanied by a large increase in apoptosis *(7)*. Estrogen treatment rapidly reverses these changes elicited by estrogen deprivation. Progesterone treatment also produces changes in uterine morphology and function, such as an increase in lipids in the luminal epithelium and increased secretion by glandular epithelium.

Progesterone normally plays a critical role in preparing the endometrium for implantation of the fertilized egg *(8)*. One of the major uterine events associated with the rising P levels after estrus is decidualization, the process in which uterine stromal cells undergo changes in proliferation, differentiation, and functional activity during pregnancy. Estrogen treatment alone does not induce as pronounced of a mitogenic increase in stroma as in epithelium. Instead, the decidual changes in stromal proliferation and differentiation, which begin at about the time of implantation in the rodent, are regulated by the coordinated actions of P and E2 *(9,10)*. Although the stromal changes involved in decidualization have been described extensively, understanding of the mechanism of this phenomenon at the cellular and molecular level is limited.

E2 and P also are critical for epithelial proliferation, development, and functional activity in the mammary gland and vagina. E2 is not required for initial mammary gland development, as shown by the rudimentary mammary glands found in estrogen receptor knockout mice at birth *(11)*. However, full ductal development of the mammary gland and initiation of secretory function require E2. Progesterone is essential for normal lobular-alveolar development in the mammary gland during pregnancy, as shown by the lack of lobular-alveolar structures in progesterone receptor knockout mice treated with E2 and P *(10)*. E2 induces proliferation of vaginal epithelium and the stratified squamous epithelial morphology typical of this organ. E2 also induces comification of the vaginal epithelium. P given in concert with a relatively low dose of E2 induces mucification of vaginal epithelium *(12)*. Vaginal mucification is characterized by a stratified epithelium with an apical cell layer of tall columnar cells whose cytoplasm is filled with mucins.

E2 and P elicit their effects by binding to their respective receptors. Estrogen receptors (ER) and progesterone receptors (PR) are ligand-activated transcription factors that are part of a large and still-growing superfamily of receptors that includes the steroid, thyroid, and retinoic acid receptors, as well as receptors for other hormones and a variety of orphan receptors for which a ligand has not yet been identified. Both forms of the estrogen receptor, the classical estrogen receptor now known as ERα and the recently discovered second form of ER, ERβ, are found in the epithelium, stroma, and myometrium of the uterus *(13)*. Likewise, PR are also present in the epithelium, stroma and myometrium of the uterus *(14)*.

A critical question is whether the observed effects elicited by E2 and P in the epithelium and other cell types are caused by direct actions of these hormones. For example, E2 induces epithelial mitogenesis in the uterus, and this effect is antagonized by P *(5,6)*. The presence of ER and PR in uterine epithelium combined with the well-documented ability of E2 and P treatment to produce effects on cell proliferation in this epithelium certainly suggests a causal link; i.e., that the effects of E2 and P on uterine epithelial proliferation are mediated directly through ER and PR in these cells. However, such a causal link between the presence of epithelial ER and PR in uterus and the effects of E2 and P on proliferation of this epithelium has never been established. In fact, a rapidly emerging body of evidence suggests that this is clearly not the case and that many effects of E2 and P on epithelium of female reproductive organs are mediated totally or at least in part by ER and PR in stromal cells.

THE ROLE OF STROMAL-EPITHELIAL INTERACTIONS IN MEDIATING RESPONSES TO ESTROGEN AND PROGESTERONE

A critical finding that initially suggested the possibility that E2 might not act directly through epithelial ER to produce uterine epithelial mitogenesis was that androgen stimulation of epithelial mitogenesis in male reproductive organs such as prostate and seminal vesicle occurred indirectly through stromal androgen receptors and that epithelial androgen receptors did not seem to be involved in this process (reviewed in ref. *1*). Was it possible that a similar indirect mechanism was responsible for the mitogenic effect of estrogen on female reproductive tract epithelia? A subsequent study by Cunha et al. *(15)* demonstrated that ER are not detectable in uterine epithelium of neonatal mice, but are present in uterine stroma. However, estrogen treatment increased proliferation of uterine epithelium in neonatal mice *(16)*, suggesting that the mitogenic effects of E2 on neonatal uterine epithelium may be indirectly mediated by ER-positive stromal cells. Consistent with this idea, numerous studies indicated that estrogen, the main mitogen for uterine, vaginal, and other female reproductive tract epithelium in vivo, is not mitogenic for epithelium isolated from these organs and cultured in vitro *(17,18)*.

The evidence that E2 induced uterine epithelial mitogenesis indirectly through stromal ER was suggestive, but not definitive. Though neonatal uterine epithelium in the mouse lacked detectable ER, it was possible that ER expression at levels below the limit of detection by present techniques could be sufficient to directly mediate mitogenic effects of E2. Similarly, the lack of a mitogenic effect of estrogen on isolated uterine, vaginal and mammary epithelia in vitro could reflect changes in these cells that made them unable to respond normally to E2 or could reflect insufficiencies in the culture environment which precluded normal mitogenic responses to estrogen. Clearly, another experimental approach was needed to definitively test the hypothesis that E2 stimulated epithelial mitogenesis or other processes indirectly through stroma.

Use of a Tissue Recombination System to Study the Mechanism of E2 and P Effects on Reproductive Epithelia

The advent of gene knockout technology, in which specific genes are inactivated or "knocked out," has provided a powerful new tool to examine the role of various genes and their corresponding proteins. One such mouse, the estrogen receptor knockout (ERKO) mouse *(11)*, in which the ERα gene has been rendered nonfunctional by gene targeting, has been used extensively to study the role of ERα in genital and other organs.

We have recently developed a new experimental system which utilizes tissues from the ERKO mouse to study the mechanism of E2 effects on female reproductive tract epithelia *(19)*. The crucial feature of this system involves enzymatically separating and recombining uterine tissue from the ERKO mouse (which lacks functional ERα in all uterine cell types) with that of the wild-type Balb/c mouse (which expresses ERα in both epithelial and stromal cells). This tissue separation/recombination technique provides a unique method for experimentally controlling the ERα status of both stroma and epithelium and allows preparation of tissue recombinations which lack ERα in both stromal and epithelial compartments (ERKO stroma + ERKO epithelium), express ERα in either epithelium or stroma (ERKO stroma + wild-type epithelium and wild-type stroma + ERKO epithelium respectively), or express ERα in both epithelium and stroma (wild-type stroma + wild-type epithelium). These tissue recombinants are then grown as kidney capsule grafts in nude mice, and their E2 responsiveness is tested following ovariectomy of the host. By analyzing the effects of a lack of stromal and/or epithelial ER on E2 responses such as epithelial mitogenesis or secretory protein production, the role of ERα in each tissue compartment can be definitively determined.

The recent development of a transgenic mouse in which the progesterone receptor (PR) has been knocked out by gene targeting *(10)* makes it possible to employ the same tissue recombination strategy as described above with the ERKO tissue to determine the role of epithelial and stromal PR in several critical effects mediated by P. Despite the critical role of P in the uterus, there is little mechanistic information on which cells types (stromal and/or epithelial) P acts on to produce its effects. The tissue recombination technique

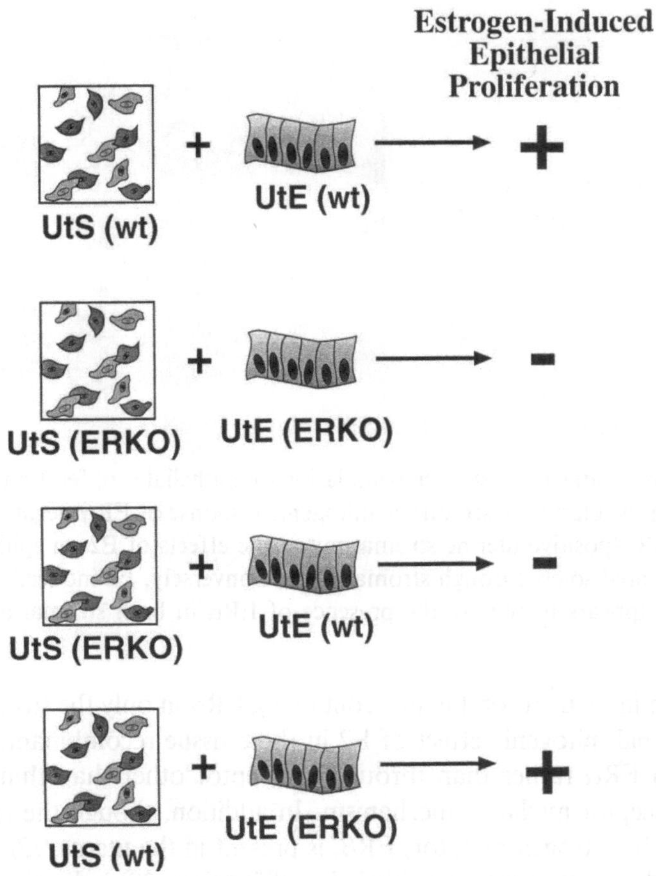

Fig. 1. Summary of tissue recombination experiments to determine how E2 induces epithelial proliferation in the uterus. E2 induced epithelial proliferation in uterine tissue recombinants where ERα was present in the stroma (wt-S+ wt-E, wt-S+ ko-E) even though the wt-S+ ko-E tissue recombinants did not express epithelial ERα. Conversely, E2 did not stimulate proliferation in tissue recombinants that lacked stromal ERα (ko-S+ wt-E and ko-S+ ko-E), even though the ko-S+ wt-E tissue recombinants expressed epithelial ERα. These results clearly indicate that the stimulatory effect of E2 on epithelial proliferation in uterine epithelium is mediated indirectly through stromal ER. (From ref. *19*)

used with tissues from the progesterone receptor knockout (PRKO) mice provides a method for obtaining unequivocal mechanistic data concerning the relative roles of epithelial and stromal PR in various effects of P in the uterus and other target tissues.

E2 Induces Epithelial Proliferation in the Uterus Indirectly Through Stromal ERα

Tissue recombination experiments utilizing uterine tissue from ERKO and wild-type animals indicated that uterine epithelium lacking ERα can respond mitogenically to E2 when associated with uterine stroma that expresses ERα *(19)*. In contrast, in uterine tissue recombinants in which ERα was expressed in the epithelium, but not the stroma, E2 did not stimulate epithelial proliferation (Fig. 1). Therefore, E2 does not stimulate epithelial proliferation in tissue recombinants that lack stromal ERα, even if epithelial ERα are present. The use of a specific estrogen receptor antagonist blocked the proliferative effect of

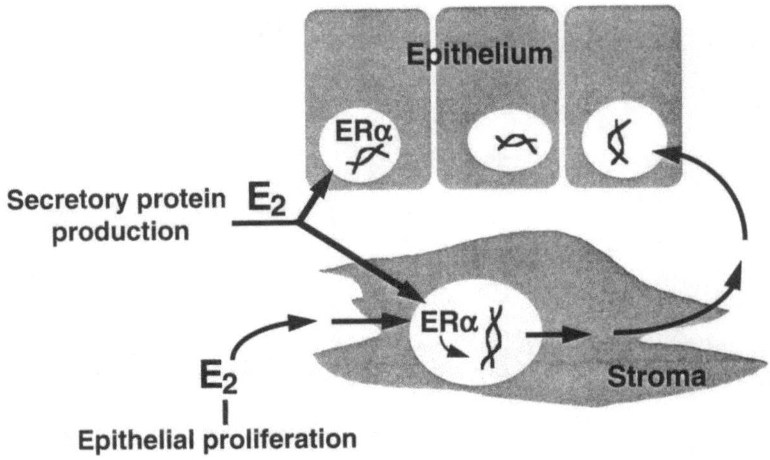

Fig. 2. Proposed mechanism of estrogen stimulation of epithelial proliferation and secretory protein production in the uterus. Based on the mitogenic response of ERα-negative UtE to E2 when associated with ERα-positive uterine stroma, mitogenic effects of E2 on epithelial proliferation appear to be mediated solely through stromal ERα. Conversely, E2-induced epithelial secretory protein secretion appears to require the presence of ERα in both stromal and epithelial cells. (From ref. *19*)

E2 on epithelium in tissue recombinants containing ERα in only the stromal cells, indicating that the normal mitogenic effect of E2 in these tissue recombinants is indeed acting through stromal ERα rather than through a receptor other than that for estrogen or through a nonreceptor mediated mechanism. In addition, though the recently described second form of the estrogen receptor, ERβ, is present in the uterus *(13)*, E2 treatment of ERKO animals does not stimulate epithelial proliferation *(20)* indicating that ERβ is not involved in this process. These results show that epithelial ERα are neither necessary nor sufficient to mediate a mitogenic response to E2 in uterine epithelium, while stromal ERα are obligatory (Figs. 1 and 2).

Similar findings were obtained in the vagina and in the mammary gland (see below). These data have led to the proposal that estrogens normally induce epithelial mitogenesis in female reproductive organs by binding to ER in mesenchymal/stromal cells, which then induces the production of paracrine factors which act on the epithelium to stimulate mitogenesis *(19,21)*.

Is E2-Induced Uterine Epithelial Secretory Protein Production Mediated by Stromal or Epithelial ER?

In addition to its effects on uterine and vaginal epithelial mitogenesis, E2 is essential for the production of major uterine epithelial secretory proteins such as lactoferrin and complement component C3 *(22,23)*. The inability of ERKO mice lacking ERα to produce lactoferrin in response to E2 treatment *(20)* indicates that it is normally ERα, rather than ERβ, which mediates the effects of E2 on secretory protein production by uterine epithelial cells. Though epithelial ERα does not appear to be involved in the induction of epithelial proliferation by E2, earlier work has indicated that epithelial ERα may be obligatory for production of E2-regulated secretory proteins by uterine epithelium *(24)*.

Using the tissue separation/recombination methodology, we have recently determined that both stromal and epithelial ERα are required for production of lactoferrin and C3 or their mRNAs in response to E2 (Fig. 2). Thus, if the tissue recombinants lack either epithelial or stromal ERα, they do not produce significant amounts of estrogen-dependent secretory proteins such as lactoferrin and C3 *(21)*. These results are in contrast to E2-induced epithelial mitogenesis, where only stromal ERα is required for the normal E2 response.

Stromal Progesterone Receptors Mediate the Inhibitory Effects of Progesterone on Estrogen-Induced Uterine Epithelial Proliferation

As stated above, E2 induces uterine epithelial proliferation *(5)*. However, pretreatment with P inhibits estrogen-induced proliferation of uterine epithelial cells in rodents *(6)*. P elicits its effects via PR, which have been detected in uterine epithelial, stromal and myometrial cells *(14,25)*. Since both epithelial and stromal tissues contain PRs, it is unclear whether uterine epithelial proliferation is down-regulated by P via epithelial or stromal PR. To resolve this issue we have used PRKO mice, which lack functional PR as a result of disruption of the PR gene by insertion of a neo-gene *(10)*. To determine whether uterine epithelial proliferation is regulated by P via epithelial versus stromal PR, uterine tissues from PR knockout (PRKO) mice and wild-type (wt) mice have been used to produce tissue recombinants in which epithelium, stroma or both are devoid of functional PR *(26)*. For this purpose, the following tissue recombinants were prepared with uterine stroma (S) and epithelium (E) from wild-type (wt) and PRKO (ko) mice: wt-S + wt-E, ko-S + ko-E, wt-S + ko-E, and ko-S + wt-E. Tissue recombinants were grown as subrenal capsule grafts in female nude mice for 4 wk, at which time all hosts were ovariectomized. Two weeks after ovariectomy, hosts received E_2 with or without P treatment. Control hosts received oil. Eighteen hours after the last hormone injection, the tissue recombinants were harvested and epithelial labeling index was determined in tissue sections using ^{3}H-thymidine autoradiography. All four types of tissue recombinants (wt-S + wt-E, ko-S + ko-E, wt-S + ko-E, and ko-S + wt-E) responded equally to E_2 and showed a several-fold increase in epithelial labeling index compared to the oil treated group. In tissue recombinants prepared with PR positive wild-type stroma (wt-S + wt-E and wt-S + ko-E), E_2 stimulation of epithelial proliferation was totally inhibited by P, even in tissue recombinants lacking epithelial PR (wt-S + ko-E), which indicates a key role of stromal PR in the inhibition of uterine epithelial proliferation (Fig. 3). In contrast, in tissue recombinants prepared with PRKO stroma (ko-S + ko-E and ko-S + wt-E), P did not inhibit epithelial proliferation, and thus epithelial labeling index was similar to that of E_2-treated tissue recombinants even in grafts containing epithelial PR (ko-S + wt-E). These results clearly indicate that stromal PR is essential and sufficient to mediate an inhibitory effect of P on uterine epithelial proliferation. Moreover, epithelial PR is neither necessary nor sufficient for P inhibition of estrogen-induced epithelial proliferation.

Stromal-Epithelial Interactions During Mammary Gland Development and Function

The mammary fat pad, along with the mammary mesenchyme, forms the connective tissue component of the mammary gland. The mesenchymally-derived fat pad is believed to play a critical role in mammary epithelial development, and the mammary fat pad appears to be the tissue responsible for inducing morphogenesis of the ductal pattern typical of the mammary gland (reviewed in ref. *2*). Based on studies with ERKO mice,

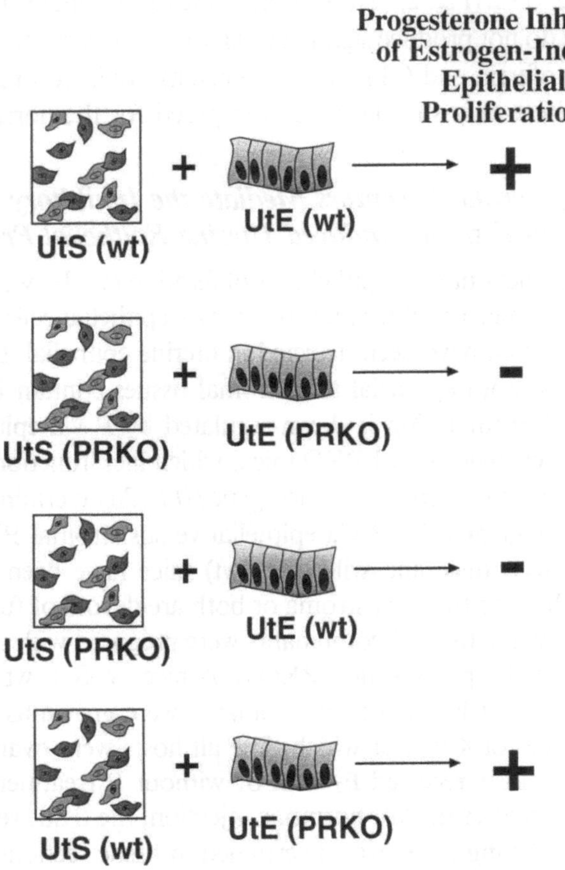

Fig. 3. Summary of tissue recombination experiments to determine how P inhibits E2-induced epithelial proliferation in the uterus. P treatment inhibited E2-induced epithelial proliferation in uterine tissue recombinants where PR was present in the stroma (wt-S+ wt-E, wt-S+ ko-E) even though the wt-S+ ko-E tissue recombinants did not express epithelial PR. Conversely, P did not inhibit E2-induced proliferation in tissue recombinants that lacked stromal PR (ko-S+ wt-E and ko-S+ ko-E), even though the ko-S+ wt-E tissue recombinants expressed epithelial PR. These results clearly indicate that the inhibitory effect of P on E2-induced proliferation in uterine epithelium is mediated indirectly through stromal PR. (From ref. *26*).

ductal growth in the mammary gland is induced by E2 acting through ERα *(11)*. To determine whether estrogen induces mammary ductal growth via ERα in the epithelium versus the stroma, tissue recombinants were prepared with mammary epithelium (MgE) and fat pad (FP) from wild-type (wt) and ERKO (ko) mice: wt-FP + wt-MgE, wt-FP + ko-MgE, ko-FP + ko-MgE, and ko-FP + wt-MgE *(27)*. All tissue recombinants were grown as kidney capsule grafts in intact nude mice for 1 mo after which ductal wholemounts were prepared. Tissue recombinants prepared with wild-type stroma (wt-FP + wt-MgE or wt-FP + ko-MgE) contained a highly branched ductal network which completely filled the FP. In contrast, ductal growth was meager in tissue recombinants prepared with ERKO stroma (ko-FP + ko-MgE and ko-FP + wt-MgE). These studies demonstrate that epithelial ER are neither necessary nor sufficient for mammary ductal growth and branching morphogenesis. Instead, estrogen stimulation of mammary epithelial growth and development is a paracrine event mediated by mammary stromal ER.

POSSIBLE ROLE OF STROMAL-EPITHELIAL INTERACTIONS IN MEDIATING ANDROGEN EFFECTS IN FEMALE REPRODUCTIVE ORGANS

Although the existence of androgen receptors in the uterus and other reproductive organs has been known for several years *(28)* and effects of androgen treatment on the uterus have been described *(29)*, the exact role of androgens in the normal female tract is not clear. However, recent work indicates that androgens may have greater importance in the uterus than previously recognized. To determine the role of androgens in the uterus, a non-aromatizable androgen, dihydrotestosterone (DHT), was administered to ovariectomized normal or ERKO female mice. A twofold increase in wet weight and tritiated thymidine incorporation was observed *(30)*. This treatment also stimulated epithelial proliferation *(30)*. The stimulatory effects of DHT are far less than observed with E2 treatment, but do suggest that androgens, acting through the androgen receptor, may normally have a role in epithelial proliferation and growth in the uterus. However, these actions may normally be obscured by the effects of the more abundant and more potent estrogens.

The importance of stromal-epithelial interactions in mediating the proliferative response of epithelium in male reproductive organs such as prostate and seminal vesicle has been well established. Androgens induce epithelial mitogenesis in these organs by acting indirectly through stromal androgen receptors to induce epithelial mitogenesis *(1)*. As in our recent work with uterus and estrogen receptor, the epithelial androgen receptor may be necessary for the production of secretory proteins in organs such as seminal vesicle and prostate *(31)*, but is not necessary for normal androgen-induced epithelial proliferation. The previous work showing that stromal androgen receptors mediate androgen-induced epithelial mitogenesis in male reproductive organs would suggest that uterine epithelial mitogenesis induced by androgen may also be mediated by stromal androgen receptors.

Female mice lacking the type 1 isozyme of 5α-reductase, the enzyme which normally converts testosterone to DHT, have decreased litter sizes and parturition defects *(32)*. The fecundity and parturition problems can be reversed by replacement therapy with 5α-reduced androgens. The fetal loss takes place during mid-pregnancy, which is normally the time of a surge in placental androgen production and increased expression of type 1 5α-reductase in the uterine decidua. These results suggest that the local production and action of 5α-reduced androgens in the uterus may be important for the maintenance of pregnancy during the last third of gestation and for parturition. Therefore, it appears that androgens may play a more critical role in the development and function of the uterus than previously recognized, and it is likely that stromal-epithelial interactions may be involved in androgen responses in the uterus.

ROLE OF EPITHELIUM IN REGULATING MESENCHYMAL/STROMAL DIFFERENTIATION

Interest in stromal-epithelial interactions has typically focused on factors that are produced in the stroma and have actions in the epithelium. However, stromal-epithelial interactions are reciprocal, and factors produced in the epithelium may also have significant effects on the differentiation and function of connective tissue. For example, in tooth development the induction of enamel production by the epithelial ameloblasts is obligatorily dependent on the presence of the underlying connective tissue, the odontoblastic layer. Similarly, full differentiation of the odontoblastic layer and its production of dentin is obligatorily dependent on the presence of the ameloblasts *(33)*. Similar reciprocal inductions have been reported to occur in kidney development *(34)*.

These same type of reciprocal interactions occur in male and female reproductive tracts. For example, uterine epithelium is apparently necessary for the normal differentiation and spatial organization of myometrial smooth muscle in the uterus *(35,36)*. Likewise, differentiation of prostatic smooth muscle from urogenital sinus mesenchyme is induced by developing prostatic epithelium *(36)*. Similarly, the decidual reaction does not occur normally in uterine stroma following removal of the uterine epithelium, indicating that this process may require or at least be regulated by epithelium *(37)*. A complete elucidation of stromal-epithelial communication and its role in mediating hormonal responses will necessitate a determination of how epithelium regulates stromal differentiation in addition to the more commonly addressed mechanisms by which stroma regulates epithelial differentiation.

MECHANISM OF STROMAL-EPITHELIAL CELL COMMUNICATION

Though the phenomenon of one tissue inducing the differentiation of another was described nearly a century ago by Spemann in his classic studies of amphibian development, relatively little mechanistic information is available about how stromal and epithelial cells communicate. A basement membrane typically separates stromal and epithelial tissue, so normal stromal-epithelial communication is thought to occur without direct cell–cell contact between the cells of the two tissue types. Thus, the communication must occur over a distance of approx 50–350 nm through the physical barrier of the basement membrane. Stromal-epithelial communication is influenced by stromal contributions to the molecular composition of the extracellular matrix (ECM). In the mammary gland, for example, many ECM components of the basement membrane are produced by stromal cells; ECM molecules, such as fibronectin, laminin, and collagen, and their integrin receptors have been reported to play important roles in cell–cell interactions *(38)*. However, most work in this area has focused on growth factors as potential candidates for mediating stromal-epithelial cell interactions. These factors would appear to possess the ideal attributes for factors involved in communication between stroma and epithelium. They can diffuse into or across basement membranes, they can produce rapid and profound changes in cell proliferation, morphology and activity, and in many cases, the expression of a growth factor in either stromal or epithelial cells and the existence of that growth factor's receptor in the other tissue type has been reported.

Stromal and epithelial cells may also communicate by mechanisms other than simple changes in growth factor production. Paracrine communication could be influenced by stromal effects on processes such as enzymatic modification (digestion, phosphorylation, or glycosylation) or changes in bioavailability (secretion, binding, and release from extracellular matrix) of growth factors themselves, their receptors, binding proteins, or enzymes that modify activity of the molecules involved. In this regard, it is important to recognize that many growth factors bind to heparan sulfate proteoglycans (HSPG) in the extracellular matrix. HSPGs may be important as "coreceptors" for presenting the ligand to the signaling receptor which in turn triggers the signaling cascade. In support of this idea, expression of several ECM molecules or proteinases appear to be under the control of steroid hormones in the uterus *(39,40)*.

A large number of growth factors have been mentioned as possible candidates for the factors involved in stromal-epithelial communication. Some of the evidence implicating various growth factors in stromal-epithelial communication is discussed below.

Epidermal Growth Factor (EGF)

The most compelling evidence linking a growth factor with stromal-epithelial cell communication has been obtained for EGF. EGF administration to ovariectomized mice resulted in a stimulation of proliferation in uterine and vaginal epithelium, uterine stroma and uterine myometrium that was similar in magnitude to that observed with E2 *(41)*. EGF also induced vaginal cornification and lactoferrin production in a manner similar to that seen with E2. Administration of antibodies to EGF attenuated the mitogenic response of uterine epithelium to E2 *(41)*, further implicating EGF as a key component in the normal sequence of events following E2 administration which ultimately leads to epithelial proliferation. Consistent with these findings, E2 treatment has been shown to stimulate increases in EGF-R and EGF bioactivity in the uterus *(42)*.

Given the above data, it would be predicted that uterine and vaginal epithelial proliferation should be impaired in EGF receptor knockout mice. Since EGFR-KO mice die in the neonatal period, their uteri and vaginae have been studied as grafts to nude mice. When wild-type and EGFR-knockout (KO) uteri and vaginae were grown as renal capsule grafts in nude mice, growth of uterine and vaginal grafts of EGFR-KO mice was reduced by approximately a third compared to their wild-type counterparts, even though differentiation of both epithelium and mesenchyme was normal in both cases. In response to E2 treatment, stromal cell labeling index (LI) as assessed by incorporation of ^{3}H-thymidine was severely depressed in EGFR-KO uterine and vaginal grafts versus stromal cell LI in wild-type uterine and vaginal grafts. Unexpectedly, epithelium of both EGFR-KO and wild-type grafts responded comparably to E2 with a marked elevation (approximately sevenfold overall) of epithelial LI in response to E2 in uterine and vaginal epithelia. These data supported the hypothesis that overall uterine and vaginal organ growth in response to estrogen requires EGFR signaling for DNA synthesis in the fibromuscular stroma, while EGFR signaling was not essential for estrogen-induced epithelial growth in the uterus and vagina *(43)*. Therefore, though EGF can mimic many of the effects of E2 on vaginal and uterine epithelium, there may be redundancy in growth factor signaling such that the absence of the EGF receptor does not impair the normal mitogenic response of vaginal and uterine epithelium to E2.

Hepatocyte Growth Factor (HGF)

Another growth factor which is receiving increasing attention as a potential mediator of stromal-epithelial communication is HGF. HGF is a mesenchymally derived heparin-binding cytokine. The HGF receptor is the product of the c-met proto-oncogene and is expressed predominately in epithelium, and HGF has been reported to stimulate epithelial mitogenesis in several organs *(44)*. The role of HGF in the female tract has not been conclusively defined. HGF and its receptor are expressed in the mammary gland, and these patterns of expression change during pregnancy, lactation and mammary involution *(45)*. In addition, HGF stimulates the proliferation and morphogenesis of cultured human endometrial and mammary epithelium *(46)*.

Keratinocyte Growth Factor (KGF)

KGF is a member of the fibroblast growth factor family (FGF-7). KGF is secreted by mesenchymal and fibroblastic cells and stimulates epithelial cell proliferation, thereby conferring its status as a paracrine mediator of epithelial cell growth *(47)*. KGF apparently plays a critical role in mediating the effects of androgens in male reproductive organs.

Testosterone has been shown to stimulate extensive growth and branching morphogenesis in neonatal rat ventral prostates grown in serum-free organ culture *(48)*. Neutralization of endogenous KGF by use of a monoclonal antibody or a peptide representing the KGF binding pocket of the KGF receptor inhibited the testosterone stimulated ductal growth and branching morphogenesis. In contrast, exogenous KGF stimulated ductal growth and branching morphogenesis of the cultured ventral prostates even in the absence of androgen. KGF is produced by the mesenchyme/stroma of several male reproductive organs, and KGF receptor is expressed in epithelial cells of a number of male reproductive tract organs *(see 48)*.

The role of KGF in the female reproductive tract is less well defined, but available evidence is consistent with the idea that it could be a mediator of stromal-epithelial interactions. KGF is expressed in the monkey and mouse uterus *(43,49)*. In addition, in the monkey its expression is stimulated by progesterone but not E2 *(49)*. KGF is produced by mammary mesenchyme and mammary epithelium expresses KGF receptor, while KGF stimulates proliferation of mammary epithelial cells *(50,51)*. Recent studies have shown that KGF injected into newborn mice profoundly stimulates proliferation of uterine and vaginal epithelial cells *(52)*. Although the exact role of KGF in the uterus and female reproductive tract has not been definitively established, it is clear that KGF is at least potentially an important paracrine regulator of epithelial growth and development.

Insulin-like Growth Factor-I (IGF-I)

IGF-I protein and mRNA are produced in relatively high amounts in uterus, preferentially in stroma *(53)*. Likewise, IGF-I receptor is present in all tissue layers of the uterus *(53)*. E2 appears to be a primary regulator of IGF-I mRNA and protein production in uterus, and E2 also stimulates IGF-I receptor mRNA expression *(54–56)*. Treatment of ovariectomized mice with P induced IGF-I expression in stromal cells, while E2 specifically induced IGF-I in uterine epithelial cells *(56)*. The combination of E2 and P further stimulated IGF-I expression in uterine stroma. Transgenic mice in which the IGF-I gene was knocked out had thin, flaccid uteri with a wet weight only 13% that of wild-type mice *(57)*. Another transgenic mouse overexpressing IGF binding protein-1 (IGFBP-I), which affects the bioavailability and activity of IGF-I, showed a significant reduction in both estradiol- and IGF-I-induced uterine DNA synthesis compared to normal mice *(58)*. Taken together, these studies suggested that IGF-I could be important as a mediator of the effects of E2 and P on uterine tissue.

Transforming Growth Factors-α and -β

The transforming growth factor-beta (TGF-β) family of growth factors may also be involved in stromal-epithelial interactions. The actions of TGF-βs are generally antagonistic to other growth factors such as TGF-α or FGF. TGF-β is a growth inhibitor for epithelial cells, but stimulates the deposition of extracellular matrix and proliferation of stromal fibroblasts *(59)*. Immunohistochemical and *in situ* hybridization studies have shown that TGF-β1, TGF-β2 and TGF-β3 are localized in uterine epithelium, stroma and myometrium *(60)*. Furthermore, TGF-β receptors and/or responsiveness to TGF-βs have been demonstrated for epithelial, stromal and myometrial cells *(60–63)*. TGF-β also plays a role in the mammary gland; TGF-β1, TGF-β2 and TGF-β3 reversibly inhibit mammary ductal growth *(64)*, consistent with growth inhibitory effects of TGF-β on mammary epithelial cells in vitro *(65)*. Initial reports have indicated that levels of TGF-β are regulated by estrogen and/or progesterone *(61,63)*, though the exact role of TGF-β in the female reproductive tract remains to be definitively established.

Transforming growth factor-alpha (TGF-α) is a member of the EGF family, which in addition to EGF includes heparin-binding EGF, amphiregululin, heregulin, crypto, and several other molecules. TGF-α binds to the EGF receptor and mimics the action of EGF in several systems, and E2 increases expression of TGF-α in the uterus *(66)*. Despite its ability to bind to the EGF receptor and the increased expression of TGF-α following E2 treatment, it is unclear if TGF-α plays a role in mediating E2-induced epithelial proliferation in female reproductive organs. Adachi et al. *(67)* showed that E2 increased both EGF and TGF-α mRNA and EGF receptor mRNA in the epithelium of the human oviduct, confirming earlier work in the uterus. An antibody against EGF decreased the E2-induced increase in epithelial proliferation, but an antibody against TGF-α had no effect, suggesting that TGF-α might not be involved in the mitogenic response to E2 in uterus and oviduct. Finally, TGF-α knockout mice have seemingly normal uteri and are fertile (Cunha, unpublished).

Other Growth Factors

There is also evidence linking other growth factors such as platelet derived growth factor (PDGF) to stromal-epithelial interactions in female reproductive organs. PDGF receptors are present in the uterus, and PDGF can mimic some of the effects of E2 on uterus. Likewise, nerve growth factor (NGF) has been shown to be involved in stromal-epithelial interactions in several organs. NGF also appears to have a role in development of organs such as prostate *(68)*, though its role in female reproduction has not been investigated. The activins and inhibins, which have diverse roles in reproductive organs, could also potentially be involved in stromal-epithelial communication. In addition to the known growth factors, it is extremely likely that there are several heretofore unknown growth factors involved in stromal-epithelial interactions and hormonal regulation of this process. In all likelihood, multiple paracrine growth factor pathways are involved in various aspects of stromal-epithelial communication in the uterus and other reproductive organs.

SUMMARY AND CONCLUSION

It is becoming increasingly evident that many important actions of E2 on epithelium of female reproductive organs, such as the effects of E2 on epithelial mitogenesis, are mediated by stromal ERα. Other processes, such as secretory protein production in the uterus and epithelial cornification in the vagina, obligatorily require epithelial ERα, but even in those cases, stromal ERα must also be present to allow the effect to occur. Similarly, it appears that certain critical P effects, such as the ability to inhibit E2-induced epithelial proliferation, are also mediated via stromal PR. A complete understanding of the roles of E2 and P in the many far-reaching changes induced by these hormones during the normal estrous and menstrual cycle and during pregnancy will necessitate a more detailed understanding of the relative function of ERα and PR in each tissue compartment. It will also be necessary to understand at the cellular and molecular level exactly how stromal and epithelial cells normally communicate and how this communication is altered by the presence of E2 and/or P. Growth factors appear to be critical mediators of stromal-epithelial cell communication, but a much more detailed understanding of how these growth factors act, alone and in concert, will be necessary to fully elucidate the basis of stromal-epithelial communication.

ACKNOWLEDGMENTS

This work supported by NIH grants AG 15500, CA 59831, DK 45861, CA 64872, AG 13784, DK 52708, and a grant from the Army Breast Cancer Program (17-96-1-6055).

REFERENCES

1. Cunha GR, Alarid ET, Turner T, Donjacour AA, Boutin EL, Foster, BA (1992) Normal and abnormal development of the male urogenital tract: role of androgens, mesenchymal-epithelial interactions, and growth factors. J Andrology 13:465–475.
2. Cunha GR, Hom YK (1996) Role of mesenchymal interactions in mammary gland development. J Mammary Gland Biol Neoplasia 1:21–35.
3. Wessels NK (1977) Tissue Interactions and Development, Benjamin/Cummings, Menlo Park, CA.
4. Finn CA, Martin J (1967) Patterns of cell division in the mouse uterus during early pregnancy. J Endocrinol 39:593–597.
5. Martin L (1980) Estrogens, anti-estrogen and the regulation of cell proliferation in the female reproductive tract in vivo, In: Estrogens in the Environment (McLachlan JA, ed.), Elsevier/North-Holland, New York, pp. 103–130.
6. Martin L, Das R, Finn C (1973) The inhibition by progesterone of uterine epithelial proliferation in the mouse. J Endocrinol 57:549–555.
7. Finn CA, Publicover M (1981) Hormonal control of cell death in the luminal epithelium of the mouse uterus. J Endocrinol 91:335–340.
8. Weitlauf HM (1994) Biology of implantation, In: The Physiology of Reproduction, Volume 1, 2nd Ed, (Knobil E, Neill JD, eds.), Raven, New York, pp. 391–440.
9. Clark BF (1973) The effect of oestrogen and progesterone on uterine cell division and epithelial morphology in spayed-hypophysectomized rats. J Endocrinol 56:341–342.
10. Lydon JP, DeMayo FJ, Funk CR, Mani SK, Hughes AR, Montgomery CA, et al. (1995) Mice lacking progesterone receptor exhibit pleiotropic reproductive abnormalities. Genes Development 9:2266–2278.
11. Lubahn DB, Moyer JS, Golding TS, Couse JF, Korach KS, Smithies O (1993) Alteration of reproductive function but not prenatal sexual development after insertional disruption of the mouse estrogen receptor gene. Proc Natl Acad Sci USA 90:11,162–11,166.
12. Rosa DG, Velardo JT (1959) Histochemical localization of vaginal oxidative enzymes and mucins in rats treated with estradiol and progesterone. Ann NY Acad Sci 83:122–144.
13. Saunders PTK, Maguire SM, Gaughan T, Millar MR (1997) Expression of oestrogen receptor beta (ERβ) in multiple rat tissues visualized by immunohistochemistry. J Endocrinol 154:R12–R16.
14. Ohta Y, Sato T, Iguchi T (1993) Immunocytochemical localization of progesterone receptor in the reproductive tract of adult female rats. Biol Reprod 48, 205–213.
15. Cunha GR, Shannon JM, Vanderslice KD, Sekkingstad M, Robboy SJ (1982) Autoradiographic analysis of nuclear estrogen binding sites during postnatal development of the genital tract of female mice. J Steroid Biochem 17:281–286.
16. Bigsby RM, Cunha GR (1986) Estrogen stimulation of deoxyribonucleic acid synthesis in uterine epithelial cells which lack estrogen receptors. Endocrinology 119:390–396.
17. Casimiri V, Tath NC, Parvey H, Psychoyos A (1980) Effect of sex steroids on rat endometrial epithelium and stroma cultured separately. J Steroid Biochem 12:293–298.
18. Iguchi T, Uchima FDA, Ostrander PL, Bern HA (1983) Growth of normal mouse vaginal epithelial cells in and on collagen gels. Proc Natl Acad Sci USA 80:3743–3747.
19. Cooke PS, Buchanan DL, Young P, Setiawan T, Brody J, Taylor J, et al. (1997) Stromal estrogen receptors (ER) mediate the mitogenic effect of estradiol on uterine epithelium. Proc Natl Acad Sci USA 94:6535–6540.
20. Couse JF, Curtis SW, Washburn TF, Lindzey J, Golding TS, Lubahn DB, et al. (1995) Analysis of transcription and estrogen insensitivity in the female mouse after targeted disruption of the estrogen receptor gene. Mol Endocrinol 9:1441–1454.
21. Cooke PS, Buchanan DL, Lubahn DB, Cunha GR (1998) Mechanism of estrogen action: lessons from the ERKO mouse. Biol Reprod (in press).
22. Sundstrom SA, Komm BS, Ponce-de-Leon H, Yi Z, Teuscher C, Lyttle CR (1989) Estrogen regulation of tissue-specific expression of complement. J Biol Chem 264:16,941–16,947.
23. Pentecost BT, Teng CT (1987) Lactotransferrin is the major estrogen inducible protein of mouse uterine secretions. J Biol Chem 262:10,134–10,139.
24. Yamashita S, Newbold RR, McLachlan JA, Korach KS (1990) The role of the estrogen receptor in uterine epithelial proliferation and cytodifferentiation in neonatal mice. Endocrinology 127: 2456–2463.
25. Brenner RM, McClellan MC, West NB (1988) Immunocytochemistry of estrogen and progestin receptors in the primate reproductive tract, In: Steroid Receptors in Health and Disease. (Moudgil VK, ed.), Plenum, New York, pp. 47–70.

26. Kurita T, Young P, Brody J, Lydon JP, O'Malley BW, Cunha GR (1998) Stromal progesterone receptors mediate the inhibitory effects of progesterone on estrogen-induced uterine epithelial proliferation. Endocrinology (submitted).
27. Cunha GR, Young P, Hem YK, Cooke PS, Taylor JA, Lubahn DB (1997) Elucidation of a role of stromal steroid hormone receptors in mammary gland growth and development by tissue recombination experiments. J Mammary Gland Biology and Neoplasia 2:393–402.
28. Stumpf W, Sar M (1976) Autoradiographic localization of estrogen, androgen, progestin, and glucocorticosteroid in "target tissues" and "non-target tissues", In: Receptors and Mechanism of Action of Steroid Hormones (Pasqualini J, ed.), Marcel Dekker, New York, pp. 41–84.
29. Schmidt W, Katzenellenbogen B (1979) Androgen-uterine interactions: an assessment of androgen interaction with the testosterone and estrogen receptor systems and stimulation of uterine growth and progesterone reseptor synthesis. Mol Cell Endocrinol 15:91–108.
30. Lindzey J, Korach KS (1997) Developmental and physiological effects of estrogen receptor gene disruption in mice. Trends Endocrinol Metabol 8:137–145.
31. Cunha GR, Young P (1991) Inability of Tfm (testicular feminization) epithelial cells to express androgen-dependent seminal vesicle secretory proteins in chimeric tissue recombinants. Endocrinology 128:3293–3298.
32. Mahendroo MS, Cala KM, Landrum CP, Russell DW (1997) Fetal death in mice lacking 5α-reductase type 1 caused by estrogen excess. Mel Endocrinol 11:917–927.
33. Kollar EJ (1983) Epithelial-mesenchymal interaction in the mammalian integument. Tooth development as a model for instructive induction, In: Epithelial-Mesenchymal Interactions in Development (Sawyer RH, Fallen JF, eds.), Praeger, New York, pp. 27–50.
34. Saxen L, Karkinen-Jaaskelainen, Lehtonen E, Nordling S, Wartiovaara J (1976) Inductive tissue interactions, In: The Cell Surface in Animal Embryogenesis and Development, (Poste G, Nicolson GL, eds.), Elsevier/North Holland, New York, pp. 331–408.
35. Cunha GR, Young P, Brody JR (1989) Role of uterine epithelium in the development of myometrial smooth muscle cells. Biol Reprod 40:861–871.
36. Cunha GR, Battle E, Young P, Brody JR, Donjacour A, Hayashi N, Kinbara H (1992) Role of epithelial-mesenchymal interactions in the differentiation and spatial organization of visceral smooth muscle. Epithelial Cell Biol 1:76–83.
37. Lejeune B, Leroy F (1980) Role of the uterine epithelium in inducing the decidual cell reaction. Prog Reprod Biol 7:92–101.
38. Xie J, Haslam SZ (1997) Extracellular matrix regulates hormone-ependent proliferation of mouse mammary epithelial cells. Endocrinology 138:2466–2473.
39. Choe YS, Shim C, Choi D, Lee CS, Lee KK, Kim K (1997) Expression of galectin-l mRNA in the mouse uterus is under the control of ovarian steroids during blastocyst implantation. Mol Reprod Dev 48:261–266.
40. Singer CF, Marbaix E, Kokorine I, Lemoine P, Donnez J, Eeckhout Y, et al. (1997) Paracrine stimulation of interstitial collagenase (MMP-1) in the human endometrium by interleukin-1alpha and its dual block by ovarian steroids. Proc Natl Acad Sci USA 94:10,341–10,345.
41. Nelson KG, Takahashi T, Bossert NL, Walmer DK, McLachlan JA (1991) Epidermal growth factor replaces estrogen in the stimulation of female genital-tract growth and differentiation. Proc Natl Acad Sci USA 88:21–25.
42. Mukku VR, Stancel GM (1985) Regulation of epidermal growth factor receptor by estrogen. J Biol Chem 260:9820–9824.
43. Hom YK, Young P, Wiesen JF, Miettinen PJ, Derynck R, Werb Z, et al. (1998) Uterine and vaginal organ growth requires epidermal growth factor receptor (EGFR) signaling from stroma. Endocrinology (in press).
44. Zarnegar R, Michalopoulos G (1995) The many faces of hepatocyte growth factor: from hepatopoiesis to hematopoiesis. J Cell Biol 129:1177–1180.
45. Pepper MS, Soriano JV, Menoud PA, Sappino AP, Orci L, Montesano R (1995) Modulation of hepatocyte growth factor and c-met in the rat mammary gland during pregnancy, lactation, and involution. Exp Cell Res 219:204–210.
46. Sugawara J, Fukaya T, Murakami T, Yoshida H, Yajima A (1997) Hepatocyte growth factor stimulates proliferation, migration, and lumen formation of human endometrial epithelial cells in vitro. Biol Reprod 57:936–942.
47. Aaronson SA, Bottaro DP, Miki T, Ron D, Finch PW (1990) Keratinocyte growth factor: a fibroblast growth factor family member with unusual target cell specificity. Ann NY Acad Sci 638: 62–77.

48. Sugimura Y, Foster BA, Rubin JS, Finch PW, Aaronson SA, Hayashi N, et al. (1996) Keratinocyte growth factor (KGF) replaces testosterone in the ductal branching morphogenesis of the rat ventral prostate. Int J Develop Biol 40:941–951.
49. Koji T, Chedid M, Rubin JS, Slayden OD, Csaky KG, Aaronson SA, Brenner RM (1994) Progesterone-dependent expression of keratinocyte growth factor mRNA in stromal cells of the primate endometrium: keratinocyte growth factor as a progestomedin. J Cell Biol 125:393–401.
50. Imagawa W, Cunha GR, Young P, Nandi S (1994) Keratinocyte growth factor and acidic fibroblast growth factor are mitogens for primary cultures of mammary epithelium. Biochem Biophys Res Comm 204:1165–1169.
51. Ulich TR, Yi ES, Cardiff R, Yin S, Bikhazi N, Biltz R, et al. (1994) Keratinocyte growth factor is a growth factor for mammary epithelium in vivo. The mammary epithelium of lactating rats is resistant to the proliferative action of keratinocyte growth factor. Am J Pathol 144:862–868.
52. Hom YK, Young P, Thomson AA, Cunha GR (1998) Keratinocyte growth factor (KGF) injected into female mouse neonates stimulates uterine and vaginal epithelial growth. Endocrinology (submitted).
53. Murphy LJ, Ghahary A (1990) Uterine insulin-like growth factor-1: Regulation of expression and its role in estrogen-induced uterine proliferation. Endocrine Rev 11:443–453.
54. Ghahary A, Chakrabarti S, Murphy LJ (1990) Localization of the sites of synthesis and action of insulin-like growth factor-I in the rat uterus. Mol Endocrinol 4:191–195.
55. Bhattacharyya N, Ramsammy R, Eatman E, Hollis VW, Anderson WA (1994) Protooncogene, growth factor, growth factor receptor, and estrogen and progesterone receptor gene expression in the immature rat uterus after treatment with estrogen and tamoxifen. J Submicrosc Cytol Pathol 26:147–162.
56. Kapur S, Tamada H, Dey SK, Andrews GK (1992) Expression of insulin-like growth factor-I (IGF-I) and its receptor in the peri-implantation mouse uterus, and cell-specific regulation of IGF-I gene expression by estradiol and progesterone. Biol Reprod 46:208–219.
57. Baker J, Hardy MP, Zhou J, Bondy C, Lupu F, Bellvé AR, et al. (1996) Effects of an Igf1 gene null mutation on mouse reproduction. Mol Endocrinol 10:903–918.
58. Rajkumar K, Dheen T, Krsek M, Murphy LJ (1996) Impaired estrogen action in the uterus of insulin-like growth factor binding protein-1 transgenic mice. Endocrinology 137:1258–1264.
59. Roberts AB, Sporn MB (1993) Physiological actions and clinical applications of transforming growth factor-beta (TGF-β). Growth Factors 8:1–9.
60. Chen HL, Yelavarthi KK, Hunt JS (1993) Identification of transforming growth factor-beta 1 mRNA in virgin and pregnant rat uteri by in situ hybridization. J Reprod Immunol 25:221–233.
61. Takahashi T, Eitzman B, Bossert NL, Walmer D, Sparrow K, Flanders KC, et al. (1994) Transforming growth factors beta 1, beta 2, and beta 3 messenger RNA and protein expression in mouse uterus and vagina during estrogen-induced growth: a comparison to other estrogen-regulated genes. Cell Growth Differ 5:919–935.
62. Rotello RJ, Lieberman RF, Purchio AJ, Gerschenson LE (1991) Coordinated regulation of apoptosis and cell proliferation by transforming growth factor beta 1 in cultured uterine epithelial cells. Proc Natl Acad Sci USA 88:3412–3415.
63. Chegini N, Zhao Y, Williams RS, Flanders A (1994) Human uterine tissue throughout the menstrual cycle expresses transforming growth factor-beta 1 (TGF beta 1), TGF beta 2, 22 TGF beta 3, and TGF beta type II receptor messenger ribonucleic acid and protein and contains [125I]TGF beta 1-binding sites. Endocrinology 135:439–449.
64. Daniel CW, Robinson SD (1992) Regulation of mammary growth and function by TGFβ. Mol Reprod Develop 32:145–151.
65. Ethier SP, Van de Velde RM (1990) Secretion of a TGFβ-like growth inhibitor by normal rat mammary epithelial cells in vitro. J Cell Physiol 142:15–20.
66. Nelson KG, Takahashi T, Lee DC, Luetteke NC, Bossert NL, Ross K, et al. (1992) Transforming growth factor-alpha is a potential mediator of estrogen action in the mouse uterus. Endocrinology 131:1657–1664.
67. Adachi K, Kurachi H, Homma H, Adachi H, Imai T, Sakata M, et al. (1995) Estrogen induces epidermal growth factor (EGF) receptor and its ligands in human fallopian tube: involvement of EGF but not transforming growth factor-α in estrogen-induced tubal cell growth in vitro. Endocrinology 136:2110–2119.
68. Pflug BR, Dionne C, Kaplan DR, Lynch J, Djakiew D (1995) Expression of a Trk high affinity nerve growth factor receptor in the human prostate. Endocrinology 136:262–268.

18 Maternal Cardiovascular and Other Physiologic Responses to the Endocrinology of Pregnancy

Ronald R. Magness, PHD

CONTENTS

Gestation is a unique ephemeral physiologic state in that it is associated with significant but reversible alternations in many systems, including the endocrine and cardiovascular systems. During normal pregnancy, these endocrine and physiologic changes are essential for normal embryo/fetal development to ultimately produce viable offspring for the propagation of species. The current review addresses steroid (estrogen and progesterone) hormonal changes throughout gestation and compares them to systemic and uterine vascular physiologic adaptations to pregnancy. It must be stressed initially, that no true "cause and effect" relationship has been definitively established between production of steroid hormones in pregnancy and these vascular changes.

This chapter reviews the pregnancy-mediated changes in:

1. Progesterone and estrogen concentrations;
2. Systemic cardiovascular parameters (e.g. blood pressure, cardiac output, heart rate, and so on);
3. Distribution of cardiac output;
4. Uterine blood flow;
5. Other nonvascular physiologic responses (e.g. respiration and metabolism); and
6. Factors such as estrogen and Nitric Oxide implicated in controlling uterine and systemic vascular changes.

PROGESTERONE AND ESTROGEN CONCENTRATIONS DURING PREGNANCY

The presence of the circulating steroid hormones progesterone and estrogen throughout normal pregnancy makes their productions substantially important to the hypothesis that these may be involved in some of the maternal adaptations of the cardiovascular system during gestation. The changes in progesterone and estrogen concentrations during pregnancy have been reviewed by others in detail *(1–3)* for the human, monkey, cow, ewe, pig, goat, mare, dog, and rabbit. Moreover the relative profiles of progesterone and estrogen have also been shown for the laboratory rat and/or mouse and guinea pig, although these data are limited *(4,6)*.

In all of the species that have been described, the corpus luteum is the main, if not the sole, source of the circulating levels of progesterone during the ovarian cycle. Moreover, during early gestation, about the time when the corpus luteum would have normally undergone regression, pregnancy "stabilizes or rescues" the corpus luteum through luteotrophic or antiluteolytic mechanisms. These luteoprotective influences of the blastocyst expressed from within the uterus therefore occur in order to maintain the ovarian source of progesterone. In "ovariectomy intolerant" species in which ovariectomy at any time during gestation terminates the pregnancy (e.g. pig, rabbit, dog, goat, rat, and mouse), progesterone of ovarian origin is necessary throughout the majority of gestation *(1,3)*. In other species in which the ovaries can be removed early in pregnancy (e.g. the human [d 30–50; term = 280 d], rhesus monkey [d 20–25; term = 168 d], mare [d 70–150; term = 345 d], guinea pig [d 38; term = 65–68 d], and sheep [d 55; term = 145 d]) or late in pregnancy (e.g. the cow [d 200; term = 278 d] and cat [d 50; term = 65 d]) the placenta takes over the major role of progesterone production *(1,3)*. In these "ovariectomy tolerant" species, such as primates and sheep there is a transition period of luteal function until the placenta emerges as the major source of progesterone production. This process has been termed the "luteal-placental shift". In women, cows, rats, and sheep, there is a progressive increase in circulating progesterone levels throughout most of gestation *(1–4,7)*. In the sheep, concentrations of progesterone increase continually, especially during the last third of pregnancy and by 90 d of gestation half of the estimated circulating progesterone levels derive from the corpus luteum and half is from the placenta *(7,8)*. Moreover, the level of progesterone production is higher in twin versus singleton ovine pregnancies *(3)*. By contrast, in other species progesterone levels peak either during the first trimester (pig and mare) or the second trimester (rabbit, dog, and goat) and decline somewhat thereafter to a plateau until term when it falls precipitously during the periparturient period *(1–3,9,10)*.

The profiles of estrogen throughout gestation have also been reviewed in humans, monkeys, cows, sheep, mares, dogs, goats, rabbits, pigs, guinea pigs, and rats *(1–7,9)*. During early gestation, at the time of maternal recognition of pregnancy, only local and not systemic changes in estrogen levels are observed in the uterine venous blood, uterine flushings, and uterine lymph *(2,11–15)*. The local production of estrogen during early pregnancy will be contrasted to early changes in uterine blood flow which are detailed in a subsequent section of this chapter. Many of the originally reported profiles of free circulating maternal estrogen levels showed a general tendency to be very low during most of gestation and peaked towards the latter part of pregnancy especially near term. The highest levels of estrogen are observed very late in the third trimester near the time of delivery in the human, mouse, cow, sheep, pig, goat, and rat, *(1–7)*. Other studies, with more sensitive estrogen assays have reported changes in the steroid profiles of the cow, sheep, and pig, which modified initial impressions of the low estrogen levels in these species in early- and mid-gestation *(2,9,16–20)*. The major difficulty with evaluating and understanding the "true" profiles of estrogens in pregnancy is that although free estrogens are found in relatively low abundance, there are considerably more estrogens found in the sulfated form, such as estrone and estradiol sulfate. Furthermore, these steroids may be compartmentalized locally to the fetal fluids as well as to the maternal circulation. Only in humans and other primates is the formation of estriol a significant factor owing to the presence of 16α hydroxylase in the fetal liver. Sulfated estrogens, predominately estrone sulfate, are the primary estrogens present in both maternal blood and fetal (chorioallantoic) fluids throughout gestation in cows *(20)*, sheep *(16)*, and pigs *(18,19)*. Although free estrogens are in considerably lower concentrations, the profiles of both free and sulfoconjugated estrogens appear to parallel each other. During normal gestation in the cow *(2,17,20)*, sheep *(10,16)*, and pig *(9,18,19)* there appear to be two individual peaks in the production of these estrogens. The first elevation of estrone sulfate is observed in fetal chorioallantoic fluids from d 52–132 in the cow *(20)* and from d 31–46 in sheep *(16)*, as well as in the circulating blood of pigs from 16–30 d of gestation *(18,19)*. The initial elevation of estrogens is then followed by a fall that is noted on d 132–170 in cows, d 46–55 in ewes, and d 30–50 in pigs. Near midgestation, there appears to be a second rise in estrogen levels. Ferrell and Ford *(17)* reported that the uterine venous-arterial levels of estrone were substantial on 140 d of gestation in the cow, but were zero at 182 d, and were reestablished on d 207 until term. As with progesterone, the level of estrogens in the plasma are increased further in ewes with twin fetuses (*3,7, for review*). Moreover, 90% or more of the circulating estradiol-17β is estimated to be secreted by the placenta on d 90 of ovine gestation *(21)*. When the ovine feto-placenta unit is treated in vivo with dehydroepiandrosterone, the C19 precusor for the placenta enzyme aromatase, not only are estrogen levels increased in the uterine venous blood, but uterine blood flow increases in a pattern and magnitude similar to that observed with estrogen treatment alone to the ewe *(22)*. Because estrogen has been shown to be vasodilatory to the uterine and systemic vasculature, much attention has been focused on this steroid for its potential role in the cardiovascular adaptations to pregnancy *(22–30)*. Progesterone alone on the other hand, has little effect to cause vasodilatation of the uterine vascular bed, however, progesterone has been suggested to modulate the actions of estrogen *(27,30–31)*.

SYSTEMIC CARDIOVASCULAR CHANGES IN PREGNANCY

There are numerous alterations in the systemic vasculature during gestation *(23,25, 31–34)* including minor decreases in systemic arterial blood pressure and substantial reductions in vascular resistance as well as increases in cardiac output, heart rate, stroke volume, and blood volume. Although these gestational changes in systemic vascular parameters do not necessarily follow a temporal pattern with the alterations in progesterone and estrogen, it is possible that long term exposure to these steroids in part directly or indirectly modulates some of these adaptations in pregnancy. This however remains to be fully determined.

Blood Pressure and Systemic Vascular Resistance

In pregnant women, hypotension commences around 8 wk of gestation and becomes significant by 12 wk which coincides with the time when many women suffer from dizziness and posture-induced syncope (Fig. 1; *32–35*). The nadir in blood pressure plateaus around 20 wk of gestation and remains low until 32–32 wk (term = 38–40 wk). After this

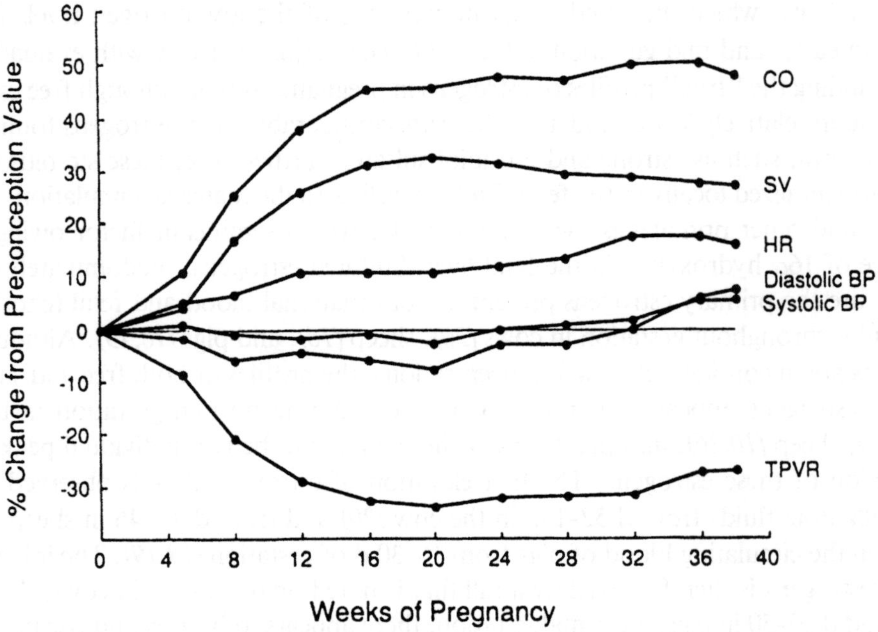

Fig. 1. Blood pressure, cross-sectional echocardiographic, and Doppler results obtained throughout gestation in women. Data were normalized as a percent change relative to the corresponding value measured during the nonpregnant state. BP, blood pressure; CO, cardiac output; HR, heart rate; SV, stroke volume; TPVR, total peripheral or systemic vascular resistance (*32,35*; with permission).

time, blood pressure slowly returns to near nonpregnant values by term *(24,26,32–35)*. Greater decreases in diastolic than systolic pressures have been reported *(32,33)*, suggesting that decreases in vascular tone may directly underlie these cardiovascular alterations. In ovine pregnancy, a decrease in mean arterial pressure is also noted early in pregnancy, but unlike women hypotension persists throughout gestation (*25,36–42*, Table 1). Guinea pigs *(43–48)* and rats *(49–56)* may also have moderate decreases in arterial blood pressure during gestation, however this is not a consistent finding.

Although there are relatively minor decreases in arterial blood pressure, relative increases in systemic blood flow measured as cardiac output are much more dramatic (Fig. 1 and Table 1). These substantial elevations in cardiac output are associated with a proportional fall in systemic vascular resistance in women *(32–35,57–67)*, sheep (*24,26,37–42,68–72*; Table 1), goats *(73)*, guinea pigs *(43–48,74,75)*, rats *(49,51,76–78)*, nonhuman primates *(79,80)*, and rabbits *(81)*. Thus pregnancy is characterized as a state of systemic vasodilation. Because systemic vascular resistance accounts for both the moderate changes in blood pressure as well as the more profound increases in total systemic flows to all vascular beds (cardiac output), it is the best physiologic index of vasodilation.

This relationship is described by the equation:

Systemic Vascular Resistance = Central Arterial Pressure – Central Venous Pressure/Cardiac Output

Because central venous pressure is generally very low (1–3 mmHg) this calculation has been estimated more easily as:

Systemic Vascular Resistance = Mean Arterial Pressure/Cardiac Output

Table 1
Systemic and Uterine Cardiovascular Measurements in Nonpregnant (n = 28) and Late Pregnant (n = 27; Days 115-135) Sheep

	Nonpregnant		*Pregnant*	%Δ
Mean arterial pressure (mmHg)	89 ± 1	**	81 ± 1	↓9
Heart rate (beats/min)	76 ± 2	**	109 ± 2	↑43
Cardiac output (mL/min)	5236 ± 84	**	7032 ± 161	↑34
Systemic vascular resistance (mmHg • min/L)	17.5 ± 0.4	**	11.9 ± 0.3	↓32
Uterine blood flow (mL/min)	22 ± 1.3	**	992 ± 103	↑4409
Uterine vascular resistance (mmHg • min/mL)	7.4 ± 0.3	**	0.12 ± 0.02	↓98

**$p < 0.01$ Nonpregnant vs pregnant; Values are means ± SE.

In view of the 30–80% fall in systemic vascular resistance that occurs in pregnancy, there has been little attention paid to the question of why substantial hypotension does not occur during normal pregnancy. We therefore *(39,68)* reversed the above equation to evaluate pressure as the dependent variable, i.e:

Mean Arterial Pressure = Systemic Vascular Resistance • Cardiac Output

This equation therefore demonstrated that as systemic vascular resistance falls, the substantial rise in the cardiac output in pregnancy will in part maintain blood pressure. Furthermore, increases in blood volume *(24,45,73,80,82–93)*, activation of both the renin-angiotensin aldosterone system *(68,94–104)* and the sympathetic division of the autonomic nervous system *(39,55,105,106)* may contribute to both maintaining blood pressure during this state of substantial vasodilation, and also to the positive chronotropism (increased Heart Rate) of pregnancy. The renin-angiotensin and sympathetic division of the autonomic nervous systems also function peripherally by vasoconstricting vascular smooth muscle of various resistance vascular beds.

Cardiac output is redistributed within the maternal cardiovascular system, such that by the end of the third trimester it greatly, but not solely reflects the growth and development of the uteroplacental vascular bed and the mammary gland vascular bed. Of particular interest is the fact that all of these cardiovascular alterations are ephemeral such that during the postpartum period they return to the nonpregnant levels within 2–5 wk *(32–35,58, 110,114)*. It is noteworthy that early in gestation the major decrease in systemic vascular resistance and the minor decline in blood pressure (Fig. 1; Table 1) begins even prior to the time that the uterine vascular bed enlarges, full placentation occurs, or uterine vascular resistance has been reduced to its greatest extent. These early events are exemplified by a recent study which demonstrated a 10–15% increase in cardiac output, a 5–7% rise in plasma volume, and a 30% decline in systemic vascular resistance during the luteal phase of the menstrual cycle immediately following conception *(107)*. Systemic vascular resistance falls in early- to mid-gestation mainly in association with increases in cardiac output in women *(32–35,57,59,60,64,90,108–116)*, sheep *(24,37–42,68–72)*, guinea pigs *(43–48, 74,75)*, goats *(73)*, rats *(49,51,76–78)*, and baboons *(80)*. Thus, these alterations in peripheral or systemic vasodilation and the rise in blood volume have been generally interpreted as "anticipating" the future major increases in uteroplacental perfusion. These results also fully dispel the misconceived theory that systemic alterations in pregnancy merely reflect the formation of a "uterine arteriovenous shunt" to account for the observed systemic vasodilation and rise in cardiac output. An alternate model described in detail by Gilson and coworkers *(51)* suggests that early in pregnancy the rise in nonreproductive blood flows, in particular renal blood flow *(35,52,53,110,118)*, may serve as a major arteriovenous shunt. Therefore these renal vascular changes may contribute to the reduced systemic vascular resistance which sets into motion the cascade of events leading to and maintaining progressive increases in cardiac output during gestation.

Cardiac Output Changes in Pregnancy

Because decreases in calculated systemic vascular resistance mainly reflect elevations in cardiac output (Fig. 1; Table 1), it is very important to evaluate factors associated with these increases in systemic blood flows. In normal pregnancy, cardiac output increases 25–60% in women *(32–35,57,59,60,64,90,108–116,119–121)*, sheep (*24,37–42,68–72*; Table 1), guinea pigs *(43–48,74,75)*, goats *(73)*, rats *(49,51,76–78)* and baboons *(80)*. In pregnant women (Fig. 1), cardiac output increases from early- to mid-gestation (5–20 wk; 1st to 2nd trimester) and then plateaus *(51,111,116)* to remain relatively unchanged *(111, 116,121)*, or even to fall slightly during the third trimester *(51,64,111)*. Definitive information in humans had been somewhat elusive because of difficulty in obtaining consistent measurements of cardiac output after the second trimester. This was a result of the increasing size of the gravid uterus, which often compresses or partially occludes both the vena cava and aorta. This causes a transient decrease in cardiac output because of decreases in venous return which reduces cardiac preload and thus end-diastolic volume. For example, average cardiac output may be 22% lower in the same women in the supine versus lateral recumbent position *(63,67,110,112)*. More definitive data have been obtained from sheep and goats in which, being a quadruped the uterus does not rest upon the "great vessels". In ovine *(26,42,69–71)*, caprine *(73)*, and rat *(51,78)* animal models, cardiac output increases progressively throughout the course of gestation (Fig. 2). For example in the sheep, cardiac output increases from nonpregnant values of 74 ± 5 to 148 ± 2.4 mL/min • kg by the end of gestation (145–150 d) *(42,71)*. This has been confirmed in numerous studies using different techniques, e.g. dye-dilution, thermal dilution, radio-labeled microspheres, 2-D echocardiography and electromagnetic flow transducers (*24,37–42, 68–72*; Table 1).

In the guinea pig, the elevation in cardiac output during pregnancy reaches a maximum (≅22% above nonpregnant values) by 20 d, which is the end of the 1st trimester and remains elevated until term (65–68 d) *(43–48,74,75)*. It is not clear why the ovine, caprine, and rat animal models have continuous increases in cardiac output and decreases in systemic vascular resistance whereas the human and guinea pig reach maximum values much earlier in pregnancy.

Because *Cardiac Output* = *Heart Rate* × *Stroke Volume,* it is important to determine which of these components is responsible for the observed increase in cardiac output during pregnancy. In both humans and sheep, relative tachycardia (increase in heart rate) of

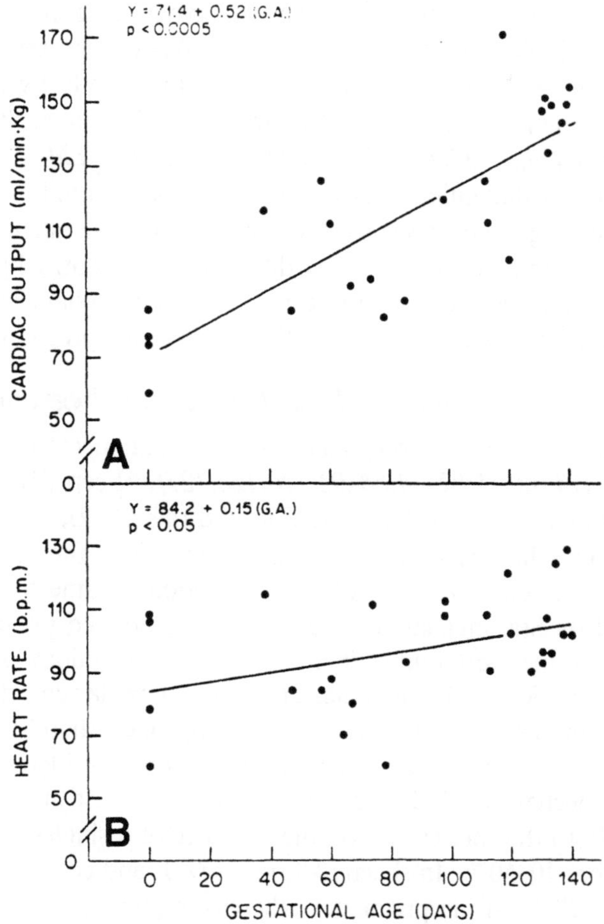

Fig. 2. Changes in cardiac output (top) and heart rate (bottom) during ovine gestation. (*71,198, 199*; with permission).

20–30% is observed (Figs. 1 and 2; Table 1). In women, heart rate increases gradually from 4–8 wk of gestation to 28–36 wk and plateaus *(32–35,66,112,119,121)*. This rise in heart rate may be attributed both to changes in the autonomic nervous system (sympathetic increases and parasympathetic decreases) and to increases in the placental steroids estrogen and/or progesterone; however, their specific roles in elevating heart rate and/or cardiac output in pregnancy remain unproven. Because the rise in heart rate is significant, but proportionately less than the relative rise in cardiac output in some but not all studies, this increase in cardiac output also reflects increases in stroke volume of 30–35% *(32–35,42, 108,112)* at midpregnancy. There is a slight decrease in cardiac output at term in women which reflects a minor decline in stroke volume rather than changes in heart rate *(32,112)*. In echocardiographic studies in women, left ventricular wall mass, left atrial dimension, and end-diastolic dimensions increase by the 12th wk of normal pregnancy and continue to increase until 20–32 wk and remain elevated through term *(32,116,117)*. Furthermore, increases in stroke volume are directly proportional to end-diastolic volume as well as ventricular diameter, implying that ventricular dilation may attenuate any dramatic change in the inotropic state of the myocardium during normal singleton pregnancies. Therefore since cardiac filling pressures are not increased greatly in pregnancy, this argues against Starling mechanisms fully controlling the changes in stroke volume. Starling mechanisms describe the direct proportionality of venous return (cardiac preload) to increase the end diastolic filling volume by "stretching" the cardiac myocytes of the ventricles and thus a greater stroke volume is ejected. However, in multifetal gestations the additional 20–30% rise in cardiac output and stroke volume occurs predominantly by increased inotropic effects as indexed by an increased fractional shortening of the ventricular diameter via true Starling mechanisms *(24,32–35,110,111,113,117,119,120,122–124)*. Similar pregnancy-mediated left ventricular dimention enlargements have been noted in the guinea pig *(45, 46,74)* and in guinea pigs and sheep treated chronically with estrogen *(45,122)*. These changes collectively suggest a decrease in "cardiac reserve" in normal pregnancy. In addition, the aorta has been observed to be larger and more compliant in pregnancy, which may contribute to the decreased afterload on the heart during pregnancy *(50,62,123,125)*.

Plasma and Blood Volume Changes in Pregnancy

The rise in cardiac output during pregnancy along with an increase in plasma and blood volume in women *(24,32–35,82–84,88–92,110,126,127)*, sheep *(24)*, goats *(73)*, cows *(84,86)*, guinea pigs *(45)*, pigs *(87)*, baboons *(80)*, and rats *(88,93,127)* relate to elevations in stroke volume. This important relationship follows from the direct proportionality between stroke volume, end-diastolic volume and blood volume to cause positive inotrophy as described by Starlings law of the heart. As described previously, echocardiographic and cardiac dimention studies in humans *(32)* and guinea pigs *(45,46,74)* have shown increases in ventricular chamber size and left ventricular end-diastolic dimensions of the heart in pregnancy *(32,46,108,121–123)*. It is improper, therefore, at least in singleton pregnancies, to "mix" this cardiac remodeling method for increasing stroke volume with "true Starling mechanisms". The magnitude of the increase in blood volume in pregnancy depends on both the species and on the presence of a singleton or multifetal pregnancy and varies from 10–50%. In sheep *(24)*, goats *(73)*, and cows *(84,86)* blood volume expands by only 10–20% during pregnancy whereas in guinea pigs *(45)* and rats *(88,93, 128)* it increases 30–50%. In multifetal gestations *(24,33,34,83)* the increase in venous return associated with the greater increase in blood volume is associated with some degree of positive inotropism suggesting that dilation (remodeling) or hypertrophic mass *(32,60, 74,117,121,123)* of the ventricular wall has finite limits.

During normal pregnancy in women, increases in plasma volume begin at about 6 wk and plateau around 30–34 wk of gestation *(82,85)*. For many years it has been thought that the fall in systemic vascular resistance and the rise in cardiac output precedes the rise in plasma volume by several weeks *(32,80,82,85)*. More recently Chapman and coworkers *(107)* reported declines in systemic vascular resistance, increases in cardiac output, with minor changes in plasma volume as early as during the luteal phase of the menstrual cycle at conception. Therefore early pregnancy should be described as initiating an underfilled cardiovascular system which requires rapid and prolonged homeostatic compensatory mechanisms. These may include rises in renin, angiotensin II, and aldosterone in association with water and electrolyte retention. With the expansion of plasma volume there must be a balance of water and electrolyte retention which accompanies this important process. For example, during the course of gestation in women, the renal system retains 500–900 mEq sodium, 300 mEq of potassium, and 30 g of calcium (*see* ref. *35 for review*). Although extra sodium is retained, osmolality falls because water retention is proportionately greater than sodium uptake in women and rats, but not in sheep. It is possible, but not proven, that the sodium retention and thus expansion of plasma volume are driven by a rise in plasma renin activity which elevates angiotensin II levels which in turn increases aldosterone secretion by the zona glomerulosa of the adrenal cortex *(29,80)*. Both estrogen and progesterone have been shown to increase plasma renin activity and aldosterone levels. Additional mechanisms may involve increased renal efferent sympathetic nerve activity *(129)*.

In pregnancy there also is enhanced erythropoiesis, presumably owing to increases in erythropoietin levels *(88,130–135)*, and thus total red blood cell volume also increases. However, the rise in plasma volume in women *(82–84,89,92,110,126,127)* and possibly goats *(73)*, but not sheep *(24)* or cows *(84,86)*, generally exceeds the increase in red cell volume which explains the so called "physiologic anemia of pregnancy" or "hemodilutional anemia of pregnancy." This is described by the equation

$$\text{Blood Volume} - \text{Plasma Volume} = \text{Red Blood Cell Volume}$$

It is unclear why plasma volume and red blood cell volume increase disproportionally in some species *(24,73,82–84,89,92,110,126,127)* and not in others *(24,84,86)*. In addition, because blood and plasma volume expansion during pregnancy are not proportional in women *(82–84,89,92,110,126,127)* and possibly goats *(73)* hematocrit falls, which also decreases the viscosity of the blood. Since viscosity is inversely proportional to systemic vascular resistance, this may also be a mechanism contributing to the rise in systemic flows in pregnancy. In humans and sheep, the decrease in systemic vascular resistance, increase in cardiac output and expansion of blood volume are greater for multifetal than singleton pregnancies *(24,33–35,136)*. This could be interpreted to mean that the maternal cardiovascular adaptation to gestation may be exacerbated by additional amounts of placental tissue. Alternatively the steroid hormones produced during gestation e.g. estrogen, progesterone, and/or aldosterone may be produced in greater quantities because of the additional placental mass *(2–4,7,10,16,17,20–22,30,80)*. Regardless, in human pregnancies with twins, there is a profound increase in the incidence of pregnancy-induced hypertension/preeclampsia suggesting that these hemodynamic adaptations exceed the normal limits set by the maternal system as dictated by the presence of the feto-placental units. Alternatively, the very large placenta is potentially subjected to ischemia/hypoxia during twin gestation which contributes to the higher incidence of pregnancy-induced hypertension/preeclampsia.

Vascular Reactivity During Pregnancy

One mechanism believed to contribute significantly to the fall in blood pressure and systemic vascular resistance during pregnancy is the generalized attenuation of blood pressure responses to a similar infused dose of a vasoconstrictor such as angiotensin II (*26,41,44,48,54,68,96–99,101,102,104–106,137–147*; Fig. 3), adrenergic agonist (norephinepherine or pheynylephrine *[38,39,54,104,106,143,148–152]*), arginine vasopressin *(148)* or prostaglandin (PG) $F_{2}\alpha$ *(153)*. This appears to be neither species nor agonist specific, although the mechanisms for the reduced pressor responses to different agonist are likely to vary somewhat. Numerous mechanisms have been theorized to account for these pregnancy-mediated attenuated pressor responses, although many of these are controversial. They include:

1. Increases in arterial and/or cardiac baroreceptor feedback control for elevations in blood pressure as was shown in the case for α adrenergic agents *(39,55,104,106,141,149,151,154,155)*, but not angiontensin II *(68,154,155)*;
2. Increases of the metabolic clearance rate of infused vasoactive agents in pregnancy *(97,98, 102,140)*, which was disproved during angiontensin II infusions (*97,98*; Fig. 3);
3. Downregulation of the number and/or functional activity of vascular smooth muscle receptors *(95,104,156–161)* that may not be the case for angiotensin II *(73,129,130)*;

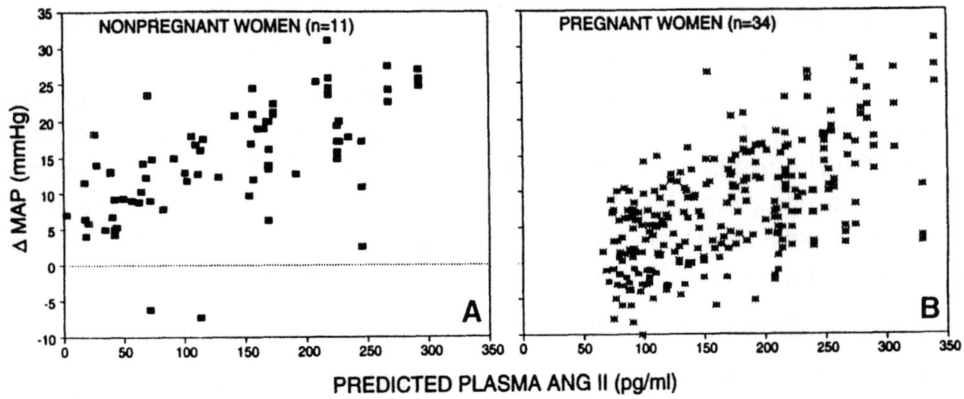

Fig. 3. Relationship between the plasma angiotensin II (*ANG II*) levels and systemic pressor responses (ΔMAP = change in mean arterial pressure) in nonpregnant (**A**) [$n = 11$] and pregnant (**B**) [$n = 34$] women, including all "stepwise" doses of infused angiotensin II. These concentration-dependent pressor response relationships are best defined by linear regression analysis ($p > 0.05$ vs quadratic regressions) and are different between groups. Nonpregnant: $\Delta MAP = 0.06\ [Concentration_{ANG\ II}] + 6.97$, $r = 0.63$ ($p < 0.001$, $n = 84$). Pregnant: $\Delta MAP = 0.07\ [Concentration_{ANG\ II}] - 4.11$, $r = 0.61$ ($p < 0.001$, $n = 276$). $p < 0.001$, y-intercept, nonpregnant vs pregnant. (*97*; with permission).

4. Release of basal vasodilating substances or in response to vasoconstrictor agents (e.g. angiotensin II) to locally antagonize pressor responses including vasodilator prostanoids (PGI_2 or PGE_2) *(40,41,54,96,97,138,139,142,146,147,159,162–170)* or Nitric Oxide *(143,164,165,167,171–179)*.

In this regard, we have recently demonstrated that the increases in vasodilator production by uterine or omental arteries treated with angiotensin II in vitro *(166–168)* occurs in association with an 8–10-fold elevation of angiotensin II (AT_1) receptors located on the uterine endothelium and a nearly twofold increase on omental artery endothelium *(158)*. Moreover the increases in vascular vasodilators (e.g. PGI_2 and Nitric Oxide) in pregnancy *(96,146,164,165,167,168,172,174)* are derived primarily from the endothelium to locally reduce vascular smooth muscle tone *(26,27,96,143,146,164,165,173,174,177,178)*. These increases in PGI_2 and Nitric Oxide in uterine artery endothelium are regulated, in part, by increases in the expression of the protein and/or mRNA for prostaglandin-H synthase-1 (cyclooxygenase-1) and endothelial cell Nitric Oxide synthase (eNOS or NOS III), respectively (*163,172,* Bird and Magness, unpublished observations). It is unclear which factors of pregnancy (e.g. estrogen, progesterone, growth factors, shear stress, and so on) increase expression of the enzymes responsible for increasing these endothelial vasodilators *(25–27, 28,29,96,142,164,165,180–189)*. A functional role for Nitric Oxide in the blunted pressor responsiveness observed during pregnancy has been reported *(143)*. The involvement of Nitric Oxide in the regulation of normal vascular alterations during pregnancy are further supported by the studies in which inhibition of Nitric Oxide synthesis, through infusion of inhibitors such as L-NAME, during pregnancy causes hypertension and fetal growth retardation and these effects can be reversed by coinfusion with L-arginine, the substrate for Nitric Oxide synthesis *(190–192)*.

DISTRIBUTION OF CARDIAC OUTPUT IN PREGNANCY

Another extremely important issue is the redistribution of the increased cardiac output during gestation. The largest relative or percentage increase in blood flow distribution

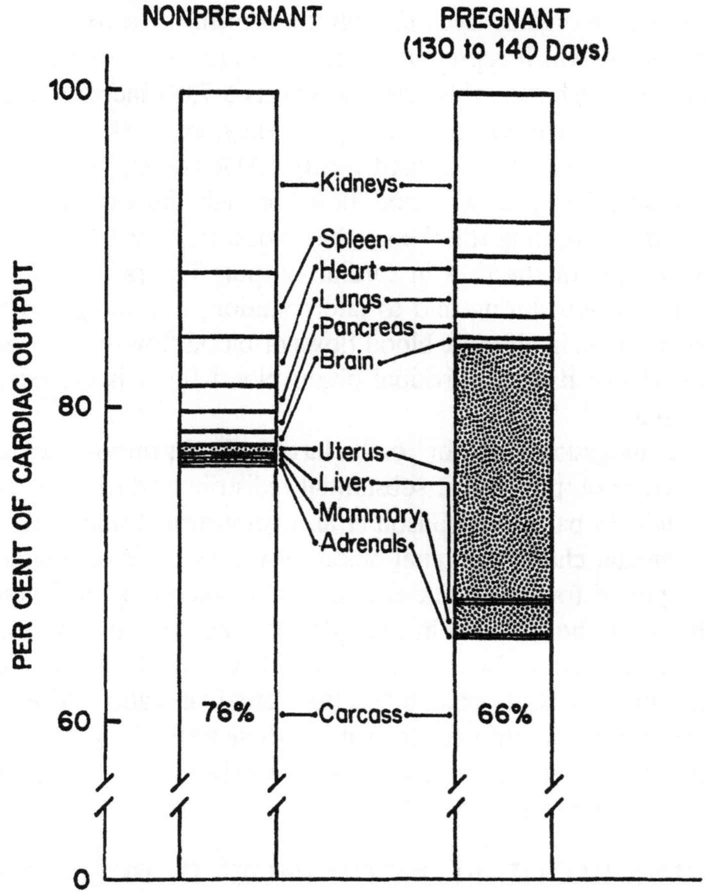

Fig. 4. Distribution of cardiac output in nonpregnant and pregnant ewes at 130–140 d of gestation. Stippled areas represent mammary gland and uterine blood flows as a percent of cardiac output. (*71,198,199*; with permission).

in pregnancy is to the dramatically developing uteroplacental vascular bed as described in women *(35,110,193–197)*, sheep *(26,40,42,71,195,198–200)*, guinea pigs *(43,46,201)*, rats *(51,76,77)*, and rabbits *(81)*. In the pregnant ewe, cardiac output increases as much as 3000–4000 mL/min by term, however, uteroplacental blood flow only increases by 800–1200 mL/min, Therefore, systemic blood flow other than that to the uterine circulation must also increase and on an absolute ml/min basis the rise in total systemic blood flow is greater than that to the uteroplacental unit. Using radiolabeled microspheres (Fig. 4), however, it was determined that the greatest relative increase in organ blood flow, i.e. the uteroplacental vascular bed, increased from 0.058 ± 0.08 (± SE) percent of cardiac output in nonpregnant ewes to 7.65 ± 0.61% and 15.7 ± 1.28% in mid- and late-gestation animals, respectively *(42,71,198,199)*. Towards the end of pregnancy, mammary gland blood flow also increased dramatically, from 0.20 ± 0.07% in nonpregnant ewes to 2.05 ± 0.25% of cardiac output at term. The increase in uterine blood flow at term as a percent of cardiac output increases 16% in sheep (*42,71,198*; Fig. 4), 16–17% in women *(35,202)*, 11–13% in guinea pigs *(43,46,201)*, and rats *(51,76,77)*, as well as 7% in rabbits *(81)*. By summing the increases in blood flow to the gravid ovine uterus and mammary gland, 40–55% of the observed increase in cardiac output can be accounted for in these species near term. Thus, 45–60% of this gestational-mediated elevation in cardiac output is diverted to other systemic or nonreproductive organs. Even though the percent of cardiac output received by nonreproductive tissues, which represent mainly, but not solely the carcass, falls from 76% to 66% in ovine pregnancy, this actually reflects a 73% increase in absolute blood flow to these tissues. Of particular interest to pregnancy, in the skin, the largest organ in the body, blood flow/g of tissue increased nearly 100% *(42,71,198)*. Women also have shown rather dramatic increases in blood flow through the extremities as pregnancy progresses *(202–208)*, supporting the theory that blood flow to the skin likely accounts for a substantial portion of the rises in cardiac output. The percent of cardiac output to other major organs falls during mid to late gestation, but compared to uterine and mammary tissues, changes in absolute blood flows or blood flow/g of tissue changes very little because the relative rise in individual organ blood flows is exceeded by the total rise in cardiac output.

During early to midgestation, prior to the largest rise in uteroplacental blood flow, the increases in cardiac output exhibit substantial redistribution to many of the systemic tissues *(51,76,77,198)*. In particular, Gilson et al. demonstrated that in the rat *(51)*, as in the human *(107)*, greater changes in renal blood flow are seen as compared to the earlier blood flow rises reported for the uterine circulation by others *(76,77)*. These investigators *(51)* suggested that since the elevation in renal flow during pregnancy was not maintained throughout the third trimester, the rises in renal and systemic flows set the stage for the largest subsequent rise in uteroplacental blood flow later in gestation. Moreover these data and others *(80,107)* underscore the need to evaluate these systemic vascular changes during early rather than late gestation. These critical comparisons early in pregnancy are not available for the ovine model *(47,71,198)*.

UTERINE BLOOD FLOW CHANGES IN PREGNANCY

The uteroplacental vascular bed undergoes the most dramatic cardiovascular alterations during gestation. These substantial alterations are unique to pregnancy and provide the only direct link between maternal and fetal blood compartments which do not mix, but are separated by the placental membrane interface. The changes that normally occur in the uterine vascular bed during gestation should be evaluated with regard to the total uterus as a single organ vascular bed, as well as with regard to the distribution of its component vascular beds, i.e., the endometrium, myometrium, and maternal placenta tissues *(23,25,26,42,70,71,79,87,198,199,209,210)*. Many of these invasive investigative studies in this area have used the ovine model.

Early Pregnancy Changes in Uterine Blood Flow

It is noteworthy that the highest rate of blood flow observed early in gestation most likely reflects the high metabolic perfusion needs of uterine tissues and the early embryo, as well as increases in the production of steroid hormones (estrogen and/or progesterone) necessary for the establishment and maintenance of pregnancy, or a combination of these factors *(2,7,11,13–15,30,45,183,209–216)*. The pattern of uterine blood flow very early in ovine, bovine and porcine pregnancies, i.e., during the perifertilization period, are similar to those during the estrous cycle, which directly correlate with the changes in estrogen/progesterone ratios mediated by the ovarian cycle *(2,11,14,15,25,30,183,211–220)*. However, the only divergence in perfusion are observed around the time of maintenance of the corpus luteum and maternal recognition of pregnancy when blood flow to the gravid uterine horns increase two- to threefold, in a transient fashion. This transient pattern

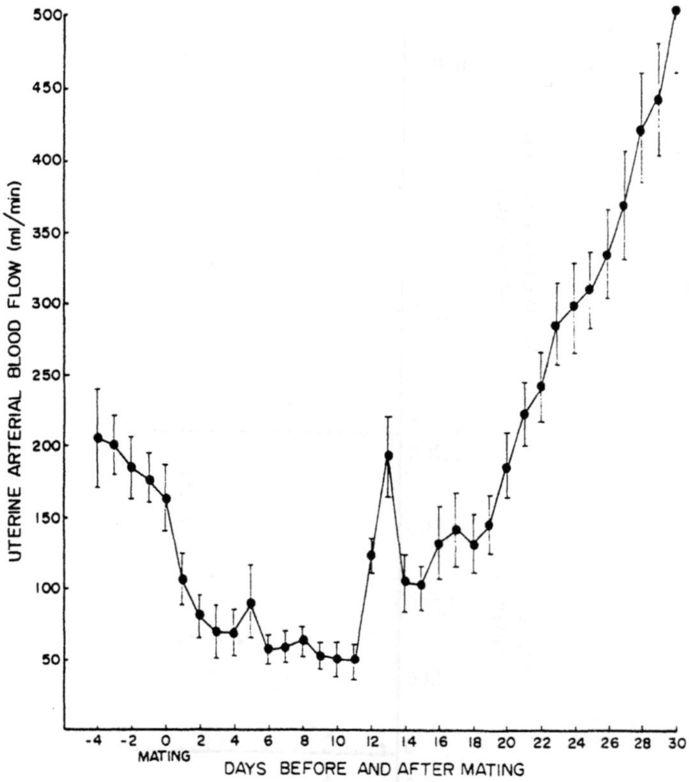

Fig. 5. Pattern of uterine blood flow of six sows throughout the first 30 d of pregnancy (day of mating = d 0). Each point represents the mean ± SE of 12 uterine arteries. (*212*; with permission).

of increase in uterine blood flow occurs on d 13–15 in sheep *(13,214)*, d 15–17 in cows *(11,12,211,213)* and d 12–13 in pigs (*11–13,209,212*; Fig. 5). Moreover, this is a strictly local event since in unilaterally pregnant pigs *(210)* or cows *(2,211,213)* uterine blood flow increases only to the gravid uterine horn. This local event was further substantiated by observations that blood flow to uterine tissues directly adjacent to elongating porcine conceptuses at this very critical time had a higher blood flow/g of tissue than uterine tissues between conceptuses *(209)*. As in the ovarian cycle, transient changes in uterine blood flow were temporally associated with increases in local estrogen/progesterone ratios in uterine flushings, uterine venous effluent, and uterine lymph *(2,11–15,25,30,219)*. As fetal attachment occurs *(221,222)* there is a sharp progressive increase in uterine blood flow from about d 17 in sheep *(2,26,214)*, d 25 in cows *(2,11,213)*, and d 19 in pigs (*2,11,212*; Fig. 5). These changes in blood flow appear to reflect the need for increased uterine oxygen and nutrient substrate delivery in early pregnancy when estrogen levels are elevated locally.

Changes in Total Uterine Blood Flow in Mid- and Late-Gestation

Total uterine blood flow increases dramatically during pregnancy, rising 50- to 70-fold above nonpregnant values during the course of normal gestation in women *(33,113, 193–197)*, sheep (*2,11,26,42,70,71,195,198–200*; Fig. 6; Table 1), cows *(2,17)*, pigs *(2,11, 212)*, and guinea pigs *(43,47,48,75,201,225,226)*. Moreover, because of the additional metabolic demands for placental and fetal growth/development, even larger increases in total uterine blood flow are observed in multifetal gestations. This increase in uteroplacental blood flow is directly related to the number of feto-placental units, e.g., triplets > twins >

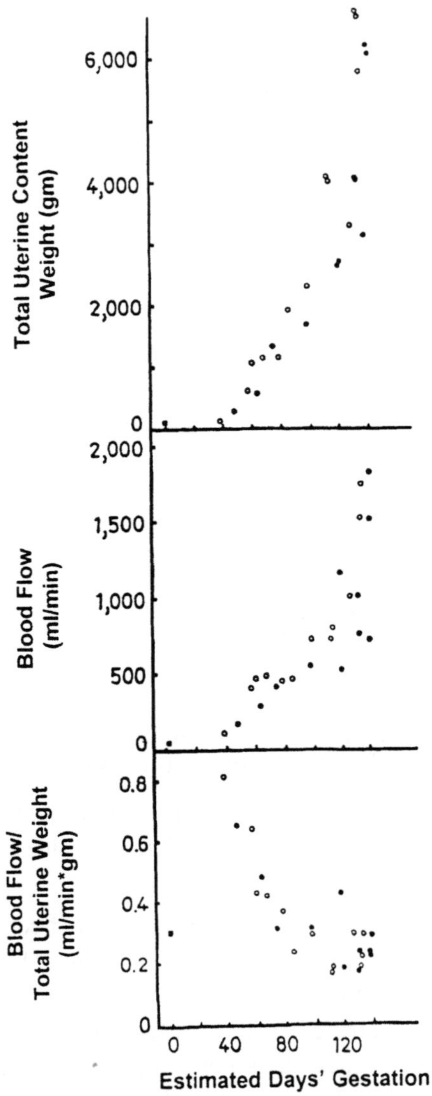

Fig. 6. Changes in the uterine weight (top), blood flow (middle), and blood flow per gram of total uterine weight (bottom) during ovine gestation. Total uterine weight is defined in the text. ■ = nonpregnant; ● = singleton pregnant; ○ = twin pregnancy. (*42,198,199*; with permission).

single, and in those species which carry litters (dogs, pigs, and so on) the total number of fetuses present. The increase in uteroplacental blood flow in pregnancy is of such a magnitude it accounts for 7–17% of cardiac output at term in sheep, guinea pigs, rabbits, and women *(35,42,43,71,81,123,201,202)*. Because blood flow to any organ including the uteroplacental vascular bed, is controlled on a minute to minute basis by relative changes in both vascular resistance and perfusion pressure, which can be estimated as mean arterial blood pressure, it should be clarified that this dramatic increase in uterine blood flow occurs while perfusion pressure falls slightly (Table 1). Thus there are substantial decreases in uterine vascular resistance, which can be estimated using the following equation:

$$\text{Uterine vascular resistance} = \text{Mean arterial pressure/Uterine blood flow}$$

However, unlike decreases in vascular resistance to most individual systemic vascular beds, the fall in uterine vascular resistance during gestation is accomplished by both vasodilation and neovascularization or angiogenesis of the developing uteroplacental unit *(26,180, 181,183)*, which is accompanied by the growth of its distributing arteries *(225,227–232)*.

During ovine pregnancy uterine vascular resistance decreases about 25-fold from non-pregnant values (4.91 ± 0.78 mmHg • min/mL) to 0.198 ± 0.0018 in mid-gestation and around 70-fold by late gestation (0.07 ± 3.5 mmHg • min/mL), providing direct evidence for profound vasodilation (*42,71,198*; Table 1). However, the increase in total uterine perfusion that occurs during normal gestation is controlled by two important mechanisms: growth of existing myoendometrial vascular beds and the development of the new placental vascular bed via angiogenesis; and vasodilation of each of these vascular beds. The angiogenic growth component of the rise in blood flow is associated with an increase in total blood flow to this organ, but not by elevations of flow/g of tissue and has been suggested to be controlled by the increases in expression of placental and/or uterine angiogenic growth factors (e.g., bFGF, VEGF, and so on), which induce both endothelial cell mitogenesis and cell migration *(26,180–183,216)*. In contrast, the vasodilatory component of the rise in blood flow reflects increases in total perfusion and blood flow/g of tissue. Neither of these mechanisms is associated with a very significant change in perfusion pressure or mean arterial pressure. These patterns of change in total uterine weight, uterine blood flow, and blood flow/g of tissue during ovine pregnancy are illustrated in Fig. 6. Total uterine weight was defined by these authors *(42,71,198,199)* as the sum of the metabolically active tissues, i.e. endometrium, myometrium, placentomes (caruncles and cotyledons), fetal membranes, and fetus even though the maternal uterine blood flow does not directly perfuse the fetal cotyledons, fetal membranes or fetus. During early gestation (first trimester) there are relatively small increases in uterine weight. Thereafter, total uterine weight increases extremely fast, continuing in a nearly logarithmic (exponential) manner throughout the remainder of pregnancy. This weight increase during the last two thirds of gestation mainly reflects growth and development of the uterine tissues and the placenta, as well as the fetus, and is accompanied by rather large increases in absolute blood flow. These patterns of the pregnancy-mediated rises in uteroplacental blood flow suggest that there are indeed two periods of rapid absolute blood flow (mL/min) increases, the first occurring during the second trimester and the second occurring during the third trimester. The mid-gestation changes can be associated with completion of the process of placentation and placental development whereas the late pregnancy increases are related temporally to very rapid fetal growth and development throughout the third trimester. It must be stressed that in all species evaluated, the placenta is formed by mid-gestation and the majority of fetal growth occurs during the latter third of gestation. Therefore, early pregnancy is the embryonic or placental attachment phase, whereas the mid-gestation is the placental development phase and late gestation is the fetal growth phase. These phases of uteroplacental development are very distinctive from the standpoint of vascular development. This is illustrated when the pregnancy-related alterations in uterine blood flow are expressed per gram of tissue (*42,71,198*; Fig. 6), to take into account not only changes in blood flow, but also changes in metabolically active (consuming) tissues, for the developmental/growth changes in both the tissue and its blood supply. In this case, an inverse pattern is observed such that there are extremely high blood flows (mL/g tissue) during early pregnancy (early implantation/attachment and initiation of placentation), followed by a gradual fall in blood flow (mL/g tissue) during mid-gestation (placental development stage). However, in late pregnancy, as the fetus grows, blood flows (mL/g tissue) remains unchanged as uteroplacental tissue blood flows keep pace with the demands for fetal growth. These results suggest that during the first two-thirds of

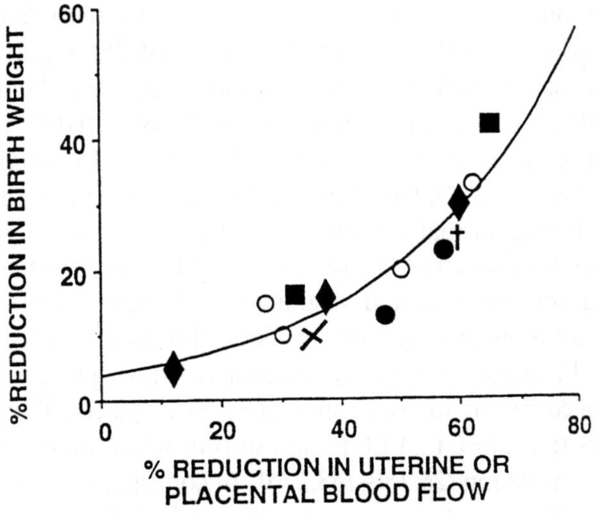

Fig. 7. The percent reduction in uteroplacental blood flow (x-axis) plotted against the percent reduction in neonatal birth weight (y-axis). The data used to predict the best fit exponential line were obtained from literature values of studies in sheep (■), rodents (○), rabbits (◆), humans (●): x = normotensive women and † = preeclamptic women at 3100 m (*224*; with permission).

pregnancy the increase in total uterine weight is dramatically greater than the increase in total uterine blood flow, whereas increases in tissue weight and blood flow are nearly proportional thereafter. The modifications in uterine blood flow during the last third of pregnancy also provide an indirect demonstration of uteroplacental vasodilation when, because of the large amount of fetal growth the most substantial fetal metabolic demands occur. In human pregnancies, Palmer et al. *(223)* observed patterns of elevations in uterine blood flow throughout gestation and blood flows/kg of fetal weight which were similar to reports in the ovine model *(26,42,71,198,199)*. The physiologic significance of the rise in uteroplacental blood flow is exemplified by the observations in women studied at high altitude (3100 m) compared to animal model studies that during the fetal growth phase of pregnancy, reductions in blood flow are associated with small for gestational age neonates (*223,224*; Fig. 7). Therefore there is a positive association between uteroplacental blood flow and newborn birth weights *(223,224)*.

Blood Flow Distribution Within The Uterus

Alterations in the pattern of total uteroplacental blood flow represent the summation of the patterns of flow to the individual uterine tissues. Radiolabeled microspheres have been used to measure blood flow to individual uterine tissues and to evaluate changes in the distribution of total uterine blood flow to individual uteroplacental tissues during ovine gestation (Fig. 8). In nonpregnant ovariectomized (to remove the source of ovarian steroids) sheep, uterine blood flow is evenly distributed amongst the endometrium, myometrium, and caruncles *(25,26,42,71,198,199)*.

In ruminants (sheep, cows, goats, deer, and so on) the caruncles are specialized sites for implantation/placentation that develop into the maternal compartment of the placentome which is in direct apposition to the fetal cotyledonary portion of the placentone. During the first trimester, the endometrium receives nearly 60% of total uterine blood flow, while the remaining blood flow is evenly distributed between the myomtrium and the enlarged caruncles, which at this stage are undergoing substantial hypertrophy and hyperplasia

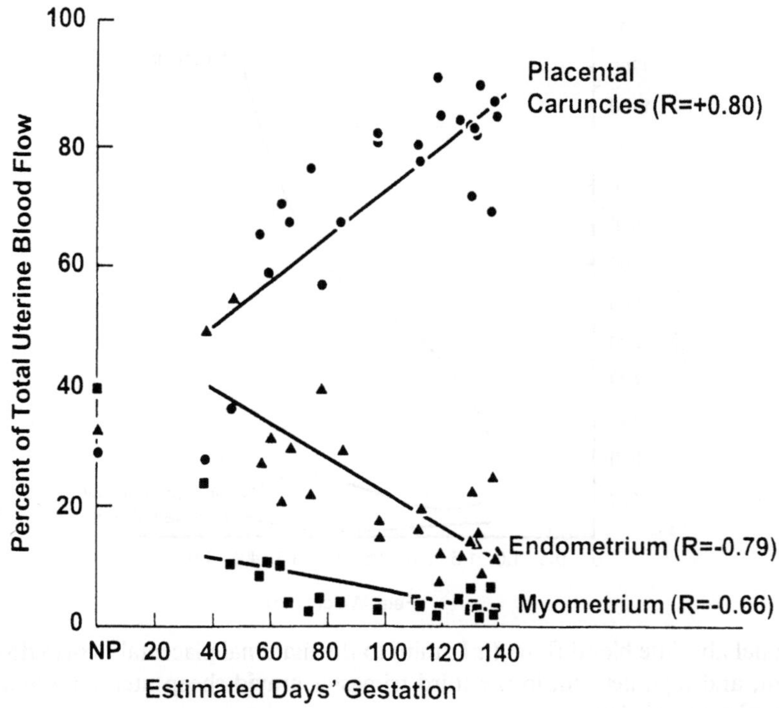

Fig. 8. Distribution of total uteroplacental blood flow during ovine pregnancy (term = 145 d). Blood flow distributions were determined by the radioactive microsphere technique. Correlation coefficients are significant at $p < 0.01$. (As modified from *25,26,42,71,198,199*).

owing to angiogenesis *(26,180,181,183,216)*. This is in preparation for the caruncles to become the maternal portion of the placentome that receives villous chorionic interdigitations from the developing fetal coyledonary portion of the placentome. These results also suggest that the profound functional and metabolic alterations which occur in the endometrium and the caruncles during the first third of gestation require increases in perfusion to be manifested, and mostly likely sets the stage for maternal placental development. Throughout the second trimester, during which time ovine placental development is being completed, there is a dramatic redistribution of uterine blood flow such that maternal placental or caruncular blood flow accounts for approx 60%, endometrial blood flow 30% and myometrial blood flow 10% of total uterine perfusion. Thereafter, the proportion of uterine blood flow to the caruncular component of the placentome continues to increase dramatically with commensurate relative decreases in the proportions perfusing the endometrium and myometrium. This substantial redistribution of uterine perfusion towards maternal placental blood flow has been hypothesized to reflect the ever increasing metabolic needs of the fetal-placental unit during fetal growth and further demonstrates that anatomically and physiologically the placenta is the main link between the separate maternal and fetal circulations. This relationship is further illustrated in Fig. 9 in which Makowski and coworkers *(210)* demonstrated the direct relationship between alterations in blood flow to the maternal placenta, endometrium, and myometrium relative to fetal weight. These investigators reported that increases in fetal weight, especially during the third trimester were correlated mainly with increases in maternal placental blood flow but not endometrial or myometrial blood flows.

As pregnancy advances, maternal placental blood flow is progressively favored and by term, it accounts for 80–85% of total uterine blood flow, whereas the endometrium

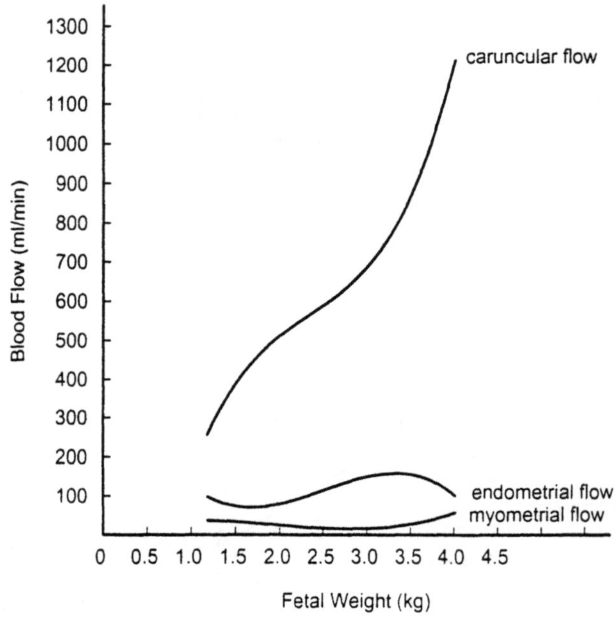

Fig. 9. Regional absolute blood flows (mL/min) to the maternal placental "cotyledon" (caruncle), endometrium, and myometrium in the third trimester gravid sheep uterus plotted against fetal weight (*210*; with permission).

receives only 10% and the myometrium only 5%, demonstrating that alterations in total uterine blood flow late in gestation (Fig. 8), for the most part reflect alterations in the placental vascular bed *(25,26,42,71,198,199,210)*. Thus experiments which only report total uteroplacental blood flow may not, in all cases, determine vascular responses of the individual tissues which comprise the gravid uterus. This is especially true in the caruncular portion of the ovine placentome in early- and mid-gestation when changes in relative blood flow are less substantial compared to late pregnancy. In the late pregnant rabbit placental blood flow accounts for 71% of total uterine blood flow *(81)*.

OTHER NONVASCULAR PHYSIOLOGIC CHANGES DURING PREGNANCY

There are numerous nonvascular changes in pregnancy which contribute to a successful pregnancy outcome by altering oxygen utilization and metabolic processes. These primarily include the respiratory and metabolic changes needed for placental and fetal growth.

Respiratory Changes in Pregnancy

Growth and development are processes which require a tremendous amount of energy utilization which because of their direct proportionality can be estimated as oxygen consumption. However the ventilatory changes noted in pregnancy can also be described by the equation for *Minute Ventilation* = *Respiratory Rate* • *Tidal Volume (35)*. During normal gestation the observed increases in oxygen consumption are associated with an even greater rise in minute ventilation in women, *(233)*, cows *(234)*, and goats *(235)* leading to a fall in end-tidal pCO_2 and/or arterial pCO_2 *(180)*. Elevations in minute ventilation during pregnancy are associated primarily with increases in tidal volume in women *(233)* or in the respiratory rate in cows *(234)* and goats *(235)*. These respiratory changes can be mimicked in the nonpregnant state with progesterone administration, but require the presence of estrogen and progesterone receptors *(236,237)*. Moore et al. *(238)* suggested that one pathway through which hormonal stimuli raise maternal ventilation is by increasing maternal ventilatory sensitivity to chemosensory stimuli as demonstrated by the rise in maternal hypoxic ventilatory responsiveness early in human pregnancy *(238)*. The rise in maternal ventilation is likely to be important for defending maternal arterial oxygen supply, particularly under circumstances of ambient hypoxia, and for fetal unloading of carbon dioxide and pH regulation *(239,240)*. Recently Evans and coworkers *(72)* evaluated the cardiopulmonary effects of normal pregnancy using the ovine animal model. They reported in the nonpregnant sheep, that decreases in cardiac output, and thus tissue oxygen delivery, leads to an increase in whole body oxygen extraction. This protective mechanism is exceeded, however, when a "critical cardiac output" is reached, i.e., oxygen consumption becomes fully dependent on the decreases in whole body flow with further incremental reductions in cardiac output. By contrast, during normal ovine pregnancy, oxygen consumption is already so high that there is no "critical cardiac output" and for each reduction in cardiac output there is a proportional decrease in oxygen consumption. We have recently shown that this can only be mimicked in part with estrogen administration to nonpregnant sheep *(241)*.

Maternal Metabolic Changes in Pregnancy

Stock and Metcalf *(35)* reviewed the maternal metabolic alterations which occur during gestation. For the purposes of the current review, the concept of metabolism has been simplified to reflect the sum total of its anabolic and catabolic processes. As expected, since pregnancy is a highly anabolic state with tremendous growth and tissue accretion, the energy and nutrient requirements are dramatically increased. This increase in energy required in pregnancy manifests from both the growth of new tissues in the fetus (placenta, membranes, and fluids), and mother (plasma, red blood cells and other whole blood elements, lipid and protein stores, uterine and mammary tissues), as well as the catabolic price it takes for these biosynthetic processes to occur. One must also factor in the metabolic cost of the maintenance of these newly formed tissues that by term is quite substantial. Estimates of the total net energy cost of pregnancy in humans is $\cong$77,000 kcal. Increases in basal maternal oxygen consumption during pregnancy, which was used to estimate this energy cost, are representative of requirements for both tissue synthesis and maintenance of the tissues in the maternal and fetal compartments. Metcalf *(242)* estimated the increase in pregnancy-mediated basal oxygen consumption to be $\cong$ 51 mL O_2/min in human pregnancy and then partitioned this to reflect the increase in oxygen consumption to be 49% by the gravid uterus (including the fetus and placenta), 20% by the muscles of ventilation, 18% by the myocardium, 10% by the kidney, and 3% by the mammary gland (i.e., before lactation). Of particular interest to this review is the increase in myocardial oxygen consumption associated with the described increases in heart rate, end-diastolic volume, as well as ventricular wall mass and contractility *(24,32–35,60,108,116,117, 121–123)*. In addition, the elevation in renal oxygen consumption relates well to the increased renal blood flow, sodium reabsorption, and glomerular filtration for plasma volume expansion *(24,51–53,82,85)*. Increases in uterine and mammary gland oxygen consumption are associated with the neovascularization, but also vasodilatation of these important vascular beds that are respectively responsible for supplying energy and nutrients to the fetus and neonate.

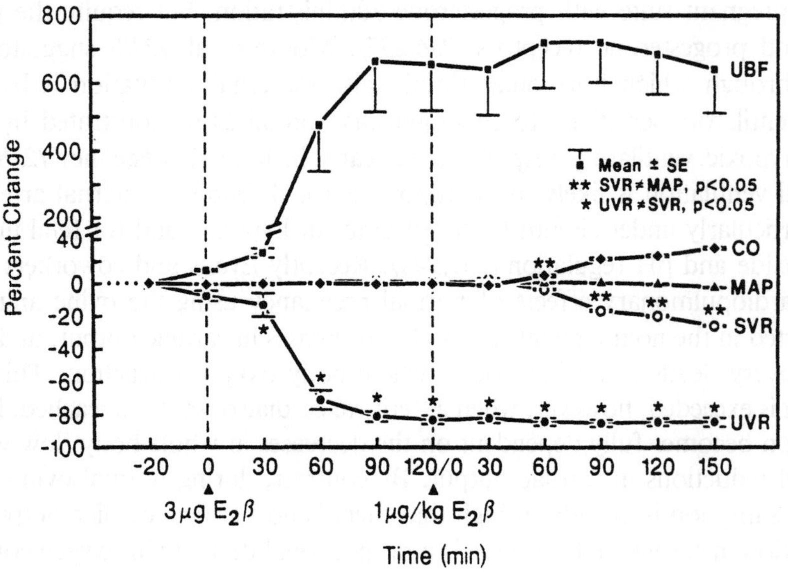

Fig. 10. Effects of local and systemic estradiol-17β (E2β) on relative (%Δ) responses of uterine blood flow (UBF), cardiac output (CO), mean arterial pressure (MAP), systemic vascular resistance (SVR), and uterine vascular resistance (UVR) in nonpregnant oophorectomized sheep (*28*; with permission).

FACTORS CONTROLLING UTERINE AND SYSTEMIC VASCULATURE IN PREGNANCY

There are many hypotheses regarding factors which control uteroplacental and systemic vascular changes during normal pregnancy. These proposed factors include estrogen, progesterone, prostaglandins, sympathetic and parasympathetic mediators of the autonomic nervous system, endothelial-derived relaxing factor (Nitric Oxide), histamine, growth factors, and even calcium channel blockade. To date, conclusive "direct cause and effect" relationships have not been established for any of these substances or pathways which can fully explain all of the pregnancy-associated alterations described in this chapter. However, based on the detailed studies by Gilson and associates *(51)* in the rat, the very early pregnancy-mediated rises in renal blood flows contribute to the reduced systemic vascular resistance and they believe that these early renal events may initiate the progressive systemic cascade of hemodynamic adaptations of pregnancy. In subsequent studies they provide convincing physiologic data also in the rat which suggests that Nitric Oxide is involved in these renal hemodynamic events during early pregnancy, while prostaglandins at best have merely a compensatory role *(52,53)*.

Endogenous estrogen production increases during gestation with the sources deriving from the feto-placental unit and/or the ovary *(1–7,10–12,14,22,25,30,195,216)*. Moreover, uterine and systemic vasodilation of pregnancy can be mimicked to some extent by estrogen administration to nonpregnant castrated sheep (*2,11,23–31,42,122,176,195,200, 215,243–246*; Figs. 10 and 11). These responses are also similar to the systemic responses of postmenopausal women to estrogen replacement therapy *(24–29,122,244,245)*. In the sheep, estrogen increases uterine blood flow, cardiac output, and blood volume while decreasing uterine and systemic vascular resistance *(24–29,122,244,245)*. We examined the acute (1–4 h) effects of estradiol-17β administered both locally into the uterine arterial

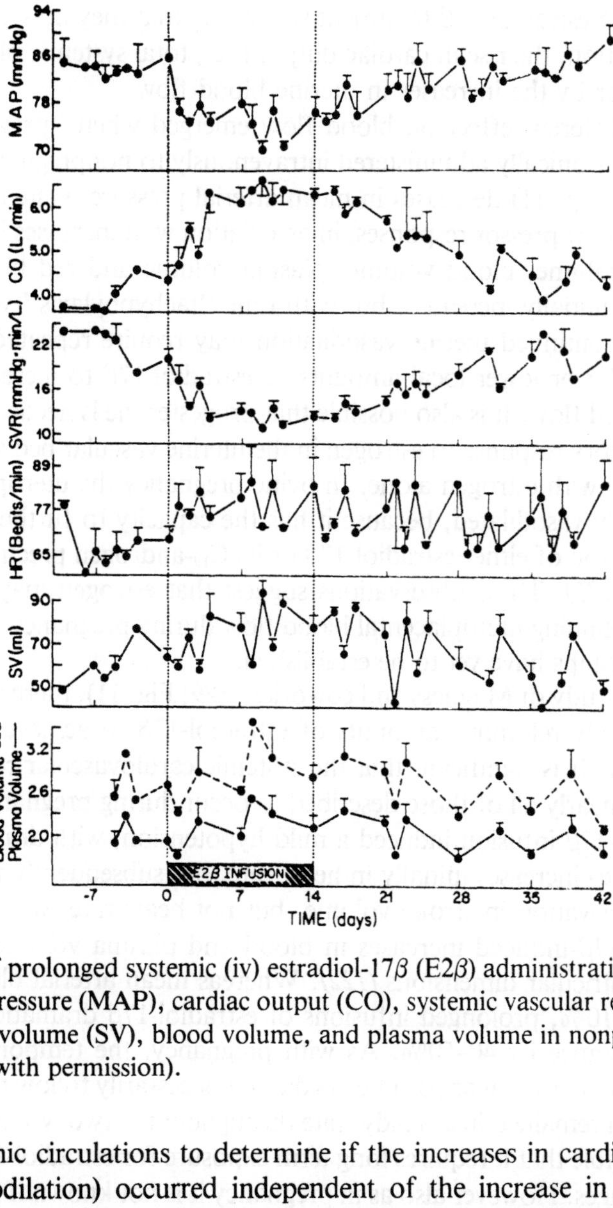

Fig. 11. Effects of prolonged systemic (iv) estradiol-17β (E2β) administration on daily responses of mean arterial pressure (MAP), cardiac output (CO), systemic vascular resistance (SVR), heart rate (HR), stroke volume (SV), blood volume, and plasma volume in nonpregnant oophorectomized sheep (*29*; with permission).

versus the systemic circulations to determine if the increases in cardiac output (systemic blood flow vasodilation) occurred independent of the increase in uterine blood flow (*28*; Fig. 10). In this study, 3 μg of estradiol-17β were injected locally as a bolus into both uterine arteries followed 120 min later by 1 μg/kg of estradiol-17β administered intravenously. Confirming results of numerous other studies *(2,11,22,23,25,27,31,70,176, 215,220)* there was a 30 min delay postlocal injection, before maximum increases in uterine blood flow, associated with decreases in uterine vascular resistance, occurred 90 min after local estradiol-17β and flow remained constant for the duration of the experiment. Uterine perfusion pressure (mean arterial pressure) was not affected by acute estrogen treatment. In contrast, systemic vascular resistance was not affected by the local administration of estradiol-17β, until 60–90 min after the systemic administration of estradiol-17β when peripheral resistance decreased gradually through 120–150 min. Therefore, in response to estrogen the uterine and systemic vascular beds undergo vasodilatation independently of each other, and on a relative percent basis the uterine vascular bed is substantially more responsive to estrogen than the systemic vascular bed (Fig. 10). We noted that the gradual rise in cardiac output directly paralleled the pattern of increase in uterine blood flow following estradiol-17β treatment suggesting that they may occur by a similar mechanism. In addition, the rise in cardiac output (i.e., total systemic blood flows) could not be accounted for by the increases in uterine blood flow.

A dramatically different effect on blood flow emerged when "pregnancy" levels of estradiol-17β were chronically administered intravenously to nonpregnant sheep for 2 wk *(29)*. These include (Fig. 11) decreases in mean arterial pressure, systemic vascular resistance and angiotensin II pressor responses, in association with increases in cardiac output, heart rate, stroke volume, blood volume, plasma volume and red blood cell volume. Uterine blood flow initially increased, but with time "tachyphylaxis" was observed. We hypothesized, that continued uterine vasodilation may require repeated higher systemic doses of estradiol-17β or lower local amounts of estradiol-17β to increase and maintain elevated uterine blood flow. It is also possible that progesterone is needed to maintain and sustain the vasodilatory response to estrogen in the uterine vascular bed as observed in the systemic vasculature with estrogen alone. In ovine pregnancy the uteroplacental vascular bed is not maximally vasodilated, because it has the capacity to further vasodilate after systemic administration of either estradiol-17β or its C_{19}-androgen precursor, dehydroepiandrosterone *(22,23,25)*. These observations suggest that estrogen may be important in modulating or maintaining uteroplacental blood flow during pregnancy, however, "cause and effect" relationships have yet to be established.

Returning to the study of Magness and coworkers (*29*; Fig. 11), there was an attempt to infuse "physiologically relevant" amounts of estradiol-17β to achieve pregnancy levels *(1–8,10,16,22,28,29)*. It is significant that the systemic cardiovascular responses to estradiol-17β mimicked nearly all of those described to occur during pregnancy. For example, prolonged estradiol-17β infusion induced a mild hypotension, with dramatic increases in cardiac output due to increases initially in heart rate, but subsequently in stroke volume. Furthermore, this elevation in stroke volume, but not heart rate, was highly correlated with the estradiol-17β-induced increases in blood and plasma volumes *(29)* as well as increases in left ventricular dimensions *(122)*. Whereas mean arterial blood pressure was reduced by only 8–10%, prolonged infusions of estradiol-17β dramatically lowered systemic vascular resistance by 40–50%. As with pregnancy, the temporal pattern of the changes in these systemic vascular parameters did not necessarily follow the blood levels of estradiol-17β, which remained in a steady state throughout the two weeks of infusion *(29)*. Therefore, it is possible that it requires long term exposure for estradiol-17β to cause these cardiovascular changes. However also as in pregnancy it is not known if estradiol-17β initiates these changes by direct action on the vasculature to cause these uterine and/or systemic changes, or if there is an intermediary vasodilator factor being induced (e.g., PGI_2 or Nitric Oxide). Although several investigators have suggested that the increase in production of vasodilator prostaglandins normally seen in pregnancy is necessary for the pregnancy-associated vasodilation in both the systemic and uteroplacental vascular beds, data are available which raise questions about this conclusion *(41,54,96,142,146)*. For example, we have shown that in ovine pregnancy decreases in PGE_2 and/or PGI_2 of 40–70% after systemic or local indomethacin infusion do not alter basal uterine blood flows or other systemic cardiovascular parameters *(41,46)*. Furthermore, estrogen-induced uterine blood flow responses are to a great extent ~60–70%) modulated by increases in Nitric Oxide production (*176,246*; Fig. 12), but not prostaglandin production *(176)*, in association with increases in uterine artery endothelial cell Nitric Oxide Synthase expression and Nitric Oxide-mediated functional activity *(174,184,247)*. The role of Nitric Oxide in pregnancy has been extensively reviewed recently *(174)*.

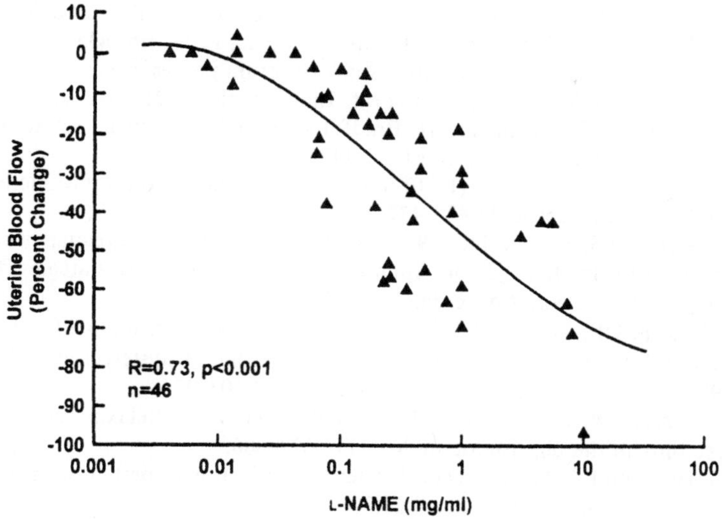

Fig. 12. Dose-response curve illustrating the relationship between the calculated uterine arterial blood concentration of L-Nitro Arginine Methyl Ester (L-NAME) infused locally into a uterine arterial catheter over 1 min and the percent change in uterine blood flow during the maximum response (90–150 min) to the systemic infusion of $E_2\beta$ (1 μg/kg) in nonpregnant sheep (*176*; with permission).

Another recently proposed mechanism includes the Calcitonin Gene-Related Peptide (CGRP)-induced cardiovascular adaptations in pregnancy. Yallampalli and coworkers *(248–251)* provide evidence that CGRP is elevated in ovine and rat pregnancy and that the vasodilator responses to CGRP are elevated during rat pregnancy and in progesterone-treated nonpregnant rats. In addition, in the absence of progesterone, CGRP-induced vasodilatory responses are blunted. These studies suggest an additional mechanism through which progesterone may exert its vascular effects, namely the CGRP system.

Other mechanisms which need to be critically evaluated in this manner include growth factors, shear stress, and progesterone. Thus the mechanisms responsible for the systemic and/or uteroplacental vasodilation in pregnancy and the interactions of these many factors remain to be further elucidated.

ACKNOWLEDGMENTS

I would like to express my gratitude to the co-investigators and technicians who worked on these projects. In particular, Ian M. Bird, PhD, Jing Zheng, PhD, Hiroaki Itoh, MD, Terrance M. Phernetton, BS, Beth Shaw, BS, as well as Cindy Goss for her help in preparing this chapter for publication. I am also grateful to Kirk P. Conrad, MD (Magee Women's Research Institute), Lorna G. Moore, PhD (University of Colorado Health Science Center), and Chandrasekhar Yallampalli (University of Texas-Medical Branch at Galveston) for their critical and expert peer review input into the final concepts presented in this book chapter. The data from our laboratory were supported by: NIH grants HL49210, HD33255, and HL57653.

REFERENCES

1. Catchpole HR (1991) Hormonal mechanisms in pregnancy and parturition, In: Reprod in Domestic Ani, Fourth Edition, Academic, pp. 361–383.
2. Ford SP (1982) Control of uterine and ovarian blood flow throughout the estrous cycle and pregnancy of the ewe, sow, and cow. J Anim Sci 55 (Suppl. II): 32–42.

3. Martal J, Cedard L (1993) Endocrine functions of the placenta, In: Reprod in Mammals and Man (Thibault C, LeVasseur MC, Hunter RHF, eds.), Ellipses, Paris, pp. 435–459.
4. Pepe GJ, Rothchild I (1974) A comparative study of serum progesterone levels in pregnancy and in various types of pseudopregnancy in the rat. Endocrinology 95:275–279.
5. Barkley MS, Michael SD, Geschwind II, Bradford GE (1977) Plasma testosterone during pregnancy in the mouse. Endocrinology 100:1472–1475.
6. Batra S, Sjoberg NO, Thorbert G. (1980) Sex steroids in plasma and reproductive tissues of the female guinea pig. Biol Reprod 22:430–437.
7. Weems CW, Weems YS, Vincent DL (1995) Maternal recognition of pregnancy and maintenance of gestation of sheep, In: Reprod and Anim Breeding: Advances and stategies (Enne G, Greppi GF, Laura D, eds.), Elsevier, Amsterdam, pp. 277–293.
8. Weems YS, Vincent DL, Tanaka Y, Miller-Patrick K, Nusser K, Ashimine D, et al. (1992) Effect of prostaglandin F2α (PGF2α) on sources of progesterone in hysterectomized intact or ovariectomized 90–100 day pregnant ewes. Prostaglandins 43:203–222.
9. Anderson LL, Adair V, Stromer MH, MacDonald WG (1983) Relaxin production and release after hysterectomy in the pig. Endocrinology 113:677–686.
10. Challis JRG, Harrison FA, Heap RB (1971) Uterine production of oestrogens and progesterone at parturition in the sheep. J Reprod Fertil 25:306–307.
11. Ford SP (1989) Factors controlling uterine blood flow during estrous and early pregnancy, In: The Uterine Circulation (Rosenfeld CR, ed.), Perinatology, Ithaca, NY. 10:113–134.
12. Ford SP, Chenault JR, Christenson RK, Echternkamp SE, Ford JJ (1981) Effects of preimplantation bovine and porcine conceptuses on blood flow and steroid content of the uterus, In: Cellular and Molecular Aspects of Implantation (Glasser SR, Bullock DW, eds.), Plenum, NY. pp 436–438.
13. Ford SP, Christenson RK, Ford JJ (1982). Uterine blood flow and uterine arterial, venous and luminal concentration of oestrogens on days 11, 13, and 15 after oestrus in pregnant and nonpregnant sows. J Reprod Fertil 64:185–190.
14. Magness RR, Ford SP (1982) Steroid concentrations in uterine lymph and uterine arterial plasma of gilts during the estrous cycle and early pregnancy. Biol Reprod 27:871–877.
15. Reynolds LP, Magness RR, Ford SP (1984) Uterine blood flow during early pregnancy in ewes: Interaction between the conceptus and the ovary bearing the corpus luteum. J Anim Sci 58:423–429.
16. Carnegie JA, Robertson HA (1978) Conjugated and unconjugated estrogens in fetal and maternal fluids of the pregnant ewe: a possible role for estrone sulfate during early pregnancy. Biol Reprod 19:202–211.
17. Ferrell CL, Ford SP (1980) Blood flow, steroid secretion, and nutrient uptake of the gravid bovine uterus. J Anim Sci 50:1113–1121.
18. King GJ, Rajamahendran R. (1988) Comparison of plasma progesterone profiles in cyclic, pregnant, pseudopregnant and hysterectomized pigs between 8 and 27 days after oestrus. J Endocrinol 119:111–116.
19. Robertson HA, King GJ (1974) Plasma concentrations of progesterone, oestrone, oestradiol-17β and of oestrone sulphate in the pig at implantation, during pregnancy and at parturition. J Reprod Fertil 40:133–141.
20. Robertson HA, King GJ (1979) Conjugated and unconjugated oestrogens in fetal and maternal fluids of the cow throughout pregnancy. J Reprod Fertil 55:463–470.
21. Weems YS, Vincent DL, Nusser KD, Tanaka Y, Miller-Patrick K, Ledgerwood KS, et al. (1994) Effects of prostaglandin F2α (PGF2α) on secretion of estradiol-17β and cortisol in 90–100 day hysterectomized, intact or ovariectomized pregnant ewes. Prostaglandins 48:139–157.
22. Rosenfeld CR, Worley RJ, Milewich L, Gant Jr NF, Parker Jr CR (1980) Ovine fetoplacental sulfoconjugation and aromatization of dehydroepiandrosterone. Endocrinology 106:1971–1979.
23. Rosenfeld CR, Morriss Jr FH, Battaglia FC, Makowski EL, Meschia G. (1976) Effect of estradiol-17β on blood flow to reproductive and nonreproductive tissues in pregnant ewes. Am J Obstet Gynecol 124:618–629.
24. Longo LD (1983) Maternal blood volume and cardiac output during pregnancy: a hypothesis of endocrinologic control. Am J Physiol 245:R720–R729.
25. Magness RR, Rosenfeld CR (1989) The role of steroid hormones in the control of uterine blood flow, In: The Uterine Circulation (Rosenfeld CR, ed.), Perinatology, Ithaca, NY, pp. 239–271.
26. Magness RR, Zheng J (1996) Maternal cardiovascular alterations during pregnancy, In: Pediatrics and Perinatology: The Scientific Basis. 2nd edition (Gluckman PD, Heymann MA, eds.), Arnold Publishing, London, pp. 762–772.

27. Magness RR (1990) Ovarian secretion and vascular function, In: Ovarian Secretions and Cardiovascular and Neurological Function (Naftolin F, Gutmann JN, Sarrell PM, DeCherney AH, eds.), Serono Foundation Symposia, USA, Norwell, MA (Raven), pp. 93–125.
28. Magness RR, Rosenfeld CR (1989) Local and systemic estradiol-17β: Effects on uterine and systemic vasodilation. Am J Physiol 256:E536–E542.
29. Magness RR, Parker CR, Rosenfeld CR (1993) Systemic and uterine responses to chronic infusion of estradiol-17β. Am J Physiol 265:E690–E698.
30. Magness RR, Rosenfeld CR, Carr BR (1991) Protein kinase C in uterine and systemic arteries during the ovarian cycle and pregnancy. Am J Physiol 98260:E464–E470.
31. Resnik R, Brink GW, Plumer MH (1977) The effect of progesterone on estrogen-induced uterine blood flow. Am J Obstet Gynecol 128, 251–254.
32. Robson SC, Hunter S, Boys RJ, Dunlop W (1989) Serial study of factors influencing changes in cardiac output during human pregnancy. Am J Physiol 256:H1060–H1065.
33. Cunningham FG, MacDonald PC, Gant NF (1989) Maternal adaptations to pregnancy, In: Chapter 7, Williams Obstetrics, Vol. 18 (Patterson L, ed.), Norwalk, CT, Appleton and Lange.
34. Duvekot JJ, Peeters LLH (1994) Maternal cardiovascular hemodynamic adaptation to pregnancy. Obstet Gynec Survey 49, S1–S14.
35. Stock MK, Metcalfe J (1994) Maternal physiology during gestation, In: The Physiology of Reproduction. Second Edition (Knobil E, Neill JD, eds.), Raven, NY. Chapter 54. 947–983.
36. Clapp JF III (1985) Maternal heart rate in pregnancy. Am J Obstet Gynecol 152:659–660.
37. Clapp JF III (1978) Cardiac output and uterine blood flow in the pregnant ewe. Am J Obstet Gynecol 130:419–423.
38. Magness RR, Rosenfeld CR (1986) Systemic and uterine responses to α-adrenergic stimulation in pregnant and nonpregnant ewes. Am J Obstet Gynecol 155:897–904.
39. Magness RR, Rosenfeld CR (1988) Mechanisms for attenuated pressor responses to α-agonists in ovine pregnancy. Am J Obstet Gynecol 159:252–261.
40. Magness RR, Mitchell MD, Rosenfeld CR (1990) Uteroplacental production of eicosanoids in ovine pregnancy. Prostaglandins 39:75–88.
41. Magness RR, Rosenfeld CR, Faucher DJ, Mitchell MD (1992) Uterine prostaglandin production during ovine pregnancy: Effects of angiotensin II and indomethacin. Am J Physiol 263:H188–H197.
42. Rosenfeld CR (1989) Changes in uterine blood flow during pregnancy, In: Reproductive and Perinatal Medicine (X) The Uterine Circulation p. 135–156.
43. Curran-Everett D, Morris KG Jr, Moore LG (1991) Regional circulatory contributions to increased systemic vascular conductance of pregnancy. Am J Physiol 261:H1842–H1847.
44. Harrison GL, Moore LG (1989) Blunted vasoreactivity in pregnant guinea pigs is not restored by meclofenamate. Am J Obstet Gynecol 160:258–264.
45. Hart MV, Hosenpud JD, Hohimer AR, Morton MJ (1985) Hemodynamics during pregnancy and sex steroid administration in the guinea pig. Am J Physiol 249:R179–R185.
46. Morton M, Tsang H, Hohimer R, Ross D, Thornburg K, Faber J, et al. (1984) Left ventricular size, output, and structure during guinea pig pregnancy. Am J Physiol 246:R40–R48.
47. Meyers SA, Tseung H-Y (1985) A longitudinal study of cardiac output in unstressed pregnant guinea pigs. Am J Physiol 243:H404–H409.
48. Hariharan S, Tseung H-Y, Myers SA (1987) A comparison of the hemodynamic responses of systemic and uteroplacental vasculature to angiotensin in conscious guinea pigs. Am J Perinatol 4:235–239.
49. Slangen BFM, Out ICM, Verkeste CM, Peeters LLH (1996) Hemodynamic changes in early pregnancy in chronically instrumented conscious rats. Am J Physiol 270: H1779–H1784.
50. Slangen BFM, Van Grop AW, Van Ingen Schenau DS, DeMey JGR, Peeters LLH (1997) Aortic distensibility and compliance in awake pregnant rats. Am J Physiol 272:H1260–H1265.
51. Gilson GJ, Mosher MD, Conrad KP (1992) Systemic hemodynamic and oxygen transport during pregnancy in chronically instrumented, conscious rats. Am J Physiol 263:H1911–H1918.
52. Danielson LA, Conrad KP (1995) Acute blockade of nitric oxide synthase inhibits renal vasodilation and hyperfiltration during pregnancy in chronically instrumented conscious rats. J Clin Invest 96:482–490.
53. Danielson LA, Conrad KP (1996) Prostaglandins maintain renal vasodilation and hyperfiltration during chronic nitric oxide synthase blockade in conscious pregnant rats. Circ Res 79:1161–1166.
54. Conrad KP, Colpoys MC (1986) Evidence against the hypothesis that prostaglandins are the vasodepressor agents of pregnancy: serial studies in chronically instrumented, conscious rats. J Clin Invest 77:236–245.

55. Conrad KP, Russ RD (1992) Augmentation of baroreflex-mediated bradycardia in conscious pregnant rats. Am J Physiol 262:R472–R477.
56. Melone PJ, Meis PJ, Blizard DA (1991) Circadian rhythms of heart rate and mean arterial pressure in chronically instrumented pregnant rats. Am J Obstet Gynecol 165:758–763.
57. Bader RA, Bader ME, Rose DJ, Braunwald E (1955) Hemodynamics at rest and during exercise in normal pregnancy as studied by cardiac catheterization. J Clin Invest 34:1524–1536.
58. Capeless EL, Clapp JF (1991) When do cardiovascular parameters return to their preconception values? Am J Obstet Gynecol 165:883–886.
59. Clapp JF, Seaward BL, Sleamaker RH, Hiser J (1988) Maternal physiologic adaptations to early human pregnancy. Am J Obstet Gynecol 159:1456–1460.
60. Duvekot JJ, Cheriex EC, Pieters FAA, Menherre PPCA, Peeters LLH (1993) Early pregnancy changes in hemodynamics and volume homeostasis are consecutive adjustments triggered by a primary fall in systemic vascular tone. Am J Obstet Gynecol 169:1382–1392.
61. Easterling RR, Benedetti TJ, Schmucker BC, Millard SP (1990) Maternal hemodynamics in normal and preeclamptic pregnancies: A longitudinal study. Obstet Gynecol 76:1061–1069.
62. Easterling TR, Benedetti TJ, Schmucker BC, Carlson K, Millard SP (1991) Maternal hemodynamics and aortic diameter in normal and hypertensive pregnancies. Obstet Gynecol 78:1073–1077.
63. Hansen JM, Ueland K (1974) Maternal cardiovascular dynamics during pregnancy and parturition. Clin Anesth 10:21–36.
64. Mashini IS, Albazzaz SJ, Fadel HE, Abdykkam AM, Hadi HA, Harp R, et al. (1987) Serial noninvasive evaluation of cardiovascular hemodynamics during pregnancy. Am J Obstet Gynecol 156:1208–1213.
65. Moutquin JM, Rainville C, Giroux L, Raynauld P, Amyot G, Bilodeau R, et al. (1985) A prospective study of blood pressure in pregnancy: Prediction of preeclampsia. Am J Obstet Gynecol 151: 191–196.
66. Palmer AJ, Walker AHC (1949) The maternal circulation in normal pregnancy. J Obstet Gynaecol Br Emp 56:537–547.
67. Vorys N, Ullery JC, Hanusek GE (1961) The cardiac output changes in various positions in pregnancy. Am J Obstet Gynecol 82:1312–1321.
68. Naden RP, Gant NF Jr, Rosenfeld CR (1984). The pressor response to angiotensin II: the roles of peripheral and cardiac responses in pregnant and nonpregnant sheep. Am J Obstet Gynecol 148: 450–457.
69. Metcalfe J, Parer JT (1966) Cardiovascular changes during pregnancy in ewes. Am J Physiol 210:821–825.
70. Greiss FC Jr (1982) Uterine blood flow in pregnancy: an overview, In: Uterine and placental blood flow (Moawad AH, Lindheimer MD, eds.), New York: Masson: pp. 19–26.
71. Rosenfeld CR (1977) Distribution of cardiac output in ovine pregnancy. Am J Physiol 232: H231–H235.
72. Evans W, Capelli SC, Edelstone DI (1996) Lack of a critical output and critical systemic oxygen delivery during low cardiac output in the third trimester in the pregnant sheep. Am J Obstet Gynecol 175:222–8.
73. Hoversland AS, Parer JT, Metcalfe J (1974) Hemodynamic adjustments in the pygmy goat during pregnancy and early postpartum. Biol Reprod 10:578–588.
74. Cha SC, Aberdeen GW, Nuwayhid BS, Quillen EW Jr (1990) Influence of pregnancy on mean systemic filling pressure and the cardiac function curve in guinea pigs. Can J Physiol Pharmacol 70:669–674.
75. Peeters LLH, Grutters G, Martin CB (1980) Distribution of cardiac output in the unstressed guinea pig. Am J Obstet Gynecol 138:1177–1184.
76. Ahokas RA, Anderson GD, Lipshitz J (1983) Cardiac ouput and uteroplacental blood flow in diet-restricted and diet replete pregnant rats. Am J Obstet Gynecol 146:6–13.
77. Bruce NW (1976) The distribution of blood flow to the reproductive organs of rats near term. J Reprod Fertil 46:359–362.
78. Lundgren Y, Karlsson K, Ljungblad U (1979) Circulatory changes during pregnancy in spontaneously and renal hypertensive rats. Clin Sci 57:337S–339S.
79. Lees MH, Hill JD, Ochsner AJ III, Thomas CL, Novy MJ (1971) Maternal placental and myometrial blood flow of the rhesus monkey during uterine contractions. Am J Obstet Gynecol 110:68–81.
80. Phippard AF, Horvath S, Glynn EM, Garner MG, Fletcher P, Duggin GG, et al. (1986) Circulatory adaptation to pregnancy-Serial studies of haemodynamics, blood volume, renin and aldosterone in the baboon. J Hypertens 4:773–779.

81. Johnson RL, Gilbert M, Meschia G, Battaglia FC (1985) Cardiac output distribution and utero-placental blood flow in the pregnant rabbit: a comparative study. Am J Obstet Gynecol 151: 682–686.
82. Chelsey LC, Duffus GM (1971) Posture and apparent plasma volume in late pregnancy. J Obstet Gynaecol Br Commonw 78:406–412.
83. Chesley LC (1972) Plasma and red cell volumes during pregnancy. Am J Obstet. Gynecol 112: 440–450.
84. Feldman H, van Donk EC, Steenbock H, Schneiders EF (1936) Hydremia as a factor in the anemia of pregnancy. Am J Physiol 115:69–77.
85. Hytten FE, Paintain DB (1963) Increase in plasma volume during normal pregnancy. J Obstet Gynaecol Br Commonw 70:402–407.
86. Reynolds M (1953) Measurement of bovine plasma and blood volume during pregnancy and lactation. Am J Physiol 175:118–122.
87. Hard DL, Anderson LL (1982) Interaction of maternal blood volume and uterine blood flow with porcine fetal development. Biol Reprod 27:79–90.
88. Del Valle GO, Mosher MD, Conrad KP (1993) Serum immunoreactive erythropoietin and red blood cell mass during pregnancy in conscious rats. Am J Physiol 265:R399–R403.
89. Hytten FE (1985) Blood volume changes in normal pregnancy. Clin Haematol 14:601–612.
90. Rovinsky JJ, Jaffin H (1965) Cardiovascular hemodynamics in pregnancy. Am J Obstet Gynecol 93:1–13.
91. Taylor DJ, Lind T (1979) Red blood cell mass during and after normal pregnancy. Br J Obstet Gynecol 86:364–370.
92. Donovan JC, Lund CJ, Hicks EL (1965) Effect of lactation on blood volume in the human female. Am J Obstet Gynecol 93:588–589.
93. Baylis C (1980) Glomerular filtration rate and plasma volume in the pregnant rat. J Physiol (Lond) 305:49P–50P.
94. Oates JN, Broughton Pipkin F, Symonds EM (1982) Angiotensin-converting enzyme and the renin-angiotensin system in normotensive primigravid pregnancy. Clin Exp Hypertens (B) 1:73–91.
95. Mackanjee HR, Shaul PW, Magness RR, Rosenfeld CR (1991) Angiotensin II vascular smooth-muscle receptors are not down-regulated in near-term pregnant sheep. Am J Obstet Gynecol 165: 1641–1648.
96. Magness RR (1993) Renin-angiotensin System and Uterine Vascular Function, In: Local Systems in Reproduction (Magness RR, Naftolin F, eds.), Serono Foundation Symposia July 6–7, 1992 Paris, France, USA, Raven, Norwell, MA, pp. 96:237–261.
97. Magness RR, Cox K, Rosenfeld CR, Gant NF (1994) Angiotensin II metabolic clearance rate and pressor responses in nonpregnant and pregnant women. Am J Obstet Gynecol 171:668–679.
98. Rosenfeld CR, Gresores A, Roy TA, Magness RR (1995) Comparison of angiotensin II in fetal and pregnant sheep: Metabolic clearance and vascular sensitivity. Am J Physiol 268:E237–E247.
99. Siddiqi TA, Austin JE, Holroyd JC, Clark KE (1983) Modulation of angiotensin II pressor responsiveness by circulating levels of angiontensin II in pregnant sheep. Am J Obstet Gynecol 145: 458–464.
100. Laragh JH (1985) Atrial natriuretic hormone, the renin-aldosterone axis, and blood pressure-electrolyte homeostasis. N Engl J Med 313:1330–1340.
101. Blair-West JR, Coghlan JP, Denton DA, Scoggins BA, Wintour EM (1972) The pressor effect of angiotensin II in pregnant sheep. Aust J Exp Biol Med Sci 50:739–744.
102. Naden RP, Coultrup S, Arant BS, Rosenfeld CR (1985) Metabolic clearance of angiotensin II in pregnant and nonpregnant sheep. Am J Physiol 249:E49–E55.
103. Conrad KP, Morganelli PM, Brinck-Johnsen T, Colpoys MC (1989) The renin-angiotensin system during pregnancy in chronically instrumented conscious rats. Am J Obstet Gynecol 161:1065–1072.
104. Paller MS (1984) Mechanism of decreased pressor responsiveness to ANG II, NE, and vasopressin in pregnant rats. Am J Physiol 247:H100–H108.
105. Chelsey LC, Talledo E, Bohler CS, Zuspan FP (1965) Vascular reactivity to angiotensin II and norepinephrine in pregnant and nonpregnant women. Am J Obstet Gynecol 91:837–842.
106. Pan Z-R, Lindheimer MD, Bailin J, Barron WM (1990) Regulation of blood pressure in pregnancy: pressor system blockaid and stimulation. Am J Physiol 258:H1559–H1572.
107. Chapman AB, Zamudio S, Woodmansee W, Merouani A, Osorio F, Johnson A, et al. (1997) Systemic and renal hemodynamic changes in the luteal phase of the menstrual cycle mimic early pregnancy. Am J Physiol 273:F777–F782.
108. Capeless EL, Clapp JF (1989) Cardiovascular changes in early phase of pregnancy. Am J Obstet Gynecol 161:1449–1453.

109. Mabie WC, DiSessa TG, Crocker LG, Sibae BM, Arheart KL (1994) A longitudinal study of cardiac output in normal human pregnancy. Am J Obstet Gynecol 170:849–856.
110. Metcalfe J, Ueland K (1974) Maternal cardiovascular adjustments to pregnancy. Prog Cardiovasc Dis 16:363–374.
111. Robson SC, Hunter S, Boys RJ, Dunlop W (1989) Hemodynamic changes during twin pregnancy. A Doppler and M-mode echocardiographic study. Am J Obstet Gynecol 161:1273–1278.
112. Ueland K, Novy MJ, Perterson EN, Metcalfe J (1969) Maternal cardiovascular dynamics: IV. The influence of gestational age on the maternal cardiovascular response to posture and exercise. Am J Obstet Gynecol 104:856–864.
113. Veille JC, Morton MJ, Burry KJ (1985) Maternal cardiovascular adaptations to twin pregnancy. Am J Obstet Gynecol 153:261–263.
114. Walters WAW, MacGregor WG, Hills M (1966) Cardiac output at rest during pregnancy and the puerperium. Clin Sci 30:1–11.
115. Atkins AF, Watt JM, Milan P, Davis P, Crawford JS (1981) A longitudinal study of cardiovascular dynamic changes throughout pregnancy. Eur J Obstet Gynecol Reprod Biol 12:215–224.
116. Lees MM, Taylor SH, Scott D.B, Kerr MG (1967) A study of cardiac output at rest throughout pregnancy. J Obstet Gynaecol Br Commonw 74:319–328.
117. Devereux RB, Reichek N (1977) Echocardiographic determination of the left ventricular mass in man. Anatomic validation of the method. Circulation 55:613–618.
118. Conrad KP (1984) Renal hemodynamics during pregnancy in chronically catheterized conscious rats. Kidney Int 26:24–29.
119. Hunter S, Robson SC (1992) Adaptation of the maternal heart in pregnancy. Br Heart J 68: 540–543.
120. Katz R, Karliner JS, Resink R (1978) Effects of a natural volume overload state (pregnancy) on left ventricular performance in normal human subjects. Circulation 58:434–441.
121. Vered Z, Poler SM, Gibson P, Wlody D, Perez JE (1991) Noninvasive detection of the morphologic and hemodynamic changes during normal pregnancy. Clin Cardiol 14:327–334.
122. Giraud GD, Morton MJ, David LE, Paul MS, Thornburg KL (1993) Estrogen-induced left ventricular chamber enlargement in ewes. Am J Physiol 264:E490–E496.
123. Hart MV, Morton MJ, Hosenpud JD, Metcalf J (1986) Aortic function during normal human pregnancy. Am J Obstet Gynecol 154:887–891.
124. Rubler S, Damani PM, Pinto ER (1977) Cardiac size and performance during pregnancy estimated with echocardiography. Am J Cardiol 40:534–540.
125. Manalo-Estrella P, Barker AE (1967) Histopathological findings in human aortic media associated with pregnancy: a study of 16 cases. Arch Pathol 83:336–341.
126. Burwell CS, Strayhorn WD, Flickinger D, Corlette MB, Bowerman EP, Kennedy JA (1938) Circulation during pregnancy. Arch Intern Med 62:979–1003.
127. Ueland K (1976) Maternal cardiovascular dynamics. VII. Intrapartum blood volume changes. Am J Obstet Gynecol 126:671–677.
128. Barron WM, Stamoulsos BA, Lindheimer MD (1984) Role of volume in the regulation of vasopressin secretion during pregnancy in the rat. J Clin Invest 73:923–932.
129. Aberdeen GW, Cha SC, Mukaddam-Daher S, Nuwayhid BS, Quillen EW Jr (1992) Renal nerve effects on renal adaptation to changes in sodium intake during ovine pregnancy. Am J Physiol 262:F823–F829.
130. Cotes PM, Canning CE, Lind T (1983) Changes in serum immunoreactive erythropoietin during the menstrual cycle and normal pregnancy. Br J Obstet Gynecol 90:304–311.
131. Gough SR, Mosher MD, Conrad KP (1995) Metabolism of erythropoietin in conscious pregnant rats. Am J Physiol 268:R1117–R1120.
132. Beguin Y, Lipscei G, Thoumsin H, Fillet G (1991) Blunted erythropoietin production and decreased erythropoiesis in early pregnancy. Blood 78:89–93.
133. Manasc B, Jepson J (1969) Erythropoietin in plasma and urine during human pregnancy. Can Med Assoc J 100:687–691.
134. Widness JA, Clemons GK, Garcia JF, Schwartz R (1984) Plasma immunoreactive erythropoietin in normal women studied sequentially during and after pregnancy. Am J Obstet Gynecol 149: 646–650.
135. Zivny J, Kobilkova J, Neuwirt J, Andrasova V (1982) Regulation of erythropoiesis in fetus and mother during normal pregnancy. Obstet Gynecol 60:77–81.
136. Campbell DM, Campbell AJ (1985) Arterial blood pressure-the pattern of change in twin pregnancies. Acta Genet Med Gemellol (Roma) 34:217–223.

137. Berssenbrugge AD, Goodfriend TL, Ball DL, Rankin JHG (1980) The effect of pregnancy on the angiotensin II pressor response in the rabbit. Am J Obstet Gynecol 136:762–767.
138. Brown CEL, Gant NF, Cox K, Spitz B, Rosenfeld CR, Magness RR (1990) Low-dose aspirin II. Relationship of angiotensin II pressor responses, circulating eicosanoids and pregnancy outcome. Am J Obstet Gynecol 163:1853–1861.
139. Spitz B, Magness RR, Cox SM, Brown CEL, Rosenfeld CR, Gant NF (1988) Low-Dose Aspirin: I. Effect on angiotensin II pressor responses and blood prostaglandin concentrations in pregnant women sensitive to angiotensin II. Am J Obstet Gynecol 159:1035–1043.
140. Ito M, Nakamura T, Yoshimura T, Koyama H, Okamura H (1992) The blood pressure response to infusions of angiotensin II during normal pregnancy: relation to plasma angiotensin II concentration serum progesterone level, and mean platelet volume. Am J Obstet Gynecol 166:1249–1253.
141. Lumbers ER (1970) Peripheral vascular reactivity to angiotensin and noradrenaline in pregnant and non-pregnant women. Aust J Exp Biol Med Sci 48:493–500.
142. Magness RR, Gant NF (1994) Control of Vascular Reactivity in Pregnancy: The Basis for Therapeutic Approaches to Prevent Pregnancy-Induced Hypertension. Sem Perinat 18:45–69.
143. Molnar M, Hertelendy F (1992) Nw-Nitro-L-arginine, an inhibitor of nitric oxide synthesis, increases blood pressure in rats and reverses the pregnancy-induced refractoriness to vasopressor agents. Am J Obstet Gynecol 166:1560–1567.
144. Novak K, Kaufman S (1991) Effects of pregnancy, estradiol, and progesterone on pressor responsiveness to angiotensin II. Am J Physiol 261:R1164–R1170.
145. Rosenfeld CR, Gant NF Jr (1981) The chronically instrumented ewe: a model for studying vascular reactivity to angiotensin II in pregnancy. J Clin Invest 67:486–492.
146. Magness RR, Rosenfeld CR (1990) Eicosanoids and the regulation of uteroplacental hemodynamics, In: Eicosanoids in Reproduction (Mitchell MD, ed.), CRC Uniscience Series, CRC Press, Inc., Boca Raton, Florida. pp. 139–167.
147. Sanches-Ramos L, O'Sullivan MJ, Garrido-Calderon J (1987) Effect of low-dose aspirin on angiotensin II pressor response in human pregnancy. Am J Obstet Gynecol 156:193–194.
148. Hines T, Barron WM (1992) Effect of sinoaortic denervation on pressor responses in pregnant rats. Am J Physiol 262:R1100–R1105.
149. Leduc L, Wasserstrum N, Spillman T, Cotton DB (1991) Baroreflex function in normal pregnancy. Am J Obstet Gynecol 165:886–890.
150. Paller MS, Gregorini G, Ferris TF (1989) Pressor responsiveness in pseudopregnant and pregnant rats: role of maternal factors. Am J Physiol 257:R866–R871.
151. McLaughlin MK, Keve TM, Cooke R (1989) Vascular catecholamine sensitivity during pregnancy in the ewe. Am J Obstet Gynecol 160:47–53.
152. Harrison GL, Moore LG (1990) Systemic vascular reactivity during high-altitude pregnancy. J Appl Physiol 69:206–210.
153. Moore LG, Reeves JT (1980) Pregnancy blunts pulmonary vascular reactivity in dogs. Am J Physiol 239:H297–H301.
154. Lee WB, Ismay MJ, Lumbers ER (1980) Mechanisms by which angiotensin II affects the heart rate of the conscious sheep. Circ Res 47:286–292.
155. Ramsay M, Broughton Pipkin F, Rubin P (1992) Comparative study of pressor and heart rate responses to angiotensin II and noradrenaline in pregnant and nonpregnant women. Clin Sci 82:157–162.
156. Annibale DJ, Rosenfeld CR, Kamm KE (1989) Alterations in vascular smooth muscle contractility during ovine pregnancy. Am J Physiol 256:H1282–1288.
157. Baker PN, Broughton Pipkin F, Symonds EM (1992) Changes in human platelet angiotensin II binding sites associated with early pregnancy. Am J Obstet Gynecol 166:255–256.
158. Bird IM, Zheng J, Cale J, Magness RR (1997) Pregnancy induces an increase in angiotensin II type-1 receptor expression in uterine but not systemic artery endothelium. Endocrinology 138: 490–498.
159. Cox BE, Rosenfeld CR, Kalinyak JE, Magness RR, Shaul PW (1996) Tissue specific expression of vascular smooth muscle angiotensin II receptor subtypes during ovine pregnancy. Am J Physiol 271:H212–H221.
160. Shaul PW, Magness RR, Muntz KH, DeBeltz D, Buja LM (1990) α-1-adrenergic receptors in pulmonary and systemic vascular smooth muscle: Alterations with development and pregnancy. Circ Res 67:1193–1200.
161. Brown GP, Venuto RC (1986) Angiotensin II receptor alterations during pregnancy in rabbits. Am J Physiol 251:E58–E64.

162. Everett RB, Worley RJ, MacDonald PC, Gant NF (1978) Effect of prostaglandin synthetase inhibitors on pressor response to angiotensin II in human pregnancy. J Clin Endocrinol Metab 46:1007–1010.
163. Janowiak MA, Magness RR, Habermehl DA, Bird IM (1997) Pregnancy increases ovine uterine artery endothelial cyclooxygenase-1 expression. Endocrinology 139:765–771.
164. Magness RR (1991) Endothelium-derived vasoactive substances and uterine blood vessels. Sem Perinatology (Chaudhuri G, Ignarro LJ, McNellis D, eds.), pp. 68–78.
165. Magness RR, Itoh H, Bird IM (1997) Endothelium-derived nitric oxide production in uterine vasculature during pregnancy, In: Blood vessels and endothelium (Sagawa N, ed.), pp. 620–635.
166. Magness RR, Osei-Boaten K, Mitchell MD, Rosenfeld CR (1985) In vitro prostacyclin production by ovine uterine and systemic arteries: Effects of angiotensin II. J Clin Invest 76:2206–2212.
167. Magness RR, Rosenfeld CR, Hassan A, Shaul PW (1996) Endothelial vasodilator production by uterine and systemic arteries: I. Effects of ANG II on PGI_2 and NO in pregnancy. Am J Physiol 270:H1914–H1923.
168. Magness RR, Rosenfeld CR (1993) Calcium modulation of uterine artery endothelium-derived prostacyclin production in ovine pregnancy. Endocrinology 132:2445–2452.
169. Yoshimura T, Magness RR, Rosenfeld CR (1990) Angiotensin II and α-agonist: II. effects on ovine fetoplacental prostaglandins. Am J Physiol 259:H473–H479.
170. Yoshimura T, Rosenfeld CR, Magness RR (1991) Angiotensin II and α-agonist: III. in vitro fetal-maternal placental prostaglandins. Am J Physiol 260:E8–E13.
171. Li P, Tong C, Eisenach JC (1996) Pregnancy and ephedrine increase release of nitric oxide in ovine uterine arteries. Anest Analg 82:288–293.
172. Magness RR, Shaw CE, Phernetton T, Zheng J, Bird IM (1997) Endothelial vasodilator production by uterine and systemic arteries: II. Pregnancy effects on NO synthase expression. Am J Physiol 272:H1730–H1740.
173. Nelson SH, Steinsland OS, Johnson RL, Suresh MS, Gifford A, Ehardt JS (1995) Pregnancy-induced alterations of neurogenic constriction and dilation of the human uterine artery. Am J Physiol 268:H1694–H1701.
174. Sladek SM, Magness RR, Conrad KP (1997) Nitric oxide and pregnancy. Am J Physiol 272: R441–R463.
175. Tong C, Eisenanch JC (1992) The vascular mechanism of ephedrine's beneficial effect on uterine perfusion during pregnancy. Anesthesiology 76:792–798.
176. Rosenfeld CR, Cox BE, Roy T, Magness RR (1996) Nitric oxide contributes to estrogen-induced vasodilation of the ovine uterine circulation. J Clin Invest 98:2158–2166.
177. Weiner C, Liu KZ, Thompson L, Herrig J, Chestnut D (1991) Effect of pregnancy on endothelium and smooth muscle: their role in reduced adrenergic sensitivity. Am J Physiol 261:H1275–H1283.
178. Weiner C, Martinez E, Zhu LK, Ghodsi A, Chestnut D (1989) In vitro release of endothelium-derived relaxing factor by acetylcholine is increased during the guinea pig pregnancy. Am J Obstet Gynecol 161:1599–1605.
179. Weiner CP, Lizasoain I, Baylis SA, Knowles RG, Charles IG, Moncada S (1994) Induction of calcium-dependent nitric oxide syntheses by sex hormones. Proc Natl Acad Sci USA 91:5212–5216.
180. Millaway DS, Redmer DA, Kirsch JD, Anthony RV, Reynolds LP (1984) Angiogenic activity of maternal and fetal placental tissues of ewes throughout gestation. J Reprod Fertil 86:689–696.
181. Zheng J, Vagnoni KE, Bird IM, Magness RR (1997) Expression of basic fibroblast growth factor, endothelial mitogenic activity, and angiotensin II type-1 receptors in the ovine placenta during the third trimester of pregnancy. Biol Reprod 56:1189–1197.
182. Cheung CY, Singh M, Ebaugh MJ, Brace RA (1995) Vascular endothelial growth factor (VEGF) gene expression in ovine placenta and fetal membranes. Am J Obstet Gynecol 173:753–759.
183. Reynolds LP, Redmer DA (1995) Utero-placental vascular development and placental function. J Anim Sci 73:1839–1859.
184. Magness RR, Zheng J, Shaw CE, Phernetton TM, Bird IM (1996) Estrogen and pregnancy inrease uterine artery endothelial nitric oxide synthase (ecNOS) protein expression. International Society for the Study of Hypertension in Pregnancy, August 4–8, 1996, Seattle Washington, Abstr #11, p. 81.
185. Rubanyi GJR, Vanhoutte P (1986) Flow-induced release of endothelium-derived relaxing factor. Am J Physiol 250:H1145–H1149.
186. Learmont JG, Poston L (1996) Nitric oxide is involved in flow-induced dilation of isolated human small fetoplacental arteries. Am J Obstet Gynecol 174:583–588.
187. Cockell AP, Poston L (1996) Isolated mesenteric arteries from pregnant rats show enhanced flow-mediated relaxation but normal myogenic tone. J Physiol 495:545–551.

188. Cockell AP, Poston L (1997) Flow mediated nitric oxide synthesis is enhanced in normal pregnancy but reduced in preeclampsia. Hypertension 30:247–251.
189. Kublickiene KR, Cockell AP, Nisell H, Poston L (1997) Role of nitric oxide in the regulation of vascular tone in pressurized and perfused resistance myometrial arteries from term pregnant women. Am J Obstet Gynecol 177:1263–1269.
190. Yallampalli C, Garfield RE (1993) Inhibition of nitric oxide synthesis in rats during pregnancy produces signs similar to those of preeclampsia. Am J Obstet Gynecol 169:1316–1320.
191. Buhimschi I, Yallampalli C, Chwalisz K, Garfield RE (1995) Preeclampsia-like conditions produced by nitric oxide inhibition: effects of L-arginine and steroid hormones. Hum Reprod 10: 2723–2730.
192. Edvards DL, Arora CP, Bui DT, Castro LC (1996) Long-term nitric oxide blockade in the pregnant rat: effects on blood pressure and plasma levels of endothelin-1. Am J Obstet Gynecol 175: 484–488.
193. Assali NS, Rauramo L, Peltonen T (1960) Measurement of uterine blood flow and uterine metabolism: VIII. Uterine and fetal blood flow and oxygen consumption in early human pregnancy. Am J Obstet Gynecol 79:86–98.
194. Assali NS, Douglass RA Jr, Baird WW, Nicholson DB, Suyemoto R (1953) Measurement of uterine blood flow and uterine metabolism: IV. Results in normal pregnancy. Am J Obstet Gynecol 66:248–253.
195. Meschia G (1983) Circulation of female reproductive organs, In: Handbook of physiology (Shepherd JT, Aboud FM, eds.), Section 2, vol. III, part 1. Washington, DC: American Physiological Society, pp. 241–269.
196. Metcalfe J, Romney SL, Ramsey LH, Reid DE, Burwell CS (1955) Estimation of uterine blood flow in normal human pregnancy at term. J Clin Invest 34:1632–1638.
197. Veille JC, Tatum K, Zaccaro D (1996) Maternal right hypogastric artery blood flow during normal pregnancy and 6 weeks postpartum. J Soc Gynecol Invest 3:191–198.
198. Rosenfeld CR, Morriss FH Jr, Makowski EL, Meschia G, Battaglia FC (1974) Circulatory changes in the reproductive tissues of ewes during pregnancy. Gynecol Invest 5:252–268.
199. Rosenfeld CR (1984) Consideration of the uteroplacental circulation in intrauterine growth. Sem Perinat 8:42–51.
200. Ladner C, Brinkman CR III, Weston P, Assali NS (1970) Dynamics of uterine circulation in pregnant and nonpregnant sheep. Am J Physiol 218:257–263.
201. Myers SA, Sparks JW, Makowski EL, Meschia G, Battaglia FC (1982) Relationship between placenta blood flow and placental and fetal size in guinea pig. Am J Physiol 243:H404–H409.
202. Lunell NO, Nylund LE, Lewander R, Sarby B (1982) Uteroplacental blood flow in pre-eclampsia measurements with indium-113m and a computer-linked gamma camera. Clin Exp Hypertens B 1:105–117.
203. Abramson DI, Flachs K, Fierst SM (1943) Peripheral blood flow during gestation. Am J Obstet Gynecol 45:666–671.
204. Burt CC (1949) Peripheral skin temperature in normal pregnancy. Lancet 2:787–790.
205. Fawer R, Dettling A, Weihs D, Welti H, Schelling JL (1978) Effect of the menstrual cycle, oral contraceptives and pregnancy on forearm blood flow, venous distensibility and clotting factors. Eur J Clin Pharmacol 13:251–257.
206. Herbert CM, Banner EA, Wakim KG (1958) Variations in the peripheral circulation during pregnancy. Am J Obstet Gynecol 76:742–745.
207. Myhrman P, Jansson I, Lundgren Y (1980) Skin blood flow in normal pregnancy measured by venous occlusion plethysmography of the hand. Acta Obstet Gynecol Scand 59:107–110.
208. Spetz S (1964) Peripheral circulation during normal pregnancy. Acta Obstet Gynecol Scand 43: 309–329.
209. Ford SP, Reynolds LP, Magness RR (1982) Blood flow to the uterine and ovarian vascular beds of gilts during the estrous cycle or early pregnancy. Biol Reprod 27:878–885.
210. Makowski EL, Meschia G, Droegmueller W, Battaglia FC (1968) Distribution of uterine blood flow in the pregnant sheep. Am J Obstet Gynecol 101:409–412.
211. Ford SP, Chenault JR (1981) Blood flow to the corpus luteum-bearing ovary and ipsilateral uterine horn of cows during the oestrous cycle and early pregnancy. J Reprod Fertil 62:555–562.
212. Ford SP, Christenson RK (1979) Blood flow to uteri of sows during the estrous cycle and early pregnancy: local effect of the conceptus on the uterine blood supply. Biol Reprod 21:617–624.
213. Ford SP, Chenault JR, Echternkamp SE (1979) Uterine blood flow of cows during the oestrous cycle and early pregnancy: effect of the conceptus on the uterine blood supply. J Reprod Fertil 56:52–62.

214. Greiss FC Jr, Anderson SG (1970) Uterine blood flow during early ovine pregnancy. Am J Obstet Gynecol 106:30–38.
215. Markee JE (1932) Rhythmic uterine vascular changes. Am J Physiol 100:32–39.
216. Reynolds LP (1986) Utero-ovarian interactions during early pregnancy: role of conceptus-induced vasodilation. J Anim Sci 62 (Suppl. 2):47–61.
217. Greiss FC Jr, Anderson SG (1969) Uterine vascular changes during the ovarian cycle. Am J Obstet Gynecol 103:629–640.
218. Harvey CA, Owens DAA (1976) Changes in uterine and ovarian blood flow during the oestrous cycle in rats. J Endocrinol 71:367–369.
219. Magness RR, Ford SP (1983) Estrone, estradiol-17β, and progesterone concentrations in uterine lymph and systemic blood throughout the porcine estrous cycle. J Anim Sci 57:449–455.
220. Prill HJ, Gotz F (1961) Blood flow in the myometrium and endometrium of the uterus. Am J Obstet Gynecol 82:102–108.
221. Amoroso EC (1952) Placentation. In: Marshall's Physiology of Reproduction, 3rd ed., Vol. II. (Parkes AS, ed.), Longmans Green and Co., London. pp. 127–131.
222. Assheton R (1906) The morphology of the ungulate placenta. Particularly the development of that organ in the sheep, and notes upon the placenta of the elephant and hyrax. Phil Trans R Soc B Biol Sci 198:143–220.
223. Palmer SK, Zamudio S, Coffin C, Parker S, Stamm E, Moore LG (1992) Quantitative estimation of human uterine artery blood flow and pelvic blood flow redistribution in pregnancy. Obstet Gynecol 80:1000–1006.
224. Zamudio S, Palmer SK, Stamm E, Coffin C, Moore LG (1995) Uterine blood flow at high altitude, In: Hypoxia and the Brain (Sutton JR, Houston CS, Coats G, eds.), Queen City Printers, Inc. Burlington, VT. Chapter 10, pp. 112–124.
225. Keyes LE, Majack R, Dempsey EC, Moore LG (1997) Pregnancy stimulation of DNA synthesis and uterine blood flow in the guinea pig. Ped Res 41:708–715.
226. Peeters LLH, Sparks JW, Grutters G, Girard J, Battaglia FC (1982) Uteroplacental blood flow during pregnancy in chronically catheterized guinea pigs. Ped Res 16:716–720.
227. Mol W, Espach R, Wrobel KH (1983) Growth of mesometrial arteries in guinea pigs during pregnancy. Placenta 4:111–124.
228. Griendling KK, Fuller EO, Cox RH (1985) Pregnancy induced changes in sheep uterine and carotid arteries. Am J Physiol 248:H658–H665.
229. Makinoda S, Moss W (1986) Deoxyribonucleic acid synthesis in mesometrial arteries of guinea pig during oestrous cycle, pregnancy and treatment with oestradiol benzoate. Placenta 7:189–198.
230. Annibale DJ, Rosenfeld CR, Stull J, Kamm KE (1990) Protein content and myosin light chain phosphorylation in uterine artery during pregnancy. Am J Physiol 259:C484–C489.
231. Cipolla M, Osol G (1994) Hypertrophic and hyperplastic effects of pregnancy on the rat uterine arterial wall. Am J Obstet Gynecol 171:805–811.
232. Keyes LE, Moore LG, Walchak SJ, Dempsey EC (1996) Pregnancy stimulated growth of vascular smooth muscle cells: importance of protein kinase C-dependent synergy between estrogen and pletelet-derived growth factor. J Cell Physiol 166:22–32.
233. Lucius H, Gahlenbeck H, Kleine H-O, Fabel H, Bartels H (1970) Respiratory functions, buffer system, and electrolyte concentrations of blood during human pregnancy. Respir Physiol 9: 311-317.
234. Gahlenbeck H, Frerking H, Rathschlag-Schaefer AM, Bartels H (1968) Oxygen and carbon dioxide exchange across the cow placenta during the second part of pregnancy. Respir Physiol 4: 119–131.
235. Hoversland AS, Metcalfe J, Parer JT (1974) Adjustments in maternal blood gases, acid-base balance, and oxygen consumpton in the pregnant pygmy goat. Biol Reprod 10:589–595.
236. Hosenpud JD, Hart MV, Morton MJ, Hohimer AR, Resko JA (1983) Progesterone-induced hyperventilation in the guinea pig. Respir Physiol 52:257–264.
237. Brodeur P, Mockus M, McCullough RE, Moore LG (1986) Progesterone receptors and ventilatory stimulation by progestin. J Appl Physiol 60:590–595.
238. Moore LG, McCullough RE, Weil JV (1987) Increased HVR in pregnancy: relationship to hormonal and metabolic changes. J Appl Physiol 62:158–163.
239. Moore LG, Rounds SS, Jahnigen D, Reeves JT, Grover RF (1982) Infant birth weight is related to maternal arterial oxygenation at high altitude. J Appl Physiol 52:695–699.
240. Moore LG, Brodeur P, Chumbe O, D'Brot J, Hofmeister S, Monge C (1986) Maternal hypoxic ventilatory response, ventilation and infant birth weight at 4300 m. J Appl Physiol 60:1401–1406.

241. Evans W, Phernetton TM, Magness RR (1998) Estradiol 17-beta increases the critical cardiac output in response to reduction in cardiac output in nonpregnant oophorectomized sheep. Am J Physiol (In Press).
242. Metcalfe J, McAnulty JH, Ueland K (1986) Burwell and Metcalfe's Heart disease and pregnancy: physiology and management, 2nd ed. Boston: Little, Brown.
243. Davis LE, Magness RR, Rosenfeld CR (1992) Role of angiotensin II and α-adrenergic receptors during estrogen-induced vasodilation in ewes. Am J Physiol 263:E837–E843.
244. Ueda S, Fortune V, Bull BS, Valenzuela GJ, Longo LD (1986) Estrogen effects on plasma volume, arterial pressure, interstitial space, plasma proteins, and blood viscosity in sheep. Am J Obstet Gynecol 155:195–201.
245. Ueland K, Parer JT (1966) Effects of estrogens on the cardiovascular system of the ewe. Am J Obstet Gynecol 96:400–407.
246. Van Buren GA, Yang DS, Clark KE (1992) Estrogen-induced uterine vasodilation is antagonized by L-nitroarginine methyl ester, an inhibitor of nitric oxide synthesis. Am J Obstet Gynecol 167: 828–833.
247. Veille JC, Li P, Eisenach JC, Massmann AG, Figueroa JP (1996) Effects of estrogen on nitric oxide biosynthesis and vasorelaxant activity in sheep uterine and renal arteries in vitro. Am J Obstet Gynecol 174:1043–1049.
248. Yallampalli C, Dong Y-L, Wimalawansa SJ (1996) Calcitonin gene-related peptide reverses the hypertension and significantly decreases the fetal mortality in preeclampsia rats induced by N^G-nitro-L-arginine methyl ester. Hum Reprod 11:895–899.
249. Gangula PRR, Supowit SC, Wimalawansa SJ, Zhao H, Hallman DM, Dipette DJ, Yallampalli C (1997) Calcitonin gene-related peptide is a depressor in N^G-nitro-L-arginine methyl ester-induced hypertension during pregnancy. Hypertension 29:248–253.
250. Gangula PRR, Wimalawansa SJ, Yallampalli C (1997) Progesterone up-regulates vasodilator effects of calitonin gene-related peptide in N^G-nitro-L-arginine methyl ester-induced hypertension. Am J Obstet Gynecol 176:894–900.
251. Gangula PRR, Magness RR, Wimalawansa SJ, Chapa MT, Fang L, Phernetton TM, Yallampalli C (1998) Pregnancy and sex steroid hormones enhance the calcitonin gene-related peptide concentration in circulation in rats and sheep. 45th Annual Meeting of the Society for Gynecological Investigation, March 11–14, Atlanta, GA. (Abstr).

19 The Endocrinology of Uterine Decidualization

Kevin G. Osteen, PHD

CONTENTS

THE DECIDUALIZATION PROCESS

Although there is a rather broad degree of species variation, initiation of implantation leads to proliferation and differentiation of steroid-primed uterine stromal cells, culminating in the formation of a morphologically and biochemically distinct endocrine tissue, the decidua *(1)*. Decidualization is common among mammals, but the complex cellular processes leading to the formation of the decidua remains poorly understood. In humans, distinct morphological changes can be seen among uterine stromal cells at focal sites during the late secretory stage of the menstrual cycle in the absence of an active implantation process. In rats and mice, the conversion of stromal cells into predecidual cells in response to progesterone exposure alone does not occur, but a pseudodecidual reaction can be induced following mechanical stimulation in a steroid-primed uterus. Establishment of normal pregnancy in these animals requires that the conceptus initiate the uterine decidual response and the full process of decidualization relies on contact with the embryo during the invasive processes of implantation and placentation. Among rodents, primates or humans, steroid priming and the more specific action of progesterone is critical to the process of decidualization. Support for this position comes from studies that demonstrate that mice lacking progesterone receptors cannot elicit a decidual response *(2)* and the use of antiprogestins such as RU-486, which rapidly terminate human pregnancies *(3)*. The ultimate success of implantation and initiation of a viable pregnancy does not rest on any single factor, but rather it rests on the establishment of complex endocrine and paracrine inter-relationships among the ovary, the conceptus, and the decidua. Failure to establish these early relationships expeditiously during the implantation process leads to a blunted decidual response, and the onset of pregnancy termination.

The complete cellular makeup of uterine decidual tissue is complex and careful analysis has revealed interactive specialized stromal cells, an abundant vascular supply, and numerous invasive cells of hemopoietic origin. Recent evidence indicates that granulocytes in particular continue to migrate into the endometrium during the secretory phase and early pregnancy, contributing to the cellular complexity of the decidual environment *(4)*. Other cells of hemopoietic origin residing within the decidua include leukocytes and macrophages that in humans, can ultimately make up 40% of the decidual cell population *(5)*. The identity and origin of cells within the decidua can be confounding even to scientists because of the involvement of so many different cell types, however, only the specialized endometrial fibroblasts are considered the precursors of true decidual cells.

Early changes in the morphology of human stromal cells as they become predecidual cells in response to progesterone include modifications in intermediate filament expression that result in a more polyploid cell shape with a distinct epithelioid appearance. The full process of decidualization occurs only after the establishment of pregnancy, resulting in cells which are significantly larger than undifferentiated fibroblasts. Decidual cells exhibit further morphological attributes of epithelial cells such as microvilli and gap junctions *(6,7)* and begin to produce a variety of endocrine products *(8,9)*. However, even within a single species, the differentiation of stromal cells into decidual cells is not uniform. A diversified morphology exists in different regions of the decidual tissue *(10)*. From a practical biological standpoint, decidual tissue function reflects the collective contribution of not only decidual cells, but also each of the interactive cell types within the tissue, which includes a plethora of bioactive substances. Given this degree of complexity, the discussion here will be limited, focusing on several emerging endocrine roles played by specialized stromal cells within the human decidua. References to other species will be offered as necessary, reflecting the fact that much pregnancy-related research has been done only in experimental animals.

THE STROMA DURING THE MENSTRUAL CYCLE

At birth, the endometrium is essentially inactive, appearing as a thin tissue with low columnar or cuboidal epithelium and little associated stromal matrix. In response to the initiation of cyclic ovarian hormone stimulation, the adult endometrium develops an extensive glandular architecture continuous with surface epithelium and a rich, highly vascular supporting stroma. Pathologists view the endometrium as having distinct functional layers: the *stratum basalis,* which lies adjacent to the myometrium, remains relatively undisturbed during the tissue loss of menstruation and cells within this "feeder" region remain rather undifferentiated, apparently under the strict control of the local paracrine environment *(11,12)*. The *stratum spongiosum* or intermediate layer and the *stratum compactum* together comprise the dynamic *stratum functionalis,* which undergoes the classically recognized patterns of coordinated growth and differentiation in response to ovarian steroids throughout each menstrual cycle *(13)*. Establishment of the hemochorial-type placenta in humans is associated with extensive decidualization of the endometrial stroma in concert with the deep penetration of the stromal bed by highly invasive trophoblast cells. After breaching the basal lamina, extra-villous trophoblast cells must traverse the stromal matrix and access the maternal blood supply that allows for an efficient exchange of nutrients and bioactive substances *(see 14)*. In preparation for both accommodating and limiting these invasive events, the endometrium reestablishes a complex organ system during each menstrual cycle that is essentially discarded in the absence of nidation.

Ovarian steroids provide essential cues that dictate appropriate endometrial growth and differentiation; both estradiol and progesterone are required to direct the full complement of cellular events leading to the successful initiation of pregnancy, including the decidual response. Patterns of steroid hormone receptor levels and distribution within the endometrium mirror the highly visible changes in endometrial proliferation and morphology which occur across each menstrual cycle. Endometrial estradiol receptor levels peak during the late proliferative stage of the cycle, and progesterone receptor levels are highest somewhat later during the early luteal phase *(15)*. Endometrial growth and cellular maturation in humans is a rather slow process and approximately three weeks of steroid priming is required for the endometrium to prepare for implantation, including the capacity of specialized stromal cells to become the decidua. Although, steroids can directly affect cellular proliferation and differentiation by regulating specific genes in both stromal and epithelial cells, the specialized fibroblasts within the stroma of the endometrium are recognized as the most steroid sensitive cell type from numerous in vitro studies *(see 16)*. Undifferentiated cells isolated from endometrial stroma readily respond to steroids in vitro and can additionally direct the proliferation and differentiation of adjacent epithelial cells via paracrine factors *(17,18)*. Similar stromal-epithelial communication appears to regulate endometrial cell response to steroids in vivo *(16)*. Therefore, despite the critical role steroids play in preparing the endometrial stroma for decidualization, the local action of growth factors and cytokines is equally important for this process. A variety of local growth factors and cytokines have been identified in the cycling human endometrium *(19–21)* that likely continue to modulate progesterone-mediated decidual development and function.

ENDOCRINE AND PARACRINE SUPPORT OF DECIDUALIZATION

The process of decidualization is a complex, steroid-driven phenomenon that is associated with the unique "local" endocrine environment established by cellular interactions during the invasive events of implantation and placentation. Numerous growth factors, cytokines, and protein hormones have been identified as important signals for initiation and maintenance of decidualization in various animal species *(see 22,23)*. For example, prostaglandins appear essential for vascular development during establishment of the decidua and prostaglandin E2 can be identified as the key active prostaglandin in the stimulation of decidualization in rats *(24)*. Prostaglandins do not appear to act alone; Acker and coworkers *(25)* observed that platelet-activating factors can induce decidualization in rats, and Halhali and coworkers *(26)* obtained similar results utilizing 1,25-dihydroxy vitamin D3. More recently, relaxin, of embryonic origin, has been proposed as an essential decidualization signal in mice *(27)*. In humans, a more central role for progesterone in the decidualization process is supported by the observations that faint signs of predecidual changes can be observed in stromal cells near vascular elements by d 23 of the normal menstrual cycle in the absence of a conceptus, or in women undergoing progestin therapy *(28)*. Additionally, decidual changes in response to progesterone can be observed within stromal cells of the eutopic endometrium when an ectopic pregnancy exists *(29)* whereas the stroma within the fallopian tube at the site of a tubal pregnancy exhibit only a limited decidual response *(30)*. Although the human decidua eventually develops the capacity to synthesize steroids *(31–33)*, locally produced paracrine factors are also critical to the complete decidualization of stromal cells as well as to the maintenance of decidual cell function *(34)*. Numerous locally produced factors thought to affect the decidualization process in humans are: epidermal growth factor (EGF) *(35)*, insulin-like growth factor (IGF) *(36)*, insulin-like growth factor binding protein-1 (IGFBP-1) *(20)*, macrophage colony-stimulating factor (M-CSF) *(37)*, prostaglandin *(38)*, relaxin *(39,40)*, renin *(41)*, transforming growth factor-β (TGF-β) *(42)* and tissue factor *(43)*.

Given the complex cellular makeup of the decidua, multiple roles are likely played by each locally produced factor, acting in concert with steroids to affect cell behavior within the decidua. For example, members of the TGF-β family have been found to modulate both endocrine and immune function within the endometrium. TGF-β1 and TGF-β2 expression is associated with rising progesterone levels during the uterine cycle *(44–46)* and in the decidua *(47)*. Progesterone-mediated production of TGF-β is required for the inhibition of matrix metalloproteinase expression during the menstrual cycle and TGF-β may act in a similar fashion during trophoblast invasion *(14,48)*. However, TGF-β is also a potent immunosuppressive agent, acting on immune cells to control cellular and humoral immune responses *(49)*. Production of a TGF-β2-related molecule accounts for the immunosuppressive properties of murine and human amniotic fluid *(50–52)* and pregnancy can be terminated in mice following treatment with anti-TGF-β2 antibodies *(53)*. The complex nature of multiple factors and multiple cell interactions within the decidua during implantation and placentation precludes any clear understanding of which factors may be key to the decidualization process. However, local cell communication at the maternal-fetal interface plays an extremely important functional role during the steroid-mediated process of decidualization (23).

ENDOCRINE FUNCTION OF THE DECIDUA

Although the decidua is both a transient and constantly changing endocrine tissue, this structure plays a central role throughout establishment and maintenance of the hemochorial placenta. Several of the most important roles ascribed to decidualized stromal cells within the decidual tissue include:

1. Production of nutrients essential to the conceptus, especially prior to development of a functional fetal-maternal circulatory system;
2. The production of numerous bioactive agents, including matrix components, hormones, growth factors, and cytokines that regulate cell behavior at the maternal embryonic interface;
3. Contributing to the unique immune status of the tissue site, which prevents immune cell-mediated rejection of the fetal allograft; and
4. Actively regulating trophoblast function, including limiting trophoblast invasion within the uterus.

Many factors and functions are necessary to address the endocrinology of the decidua (*see* Table 1) and the regulation of each factor may be multifactorial. Choosing any single functional marker to study the decidua is a difficult task, however, prolactin production has been used for some time in human studies as an indicator of stromal cell differentiation and decidual cell function in vivo *(54)* and in vitro *(see 35)*. Multiple prolactin-related proteins appear essential to decidual and placental function in rodents *(55)* and prolactin in humans has been implicated in the osmoregulation of the fetal environment *(56)*, the control of prostaglandin synthesis, and myometrial contractility *(57)*. However, determining the precise role(s) played by steroids and local factors in regulating prolactin production during the process of decidualization remains difficult since in vitro data often conflict among laboratories as well as with in vivo observations. For example, Irwin and coworkers *(35)* found that treatment of endometrial stromal cells with progesterone and EGF in vitro

Table 1
Products of the Human Decidua

Hormones	*Cytokines*	*Growth factors*	*Proteases; protease inhibitors*	*Other*
Estrogen	CSF-1	TGF-β1; TGF-β2	MMP-1; MMP-2; MMP-3; MMP-9	Retinol Binding Proteins (RBP)
Progesterone	IL-1β; IL-2; IL-3; IL-6	TGF-α	TIMP-1; TIMP-2; TIMP-3	Retinoic acid and its binding proteins
Prolactin	TNF-α	EGF	uPA; PAI-1; PAI-2	CRABP-I; CRABP-II
Prostaglandins	IFN-α; IFN-γ	IGF-1; IGFBP-I	α2M	Collagen I, III, V
	Renin	LIF		Fibronectin
				Laminin (A and B chain)

Each of these substances have been identified as being produced during the decidualization process. Specific references are cited within the text.

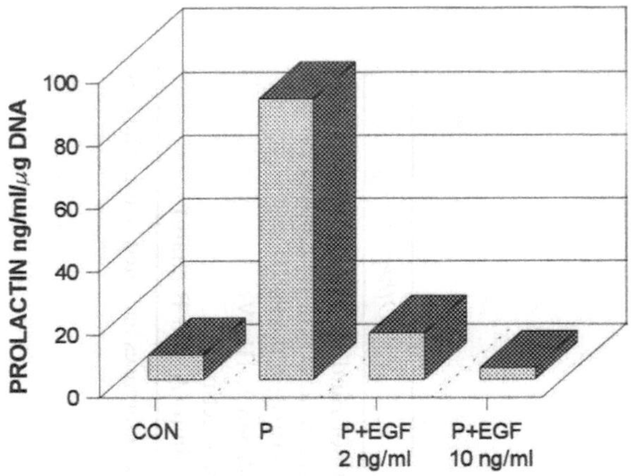

Fig. 1. Isolated normal human endometrial stromal cells exposed to progesterone (P) secrete prolactin, a distinct marker of decidualization, at an eightfold increase compared to control (steroid free) cells. Addition of EGF in the presence of progesterone, markedly reduces the amount of prolactin secreted by these cells in a dose dependent manner.

results in an increase in cell proliferation and secretion of prolactin. Using more differentiated decidual cells obtained from early human pregnancy, Saji and coworkers *(58)* found that EGF increased cell proliferation, but decreased prolactin secretion. In our experience, treatment of stromal cells obtained from either proliferative or secretory endometrial specimens with EGF suppresses progesterone-induced prolactin secretion in vitro (Fig. 1). Although the secretion of prolactin was suppressed by EGF treatment, no differences in cellular ultrastructure could be detected between cells treated with progesterone alone vs progesterone and EGF (Fig. 2). It is somewhat difficult to explain the different effects of EGF treatments on in vitro prolactin synthesis observed among several laboratories. Perhaps the differences reflect that the regulation of stromal cell decidualization is complex and that cytokines and growth factors can affect cell function differently, depending on the differentiated state of the cell being examined, the presence or absence of other cytokines and the concentration of the cytokine being used *(59)*. Another example of this phenomenon is demonstrated by TGF-β, which is known for its ability to inhibit or modify EGF action, depending on the type of uterine cell being examined *(16)*. TGF-β treatment increases expression of prolactin *(60)* and leukemia inhibitory factor, another marker of decidualization, in cultures of human stromal or decidual cells *(61)*. In contrast, Kubota and coworkers *(62)* demonstrated that TGF-β suppressed prolactin expression in isolated decidual cells.

Although the in vitro analysis of any single paracrine factor on either morphological or biochemical aspects of the decidualization process is complex, such studies remain necessary to approach an understanding of the intricate biology of decidualization. Our laboratory has begun to explore the possibility that retinoic acid, a vitamin A derivative, may modulate decidual cell sensitivity to other locally produced growth factors and cytokines. Vitamin A deficiency has been recognized for many years to decrease fertility *(63)*, but recent studies indicate more clearly the importance of retinoic acid as a uterine endocrine factor *(64)*. Retinoic acid has been shown to inhibit cell proliferation and promote differentiation of epithelium via a stromal mediated mechanism during the endometrial cycle *(65)* and retinol binding protein levels increase at implantation sites in baboons during early establishment of pregnancy *(66)*. Our group recently demonstrated the local in vitro synthesis of retinoic acid in human endometrial stromal cells and that its expression is under

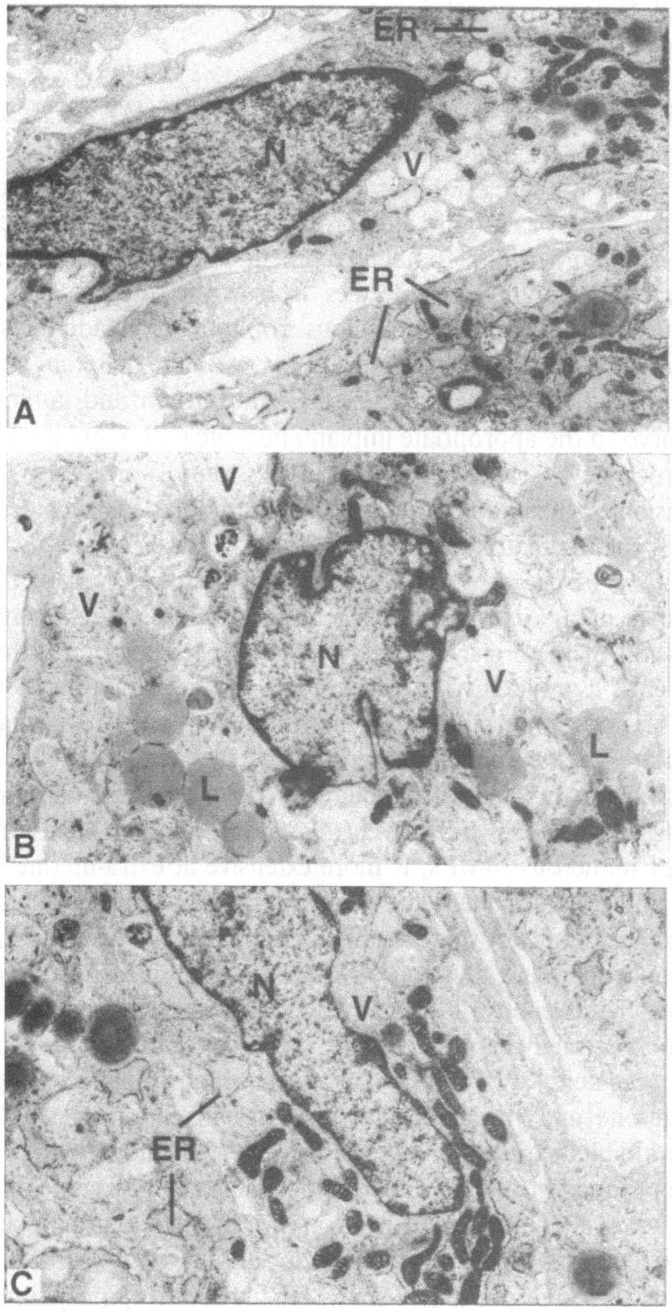

Fig. 2. Morphological characterization of cultured human endometrial cells exposed to progesterone (**A**), steroid free (**B**), and EGF in the presence of progesterone (**C**). Either progesterone or EGF plus progesterone treated cells display prominent endoplasmic reticulum (ER) with swollen cisternae suggesting secretory activity. In contrast, cells cultured under steroid free conditions display more vacuoles (V), lipid droplets (L) and a less prominent ER. Final magnification 12,000X.

the strict regulation of progesterone *(67)*. The role(s) played by retinoic acid as a regulator of endocrine factors that may be produced during decidualization is not clear at this time. Retinoic acid can regulate EGF receptors *(68)* and change cellular response to TGF-β *(69)*, but appears to decrease prolactin production by isolated stromal cells *(70)*. However complex, it is becoming increasingly clear that in addition to steroid support, a multitude of locally produced factors may act in concert or in opposition to steroids during the development and function of the decidua.

REGULATION OF INVASIVE PROCESSES BY THE DECIDUA

The degree of endometrial invasion that occurs during placentation is highly variable among species. In the human, establishment of the maternal-fetal relationship is a highly invasive event that occurs as a multi-step process requiring a coordinated effort between the blastocyst and endometrium. Initial attachment of the implanting embryo appears to be mediated by cellular adhesion molecules such as the integrins *(71)*. However, after breaching the surface epithelium, extra-villous trophoblasts invade the stromal matrix of the endometrium and eventually penetrate and fuse with the maternal vasculature. Matrix components produced by the decidua, such as fibronectin and laminin, may assist in guiding the embryo to the appropriate implantation site *(72)*, regulate cell motility during the invasive process *(73)*, and affect the expression of proteases *(74)*. Like tumor metastasis, invasion of the endometrium by the trophoblasts is accomplished via expression of proteases, such as matrix metalloproteinases (MMPs) *(14,75,76)*. Numerous MMPs have been found to be expressed by the invading blastocyst and/or maternal decidua, including members of the interstitial collagenase, gelatinase, and stromelysin subclasses *(77–79)*. Expression of these enzymes allows ECM degradation and the extensive tissue remodeling which is associated with placentation and implantation. Although it is clear that these enzymes are important for normal implantation, the mechanisms regulating their expression are not well understood.

Clinical conditions associated with impaired stromal cell decidualization are associated with more extensive trophoblast invasiveness *(80)*. Trophoblast invasion, which requires the expression of numerous MMPs, is more extensive at extra-uterine sites (i.e., kidney and spleen) and in the nondecidualized endometrium than in the decidualized endometrium *(81)*. Taken together, results of these studies indicate that the decidua plays an important role in controlling trophoblast invasion *(14)*. This position is further supported by studies in our laboratory that demonstrated that MMP-7, an enzyme associated with epithelial cells, is much more strongly expressed at the site of an ectopic pregnancy compared to a normal eutopic pregnancy *(21)*. During the normal menstrual cycle, increasing levels of ovarian progesterone and the associated increases in endometrial TGF-β during the secretory phase inhibits expression of several MMPs, including MMP-7 *(18,45,82–84)*. Increases in the production of TGF-β by the decidua *(47)* may control trophoblast function by limiting MMP-mediated tissue invasion. For example, Graham and Lala *(14)* have shown that production of TIMP-1, which binds and inactivates MMPs, is normally produced by decidual cells in response to TGF-β. Highly invasive, malignant trophoblasts are resistant to both TGF-β-mediated suppression of MMPs and induction of TIMP-1 *(85)*. Interestingly, isolated endometrial stromal cells, which are not responsive to TGF-β-mediated suppression of MMP-3, are responsive to retinoic acid (Fig. 3). These results suggest that retinoic acid, like TGF-β, may play an important role in inhibiting trophoblast invasion. Multiple products of the human decidua appear to act in concert with progesterone to regulate MMP expression in the endometrium during the establishment and maintenance of pregnancy.

SUMMARY

Both morphological and biochemical changes occur in specialized endometrial stromal cells in response to a complex array of hormones and cytokines as well as cellular disrup-

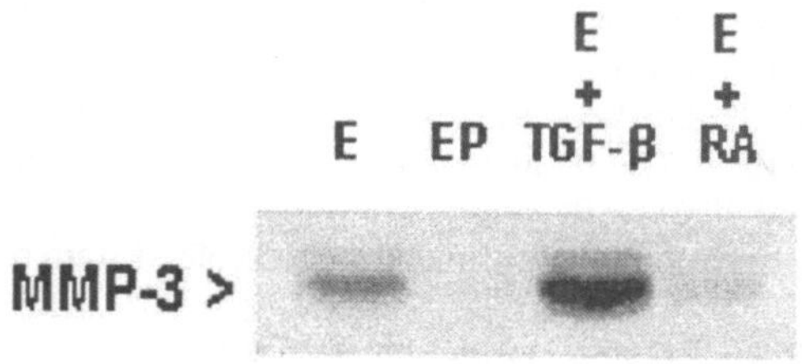

Fig. 3. Regulation of MMP-3 in isolated human endometrial stromal cells from proliferative phase of the cycle in the presence of steroids, transforming growth factor-β (TGF-β), or retinoic acid (RA). Cells were cultured under serum-free conditions in the presence of estradiol (10^{-8} *M*), E (10^{-9} *M*) plus progesterone (5×10^{-7} *M*), E (10^{-9} *M*) plus TGF-β (2ng/mL) or E (10^{-9} *M*) plus RA (10^{-6} *M*). During the final 18 h of culture, the cells were labeled with ^{35}S-methionine; secreted proteins were collected and immunoprecipitated with anti-MMP-3. The secretion of MMP-3 was suppressed by P and RA, whereas the presence of TGF-β in the culture resulted in upregulation of MMP-3.

tions that are associated with the establishment of pregnancy. Accompanying these dramatic stromal cell changes is the influx of hemopoietic cells and the development of an extensive vascular supply. Together these events lead to the formation of the decidua, a functionally and structurally unique endocrine tissue with many, but poorly defined, functions. A primary nutritional role for the decidua has been assumed for some time but it has also been suggested that the decidua prevents rejection of the fetal allograft and restricts trophoblast penetration of the endometrium in some species, especially the human. New techniques at the cellular and molecular level will enhance our ability to dissect the relative roles of steroids and growth factors in both endometrial differentiation and the process of decidualization. Clearly, both in vivo and in vitro studies will be needed to fully understand which factors, of embryonic or maternal origin, participate in the unique processes of decidualization.

REFERENCES

1. O'Rahilly R, Miller F (1987) Developmental stages in human embryos. Carnegie Institution of Washington, Publ. No. 637, Washington, D.C.
2. Lydon JP, DeMays FJ, Funk CR, Mani SK, Hughes AR, Montgomery CA, Gopala-Shymala, Connely OM, O'Malley BW (1995) Mice lacking progesterone receptor exhibit pleitropic reproductive abnormalities. Gene Develop 9:2266–2278.
3. Jannet D, Aflak N, Abankwa A, Carbonne B, Marpeau L, Milliez J (1996) Termination of 2nd and 3rd trimester pregnancies with mifepristone and misoprostol. Eur J Obstet Gynec Rep Biol 70: 159–163.
4. Loke YW, King A, Burrows D (1995) Decidua in human implantation. Hum Reprod (10 Suppl) 2:14–20.
5. Bulmer JN, Longfellow M, Ritson A (1991) Leukocytes and resident blood cells in endometrium. Ann NY Acad Sci 622:57–68.
6. Enders AC (1991) Current topic: structural responses of the primate endometrium to implantation. Placenta 12:309–325.
7. Parr MB, Parr EL (1990) The implantation reaction, In: Biology of the Uterus (Wynn RM, Jollie WP, eds.), Plenum, New York, pp. 233–278.
8. Riddick DH, Luciano AA, Kusmik WF, Moslar IA (1978) De novo synthesis of prolactin by human decidua. Life Sci 23:1913–1917.
9. Loke YW, King A (1995) Cytokines and their receptors during implantation, In: Human Implantation: Cell Biology and Immunology. Cambridge University Press, Cambridge, pp. 180–223.

10. Abrahamsohn PA (1989) Morphology of the decidua, In: Blastocyst Implantation (Yoshinaga K, ed.), Adams Publishing Group, Ltd., Serono Symposia USA.
11. Padykula HA, Coles LG, Okulicz WC, Rapaport SI, McCracken JA, King NW Jr., Longcope C, Kaiserman-Abramof IR (1989) The basalis of the primate endometrium: a bifunctional germinal compartment. Biol Reprod 40:681–690.
12. Padykula HA (1991) Regeneration in the primate uterus: role of stem cells. Ann NY Acad Sci 622: 47–56.
13. Noyes RA, Hertig AT, Rock J (1950) Dating the endometrial biopsy. Fertil Steril 1:3–25.
14. Graham CH, Lala PK (1992) Mechanisms of placental invasion of the uterus and their control. Biochem Cell Biol 70:867–874.
15. Lessey BA, Killam AP, Metzger DA, Haney AF, Greene GL, McCarty KD (1988) Immunohistochemical analysis of human uterine estrogen and progesterone receptors in the normal human uterus throughout the menstrual cycle. J Clin Endocrinol Metab 67:334–340.
16. Anderson TL, Gorstein F, Osteen KG (1990) Stromal-epithelial cell communication, growth factors and tissue regulation. Lab Invest 62:519–521.
17. Cunha GR, Young P (1992) Role of stroma in oestrogen induced epithelial proliferation. Cell Biol 1:18–31.
18. Osteen KG, Rodgers WH, Gaire M, Hargrove JT, Gorstein F, Matrisian LM (1994) Stromal-epithelial interaction mediates steroidal regulation of matrix metalloproteinases in the human endometrium. Proc Natl Acad Sci USA 91:10,129–10,133.
19. Tabibzadeh S (1991) The human endometrium: an active site of cytokine production and action. Endocrine Rev 1991; 12:272–290.
20. Giudice L (1997) Multi-faceted roles for IGFBP-I in human endometrium during implantation and pregnancy. Ann NY Acad Sci 828:146–156.
21. Osteen KG, Sierra-Rivera E, Keller NR, Fox DB (1997) Interleukin-1α opposes progesterone-mediated suppression of MMP-7: a possible role for this cytokine in human implantation. Ann NY Acad Sci 828:137–145.
22. Kennedy TG (1994) Involvement of local mediators in blastocyst implantation, In: Endocrinology of Embryo-Endometrial Interactions (Glasser SR, ed.), Plenum, New York, pp. 183–194.
23. Loke YW, King A (1995) Decidualisation, In: Human Implantation: cell Biology and Immunology. Cambridge University Press, Cambridge, pp. 18–31.
24. Yee GM, Kennedy TG (1991) Role of cyclic adenosine 3′5′monophosphate in mediating the effect of PGE2 on decidualization in vitro. Biol Reprod 45:163–171.
25. Acker GM, Braquet P, Mencia-Huerta JM (1988) Role of platelet-activating factor (PAF) in ovo-implantation and decidualization process in the rat. J Reprod Fertil Abstract Series 2:38.
26. Halhali A, Acker GM, Garabedian M (1991) 1,25-Dihydroxyvitamin D3 induces in vivo decidualization of rat endometrial cells. J Reprod Fertil 91:59–64.
27. Bani G, Maurizi, M, Bigazzi M, Bani Sacchi T (1995) Effect of relaxin on the endometrial stroma: studies in mice. Biol Reprod 52:253–262.
28. Nilsson CG, Luukkainen T, Arko H (1978) Endometrial morphology of women using a D-norgestrel-releasing intrauterine device. Fertil Steril 29:394–401.
29. Albert F, Teiltman A (1986) Endometrium in term extrauterine pregnancey. Human Pathol 17: 865–901.
30. Spornitz UM (1993) Pseudo-decidualization at the site of implantation in tubal pregnancy. Arch Obstet Gynecol 253:85–95.
31. Tseng L, Mazella J, Mann WJ, Chumas J (1982) Estrogen synthesis in normal and malignant human endometrium. J Clin Endocrinol Metab 55:1029–1031.
32. Chibbar R, Mitchell BF (1990) Steroid sulfohydrolase in human chorion and decidua: studies using pregnenolone sulfate and dehydroepiandrosterone sulfate as substrate. J Clin Endocrinol Metab 70:1693–1701.
33. Mitchell BF, Challis JR, Lukash L (1987) Progesterone synthesis by human amnion, chorion, and decidua at term. Amer J Ob Gyn 157:349–353.
34. Irwin JC, da las Fuentes L, Giudice LC (1994) Growth factors and decidualization in vitro. Ann NY Acad Sci 734:7–18.
35. Irwin JC, Utian WH, Eckert RL (1991) Sex steroids and growth factors differentially regulate the growth and differentiation of cultured human endometrial stromal cells. Endocrinology 129: 2385–2392.

36. Han VK, Basset N, Walton J, Challis JR (1996) The expression of insulin-like growth factor (IGF) and IGF-binding proteins (IGFBP) genes in the human placenta and membranes: evidence for IGF-IGFBP interactions at the feto-maternal interface. J Clin Endocrinol Metab 81:2680–2693.
37. Kanzaki H, Mori T (1995) Immunological regulation of endometrial function: cytokine production in the human endometrium, In: Molecular and Cellular Aspects of Peri-implantation Process (Dey SK, ed.), Springer, New York, pp. 288–300.
38. Barkai U, Kraicer PF (1996) Intauterine signaling and embryonic implantation. Biol Signals 5: 111–121.
39. Zhu HH, Huang JR, Mazella J, Elias J, Tseng L (1992) Progestin stimulates the biosynthesis and accumulation of mRNA of fibronectin in human endometrial stromal cells. Hum Rep 7:141–146.
40. Lane B, Oxberry W, Mazella J, Tseng L (1994) Decidualization of human endometrial stromal cells in vitro: effects of progestin and relaxin on the ultrastructure and production of decidual secretory proteins. Human Reprod 9:259–266.
41. Shah DM, Higuchi K, Inagami T, Osteen KG (1991) Effect of progesterone on renin secretion in endometrial stromal, chorionic trophoblast, and mesenchymal monolayer cultures. Am J Obstet Gyncol 164:1145–1150.
42. Graham CH, Lysiak JJ, McCrae KR, Lala PK (1992) Localization of transforming growth factor β (TGFβ) at the human fetomaternal interface: role on trophoblast growth and differentiation. Biol Reprod 46:561–572.
43. Lockwood CJ, Nemerson Y, Guller S, Krikun G, Alvarez M, Hausknecht V, Gurpide E, Schatz F (1993) Progestational regulation of human endometrial stromal cell tissue factor expression during decidualization. J Clin Endocrinol Metab 76:231–236.
44. Ace CI, Okulicz WC (1995) Differential gene regulation by estrogen and progesterone in the primate endometrium. Mol Cell Endocrinol 115:95–103.
45. Bruner KL, Rodgers WH, Korc M, Gold LI, Hargrove JT, Matrisian LM, Osteen KG (1995) Transforming growth factor-β mediates progesterone suppression of an epithelial metalloproteinase by adjacent stroma in human endometrium. Proc Natl Acad Sci USA 92:7362–7366.
46. Okulicz WC, Ace CI, Longcope C, Tast J (1996) Analysis of differential gene regulation in adequate versus inadequate secretory-phase endometrial cDNA populations from the rhesus monkey. Endocrinology 137:4844–4850.
47. Kauma S, Matt D, Stephen S, Eierman D, Turner T (1990) IL-1b, human leukocyte antigen HLA-Dra and TGF-β expression in endometrium, placenta and placental membranes. Am J Obstet Gynecol 163:1430–1437.
48. Osteen KG, Hargrove JT, Gorstein F (1992) Transforming growth factor-β enhances progestin-induced in vitro decidualization of human endometrial stroma. (Abstr) Biol Reprod 46 (Suppl 1):140.
49. Border WA, Rouslahti E (1992) Transforming growth factor-β in disease: the dark side of tissue repair. J Clin Invest 90:1–7.
50. Clark DA, Falbo M, Rowley RB, Banwatt D, Stedronka-Clark J (1988) Active suppression of host-vs graft reaction in pregnant mice. J Immunol 141:3833–3840.
51. Altman DJ, Schneider SL, Thompson DA, Cheng H, Tomasi TB (1990) A transforming growth factor-β2 (TGF-β2)-like immunosuppressive factor in amniotic fluid and localization of TGF-β2 mRNA in the pregnant uterus. J Exp Med 172:1391–1401.
52. Merali FS, Arck PC, Beaman K, Clark DA (1996) Transforming growth factor-β2-related decidual suppressor factor is not related to TJ6 protein. Am J Reprod Immunol 35:342–347.
53. Clark, DA (1992) Animal models of recurrent pregnancy loss, In: Immunological Obstetrics (Coulam CB, Farek WB, McIntyre JA, eds.), Norton, New York, pp. 428–436.
54. Healy DL (1984) The clinical significance of endometrial prolactin. Austral New Zeal J Obstet Gynecol 24:111–116.
55. Soares MJ, Faria TN, Roby KF, Deb S (1991) Pregnancy and the prolactin family of hormones: coordination of anterior pituitary, uterine and placental expression. Endocrine Rev 12:402–423.
56. Leontic EA, Tyson JE (1977) Prolactin and fetal osmoregulation: water transport across isolated human amnion. Am J Physiol 232:R124.
57. Healy D, Hodgen G (1983) The endocrinology of the human endometrium. Obstet Gynecol Survey 38:509–530.
58. Saji M, Taga M, Minaguchi H (1990) Epidermal growth factor stimulate cell proliferation and inhibits prolactin secretion of the human decidual cells in culture [Japanese]. Endocrinologia Japonica 37:177–182.

59. Tang XM, Zhao Y, Rossi MJ, Abu-Rustum RS, Ksander GA, Chegini N (1994) Expression of transforming growth factor-β (TGF-β) isoforms and TGF-β type II receptor messenger ribonucleic acid and protein, and the effect of TGF-βs on endometrial stromal cell growth and protein degradation in vitro. Endocrinology 135:450–459.
60. Vicovac LM, Starkey PM, Alpin JD (1994) Comment: effect of cytokines on prolactin production by human decidual stromal cells in culture: studies using cells freed of bone marrow-derived contaminants. J Clin Endocrinol Metab 79:1877–1882.
61. Sawai K, Matsuzaki N, Okada T, Shimoya K, Koyama M, Azuma C, Saji F, Murata Y (1997) Human decidual cell biosynthesis of leukemia inhibitory factor: regulation by decidual cytokines and steroid hormones. Biol Reprod 56:1274–1280.
62. Kubota T, Taguchi M, Kobayashi K, Masuda M, Aso T (1997) Relationship between the release of prolactin and endothelin-1 in human decidualized endometrial cells. Eur J Endocrinol 137:200–204.
63. Wolbach SB, Howe PR (1925) Tissue changes following deprivation of fat-soluble vitamin A in the rat. J Exp Med 43:753–777.
64. Loughney AD, Kumarendran MD, Thomas EJ, Redfern CPF (1995) Variation in the expression of cellular retinoid binding proteins in human endometrium throughout the menstrual cycle. Hum Reprod 10:1297–1304.
65. Loughney AP, Redfern CPF (1995) Menstrual cycle related differences in the proliferative response of cultured human endometrial stromal cells to retinoic acid. J Reprod Fertil 105:153–159.
66. Fazleabas AT, Hild-Petito S, Verhage HG (1994) Secretory peptides and growth factors of the baboon (Papio anubis) uterus: potential roles in pregnancy. Cell Biol International 18:1145–1153.
67. Sierra-Rivera E, Zheng WL, Bucco RA, Ong DE, Osteen KG (1997) Local synthesis of retinoic acid by normal human endometrial cells may regulate MMP-3 and MMP-7 expression. (Abstr) Am Assoc Cancer Res, April, 1997.
68. Roulier S, Rochette-Egly C, Rebut-Bonneton C, Porquet D, Evain-Brion D (1994) Nuclear retinoic acid receptor characterization in cultured human trophoblast cells: effect of retinoic acid on EGF receptor expression. Mol Cell Endocrinol 105:165–173.
69. Giguere V (1994) Retinoic acid receptors and cellular retinoid binding proteins: complex interplay in retinoid signalling. Endocrine Rev 15:61–97.
70. Brar AK, Kessler CA, Meyer AJ, Cedars MI, Jikihara H (1996) Retinoic acid suppresses in vitro decidualization of human endometrial stromal cells. Mol Hum Reprod 2:185–193.
71. Moore KL (1988) The developing human. W.B. Saunders, Philadelphia, pp. 33–38.
72. Edwards RG (1995) Physiological and molecular aspects of human implantation. Hum Reprod 10 Suppl 2:1–13.
73. Damsky CH, Librach C, Lim KH, Fitzgerald ML, McMaster MT, Janatpour M, Zhou Y, Logan SK, Fisher SJ (1994) Integrin switching regulates normal trophoblast invasion. Development 120: 3657–3666.
74. Bischof P, Martelli M, Campana A (1994) The regulation of endometrial and trophoblastic metalloproteinases during blastocyst implantation [French]. Contraception Fertilite Sexualite 22:48–52.
75. Ray JM, Stetler-Stevenson WG (1994) The role of matrix metalloproteases and their inhibitors in tumor invasion, metastasis and angiogenesis. Eur Resp J 7:2062–2072.
76. Librach CL, Werb Z, Fitzgerald ML, Chui K, Corwin NM, Esteves RA, Grobelny D, Galardy R, Damsky CH, Fisher SJ (1991) 92 kDa type-IV collagenase mediates invasion of human cytotrophoblasts. J Cell Biol 113:437–449.
77. Vettraino IM, Roby J, Tolley T, Parks WC (1996) Collagenase-I, stromelysin-I and matrilysin are expressed within the placenta during multiple stages of human pregnancy. Placenta 17:557–563.
78. Polette M, Nawrocki B, Pintiaux A, Massenat C, Maquoi E, Volders L, Schaaps JP, Birembaut P, Foidart JM (1994) Expression of gelatinases A and B and their tissue inhibitors by cells of early and term human placenta and gestational endometrium. Lab Invest 71:838–846.
79. Maquoi E, Polette M, Nawrocki B, Bischof P, Noel A, Pintiax A, Santavicca M, Schaaps JP, Pijnenborg R, Birembaut P, Foidart JM (1997) Expression of stromelysin-3 in the human placenta and placental bed. Placenta 18:277–285.
80. Billington WD (1971) Biology of the trophoblast. Adv Reprod Physiol 5:39–42.
81. Kirby DRS (1967) The "invasiveness" of the trophoblast, In: The early conceptus: normal and abnormal (Park WW, ed.), University of St Andrews Press, Edinburgh, pp. 68–74.
82. Rodgers WH, Osteen KG, Matrisian LM, Navre M, Gorstein F (1993) Expression and localization of matrilysin (Pump-1, MMP-7) a matrix metalloproteinase in the human endometrium. Am J Obstet Gynecol 168:253–260.

83. Rodgers WH, Matrisian LM, Giudice LC, Dsupin B, Cannon P, Svitek C, Gorstein F, Osteen KG (1994) Patterns of matrix metalloproteinase expression in cycling endometrium imply differential functions and regulation by steroids. J Clin Invest 94:946–953.
84. Schatz F, Papp C, Toth-Pal E, Lackwood CJ (1994) Ovarian steroid-modulated stromelysin-1 expression in human endometrial stromal and decidual cells. J Clin Endocrinol Metab 78: 1467–1472.
85. Graham CH, Connelly I, MacDougal JR, Kerbel RS, Stetler-Stevenson WG, Lala PK (1994) Resistance of malignant trophoblast cells to both the anti-proliferative and anti-invasive effects of transforming growth factor-β. Exp Cell Res 214:93–97.

20 Endocrine Regulation of Maternal Behavior Postpartum

Gary L. Williams, PHD

Contents

INTRODUCTION

Mammalian maternal behavior is one of the most complex, highly integrated, and essential behaviors observed in nature. Clearly, maternal care and the maternal-offspring bond represent the true final measures of reproductive success. Without this behavior, the mammalian neonate could not survive under natural conditions and the evolution of mammalian species would not have been possible. During the last two decades, investigations to determine the physiological basis of maternal behavior have placed the endocrine system at the core of many of the processes governing its development and maintenance. To a large degree, these investigations have been conducted with rodents and sheep. Hence, the information in this review will focus primarily on what has been learned in these species.

BEHAVIORAL ELEMENTS OF MATERNAL CARE

What is Maternal Behavior?

At parturition, a dramatic behavioral transformation occurs in all female mammals that is characterized by a change from total disregard of, or even aggressiveness toward, a neonate before parturition to one of intense interest immediately after parturition. This is followed by a highly motivated sequence of proceptive or "maternal" activities, including smelling, licking, vocalization, and a desire for close and sustained interaction *(1–3)*. Eventually, this behavior culminates in the dam allowing the offspring to suckle, in the exhibition of protective acts against intruders, and in the development of selectivity. Proceptive behaviors actually begin prepartum in some species, and include activities such as nest building and increased interest toward neonates. In litter-bearing animals, pup-searching and retrieval are elements of maternal care, and this behavior can be induced to some

Table 1
Endocrine Support of Maternal Behavior in Mammals

Hormone	*Effects*	*Timing*	*Mechanisms*
Estradiol	CNS priming, proception	Prepartum	↑OT gene promoter activity, ↑OT receptor affinity
Progesterone	CNS priming, proception	Prepartum	↑OT receptor number
Glucocorticoids	CNS priming	Prepartum	Facilitate P4 Effects??
Lactogens	CNS priming, proception	Prepartum	Unknown
Oxytocin	Acute proceptive arousal	Parturition; Sensitive period	Anxiolytic; ↓aggression
Opiates	Intensifies OT effects (sheep)	Parturition	Anxiolytic; Facilitate OT effects

Lactogens are prolactin (PRL) and placental lactogens (PL); Opiates are β-endorphin, metenkephalin, and dynorphins; OT, oxytocin; P4, progesterone.

degree in rodents by chronic exposure of nonparturient adults, including males, to neonates *(4–6)*. This has been termed "concaveation," and adult reactions appear to be in response to ultrasonic vocalization by pups *(7,8)*. The response can be markedly enhanced by pretreatment of test animals with estrogen *(8)*. Limited elements of maternal behavior unrelated to pregnancy or parturition have also been observed in other species, including sheep and goats, in which a heightened interest in neonates is observed during estrus *(9)*. Indeed, there are a number of hormonal, tactile, olfactory, visual, and cognitive functions that contribute to the full development of maternal behavior. Although the endocrine system is not absolutely essential for the development and maintenance of maternal behavior *(1)*, the rapid onset and expression of the full repertoire of maternal care following parturition are clearly dependent upon endocrine support (Table 1).

PHYSIOLOGICAL BASIS OF MATERNAL BEHAVIOR

Sensory and Hormonal Control Systems

Hormonal Steroids. The onset of maternal behavior is associated with increases in circulating concentrations of both progestogens and estrogens during late pregnancy *(9,10)*. In nature, a commonly-observed example of this behavior is the near-term female attempting to claim or "mother" a new-born neonate belonging to a herdmate. Experimentally, a degree of maternal behavior has been induced in up to 50% of nonlactating ewes with previous maternal experience using injections of estradiol and progesterone, either alone or in combination. Estradiol alone was more potent than progesterone alone *(9)*; however, estradiol treatment either concurrently with or following progesterone exposure resulted in the greatest maternal behavior response in sheep *(9)* and rats *(11)*. These responses occur within hours of treatment and are independent of lactation. The effects of estrogen are dependent in part upon maternal experience, as primigravid and primiparous ewes responded poorly to estrogen stimulation compared to the response obtained with more experienced, pluriparous females *(12)*. Similarly, in female rats the expression of estrogen-induced, short-latency maternal behavior requires a much higher dose of

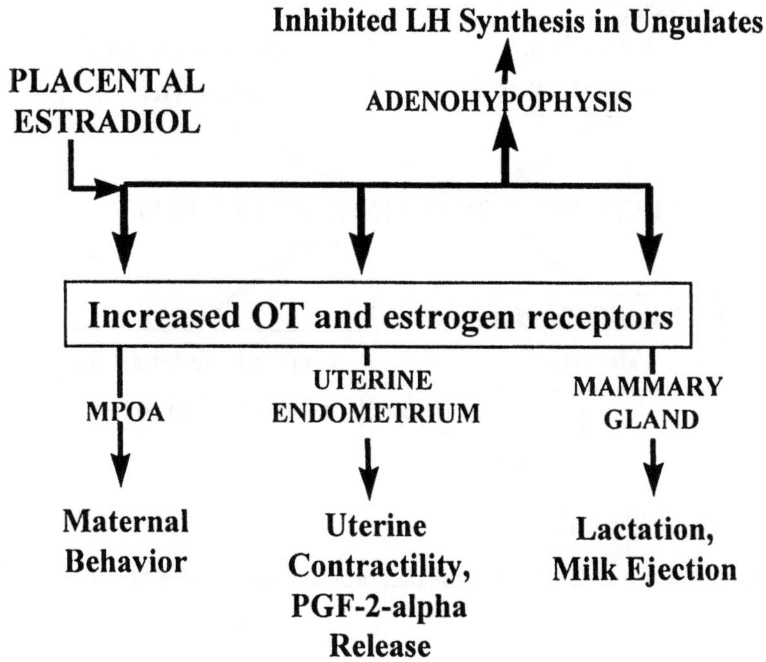

Fig. 1. Multi-targeted effects of placental-derived estradiol during late gestation. With the exception of effects on the anterior pituitary (adenohypophysis) in ungulates, many of the effects of estradiol are mediated by modulation of the oxytocin receptor.

estrogen in nonpregnant than in pregnant females hysterectomized on d 16 of pregnancy *(13,14)*. In addition to their role in maternal behavior, placental-derived estrogens simultaneously modulate several other aspects of peripartum and puerperal reproduction at a number of target sites. These effects vary somewhat among species, but collectively include effects on the uterus (fetal delivery), mammary gland (lactation), and adenohypophysis (reduced LH synthesis in ungulates). Coincident, multitargeted effects of estradiol demonstrate the wide influence that estrogens and the estrogen receptor have on reproductive biology, including maternal behavior. Many of these effects are subsequently mediated through the neuropeptide, oxytocin (Fig. 1).

Role of Estradiol in Establishment of the Sensitive Period. A host of studies has shown that estradiol acts as an essential primer for the induction of maternal behavior and the establishment of a specific bond by other hormonal and sensory stimuli *(9–14)*. The initiation and maintenance of the so-called "sensitive period" for the establishment of these behaviors around the time of parturition has received extensive attention. The sensitive period is defined as the period during which a new maternal bond can be formed, and may last up to 6 or more hours *(1–3,15)*. However, the minimum time required for a female to form a specific bond with a neonate with full recognition at later times may be as little as a few minutes *(2)*. A lengthening of the sensitive period can be accomplished in ewes by treating them with estradiol benzoate before parturition *(16)*, which increases synthesis and release of central oxytocin. As discussed later in this chapter, intracerebral oxytocin plays an integral role in the induction of maternal behavior.

Genital Stimulation and Central Oxytocin Release. Genital stimulation, particularly vaginal, uterine, and cervical distension, facilitates maternal behavior *(9,17–19)*. However, these stimuli are only effective if the animal has been primed naturally or experimentally with estradiol *(20)* and is most critical in the primigravid female. The action of

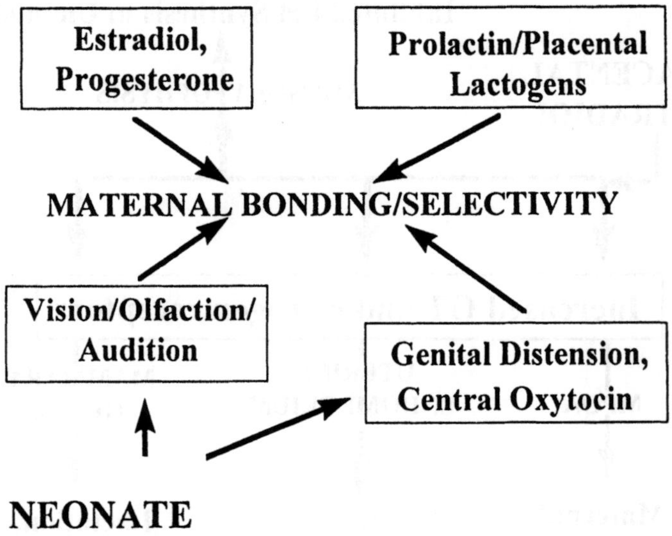

Fig. 2. Hormonal, genital, and sensory factors that promote maternal behavior in female mammals.

genital stimulation appears to be mediated through central oxytocin release. Although neurohypophyseal release of oxytocin into the peripheral circulation often occurs coincident with central release, peripheral circulating oxytocin does not cross the blood-brain barrier *(21–23)*. However, oxytocin is clearly liberated within the brain, with a dense network of non-pituitary projections arising from small cells in the paraventricular nucleus (PVN) and extending into the limbic system and brainstem *(24)*. In sheep, concentrations of oxytocin increase in cerebrospinal fluid collected through the lateral ventricles at parturition and following genital stimulation *(21–23)*, and oxytocin receptors are found throughout the central nervous system *(25)*. Epidural anesthesia blocks the release of oxytocin and attenuates development of maternal behavior in sheep *(20,26)*, and intracerebroventricular infusions of oxytocin stimulate the expression of maternal behavior *(23)*. In rats, the response to central administration of oxytocin is dependent upon the amount of time females are habituated to the maternal observation cages prior to pup presentation. Thus, in rats, estrogen and oxytocin can only induce maternal behavior if cage novelty is of appropriate duration (approx 2 h) to permit the response *(27)*. A sequence of estrogen priming, genital stimulation (oxytocinergic effect) and olfaction serve as powerful signals for the full establishment of maternal behavioral responses in sheep, rats, and other species *(1,12,15,16,20–23,25*; Fig. 2).

The temporal sequence of events through which sensory and hormonal factors influence maternal behavior also appear to differ markedly among species. In both rats *(28)* and cattle *(29)*, hormonal signals present before the onset of parturition make lasting contributions to the development of maternal behavior, and the creation of pelvic sensory deficits using epidural anesthesia immediately before and during parturition fail to prevent its establishment. However, similar to observations in sheep, central infusion of oxytocin into the cerebroventricles of the estrogen-primed rat rapidly stimulates maternal behavior *(30)*.

Interaction of Hormonal Steroids and Extrahypothalamic Oxytocin Neurons in the Brain. *Ewe Model.* The medial preoptic area (MPOA) is a major site of action for estrogen-mediated effects on maternal behavior, and lesions of the MPOA prevent maternal behavior *(31,32)*. Estradiol implanted directly into the MPOA is as effective as parenteral administration in stimulating maternal behavior in rats, and immunocytochemical studies indicate an increase in both immunoreactive oxytocin *(33)* and oxytocin mRNA *(32)*. Indeed, late pregnant females and estrogen-treated, hysterectomized females exhibit high levels of cytosolic estrogen receptors in the POA that correlate with induced maternal behavior. Caldwell and coworkers *(32,33)* have provided evidence of differential roles for progesterone, estrogen, and the corticosteroids in the MPOA in relation to oxytocin's effect on sexual behavior in rodents. Estrogens increase oxytocin receptor affinity in the MPOA, whereas progesterone may alter oxytocin release patterns by acting at the level of the neuronal membrane and increasing oxytocin receptor density. Glucocorticoids, on the other hand, may act permissively to facilitate the action of progesterone on sexual receptivity. Behaviorists suggest a close association between the "satisfaction" of sexual arousal and that related to the mother-infant bond, and both are probably related to increased production and release of endogenous opioid peptides. Therefore, it is possible that the interactions of ovarian steroids in modulating oxytocin synthesis, secretion, and action are closely associated to those that control maternal behavior as well. Indeed, the endogenous opioid peptides increase in the brain at parturition, and facilitate vaginocervical stimulation-mediated maternal behavior in ewes *(12)*. While genital stimulation and intracerebroventricular infusion of oxytocin have both been shown to induce marked proceptive behavior in the steroid-primed ewe, neither are able to reproduce the intensity of maternal behavior and bonding that occurs naturally. However, if ewes are treated simultaneously with opiates *(12)*, the resulting behavior is purported to have the quality and intensity of that observed postpartum.

Rat Model. In direct contradiction to the above findings are data in the rat indicating that the opiates serve as internal brakes to prevent maternal behavior until after parturition *(1,34)*. Both systemic and central administration of morphine into rats suppresses central oxytocin release and disrupts maternal behavior. This effect is reversed by concurrent naloxone treatment *(35)*. During late pregnancy and following estradiol treatment, concentrations of β-endorphins increase in hypothalamus, midbrain, and amygdala of the rat, and fall during the first 2 wk postpartum *(36)*. Hence, there is an inverse relationship between brain levels of endogenous opioids and maternal behavior in the rat.

Localization, Activity, and Control of Oxytocin-Containing Neurons and Oxytocin Receptors in the Central Nervous System. *Synthesis and Release of Oxytocin.* Oxytocin neurons and receptors have been identified in virtually every part of the brain in which maternal behavior is thought to be controlled. A variety of techniques have been employed in sheep by Kendrick and coworkers *(37)* to establish the location, secretory activity, and control of oxytocin-containing neurons in the ewe. Using immunocytochemistry and *in situ* hybridization, cells and fibers containing immunoreactive hormone and/or mRNA have been observed in the paraventricular nucleus (PVN) of the hypothalamus, MPOA, and within the bed nucleus of the stria terminalis (BNST). Oxytocin immunoreactivity increases in all of the foregoing at parturition *(37)*, as well as in the CSF *(21–23,29)*.

Gene Structure for Oxytocin. Genes for oxytocin and the related peptide, vasopressin, are located on the same chromosomal locus, in opposite transcriptional orientations, and are separated by different lengths of intergenic sequences, depending on species (*38*; Fig. 3). It has been noted that the first 2–300 bases in the 5′ upstream promoter region of both the oxytocin and vasopressin genes are highly conserved among the species studied. However, the same region shows very low sequence homology between the two peptides *(39)*.

The Oxytocin Receptor in CNS. Pedersen and coworkers *(30)* reported increased oxytocin binding at parturition in the amygdala, MPOA, and ventral tegmental area and substantia nigra of the rat. In other studies, the highest densities of high affinity oxytocin

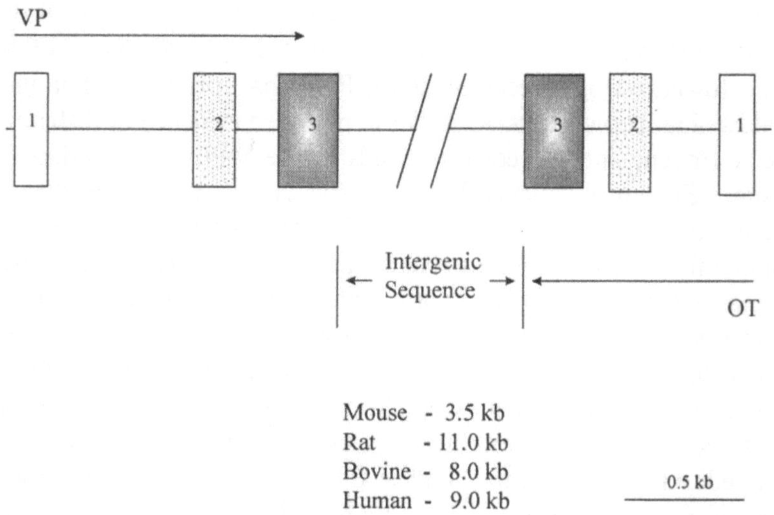

Fig. 3. Diagram of vasopressin (VP) and oxytocin (OT) gene structures illustrating their three exons (boxes 1, 2, and 3) and two introns present on the same chromosome locus in opposite transcriptional directions (arrows). Similar gene structures but with variable lengths of intergenic sequences have been found in four mammalian species (Adapted from ref. *38* with permission).

receptors in the rat were found in the anterior olfactory nucleus, the islands of calleja and other cell groups of the olfactory tubercle belonging to the ventral pallidum, the hypothalamic ventromedial nucleus, amygdala, and the ventral subiculum and BNST *(24,40)*. The affinity and ligand specificity of the brain oxytocin receptor does not appear to differ from that found in the uterus, mammary gland, or fat cells. Peripheral oxytocin receptors are functionally coupled to a phosphoinositidase/protein kinase C signal transduction system, and the latter has been exploited as a means of monitoring oxytocin-receptor activity in uterus *(41)* of sheep and other animals. However, it is not known whether brain oxytocin receptors operate similarly. Mapping studies in other species, such as the guinea pig, hamster, rabbit, marmoset, and human, have revealed enigmas related to differential distributions of oxytocin binding sites *(40)*. Moreover, it is not known whether these binding sites represent true high affinity receptors in all cases, since most of the studies utilized simple autoradiography. Neuronal recordings in rats and guinea pigs indicate that oxytocin binding sites correlate well with differences in neuronal sensitivity to oxytocin, providing evidence that these sites are indeed functional receptors. Recently, Adan and coworkers *(42)* determined the partial sequence and immunocytochemical localization of the rat oxytocin receptor in brain, pituitary, mammary gland and uterus. Results demonstrated that the same receptor type is expressed in both peripheral oxytocin target tissues and the brain, and suggested the possibility that a different oxytocin subtype may be present in some areas of the brain. Table 2 summarizes the distribution and relative intensities of oxytocin binding sites in the adult and infant rat brain based on autoradiographic analyses *(40)*.

Lactogenic Hormones. Perhaps the earliest experimental observations on the association of the endocrine system to maternal behavior were made by Riddle et al. *(43)*, who suggested a role for prolactin in maternal behavior induction. A period of controversy then followed as an increasing number of experiments either supported or failed to support a role for this hormone in maternal behavior *(1)*. However, in recent years there has been a renewed interest in the lactogenic hormone gene family, which includes prolactin

Table 2
Distribution and Relative Densities of OT-Binding Sites in the Adult (PN90) and the Infant (PN10) Rat Brain[a]
(Adapted from ref. *40* with permission)

	Adult	*Infant*
Cortical Areas		
Dorsal peduncular cortex	3	2
Insular cortex	1	1
Perirhinal cortex	1	1
Cingulate cortex	0	4
Retrosplenial cortex	0	4
Olfactory System		
Anteroventral olfactory nucleus	2	2
Basal Ganglia		
Caudoputamen	1	3
Islands of Calleja	4	0
Ventral pallidum cell groups	4	0
Hypothalamus		
Ventromedial nucleus	4	0
Medial tuberal nucleus	2	2
Supramammillary nucleus	1	1
Lateral mammillary nucleus	1	3
Medial mammillary nucleus	0	3
Limbic System		
Bed nucleus of the stria terminalis	3	2
Lateral septal nucleus, intermediate	1	1
Central amygdaloid nucleus	3	2
Medial amygdaloid nucleus	1	1
Basolateral amygdaloid nucleus	1	1
Dorsal subiculum	1	4
Ventral subiculum	4	1
CA1	1	1
Amygdalohippocampal area	1	1
Parasubiculum	2	2
Presibiculum	2	2
Thalamus		
Anteroventral thalamic nucleus	0	1
Periventricular thalamic nucleus	1	2
Brainstem		
Dorsal motor nucleus of the vagus nerve	1	1
Inferior olive	1	1
Substantia gelatinosa of the trigeminal nucleus	1	4
Spinal Cord		
Substantia gelatinosa	1	4

[a] Just detectable (1) to highest density observed (4). No binding, (0). PN90, postnatal d 90.

(PRL) and the placental lactogens (PL), as modulators of maternal behavior. Recent findings using hypophysectomized female rats indicate the PRL and PL-like molecules play major roles in stimulating the onset of maternal behavior, particularly in rodents *(44)*. Effects of PRL and rat PL (rPL) occur rapidly, are dependent upon prior exposure to progesterone concurrently with estrogen exposure, and act at the level of the MPOA.

Other nonlactogenic protein hormones do not share these properties *(11)*. Rat PRL and rPL exhibit essentially equal potencies relative to their effects on maternal behavior once reaching the brain. Bridges et al. *(11,45)* suggest that PRL and rPL prime the maternal brain over a prolonged period of time during pregnancy, and this priming appears to complement the more acute regulatory actions of the neuropeptides, oxytocin and β-endorphin. Moreover, rPL-I and rPL-II are the predominant lactogens present in the cerebrospinal fluid during the second half of gestation *(11,45)*, and transport of these molecules across the blood-brain barrier exceeds that of PRL at this time. Hence, rPL's would seem to be of greater import than PRL during this critical period because of their ability to reach the brain itself. One mode of action through which the lactogens may affect behavior is through their effects on dopamine turnover and the dopamine D_2 receptor *(46)*. Within the cell, PRL and PL's have been hypothesized to influence nurturing through either the JAK-STAT (Janus kinase-signal transducer and activator of transcription) pathway *(47)* or directly at the FosB gene *(48)*.

Vision, Olfaction, and Audition

That olfaction plays an important role in maternal behavior has been known by practical husbandmen for centuries, and the fostering of orphaned offspring to unrelated dams by transferring odors from own to unrelated offspring is a well-documented fostering technique *(49)*. Although sensory perception plays a prominent role in the establishment of maternal behavior and the maternal bond, there is a paucity of information relating these phenomena to the endocrine system. However, we would be remiss if we did not accentuate the importance of these systems in the total integration of the maternal behavior response and their interaction with hormone-dependent pathways. Moreover, as will be discussed later, there now appear to be several neurotransmitters in the brain, such as glutamate and γ-aminobutyric acid (GABA), that are involved in pathways common to both neuroendocrine and non-endocrine neural systems via nitric oxide.

Vision and Olfaction During the Sensitive Period. Sensory information from the neonate is critical for development of maternal behavior in the sheep model, and olfactory cue deprivation during the sensitive period disturbs maternal acceptance in this species *(9,50–53)*. Vision has been said to play a minor role in development of a maternal bond in many species *(3)*; however, in domestic cattle, vision is used effectively to identify own offspring after a bond has been formed *(54)*. In the rat, olfactory deficits actually facilitate maternal behavior during the early peurperium, apparently by eliminating aversive olfactory stimuli from the pups *(1)*. Moreover, in rats elimination of vision or audition failed to eliminate maternal behavior, and losses of one sense are clearly compensated for by increased utilization of the remaining sense(s). In postparturient ewes, development of a selective maternal bond requires only about 2 h *(9)*. The minimum time required for sensitization may be as little as 5 min in cattle, with the period of receptivity lasting for up to 5 h in the absence of the calf *(55)*. Interestingly, ablation of olfactory bulbs or peripherally-induced anosmia during gestation in ewes leads to the absence of selectivity during lactation *(53)*, but does not impede maternal responsiveness per se. These ewes allow any lamb to suckle. Hence olfaction is not essential for maternal responsiveness in sheep, but is essential for development of an exclusive mother–infant bond. In parturient ewes, amniotic fluid is repulsive to ewes, whereas following appropriate hormonal priming, amniotic fluid is highly attractive to them *(15)*. In pluriparous cows, anosmia during parturition and for up to 2 h postpartum attenuated proceptive behavior. Calves were removed and returned 12 h later, at which time all cows exhibited normal maternal behavior and acceptance of

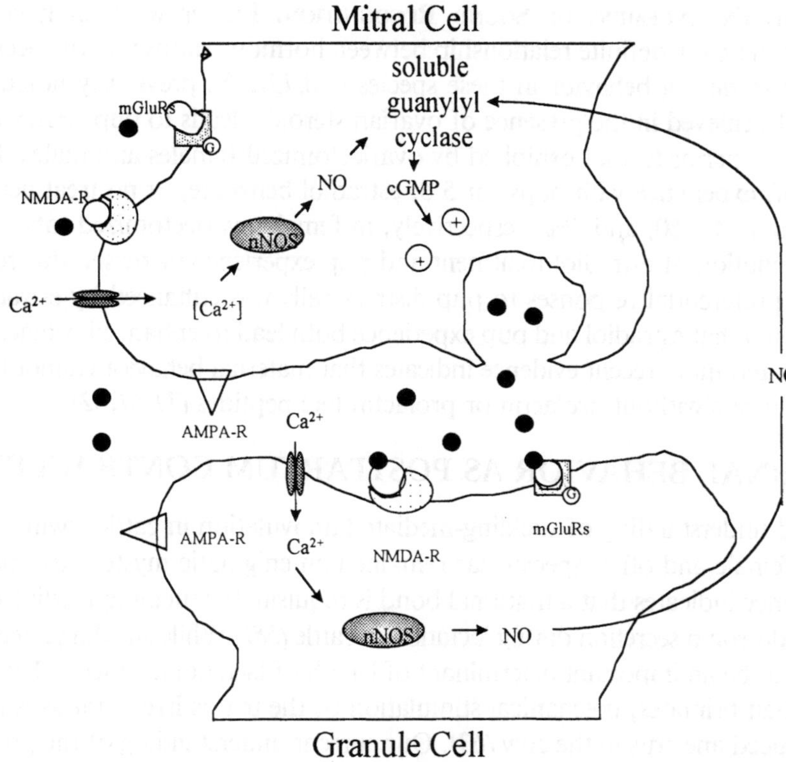

Fig. 4. Organization of mitral and granule cell activity in the olfactory bulb of sheep during formation of olfactory memory as presented by Kendrick and coworkers *(60)*. Diagram shows the proposed interactions between glutamate receptors and the NO/cyclic GMP pathway at the mitral-to-granule cell synapses during memory formation (AmPA-R = (2-aminomethyl)-phenylacetic acid) receptors); G, G protein; mGluRs, metabotropic glutamine receptors; NMDA-R, *N*-methyl-D-aspartate (Adapted from ref. *60* with permission).

the calf at the udder (GL Williams, unpublished observations). Ewes rendered anosmic after a selective bond has formed can recognize their own lamb visually, but will not allow it or any other lamb to suckle *(53)*, but this model has not been duplicated in other animals. Cows rendered anosmic after maternal bonding recognized their calves visually and allowed them to suckle *(54)*. This was accompanied by continued suppression of LH secretion, a hallmark of the maternal-offspring bond in cattle during early lactation *(56–59)*.

Olfactory Memory and Nitric Oxide. In 1997, Kendrick and coworkers *(60)* reported that the recognition of lamb odor by ewes involves synaptic changes in the olfactory bulb, with mitral cells becoming increasingly responsive to learned odor. Synaptic transmission between excitatory mitral cells and inhibitory granule cells is mediated via glutamate and GABA, and nitric oxide synthase (nNOS) is expressed in both mitral and granule cells. However, guanylyl cyclase subunits that are required for NO stimulation of cGMP formation are expressed only in mitral cells. Immediately after birth, glutamate levels rise, induce formation of NO and cGMP, and this potentiates glutamate release at the mitral-to-granule cell synapses (Fig. 4). If this system is attenuated via inhibition of nNOS or guanylyl cyclase activity, olfactory memory is prevented. Effects of nNOS inhibition can be reversed by infusion of NO into the olfactory bulb. Although NO acts indirectly to influence memory formation through increased sensitivity of mitral-to-granule cell synapses to glutamate, it does not appear to be required for memory recall or odor perception per se *(60)*.

Hormonal Enhancement of Sound Recognition. Earlier work in mice and rats revealed that there is a definite relationship between hormone status and the occurrence of parental pup-retrieving behavior in these species *(1,8,13)*. As previously noted, parental experience, if achieved in the presence of ovarian steroids, leads to pup-retrieving performance that is superior to that exhibited by ovariectomized females and males. Individual treatments of: experience with pups for 5 d; estradiol benzoate; or no treatment induced pup-retrieving in 40, 60, and 0%, respectively, in female ovariectomized rats.

The combination of estradiol treatment and pup experience increased this response to 90.5%, and preferential responses to pup distress calls was enhanced by estradiol *(8)*. It should be noted that estradiol and pup experience both lead to enhanced prolactin release, and previous and more recent evidence indicates that maternal behavior cannot be induced by estrogen in rats without prolactin or prolactin-like peptides *(11,61,62)*.

MATERNAL BEHAVIOR AS POSTPARTUM CONTRACEPTIVE

A detailed understanding of suckling-mediated anovulation in cattle, swine, monkeys, the human female and other species has remained an enigmatic mystery for many years. Recent evidence indicates that a maternal bond is requisite for suckling-mediated suppression of gonadotropin secretion during lactation in cattle *(58)*. While suckling intensity of the teat appears to be an important determinant of length of lactational amenorrhea in human and nonhuman primates, mechanical stimulation of the teat is irrelevant as it pertains to suckling-induced anestrus in the cow *(63)*. Our current understanding of the phenomenon of suckling-mediated inhibition of LH secretion in this species involves a complex array of sensory, behavioral, and spatial interactions between dam and neonate. These factors are physiologically related to those necessary for the expression of maternal behavior and selectivity *(54,56–59)*.

A Maternal Bond is Required for Suckling-Mediated Anovulation in Cattle

As discussed previously, both central oxytocin and the opioid peptides act synergistically to facilitate the onset and maintenance of maternal responsiveness in sheep. Although it has been known for some time that peripherally-released oxytocin is not involved in the induction of maternal behavior or inhibition of gonadotropin secretion *(64)*, we now have limited experimental evidence suggesting that intracerebral oxytocin release may attenuate LH secretion *(65)*. Moreover, there is clear evidence for an inverse association between factors that facilitate maternal behavior and those that negatively modulate gonadotropin secretion in cattle *(56,57,59)*. Enhanced opioid tone within the brain is a feature of both maternal behavior and suckling-induced anestrus. Messenger RNA levels of pro-enkephalin in the paraventricular nucleus, BNST, and the MPOA are correspondingly increased in sheep *(37)*, and Leshin et al. *(66)* has shown that the distribution of the generic precursor of the β-endorphins, pro-opiomelanocortin (POMC), are found in the same neuroendocrine locations in cattle. All of these anatomical sites have been implicated in the integration of maternal behavior. Moreover, both POMC and GnRH fibers are closely intermingled at the portal capillaries and in the POA, and an increase in oxytocin mRNA is observed in the POA during lactation *(67)*. Hence, we have hypothesized that enforced suckling in the absence of a maternal bond is unable to maintain an inhibited pattern of gonadotropin secretion. Indeed, an abrupt increase in LH pulsatility and return to cyclicity in postpartum cows was observed if cows were forced to suckle an alien for four to six days *(54,58)*. Based

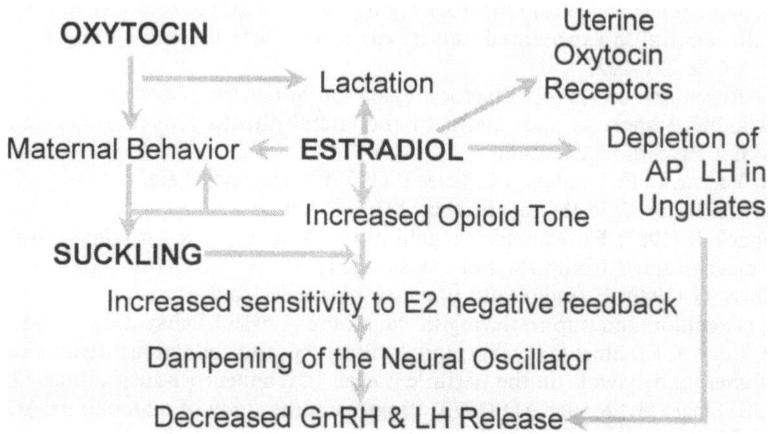

Fig. 5. Conceptual illustration of how hormonal and sensory factors that regulate maternal behavior also impinge on GnRH and LH synthesis/secretion, lactation, and uterine oxytocin receptor populations during the puerperium.

upon these collective observations, we believe there is a requisite link between physiological variables that modulate maternal behavior, opiatergic tone, and the GnRH pulse generator during suckling-mediated anovulation in cows. Figure 5 is a conceptual illustration of how hormonal and sensory factors interact to regulate both maternal behavior and gonadotropin secretion, and ultimately, length of postpartum anestrus in cattle. The degree to which the "maternal state" of the brain regulates suckling-induced anovulation in other species is unknown, but merits investigation.

SUMMARY

The onset of maternal behavior in mammalian females is closely associated with parturition. This association is characterized by increased circulating concentrations of progesterone and estradiol, heightened opioid and adrenergic tone within the MPOA, hypersecretion of PRL, and brain exposure to PL's. Heightened levels of ovarian steroids at parturition act to sensitize or prime the brain to the effects of PRL, PL, and oxytocin. Genital distension evokes an acute release of intracerebral oxytocin, and the latter neuropeptide, acting as a neurotransmitter, has acute and potent effects on proceptive behaviors. Sensory cues from the neonate are also of great importance, particularly olfactory and auditory cues, and in some species, visual. Learning results from maternal experience, and experienced females are much less dependent upon hormonal and sensory cues for the expression of maternal behavior. Collectively, the mechanisms that control maternal behavior in animals are complex, closely integrated, and in the absence of human intervention, exquisitely efficient.

REFERENCES

1. Numan M (1994) Maternal Behavior, In: The Physiology of Reproduction, second edition, (Knobil E, Neill JD, eds.), Raven, New York, pp. 221-302.
2. Lent PC (1974) Mother-infant relationships in ungulates, In: The Behavior of Ungulates and its Relation to Management (Geist V, Walther F, eds.), IUCN, Morges, Switzerland, pp. 14–55.
3. Gubernick DJ, Klopfer PH (1981) Parental Care in Mammals. Plenum, New York.

4. Fleming AS, Rosenblatt JS (1974) Olfactory regulation of maternal behavior in rats. I. Effects of olfactory bulb removal in experienced and inexperienced lactating and cycling females. J Comp Physiol Psychol 86:221–232.
5 Fleming AS, Rosenblatt JS (1974) Olfactory regulation of maternal behavior in rats. II. Effects of peripherally induced anosmia and lesions of the lateral olfactory tract in pup-induced virgins. J Comp Physiol Psychol 86:233–246.
6. Fleming AS, Vaccarino F, Tambosso L, Chee P (1979) Vomeronasal and olfactory system modulation of maternal behavior in the rat. Science 203:372–374.
7. Ehret G, Haack B (1982) Ultrasound recognition in house mice: key-stimulus configuration and recognition mechanism. J Comp Physiol 148:245–251.
8. Koch M, Ehret G (1988) Estradiol and parental experience, but not prolactin are necessary for ultrasound recognition and pup-retrieving in the mouse. Physiol Behav 45:771–776.
9. Poindron P, Levy F, Krehbiel D (1988) Genital, olfactory, and endocrine interactions in the development of maternal behaviour in the parturient ewe. Psychoneuroendocrinology 13:99–125.
10. Rosenblatt JS, Siegel HI, Mayer AD (1979) Progress in the study of maternal behavior in the rat: hormonal, nonhormonal, sensory, and developmental aspects. Adv Study Behav 10:225–311.
11. Bridges RS, Robertson MC, Shis RPC, Sturgis JD, Henriquez BM, Mann PE (1997) Central lactogenic regulation of maternal behavior in rats: steroid dependence, hormone specificity, and behavioral potencies of rat prolactin and rat placental lactogen I. Endocrinology 138:756–763.
12. Keverne EB, Kendrick KM (1992) Oxytocin facilitation of maternal behavior in sheep, In: Oxytocin in Maternal, Sexual, and Social Behaviors (Pedersen CA, Caldwell JD, Jirkowski GE, Insel TR, eds.), Ann NY Acad Sci 652:83–99.
13. Rosenblatt JS, Mayer AD, Siegel HI (1985) Maternal behavior among the nonprimate mammals, In: Handbook of Behavioral Neurobiology, Vol v (Adler N, Pfaff D, Goy RW, eds.), Plenum, New York, pp. 229–298.
14. Siegel HI, Doerr HK, Rosenblatt JS (1978) Further studies on estrogen-induced maternal behavior in hysterectomized-ovariectomized virgin rats. Physiol Behav 21:99–103.
15. Poindron P, Levy F, Le Neindre P, Keverne EB (1986) The roles of genital stimulation, oestrogens and olfaction in the maternal bonding of sheep and other mammals, In: Hormones and Behaviour (Dennerstein L, Fraser I, eds.), Elsevier, Amsterdam, pp. 538–548.
16. Poindron P, Martin GB, Hooley RD (1979) Effects of lambing induction on the sensitive period for the establishment of maternal behavior in sheep. Physiol Behav 23:1081–1087.
17. Rosenblatt JS, Siegel HI (1981) Factors governing the onset and maintenance of maternal behavior among nonprimate mammals: The role of hormonal and nonhormonal factors, In: Parental Care in Mammals (Gubernick DJ, Klopfer PH, eds.), Plenum, New York, pp. 13–76.
18. Poindron P, Rempel N, Troyer A, Krehbiel D (1989) Genital stimulation facilitates maternal behavior in estrous ewes. Horm Behav 23:305–316.
19. Keverne EB, Levy F, Poindron P, Lindsay DR (1983) Vaginal stimulation: an important determinant of maternal bonding in sheep. Science 219:81–83.
20. Poindron P, Le Neindre P (1980) Endocrine and sensory regulation of maternal behavior in the ewe, In: Advances in the Study of Behavior, Volume 1 (Rosenblatt JS, Hinde RA, Beer C, Busnel MC, eds.), Academic, New York, pp. 75–119.
21. Kendrick KM, Keverne EB (1992) Control of synthesis and release of oxytocin in the sheep brain, In: Oxytocin in Maternal, Sexual and Social Behaviors (Pedersen CA, Caldwell JD, Jirkowski GF, Insel TR, eds.), Ann NY Acad Sci 652:102–121.
22. Kendrick KM, Keverne EB, Baldwin BA, Sharman DF (1986) Cerebrospinal fluid levels of acetylcholinesterase, monoamines and oxytocin during labor parturition, vaginocervical stimulation, lamb separation and suckling in sheep. Neuroendocrinology 46:56–61.
23. Kendrick KM, Keverne EB, Baldwin BA (1987) Intracerebroventricular oxytocin stimulates maternal behavior in sheep. Neuroendocrinology 46:56–61.
24. Insel TR, Shapiro LE (1992) Oxytocin receptors and maternal behavior, In: Oxytocin in Maternal, Sexual, and Social Behaviors (Pedersen CA, Caldwell JD, Jirikowski GF, Insel TR, eds.), Ann NY Acad Sci 652:122–141.
25. Insel TR, Young L, Wang Z (1997) Central oxytocin and reproductive behaviors. Rev Reprod 2:28–37.
26. Krehbiel D, Poindron P, Levy F, Prud'homme MJ (1997) Peridural anesthesia disturbs maternal behavior in primiparous and multiparous parturient ewes. Physiol Behav 40:463–472.
27. Fahrbach SE, Morrell JI, Pfaff DW (1986) Effect of varying the duration of pre-test cage habituation on oxytocin induction of short-latency maternal behavior. Physiol Behav 37:135–139.

28. Moltz H, Robbins D, Parks M (1996) Caesarean delivery and the maternal behavior of primiparous and multiparous rats. J Comp Physiol Psychol 61:382–387.
29. Guzman Vega GA, Gazal OS, Zocchi C, Leshin SL, Anderson LL, Williams GL (1996) Roles of estradiol-17β, genital stimulation, and central oxytocin release in the development of maternal behavior in heifers. J Anim Sci 74 (suppl 1):224.
30. Pedersen CA, Caldwell JD, Peterson G, Walker CH, Mason GA (1992) Oxytocin activation of maternal behavior in the rat, In: Oxytocin in Maternal, Sexual, and Social Behaviors (Pedersen CA, Caldwell JD, Jirikowski GF, Insel TR, eds.), Ann NY Acad Sci 652:58–69.
31. Giordano AL, Siegel HI, Rosenblatt JS (1989) Nuclear estrogen receptor binding in the preoptic area and hypothalamus of pregnancy-terminated rats: correlation with the onset of maternal behavior. Neuroendocrinology 50:248–258.
32. Caldwell JD (1992) Central oxytocin and female sexual behavior, In: Oxytocin in Maternal, Sexual, and Social Behaviors (Pedersen CA, Caldwell JD, Jirikowski GF, Insel TR, eds.), Ann NY Acad Sci 652:166–179.
33. Caldwell JD, Brooks PJ, Barakat AS, Lund PK, Pedersen CA (1989) Estrogen alters oxytocin gene expression in the preoptic area. J Neuroendocrinol 1:273–278.
34. Numan M (1988) Neural basis of maternal behavior in the rat. Psychoneuroendocrinology 13: 47–62.
35. Bridges RS, Grimm CT (1982) Reversal of morphine disruption of maternal behavior by concurrent treatment with the opiate antagonist naloxone. Science 218:166–168.
36. Wardlaw SL, Frantz AG (1983) Brain β-endorphin during pregnancy, parturition, and the postpartum period. Endocrinology (vol 113), pp. 1664–1668.
37. Kendrick KM, Keverne EB (1992) Control of synthesis and release of oxytocin in the sheep brain, In: Oxytocin in Maternal, Sexual, and Social Behaviors (Pedersen CA, Caldwell JD, Jirikowski GF, Insel TR, eds.), Ann NY Acad Sci 652:102–121.
38. Gainer H, Wray S (1992) Oxytocin and vasopressin: from genes to peptides, In: Oxytocin in Maternal, Sexual, and Social Behaviors (Pedersen CA, Caldwell JP, Jirikowski GF, Insel TR, eds.), Ann NY Acad Sci 652:14–28.
39. Sausville E, Carney D, Battey J (1985) The human vasopressin gene is linked to the oxytocin gene and is selectively expressed in a cultured lung cancer cell line. J Biol Chem 260:10,236–10,241.
40. Tribollet E, Dubois-Dauphin M, Dreifuss JJ (1992) Oxytocin receptors in the central nervous system: distribution, development, and species differences, In: Oxytocin in Maternal, Sexual, and Social Behaviors (Pedersen CA, Caldwell JD, Jirilowski GF, Insel TR, eds.), Ann NY Acad Sci 652:29–38.
41. Mirando MA, Ott TL, Vallet JL, Davis M, Bazer FW (1990) Oxytocin-stimulated inositol phosphate turnover in endometrium of ewes is influenced by stage of the estrous cycle, pregnancy, and intrauterine infusion of ovine conceptus secretory proteins. Biol Reprod 42:98–105.
42. Adan RAH, Van Leeuwen FW, Sonnemans MAF, Brouns M, Hoffman G, Verbalis JG, Burbach JPH (1995) Rat oxytocin receptor in brain, pituitary, mammary gland, and uterus: partial sequence and immunocytochemical localization. Endocrinology 136:4022–4028.
43. Riddle O, Lahr EL, Bates RW (1935) Maternal behavior induced in virgin rats by prolactin. Proc Soc Exp Biol Med 32:730–734.
44. Bridges RS, Ronsheim PM (1990) Prolactin (PRL) regulation of maternal behavior in rats: bromocriptine treatment delays and PRL promotes the rapid onset of behavior. Endocrinology 126: 837–848.
45. Bridges RS, Robertson MC, Shiu RPC, Friesen HG, Stuer AM, Mann PE (1996) Endocrine communication between conceptus and mother: a role for placental lactogens in the induction of maternal behavior. Neuroendocrinology 64:57–64.
46. Clarke-Hall YM, Rosenblatt JS, Creese I (1995) A role for dopamine D_2 receptors in lactating rats. 25th Annual Meeting of the Society for Neuroscience, San Diego, CA (Abstract 149.7).
47. Horseman ND, Yu-Lee L-Y (1994) Transcriptional regulation by the helix bundle hormones: growth hormone, prolactin, and hematopoietic cytokines. Endocr Rev 15:627–649.
48. Brown JR, Ye H, Bronson RT, Dikkes P, Greenberg ME (1996) A defect in nurturing in mice lacking the immediate early gene, FosB. Cell 86:297–309.
49. Hudson SJ (1977) Multiple fostering of calves onto nurse cows at birth. Appl Anim Ethol 3:57–63.
50. Gandelman R, Zarrow MX, Denenberg VH, Myers M (1971) Olfactory bulb removal eliminates maternal behavior in the mouse. Science 171:210–212.
51. Alexander G, Shillito Walser EE (1978) Visual discrimination between ewes by lambs. Appl Anim Ethol 4:81–85.

52. Alexander G, Shillito EE (1977) The importance of odour, appearance and voice in maternal recognition of the young in Merino sheep (*Ovis aries*). Appl Anim Ethol 3:127–135.
53. Baldwin BA, Shillito EE (1974) The effects of ablation of the olfactory bulbs on parturition and maternal behavior in Soay sheep. Anim Behav 22:220–223.
54. Griffith MK, Williams GL (1996) Roles of maternal vision and olfaction in suckling-mediated inhibition of luteinizing hormone secretion, expression of maternal selectivity, and lactational performance of beef cows. Biol Reprod 54:764–768.
55. Hudson SJ, Mullord MM (1977) Investigations of maternal bonding in dairy cattle. Appl Anim Ethol 3:271–276.
56. Williams GL, Griffith MK (1995) Sensory and behavioral control of gonadotrophin secretion during suckling-mediated anovulation in cows. J Reprod Fertil (suppl) 49:463–475.
57. Williams GL, Griffith MK (1992) Maternal behavior and neuroendocrine regulation of suckling-mediated anovulation in cows. J Phys Pharm 43 (suppl 1):165–177.
58. Silveira PA, Spoon RA, Ryan DP, Williams GL (1993) Evidence for maternal behavior as a requisite link in suckling-mediated anovulation in cows. Biol Reprod 49:1338–1346.
59. Williams GL, Gazal OS, Guzman Vega GA, Stanko RL (1996) Mechanisms regulating suckling-mediated anovulation in the cow. Anim Reprod Sci 42:289–297.
60. Kendrick KM, Guevara-Guzman R, Zorrilla J, Hinton MR, Broad KD, Mimmack M, Ohkura S. (1997) Formation of olfactory memories mediated by nitric oxide. Nature 388:670–673.
61. Bridges KS, DiBiase R, Loundes DD, Doherty PC (1985) Prolactin stimulation of maternal behavior in female rats. Science 227:782–784.
62. Bridges RS, Dunckel PT (1987) Hormonal regulation of maternal behavior in rats: stimulation following treatment with ectopic pituitary grafts plus progesterone. Biol Reprod 37:518–526.
63. Williams GL, McVey WR, Jr, Hunter JF (1993). Mammary somatosensory pathways are not required for suckling-mediated inhibition of luteinizing hormone secretion and delay of ovulation in cows. Biol Reprod 49:1328–1337.
64. Fletcher IC (1973). Effects of lactation, suckling and oxytocin on postpartum ovulation and estrus in ewes. J Reprod Fert 33:293–298.
65. Williams GL, Gazal OS, Stanko RL (1997) Relationships of β-endorphin, excitatory amino acids, and oxytocin in cerebrospinal fluid of the third ventricle to hypothalamic GnRH secretion in cows. Biol Reprod 56 (suppl. 1):306.
66. Leshin LS, Rund LA, Crim JW, Kiser TE (1988) Immunocytochemical localization of luteinizing hormone-releasing hormone and proopiomelanocortin neurons within the preoptic area and hypothalamus of the bovine brain. Biol Reprod 39:963–975.
67. Brooks PJ (1992) The regulation of oxytocin mRNA levels in the medial preoptic area: relationship to maternal behavior in the rat, In: Oxytocin in Maternal, Sexual and Social Behaviors (Pedersen CA, Caldwell JD, Jirkowski GF, Insel TR, eds.), Ann NY Acad Sci 652:271–285.

INDEX

K

L

MIX
Papier aus verantwortungsvollen Quellen
Paper from responsible sources
FSC® C105338

If you have any concerns about our products,
you can contact us on
ProductSafety@springernature.com

In case Publisher is established outside the EU,
the EU authorized representative is:
Springer Nature Customer Service Center GmbH
Europaplatz 3, 69115 Heidelberg, Germany

Printed by Libri Plureos GmbH
in Hamburg, Germany